COMPLETE GUIDE TO
SYMPTOMS, ILLNESS & SURGERY

Revised Fourth Edition

By H. Winter Griffith, M.D.

**Revised and updated by
Stephen Moore, M.D.
and
Kenneth Yoder, M.D.**

**Surgical Illustrations
by Mark Pederson**

A Perigee Book

A Perigee Book
Published by The Berkley Publishing Group
A division of Penguin Putnam Inc.
375 Hudson Street
New York, New York 10014

Library of Congress Cataloging-in-Publication Data

Griffith, H. Winter (Henry Winter), 1926–1993
    Complete guide to symptoms illness & surgery / H. Winter Griffith ;
surgical illustrations by Mark Pederson.—4th ed.
    p.
    Includes index.
    ISBN 0-399-52610-2
    1. Medicine, Popular—Handbooks, manuals, etc.
2. Symptoms—Handbooks, manuals, etc. 3. Surgery—
Handbooks, manuals, etc. I. Title.
RC81.G834   2000
616—dc21   00-036049
ISBN 0-399-52609-9

First printing: July 1995
Text © 1985, 1989, 1995, 2000 Penguin Putnam Inc.
Surgical Illustrations © 1989, 1995, 2000 Mark Pederson

The Penguin Putnam Inc. World Wide Web site address is
http://www.penguinputnam.com

Printed in The United States of America
10 9 8 7 6 5 4 3 2

Contents

About the Author

H. Winter Griffith, M.D., authored many medical books, including the best-selling *Complete Guide to Prescription & Nonprescription Drugs, Complete Guide to Symptoms, Illness & Surgery for People Over 50, Complete Guide to Sports Injuries,* and *Complete Guide to Pediatric Symptoms, Illness & Medications,* all from Perigee Books. Others include *Instructions for Patients, Drug Information for Pediatric Patients, Vitamins, Minerals and Supplements* and *Medical Tests—Doctor-Ordered and Do-It-Yourself.*

Dr. Griffith received his medical degree from Emory University in 1953. After 20 years in private practice, he established a basic medical-science program at Florida State University. He subsequently became an Associate Professor of Family and Community Medicine at the University of Arizona College of Medicine. Until his death in 1993, Dr. Griffith lived in Tucson, Arizona.

Technical Consultants

Isaac B. Paz, M.D.
Chief Surgical Resident, University of Arizona College of Medicine.

Daniel Levinson, M.D.
Associate Professor of Family and Community Medicine, University of Arizona College of Medicine. Fellow of the American Board of Family Practice.

Evan W. Kligman, M.D.
Medical Director, Geriatrics Primary Care Centers, Department of Family and Community Medicine, University of Arizona College of Medicine. Diplomate of the American Board of Family Practice.

Donald J. McFarlane, M.D.
Clinical Professor, University of Arizona College of Medicine. Fellow of the American College of Surgeons.

Sally Watkins, R.N.
Head Nurse, Family Practice Residency Program, University of Arizona College of Medicine.

Stephen Moore, M.D.
Family Physician, Tucson, Arizona.

Donald D. Ewing, M.D.
Surgeon, Tucson, Arizona.

Kenneth Yoder, M.D.
Surgeon, Tucson, Arizona.

Preface

I first came across Winter Griffith's name when asked to take over the U.S. Food and Drug Administration's patient information program. When reviewing correspondence from the 1960s, I found a letter from a Florida doctor asking if there was any problem in distributing written drug information to patients.

As far as I know, no one had previously thought of providing specific written information to patients. This was Dr. Griffith's idea and goal, and it became his lifelong mission.

Until the 1970s, patient education consisted of doctors patting patients on their heads and telling them to call if they had problems. Doctors did not discuss risks and side effects of drugs for fear of how patients would react.

Some doctors still have this attitude. But most doctors and patients recognize that information about risks and benefits of drug treatment is not only a patient's right, it is a patient's responsibility. Taking care of oneself means active participation in treatment decisions. Promoting participation between doctors and patients is the purpose of this book.

Winter Griffith is the godfather of patient education. His first books were compilations of simple instruction sheets that doctors hand out to patients. The sheets contained information the doctor wanted patients to know about illness and treatment. These instruction sheets are still copied an average of 16 million times a year and distributed to patients.

Dr. Griffith's later books have evolved to contain information the patient wants to know! Over the years, Dr. Griffith has come to understand people's needs for accurate, understandable information.

Some doctors think patients want to make their own decisions about health care, so they try to control the amount of information patients receive. Dr. Griffith understands that people want to decide with their doctors about treatment and other decisions affecting their health.

This book is a patient-advocate bible. It provides the information people want about symptoms, illnesses and surgeries.

The beauty of this book is that it explains what happens to the patient, why it happens, what risks are involved, what to expect in diagnosis and treatment, and how to monitor treatment.

The book is chock-full of usable information. Dr. Griffith has mastered the art of transmitting technical information. There is no medical jargon—just solid, helpful facts.

Louis A. Morris, Ph.D.
Head, Patient Education, Research, and Labeling Branch
U.S. Food and Drug Administration

Take Care of Yourself

As a patient, you can and should share responsibility with your doctor for your medical care. Knowing the "what," "why," and "how" of an illness enables you to get maximum benefit from your medical treatment.

Several years ago, I set a personal goal to translate complicated, technical medical information into up-to-date, easily understood information that any interested layman could use. *Complete Guide to Prescription and Nonprescription Drugs* was a major step toward that goal. The public's response to that effort has been overwhelmingly positive.

This book is another major step. It has evolved out of more than 25 years as a family doctor and teacher, answering questions of patients and medical students.

CHANGING TIMES

Early in my practice, patients would come to me for help with the attitude, "Do something to make me better." At that time, my attitude—and that of most colleagues—was, "Do what I tell you and things will get better—but don't ask too many questions. A little knowledge is a dangerous thing." We had been trained to be authoritarian in our dealings with patients.

These attitudes are self-defeating. Fortunately, they are changing, and enlightened medical professionals welcome this change as an important way to improve health care.

Many thoughtful and assertive patients have taught us they wish to be more involved. They don't want to be passive and powerless in matters that affect their own bodies. They don't want instructions or advice that is incomplete or lacking in credibility. They seek—and sometimes demand—enough information so they can think for themselves and participate in important medical decisions affecting them.

I wrote this book—with the help of many friends—for those persons who want additional responsibility for their own health and that of their families.

THE INFORMATION GAP

The information in this book barely scratches the surface of all information in medical literature. It is a scant amount of the knowledge doctors have acquired. In addition to a medical education, most doctors have extensive clinical experience—and ideally, a great deal of wisdom and compassion.

But somehow, and sometimes for justifiable reason, a doctor's medical information does not get translated and transmitted into usable form for the most important member of the health-care team—the patient.

Even when information *is* competently conveyed to the patient by a doctor, nurse or other health professional, the patient has no follow-up written checklist to remind and reinforce what he or she has learned. This book is intended to provide you with the missing checklist and to supplement information you have received from your doctor.

SIMPLE, CONCISE INFORMATION

Condensing the available mass of medical and surgical knowledge into one volume has required much simplification. I have tried not to omit major facts and concepts, but of necessity, many details have been left out.

It is impossible to include all the factors and circumstances that affect each individual's health. Thus, your doctor may take into account other factors not included here when he or she makes a precise diagnosis and recommends treatment for you.

WHAT YOU CAN FIND IN THIS BOOK

This book contains three major sections: Symptoms, Illnesses and Disorders, and Surgeries. Information for each is organized in chart form. The three chart formats vary somewhat, and each format is explained in detail in the following pages.

The book contains an appendix section to supplement information in the charts. The appendix entries cover a variety of topics that do not fit into the chart format used in the other sections. The topics include: a number of special diets; suggestions to reduce stress; instructions for breast, skin and testicle self-exams; guidelines for safe drug use; information about sexually transmitted diseases as well as other subjects.

A special feature of the book is a list of resources for additional information. If you want more, in-depth information about symptoms, illnesses, surgeries or other medical problems discussed in this book, the list provides a starting place to find that type of information. The resource list contains names, addresses and, where available, telephone numbers of organizations and government health agencies devoted to specific disorders.

A glossary section of medical-related terms is also included. This includes definitions of medical tests and medical terms that are used throughout the book. In addition, it will give a brief description of some rare illnesses and disorders that are not covered in the Illness section due to lack of space.

WHAT YOU CAN'T FIND IN THIS BOOK

This book will not help you diagnose or treat your own illnesses very often. Printed words cannot replace the knowledge and expertise that your doctor provides.

A book is no substitute for communication between you and your doctor. Only your doctor knows your medical history and special circumstances about your health. Only you know the intensity and exact quality of your symptoms. The printed page cannot capture or convey the *feelings* that accompany illness.

HOW YOU WILL BENEFIT

Yet, armed with introductory knowledge about diseases and surgical procedures discussed in this book, you are in a strong position in the following ways:
• You can better understand the nature of your illness.
• You can more easily recognize circumstances when a doctor's help is necessary.
• You can learn useful facts about how to prevent disease and injury.
• You can confirm, refresh your memory and help your family learn and understand the facts regarding your illness.
• You can review a checklist of ways to make yourself better if you are ill.
• You can discuss issues with your doctor if treatment steps outlined in the book differ from what your doctor advises. Doctors do not always agree on the best course of treatment for a particular illness. When information from different medical sources has varied, I have tried to provide the general, up-to-date medical consensus.

If your doctor's recommendations differ, they may be very valid. However, you should feel free to explore the options with your doctor. He or she should welcome and answer your questions. If not, consider consulting another doctor.

I believe your best chance to achieve and maintain optimal health is to participate fully in taking care of yourself. I hope this book provides a tool to help you reach that goal.

Guide to Symptom Charts

The symptom charts are designed to suggest one or more illnesses and disorders that a specific symptom might indicate. Each chart focuses on one common symptom as shown on the list at the beginning of the section. The chart for *excessive sweating* appears on the facing page.

These charts do not include every possible *sign* or *symptom* the human body can exhibit, but they represent the most familiar and easily recognizable ones. *Signs* are observed. *Symptoms* are felt or experienced. A sign may be observed by the patient or by someone else. Symptoms are feelings only the patient can describe.

The charts provide a guide for how serious symptoms are. They give you clues as to what symptoms can mean. They refer you to other sections of the book for further information. *However, they are not intended as self-diagnosis charts.* No book should replace a competent doctor's diagnosis! The charts are only to help you decide how to proceed when you or someone else develops symptoms.

Refer to the numbers on the sample chart for an explanation of each heading described below.

1—SYMPTOM NAME

Charts are titled and arranged alphabetically by the name that is most common or that best describes the symptom (**SWEATING, EXCESSIVE**).

In cases where the symptom name is ambiguous, or the symptom can apply to several parts of the body, the body part is part of the title. For example, **SWELLING** (a symptom) appears as separate charts titled: **ABDOMINAL SWELLING; ANKLES, SWOLLEN; SWELLING OR LUMP**; and **TESTICLES OR PENIS, PAINFUL OR SWOLLEN**. One chart is alphabetized by the symptom name, **SWELLING OR LUMP**. The rest are alphabetized by the body part the swelling affects.

If you can't find your symptom under its own name, refer to the list at the start of the section and check alphabetically for the main part of the body it affects.

2—SYMPTOMS & FACTORS

The main symptom is grouped in the first column with other symptoms or factors that frequently accompany it. Each group represents one or more separate illnesses or disorders that the symptom can indicate.

For instance, excessive sweating can mean many things, depending on what other symptoms appear with it. When accompanied by chest pain, excessive sweating can be a sign of heart attack. When accompanied instead by weight

SWEATING, EXCESSIVE

SYMPTOMS & FACTORS	POSSIBLE PROBLEM	WHAT TO DO*
• Excessive sweating. • Anxiety or excitement.	Normal occurrence with stress.	See Anxiety.
• Excessive sweating. • Overweight.	Effect of excess weight.	See Obesity.
• Excessive sweating in woman older than 38. • Irregular menstrual periods.	Hormone changes; end of menstrual cycles approaching.	See Menopause.
• Excessive sweating in woman during menstrual period. OR • Excessive sweating due to tension or apprehension. OR • Excessive sweating following coffee consumption.	No underlying disorder.	Nothing.
Excessive sweating in teenager.	Normal occurrence during adolescence.	Nothing.
• Sweating. • Palpitations; tremors; flushing. • Symptoms of anxiety when exposed to, or thinking of, a particular stimulus.	Fears.	See Phobias.
• Excess sweating. • Unpleasant body odor.	Several disorders.	See Hyperhidrosis.
• Skin is cool and moist. • Prolonged exposure to hot temperature.	Excessive fluid loss.	See Heatstroke or Heat Exhaustion.
• Excessive sweating. • Chest pain.	Heart attack.	• Call doctor now! • See Heart Attack. • See Coronary-Artery Disease.
• Excessive sweating at night. • Weight loss. • Persistent cough with blood in sputum. • Fever. • Fatigue.	• Lung inflammation or infection. • Cancer.	• See Tuberculosis. • See Hodgkin's Disease. • See Lung Cancer.
• Excessive sweating, plus 2 or more of following: • Weight loss. • Increased appetite. • Anxiety. • Sleeping problems.	Overactive thyroid gland.	See Hyperthyroidism.
• Excessive sweating. • Use of prescription, non-prescription or illegal drug.	Adverse reaction or side effect of drug.	• Consult doctor about prescription drug. • Discontinue use of non-prescription or illegal drug.
• Excessive sweating. • Fever.	Normal occurrence with fever.	See Fever charts (in Symptoms section).

*All references are to Illness section unless noted otherwise.

loss, coughing with blood, fever and fatigue, it can be a strong indication of serious lung disorders. Another entry relating to a disorder of the thyroid gland presents yet another possibility.

Often, none of the symptom groups will match your present problem. Your doctor knows your medical history and can perform a physical examination and use laboratory tests to diagnose your condition.

3—POSSIBLE PROBLEM

The center column provides a short description of what a symptom group can indicate and may briefly define the illness or disorder to which you are referred in the third column.

In some cases, a group of symptoms can indicate more than one illness—sometimes they are totally unrelated. In that event, each description is listed next to an editor's bullet. For instance, one group of symptoms that we have discussed can indicate lung inflammation or infection, *or* cancer.

No attempt has been made to include every possible illness or disorder signaled by a symptom group. The identifications are based on illnesses that are *more obvious, most common or most serious.* For similar reasons, some rare illnesses described on illness charts in this book may not be referred to on symptom charts.

4—WHAT TO DO

The more serious medical problems that require immediate help are usually preceded by directions to call your doctor *now*. Below that, you will often be directed to the illness chart in this book that explains the problem. For instance, one entry has the instructions:

- Call doctor now.
- See Heart Attack.
- See Coronary Artery Disease.

All "See . . ." instructions refer to illness charts. Exceptions to this rule will be noted on the symptom chart.

If the chart says "Call doctor now," don't waste precious time looking up the illness in this book. Wait to read more about it when the crisis has passed. Call your doctor immediately!

If anyone develops dramatic symptoms that you think represent life-threatening danger, call for *emergency help*. Dial 911 or 0 operator and report your address or location (with directions).

In extreme situations, render what first aid you can, such as giving cardiopulmonary resuscitation (CPR). Yell for help from anyone within range.

Additional emergency information appears on the pages just before the index.

Guide to Illness & Disorder Charts

The information about illnesses and disorders is organized in condensed, easy-to-read charts.

Each one is described in a one-page format shown in the sample chart, **HYPERTHYROIDISM**.

Major sections of the chart format are numbered and explained in the next few pages.

Most of the charts in this section refer to an illness. In some cases, however, charts refer to disorders or problems that are not really illnesses. The chart, **TEETHING**, is not about a disease—or even a disorder. It deals with a normal process that all people experience. It would be a disorder only if it did *not* occur.

But teething can be a medical problem. It often affects an infant's sense of well-being, and it may require treatment. Because teething is so common, and because some treatments for it are appropriate and others are not, it is included with illness charts.

1—CHART NAME

Charts are arranged alphabetically by the most-common name for the illness, disorder or medical problem. Other names or terms for these appear in parentheses below the main heading. Hyperthyroidism may also be referred to as thyrotoxicosis; toxic goiter or Graves' disease.

Sometimes names for various medical problems vary in different geographic regions. All names in this book, including alternate names, are cross-referenced in the index.

To find information about a medical problem, check the index. You may also look up its major symptom in the symptom charts. If you can't find the illness chart you want, ask your doctor or nurse for alternate names by which the disorder is known.

2—GENERAL INFORMATION

This section includes seven topics: *Definition; Body Parts Involved; Sex or Age Most Affected; Signs and Symptoms; Causes; Risk Increases With;* and *How to Prevent.* Each is discussed separately.

3—DEFINITION

A short definition of the problem or disease is provided. Sometimes the definition must include information from other categories, such as causes, body parts involved and others. The definition may also include information of general interest, such as how common a disease is, or whether it is contagious, cancerous or inherited.

4—BODY PARTS INVOLVED

This is usually a list of specific body parts or organs, such as bones, skin or liver. Sometimes general body systems, such as central nervous system, genitourinary system or gastrointestinal system, will be listed. The list usually includes body parts affected at the beginning of the disease, as many diseases spread to other body parts as they progress.

Of course, some illnesses involve all body cells—even from the beginning. Then the words "Total body" appear.

5—SEX OR AGE MOST AFFECTED

Some medical problems affect specific population groups only. Others affect all ages and both sexes indiscriminately. This section explains whether the medical problem occurs more often in males or females, or whether the incidence is about equal in either sex. It also lists the age group usually affected. These are generalizations, and variations can occur with specific individuals.

Sometimes labels, such as "newborns" or "adolescents," are used to describe age ranges. These labels are arbitrary names for specific ages, but they are commonly used in medical texts. Following are the age classifications:
• Newborns (0 to 2 weeks)
• Infants (2 weeks to 1 year)
• Young children (1 to 5 years)
• Older children (5 to 12 years)
• Adolescents (12 to 20 years)
• Young adults (20 to 40 years)
• Middle-aged adults (40 to 60 years)
• Older adults (over 60 years).

6—SIGNS AND SYMPTOMS

Signs are observed. *Symptoms* are felt or experienced.

A sign may be observed by the patient or by someone else, or it may represent physical findings determined by laboratory tests, x-rays and other diagnostic measures. Symptoms are feelings only the patient can describe.

Refer to the chart. The first item under this heading—hyperactivity—is a sign. It can be observed by the patient and others around him or her. The next three items—feeling warm or hot all the time, tremors and sweating—are signs *and* symptoms. They can be observed by others and they can be felt by the patient. The fifth—itching skin—is a symptom that only the patient can feel and describe.

Signs and symptoms are listed together in this book; no attempt is made to separate the two. On most charts, a wide range of possible signs and symptoms are listed. *It is unlikely that any patient will have all, or even most, of the possible signs and symptoms.* The presence or absence of signs and symptoms may vary according to:
• The age and sex of the patient.
• Extent of the illness.
• The stage of the illness.
• Medical and family history.
• Current state of health.

7—CAUSES

Many times the cause of a disorder is unknown. Causes for most medical problems include the following:
• Inherited (congenital) defects.
• Infections from bacteria, viruses, parasites, yeasts or fungi. All of these are sometimes referred to as "germs," but most people associate "germs" with bacteria only.
• Physical injury.
• Toxins (poisons) from a wide range of sources, such as contaminated food, environmental pollution and bites from poisonous snakes or insects.
• Allergies.
• Tumors. These may be benign or malignant. Benign tumors do not spread to adjacent or distant organs and threaten

HYPERTHYROIDISM
(Thyrotoxicosis; Toxic Goiter; Graves' Disease)

GENERAL INFORMATION

DEFINITION—Overactivity of the thyroid, an endocrine gland that regulates all body functions. The most common form of hyperthyroidism is called Graves' disease.

BODY PARTS INVOLVED—Thyroid gland and most other body organs, especially the endocrine system, which includes the pituitary gland, parathyroid glands, pancreas, adrenal glands, and ovaries or testicles.

SEX OR AGE MOST AFFECTED—Adults between ages 20 and 50, mostly women.

SIGNS & SYMPTOMS
- Hyperactivity.
- Feeling warm or hot all the time.
- Tremors.
- Sweating.
- Itching skin.
- Pounding, rapid, irregular heartbeat.
- Weight loss, despite overeating. Older persons may gain weight.
- Marked anxiety and restlessness.
- Sleeplessness.
- Fatigue and weakness.
- Protruding eyes (exophthalmos) and double vision (sometimes).
- Diarrhea (sometimes).
- Hair loss (sometimes).
- Goiter (enlarged thyroid) (sometimes).

CAUSES
- Autoimmune disorder (body develops antibodies that stimulate excessive amounts of thyroid hormone).
- Thyroid nodules or tumors.
- Thyroiditis (inflammation of thyroid gland).

RISK INCREASES WITH
- Family history of hyperthyroidism.
- Stress.
- Female gender.
- Other autoimmune disorders.

HOW TO PREVENT—No specific preventive measures.

WHAT TO EXPECT

DIAGNOSTIC MEASURES
- Your own observation of symptoms.
- Medical history and physical exam by a doctor.
- Laboratory blood studies.
- ECG (see Glossary).
- Radioactive studies such as I-131 uptake (see Glossary).

APPROPRIATE HEALTH CARE
- Self-care after diagnosis.
- Doctor's treatment.
- Appropriate treatment will depend on the size of the goiter, the causes, your age and how long surgery may be delayed (if you are a candidate for it).
- Medication controls the problem in most patients.
- Surgery to remove part of the thyroid (see Thyroid-Gland Removal in Surgery section) if needed.

POSSIBLE COMPLICATIONS
- Congestive heart failure.
- "Thyroid storm"—a sudden worsening of all symptoms. This is a life-threatening emergency.
- Misdiagnosis as a psychiatric anxiety reaction.

PROBABLE OUTCOME—Usually curable with medication or surgery. Allow 6 months of treatment for the condition to stabilize. Some forms may return to normal without treatment.

HOW TO TREAT

GENERAL MEASURES
- Since this condition develops gradually, symptoms may be difficult to recognize. If family and friends mention changes in your behavior or appearance, consult your doctor.
- It is important for your doctor to monitor the treatment. Be sure to keep follow-up appointments.

MEDICATION—Your doctor may prescribe:
- Antithyroid drugs to depress thyroid activity.
- Beta-adrenergic blockers to decrease a rapid heartbeat.
- Radioactive iodine, which selectively destroys thyroid cells.

ACTIVITY—Limit activity as much as possible until the disorder is controlled. Modify activities according to disease severity.

DIET
- Eat a diet high in protein to replace tissue lost from thyroid overactivity.
- Weight loss diet if you are overweight (see Weight-Loss Diet in Appendix).

CALL YOUR DOCTOR IF

- You have symptoms of hyperthyroidism.
- Symptoms worsen suddenly, especially after surgery.
- New, unexplained symptoms develop. Drugs used in treatment may produce side effects.

life. Malignant (cancerous) tumors can.
• Endocrine disorders. This means too many or too few hormones are produced from the pituitary gland, thyroid gland, parathyroid gland, pancreas, adrenal glands, ovaries, testicles or thymus gland.
• Mental or emotional disorders, such as anxiety, depression or schizophrenia.
• Diseases caused by defects in the body's immune system. These include disorders of hypersensitivity, such as rheumatic fever, rheumatoid arthritis, systemic lupus erythematosus and many others.

8—RISK INCREASES WITH

Many disorders have known risk factors that can trigger the problem, make it more likely to occur or increase its duration and intensity. The most common risk factors include:
• Age, especially older persons or newborns and infants.
• Stress—either physical or emotional.
• Anxiety, depression and other mental or emotional problems.
• Fatigue or overwork.
• Poor nutrition due to improper diet or disease.
• Obesity.
• Recent or chronic illness that can lower resistance to other diseases.
• Recent surgery or injury.
• Genetic factors, such as family or ethnic tendency toward a disease.
• Use of drugs, such as alcohol, tobacco, caffeine, narcotics, psychedelics, hallucinogens, marijuana, sedatives, hypnotics or cocaine.
• Use of medications, whether prescription or nonprescription. Even necessary drugs cause adverse reactions and side effects that can complicate treatment and outcome of medical problems.
• Exposure to allergens, environmental pollutants or poisons.
• Geographic areas.
• Crowded or unsanitary living conditions.
• Socioeconomic factors.

9—HOW TO PREVENT

Prevention can be of two types—prevention of the initial disease or prevention of a relapse or recurrence after recovery.

Prevention of any medical problem is the *best treatment*. Researchers continue to discover ways to prevent, delay or diminish some illness, pain, disability and untimely deaths. These are included whenever available.

The causes and risk factors for a disease often provide the best clues for prevention. Many diseases, however, cannot be prevented at present.

10—WHAT TO EXPECT

This section includes four topics: *Diagnostic Measures; Appropriate Health Care; Possible Complications;* and *Probable Outcome*. Each is discussed separately below.

11—DIAGNOSTIC MEASURES

Your own observation of symptoms is usually the first—and often, most important—diagnostic measure. It is the first step toward medical treatment. For that reason, it is listed under this heading on almost all illness charts. Exceptions are made for a few medical problems, such as those that are signaled by unconsciousness, in which case self-observation is impossible.

A medical history and physical exam by a doctor are also almost universal requirements before treatment for any disorder can begin. Even if a medical problem is usually treated at home, a history and exam will be necessary if complications develop that require medical treatment.

Additional diagnostic measures include laboratory studies and other medical tests. The most-common include:
• Studies of body fluids, such as blood, serum, plasma or spinal fluid.
• Microscopic and chemical examination of excreted material, such as urine or stools.
• CAT (computerized axial tomography) scans or x-rays of the affected body part.
• ECG (electrocardiogram), EEG (electroencephalogram) and EMG (electromyogram).
• Therapeutic trial of medication. This is used sometimes for a critically ill patient without a specific diagnosis while awaiting laboratory results.

You may not undergo every diagnostic test listed on the chart, and conversely, you may undergo tests not listed. Some tests are performed only if previous tests have not provided enough information. Others are performed only when complications develop. All medical diagnostic tests mentioned in this book are defined in the Glossary.

12—APPROPRIATE HEALTH CARE

Self-care or home care is often listed as the first form of appropriate health care. It is an important part of care for almost all disorders. Sometimes total self-care suffices if you have previous experience with a medical problem and a source to review important points in treatment.

Usually, however, a medical problem should be diagnosed by a doctor before you attempt self-care. Once your doctor diagnoses an illness and outlines a treatment program, self-care or home care is often important. Treatment measures outlined in this book are designed to guide you, whether you are caring for yourself or taking care of someone else.

Effective self-care includes maintaining a positive attitude about yourself and being determined to improve or heal. During illness, a sense of humor and a positive outlook are just as helpful as medication or other treatments.

A doctor's care is often necessary, not only to diagnose and prescribe treatment for a medical problem, but to supervise self-care (or hospitalization, when necessary) and to provide additional medical treatment such as surgery.

In addition, even the simplest medical problems sometimes develop complications and require a doctor's care. In those cases, a doctor's treatment can be appropriate even though it applies to a small fraction of cases.

Find a competent personal physician who communicates well with you and with whom you can establish a good rapport and mutual respect.

Psychotherapy, counseling or biofeedback training may be the only useful health care for a medical problem caused mainly by stress or emotional problems.

Counseling and therapy are also helpful in providing personal and family support, especially with illnesses that are terminal or represent major lifestyle adjustments.

Rehabilitation is often helpful for illnesses or injuries that cause temporary or permanent disability. Rehabilitation may be provided by trained physical therapists or physiatrists (medical doctors who specialize in physical therapy). If rehabilitation is mentioned as appropriate health care, ask your doctor for information specific to your disability.

13—POSSIBLE COMPLICATIONS

Complications are additional medical problems triggered by or as a result of the original illness. Complications sometimes occur, despite accurate diagnosis and competent treatment. Some are preventable, a few are inevitable—but most are rare.

14—PROBABLE OUTCOME

A very important concern in any illness is the patient's question, "What is going to happen to me? How will this disease or injury affect my life?"

No one can completely predict the outcome of an accident or illness. The predictions in this section are guesses based on averages.

Patients and doctors work toward optimal results, but medicine is an inexact science. Response to treatment depends on many variables, and there are many unanswered questions about health and disease.

Some illnesses are considered incurable at present. The term "incurable" is a general one that includes everything from insignificant conditions that are mere annoyances to fatal diseases that bring certain death in a short time. For that reason, additional information about life expectancy is usually included for incurable illnesses. Again, individual variations are common, but the predictions are an attempt to answer a patient's most important questions. They help you adopt optimistic but realistic expectations.

In almost all cases—no matter how serious the illness—symptoms can be relieved or controlled to minimize pain and discomfort.

15—HOW TO TREAT

This section provides the checklist mentioned earlier that reminds you of instructions your doctor has given you. The information should not replace your doctor's instructions, because treatments vary a great deal between individuals.

If the instructions don't seem to fit your problem, ask your doctor or nurse for answers that apply uniquely to you.

The four major headings include: *General Measures; Medication; Activity;* and *Diet.*

16—GENERAL MEASURES

The instructions under this heading apply to home treatment. They cover common matters, such as soaks for skin problems, use of crutches, appropriate clothing, bandages or bathing.

They are not complete and may not apply to everybody, but they provide a good review of general measures helpful for most patients.

17—MEDICATION

Information under this heading is generally of two types—drugs your doctor may prescribe, and nonprescription drugs you can take safely.

Prescription drugs are named by generic name or drug class. A brief description of a drug's purpose and effect is given. For more information about a specific drug, see the Glossary. It contains entries for generic drugs and drug classes mentioned in this book.

Additionally, you may refer to my book, *Complete Guide to Prescription and Nonprescription Drugs*.

For general instructions about safe use of medicine, see the Appendix section.

18—ACTIVITY

Patients are often confused about whether they must stay in bed during an illness. They are often concerned with returning to work or school, and whether activity will be restricted after recovery.

These questions are answered under this heading.

In some topics, guidelines are given for resuming sexual relations—an important area that patients are sometimes reluctant to mention. If the illness has been life-threatening, as with a heart attack, or if it involves abdominal or genital organs, this is particularly pertinent information.

Exercise references are often included, and when not specified otherwise, references to regular physical exercise mean an *aerobic* exercise such as walking.

19—DIET

Diet information can vary from "no special diet" to references to the special diets included in the Appendix section.

For additional specialized diets, consult your doctor or a dietitian.

20—CALL YOUR DOCTOR IF

For most medical problems, a phone call or visit to your doctor is recommended to establish a diagnosis.

After diagnosis, when the course of an illness differs from what is expected, your doctor wants to know. Many developing complications can be averted with prompt medical treatment. Specific symptoms are usually listed that indicate complications.

Of course, if any other symptoms begin that you believe are related to your illness or the drugs you take, call your doctor about them, too.

Guide to Surgery Charts

The information about common surgeries is organized in charts with a format similar to that for illness and disorder charts (see sample chart on facing page).

Generally, surgeries discussed in this section are those commonly performed as treatment for a disorder, such as thyroid-gland removal, or as a diagnostic procedure, such as dilatation and curettage. The surgery topics may be about a minor procedure such as a toenail removal, or a major lifesaving procedure such as a heart transplant.

Sometimes a surgery is mentioned on an illness chart as part of treatment for that disorder. For instance, thyroid-gland removal is mentioned on the chart for hyperthyroidism (the previous sample chart) as a treatment for patients whose disorder does not respond to other treatment.

Each major heading on the surgery charts is numbered in the sample chart, and the numbered sections are explained in the next few pages.

1—NAME OF SURGERY
Charts are arranged alphabetically by the name that most simply describes the surgical procedure. In some cases, medical professionals refer to the surgery by a more technical name. The technical name appears in parentheses below the main title.

Thyroid-gland removal is clearly understood by everyone, but your surgeon may refer to it as *thyroidectomy*. Both names are included on the chart, and the surgery appears in the index under both names.

2—GENERAL INFORMATION
This section contains four topics: *Definition; Body Parts Involved: Reasons for Surgery* and *Surgical Risk Increases With*. Each topic is discussed separately.

3—DEFINITION
A short definition of the surgery may include information about how common the procedure is and whether or not the medical problem requiring surgery is caused by congenital defects or is the result of disease or injury.

4—BODY PARTS INVOLVED
Body parts can refer to specific organs, such as the brain, or to body systems, such as the central nervous system.

Body parts are often defined in the text, if space permits. If you are not familiar with the body parts involved in a procedure, and the parts are not defined in text, refer to the Glossary for information.

5—REASONS FOR SURGERY
This section lists the most common reasons for a surgical procedure. (Of course, it cannot include *all* possible reasons.)

If the medical problems listed are unfamiliar to you, refer to the index. Some have separate illness charts, and the rest may be explained in the Glossary.

6—SURGICAL RISK INCREASES WITH
Risk factors make a surgery more complicated or delay healing. Following are common risk factors for most surgeries:
• Stress, anxiety, depression or other emotional problems.
• Poor nutrition from any cause.

THYROID GLAND REMOVAL
(Thyroidectomy)

GENERAL INFORMATION

DEFINITION—Removal of part or all of the thyroid gland.

BODY PARTS INVOLVED—Thyroid gland, the organ in the neck below the Adam's apple that controls the body's metabolism; lymph nodes in the neck.

REASONS FOR SURGERY
- Hyperthyroidism.
- Benign or cancerous tumors of the thyroid.
- Goiter (see Glossary).

SURGICAL RISK INCREASES WITH
- Adults over 60.
- Obesity; poor nutrition.
- Smoking.
- Untreated hyperthyroidism (see Glossary).
- Diabetes mellitus.
- Use of some prescription and nonprescription drugs. Inform your doctor of any drugs, medications, or vitamin and herb supplements you are using or have used in the last month.

WHAT TO EXPECT

WHO OPERATES—General surgeon.

WHERE PERFORMED—Hospital.

DIAGNOSTIC TESTS
- Before surgery: Blood studies; ultrasound; CT scan; needle biopsy; radioactive-iodine uptake and scan (see Glossary for all).
- After surgery: Blood studies.

ANESTHESIA—General anesthesia by injection and inhalation with an airway tube placed in the windpipe.

DESCRIPTION OF OPERATION
- An incision is made in the neck following natural skin lines.
- Neck muscles are cut or retracted.
- Blood supply to the thyroid gland is clamped.
- The thyroid gland is cut free and removed, and a drain is left in place. In certain cases, some normal thyroid gland tissue is left intact.
- If cancer is present, some lymph nodes may be removed around the thyroid.
- The muscles are closed and the skin is closed with sutures or clips, which can usually be removed in 2 to 10 days after surgery.

POSSIBLE COMPLICATIONS
- Hoarseness or loss of voice, if vocal-cord nerves are damaged during surgery.
- Hypothyroidism (see Glossary).
- Hypoparathyroidism (see Glossary).
- Excessive bleeding.
- Surgical-wound infection.

AVERAGE HOSPITAL STAY—1 to 3 days.

PROBABLE OUTCOME—Underlying problem cured in most patients. Cancer that is present but has not spread may require radiation treatment. Allow about 6 weeks for recovery from surgery.

POSTOPERATIVE CARE

GENERAL MEASURES
- A hard ridge should form along the incision. As it heals, the ridge will gradually recede.
- Use an electric heating pad, a heat lamp or a warm compress to relieve incisional pain.
- Bathe and shower as usual. You may wash the incision gently with mild, unscented soap. After bathing, replace any wet dressings with clean, dry ones.

MEDICATION
- Your doctor may prescribe:
  Pain relievers. Don't take prescription pain medication longer than 4 to 7 days. Use only as much as you need.
  Thyroid hormones.
  Antibiotics to fight or prevent infection.
- You may use nonprescription drugs, such as acetaminophen, for minor pain. Avoid aspirin.

ACTIVITY
- Return to daily activities and work as soon as possible to promote healing.
- Resume driving 2 weeks after you return home.
- Resume sexual relations when able.

DIET—No special diet.

CALL YOUR DOCTOR IF

- Pain, swelling, redness, drainage or bleeding increases in the surgical area.
- You develop signs of infection, including headache, muscle aches, dizziness or a general ill feeling and fever.
- You develop symptoms of hypothyroidism, including excessive weakness, fatigue, intolerance to cold, menstrual irregularities, constipation, or dry and coarse skin and hair.
- You develop symptoms of hypoparathyroidism (see Glossary), including dry hair, brittle fingernails; dry, scaly skin or irregular heartbeat.
- New, unexplained symptoms develop. Drugs used in treatment may produce side effects.

- Chronic illness.
- Recent illness, surgery or injury.
- Genetic factors.
- Obesity.
- Smoking.
- Alcoholism.
- Age, especially newborns and infants or older adults.
- Use of drugs of abuse, such as narcotics, psychedelics, hallucinogens, marijuana, sedatives, hypnotics or cocaine.
- Use of some drugs or medications, whether prescription or nonprescription. Medicines most likely to increase surgical risk include antihypertensives, muscle relaxants, tranquilizers, sleep inducers, insulin, sedatives, cortisone, beta-adrenergic blockers, calcium-channel blockers and antibiotics.

These same drugs, of course, are lifesaving for some serious illnesses, but they can complicate treatment and outcome of other medical or surgical problems.

7—WHAT TO EXPECT

This section includes eight topics: *Who Operates; Where Performed; Diagnostic Tests; Anesthesia; Description of Operation; Possible Complications; Average Hospital Stay;* and *Probable Outcome*. Each topic is discussed separately.

8—WHO OPERATES

A routine surgery is often performed by a general surgeon or by a doctor who specializes in the body system involved. For instance, either a general surgeon or an obstetrician-gynecologist might remove an ovarian cyst.

Highly complicated surgeries, such as a heart transplant, are usually done by surgeons with additional specialized training.

We have included the type of surgeon most likely to perform the procedure, but variations can occur. In many communities general surgeons perform operations that are customarily performed elsewhere by a surgical subspecialist.

Your surgeon should not be uneasy about discussing with you before surgery his or her previous experience and education. Most competent surgeons welcome and sometimes recommend a second opinion when the surgery to be performed is elective rather than an emergency.

9—WHERE PERFORMED

A surgical procedure may be performed in any of the following places:
- A doctor's office.
- An independent, outpatient surgical facility.
- A hospital outpatient surgical facility.
- The operating room of a hospital.
- An emergency room.

10—DIAGNOSTIC TESTS

Diagnostic tests related to surgery can occur before, during or after the surgical procedure.

Laboratory studies are helpful in diagnosis and in providing necessary anatomical information prior to surgery. Many tests are the same as those discussed earlier in diagnosis of illnesses.

Some tests are especially useful in surgery. Examples include:
- Special x-ray studies of the gastrointestinal tract (upper GI series or lower GI series).

• Intravenous studies of the kidney and urinary tract (intravenous pyelogram and retrograde pyelogram).

• Coronary angiography (x-ray studies of the coronary arteries performed during a cardiac catheterization procedure).

• Biopsy (microscopic study of tissue) before surgery to establish a diagnosis prior to extensive surgery (usually for cancer) and biopsy afterward of tissue removed during the surgical procedure.

11—ANESTHESIA

Anesthesia makes surgery possible without pain. Prior to giving anesthesia, most surgeons prescribe preoperative medications. These generally consist of:

• Tranquilizers or sedatives to help reduce apprehension.

• Pain relievers (frequently a narcotic drug such as morphine). This medication also reduces apprehension and decreases the amount of anesthesia needed.

• An anticholinergic drug, such as scopolamine or atropine, to decrease secretions from the nose, throat and lungs during the operation.

The type of anesthesia used depends on the surgical problem, the age and general condition of the patient, and sometimes on the availability of personnel to administer the anesthesia.

If an operation can be performed with any of several types of anesthesia, you have a right to know the advantages and disadvantages of each. If you wish, you have the right to participate in the selection. Don't hesitate to ask questions.

Before you have any anesthesia, tell your doctor or dentist about any allergic responses you have had to anesthesia in the past. Also inform him or her about any prescription or nonprescription drugs you take, and about any cardiovascular disease, heartbeat irregularities or peripheral vascular disease you have.

If a chart lists several anesthesia options for a surgery, you will have one of them, but not all.

The various types of anesthesia include:

Local Anesthesia—This is usually an injectable form of a drug ending in "caine," such as novocaine or lidocaine.

Local anesthesia is frequently injected into an injury site, such as a fracture, and bleeding from the injury disperses the anesthetic to all pain-sensitive parts of the injury. Local anesthesia may also be used to block a specific nerve bundle, allowing a pain-free procedure such as a tooth extraction.

Regional Anesthesia—This is used when it is desirable for the patient to remain conscious during the operation. Regional anesthesia works only on the part of the body upon which surgery is performed. Types of regional anesthesia includes: Spinal or epidural anesthesia.

Spinal anesthesia involves an injection of local anesthetic into the spinal canal, above the level of the surgery site. It relieves pain satisfactorily for many procedures below the waist, such as surgery of the rectum, genitourinary tract or lower extremities.

A special type of low-spinal anesthesia is called caudal anesthesia or "saddle block" (it affects the body area that comes into contact with a horse saddle).

Epidural anesthesia involves an injection of local anesthetic into the extradural (epidural) space in the lower back. It is used to block pain for the abdominal region.

General Anesthesia—This form of anesthesia is generally administered by inhalation or injection, or a combination of the two.

A short-acting hypnotic or sedative is injected into a vein, followed by a muscle relaxer. This quickly produces light sleep and allows placement of an airway tube (endotracheal tube) without discomfort. The tube is connected to hoses that lead to gas machines.

The anesthesiologist controls the flow of anesthesia gases and monitors many body functions, such as blood pressure, breathing rate, pulse and ECG, while the patient sleeps.

When you awaken, the endotracheal tube may still be in place or may have been removed. Unless your respiration needs continued machine support, the endotracheal tube is usually removed in the recovery room.

The tube will make your throat sore for about 24 hours. This is normal and requires no treatment.

12—DESCRIPTION OF OPERATION

The surgical procedure is described in brief, nontechnical terms. Individual surgeons may use slightly varying techniques, but the basic steps are included and only details vary.

If you want additional information, your surgeon can give more details or a librarian can suggest resource materials with fuller descriptions and explanations.

During some surgeries of the gastrointestinal tract, a hollow tube (Levin tube) is passed through your nose into your stomach after you are asleep. The tube will probably be in place when you awaken in the recovery room. The purpose of the tube is to keep the stomach empty to prevent vomiting or aspiration of material while you are asleep. It also keeps the stomach decompressed until normal muscular movement of the gastrointestinal tract can resume after surgery. An empty stomach is more comfortable and helps prevent complications that may arise if the stomach becomes distended with air or gas.

The average time in surgery and in the recovery room are left out because variations are too great. Factors that affect the time limits depend upon:
• The exact techniques chosen.
• The experience and preference of the surgeon.
• The availability and experience of assistants and operating room personnel.
• The presence or absence of complications during surgery.
• The age and condition of the patient prior to surgery.

Don't hesitate to ask your surgeon to estimate the time your operation will require.

13—POSSIBLE COMPLICATIONS

Complications are additional medical problems related to the surgery that occur during or after the procedure. They sometimes happen despite accurate diagnosis, skillful surgery, competent assistance and well-equipped operating rooms. Some complications are preventable, and some occur frequently—but most are rare.

14—AVERAGE HOSPITAL STAY

This estimate is based on an average. It varies according to how healing and recuperation progress and whether complications develop before, during or after surgery. It is also influenced by the amount insurance companies will allow as reimbursement of specific procedures.

15—PROBABLE OUTCOME

This heading relates to the surgery's effect on the underlying disorder and the average length of time required to recover from surgery. Estimates are based on the assumption that complications do not occur and healing proceeds normally. Complications can alter the course of healing dramatically. A positive outlook following surgery is an important factor in good outcome and rapid healing.

16—POSTOPERATIVE CARE

This section generally provides instructions for self-care during recuperation after hospitalization. It should serve as a reminder for instructions given you by your surgeon. It should not replace your doctor's instructions.

The section has four major topics: *General Measures; Medication; Activity;* and *Diet.*

17—GENERAL MEASURES

Some questions are almost universal following surgery. Most patients are unsure how to care for a surgical wound. They have questions about pain, bathing, stitches, clothing and other matters. These questions are answered in this section.

18—MEDICATION

Drugs usually prescribed after surgery are described, along with brief instructions for their use.

See Safe Use of Medicine (in Appendix) for general instructions.

19—ACTIVITY

Resumption of activity is a strong area of concern for postsurgical patients. Guidelines are provided for when to return to school or work, when to resume driving, when to resume sexual relations and what types of exercise are appropriate. Again, it should serve as a reminder for instructions given you by your surgeon. It should not replace your doctor's instructions.

20—DIET

During surgery with general anesthesia, the gastrointestinal tract is kept empty. After the patient awakens, clear liquids are usually provided until the gastrointestinal tract begins to function again. When appropriate, this information is included in the surgery charts. Additional diet instructions often refer to special diets in the Appendix section.

21—CALL YOUR DOCTOR IF

Call your doctor if healing and recuperation after surgery don't follow the usual course of events. Excessive bleeding and general or surgical-wound infection are common dangers after most surgical procedures, and these are always mentioned on surgery charts when appropriate.

Other reasons listed can serve as reminders of possible complications. If you develop symptoms you believe are related to your illness—even if they don't appear on the chart—call your doctor about them.

Symptoms

Symptom Charts

Find your main symptom on this list and then look at that chart for additional symptoms you may have.

Abdominal Pain, Recurrent Attacks
Abdominal Pain, Sudden Attack
Abdominal Swelling
Ankle Pain
Ankles, Swollen
Anxiety and Nervousness
Appetite Loss
Arm or Hand Pain
Backache
Behavioral or Emotional Changes
Bleeding, Rectal
Bowel, Lack of Control
Breast Pain or Lumps
Breath, Bad
Breathing Difficulty
Bruising or Blood Spots Under the Skin,
    Unexplained
Burping or Gas
Chest Pain
Confusion (Person Over Age 65)
Confusion (Person Under Age 65)
Constipation
Cough
Cough With Blood
Coughing In Children
Crying, Excessive (Infant 0 To 6 Months)
Depression
Diarrhea (Infant 0 To 6 Months)
Diarrhea (Person Over 6 Months)
Dizziness
Ear, Ringing or Buzzing Sounds
Earache
Eye Pain; Swelling; Dryness; Itching;
    Tearing
Face Pain
Facial Skin Problems
Faintness or Fainting
Fatigue or Tiredness
Fever (Child 0 To 2 Years)
Fever (Child Over 2 Years)
Fever (Person Over Age 12)
Foot Problems
Genital Sores, Blisters, Warts or Boils
Hair Growth In Women, Excessive
Hair Loss
Headache
Hearing Loss
Heartbeat Irregularity

Impotence, Male Sexual
Itching
Knee Pain
Leg Pain
Memory Problems
Menstrual Periods, Late or Absent
Menstrual Periods, Painful or Heavy
Mouth, Sore; Tingling; Dry
Muscle Cramp; Ache; Weakness
Neck Pain
Nose, Stuffy or Runny
Numbness, Tingling or Prickling
Rash With Fever
Rash Without Fever
Sexual Intercourse, Painful For Man
Sexual Intercourse, Painful For Woman
Shoulder Pain
Skin, Bumps on
Skin Problems (Child Under Age 2)
Skin Problems (Person Over Age 2)
Sleeping Problems
Speaking Difficulty
Stool, Abnormal Appearance
Swallowing Difficulty
Sweating, Excessive
Swelling or Lump
Testicles or Penis, Painful or Swollen
Throat, Sore
Tongue, Sore
Toothache
Trembling or Twitching
Urination, Frequent
Urination, Lack of Control
Urination, Painful
Urine, Abnormal Color
Vaginal Bleeding, Unexpected
Vaginal Discharge, Abnormal
Vaginal Itching
Vision Disturbance or Loss
Voice Loss or Hoarseness
Vomiting (Infant 0 To 6 Months)
Vomiting, Recurrent Attacks
Vomiting, Sudden Attack
Weight Gain
Weight Gain, Slow (Child 0 To 5 Years)
Weight Loss
Wheezing

ABDOMINAL PAIN, RECURRENT ATTACKS

SYMPTOMS & FACTORS	POSSIBLE PROBLEM	WHAT TO DO*
• Recurrent pain in upper right abdomen that may spread to chest, back or shoulders. • No fever.	Gallbladder disorder.	See Gallstones.
• Recurrent pain in lower abdomen. • Nausea. • Recurrent diarrhea. • General ill feeling. • Fever during attacks. • Blood or mucus in stool.	• Inflammatory disease of large intestine.	See Colitis, Ulcerative.
• Pain or cramping in the upper abdomen. • Appetite loss. • Weight loss.	• Inflammation. • Peptic-ulcer disease.	• See Gastritis. • See Ulcer, Peptic.
• Cramping pain in lower left abdomen (male). • Constant urge to have a bowel movement.	Rectum inflammation.	See Proctitis.
• Recurrent pain in upper abdomen. • Poor appetite. • Unexplained weight loss.	• Tumor. • Disorder of pancreas	• See Stomach Cancer. • See Pancreatitis. • See Pancreas Cancer.
• Recurrent pain in lower abdomen. • No fever. • Recurrent diarrhea, usually without blood.	• Inflammation of large intestine. • Tumor.	• See Diverticular Disease. • See Large Intestine Cancer.
• Recurrent pain in lower abdomen. • Recurrent diarrhea, usually without blood or mucus in stool. • General ill feeling. • Fever during attacks.	Inflammation of small intestine.	See Crohn's Disease.
• Recurrent pain in upper right abdomen. • Vomiting. • Fever during attacks.	Gallbladder inflammation.	See Cholecystitis or Cholangitis.
• Recurrent pain in lower abdomen. • Alternating diarrhea and constipation. • Recurrent, burning pain in upper abdomen, especially when bending forward or lying down.	• Disorder of muscle contractions in colon. • Stomach acid in esophagus.	• See Irritable Bowel Syndrome. • See Gastroesophageal Reflux Disease.
• Pain in upper abdomen. • Loss of appetite and weight loss. • Tender mass in upper right abdomen.	Cancer.	See Liver Cancer.

*All references are to Illness section unless noted otherwise.

ABDOMINAL PAIN, SUDDEN ATTACK
(continued on next page)

SYMPTOMS & FACTORS	POSSIBLE PROBLEM	WHAT TO DO*
Abdominal pain following excessive consumption of alcohol or food.	Stomach inflammation.	• See Indigestion. • See Gastritis.
• Abdominal pain. • Diarrhea. • Vomiting.	• Infections of digestive tract. • Food poisoning.	• See Gastroenteritis. • See Food Poisoning. • See Salmonella Infections.
• Abdominal pain. • Diarrhea. • Flatulence and bloating.	Reaction to swallowed substance.	See Food Allergy and Intolerance.
• Abdominal pain that began in small of back, spreading to genital area. • Fever. • Frequent, painful, occasionally bloody urination.	Infection in urinary tract.	• See Cystitis. • See Kidney Infection, Acute.
• Mild pain in lower abdomen. • Constipation or gas. • Recent diet change, such as adding more fiber.	Intestinal disturbance caused by diet change.	Consult doctor if discomfort persists longer than 3 hours.
• Severe abdominal pain, plus any of following: • Temperature of 100F (37.8C) or higher. • Constipation. • Abdominal swelling. • Vomiting.	Serious abdominal disorder.	• Call doctor now. • See Intestinal Obstruction. • See Appendicitis. • See Aneurysm. • See Peritonitis.
• Severe abdominal pain. • Menstrual period late 4 or more weeks. • Shoulder pain. • Abdominal pain that began in small of back, spreading to genital area. • No fever at onset of pain. • Smoky or bloody urine.	• Pregnancy developing outside uterus. • Kidney colic.	• See Ectopic Pregnancy. • See Urinary Calculi.
• Pain in lower abdomen in woman. • Green-yellow, heavy or bad-smelling vaginal discharge.	Infection of reproductive organs.	• See Pelvic Inflammatory Disease. • See Ovarian Tumor Benign.
• Burning pain of abdominal skin with tenderness along pain route. • Skin blisters.	Virus infection of sensory nerves.	See Herpes Zoster.
• Pain in upper right abdomen that may spread to chest, back or shoulders. • Nausea or vomiting.	• Gallbladder disorder. • Heart problem.	• See Gallstones. • See Pancreatitis. • See Heart Attack.

*All references are to Illness section unless noted otherwise.

ABDOMINAL PAIN, SUDDEN ATTACK
(continued from previous page)

SYMPTOMS & FACTORS	POSSIBLE PROBLEM	WHAT TO DO*
• Pain in lower abdomen in females. • Unexplained vaginal bleeding.	Several disorders.	See Vaginal Bleeding, Unexpected (in Symptoms section).
Recurrent abdominal pain for 1 week or more.	Several disorders.	See Abdominal Pain, Recurrent (in Symptoms section).
• Abdominal cramps. • Intermittent diarrhea. • Gas and abdominal bloating.	Parasitic infection.	See Amebiasis.

*All references are to Illness section unless noted otherwise.

ABDOMINAL SWELLING

SYMPTOMS & FACTORS	POSSIBLE PROBLEM	WHAT TO DO*
• Lower abdominal swelling that is slowly increasing. • No signs of pregnancy. • Persistent constipation.	• Intestinal disorder. • Tumor.	• See Constipation. • See Ovarian Tumor Benign.
Abdominal swelling in woman 1 to 5 days before or during menstrual period.	Fluid retention caused by hormone changes.	See Premenstrual Syndrome.
• Abdominal swelling; bloated and full feeling. • Gas or belching. • Abdominal pain or discomfort.	• Heartburn. • Stones in gallbladder.	• See Indigestion. • See Gallstones.
• Abdominal swelling in last 24 hours. • Severe abdominal pain. • Fever. • Diarrhea or constipation. • Vomiting.	Serious abdominal disorder.	• Call doctor now. • See Intestinal Obstruction.
• Abdominal swelling. • Swollen ankles. • Breathing difficulty, especially at night.	Fluid in abdomen and other body parts caused by heart condition.	• Consult doctor. • See Congestive Heart Failure.
• Abdominal swelling. • Puffy ankles that hold a dent when pressed with finger. • Decreased urination	Kidney disorder.	• Consult doctor. • See Glomerulonephritis. • See Wilm's Tumor (children only).
• Abdominal swelling. • Yellow skin and eyes.	Liver disorder.	• Consult doctor. • See Cirrhosis of the Liver.
• Abdominal swelling. • Overweight.	Effect of excess weight.	See Obesity.
• Abdominal swelling in woman of childbearing age. • Tender, enlarged breasts. • Morning nausea. • No menstrual period for 2 months or longer.	Pregnancy.	Consult doctor to confirm pregnancy.
• Swollen abdomen in an infant. • Weight loss or slow weight gain. • Loose, pale, bad-smelling stools.	Gluten intolerance.	See Celiac Disease.

*All references are to Illness section unless noted otherwise.

ANKLE PAIN

SYMPTOMS & FACTORS	POSSIBLE PROBLEM	WHAT TO DO*
• Severe pain in ankle following injury. • Ankle can't move or bear weight. • Ankle swells rapidly and turns blue.	• Severe injury. • Broken bone.	• See Sprains & Strains. • See Bone Fracture.
• Pain in ankles or other joints, such as knees or fingers. • Affected joints red, warm, swollen. • No fever.	• Joint inflammation. • Degenerative condition of joints.	• See Arthritis, Rheumatoid. • See Arthritis, Juvenile Rheumatoid (children only). • See Gout. • See Osteoarthritis.
• Moderate pain in ankle following injury. • Ankle can move and bear weight.	Mild ligament injury.	See Sprains & Strains.
• Pain in ankle. • Ankle swollen, red and hot. • Fever. • Recent infection, such as gonorrhea.	Joint infection.	See Arthritis, Infectious.
• Pain in ankles or other joints. • Affected joints red, warm, swollen. • Fever. • General ill feeling. • Recent illness, such as sore throat or skin infection.	Complication of prior streptococcal infection.	• Consult doctor. • See Rheumatic Fever.
• Acute attack of swelling and pain in one or more joints. • Attacks may last for 2 or more days.	Joint disorder.	See Pseudogout.

*All references are to Illness section unless noted otherwise.

ANKLES, SWOLLEN

SYMPTOMS & FACTORS	POSSIBLE PROBLEM	WHAT TO DO*
• Swollen ankle. • Injury to ankle in last 4 months.	Normal swelling following injury.	If ankle becomes painful, consult doctor.
• Swollen ankles. • Recent confinement for several hours, such as car, bus, train, airplane. • No pain.	Normal occurrence.	• Elevate legs. When possible, avoid prolonged sitting or standing—move around frequently. • If swelling persists more than 48 hours, consult doctor.
Swollen, painful ankle.	Several disorders.	See Ankle Pain (in Symptoms section).
• Swollen ankles. • Use of prescription or nonprescription drug.	Adverse reaction or side effect of drug.	• Consult doctor about prescription drug. • Discontinue use of nonprescription drug.
• Swollen ankles. • Menstrual period due in a few days.	Fluid retention caused by hormone changes or excess salt intake.	See Premenstrual Syndrome.
Swollen or distended veins in ankles.	Dilated, twisted or blocked veins.	• See Varicose Veins. • See Thrombophlebitis, Superficial.
• Swollen ankles. • Pregnancy.	Common occurrence during pregnancy, but may be sign of high blood pressure.	See Toxemia of Pregnancy.
• Swollen ankle. • Calf of swollen leg is tender. • Pain when flexing ankle.	Blood clot in deep vein.	• Call doctor now. • See Thrombosis, Deep-Vein.
• Swollen ankles. • Chronic breathing difficulty that is worsening. • Cough that is worse when lying down.	Fluid in lungs and other body parts caused by heart condition.	• See Congestive Heart Failure. • See Glomerulonephritis.
• Swollen ankles. • Use of oral contraceptives, cortisone drugs or nonsteroidal anti-inflammatory drugs.	• Adverse reaction or side effect of drug. • Blood clot in deep vein.	• Consult doctor. • See Thrombosis, Deep-Vein.

*All references are to Illness section unless noted otherwise.

ANXIETY AND NERVOUSNESS
(continued on next page)

SYMPTOMS & FACTORS	POSSIBLE PROBLEM	WHAT TO DO*
• Anxiety, plus any of following: • Inability to listen attentively and remember. • Clinging dependency. • Cold or hot flashes. • Cool, sweaty hands. • Abdominal cramps. • Diarrhea or constipation. • Dizziness. • Dry mouth. • Lack of concentration. • Faintness. • Rapid heartbeat. • Impotence in men. • Low frustration level. • Muscle tension and pain (backache, neck ache, headache). • Painful menstruation. • Painful sexual intercourse. • Pale or flushed skin. • Restlessness. • Tightness in chest. • Frequent urination.	Effect of stress or unrecognized fear.	See Anxiety.
Anxiety about any of following: enclosed spaces; airplanes; crowds; heights; "going crazy"; infection; or death.	Psychological disorder.	See Phobias.
• Anxiety, plus 2 or more of following: • Weight loss. • Bulging eyes. • Excessive sweating. • Fatigue. • Rapid or irregular heartbeat.	Overactive thyroid gland.	See Hyperthyroidism.
Persistent anxiety without other symptoms.	Effect of stress.	See Anxiety.
• Anxiety. • Dizziness or lightheadedness. • Rapid breathing. • Frequent sighing.	Decreased carbon dioxide in blood.	See Panic Disorder.
• Anxiety. • Use of prescription or nonprescription drug.	Adverse reaction or side effect of drug.	• Consult doctor about prescription drug. • Discontinue use of nonprescription drug if symptoms persist.
• Nervousness and irritability in a female. • Menstrual period is due in 7 to 14 days.	Hormone fluctuation.	See Premenstrual Syndrome.

*All references are to Illness section unless noted otherwise.

ANXIETY AND NERVOUSNESS
(continued from previous page)

SYMPTOMS & FACTORS	POSSIBLE PROBLEM	WHAT TO DO*
• Anxiety. • Recent withdrawal from tobacco, alcohol or drug, such as sleeping pills.	Withdrawal symptom.	• Consult doctor about drug withdrawal. • See Drug Abuse & Addiction. • See Alcoholism.
• Anxiety behavior in a child. • Restlessness; inability to be still. • Unable to pay attention to directions.	Psychological disorder.	See Attention Deficit Hyperactivity Disorder.
• Anxiety involving recurrent, intrusive and distressing recollection of an event. • Reliving of an event.	Psychological disorder.	See Post-Traumatic Stress Disorder.

*All references are to Illness section unless noted otherwise.

APPETITE LOSS (continued on next page)

SYMPTOMS & FACTORS	POSSIBLE PROBLEM	WHAT TO DO*
• Appetite loss. • Nausea and vomiting • Fever.	Irritation or infection of digestive tract.	See Gastroenteritis.
• Appetite loss. • Use of vitamins or prescription or nonprescription drug, especially: anticancer drugs; digitalis; aminophylline; narcotics; antihistamines; ephedrine; methylphenidate; diphenyl-hydantoin; or amphetamines.	Adverse reaction or side effect of drug.	• Consult doctor about prescription drug. • Discontinue use of nonprescription drugs.
• Appetite loss, plus 2 or more of following: • Fever. • Sore throat. • Headache. • Painful swelling in neck, armpit or groin. • Fatigue. • Jaundice (yellow skin and eyes). • Pain in upper right abdomen.	Virus infection.	See Mononucleosis, Infectious.
• Appetite loss. • Pain or pressure in stomach. • Excessive consumption of alcohol or food.	Stomach inflammation caused by alcohol or spices.	See Gastritis.
• Appetite loss. • Depression or anxiety.	Effect of stress.	• See Depression. • See Anxiety. • See Anorexia Nervosa.
• Decrease in appetite (especially in a child). • Low-grade fever. • Runny nose. • Cough.	Virus infection.	See Respiratory Syncytial Virus.
• Appetite loss. • Emotional upset such as grief.	Temporary emotional situation.	Appetite will return in time. Drink plenty of fluids.
• Appetite loss (sudden). • Headache. • Nausea or vomiting. • Bloody urine. • Decreased urination. • Puffy face.	Kidney disorder.	See Glomerulonephritis.
• Appetite loss. • Nausea at sight of food, plus 2 or more of following: • Jaundice (yellow skin and eyes). • Vomiting. • Tenderness over liver area. • Fever. • Weakness and fatigue.	Liver disorder.	• See Hepatitis, Viral. • See Cirrhosis of the Liver.
• Appetite loss. • Weight loss. • Vague feeling of illness or fatigue.	Early signs of cancer or other disorder.	Consult doctor.

*All references are to Illness section unless noted otherwise.

SYMPTOMS & FACTORS	POSSIBLE PROBLEM	WHAT TO DO*
• Appetite loss. • Fatigue. • Weight loss. • Hair loss. • Craving for salt. • Skin that darkens. • Dizziness on standing.	Inadequate cortisone hormone.	See Addison's Disease.
• Appetite loss with weight gain. • Loss of energy, fatigue. • Puffy face. • Decreased sex drive. • Dry skin and hair. • Constipation. • Low voice.	Underactive thyroid gland.	See Hypothyroidism.
• Appetite loss. • Excessive alcohol consumption.	Vitamin deficiency caused by alcohol.	See Alcoholism.
• Appetite loss. • Weight loss, plus 2 or more of following: • Paleness. • Sore, red, smooth, burning tongue. • Yellowish skin	Vitamin B-12 and folic-acid deficiency.	See Anemia, Pernicious.
• Gradual appetite loss in woman 45 or older. • Fatigue. • Menstrual changes.	Normal occurrence with the decreasing estrogen level of menopause.	See Menopause.
• Appetite loss. • Fluid retention. • Reduced urine production.	Kidney disease.	See Nephrotic Syndrome.
• Appetite loss in child. • Irritability. • Paleness.	Disorder of red-blood cells.	See Anemia, Iron Deficiency.
• Appetite loss. • Nausea. • Pregnancy or possible pregnancy.	Effect of hormone change during pregnancy.	Eat small, frequent meals.
Appetite loss in child around age 2.	Normal occurrence caused by slowed growth rate.	Nothing. Appetite will return when growth accelerates.
• Poor appetite. • Sleeping problems. • Lack of energy. • Feelings of hopelessness; self-pity.	Chronic mild depression.	See Dysthymia.
• Appetite loss and weight loss. • Tender mass in upper right abdomen. • Pain in upper right abdomen.	Cancer.	See Liver Cancer.

*All references are to Illness section unless noted otherwise.

ARM OR HAND PAIN

SYMPTOMS & FACTORS	POSSIBLE PROBLEM	WHAT TO DO*
• Pain in elbow, wrist or finger joint when bending arm or hand. • No redness or swelling.	Tendon inflammation.	• See Tendinitis. • See Tennis Elbow.
• Pain in arm or hand • Numbness or tingling in arm or hand, especially at night. • No recent injury.	Pressure on nerves in wrist.	See Carpal Tunnel Syndrome.
• Severe pain in arm following injury. • Arm not misshapen.	Muscle or ligament injury.	See Sprains & Strains.
• Pain in arm during exercise. • Feeling of pressure in chest.	Temporary lack of oxygen to heart.	• Call doctor if pain lasts longer than 5 minutes. • See Angina Pectoris. • See Coronary Artery Disease.
• Pain in elbow, wrist or finger joint. • Affected joint red and swollen. • Fever. • General ill feeling.	Bone or joint infection.	• Consult doctor. • See Osteomyelitis. • See Arthritis, Infectious.
• Severe pain in arm following injury. • Arm misshapen.	Broken bone.	• Call doctor now. • See Bone Fracture.
• Pain in elbow, wrist or finger joints. • Affected joints red, warm, swollen. • Fever. • Recent illness, such as sore throat, gonorrhea or skin infection.	Complication of prior streptococcal infection.	See Rheumatic Fever.
• Discomfort in fingers. • Fingers turn pale, then bluish, then red, when exposed to cold.	Circulation disorder.	See Raynaud's Phenomenon.
• Pain in elbow, wrist or finger joint. • Affected joint red, warm, swollen.	Joint inflammation.	• See Osteoarthritis. • See Arthritis, Rheumatoid. • See Arthritis, Juvenile Rheumatoid (children only). • See Bursitis. • See Gout. • See Psoriatic Arthritis.
• Pain in arm or hand. • Numbness or tingling in arm or hand. • Stiff neck and cracking sound with neck movement.	Pressure on nerves in neck.	See Cervical Spondylosis.
Pain around fingernails.	Tissue inflammation.	See Paronchia.
• Redness, swelling, warmth around a nail. • Sudden pain around the nail.	Herpes infection of the skin.	See Herpetic Whitlow.

*All references are to Illness section unless noted otherwise.

BACKACHE
(continued on next page)

SYMPTOMS & FACTORS	POSSIBLE PROBLEM	WHAT TO DO*
• Sudden backache. • Recent fall or injury to back. • Pain only at injury site.	Muscle injury or muscle spasm.	• See Sprains & Strains. • See Back Pain. • See Disk, Ruptured.
• Sudden sharp pain down back of leg. • Recent heavy lifting or strenuous exercise.	Pressure on large nerve in leg.	See Back Pain.
• Sudden backache in person over age 60. • Sharp pain in one place over the spine. OR • Recent confinement to bed or wheelchair.	Bone damage caused by softening of bones.	• Consult doctor. • See Osteoporosis.
• Backache. • Fever. • Painful urination.	• Kidney infection. • Virus infection.	• See Kidney Infection, Acute. • See Influenza.
• Backache in person older than 60. • Pain in other joints.	Degenerative condition.	See Osteoarthritis.
• Backache. • Overweight plus any of the following: • Use of chair too high or too low for desk. • Recent heavy lifting or strenuous exercise. • Recent use of jackhammer or other heavy equipment.	Strain of back muscle or ligament.	• See Back Pain. • See Obesity.
• Chronic backache. • Numbness or tingling in extremities that is worsening.	Pressure on spinal cord.	See Spinal-Cord Tumor.
• Sudden backache. • Recent fall or injury to back, plus any of following: • Difficulty moving arm or leg. • Loss of bladder or bowel control. • Numbness or tingling in extremities.	Damaged spinal cord.	• Call doctor now. • Don't move injured person.
• Backache in female. • Wearing high heels.	Poor weight distribution.	Wear lower heels.
• Chronic backache. • Repetitive work such as computer use or typing.	Poor posture, incorrect chair or desk height.	• Correct problem with posture or equipment. • See Back Pain.
Backache that is worse in morning.	• Lack of adequate back support during sleep. • Chronic inflammation.	• Sleep on back or side. • Use mattress that is neither too firm or too soft. • See Ankylosing Spondylitis.

*All references are to Illness section unless noted otherwise.

BACKACHE
(continued from previous page)

SYMPTOMS & FACTORS	POSSIBLE PROBLEM	WHAT TO DO*
• Backache that worsens with lifting. • Lump in back or front of the vagina or projecting outside of it.	Fallen uterus.	See Uterine Prolapse.
• Pain in bones in back. • Weight loss. • Symptoms of anemia.	Cancer.	See Multiple Myeloma.
• Back pain in female. • Pain with sexual intercourse. • Blood in the urine.	Disorder of the uterus.	See Endometriosis.
• Back pain. • Visible curving of the upper body.	Curvature of the spine.	See Scoliosis.

*All references are to Illness section unless noted otherwise.

BEHAVIORAL OR EMOTIONAL CHANGES
(continued on next page)

SYMPTOMS & FACTORS	POSSIBLE PROBLEM	WHAT TO DO*
• Behavior that involve thoughts of failure, inadequacy and negative thoughts. • Lack of energy. • Sleeping problems. • Poor appetite.	Mild or clinical depression.	• See Dysthymia. • See Depression.
• Behavioral changes. • Use of a prescription or nonprescription drug.	Adverse reaction or side effect of drug.	• Consult doctor about prescription drug. • Discontinue nonprescription drug.
Obsessions and/or compulsive behaviors that consume more than an hour a day.	Psychological disorder.	See Obsessive Compulsive Disorder.
Anxiety symptoms when exposed to, or thinking of, a particular stimulus.	Psychological disorder.	See Phobias.
• Recurrent, intrusive and distressing recollection of an event. • Reliving of an event.	Psychological disorder.	See Post-Traumatic Stress Disorder.
• Start of winter season. • Depression. • Irritability. • Tiredness.	Lack of light.	See Seasonal Affective Disorder.
• Fear of going crazy. • Fear of dying. • Sense of terror or doom. • Palpitations. • Rapid heartbeat.	Severe anxiety.	See Panic Disorder.
• Behavioral changes in a female. • Week to 14 days before menstrual period. OR • Beginning of menopause.	Hormone fluctuations.	• See Premenstrual Syndrome. • See Menopause.
• Young child. • Easily distracted. • Squirms in seat.	Behavioral problem.	See Attention Deficit Hyperactivity Disorder.
• Irritability. • Paleness, fatigue, lethargy. • Abdominal discomfort. • Headache. • Tremor.	Inhalation or ingestion of lead.	See Lead Poisoning.
Behavioral changes in an elderly person.	Mental deterioration.	• See Alzheimer's Disease. • See Dementia.

*All references are to Illness section unless noted otherwise.

BEHAVIORAL OR EMOTIONAL CHANGES
(continued from previous page)

SYMPTOMS & FACTORS	POSSIBLE PROBLEM	WHAT TO DO*
• Behavioral changes. • Recent withdrawal from tobacco, alcohol or drug, such as sleeping pills.	Withdrawal symptom.	• Consult doctor about drug withdrawal. • See Drug Abuse & Addiction. • See Alcoholism.
• Behavioral or personality changes. • Stiff neck. • General ill feeling. • Headache; vomiting; fever.	Brain inflammation.	See Encephalitis, Viral.
• Confusion. • Restlessness and anxiety. • Weakness. • Muscle cramps.	Electrolyte disorder.	See Sodium Imbalance.
In infant: Restlessness, poor sleep habits, profuse sweating, delayed motor skills.	Vitamin deficiency.	See Vitamin D Deficiency.

*All references are to Illness section unless noted otherwise.

BLEEDING, RECTAL

SYMPTOMS & FACTORS	POSSIBLE PROBLEM	WHAT TO DO*
• Bright red bleeding. • Rectal pain and itching.	Dilated rectal and anal veins.	See Hemorrhoids.
• Rectal bleeding. • Pain with bowel movements. • Discomfort when cleaning after bowel movements.	Tear in the skin or sphincter muscle surrounding the rectum.	See Anal Fissure.
Bright red rectal bleeding following injury, insertion of foreign object in the rectum, or anal sex.	Traumatic tear in the skin or sphincter muscle surrounding the rectum.	Consult doctor immediately.
• Rectal bleeding. • Abdominal cramps. • Severe abdominal pain. • Vomiting.	• Intestinal adhesions. • Intestinal tumors and cancers. • Twisted bowel.	See Intestinal Obstruction.
Rectal bleeding in a child with severe abdominal pain.	Telescoping of intestine into itself.	See Intussusception.
Rectal bleeding plus unexplained bleeding from other body orifices.	Bleeding disorder.	• See Renal Failure, Acute. • See Anemia, Aplastic. • See Leukemia, Acute.
• Blood in stool. • Vomiting blood.	Ulceration of stomach lining.	See Gastric Erosion.
• Bloody diarrhea with mucus. • Abdominal pain.	Inflammation of bowel.	See Colitis, Ulcerative.
• Blood, mucus or pus in stool. • Diarrhea and abdominal cramps. • Fever.	Bacteria infection.	See Dysentery, Bacillary.
Blood in stool that is mixed with feces and appears black or dark red.	Bleeding from an abnormality in the stomach, duodenum or colon.	• Consult doctor. • See Stomach Cancer. • See Ulcer, Peptic. • See Diverticular Disease. • See Large Intestine Polyp. • See Crohn's Disease. • See Large Intestine Cancer. • See Small Intestine Tumor.
• Mucous discharge, sometimes tinged with blood. • Sense of fullness in abdomen or rectal area. • Tissue mass that can be felt after bowel movement.	Rectal tissue disorder.	See Rectal Prolapse.

*All references are to Illness section unless noted otherwise.

BOWEL, LACK OF CONTROL

SYMPTOMS & FACTORS	POSSIBLE PROBLEM	WHAT TO DO*
• Lack of bowel control, plus any of following: • Recent childbirth with episiotomy. • Recent surgery of vagina. • History of rectal surgery. • Anal fissure or fistula. • Hemorrhoids.	Rectal or anal abnormalities caused by any of several factors.	Consult doctor.
• Lack of bowel control. • Convulsions or unconsciousness.	Brain abnormality, such as tumor or stroke.	Call doctor now.
• Lack of bowel control. • Lump just inside anus.	Rectal tumor.	See Large Intestine Cancer.
• Lack of bowel control, plus any of following: • Slurred speech. • Weakness or paralysis of any part of body. • Unconsciousness. • Blurred vision.	• Decreased blood supply to brain. • Pressure on spinal cord.	• See Stroke. • See Spinal-Cord Tumor.
• Lack of bowel control. • Acute diarrhea.	Powerful, uncontrollable bowel function.	See Diarrhea, Acute.
• Frequent leakage of small amounts of stool. • Chronic constipation, especially in child or person over 65.	Stretched anus caused by constipation.	See Fecal Impaction.
Lack of bowel control in a young child who once was toilet-trained.	• Regressive behavior. • Emotional disturbance caused by factors such as: new siblings; change in home or school; divorce of parents; parental withdrawal, neglect or abuse.	See Encopresis.
• Lack of bowel control. • Mental retardation.	Failure to achieve control due to intellectual deficit.	Continue attempts to toilet train. Place person on toilet at regular times. Provide rewards for success.

*All references are to Illness section unless noted otherwise.

BREAST PAIN OR LUMPS

SYMPTOMS & FACTORS	POSSIBLE PROBLEM	WHAT TO DO*
Breast pain or lump that can be felt or seen.	• Cyst. • Tumor.	• Consult doctor. • See Fibrocystic Breast Disease. • See Breast Cancer.
• Pain or tenderness in breasts before menstrual periods. • Irregular periods. • Woman over age 38.	Thickening of gland tissue in breasts caused by hormonal changes.	See Menopause.
• Throbbing pain in breast of new mother. • Hard, tender, red lump on breast, or inflamed nipple. • Fever.	Breast infection.	See Mastitis.
• Breast pain. • Use of estrogen medications.	Adverse reaction or side effect of drug.	Consult doctor.
• Pain or tenderness in breasts. • Possible pregnancy.	Common sensitivity during pregnancy.	Wear a support bra as breasts enlarge.
Swollen, tender, hard breasts within 4 days of delivering baby.	Engorgement of breast tissue with milk.	Consult doctor.
• Sore nipples in woman who is breast-feeding. OR • Sharp pain in nipple of nursing mother when breast-feeding baby. • No fever. • No other symptoms related to breast.	Cracked or sore nipples. Common occurrence during first weeks of breast-feeding.	• Wash nipples and apply lanolin cream after breast-feeding. • Consult doctor if fever develops.
• Pain or tenderness in breasts. • Menstrual period due in a few days.	Discomfort caused by hormone changes.	See Premenstrual Syndrome.

*All references are to Illness section unless noted otherwise.

BREATH, BAD

SYMPTOMS & FACTORS	POSSIBLE PROBLEM	WHAT TO DO*
• Bad breath. • Bleeding gums. OR • Aching teeth and gums when eating hot, cold or sweet foods.	Gum inflammation.	• See Gingivitis. • See Periodontitis.
• Bad breath. • Dentures.	Food particles trapped in dentures.	Consult dentist if home-cleaning techniques fail.
• Bad breath. • No visit to dentist in last 6 months or poor dental hygiene.	Tooth decay or plaque deposits.	• Consult dentist. • See Tooth Decay.
• Bad breath. • Recent consumption of garlic, onions or alcohol.	Metabolism of these substances.	Nothing. Breath will return to normal.
• Bad breath. • Cold or sore throat.	Symptom of infection.	Nothing. Breath will return to normal.
• Bad breath caused by dry mouth. • Use of drugs causing dry mouth, such as diuretics, antihistamines, some drugs for high-blood pressure, cancer and angina.	Effects of dry mouth on odor control.	• Drink plenty of water or citrus juices; chew sugarless gum or suck on hard candies. • Consult doctor if problem is causing concern.
• Bad breath. • Persistent cough with bad-smelling sputum.	Chronic lung infection.	• See Bronchiectasis. • See Lung Abscess.
• Bad breath. • Fever.	Common occurrence with fever and illness.	See Fever charts (in Symptoms section).
Bad breath that smells like oranges.	Sugar in the urine.	• See Diabetes Mellitus, Insulin Dependent. • See Diabetes Mellitus, Non-Insulin Dependent.
• Bad breath that smells like ammonia. • Kidney disease.	Kidney failure.	• See Renal Failure, Acute. • See Renal Failure, Chronic.
• Bad breath. • Sore mouth or tongue.	Infection or sores in mouth or tongue.	See Sore Mouth (in Symptoms section).

*All references are to Illness section unless noted otherwise.

BREATHING DIFFICULTY
(continued on next page)

SYMPTOMS & FACTORS	POSSIBLE PROBLEM	WHAT TO DO*
• Breathing difficulty. • Fever. • Cough with green-yellow or brownish sputum.	Infection of breathing passages.	• See Pneumonia (all charts). • See Bronchitis, Acute.
• Breathing difficulty. • Lightheadedness. • Numbness or tingling in hands and feet. • Stress, fear or anxiety.	Decreased carbon dioxide in blood.	• See Panic Disorder. • See Anxiety.
• Mild breathing difficulty. • Noisy breathing.	Spasm of bronchial tubes.	See Wheezing (in Symptoms section).
• Chronic breathing difficulty that is worsening. • Persistent cough with sputum. • Dusty working conditions.	Lung inflammation.	• See Pneumoconiosis. • See Silicosis. • See Asbestosis.
• Chronic breathing difficulty that is worsening. • Persistent cough with sputum. • No dusty working conditions.	Chronic inflammation or infection of breathing passages.	• See Bronchitis, Chronic. • See Chronic Obstructive Pulmonary Disease. • See Bronchiectasis.
• Shortness of breath. • Chest pain. • Shock.	Lung collapse.	See Atelectasis.
• Shortness of breath. • Ascent to high altitude. • Headache; nausea.	Lack of oxygen.	See Altitude Illness.
• Trouble breathing. • Dizziness. • Headache. • Nausea and vomiting.	Gas inhalation.	See Carbon Monoxide Poisoning.
• Difficult breathing in child under 6. • Barking cough. OR • Wheezing with rapid, shallow breathing.	Inflammation or infection.	• See Croup. • See Bronchiolitis.
• Shortness of breath. • Tiredness and weakness. • Paleness.	Lack of red blood cells.	See Anemia (all charts).
• Shortness of breath. • Fatigue. • Irregular heartbeat.	Heart inflammation.	See Myocarditis.
• Difficult breathing. • Tingling or numbness. • Sneezing, wheezing or itching.	Allergic reaction.	• Call doctor now or seek emergency help. • See Anaphylaxis.

*All references are to Illness section unless noted otherwise.

BREATHING DIFFICULTY
(continued from previous page)

SYMPTOMS & FACTORS	POSSIBLE PROBLEM	WHAT TO DO*
• Rapid breathing. • Dull or sharp pain in front of chest. • Cough; fever; chills.	Heart inflammation.	See Pericarditis, Acute.
• Sudden breathing difficulty. • Severe chest pain spreading to jaw, neck or arms.	Heart attack or other heart problem.	• Call doctor now. • See Heart Attack. • See Coronary Artery Disease. • See Heart Rhythm Irregularity. • See Heartbeat, Rapid.
• Sudden breathing difficulty. • Sharp chest pain that worsens with inhalation.	• Blood clot in lung. • Collapsed lung.	• Call doctor now. • See Pulmonary Embolism. • See Pneumothorax.
• Sudden breathing difficulty. • Chest pain.	Temporary lack of oxygen to heart.	See Angina Pectoris.
• Chronic breathing difficulty that is worsening. • Swollen ankles.	Fluid in lungs and other body parts caused by heart condition.	See Congestive Heart Failure.
• Extreme shortness of breath. • Congestive heart failure.	Lack of oxygen in blood.	• Call doctor now. • See Pulmonary Edema.

*All references are to Illness section unless noted otherwise.

BRUISING OR BLOOD SPOTS UNDER THE SKIN, UNEXPLAINED

SYMPTOMS & FACTORS	POSSIBLE PROBLEM	WHAT TO DO*
• Unexplained blood spots under skin. • Fever. • Pain in affected area. • Headache. • Weakness. • General ill feeling.	Bacterial, viral or parasitic infection.	Consult doctor
• Unexplained bruising or blood spots under skin. • Use of prescription or nonprescription drug, such as: anticoagulants; aspirin; sulfa drugs; Digitoxin; quinine; quinidine; antihistamines; phenothiazines; antidepressants; local anesthetics; penicillin; mercury; bismuth; cortisone drugs; or anticonvulsants.	Adverse reaction or side effect of drug.	Consult doctor.
Unexplained bruising in healthy child.	Child abuse.	Notify authorities.
• Unexplained bruising or blood spots under skin. • Swollen gums that bleed occasionally.	Poor nutrition.	• Consult doctor. • See Vitamin C Deficiency. • See Vitamin K Deficiency.
Unexplained blood spots under skin following violent coughing, vomiting or choking.	Raised pressure in blood vessels of head and neck.	Consult doctor.
• Unexplained bruising in newborn. • Jaundice (yellow skin and eyes).	Blood disorder.	See Rh Incompatibility.
• Unexplained bruising or blood spots under skin. • Recent virus infection.	Blood disorder.	• Call doctor now. • See Thrombocytopenia.
• Unexplained bruising on lower extremities. • Abdominal pain. • Red, swollen and tender joints.	Allergic disorder.	See Purpura, Allergic.
• Frequent bruises. • Painful, swollen joints. • Excessive bleeding from minor cuts.	Blood disorder.	See Hemophilia.
• Unexplained bruising or blood spots under skin. • Kidney or liver disorder.	Abnormal platelet function.	See Renal Failure, Chronic.
• Easy bruising and spontaneous bleeding. • Fever; tiredness; paleness. • General ill feeling.	Cancer.	See Leukemia, Acute.

*All references are to Illness section unless noted otherwise.

BURPING OR GAS

SYMPTOMS & FACTORS	POSSIBLE PROBLEM	WHAT TO DO*
• Burping. • Discomfort and fullness after eating.	Air swallowed while eating.	See Indigestion.
• Burping that worsens after eating fatty foods. • Pain in upper right abdomen that may spread to back.	Gallbladder disorder.	See Gallstones.
• Gas or bloating. • Consumption of cow's milk or other dairy product.	Inability to digest lactose.	See Lactose Intolerance.
• Gas. • Pale, bad-smelling stool. • Unexplained weight loss.	Poor digestion.	See Malabsorption.
Burping that worsens when bending or lying down	Stomach acid in esophagus.	See Gastroesophageal Reflux Disease.
Burping excessively plus any of the following: drinking carbonated beverages; eating too quickly; not chewing food properly; chewing gum or sucking hard candies.	Swallowed air.	Change eating habits. Avoid causative agent.
• Gas. • Alternating constipation and diarrhea. • Lower abdominal pain that is relieved by passing gas or bowel movements.	Disorder of muscle contractions in colon.	See Irritable Bowel Syndrome.
• Burping. • Discomfort and fullness after eating. • Nausea; poor appetite.	Tumor.	See Stomach Cancer.
• Gas. • High-fiber diet or consumption of gas-causing foods.	Effect of diet.	Nothing. Improves eventually.
• Indigestion symptoms (burping). • Pain in upper abdomen. • Pain comes and goes.	Ulcer.	See Ulcer, Peptic.
• Gas and abdominal bloating. • Abdominal cramps. • Intermittent diarrhea.	Parasitic infection.	See Amebiasis.

*All references are to Illness section unless noted otherwise.

CHEST PAIN
(continued on next page)

SYMPTOMS & FACTORS	POSSIBLE PROBLEM	WHAT TO DO*
• Severe chest pain beneath breastbone, spreading to jaw, neck or arms. • Sweating. • Anxious feeling. • Sudden breathing difficulty. • Nausea, vomiting.	Life-threatening heart attack.	• Call doctor now. • See Heart Attack. • See Heartbeat, Rapid. • See Coronary Artery Disease.
• Chest pain. • Sudden breathing difficulty. • Recent surgery. OR • Recent injury or illness requiring bed confinement.	Blood clot from leg or pelvis that has lodged in lung.	• Call doctor now. • See Pulmonary Embolism. • See Atelectasis.
• Severe chest pain, spreading to jaw, neck or arms. • No other symptoms.	• Temporary lack of oxygen to heart. • Life-threatening heart damage.	• Call doctor now. • See Angina Pectoris. • See Coronary Artery Disease.
• Sharp chest pain that worsens with inhalation. • Sudden breathing difficulty. • No other factors.	Collapsed lung.	• Call doctor now. • See Pneumothorax.
• Chest pain. • Shortness of breath. • Cough. • Fever.	• Lung infection. • Inflammation of membranes around lungs. • Fungal infection.	• See Pneumonia (all charts). • See Pleurisy. • See Blastomycosis.
• Chest pain on one side. • Burning feeling at pain site. • Pain unaffected by breathing. • Skin rash at pain site.	Virus infection of sensory nerves.	See Herpes Zoster.
• Chest pain. • Cough with green or gray-yellow sputum.	Infection of bronchial tubes.	See Bronchitis, Acute.
• Chest pain on one side. • Recent chest injury, chest surgery or severe cough.	Pulled muscle or broken rib.	• See Sprains & Strains. • See Bone Fracture.
• Pain in the chest or upper abdomen. • Heartburn.	Digestive disorder.	• See Indigestion. • See Gastroesophageal Reflux Disease. • See Hiatal Hernia.
Chest pain that worsens when swallowing.	Several disorders.	See Swallowing Difficulty (in Symptoms section).
• Pain in chest wall. • Affected area sensitive to touch.	Cartilage inflammation.	See Costochondritis.
• Chest pain (sharp, dull or pressing). • Fatigue, shortness of breath. • Dizziness. • Anxiety.	Heart disorder.	See Mitral Valve Prolapse.

*All references are to Illness section unless noted otherwise.

CHEST PAIN
(continued from previous page)

SYMPTOMS & FACTORS	POSSIBLE PROBLEM	WHAT TO DO*
• Chest pain; palpitations. • Rapid heartbeat. • Shortness of breath. • Numbness or tingling around mouth, hands or feet. • Emotional changes.	Severe anxiety.	See Panic Disorder.
• Dull or sharp pain in front of chest. • Rapid breathing. • Cough; fever; chills.	Heart inflammation.	See Pericarditis, Acute.
Chest pain without symptoms or factors listed on this chart.	Many disorders, including stress and anxiety.	Consult doctor. Chest pain should never be ignored.

*All references are to Illness section unless noted otherwise.

CONFUSION (PERSON OVER AGE 65)

SYMPTOMS & FACTORS	POSSIBLE PROBLEM	WHAT TO DO*
• Confusion. • Use of drugs, including: antihistamines; appetite suppressants; muscle relaxants; pain killers; sedatives; tranquilizers; or mind-altering drugs, such as marijuana, cocaine, LSD and heroin.	• Adverse reaction or side effect of drug. • Drug interaction.	Consult doctor.
• Confusion. • Slurred speech. • Weakness in extremities.	Decreased blood supply to brain.	• Call doctor now. • See Stroke. • See Transient Ischemic Attack.
• Sudden confusion. • Unusually long time since eating. OR • Use of insulin or oral hypoglycemic drug.	Low blood sugar.	Drink sweet drink or eat sweet snack. If confusion lasts longer than 10 minutes, call doctor.
• Confusion appearing over several weeks. • Fall or head injury in last 2 months.	Effect of injury.	• Call doctor now. • See Subdural Hemorrhage & Hematoma.
• Sudden confusion. • Signs of physical illness, such as fever, cough or loss of bladder control.	Effect of illness.	Call doctor now.
• Sudden confusion. • Cold abdomen. • Recent chill.	Drop in body temperature.	See Hypothermia.
• Sudden confusion. • Use of prescription drug. OR • Use of mind-altering drugs, such as marijuana or cocaine.	Adverse reaction or side effect of drug.	Consult doctor.
• Confusion appearing over several weeks, plus 2 or more of following: • Inability to remember recent events. • Decline in attention to personal appearance or cleanliness. • Personality change.	• Poor nutrition. • Mental deterioration.	• See Vitamin C Deficiency. • See Vitamin B Deficiencies. • See Dementia. • See Alzheimer's Disease.

*All references are to Illness section unless noted otherwise.

CONFUSION (PERSON UNDER AGE 65)

SYMPTOMS & FACTORS	POSSIBLE PROBLEM	WHAT TO DO*
• Confusion. • Use of drugs, including: antihistamines; appetite suppressants; muscle relaxants; pain killers; sedatives; tranquilizers; or mind-altering drugs, such as marijuana, cocaine, LSD and heroin.	• Adverse reaction or side effect of drug. • Drug interaction.	Consult doctor.
• Confusion, plus any of following: • Blurred vision. • Dizziness. • Numbness or tingling in any part of body. • Speaking difficulty. • Weakness in extremities.	Decreased blood supply to brain.	• Call doctor now. • See Stroke. • See Transient Ischemic Attack.
• Confusion in a child. • Lethargy; weakness; paralysis in an arm or leg. • Personality changes.	Brain and liver infection.	See Reye's Syndrome.
• Confusion. • Alcohol consumption either alone or with drug.	• Adverse reaction or side effect of alcohol. • Drug interaction.	• Consult doctor. • Stop drinking alcohol.
• Sudden confusion. • Recent head injury.	Brain injury.	• Call doctor now. • See Head Injury.
• Confusion. • Excessive dieting.	Vitamin deficiency.	Consult doctor for proper method of weight control.
• Confusion in a woman of childbearing age. • Sudden fever of 101F (38.3C) or higher. • Vomiting. • Skin rash.	Infection.	• Call doctor now. • See Toxic Shock Syndrome.
• Confusion. • Fever of 103F (39.4C) or higher.	Effect of fever.	• Call doctor now. • See Fever of Unknown Origin.
• Confusion, plus any of following: • Heart disease. • Lung disease. • Diabetes.	Complication of underlying disorder.	Call doctor now.
• Confusion, plus any of following: • Agitation. • Delirium. • Disorientation. • Inability to recognize others. • Hallucinations.	• Mental illness. • Sugar in the urine. • Bleeding inside skull. • Tumor.	• Call doctor now. • See Diabetes Mellitus, Insulin Dependent. • See Diabetes Mellitus, Non-Insulin Dependent. • See Diabetic Hypoglycemia. • See Subdural Hemorrhage & Hematoma. • See Brain Tumor.

*All references are to Illness section unless noted otherwise.

CONSTIPATION

SYMPTOMS & FACTORS	POSSIBLE PROBLEM	WHAT TO DO*
• Constipation. • Pain with bowel movements. • Occasional blood in stool.	• Varicose veins in anus. • Split in skin around anus.	• See Hemorrhoids. • See Constipation.
• Constipation. • Use of prescription or nonprescription drug.	Adverse reaction or side effect of drug.	• Consult doctor about prescription drug. • Discontinue use of nonprescription drug.
• Constipation. • Pain in lower abdomen within last week.	Inflammation of large intestine.	• See Diverticular Disease. • See Intestinal Obstruction. • See Large Intestine Cancer.
• Chronic constipation. • Recurrent pain in lower abdomen.	Disorder of muscle contractions in colon.	See Irritable Bowel Syndrome.
• Constipation, plus 2 or more of following: • Fatigue. • Unexplained weight gain. • Dry skin or hair. • Decreased tolerance to cold.	Underactive thyroid gland.	See Hypothyroidism.
• Chronic tendency toward constipation. • Frequent suppression of urge for bowel movement. OR • Regular laxative use.	Poor bowel reflexes.	See Constipation.
Constipation while dieting.	Lack of adequate water or fiber in diet.	Include more fiber in your diet.
• Chronic tendency toward constipation. • No other symptoms.	Lack of adequate water or fiber in diet.	See Constipation.
• In male, constant urge to have a bowel movement when little or no stool present. • Rectal pain. • Cramping pain in lower abdomen.	Rectum inflammation.	See Proctitis.

*All references are to Illness section unless noted otherwise.

COUGH
(continued on next page)

SYMPTOMS & FACTORS	POSSIBLE PROBLEM	WHAT TO DO*
• Recent cough. • Stuffy or runny nose. • Sore throat.	Virus infection.	See Cold, Common.
• Recent cough. • Fever.	Inflammation or infection of breathing passages.	• See Bronchitis, Acute. • See Influenza.
• Persistent cough following cold or flu. • History of persistent cough during previous cold or flu seasons.	Chronic inflammation or infection.	• See Bronchitis, Chronic. • See Sinusitis.
• Persistent cough with sputum. • Chronic breathing difficulty that is worsening. • No dusty working conditions.	Chronic inflammation or infection of breathing passages.	• See Chronic Obstructive Pulmonary Disease.
• Chronic cough. • Smokers in the home.	Effect of second-hand smoke.	Encourage smoker to quit or stop smoking inside the house.
• Recent cough with green-yellow or rusty sputum. • Fever. • Breathing difficulty.	Lung infection.	• See Pneumonia (all charts). • See Histoplasmosis. • See Valley Fever. • See Psittacosis.
• Persistent cough with sputum that is worsening. • Fever. • Unexplained weight loss. • Fatigue. • Excessive sweating at night.	Lung infection or inflammation.	• See Tuberculosis. • See Bronchiectasis. • See Lung Abscess.
• Sudden cough without sputum. • Inhalation of irritating substance or fumes such as smog.	Irritation of breathing passages.	Avoid exposure to chemicals, dust and cigarettes.
• Recent cough without sputum. • Hoarseness or voice loss.	Inflammation of vocal cords.	See Voice Loss or Hoarseness (in Symptoms section).
• Cough. • Chest pain. • Chills; fever; sweats. • Shortness of breath.	Fungal infection.	See Blastomycosis.
• Sudden violent cough. • Inhalation of foreign object.	Normal coughing to expel object from lungs.	Consult doctor if cough lasts longer than 1 hour.
Persistent cough without sputum.	• Tumor. • Heart disorder. • Spasm of bronchial tubes. • Irritation of bronchial tubes from smoking.	• Request chest X-ray. • See Lung Cancer. • See Congestive Heart Failure. • See Asthma.

*All references are to Illness section unless noted otherwise.

COUGH
(continued from previous page)

SYMPTOMS & FACTORS	POSSIBLE PROBLEM	WHAT TO DO*
• Cough. • Shortness of breath.	Several disorders.	See Breathing Difficulty (in Symptoms section).
• Slow onset of dry, nonproductive cough. • Fever. • Shortness of breath. • Immune disorder such as HIV or AIDS.	Protozoan infection.	See Pneumonia, Pneumocystis Carinii.
• Cough; sore throat; increased saliva. • Fatigue; slight fever. • Recent animal bite.	Virus infection.	See Rabies.

*All references are to Illness section unless noted otherwise.

COUGH WITH BLOOD

SYMPTOMS & FACTORS	POSSIBLE PROBLEM	WHAT TO DO*
• Cough with blood. • Recent surgery. OR • Recent bed confinement because of illness or injury.	Blood clot in lung.	• Call doctor now. • See Pulmonary Embolism.
• Cough with blood. • Persistent cough following recent cold or flu.	Bleeding in breathing passages.	Call doctor now.
• Persistent cough with blood for several weeks. • Fever of 100F (37.8C) or higher. • Unexplained weight loss. • Fatigue. • Excessive sweating at night.	• Bacterial inflammation or infection of lung. • Tumor.	• Call doctor now. • See Tuberculosis. • See Lung Cancer. • See Lung Abscess.
• Cough with blood or frothy pink or brownish sputum. • Breathing difficulty. • History of high blood pressure or heart disorder.	Fluid in lungs.	• Consult doctor. • See Pulmonary Edema.
• Cough with blood or brownish sputum. • Fever of 102F (38.9C) or higher.	Lung infection.	• Call doctor now. • See Pneumonia (all charts).

*All references are to Illness section unless noted otherwise.

COUGHING IN CHILDREN

SYMPTOMS & FACTORS	POSSIBLE PROBLEM	WHAT TO DO*
• Cough. • Fever.	Virus infection.	• See Cold, Common. • See Influenza.
• Cough, sometimes with wheezing. • Runny nose. • Low grade fever. • Decrease in appetite. • Lethargy. • Infant or child may refuse to eat. • Ear ache.	Virus infection.	See Respiratory Syncytial Virus.
• Cough. • Severe breathing difficulty. • Wheezing. OR • Bluish face or fingertips.	• Spasm of bronchial tubes. • Swelling in vocal cords.	• Call doctor now. • See Asthma. • See Croup.
• Cough. • Use of prescription or nonprescription drug.	Adverse reaction or side effect of drug.	• Consult doctor about prescription drug. • Discontinue use of non prescription drug.
• Cough. • Fever. • Rapid or difficult breathing.	Infection of breathing passages.	• Call doctor now. • See Bronchitis, Acute. • See Bronchiolitis. • See Pneumonia (all charts).
• Severe uncontrollable cough. • Noisy "whooping" gasps for air following cough.	Bacterial lung infection.	See Whooping Cough.
• Cough. • Noisy breathing with wheezing. • Possible inhalation of small foreign object, such as peanut.	Coughing to expel object from lung.	Call doctor now or seek emergency help.
• Cough. • Sore throat.	Several disorders.	See Throat, Sore (in Symptoms section).
• Persistent cough in an infant. • Abdominal swelling. • Frequent, bad-smelling stools.	Inherited disorder.	See Cystic Fibrosis.
• Cough. • Chronic runny or stuffy nose.	Enlarged adenoids.	Consult doctor.
• Cough. • Adult smokers in house or child may have smoked.	Irritation caused by tobacco smoke.	• Adult smokers should smoke outside. • Talk to child about hazards of smoking.
• Sudden "barking" cough. • Sore throat; fever. • Odd head posture.	Bacterial infection.	See Epiglottitis, Acute.

*All references are to Illness section unless noted otherwise.

CRYING, EXCESSIVE (INFANT 0 TO 6 MONTHS)

SYMPTOMS & FACTORS	POSSIBLE PROBLEM	WHAT TO DO*
• Excessive crying. • Irritability. • Lethargy. • Poor appetite. • Fever.	Infection.	• Consult doctor. • See Fever (Child 0 to 2 Years) in Symptoms section.
• Excessive crying. • Irritability. • Lethargy. • Poor appetite.	Minor illness.	Consult doctor if symptoms persist longer than 1 day.
Excessive crying in infant younger than 3 months usually after feeding.	Irritation of digestive tract.	See Colic in Infants.
• Excessive crying. • Crying stops after feeding. • Crying resumes less than 2 hours after feeding.	• Inadequate nourishment. • Thirst.	• If breast-feeding, feed on demand and increase sucking time. • If bottle-feeding, increase amount offered. • Offer water between feedings. • See Colic in Infants.
• Excessive crying. • Rash in diaper area.	Chemical skin irritation.	See Diaper Rash.
Crying until picked up.	Boredom or loneliness.	• Touch and talk to infant more. • Place infant within sight of you.
• Crying. • Cool or chilly environment.	Cold.	• Dress infant warmly. • Move infant into warm room.
Crying in infant younger than 3 months before falling asleep.	Muscle jerks and twitches when falling asleep.	Wrap infant firmly in blanket before putting to bed.
• Crying and other fussy behavior. • Excess saliva and drooling.	Eruption of new teeth.	See Teething.

*All references are to Illness section unless noted otherwise.

DEPRESSION

SYMPTOMS & FACTORS	POSSIBLE PROBLEM	WHAT TO DO*
• Depression. • Chronic illness, especially rheumatoid arthritis, multiple sclerosis and chronic heart disease.	Any illness, severe or mild, can cause significant depression.	• Consult doctor. • See Depression. • See chart in Illness section for the particular disorder.
• Depression. • Use of prescription or nonprescription drug. OR • Excessive alcohol consumption.	Adverse reaction or side effect of drug or alcohol.	• Consult doctor. • See Alcoholism.
• Depression. • Recent virus infection with fever such as flu, infectious mononucleosis or hepatitis.	Common occurrence following infection.	Consult doctor if depression worsens or lasts longer than 2 weeks.
Depression following traumatic or sad event, such as death in family.	Normal occurrence for 3 to 6 months following such experiences.	Feelings are a normal part of mourning and will gradually improve over time. Seek medical help if depression worsens.
Depression experienced at the start of winter season.	Lack of light.	See Seasonal Affective Disorder.
Chronic depressive mood.	Mild depression.	See Dysthymia.
Depression in a woman following childbirth.	Common occurrence for several weeks after delivery.	See Postpartum Depression.
• Depression. • Persistent fatigue over the last 6 months.	Unknown cause.	See Chronic Fatigue Syndrome.
• Depression and anxiety. • Sadness, numbness, pain or anger.	Emotional reaction following loss of a loved one or other significant loss.	See Grief.

*All references are to Illness section unless noted otherwise.

DIARRHEA (INFANT 0 TO 6 MONTHS)

SYMPTOMS & FACTORS	POSSIBLE PROBLEM	WHAT TO DO*
• Diarrhea. • Fever. • Vomiting.	• Infection of digestive tract.	• See Gastroenteritis. • See Diarrhea, Acute. • See Dehydration.
• Diarrhea. • Baby content, alert and feeding well. • Baby taking nonprescription drug.	Adverse reaction or side effect of drug.	• Consult doctor. • Discontinue use of drug unless recommended by doctor.
• Diarrhea. • Baby taking prescription drug for some other disorder.	Adverse reaction or side effect of drug.	Consult doctor. Dose may need adjustment, substitution or discontinuation.
• Diarrhea. • Itching at night. OR • Worms in stool.	Parasites.	• See Pinworms. • See Roundworms.
• Diarrhea. • Recent addition of solids to diet.	Baby too young to digest solid food.	• Consult doctor. • Wait until age 4 months before trying solids.
• Diarrhea. • Pulling at the ear.	Ear infection.	See Ear Infection, Middle.
• Diarrhea. • Baby seems content, alert and feeds well on bottle feedings. • Sugar added to any formula or water OR • Less than recommended amount of water added to baby's orange juice. OR • Fruit juice sweetened with sugar.	Upset digestion due to excess sugar.	• Consult doctor. • Don't add sugar to baby's food. • Use recommended amounts of water to dilute juice.
Chronic, frequent loose stools in young child.	Intestinal problem.	See Diarrhea, Chronic, Non-Specific of Childhood.
• Diarrhea. • Abdominal pain. • Flatulence and bloating.	Reaction to a swallowed substance.	• See Food Allergy & Intolerance. • See Lactose Intolerance.
• Diarrhea. • Vomiting.	Several disorders.	See Vomiting (Infant 0 to 6 months) (in Symptoms section).
• Loose, pale, bad-smelling stools. • Weight loss or slow weight gain. • Swollen abdomen; abdominal pain.	Gluten intolerance.	See Celiac Disease.

*All references are to Illness section unless noted otherwise.

DIARRHEA (PERSON OVER 6 MONTHS)

SYMPTOMS & FACTORS	POSSIBLE PROBLEM	WHAT TO DO*
• Diarrhea. • Nausea or vomiting.	Viral, bacterial or parasitic infection of digestive tract.	• See Gastroenteritis. • See Dysentery, Bacillary. • See Diarrhea, Acute.
• Diarrhea for 24 hours or longer. • Vomiting. • Abdominal pain. • Consumption of spoiled food or contaminated food or water.	Effect of toxins in food.	• See Food Poisoning. • See Salmonella Infections. • See Typhoid.
• Recurrent attacks of diarrhea. • Pain in lower abdomen.	• Intestinal parasites. • Several disorders.	• See Amebiasis. • See Giardiasis. • See Recurrent Abdominal Pain (in Symptoms section).
• Diarrhea. • Use of prescription or nonprescription drug.	Adverse reaction or side effect of drug.	• Consult doctor about prescription drug. • Discontinue use of nonprescription drug.
• Diarrhea. • Blood in stool.	Inflammation of large intestine.	See Colitis, Ulcerative.
Recurrent attacks of diarrhea during periods of stress.	Effect of stress.	• See Anxiety. • See Irritable Bowel Syndrome.
• Diarrhea. • Use of sorbitol, a common sweetener found in many diet products.	The sugar is not absorbed by the small intestine.	Discontinue use of the product with sorbitol.
• Diarrhea. • Abdominal pain. • Flatulence and bloating.	Reaction to a swallowed substance.	See Food Allergy & Intolerance.
• Explosive diarrhea. • Weakness and faintness. • Recent stomach surgery.	Intestinal disorder.	See Dumping Syndrome.

*All references are to Illness section unless noted otherwise.

DIZZINESS

SYMPTOMS & FACTORS	POSSIBLE PROBLEM	WHAT TO DO*
• Dizziness. • Use of prescription or nonprescription drug.	Adverse reaction or side effect of drug.	• Consult doctor about prescription drug. • Discontinue use of nonprescription drug.
• Dizziness. • Decreased hearing. • Noises in ear. OR • Earache.	Infection or disorder of inner ear.	• See Labyrinthitis. • See Meniere's Disease.
Dizziness when turning head in person over age 50.	Pressure on nerves in neck.	See Cervical Spondylosis.
Dizziness when standing suddenly.	• Temporary drop in blood pressure. • Disorder of red blood cells.	• Avoid rising suddenly. • See Anemia, Iron Deficiency.
• Dizziness. • Stress or anxiety.	Hyperventilation.	• See Anxiety. • See Panic Disorder. • See Phobias.
Dizziness (spinning sensation).	Travel by air, sea or motor vehicle.	See Motion Sickness.
• Dizziness. • Headache. • Faintness. • Nausea, vomiting.	Toxic gas inhalation.	See Carbon Monoxide Poisoning.
• Dizziness. • Excess sun or heat exposure.	Body overheated.	See Heatstroke or Heat Exhaustion.
• Dizziness, plus any of following: • Speaking difficulty. • Blurred vision. • Numbness or tingling in any part of body. • Weakness or paralysis in extremities.	Decreased blood supply to brain.	• Call doctor now. • See Stroke. • See Transient Ischemic Attack. • See Subarachnoid Hemorrhage.
• Dizziness. • Recurrent morning headache. • Nausea or vomiting.	• Bleeding inside skull. • Tumor.	• Call doctor now. • See Subdural Hemorrhage & Hematoma. • See Brain Tumor.
• Dizziness. • Irregular heartbeat.	Heart rhythm disorder.	• See Atrial Fibrillation. • See Heart Rhythm Irregularity. • See Heart Block.

*All references are to Illness section unless noted otherwise.

EAR, RINGING OR BUZZING SOUNDS

SYMPTOMS & FACTORS	POSSIBLE PROBLEM	WHAT TO DO*
• Ear noises. • Use of prescription or nonprescription drug.	Adverse reaction or side effect of drug.	• Consult doctor about prescription drug. • Discontinue use of nonprescription drug.
• Ear noises. • Hearing loss.	Damaged auditory nerve.	See Hearing Impairment or Loss.
• Noises in the ear. • Dizziness.	Fluid in the ear.	See Meniere's Disease.
• Strange, loud ear noises. • Severe, uncomfortable tickling in ear.	Insect in outer-ear canal.	Consult doctor.
Ear noises after airplane flight.	Middle-ear problem caused by change in air pressure.	See Barotitis Media.
Noise in ear (ringing, buzzing, roaring, whistling or hissing).	Damaged auditory nerve.	See Tinnitus.
• Ringing in ear. • Slow, progressive hearing loss.	Abnormal bone growth in middle ear.	See Otosclerosis.

*All references are to Illness section unless noted otherwise.

EARACHE

SYMPTOMS & FACTORS	POSSIBLE PROBLEM	WHAT TO DO*
• Earache. • Sticky, green-yellow discharge from ear canal or middle ear.	Infection of outer-ear.	• See Ear Infection, Outer. • See Ear Infection, Middle. • See Eardrum, Ruptured.
• Earache. • Fever.	Infection of middle ear.	See Ear Infection, Middle.
• Earache. • Stuffy nose.	Common occurrence with cold or allergy.	See Ear Infection, Middle.
Earache that worsens when earlobe is pulled.	Infection of outer-ear canal.	See Ear Infection, Outer.
• Earache. • Pain in tooth or jaw.	• Tooth or gum infection. • Inflammation of joint in jaw.	• Consult dentist. • See Tooth Abscess. • See Temporomandibular Joint Syndrome.
• Earache. • Blocked feeling in ear that cannot be cleared by swallowing. • Diminished hearing.	Wax in ear canal.	See Earwax Blockage.
• Earache that began during airplane flight. • Blocked feeling in ear that cannot be cleared by swallowing.	Middle-ear damage caused by change in air pressure.	See Barotitis Media.

*All references are to Illness section unless noted otherwise.

EYE PAIN; SWELLING; DRYNESS; ITCHING; TEARING (continued on next page)

SYMPTOMS & FACTORS	POSSIBLE PROBLEM	WHAT TO DO*
• Eye pain. • Eye injury without visible damage.	Minor injury.	See Eye Contusion or Laceration.
• Pain behind eye. • Area of tenderness over nose or cheekbones. • Pain that worsens when bending forward. • Recent cold or nasal allergies.	Sinus infection.	See Sinusitis.
• Itching, watery eyes. • Frequent sneezing; stuffy nose; with clear discharge.	Allergy.	See Hay Fever.
• Eye pain. • Watery, red eye.	Foreign object in eye.	See Eye, Foreign Body in.
• Eye pain. • Red, swollen bump on eyelid. • Red eye.	Infection of hair follicle on eyelid.	See Stye.
• Eye pain. • Red eye. • Gritty feeling in eye. • Stickiness around eye.	Infection of eye membrane.	See Conjunctivitis.
• Eye pain. • Red eye. • Gritty feeling in eye.	Inadequate tear production.	Use nonprescription artificial tears. Consult doctor if discomfort lasts longer than 2 days.
• Eye pain. • Eyelid curls inward. • Red eyelid and eye.	Disorder of eyelid.	See Entropion and Ectropion.
Swelling on eyelid.	Eye infection.	See Chalazion.
• Redness and greasy scales on the eyelid edges. • Eyelashes that fall out.	Infection.	See Blepharitis.
• Pain around eye. • Sudden onset of headache. • Headache appears at same time on consecutive days.	Chronic headache disorder.	See Headache, Cluster.
• Eye pain. • Sensitivity to light. • Tearing.	Inflammation of the cornea.	See Keratitis.
• Eye pain. • Purple-red inflamed area in one or more areas of the white of the eye.	Eye inflammation.	See Scleritis.
• Bulging eyes. • Double vision.	Tissue swelling.	See Exophthalmos.

*All references are to Illness section unless noted otherwise.

EYE PAIN; SWELLING; DRYNESS; ITCHING; TEARING (continued from previous page)

SYMPTOMS & FACTORS	POSSIBLE PROBLEM	WHAT TO DO*
• Whitish light reflection in pupil. • Gradual loss of vision.	Tumor.	See Eye Tumor.
• Dryness of eyes. • Foreign body sensation. • Dryness of mouth. • Parotid gland enlargement (chipmunk look).	Autoimmune disorder.	See Sjögren's Syndrome.
Sudden appearance of blood in the white of the eye.	Spontaneous bleeding.	See Subconjunctival Hemorrhage.
• Persistent tearing of one or both eyes. • Drainage of mucous and pus from tear duct.	Obstructed tear duct.	See Tear Duct Infection or Blockage.
• Severe eye pain. • Recent eye injury with visible damage. • Loss of vision.	Serious injury.	Call doctor now.
• Pain behind eye. • Tenderness in temple on affected side.	Inflammation of arteries in temples.	• Call doctor now. • See Polymyalgia Rheumatica or Temporal Arteritis.
• Pain behind eye, plus any of following: • Eyes sensitive to light. • Lethargy. • Confusion. • Pain that worsens when bending head forward. • Severe headache.	• Inflammation of membranes around brain. • Bleeding in membrane around brain.	• Call doctor now. • See Meningitis, Aseptic. • See Meningitis, Bacterial. • See Subarachnoid Hemorrhage.
• Eye pain in one eye. • Blurred vision. • Eye sensitive to light.	• Excess pressure in eye. • Inflammation of iris. • Eye injury.	• See Glaucoma, Primary Angle Closure. • See Uveitis. • See Corneal Abrasion & Ulcer.
• Eye pain • Sensitivity to light. • Eye redness • Tears, blurred vision. • Smaller pupil in affected eye.	Infection.	See Iritis.

*All references are to Illness section unless noted otherwise.

FACE PAIN

SYMPTOMS & FACTORS	POSSIBLE PROBLEM	WHAT TO DO*
• Pain on one side of face or all over head. • Tight feeling around head.	Headache.	• See Migraine. • See Headache, Tension.
• Pain or tenderness around eyes and cheekbones that worsens when bending head forward. • Recent cold or nasal allergies.	Sinus infection.	See Sinusitis.
Throbbing pain on one side of face that worsens at night, when eating or when touching a particular tooth.	Infection around tooth.	Consult doctor or dentist.
• Aching pain over or around jaw joint. • Jaw that sometimes clicks when opening. • Frequent headaches.	Inflammation of joint in jaw.	See Temporomandibular Joint Syndrome.
• Pain around ear. • Sudden paralysis on one side of face.	Facial paralysis.	See Bell's Palsy.
• Parotid gland enlargement (chipmunk look). • Dryness of eyes and mouth.	Autoimmune disorder.	See Sjögren's Syndrome.
• Face pain. • Recent rash at site of pain.	Virus infection of sensory nerves.	See Herpes Zoster.
• Frequent contractions of muscles on the side of the face. • Tooth-grinding noises at night.	Tooth problem.	See Tooth Grinding.
• Severe pain on one side of face over eye. • Redness of white of eye. • Blurred vision.	Excess pressure in eye.	See Glaucoma, Primary Angle Closure.
Sharp pain on one side of face when face is touched or when chewing.	Damaged nerve.	See Trigeminal Neuralgia.
• Sudden, throbbing pain in temple. • General ill feeling. • Tender scalp.	Inflammation of arteries in temples.	See Polymyalgia Rheumatica or Temporal Arteritis.
• Face pain, plus any of following: • Chest pain. • Neck pain. • Shoulder pain. • Arm pain.	Heart attack.	• Call doctor now. • See Heart Attack. • See Coronary Artery Disease. • See Atherosclerosis.

*All references are to Illness section unless noted otherwise.

FACIAL SKIN PROBLEMS

SYMPTOMS & FACTORS	POSSIBLE PROBLEM	WHAT TO DO*
• Any of following conditions on face: • Painful, red bumps. • Bumps with white or yellow centers. • Blackheads.	Skin disorder beginning after puberty.	See Acne.
• Flushed face that may last minutes or hours to several days. • Facial tenderness.	Disorder of tiny blood vessels.	See Acne Rosacea.
Blister or red, rough or painful area around mouth.	Virus infection.	See Herpes Simplex.
Sore on face or lip that doesn't heal in 3 weeks.	Skin cancer.	• See Skin Cancer, Basal-Cell. • See Skin Cancer, Squamous-Cell.
• Blister-like rash on one side of face. • Painful, burning sensation at site 1 or 2 days before rash appears.	Virus infection of sensory nerves.	See Herpes Zoster.
Blisters that burst and become crusty.	Skin infection.	See Impetigo.
Red, itching, scaling rash on face.	Allergic reaction.	See Eczema.
• Rash (usually on the cheeks). • Fatigue. • Fever. • Joint pain.	Autoimmune disorder.	See Lupus Erythematosus, Systemic.
Red bumps on cheeks, on either side of nose and on scalp (sometimes).	Autoimmune disorder.	See Lupus Erythematosus, Discoid.
• Rough, red patch on cheek, nose or forehead. • Person over age 35.	Skin damage caused by sun exposure.	• See Sunburn. • See Keratosis, Actinic.
Patch of skin on face that is lighter or darker than surrounding skin.	Disorder of skin pigment.	See Vitiligo.
• Rash (especially in children) starting on cheeks, then spreading to other body parts. • Slight tiredness or fatigue.	Virus infection.	See Fifth Disease.
• Change in face mole's size, color or sensitivity. OR • A new mole or lump on face.	Skin cancer.	See Melanoma.

*All references are to Illness section unless noted otherwise.

FAINTNESS OR FAINTING
(continued on next page)

SYMPTOMS & FACTORS	POSSIBLE PROBLEM	WHAT TO DO*
Fainting.	No underlying disorder.	See Fainting.
• Faintness when standing suddenly. OR • Faintness following bed confinement.	Temporary drop in blood pressure.	Avoid rising suddenly.
• Faintness. • Breathing deeply, rapidly or sighing before faintness.	Effect of stress. No underlying disorder.	• See Panic Disorder. • See Anxiety. • Consult doctor if happens repeatedly.
• Faintness. • Use of drug for high blood pressure.	Adverse reaction or side effect of drug.	Consult doctor.
• Faintness. • Dizziness.	Several disorders.	See Dizziness (in Symptoms section).
• Faintness or fainting. • Feeling that heart speeds or slows before faintness. • Known heart disease.	Heart rhythm disorder.	• Call doctor now. • See Heart Block. • See Heart Rhythm Irregularity. • See Atrial Fibrillation. • See Cardiac Arrest.
• Faintness, plus any of following: • Blurred vision. • Speaking difficulty. • Confusion. • Numbness or tingling in any part of body. • Weakness or paralysis in extremities.	Decreased blood supply to brain.	• Call doctor now. • See Transient Ischemic Attack. • See Stroke.
• Fainting. • Seizure disorder.	Minor seizure.	See Seizure Disorder.
Faintness after several hours in strong sunshine or hot environment.	Excess heat exposure.	• Call doctor now. • See Heatstroke or Heat Exhaustion.
• Faintness. • Diabetes.	Low blood sugar.	• Drink sweetened juice or beverage or eat something sugary or starchy. • See Diabetic Hypoglycemia.
• Faintness. • Fatigue. • Shortness of breath. • Person older than 50.	• Heart disease. • Disorder of red blood cells.	• See Congestive Heart Failure. • See Anemia, Pernicious.
Faintness when turning head (in person older than 50).	Pressure on nerves in neck.	See Cervical Spondylosis.

*All references are to Illness section unless noted otherwise.

FAINTNESS OR FAINTING
(continued from previous page)

SYMPTOMS & FACTORS	POSSIBLE PROBLEM	WHAT TO DO*
• Fainting. • Shortness of breath before faintness. • Recent strenuous exercise.	Temporary change in blood chemistry.	Consult doctor if happens repeatedly.
• Fainting and weakness. • Sweating; irregular heartbeat. • Recent stomach surgery. • Diarrhea.	Intestinal disorder.	See Dumping Syndrome.
• Faintness. • Headache; dizziness; nausea and vomiting.	Toxic gas inhalation.	See Carbon Monoxide Poisoning.
• Fainting and weakness. • Sweating, headache, confusion. • Excessive hunger	Low blood sugar.	See Hypoglycemia, Functional.

*All references are to Illness section unless noted otherwise.

FATIGUE OR TIREDNESS
(continued on next page)

SYMPTOMS & FACTORS	POSSIBLE PROBLEM	WHAT TO DO*
• Fatigue. • Appetite loss. • Weight loss.	• Cancer. • Disorder of red blood cells.	• Consult doctor. • See Anemia (all charts).
• Fatigue, plus 2 or more of following: • Appetite loss. • Fever. • Headache. • Painful swelling in neck, armpit or groin. • Jaundice (yellow skin and eyes). • Sore throat.	Virus infection.	See Mononucleosis, Infectious.
• Fatigue. • Use of prescription or nonprescription drug.	Adverse reaction or side effect of drug.	• Consult doctor about prescription drug. • Discontinue use of nonprescription drug.
• Fatigue. • Coarse skin and hair. • Low voice. • Loss of sex drive. • Puffy face.	Underactive thyroid gland.	See Hypothyroidism.
• Fatigue. • Fever. • Headache, plus any of following: • Nausea, vomiting or diarrhea. • Drowsiness. • Cough. • Sore throat. • Pain in neck. • Aches in bones or joints. • Skin rash. • Pain in back. • Painful urination.	Bacterial or viral infection.	Consult doctor.
• Fatigue in woman at menopause. • Appetite loss.	Normal occurrence with decreasing estrogen level of menopause.	• See Menopause.
• Fatigue. • Pregnancy. • Shortness of breath.	Dietary deficiency of pregnancy, particularly of protein, calcium, vitamins or iron.	• Consult doctor. • Eat extra protein foods. • Drink 2 extra glasses of skim milk daily. • Take iron supplement and prenatal vitamin supplement.
• Fatigue. • Depression or anxiety.	Effect of stress.	• See Depression. • See Anxiety.
• Ongoing fatigue for several months. • Numerous other symptoms.	Unknown infection or problem.	See Chronic Fatigue Syndrome.

*All references are to Illness section unless noted otherwise.

FATIGUE OR TIREDNESS
(continued on next page)

SYMPTOMS & FACTORS	POSSIBLE PROBLEM	WHAT TO DO*
• Fatigue. • Chest discomfort with exertion that is relieved by rest.	Narrowing of coronary arteries.	• Consult doctor. • See Atherosclerosis. • See Coronary Artery Disease. • See Heart Valve Disease.
• Tiredness. • Depression. • Increased appetite. • Beginning of winter.	Lack of light.	See Seasonal Affective Disorder.
• Fatigue and weakness. • Intermittent fever, chills, sweating. • Weight loss.	Heart valve or heart lining infection.	See Endocarditis.
• Fatigue. • Fever; rash (usually on the cheeks). • Joint pain.	Autoimmune disorder.	See Lupus Erythematosus, Systemic.
• Fatigue. • Appetite loss. • Weight loss. • Hair loss. • Craving for salt. • Skin that darkens.	Inadequate cortisone hormone.	See Addison's Disease.
• Fatigue. • Cough. • Fever. • Weight loss. • Shortness of breath.	• Lung infection. • Tumor.	• See Tuberculosis. • See Bronchiectasis. • See Pneumonia (all charts). • See Influenza. • See Lung Cancer.
• Fatigue. • Headache and nausea. • Recent travel to foreign country.	Parasite infection.	See Malaria.
• Fatigue. • Shortness of breath. • Irregular heartbeat.	Heart inflammation.	See Myocarditis.
• Fatigue, slight fever. • Restlessness and irritability. • Cough; sore throat; increased saliva. • Animal bite.	Virus infection.	See Rabies.
• Fatigue. • Chills; fever; sweating. • Tenderness along spine.	Bacterial infection.	See Brucellosis.

*All references are to Illness section unless noted otherwise.

FATIGUE OR TIREDNESS
(continued from previous page)

SYMPTOMS & FACTORS	POSSIBLE PROBLEM	WHAT TO DO*
• Fatigue and lethargy. • Paleness. • Behavioral changes. • Abdominal discomfort.	Inhalation or ingestion of lead.	See Lead Poisoning.
• Tiredness. • Fever. • Swollen lymph glands.	Protozoan infection.	See Toxoplasmosis.
• Fatigue and weakness. • Tingling sensation in arms, hands, legs and feet. • Urinary frequency.	Endocrine disorder.	Hyperaldosteronism.
• Lethargy; weakness; paralysis in an arm or leg (in a child). • Confusion. • Personality changes.	Brain and liver infection.	See Reye's Syndrome.
• Fatigue in a child who fails to grow normally. • Shortness of breath. • Blueness under fingernails.	Congenital heart disease.	Consult doctor.
• Fatigue. • Appetite loss. • Nausea at sight of food, plus 2 or more of following: • Jaundice (yellow skin and eyes). • Vomiting. • Tenderness over liver. • Fever. • Weakness.	Liver disorder.	• See Hepatitis, Viral. • See Cirrhosis of the Liver.
• Fatigue. • Sleep disturbances, malaise. • Loss of concentration.	Disturbance in the body's physiological processes.	See Jet Lag.

*All references are to Illness section unless noted otherwise.

FEVER (CHILD 0 TO 2 YEARS)

SYMPTOMS & FACTORS	POSSIBLE PROBLEM	WHAT TO DO*
• Fever. • Runny nose. • Recent exposure to contagious disease, such as measles, mumps or chickenpox.	Early stage of contagious illness.	Consult doctor.
• Fever. • Diarrhea.	Infection of digestive tract.	• Consult doctor. • See Gastroenteritis.
• Fever. • Runny nose.	Virus infection.	• See Cold, Common. • See Respiratory Syncytial Virus. • Consult doctor if temperature rises.
• Fever. • Infant overdressed. • Hot weather or environment.	Overheating.	• Remove some of infant's clothing. • Offer water to drink. • Give cool sponge bath.
• Fever. • Crying as if in pain. • Pulling at ear.	Infection of middle ear.	• Consult doctor. • See Ear Infection, Middle.
• Fever. • Convulsions.	Effect of high fever.	• Call doctor now. • See Convulsion, Febrile.
• Fever. • Infant of 3 months or younger.	Many possibilities. Signs of illness at this age require prompt medical evaluation.	Consult doctor.
• Fever. • Rash.	Several disorders.	See Rash with Fever (in Symptoms section).
• Fever. • Noisy breathing.	Swelling in vocal cords.	• Consult doctor. • See Croup.
• Fever. • Rapid or difficult breathing.	Infection of breathing passages.	• Call doctor now. • See Bronchitis, Acute • See Bronchiolitis. • See Pneumonia (all charts).

*All references are to Illness section unless noted otherwise.

FEVER (CHILD OVER 2 YEARS)

SYMPTOMS & FACTORS	POSSIBLE PROBLEM	WHAT TO DO*
• Fever. • Diarrhea.	Infection of digestive tract.	See Gastroenteritis.
• Fever. • Earache. • Child pulls at ear.	Infection of middle ear.	See Ear Infection, Middle.
• Fever. • Cough. • Runny nose.	Virus infection.	• See Cold, Common. • See Influenza. • See Respiratory Syncytial Virus. • Consult doctor if temperature rises.
• Fever. • Convulsions.	Several disorders.	• Call doctor now. • See Convulsion, Febrile.
• Fever of 102F (38.9C) or higher. • No other symptoms.	Infection.	Consult doctor.
• Fever. • Cough. • Rapid or difficult breathing.	Infection of breathing passages.	See Pneumonia (all charts).
• Fever. • Rash.	Several disorders.	See Rash with Fever (in Symptoms section).
• Fever. • Abdominal pain.	Several disorders.	See Abdominal Pain, Sudden Attack (in Symptoms section).
• Fever. • Swelling between ear and jaw.	Virus infection.	See Mumps.
• Fever. • Sore throat or hoarseness.	Infection of upper respiratory tract.	• See Tonsillitis. • See Pharyngitis. • See Laryngitis.
• Fever. • Runny nose. • Recent exposure to contagious disease, such as measles, mumps or chickenpox.	Early stage of contagious illness.	Consult doctor.
• Fever. • Child seems very ill, plus any of following: • Stiff neck. • Pain when bending head forward. • Eyes sensitive to light. • Headache. • Vomiting.	Infection of membranes around brain.	• Call doctor now. • See Meningitis, Aseptic.
• Fever. • Chills; muscle aches, cough. • Listlessness. • Exposure to field mice or other rodents.	Virus infection.	See Hantavirus.

*All references are to Illness section unless noted otherwise.

FEVER (PERSON OVER AGE 12)
(continued on next page)

SYMPTOMS & FACTORS	POSSIBLE PROBLEM	WHAT TO DO*
• Fever. • Cough. • Headache. • Aches in bones or joints. • Stuffy or runny nose.	Virus infection.	• See Cold, Common. • See Influenza.
• Fever for 24 hours without other symptoms. OR • Recurrent fever with normal temperature between fevers.	Several disorders.	• Consult doctor. • See Fever of Unknown Origin.
• Fever. • Nausea or vomiting. • Diarrhea.	Infection of digestive tract.	See Gastroenteritis.
• Fever. • Pain in back below last rib.	Infection of urinary tract.	See Kidney Infection, Acute
Fever after several hours in strong sunshine or hot environment.	Excess heat exposure.	• See Heatstroke or Heat Exhaustion. • See Sunburn.
• Fever. • Cough. • Shortness of breath, even when resting.	Lung infection.	See Pneumonia (all charts).
• Fever. • Cough with gray-yellow sputum. OR • Wheezing.	Infection of bronchial tubes.	See Bronchitis, Acute.
• Fever. • Use of prescription or nonprescription drug.	Adverse reaction or side effect of drug.	• Consult doctor about prescription drug. • Discontinue use of nonprescription drug.
• Fever. • Painful urination. • Frequent urination.	Urinary-tract infection.	• See Cystitis. • See Kidney Infection, Acute.
• Fever. • Sore throat.	Infection.	• See Tonsillitis. • See Pharyngitis. • See Agranulocytosis.
• Fever. • Rash.	Several disorders.	See Rash with Fever (in Symptoms section).
• Sudden high fever. • Vomiting and watery diarrhea. • Rash resembling sunburn.	Blood poisoning.	See Toxic Shock Syndrome.

*All references are to Illness section unless noted otherwise.

SYMPTOMS

FEVER (PERSON OVER AGE 12)
(continued from previous page)

SYMPTOMS & FACTORS	POSSIBLE PROBLEM	WHAT TO DO*
• Fever. • Other symptoms similar to cold (cough, tiredness, chills).	Fungal infection or tick caused disorder depending on location in U.S.	• See Valley Fever (Southwest). • See Rocky Mountain Spotted Fever (West; Northwest; Middle Atlantic). • See Blastomycosis (Mississippi Valley). • See Lyme Disease (Northeast). • See Histoplasmosis (East and Midwest).
• Fever. • Headache, plus any of following: • Pain bending forward. • Lethargy. • Confusion. • Nausea or vomiting.	Infection of membranes around brain.	• Call doctor now. • See Meningitis, Aseptic.
• Intermittent fever and chills. • Fatigue and weakness. • Weight loss. • Vague aches and pains.	Heart valve or lining infection.	See Endocarditis.
• Fever and chills. • General ill feeling. • Headache. • Muscle ache.	Bacterial or viral infection.	• See Legionnaire's Disease. • See Encephalitis, Viral
• Low-grade fever. • Weight loss. • Recurrent respiratory and skin infections.	Virus infection.	See HIV Infection and AIDS.
• Fever (rapid temperature rise). • Shaking chills. • Pounding heartbeat. • General ill feeling.	Severe bacterial infection.	See Blood Poisoning.
• Intermittent fever. • Chills. • Marked fatigue. • Enlarged lymph glands.	Bacterial infection.	See Brucellosis.
• Fever. • Chills; muscle aches, cough. • Listlessness. • Exposure to field mice or other rodents.	Virus infection.	See Hantavirus.
• Fever. • Tiredness. • Swollen lymph glands.	Protozoan infection.	See Toxoplasmosis.

*All references are to Illness section unless noted otherwise.

FOOT PROBLEMS
(continued on next page)

SYMPTOMS & FACTORS	POSSIBLE PROBLEM	WHAT TO DO*
Excessively sweaty feet.	No underlying disorder.	• Wash and dry feet twice a day. Apply talcum powder. • Wear cotton socks.
• Foot pain. • Big toe turned inward.	Bony protrusion.	See Bunion.
Small blisters on toes or soles.	Effect of stress.	See Dyshidrosis.
Pain in foot following injury.	• Broken bone. • Ligament injury.	• See Bone Fracture. • See Sprains & Strains.
• Pain in foot joint, especially big toe. • Affected joint red, warm, swollen.	Joint inflammation.	See Gout.
• Pain on bottom of foot. • Small growth or area on sole that hurts when walking.	Skin growth caused by virus.	See Warts.
• Itching foot. • Skin between toes red, soft and peeling.	Fungus infection.	See Athlete's Foot.
• Pain in toe joints. • Affected joints red, warm, swollen. • Fever. • Recent illness, such as sore throat or skin infection.	Complication of prior streptococcal infection.	See Rheumatic Fever.
Pain in foot after walking or running.	• Circulatory disorder. • Bone injury.	• See Atherosclerosis. • See Buerger's Disease.
• Pain on bottom of foot. • Red, swollen area on sole.	Infection caused by a penetrating wound or splinter.	Consult doctor. You may need tetanus protection.
• Pain in toe joints. • Affected joints red, warm, swollen.	Inflammatory disease of joints.	See Arthritis, Rheumatoid.
• Pain or tenderness in foot joint, especially big toe. • Affected joint red, warm, swollen. • Use of prescription drug to prevent fluid retention (diuretic).	Adverse reaction or side effect of diuretic drug.	• Consult doctor. • See Gout.
• Aching feet. • Significantly overweight.	Effect of excess weight.	See Obesity.
• Pain in toe joints, ankles, knees or hips. • Person over age 50.	Degenerative condition of joints.	See Osteoarthritis.

*All references are to Illness section unless noted otherwise.

FOOT PROBLEMS
(continued from previous page)

SYMPTOMS & FACTORS	POSSIBLE PROBLEM	WHAT TO DO*
Numbness, hardness or paleness in skin exposed to subfreezing temperatures.	Tissue injury.	See Frostbite.
Pain and tenderness in the sole of the foot under the heel.	Tissue inflammation.	See Heel Spur.
• Tingling and numbness in feet or hands. • Shooting pain that may worsen at night.	Nerve disorder.	See Peripheral Neuropathy.

*All references are to Illness section unless noted otherwise.

GENITAL SORES, BLISTERS, WARTS OR BOILS

SYMPTOMS & FACTORS	POSSIBLE PROBLEM	WHAT TO DO*
Painless blister on genitals.	Sexually transmitted disease.	See Granuloma Inguinale.
• Painless red sore on genitals. • Enlarged lymph glands in neck, armpit, or groin. • Headache. • Rash on skin.	Sexually transmitted disease.	See Syphilis.
• Small flesh colored bumps or tiny cauliflower like bumps. • Warts may produce no symptoms, or cause itching, burning, tenderness or pain.	Sexually transmitted disease.	See Warts, Venereal.

*All references are to Illness section unless noted otherwise.

HAIR GROWTH IN WOMEN, EXCESSIVE

SYMPTOMS & FACTORS	POSSIBLE PROBLEM	WHAT TO DO*
• Excessive hair growth over 4 or 5 months. • Unexplained weight gain. • Menstrual changes or absent periods. • Deep voice.	Disorder or tumor of ovaries or adrenal gland.	• See Ovarian Tumor, Benign. • See Ovarian Cancer. • See Cushing's Syndrome. • See Polycystic Ovarian Syndrome.
• Excessive hair growth over 2 months or less. • Use of prescription drug, such as hormones, cortisone drugs or anticonvulsants.	Adverse reaction or side effect of drug.	Consult doctor.
• Excessive hair on face or body that developed before age 20. • Similar hairiness in other female family members.	Genetic causes; no underlying disorder.	Consult cosmetologist for removal of unwanted hair.
Excessive hair growth, especially on face, in woman who has had ovaries removed or is over age 40.	Normal occurrence with decreasing estrogen level of menopause.	• Consult doctor. • Consult cosmetologist for removal of unwanted hair.
Excessive hair growth during pregnancy.	Hormone changes of pregnancy.	Nothing. Hair growth decreases after delivery.
• Excessive hair growth on the face and body of a woman. • Irregular or no menstruation. • Acne.	Excessuve production of male hormones.	See Hirsutism.

*All references are to Illness section unless noted otherwise.

HAIR LOSS

SYMPTOMS & FACTORS	POSSIBLE PROBLEM	WHAT TO DO*
• Hair loss. • Use of prescription drug or radiation therapy, especially for cancer or circulatory disorders.	Adverse reaction or side effect of drug.	Consult doctor.
Sudden hair loss in patches on head.	Skin disorder.	• See Lichen Planus. • See Alopecia Areata. • See Ringworm. • See Telogen Effluvium.
Hair thinning in a woman within 2 to 3 months following childbirth.	Effect of hormonal changes.	Nothing. Hair growth will return to normal.
Gradual hair loss in women, especially thinning of hair on top of head.	Normal occurrence with aging.	See Baldness, Pattern, Male & Female.
Receding front hairline or thinning of hair on top of head in men.	Hereditary baldness occurring in men at any age.	See Baldness, Pattern, Male & Female.
• Hair loss. • Frequent use of any of following hair-care products or styles: permanent waves; dyes; bleaches; curling irons or hot rollers; straighteners; tight braids; ponytails; or cornrows.	Hair damage.	• Change hair style; avoid damaging products or styles. • Consult doctor if hair loss persists.
• Hair loss. • Unconscious pulling on hair.	Effect of stress.	See Anxiety.
Hair loss in 2 to 3 months following serious illness.	Temporary effect of illness and high fever.	Nothing. Hair should return to normal within few months.
Pulling out of hair.	Psychological disorder called trichotillomania.	Consult doctor.

*All references are to Illness section unless noted otherwise.

SYMPTOMS

HEADACHE
(continued on next page)

SYMPTOMS & FACTORS	POSSIBLE PROBLEM	WHAT TO DO*
• Headache. • Use of prescription or nonprescription drug.	Adverse reaction or side effect of drug.	• Consult doctor about prescription drug. • Discontinue use of nonprescription drug.
• Severe headache. • Fever.	Common occurrence with infection.	See Fever charts (in Symptoms section).
• Headache. • Recent head injury. • No other symptoms.	Common occurrence after head injury.	See Head Injury.
• Headache. • Vision disturbance before headache. • Nausea or vomiting.	Severe vascular headache.	See Migraine.
• Headache in forehead or back of head. • Tense, stressed feeling. • Sleeping difficulty.	Effect of stress.	• See Anxiety. • See Headache, Tension. • See Depression.
• Sudden onset of headache. • Pain around eyes. • Headache occurs at same time every day.	Chronic headache disorder.	See Headache, Cluster.
• Pain or tenderness around eyes and cheekbones that worsens when bending head forward. • Recent cold or nasal allergies.	Sinus infection.	See Sinusitis.
• Headache without pain around eyes and cheekbones. • Runny or stuffy nose.	Virus infection.	See Cold, Common.
• Headache. • Decreased consumption of caffeine-containing beverages (coffee, colas, cocoa, tea).	Caffeine withdrawal.	• Reduce consumption of caffeine gradually. • Use a nonprescription pain reliever, such as acetaminophen.
• Headache, plus any of following: • Unusually long time since eating. • Excessive alcohol consumption. • Stuffy, smoky or noisy room. • Exposure to strong sunlight.	Circumstantial headache. No underlying disorder.	Use a nonprescription pain reliever, such as acetaminophen.
• Headache after excessive alcohol consumption. • Nausea or vomiting.	"Hangover."	Use a nonprescription pain reliever, such as acetaminophen.

*All references are to Illness section unless noted otherwise.

HEADACHE
(continued from previous page)

SYMPTOMS & FACTORS	POSSIBLE PROBLEM	WHAT TO DO*
• Severe headache that worsens when bending head forward. • Eyes sensitive to light. • Lethargy. • Confusion. • No recent head injury.	Bleeding in membrane around brain.	• Call doctor now. • See Subarachnoid Hemorrhage. • See Brain or Epidural Abscess.
• Headache that worsens when bending head forward. • Fever. • Eyes sensitive to light.	Infection of membranes around brain.	• Call doctor now. • See Meningitis, Aseptic. • See Meningitis, Bacterial.
• Headache. • Eye pain. • Blurred vision. • Nausea or vomiting. • No injury to eye.	Excess pressure in eye.	• Call doctor now. • See Glaucoma, Primary Angle Closure.
• Habitual headache on waking; no excessive alcohol consumption. • Double vision. • Nausea or vomiting.	• High blood pressure. • Brain tumor.	• See Hypertension. • See Brain Tumor.
Headache after reading or straining to see.	Strain on neck muscles (not strain on eyes).	See Headache, Tension.
• Headache; nausea; vomiting. • Ascent to higher altitude.	Lack of oxygen.	See Altitude Illness.
• Headache. • Dizziness. • Nausea; vomiting. • Faintness.	Gas inhalation.	See Carbon Monoxide Poisoning.
• Headache. • Stiff neck. • Fever.	Fungal infection.	See Cryptococcosis.
• Headache. • General ill feeling. • Chills and fever. • Muscle aches.	Bacterial infection.	See Legionnaire's Disease.
• Headache. • Fatigue and nausea. • Travel to foreign country.	Parasite infection.	See Malaria.

*All references are to Illness section unless noted otherwise.

HEARING LOSS

SYMPTOMS & FACTORS	POSSIBLE PROBLEM	WHAT TO DO*
• Hearing loss. • Use of prescription or nonprescription drug.	Adverse reaction or side effect of drug.	• Consult doctor about prescription drug. • Discontinue use of nonprescription drug.
• Hearing loss. • Sticky, green-yellow discharge from ear.	• Infection of outer-ear canal or middle ear. • Injury to eardrum.	• See Ear Infection, Outer. • See Ear Infection, Middle. • See Eardrum, Ruptured.
• Hearing loss. • Dizziness.	Disorder or infection of inner ear.	• See Labyrinthitis. • See Meniere's Disease.
• Hearing loss, especially of high-pitched sounds. • Exposure to excessive noise, such as a jackhammer.	Damage caused by exposure to harmful noise levels.	See Hearing Impairment or Loss.
• Hearing loss. • Earache.	Infection or blockage.	See Earache (in Symptoms section).
Gradual hearing loss in person over age 60.	Common occurrence with aging.	Consult doctor.
• Gradual hearing loss over several weeks or months. • History of similar hearing loss in other family members.	Poor function of middle-ear bones.	See Otosclerosis.
• Hearing loss. • Recent cold or sore throat.	Blockage of canal between middle ear and back of throat (eustachian tube).	• See Cold, Common. • Consult doctor if hearing loss lasts longer than 3 days.
Gradual hearing loss over several weeks or months without other symptoms.	Earwax blockage.	See Earwax Blockage.
Noise in ear (ringing, buzzing, roaring, whistling or hissing).	Acoustic nerve disorder.	See Tinnitus.
• Hearing loss. • Plugged feeling in ear. • Change in air pressure (flying, diving).	Ear damage.	See Barotitis Media.

*All references are to Illness section unless noted otherwise.

HEARTBEAT IRREGULARITY

SYMPTOMS & FACTORS	POSSIBLE PROBLEM	WHAT TO DO*
• Irregular heartbeat. • General ill feeling. • History of heart disease.	Disorder of heart rate or rhythm.	• Call doctor now. • See Atrial Fibrillation. • See Heart Rhythm Irregularity. • See Heart Block. • See Heartbeat, Rapid. • See Potassium Imbalance. • See Aneurysm. • See Heart Valve Disease. • See Calcium Imbalance. • See Idiopathic Hypertrophic Subaortic Stenosis.
• Irregular heartbeat. • Use of prescription or nonprescription drugs, such as: thyroid medication; digitalis preparations; diuretics; diet pills; stimulants; caffeine; decongestants; cold remedies, including nasal sprays; illegal drugs, including marijuana, cocaine, psychedelics, amphetamines.	Adverse reaction or side effect of drug.	• Consult doctor about prescription drug. • Discontinue use of nonprescription or illegal drug.
• Irregular heartbeat. • Unexplained weight loss. • Anxiety. • Excessive sweating. • Fatigue.	Overactive thyroid gland.	See Hyperthyroidism.
• Rapid or irregular heartbeat. • Recent tension or worry.	Effect of stress.	• See Anxiety. • See Panic Disorder. • See Phobias.
• Irregular heartbeat. • Excessive smoking. OR • Excessive consumption of caffeine-containing beverages such as coffee, cola, tea or cocoa.	Effect of nicotine or caffeine.	Decrease nicotine or caffeine use.
• Rapid or irregular heartbeat. • Fever.	Infection.	See Fever charts (in Symptoms section).
• Heartbeat irregularity. • Shortness of breath. • Fatigue.	Heart inflammation.	See Myocarditis.
• Rapid heartbeat following exercise, emotional upset or exposure to cold. • Tremors and nervousness. • Feelings of doom.	Adrenal tumor.	See Pheochromocytoma.

*All references are to Illness section unless noted otherwise.

IMPOTENCE, MALE SEXUAL
(Erectile Dysfunction)

SYMPTOMS & FACTORS	POSSIBLE PROBLEM	WHAT TO DO*
• Sexual impotence. • Use of prescription or nonprescription or mood-altering drugs, such as: antihypertensives; narcotics; cocaine; antidepressants; antihistamines; antiulcer medicines; diuretics; hormones including birth-control pills; beta-adrenergic blockers; tranquilizers; reserpine; marijuana; digitalis; skeletal-muscle relaxants; sedatives; hypnotics; or phenothiazines	Adverse reaction or side effect of drug.	• Consult doctor about prescription drug. • Discontinue use of nonprescription drug.
• Sexual impotence. • Chronic illness.	• Low level of testosterone (male sex hormone). • Diminished blood circulation to genitals.	• Consult doctor. • See Atherosclerosis. • See Diabetes Mellitus, Insulin Dependent. • See Diabetes Mellitus, Non-Insulin Dependent. • See Cirrhosis of the Liver. • See Hypothyroidism. • See Multiple Sclerosis. • See Prostate, Enlarged. • See Pituitary Gland, Underactive.
• Sexual impotence. • Excessive alcohol consumption.	Effect of alcohol.	See Alcoholism.
• Sexual impotence. • Anxiety or depression.	Effect of stress.	• See Anxiety. • See Depression.
• Sexual impotence. • History of sexually transmitted disease.	Scarring or other effect of infection.	• See Syphilis. • See Gonorrhea. • See Urethritis. • See HIV Infection and AIDS. • See Herpes, Genital. • See Reiter's Syndrome. • See Warts, Venereal. • See Lymphogranuloma Venereum.
• Sexual impotence. • History of premature ejaculation or other sexual dysfunction.	Psychosexual problem.	• See Impotence, Male Sexual. • See Premature Ejaculation.
• Sexual impotence. • Acute illness with fever.	Temporary effect of illness.	Nothing. Sexual function will return when illness subsides.

*All references are to Illness section unless noted otherwise.

ITCHING

SYMPTOMS & FACTORS	POSSIBLE PROBLEM	WHAT TO DO*
• Itching hands. • Hands are frequently wet or exposed to chemicals.	Effect of chemicals or moisture.	See Dermatitis, Contact.
• Itching on head or between toes. • Small bald patches on scalp.	Fungus infection.	• See Ringworm. • See Athlete's Foot.
• Itching on head. • Tiny white spots on hair that won't come off.	Parasites.	See Lice.
• Itching. • Insect bite or sting.	Reaction.	See Insect Bites & Stings.
• Itching or bleeding around anus. • Painful bowel movements.	• Varicose veins in anus. • Split in skin around anus.	• See Hemorrhoids. • See Anal Fissure.
Itching around anus following severe diarrhea.	Normal response to irritation.	Apply ointment containing zinc oxide.
• Itching. • Diarrhea. • Abdominal pain. • Flatulence and bloating. • Rash.	Reaction to a swallowed substance.	See Food Allergy and Intolerance.
• Intense itching and burning. • Bright red skin rash. • Contact with poisonous plant.	Allergic reaction to plant.	See Poison Ivy, Oak, Sumac.
• Itching. • Fluid-filled blisters. • Skin disorder elsewhere on body.	Allergic reaction.	See Id Reaction.
• Itching. • Yellow skin and eyes.	• Liver disorder. • Blood disorder.	Call doctor now.
• Itching. • General ill feeling.	• Blood disorder. • Kidney disorder. • Overactive thyroid gland. • Adverse reaction or side effect of drug. • Cancer.	• Consult doctor. • See Polycythemia. • See Renal Failure, Acute. • See Hyperthyroidism. • See Drug Hypersensitivity.
• Itching. • Rash. • No fever.	Several skin disorders.	See Rash without Fever (in Symptoms section).
Itching in genital area in females.	Irritation or infection.	See Vaginal Itching (in Symptoms section).
Itching around anus, especially at night.	• Parasites. • Several causes.	• See Pinworms. • See Pruritis Ani.
• Itching. • Wheezing; coughing; sneezing. • Swelling around face and hands. • Difficult breathing.	Allergic reaction.	• Call doctor now. • See Anaphylaxis.

*All references are to Illness section unless noted otherwise.

KNEE PAIN

SYMPTOMS & FACTORS	POSSIBLE PROBLEM	WHAT TO DO*
• Pain in knee. • Knee "catches" or won't bear weight.	Injured knee cartilage.	See Sprains & Strains.
• Pain in knee following injury. • Knee won't bear weight. • Knee misshapen.	Broken bone or dislocation.	• Call doctor now. • See Bone Fracture. • See Dislocation or Subluxation.
• Pain in knee. • Knee red, warm, swollen. • Fever. • General ill feeling.	Bone or joint infection.	See Osteomyelitis.
• Pain in knee and other joints. • Affected joints red, warm, swollen. • Fever. • Recent illness such as sore throat, gonorrhea or skin infection.	Complication of prior infection.	• See Rheumatic Fever. • See Arthritis, Infectious.
• Pain in knee or other joints. • Affected joints red, warm, swollen. • No fever.	Joint inflammation.	• See Bursitis. • See Gout. • See Arthritis, Rheumatoid. • See Arthritis, Juvenile Rheumatoid (children only). • See Osgood-Schlatter Disease (older children and adolescents only). • See Psoriatic Arthritis.
• Chronic pain in knee. • Knee sometimes "catches" or won't support weight. OR • Persistent discomfort in knee, fingers or other joints without other symptoms.	Degenerative joint disease.	See Osteoarthritis.
• Pain in knee in child under 12. • Hip pain. • Limp.	Degenerative condition of hip joint in children.	See Legg-Perthes Disease.
• Acute attack of swelling and pain in the knee. • Attack lasts for 2 or more days.	Joint disorder.	See Pseudogout.

*All references are to Illness section unless noted otherwise.

LEG PAIN

SYMPTOMS & FACTORS	POSSIBLE PROBLEM	WHAT TO DO*
• Leg pain. • Back pain.	Muscle strain or sciatica.	See Back Pain.
• Leg pain following strenuous exercise or following injury. • Leg can bear weight.	Muscle injury.	See Sprains & Strains.
• Leg pain. • Restricted movement, tenderness and swelling around a tendon.	Tendon inflammation.	See Tendinitis.
• Leg pain following injury. • Leg won't bear weight.	Broken bone.	• Call doctor now. • See Bone Fracture.
Sharp pain down back of leg, especially when coughing, sneezing or laughing hard.	Pressure on large nerve in leg.	• See Disk, Ruptured. • See Backache (in Symptoms section).
• Leg pain. • Muscles tighten briefly— usually while asleep—then return to normal.	Several disorders.	See Muscle Cramp, Ache or Weakness (in Symptoms section).
• Leg ache, especially after standing a long time. • Prominent veins in legs.	Disorder of veins.	See Varicose Veins.
• Shooting pain in leg. • Tingling and numbness that begins in hands or feet. • Gradual muscle weakness.	Nerve disorder.	See Peripheral Neuropathy.
• Pain in calf. • One vein red, hot and hard.	Blood clot in superficial vein.	See Thrombophlebitis, Superficial.
• Pain in calf when flexing ankle. • Swollen, tender calf.	Blood clot in deep vein.	• Call doctor now. • See Thrombosis, Deep Vein.
• Persistent pain in one part of leg. • Fever. • General ill feeling.	• Bone infection. • Cancer.	• See Osteomyelitis. • See Multiple Myeloma.
• Pain in calf after walking. • Pain disappears with rest.	Circulatory disorder.	• See Atherosclerosis. • See Buerger's Disease. • See Claudication. • See Thrombosis & Embolus, Arterials.
• Leg pain. • Painful or stiff hip on same side as leg pain.	Degenerative condition of joints.	See Osteoarthritis.
• Leg pain along sciatic nerve. • Recurrent low backache. • Stiffness.	Joint disease.	See Ankylosing Spondylitis.

*All references are to Illness section unless noted otherwise.

MEMORY PROBLEMS

SYMPTOMS & FACTORS	POSSIBLE PROBLEM	WHAT TO DO*
Gradual decline over past 10 years in ability to remember everyday things in person over age 50.	Common occurrence with aging; no underlying disorder.	• Consult doctor at next appointment. • Write lists to help your memory. This is not the beginning of serious mental decline.
• Inability to remember everyday things, such as location of keys, pens, glasses, or forgetting items on shopping list. • Depression or tension.	Effect of stress.	• See Depression. • See Anxiety.
• Inability to remember a period of time. • Use of prescription or nonprescription drug, especially for sleeping difficulty.	Adverse reaction or side effect of drug.	Consult doctor.
Total memory loss.	Psychological disorder.	Consult doctor.
• Inability to remember a period of time. • Recent head injury.	Brain injury.	• Call doctor now. • See Head Injury.
Inability to remember episodes of excessive-alcohol consumption.	Effect of alcohol.	• Consult doctor. • See Alcoholism.
• Inability to remember recent events while remembering long-ago events, plus 2 or more of following: • Poor attention span in conversations or with instructions. • Decline in attention to personal appearance or cleanliness. • Personality change. • Decline in ability to cope with everyday matters.	Mental deterioration.	• See Dementia. • See Vitamin B Deficiencies. • See Alzheimer's Disease.
• Inability to remember a period of time, plus events surrounding any of the following: • Epileptic seizure. • Diabetic coma. • Period before and after surgery. • Severe, feverish, illness such as meningitis or pneumonia.	Common occurrence following these situations.	Nothing.
• Memory problems and confusion. • Inability to speak or move part of body. OR • Low body temperature.	• Decrease in blood supply to brain. • Prolonged exposure to cold, especially in the elderly.	• Call doctor now. • See Stroke. • See Hypothermia.
• Memory loss. • Headaches; vomiting. • Vision changes.	Tumor.	• Call doctor now. • See Brain Tumor.
• Memory problems. • Recent surgical procedure with general anesthetic.	Often occurs.	Memory should return to normal.

*All references are to Illness section unless noted otherwise.

MENSTRUAL PERIODS, LATE OR ABSENT

SYMPTOMS & FACTORS	POSSIBLE PROBLEM	WHAT TO DO*
• Menstrual periods absent, plus 2 or more of following: • Unexplained weight gain. • Masculine voice. • Abnormal hairiness.	Hormone imbalance.	Consult doctor.
Menstrual periods absent in woman over age 38.	Normal menstrual irregularities at this age.	See Menopause.
• Menstrual periods absent. • Recent quick weight loss from drastic dieting. OR • Current participation in strenuous exercise program. OR • Recent illness. OR • Tension or worry. OR • Change in lifestyle such as new job or new home. OR • Menstrual periods absent since discontinuing use of oral contraceptives.	• Hormone changes. • Effect of stress. • Hormone changes caused by discontinuing pill.	See Amenorrhea.
• Menstrual periods absent. • Use of prescription drug.	Adverse reaction or side effect of drug.	• Consult doctor. • See Amenorrhea.
• Menstrual period late by 2 or more weeks. • Sexual intercourse within last month.	Pregnancy.	• Consult doctor to confirm pregnancy. • Take home pregnancy test.
Menstrual periods absent since delivery of baby.	Normal occurrence caused by hormone changes following childbirth.	• If bottle-feeding, consult doctor if periods do not resume within 8 weeks after delivery. • If breast-feeding, consult doctor if periods do not resume within 4 weeks after weaning.
Menstrual periods have never started.	Hormone changes of puberty have not occurred.	• Consult doctor if older than 16. • See Amenorrhea.
• Irregular menstrual periods. • Gastrointestinal upsets. • Discomfort or pain in lower abdomen.	• Cyst. • Cancer.	• See Polycystic Ovarian Syndrome. • See Ovarian Cancer.

*All references are to Illness section unless noted otherwise.

MENSTRUAL PERIODS, PAINFUL OR HEAVY

SYMPTOMS & FACTORS	POSSIBLE PROBLEM	WHAT TO DO*
• Excessive menstrual flow. • Menstrual period lasts more than 7 days.	Menstrual irregularity.	See Menorrhagia.
Menstrual period more painful or heavier than usual, especially during last days of period.	Disorder of lining of pelvic organs.	• See Endometriosis. • See Dysmenorrhea.
• Current menstrual period more painful or heavier than usual. • Period arrived one week or more late.	• Early pregnancy and miscarriage. • Pregnancy outside uterus.	• Consult doctor. • See Miscarriage. • See Ectopic Pregnancy.
Menstrual periods more painful or heavier since receiving intrauterine contraceptive device (IUD).	Common side effect of using IUD.	Consult doctor.
• Menstrual periods more painful or heavier than usual. • No other pelvic or genital symptoms.	Benign growth in uterus.	See Fibroid Tumors of the Uterus.
Menstrual periods painful or heavy since discontinuing use of oral contraceptives.	Hormone changes caused by discontinuing pill.	Consult doctor.
• Menstrual periods painful. • Periods began within last 3 years. • Healthy otherwise.	No disease.	See Dysmenorrhea.
Menstrual period heavy in woman who has recently delivered a baby.	Normal occurrence during first 2 menstrual periods following childbirth.	Consult doctor if heavy periods persist.
Menstrual flow always heavy.	No underlying disorder.	Consult doctor for blood test for anemia.
• Heavy menstrual flow. • Bleeding between normal menstrual periods.	Excessive estrogen.	See Endometrial Hyperplasia.
Painful, prolonged or irregular bleeding through the vagina.	Several causes.	See Uterine Bleeding, Dysfunctional.
• Menstrual periods more painful or heavier than usual. • Bad-smelling vaginal discharge. • Fever.	Infection of reproductive organs.	• Call doctor now. • See Pelvic Inflammatory Disease.

*All references are to Illness section unless noted otherwise.

MOUTH, SORE; TINGLING; DRY
(continued on next page)

SYMPTOMS & FACTORS	POSSIBLE PROBLEM	WHAT TO DO*
• Sore mouth. • Blisters or red, rough or painful areas on lips or in mouth.	Virus infection.	• See Herpes Simplex. • See Hand, Foot & Mouth Disease.
• Sore mouth. • Creamy-white patches in mouth or tongue.	Fungus infection.	See Thrush.
• Dry mouth. • Use of prescription or nonprescription medication.	Adverse reaction or side effect of medication.	• Consult doctor about prescription drug. • Discontinue nonprescription drug if dry mouth is causing problems.
• Sore mouth. • Fever. • Sores in mouth. • Use of prescription or nonprescription drugs.	Adverse reaction or side effect of drug.	Call doctor now.
• Sore mouth. • Red, painful gums that bleed easily. • Bad breath.	Bacterial infection.	See Trench Mouth.
• Sore mouth. • Painful ulcers in the mouth.	Infection or inflammation.	See Canker Sores.
• Sore mouth. • Use of new cosmetics.	Allergic reaction caused by chemical.	Discontinue use of new cosmetic.
• Dry mouth. • Stress or apprehension.	Normal occurrence.	Dry mouth will disappear when stress is diminished.
• Small white patch in the mouth that feels firm, rough and stiff. • Sensitivity to hot and spicy foods.	Several causes.	See Leukoplakia.
• Small bumps or sores in the mouth. • Sores form an irregular whitish line in the mouth.	Infection.	See Lichen Planus.
• Dry mouth. • Decreased urination. • Severe thirst.	Electrolyte disorder.	See Dehydration.
• Sore mouth. • Rough or split corners of mouth.	Vitamin or mineral deficiency.	• See Vitamin B Deficiencies. • See Anemia, Folic Acid Deficiency. • See Anemia, Aplastic.
• Bleeding from the gums. • Easy bruising. • Tiredness; low fever; anemia.	Cancer.	See Leukemia, Acute.

*All references are to Illness section unless noted otherwise.

MOUTH, SORE; TINGLING; DRY (continued from previous page)

SYMPTOMS & FACTORS	POSSIBLE PROBLEM	WHAT TO DO*
• Pale, painless lump in mouth. • Lump may enlarge, ulcerate and bleed.	Cancer.	See Oral Cancer.
• Mouth tingling. • Sneezing, coughing, wheezing. • Watery eyes. • Difficult breathing.	Allergic reaction.	• Call doctor now. • See Anaphylaxis.
• Dryness of mouth. • Dryness of eyes. • Parotid gland enlargement (chipmunk face).	Autoimmune disorder.	See Sjögren's Syndrome.
• Numbness and tingling around the mouth. • Palpitations; rapid heartbeat. • Shortness of breath. • Emotional fears.	Severe anxiety.	See Panic Disorder.

*All references are to Illness section unless noted otherwise.

MUSCLE CRAMP; ACHE; WEAKNESS
(continued on next page)

SYMPTOMS & FACTORS	POSSIBLE PROBLEM	WHAT TO DO*
Muscle cramp while relaxed or resting in bed. OR • Muscle cramp in arm or leg during or after exercise. OR • Muscle cramp after sitting in awkward position.	Common occurrence; usually no underlying disorder.	• Massage muscle and use heat to relieve pain. • See Sprains & Strains. • See Tendinitis.
Recurrent leg cramps when walking.	Circulatory disorder.	• See Atherosclerosis. • See Buerger's Disease. • See Thrombosis & Embolus, Arterial. • See Claudication.
Muscle cramp following exposure to heat.	Heat exhaustion.	See Heatstroke or Heat Exhaustion.
Pain, tenderness and limited movement in muscle.	Inflammation.	See Bursitis.
• Recurrent muscle cramps. • Tender nodules on skin. • Stiffness and weakness.	Inflammation of connective tissue.	See Fibrositis.
• Muscle cramp. • Use of diuretic drug for high blood pressure or heart disorder.	Adverse reaction or side effect of drug.	Consult doctor.
• Muscle cramp. • Numbness, tingling in arms or legs. • Irregular heartbeat.	Electrolyte disorder.	See Calcium Imbalance.
• Muscle aches. • Chills; fever; cough. • Exposure to field mice or other rodents.	Virus infection.	See Hantavirus.
• Muscle aches. • Fever; tiredness. • Exposure to cats; cat litter or dirt soiled by cats.	Protozoan disorder.	See Toxoplasmosis.
• Muscle weakness in hands, feet and arms. • Weakness spreads within 72 hours. • Shock.	Inflammatory nerve condition.	See Guillain-Barré Syndrome.
• Weakness. • Ducklike gait. • Falling; difficulty in getting up after falling.	Muscle deterioration.	See Muscular Dystrophy.
• Weakness in the pelvic or shoulder muscles. • Skin rash on the face, shoulders, arms, and over joints.	Connective tissue disorder.	See Polymyositis.

*All references are to Illness section unless noted otherwise.

MUSCLE CRAMP; ACHE; WEAKNESS
(continued from previous page)

SYMPTOMS & FACTORS	POSSIBLE PROBLEM	WHAT TO DO*
• Muscle cramps (usually in the legs). • Confusion; restlessness; anxiety. • Weakness.	Electrolyte disorder.	See Sodium Imbalance.
• Muscle weakness or cramps (in infants). • Swelling of ankles, abdomen and face. • Anemia in premature infant.	Vitamin deficiency.	See Vitamin E deficiency.
• Weakness of arm and leg muscles. • Weakness of facial muscles.	Autoimmune disorder.	See Myasthenia Gravis.

*All references are to Illness section unless noted otherwise.

NECK PAIN

SYMPTOMS & FACTORS	POSSIBLE PROBLEM	WHAT TO DO*
• Stiffness or severe neck pain on waking. • No pain before going to bed.	Uncomfortable sleeping position.	Consult doctor if pain lasts longer than 24 hours.
• Sudden, severe neck pain. • Injury to neck.	Muscle injury.	See Sprains & Strains.
• Neck pain. • Stressful situation.	Muscle tension.	Take a hot shower or have someone massage your neck muscles to relieve tension.
• Severe neck pain. • Sharp pain in shoulders or arms when moving head.	• Slipped disk in neck. • Neck-muscle injury.	• See Disk, Ruptured. • See Whiplash. • See Torticollis.
• Neck and shoulder pain. • Working at computer or other repetitive task for many hours.	Muscle spasm.	• Be sure computer screen is at proper eye level and chair is at correct height. • Take a break every hour.
• Sudden neck pain, especially when bending head forward, plus any of following: • Lethargy. • Confusion. • Eyes sensitive to light. • Nausea or vomiting. • Severe headache.	Infection or bleeding in membrane around brain.	• Call doctor now. • See Meningitis, Aseptic. • See Subarachnoid Hemorrhage.
• Sudden, severe neck pain. • Recent strong jolt. • Difficulty controlling arms or legs. • Loss of bowel or bladder control.	Damaged spinal cord.	Call doctor now.
• Stiff neck. • Behavioral or personality changes. • General ill feeling. • Headache; vomiting; fever.	Brain inflammation.	See Encephalitis, Viral.
Swelling or lump in neck.	Several disorders.	See Swelling or Lump (in Symptoms section).
• Chronic neck pain that is worsening. • Numbness or tingling in arm or hand. • Person over age 40.	Pressure on nerves in neck.	See Cervical Spondylosis.

*All references are to Illness section unless noted otherwise.

NOSE, STUFFY OR RUNNY

SYMPTOMS & FACTORS	POSSIBLE PROBLEM	WHAT TO DO*
• Stuffy or runny nose (clear, watery discharge) plus any of following: • Fever. • Cough. • Headache. • Aches in bones or joints. • Sore throat.	Virus infection.	• See Cold, Common. • See Influenza.
• Stuffy or runny nose (clear, watery discharge). • Itching eyes. • Sneezing.	Nasal allergy.	See Hay Fever.
• Runny nose. • Low-grade fever. • Decrease in appetite. • Cough; lethargy.	Virus infection.	See Respiratory Syncytial Virus.
• Stuffy or runny nose (thick, cloudy, yellow-green discharge). • Pain or tenderness around eyes and cheekbones that worsens when bending head forward.	Sinus infection.	See Sinusitis.
• Chronic "stuffy nose" feeling. • Impaired sense of smell. • Feeling of fullness in the face.	Growth in nasal cavity.	See Nasal Polyps.
• Obstruction of air through the nostrils. • Nasal discharge.	Septum problem.	See Nasal Septum, Deviated.
• Chronic "stuffy nose" feeling. • Use of nasal decongestants for more than 3 days.	Decongestant is suddenly withdrawn after extended use or they are overused.	Consult doctor.

*All references are to Illness section unless noted otherwise.

NUMBNESS, TINGLING OR PRICKLING
(continued on next page)

SYMPTOMS & FACTORS	POSSIBLE PROBLEM	WHAT TO DO*
• Numbness or tingling in feet or hands after sitting in one position a long time or waking from deep sleep. • No underlying disorder.	• Stretching of, or pressure on, a nerve. • Temporary decrease in blood supply to a nerve.	Nothing. Feeling returns in a few minutes.
• Numbness or tingling in any part of body. • Use of prescription drug.	Adverse reaction or side effect of drug.	Consult doctor.
• Numbness or tingling in hands and fingers, especially at night. • Sharp pain in hand or arm, especially at night. • Weak grip.	Pressure on nerves in wrist.	See Carpal-Tunnel Syndrome.
• Numbness and tingling in injured area of the skin. • Formation of scar tissue.	Normal occurrence.	Nothing.
• Numbness or tingling on one side of body, plus any of following: • Weakness in extremities. • Dizziness. • Confusion. • Blurred vision. • Speaking difficulty.	Decreased blood supply to brain.	• Call doctor now. • See Stroke. • See Transient Ischemic Attack.
• Numbness or tingling in an arm or leg. • Weakness in the affected side. • Recent heavy lifting or strenuous exercise.	Pressure on nerves.	See Disk, Ruptured.
• Numbness or tingling in fingers or toes. • Blue fingers or toes in cold weather. • Redness and pain when numbness subsides and feeling returns.	Disorder of blood circulation in fingers and toes.	See Raynaud's Phenomenon.
• Numbness or tingling in hands. • Stiff neck. • Person over age 35.	Pressure on nerves in neck.	• See Cervical Spondylosis. • See Thoracic-Outlet-Obstruction Syndrome.
• Numbness or tingling in hands and face, especially around lips. • Dizziness.	Decreased carbon dioxide in blood.	See Panic Attack.
• Numbness, tingling in arms or legs. • Muscle cramps. • Irregular heartbeat.	Electrolyte disorder.	See Calcium Imbalance.

*All references are to Illness section unless noted otherwise.

NUMBNESS, TINGLING OR PRICKLING
(continued from previous page)

SYMPTOMS & FACTORS	POSSIBLE PROBLEM	WHAT TO DO*
• Numbness and tingling that begins in hands and feet. • Shooting pain that may worsen at night.	Nerve disorder.	See Peripheral Neuropathy.
• Fatigue and weakness. • Tingling sensation in arms, hands, legs and feet. • Frequent urination.	Endocrine disorder.	See Hyperaldosteronism.
• Tremors and nervousness. • Rapid heartbeat following exercise, emotional upset or exposure to cold. • Feelings of doom.	Adrenal tumor.	See Pheochromocytoma.

*All references are to Illness section unless noted otherwise.

RASH WITH FEVER
(continued on next page)

SYMPTOMS & FACTORS	POSSIBLE PROBLEM	WHAT TO DO*
• Raised, red, itching bumps that become blisters on face, trunk and genitals. • Fever.	Virus infection.	See Chickenpox.
• Red rash. • Fever. • Swelling on both sides of neck or at base of skull.	Virus infection.	See Rubella.
• Rash starting on cheeks and then spreading. • Fever. • Young child.	Virus infection.	See Fifth Disease.
• Rash in child age 1-3. • Fever. • Irritability.	Childhood disorder.	See Roseola Infantum.
• Red spots or blotches on face or trunk. • Fever, plus 2 or more of following: • Dry cough. • Sore, red eyes. • Runny nose. • Sore throat. • Headache.	• Virus infection. • Rickettsia infection.	• See Measles. • See Hand, Foot & Mouth Disease. • See Rocky Mountain Spotted Fever.
• Painful red, blister-like rash on body. • Fever. • General ill feeling.	Virus infection.	See Herpes Zoster.
• Purple spots, plus 2 or more of following: • Fever. • Headache. • Pain when bending head forward. • Eyes sensitive to light. • Vomiting.	Infection of membranes around brain.	• Call doctor now. • See Meningitis, Bacterial.
• Red rash in woman of childbearing age. • Fever of 101F (38.3C) or higher. • Rapid heartbeat. • Fatigue and weakness. • Excessive thirst.	Bacterial infection.	• Call doctor now. • See Toxic Shock Syndrome.
• Purple rash. • Fever.	Allergic disorder.	• Call doctor now. • See Purpura, Allergic.

*All references are to Illness section unless noted otherwise.

RASH WITH FEVER
(continued from previous page)

SYMPTOMS & FACTORS	POSSIBLE PROBLEM	WHAT TO DO*
• Red rash. • Paleness around mouth. • Fever of 102F (38.9C) or higher. • Bright red, sore throat. • Swollen tonsils. • Enlarged glands in neck.	Complication of preceding streptococcal infection.	• Call doctor now. • See Scarlet Fever.
• Mild skin rash on chest, back and abdomen. • Fever; fatigue and paleness. • Pain caused by joint inflammation.	Complication of preceding streptococcal infection.	See Rheumatic Fever.
• Red rash or spots that begins on palms, soles, arms and legs. • Rash develops into blisters. • Fever (sometimes).	Inflammatory disorder.	See Erythema Multiforme.

*All references are to Illness section unless noted otherwise.

RASH WITHOUT FEVER
(continued on next page)

SYMPTOMS & FACTORS	POSSIBLE PROBLEM	WHAT TO DO*
• Light-red bumps with raised edges. • Severe itching.	Allergic reaction.	See Hives.
• Itching rash. • Use of prescription or nonprescription drug.	Adverse reaction or side effect of drug.	• Call doctor now. • See Drug Hypersensitivity.
Itching, red, scaling or moist rash under cosmetics, jewelry or new clothing.	Allergic reaction.	See Dermatitis, Contact.
Itching, red, scaling or moist rash, especially on hands.	Skin disorder aggravated by stress.	See Dermatitis, Atopic.
• Itching, red, scaling or moist rash, plus: • Recent contact with plant, such as poison ivy, poison oak, poison sumac, primrose or mango. OR • Recent contact with irritating detergents or other chemicals.	Allergic reaction.	• See Poison Ivy, Oak, Sumac. • See Dermatitis, Contact.
• Itching rash around genitals or anus. • No other symptoms or factors.	• Sugar in urine. • Vaginal infection.	• See Diabetes Mellitus, Insulin Dependent. • See Diabetes Mellitus, Non-Insulin Dependent. • See Vaginitis, Monilial.
Red bumps in a small area without other symptoms.	Insect bites.	See Insect Bites & Stings.
• Red rash. • Rash is located in areas of heavy perspiration.	Obstruction of sweat glands.	See Prickly Heat.
• Red rash scattered over body. • Severe itching at night. • Gray lines or red, sore spots between fingers or on wrists.	Parasites.	See Scabies.
• Rash that consists of small, white blisters with pus inside. • Blisters are located in hair follicles of the skin.	Bacterial or fungal skin infection.	See Folliculitis.
Red, scaling patch that spreads into a ring.	Fungus infection.	See Ringworm.
Rash without fever in child under 2.	Several disorders.	See Skin Problems (Child Under Age 2) (in Symptoms section).
• Red rash that begins on palms, soles, arms and legs. • Rash develops into blisters.	Inflammatory disorder.	See Erythema Multiforme.

*All references are to Illness section unless noted otherwise.

RASH WITHOUT FEVER
(continued from previous page)

SYMPTOMS & FACTORS	POSSIBLE PROBLEM	WHAT TO DO*
• Red, raised rash or skin lesions. • Rash appears on cheeks in a "butterfly" appearance.	Autoimmune disorder.	• See Lupu Erythematosus, Discoid. • See Lupus Erythematosus, Systemic.
• Rash starting on cheeks then spreading. • Slight tiredness or fatigue. • Young child.	Virus infection.	See Fifth Disease.
• Skin rash, progressing to thin, raised lines on the skin. • Contact with soil or sand.	Hookworm infestation.	See Larva Migrans Cutaneous.
• Skin rash (that may itch) on face, shoulders, arms and over joints. • Weakness in the pelvic or shoulder muscles.	Connective tissue disorder.	See Polymyositis.
• Red skin rash, sometimes with small blisters. • A burning reaction similar to those that follow prolonged sun exposure. • Dizziness, nausea, vomiting. • Brief sun exposure.	Sensitivity to sun.	See Photosensitivity.

*All references are to Illness section unless noted otherwise.

SEXUAL INTERCOURSE, PAINFUL FOR MAN

SYMPTOMS & FACTORS	POSSIBLE PROBLEM	WHAT TO DO*
• Pain during ejaculation. • Burning when urinating. • Discharge from penis.	Infection of urethra or prostate gland.	• See Urethritis. • See Prostatitis. • See Gonorrhea.
• Pain in penis during intercourse. • Red, swollen, tender bumps or sores on skin or tip of penis.	Skin inflammation or infection.	• See Herpes, Genital. • See Balanitis.
• Pain in penis during intercourse. • Partner tense, difficult to arouse or uncomfortable during intercourse.	Lack of lubrication in partner's vagina.	• See Dyspareunia. • See Vaginismus.
• Pain in tip of penis after intercourse. • Use of latex condom. OR • Partner uses contraceptive cream or douching solution.	Allergic reaction to cream, solution or condom.	See Dyspareunia.
• Pain in penis before, during or after intercourse. • No other symptoms or factors.	Psychosexual problem.	• See Dyspareunia. • See Impotence, Male Sexual.
A prolonged, painful, tender erection unaccompanied by sexual arousal.	Penis disorder.	• Call doctor now or seek emergency care. • See Priapism.

*All references are to Illness section unless noted otherwise.

SEXUAL INTERCOURSE, PAINFUL FOR WOMAN

SYMPTOMS & FACTORS	POSSIBLE PROBLEM	WHAT TO DO*
• Painful intercourse only when partner penetrates vagina deeply. • Heavy, painful periods.	Disorder of lining of pelvic organs.	See Endometriosis.
• Painful intercourse. • Abnormal vaginal discharge.	Several disorders.	• See Abnormal Vaginal Discharge (in Symptoms section). • See Vaginitis (all charts).
• Painful intercourse. • Tenderness over bladder. • Frequent, painful urination.	Bladder inflammation.	See Cystitis.
Painful intercourse in woman past menopause or over age 45.	Normal occurrence caused by decreased vaginal secretions.	• See Vaginismus. • See Dyspareunia. • See Menopause.
• Painful intercourse. • Recent childbirth.	Inflammation or scarring caused by a stretched or torn vagina or episiotomy repair.	• Wait at least 3 weeks before resuming sexual relations after childbirth. • Consult doctor if pain lasts longer than 8 weeks.
• Painful intercourse. • Vaginal itching.	Several disorders.	See Vaginal Itching (in Symptoms section).
• Painful intercourse. • Vagina seems too tight.	Muscle spasm.	• See Vaginismus. • See Dyspareunia.
• Painful intercourse. • Recent start or increase in sexual activity.	No underlying disorder.	• Wait 2 to 3 days for symptoms to disappear before resuming sex. • See Vaginismus. • See Dyspareunia.
• Dryness of vagina causing painful intercourse. • Dryness of eyes and mouth.	Autoimmune disorder.	See Sjögren's Syndrome.
• Pain with intercourse. • Bad smelling vaginal discharge. • Frequent, painful urination.	Infection.	See Pelvic Inflammatory Disease.
• Pain with intercourse. • Lump in back of the vagina or projecting outside of it. • Vague backache.	Fallen uterus.	See Uterine Prolapse.
• Painful intercourse. • Swelling without pain in lower abdomen or severe abdominal pain. • Stinging or burning with urination.	Cysts.	See Polycystic Ovarian Syndrome.
• Painful intercourse. • No other symptoms or factors.	• Vaginal malformation. • Lack of experience and education.	Consult doctor.

*All references are to Illness section unless noted otherwise.

SHOULDER PAIN

SYMPTOMS & FACTORS	POSSIBLE PROBLEM	WHAT TO DO*
• Pain in shoulder following injury. • Shoulder misshapen. • Bruising in affected area. • Inability to move shoulder.	Broken bone or dislocation.	• Call doctor now. • See Bone Fracture. • See Dislocation or Subluxation.
• Pain in shoulder following injury. • Shoulder appearance normal. • Shoulder movement uncomfortable.	Injury to shoulder-cuff muscle or ligament.	• See Sprains & Strains. • See Tendinitis.
• Pain in shoulder, especially when moving arm. • No other symptoms.	Shoulder inflammation.	See Bursitis.
• Pain in shoulder and other joints. • Affected joints red, warm, swollen.	Inflammatory disease of joints.	• See Arthritis, Rheumatoid. • See Psoriatic Arthritis.
• Sudden pain in shoulder. • No fever.	Shoulder inflammation.	• See Gout. • See Pseudogout.
• Shoulder and neck pain. • Working at computer or typing for many hours.	Muscle spasm.	• Be sure computer screen is at proper eye level and chair is at correct height. • Take a break every hour.
• Sudden pain in shoulder or other joint. • Affected joint red, warm, swollen. • Fever. • Recent illness, such as sore throat or skin infection.	Complication of prior streptococcal infection.	See Rheumatic Fever.
• Pain in shoulder when moving arm. • Stiffness and severity of pain increasing.	Severe shoulder inflammation.	See Shoulder, Frozen.
• Pain between shoulder blades. • Tightness, pressure, squeezing, or mild ache in the chest. • Heart disorder.	Lack of blood to heart.	• Consult doctor. • See Angina Pectoris.

*All references are to Illness section unless noted otherwise.

SKIN, BUMPS ON
(continued on next page)

SYMPTOMS & FACTORS	POSSIBLE PROBLEM	WHAT TO DO*
Thickened bump on toe.	Skin thickening caused by pressure.	See Corn or Callus.
Bumps on skin that are cysts, blisters, scaly patches, white patches or sores.	Several disorders.	See Skin Problems (in Symptoms section).
Rough, hard bump on hand or foot with tiny black dots in bump.	Skin growth caused by virus.	See Warts.
Painful, red bump with white or yellow center in part of body with hair.	Infected hair follicle.	See Boils.
• Small raised bumps that are firm, white and have a dry sandpaper feel. • Bumps are in clusters in hair follicles.	Common skin disorder.	See Keratosis Pilaris.
• Bumps or rash. • Fever.	Several disorders.	See Rash with Fever (in Symptoms section).
• Papules (small, raised bumps) that are flat-topped with well-defined borders. • Papules don't itch or hurt.	Inflammatory skin disorder.	See Keratoses, Seborrheic.
• Nodules under the skin that are dome-shaped. • Nodules feel "doughy," smooth and are easily movable.	Benign fat-cell tumors.	See Lipomas.
Rough, small bumps on skin of anus, vagina or penis.	Skin growth caused by virus.	See Warts, Venereal.
• Light-red bumps with raised edges. • Severe itching.	Allergic reaction.	See Hives.
• Dark, slow-growing lump. OR • Change in mole size or color. • Borders of mole become irregular. • Bleeding or pain in mole.	Skin cancer or precancerous lesion.	• See Melanoma. • See Dysplastic Nevi.
Single lump that grows.	• Skin growth caused by virus. • Skin cancer, especially if center is an open sore. • Spread of cancer from other body parts.	• Consult doctor. • See Skin Cancer, Basal-Cell. • See Skin Cancer, Squamous-Cell.
Red bumps on cheeks, on either side of nose and on scalp (sometimes).	Autoimmune disorder.	See Lupus Erythematosus, Discoid.

*All references are to Illness section unless noted otherwise.

SKIN, BUMPS ON
(continued from previous page)

SYMPTOMS & FACTORS	POSSIBLE PROBLEM	WHAT TO DO*
• Nodules in the armpit. • Nodules are firm, tender and domed.	Blocked glands.	See Hidradenitis Suppurativa.
• Small red, raised bumps (papules) on the skin of the thighs, buttocks or armpits. • Followed by other symptoms: muscle aches, fatigue, chills, fever, stiff neck, headache, backache, nausea and vomiting.	Tick bite.	See Lyme Disease.
• Small, raised bumps (papules) on the skin. • Bumps are firm, smooth, domed with a central pit, and skin-colored or white.	Virus infection of the skin.	See Molluscum Contagiosum.

*All references are to Illness section unless noted otherwise.

SKIN PROBLEMS (CHILD UNDER AGE 2)

SYMPTOMS & FACTORS	POSSIBLE PROBLEM	WHAT TO DO*
Rash in diaper area.	Chemical skin irritation.	See Diaper Rash.
• Rash or blotches. • Hot weather or environment.	Sweat retention.	• Remove excess clothing. • Consult doctor if rash lasts longer than 24 hours or child seems ill. • See Prickly Heat.
Greasy, scaling, crusty patches on scalp.	Cradle cap.	Use half-strength coal-tar cream on affected areas. Your pharmacist can provide this. Cradle cap usually disappears when hair grows.
• Rash. • Fever.	Several disorders.	See Rash with Fever (in Symptoms section).
Rash, spots, blisters or discoloration in infant 3 months or younger.	Several disorders.	Consult doctor.
Inflamed skin with itching, flaking patches.	Allergic skin disorder.	See Eczema.
Blisters on face that burst and become crusty.	Skin infection.	See Impetigo.
Patch of skin that is lighter or darker than surrounding skin.	• Disorder of skin pigment. • Inherited skin lesion.	• See Pityriasis Alba. • See Skin Lesions, Benign.
• Small, itching blisters, usually in a thin line. • Broken blisters leave scratch marks.	Disease of the skin.	See Scabies.
Dark red or purple spots that don't fade when skin is pressed or stretched.	Allergic disorder.	• Call doctor now. • See Purpura, Allergic.
• Small raised bumps on the skin (often on the face). • Bumps don't hurt or itch.	Virus infection.	See Molluscum Contagiosum.
• Small, raised itch bumps. • Bumps swell and produce pink or red lesions (wheals). • Wheals form larger areas of redness.	Allergic disorder.	See Hives.

*All references are to Illness section unless noted otherwise.

SKIN PROBLEMS (PERSON OVER AGE 2)
(continued on next page)

SYMPTOMS & FACTORS	POSSIBLE PROBLEM	WHAT TO DO*
• Red, circular, flat, scaling lesions. • May be on the scalp, skin, nails and bearded area of the face.	Fungal infection.	• See Ringworm.
• Rash. • Use of prescription or nonprescription drug.	Adverse reaction or side effect of drug.	• Call doctor now about prescription drug. • Discontinue use of nonprescription drug.
Red skin areas covered with silvery scales.	Chronic skin disorder.	See Psoriasis.
Flaking, white scales over reddish patches on the skin where hair grows.	Dandruff or cradle cap.	See Dermatitis, Seborrheic.
Painful, red bump with white or yellow center in part of body with hair.	Infected hair follicle.	See Boils.
Patch of skin that is lighter or darker than surrounding skin.	• Disorder of skin pigment. • Yeast infection of skin.	• See Vitiligo. • See Pityriasis Alba. • See Tinea Versicolor.
Yellow or greenish-yellow tint to the skin (jaundice).	Can be caused by numerous disorders or drugs.	Call doctor now.
• Yellow-orange tint to the skin. • Consumption of large amounts of carrots or yellow vegetables containing beta-carotene.	Excess of carotene in the system.	Stop eating offending food for 2 to 6 weeks. Resume eating it in moderation.
• A new mole or dark lump. OR • Change in a mole or skin lesion that has been present since childhood in person over age 12.	Skin cancer or precancerous lesion.	• See Melanoma. • See Dysplastic Nevi.
• Dome-shaped cyst. • Cyst is whitish or skin-colored.	Infected cyst.	See Sebaceous Cyst.
• Blister-like rash. • Burning sensation at site 1 or 2 days before rash appears.	Virus infection of sensory nerves.	See Herpes Zoster.
Small blisters on fingers, toes, palms and soles.	Bacterial or fungal skin infection.	See Folliculitis.
Reddish, scaly, oval patches on chest, back or abdomen without fever or other symptoms.	Inflammatory skin disorder.	See Pityriasis Rosea.
Itching rash without fever.	Several disorders.	See Rash Without Fever (in Symptoms section).

*All references are to Illness section unless noted otherwise.

SKIN PROBLEMS (PERSON OVER AGE 2) (continued from previous page)

SYMPTOMS & FACTORS	POSSIBLE PROBLEM	WHAT TO DO*
• Redness, swelling and tenderness in skin. • Fever. • General ill feeling.	Skin infection.	See Cellulitis.
• Skin lesions (blue-red nodules) on face, arms and trunk. • HIV infection.	Skin cancer.	See Kaposi's Sarcoma.
Numbness, hardness or paleness in skin exposed to subfreezing temperature.	Tissue injury.	See Frostbite.
• Painless blister on genitals that ulcerates and heals quickly. • Enlarged lymph glands in the groin that form large, red, tender masses.	Sexually transmitted disease.	See Lymphogranuloma Venereum.
Pain, redness, and tenderness at the base of the spine.	Infected cyst.	See Pilonidal Cyst.
• Small, movable, nontender nodule that appears under the skin of the finger. • The nodule enlarges and becomes pink and ulcerates.	Fungal infection.	See Sporotrichosis.
New scars on the skin that arise in an area of injury, burn or other skin problem.	Defective healing process.	See Keloids.
• Clusters of small, itching blisters. • Clusters appear on both sides of the body in the same place.	Inflammation of skin.	See Dermatitis, Herpetiformis.
• Sudden appearance of warm, painful or tender nodules. • Nodules usually start on front of leg. • Color changes from pink to red to blue to brown.	Inflammatory skin disease.	See Erythema Nodosum.
• Small, raised bumps on the skin in the shape of a ring. • Pink or violet color with a dome or slightly flat shape.	Chronic benign skin disorder.	See Granuloma Annulare.
• Small raised bumps on the skin that appear first as pinhead size, but grow rapidly. • Bumps bleed easily if injured.	Skin disorder of unknown cause.	See Granuloma, Pyogenic.
• Redness, swelling, warmth around a nail. • Sudden pain around the nail.	Herpes infection of the skin.	See Herpetic Whitlow.

*All references are to Illness section unless noted otherwise.

SKIN PROBLEMS (PERSON OVER AGE 2)
(continued from previous page)

SYMPTOMS & FACTORS	POSSIBLE PROBLEM	WHAT TO DO*
• Rash. • Fever.	Several disorders.	See Rash with Fever (in Symptoms section).
Skin problems in child under 2.	Several disorders.	See Skin Problems (Person Under Age 2) (in Symptoms section).
Skin problem on feet.	Several disorders.	See Foot Problems (in Symptoms section).
Skin problem on face.	Several disorders.	See Facial Skin Problems (in Symptoms section).
Itching without change in skin appearance.	Several disorders.	See Itching (in Symptoms section).
Bumps on skin.	Several disorders.	See Skin, Bumps on (in Symptoms section).
• Plaques (Flat areas with the following characteristics: • Bright red patches with poorly defined borders. • Some are weeping or oozing. • Skin appears moist or crusted. • Severe itching.	Yeast infection of the skin.	See Candidiasis of Skin.

*All references are to Illness section unless noted otherwise.

SLEEPING PROBLEMS
(continued on next page)

SYMPTOMS & FACTORS	POSSIBLE PROBLEM	WHAT TO DO*
Sleep disturbance (difficulty falling asleep, staying asleep or remaining asleep).	Many causes.	See Insomnia.
• Sleeping problems (sleepiness or insomnia). • Use of prescription or nonprescription drug, such as appetite suppressants, decongestants ordiuretics.	Adverse reaction or side effect of drug.	Consult doctor.
Sleeping problems following late, heavy dinner or consumption of 3 or more alcoholic beverages at night.	Common occurrence.	• Eat lighter or earlier dinner. • Decrease alcohol consumption.
• Sleeping problems. • Use of caffeine-containing beverage or drug.	Stimulant effect of caffeine.	Decrease use of caffeine, especially during late afternoon or evening.
• Sleeping problems. • Sedentary lifestyle.	Common occurrence.	Begin an exercise program. Consult your doctor first if you have any chronic illness or are at risk for heart disease.
Change in sleep pattern in person over age 60.	Normal occurrence; less sleep may be needed with aging.	Nothing.
• Inability to fall asleep. • Daytime tension.	Effect of stress.	See Anxiety.
• Wakefulness during night, plus 2 or more of following: • Reduced sex drive. • Inability to concentrate. • Lowered self-esteem. • Feelings of guilt, worthlessness, self-reproach. • Fatigue. • Loss of pleasure in usual activities. • Poor appetite or overeating.	Depression.	See Depression.
• Sleeping problems. • Recent withdrawal from narcotics, sleeping pills, tranquilizers or alcohol.	Withdrawal symptom.	Nothing. Normal sleep pattern should return within several weeks.
• Sleeping problems. • Use of illegal drug.	Adverse reaction or side effect of drug.	• Discontinue use of drug. • See Drug Abuse & Addiction.

*All references are to Illness section unless noted otherwise.

SLEEPING PROBLEMS
(continued from previous page)

SYMPTOMS & FACTORS	POSSIBLE PROBLEM	WHAT TO DO*
• Sleeping problems, plus 2 or more of following: • Excessive sweating. • Unexplained weight loss. • Increased appetite. • Anxiety. • Rapid or irregular heartbeat.	Overactive thyroid gland.	See Hyperthyroidism.
• Sleep problems. • Poor appetite. • Self-pity and pessimism.	Chronic mild depression.	See Dysthymia.
Sleep attacks that may occur up to 10 times a day.	Sleep disorder.	See Narcolepsy.
• Sleepiness. • Constipation. • Decreased tolerance for hot or cold.	Underactive thyroid gland.	See Hypothyroidism.
• Fitful sleep. • Shortness of breath when awake.	Fluid in lungs caused by heart condition.	See Congestive Heart Failure.
• Long periods of not breathing when asleep. • Choking while sleeping. • Snoring.	Breathing problem.	See Sleep Apnea.
• Poor sleep habits in infants, such as restlessness and profuse sweating. • Delayed motor skills.	Vitamin deficiency.	See Vitamin D Deficiency.
• Difficulty in remaining asleep. • Stiffness and weakness. • Sudden, painful muscular spasms.	Muscle inflammation.	See Fibrositis.
• Child has sleepless nights. • Child is restless during day.	Behavior disorder.	See Attention Deficit Hyperactivity Disorder.

*All references are to Illness section unless noted otherwise.

SPEAKING DIFFICULTY

SYMPTOMS & FACTORS	POSSIBLE PROBLEM	WHAT TO DO*
• Speaking difficulty. • Use of prescription or nonprescription drug.	Adverse reaction or side effect of drug.	Consult doctor.
• Inability to complete words without repeating first consonants. OR • Inability to speak when ready to say something.	Stammering or stuttering in children, and stress in adults.	Consult doctor or speech therapist.
• Expressionless speech with abnormal tone and phrasing. • Trembling that is worse at rest. • Shuffling walk.	Disorder of central nervous system.	See Parkinson's Disease.
Normal pronunciation, but confused words or ideas in person under age 45.	Psychiatric disorder.	Consult doctor.
• Normal pronunciation but confused words or ideas, plus 1 or more of following: • Poor attention span with conversations or instructions. • Decline in attention to personal appearance or cleanliness. • Personality changes.	Mental deterioration.	• See Alzheimer's Disease. • See Dementia.
Speaking difficulty because of inability to move muscles on one side of face.	Disorder of facial nerves.	See Bell's Palsy.
• Speaking difficulty. • Vague eye problems. • Weakness; difficulty in walking and balance.	Nervous system disorder.	See Multiple Sclerosis.
Speaking difficulty because of pain in mouth or tongue.	Infection or sores in mouth or tongue.	See Mouth, Sore; Tingling; Dry (in Symptoms section).
• Speaking difficulty, plus any of following: • Blurred vision. • Numbness or tingling in any part of body. • Weakness in extremities. • Dizziness.	Decreased blood supply to brain.	• Call doctor now. • See Stroke. • See Transient Ischemic Attack. • See Aneurysm. • See Thrombosis & Embolism, Arterial.

*All references are to Illness section unless noted otherwise.

STOOL, ABNORMAL APPEARANCE

SYMPTOMS & FACTORS	POSSIBLE PROBLEM	WHAT TO DO*
• Stool that is very dark, black or contains black material, plus any of following: • Recent consumption of green, leafy vegetables; licorice; chocolate; grapes, raisins and cranberries. • Current use of iron-supplement tablets. • Recent use of Pepto-Bismol.	No underlying disorder.	Nothing. If discoloration continues, consult doctor.
• Red-looking stools. • Recent consumption of beets, tomatoes, red-colored drinks or cereal, cherry-flavored medicines.	Stools are reddish due to something you ate or drank.	Nothing. If discoloration continues, consult doctor.
• Dark or black stool. • Use of prescription or nonprescription drug.	Adverse reaction or side effect of drug.	• Consult doctor about prescription drug. • Discontinue use of nonprescription drug.
Light colored or almost white stool.	• Jaundice. • May be a symptom of numerous disorders.	Consult doctor.
• Blood in stool. OR • Stool has a black or dark-red color.	Several disorders.	See Bleeding, Rectal (in Symptoms section).
Worms in stool.	Parasitic infection.	• Call doctor now. • See Pinworms. • See Roundworms.
• Pale stool. • Yellow skin and eyes (jaundice).	Gallbladder or liver disorder.	• Call doctor now. • See Cholecystitis or Cholangitis. • See Hepatitis, Viral.
• Pale, foamy, bulky, bad-smelling stool. • No jaundice.	Poor digestion.	See Malabsorption.

*All references are to Illness section unless noted otherwise.

SWALLOWING DIFFICULTY

SYMPTOMS & FACTORS	POSSIBLE PROBLEM	WHAT TO DO*
• Swallowing difficulty. • Sensation that food is stuck high in chest. • Occasional chest pain, especially when bending forward or lying down.	Discomfort in upper digestive tract.	See Gastroesophageal Reflux Disease.
Normal swallowing with sensation that food is stuck.	Effect of stress.	• Increase fluid intake when eating. • See Anxiety.
• Swallowing difficulty. • Sore throat. • Fever.	Throat infection.	• Request throat culture. • See Strep Throat. • See Tonsillitis. • See Pharyngitis. • See Herpangina. • See Diphtheria.
• Swallowing difficulty. • Recent swallowing of foreign object, such as fish bone. • Sore throat.	Object stuck in throat.	Call doctor now.
• Swallowing difficulty that is chronic or worsening. • Sensation that food is stuck high in chest.	Esophagus muscle disorder.	• See Hiatal Hernia. • See Dysphagia.
• Swallowing difficulty. • Pain with swallowing. • Bloody mucus regurgitation.	Tumor or esophagus disorder.	• See Esophagus, Cancer of. • See Esophageal Stricture or Corrosive Esophagitis.
• Swallowing difficulty. • Drooping eyelids. • Arm and leg weakness.	Autoimmune disorder.	See Myasthenia Gravis.
• Severe swallowing difficulty. • Muscle pain and spasms. • Fever. • Difficulty in using chest muscles to breathe.	Infection in a wound or injury site.	See Tetanus.
• Swallowing difficulty. • Hardening and thickening of the skin of the fingers and face.	Connective tissue disease.	See Scleroderma.
• Swallowing difficulty. • Muscle weakness of neck, chest and extremities. • Drooping eyelids. • Double vision. • No fever.	Toxin from contaminated food.	• Call doctor now. • See Botulism.

*All references are to Illness section unless noted otherwise.

SWEATING, EXCESSIVE

SYMPTOMS & FACTORS	POSSIBLE PROBLEM	WHAT TO DO*
• Excessive sweating. • Anxiety or excitement.	Normal occurrence with stress.	See Anxiety.
• Excessive sweating. • Overweight.	Effect of excess weight.	See Obesity.
• Excessive sweating in woman older than 38. • Irregular menstrual periods.	Hormone changes; end of menstrual cycles approaching.	See Menopause.
• Excessive sweating in woman during menstrual period. OR • Excessive sweating due to tension or apprehension. OR • Excessive sweating following coffee consumption.	No underlying disorder.	Nothing.
Excessive sweating in teenager.	Normal occurrence during adolescence.	Nothing.
• Sweating. • Palpitations; tremors; flushing. • Symptoms of anxiety when exposed to, or thinking of, a particular stimulus.	Fears.	See Phobias.
• Excess sweating. • Unpleasant body odor.	Several disorders.	See Hyperhidrosis.
• Skin is cool and moist. • Prolonged exposure to hot temperature.	Excessive fluid loss.	See Heatstroke or Heat Exhaustion.
• Excessive sweating. • Chest pain.	Heart attack.	• Call doctor now! • See Heart Attack. • See Coronary Artery Disease.
• Excessive sweating at night. • Weight loss. • Persistent cough with blood in sputum. • Fever. • Fatigue.	• Lung inflammation or infection. • Cancer.	• See Tuberculosis. • See Hodgkin's Disease. • See Lung Cancer.
• Excessive sweating, plus 2 or more of following: • Weight loss. • Increased appetite. • Anxiety. • Sleeping problems.	Overactive thyroid gland.	See Hyperthyroidism.
• Excessive sweating. • Use of prescription, nonprescription or illegal drug.	Adverse reaction or side effect of drug.	• Consult doctor about prescription drug. • Discontinue use of nonprescription or illegal drug.
• Excessive sweating. • Fever.	Normal occurrence with fever.	See Fever charts (in Symptoms section).

*All references are to Illness section unless noted otherwise.

SWELLING OR LUMP
(continued on next page)

SYMPTOMS & FACTORS	POSSIBLE PROBLEM	WHAT TO DO*
Firm swelling in groin that does not disappear when pressed.	• Infection in leg or genitals. • Protruding intestinal tissue.	• Consult doctor. • See Hernia.
• Nodule or bump under the skin. • Nodule feels "doughy," smooth and easily movable.	Benign fat-cell tumor.	See Lipomas.
• Painful, red lump or swelling. • Recent injury to area.	Bleeding under skin.	• See Sprains & Strains. • See Tendinitis.
Lump in breast.	• Cyst. • Cancer.	• Consult doctor. • See Fibrocystic Breast Disease. • See Breast Cancer.
Soft lump or swelling in groin or near navel that disappears when pressed or enlarges with cough.	Protruding intestinal tissue.	See Hernia.
Swelling between ear and jaw.	• Virus infection of glands. • Infection around tooth. • Disorder or tumor of salivary gland.	• See Mumps. • See Tooth Abscess. • See Salivary-Gland Disorders.
• Lump or swelling in neck, armpit or groin. • Fever.	Virus infection.	See Mononucleosis, Infectious.
Swelling or lump in child 3 months or younger.	Several disorders.	Consult doctor.
• Swelling on both sides of neck, toward front. • Sore throat.	Bacterial or viral infection.	• See Tonsillitis. • See Pharyngitis. • See Mononucleosis, Infectious.
• Swelling at both sides of back of neck. • Pink rash. • Fever.	Virus infection.	See Rubella.
• Tender swelling in armpit, groin, elbow or base of neck. • Sore, cut or bite on hand, arm, leg or shoulder on same side as swelling.	Infected bite or wound.	Consult doctor.
Tender or hard lump in neck just below Adam's apple.	Inflammation or tumor of thyroid.	• See Thyroiditis. • See Thyroid Nodule.
• Tender lump on elbow or in armpit. • Fever. • Exposure to cats.	Virus infection.	See Cat-Scratch Disease.
Swelling in front of neck with movement when swallowing.	Thyroid goiter.	Consult doctor.

*All references are to Illness section unless noted otherwise.

SWELLING OR LUMP
(continued from previous page)

SYMPTOMS & FACTORS	POSSIBLE PROBLEM	WHAT TO DO*
• Swelling in neck, armpit or groin. • Recent vaccination, such as tetanus or typhoid.	Swelling caused by vaccination.	Consult doctor.
Painless swelling near joint that is overused.	Ganglion cyst.	Consult doctor.
• Mass in abdomen that can be felt, especially in young child. • Cramping abdominal pain.	Intestinal obstruction.	• Call doctor now. • See Intussusception.
Lump or swelling in neck, armpit or groin without other symptoms or factors.	• Infection. • Tumor.	• See Hodgkin's Disease. • See Lymphoma, Non-Hodgkin's.
• Lump or swelling in neck, armpit or groin. • Use of prescription drug, especially for epilepsy or thyroid disorder.	Adverse reaction or side effect of drug.	Consult doctor.
• Swollen lymph nodes. • Low-grade fever. • Weight loss. • Recurrent respiratory and skin infections.	Virus infection.	See HIV Infection and AIDS.
• Hard mass in right, upper abdomen. • Unexplained weight loss and appetite loss. • Bleeding tendency.	Liver tumor.	• See Hepatoma. • See Liver Cancer.
• Swelling in superficial abscesses. • Rectal redness. • Throbbing pain. • Pain during bowel movement.	Swelling caused by bacteria or fungus.	See Anorectal Abscess.

*All references are to Illness section unless noted otherwise.

TESTICLES OR PENIS, PAINFUL OR SWOLLEN

SYMPTOMS & FACTORS	POSSIBLE PROBLEM	WHAT TO DO*
Painless swelling of testicles.	• Fluid accumulation. • Enlarged veins in testicle. • Protruding intestinal tissue.	• Consult doctor. • See Hernia.
• Sudden, painful swelling in testicle. • Recent injury to genital area.	Internal injury.	Call doctor now.
• Sudden, painful swelling in testicle. • No injury to genital area.	• Twisted testicle. • Infection of glands in testicle.	• Call doctor now. • See Testicle Torsion. • See Epididymitis.
Swelling or lump on one testicle.	Cyst or tumor.	• Consult doctor. • See Testicle Cancer.
• Pain in testicles. • Painless, rubbery strands extending up scrotum. • No injury to testicles.	Enlarged veins in testicle.	Consult doctor.
• Pain in testicles or penis. • Forceful blow, injury or wound in lower abdomen or genitals.	Injury to genitourinary tract.	See Genitourinary Injury.
• Pain in testicles. • Swelling between ear and jaw. • Fever.	Virus infection of glands.	• Consult doctor. • See Mumps.
• Soft, painless swelling in the scrotum (skin covering the testicles) filled with fluid. OR Swollen, painful veins surrounding testicle.	• Inflammation, infection or injury. • Varicose veins. • Dilated vein within the sac.	• See Hydrocelectomy (in Surgery section). • See Varicocele Removal (in Surgery section).

*All references are to Illness section unless noted otherwise.

THROAT, SORE

SYMPTOMS & FACTORS	POSSIBLE PROBLEM	WHAT TO DO*
• Sore throat. • Fever. • Swelling on both sides of neck toward front. • Red, swollen tonsils with specks of pus on surface.	Bacterial or viral infection.	• Request throat culture. • See Tonsillitis. • See Strep Throat. • See Diphtheria. • See Mononucleosis, Infectious.
• Sore throat. • Excessive smoking or alcohol consumption. OR • Smoke-filled environment.	Throat irritation or inflammation.	See Pharyngitis.
• Sore throat. • Dripping nose. • Itching eyes.	Allergic reaction.	See Hay Fever.
• Sore throat. • Hoarseness or voice loss.	Several disorders.	• See Laryngitis. • See Voice Loss or Hoarseness (in Symptoms section).
• Sore throat. • Fever, plus any of following: • Aches in bones or joints. • Cough. • Headache. • Stuffy or runny nose.	Virus infection.	• See Cold, Common. • See Influenza.
• Sore throat. • Fever. • Swelling or tenderness between ear and jaw.	Virus infection of glands.	See Mumps.
• Sore throat. • Sudden "barking" cough. • Young child.	Bacterial infection of epiglottis.	See Epiglottitis, Acute.
• Sudden sore throat with redness, inflammation and painful swallowing. • Fever. • General ill feeling.	Virus infection.	See Herpangina.
• Sore throat. • Cough; chills; fever. • Muscle and joint aches. • Skin rash.	Fungal infection.	See Valley Fever.

*All references are to Illness section unless noted otherwise.

TONGUE, SORE

SYMPTOMS & FACTORS	POSSIBLE PROBLEM	WHAT TO DO*
• Sore tongue. • Use of prescription or nonprescription drugs.	Adverse reaction or side effect of drug.	Consult doctor.
• Sore tongue. • Discomfort confined to one spot.	Abrasion from denture or irregular tooth.	Consult dentist.
• Sore tongue. • Pain one one side of face.	Nerve inflammation or damage.	See Trigeminal Neuralgia.
• Sores on tongue. • Sores are small, very painful and shallow.	Several causes.	See Canker Sores.
• Sore tongue. • Hard lump on tongue or in mouth.	• Infection. • Tumor.	• Call doctor now. • See Mouth or Tongue Tumor, Benign. • See Oral Cancer.
• Sore tongue. • Diarrhea with loose, bulky, bad-smelling stool. • Retarded growth.	Poor digestion.	See Malabsorption.
• Sore tongue. • Discomfort involves whole tongue.	• Anemia. • Inflammation or infection.	• See Anemia, Pernicious. • See Anemia, Iron-Deficiency. • See Anemia During Pregnancy. • See Tongue Inflammation.
• Sore tongue. • Cracked, fissured, red tongue. • Mouth ulcers.	Poor nutrition.	• Consult doctor. • See Vitamin B Deficiencies.

*All references are to Illness section unless noted otherwise.

TOOHACHE

SYMPTOMS & FACTORS	POSSIBLE PROBLEM	WHAT TO DO*
• Toothache, plus any of following: • Fever. • Swollen face or gums. • Continual pain that interferes with sleep.	• Advanced tooth decay. • Infection around tooth.	• Call dentist now. • See Tooth Decay. • See Tooth Abscess.
• Toothache over several teeth.. • Red, swollen, bleeding gums.	Gum infection.	• See Gingivitis. • See Periodontitis.
• Recurrent toothache. • No other symptoms.	Tooth decay.	• Consult dentist. • See Tooth Decay.
• Toothache when biting food. • Recent tooth filling.	• Common occurrence following a filling. • Filling not level.	Consult dentist if pain lasts longer than 1 week.
• Cheek pain that resembles a toothache. • Nasal condition. • Feeling of pressure inside the head.	Sinus infection.	See Sinusitis.
• Gnawing pain in lower teeth and neck. • Chest discomfort beneath breastbone. • Shoulder or arm pain. • Sweating.	Insufficient oxygen to heart.	• Call doctor now. • See Angina Pectoris. • See Coronary Artery Disease.

*All references are to Illness section unless noted otherwise.

TREMBLING OR TWITCHING

SYMPTOMS & FACTORS	POSSIBLE PROBLEM	WHAT TO DO*
• Trembling or twitching, especially of tongue and face muscles. • Use of prescription or nonprescription drug, especially phenothiazine.	Adverse reaction or side effect of drug.	• Consult doctor about prescription drug. • Discontinue use of nonprescription drug.
Trembling in one part of body, especially when affected part is at rest.	Disorder of central nervous system.	See Parkinson's Disease.
• Trembling. • Alcohol withdrawal.	Withdrawal symptom.	See Alcoholism.
• Trembling. • Excessive consumption of coffee or tea. OR • Use of nonprescription drug containing caffeine.	Adverse effect of caffeine.	Decrease use of caffeine.
• Trembling, plus 2 or more of following: • Weight loss. • Fatigue. • Excessive sweating.	Overactive thyroid gland.	See Hyperthyroidism.
• Painful twitching on side of face. • Pain is triggered by stroking or touching the face.	Nerve disorder.	See Trigeminal Neuralgia.
Twitching in one small part of body, such as eyelid.	Fatigue or tension. Usually no underlying disorder.	• Nothing. • Consult doctor if you feel ill or if muscles seem weak.
Trembling in any part of body without other symptoms or factors.	Inherited tendency to tremble, especially from anxiety or stress.	Consult doctor to confirm diagnosis.
Unexpected body jerks when falling asleep.	Involuntary muscle spasms. No underlying disorder.	Nothing.

*All references are to Illness section unless noted otherwise.

URINATION, FREQUENT
(continued on next page)

SYMPTOMS & FACTORS	POSSIBLE PROBLEM	WHAT TO DO*
• Frequent urination, especially at night. • Increased urine production. • Excessive consumption of tea, coffee, cola or alcohol.	Effect of caffeine or alcohol.	Decrease consumption of caffeine or alcohol.
• Frequent urination, especially at night. • Increased urine production. • Use of diuretic drug for heart disease or high blood pressure.	Effect of diuretic drug.	Consult doctor if uneasy.
• Frequent urination. • Anxiety or excitement. OR • Cold weather.	Normal occurrence.	Nothing.
• Frequent urination. • Burning and stinging on urination. • Increased urge to urinate.	Bladder infection.	See Cystitis.
• Frequent urination. • Painful urination. • Blood in urine.	Stones.	See Urinary Calculi.
• Frequent urination. • Possible pregnancy.	Normal occurrence during first 3 months and last 3 months of pregnancy.	Consult doctor to confirm pregnancy.
• Frequent urination. • Pain with urination.	Several disorders.	See Urination, Painful (in Symptoms section).
• Frequent urination, especially at night. • Increased urine production, plus 2 or more of following: • Increased hunger and thirst. • Itching around genitals or anus. • Fatigue. • Weight loss.	Sugar in urine.	• See Diabetes Mellitus, Insulin Dependent. • See Diabetes Mellitus, Non-Insulin Dependent.
• Frequent urination in man older than 50, plus 2 or more of following: • Involuntary urine leak after urination. • Weak urinary stream. • Difficulty starting urination. • Increased waking at night to urinate.	Disorder of prostate gland.	• See Prostate, Enlarged. • See Prostatitis.
• Frequent urination in a woman. • Intense urge to urinate followed quickly by uncontrollable urine leak.	Urge incontinence.	See Incontinence.
• Frequent urination. • Difficulty controlling bladder.	Several disorders.	See Urination, Lack of Control (in Symptoms section).

*All references are to Illness section unless noted otherwise.

URINATION, FREQUENT
(continued from previous page)

SYMPTOMS & FACTORS	POSSIBLE PROBLEM	WHAT TO DO*
• Frequent urination. • Discharge from urethra. • Small ulcers on mouth, tongue and tip of penis.	Inflammatory disease.	See Reiter's Syndrome.
• Passage of large amounts of urine. • Colorless urine. • Excessive thirst.	Hormone disorder.	See Diabetes Insipidus.
• Frequent urination. • Pelvic pain and pressure. • Sensation of incomplete emptying of bladder. • Pain during intercourse. • Burning on urination.	Inflammation in area of bladder.	See Interstitial Cystitis.

*All references are to Illness section unless noted otherwise.

URINATION, LACK OF CONTROL

SYMPTOMS & FACTORS	POSSIBLE PROBLEM	WHAT TO DO*
Small urine leak in female when coughing, sneezing, laughing or running.	Stress incontinence.	See Incontinence.
• Lack of urinary control. • Use of prescription drug.	Adverse reaction or side effect of drug.	Consult doctor.
• Lack of urinary control. • Cloudy, bad-smelling urine.	Infection of urinary tract.	• See Cystitis. • See Urethritis.
Dribbling of urine after urination in male over age 50.	• Disorder of prostate gland. • Inflammation of urethra.	• See Prostate, Enlarged. • See Urethritis.
• Lack of urinary control. • Lack of bowel control.	Decreased blood supply to brain.	• Call doctor now. • See Stroke.
• Lack of urinary control. • Constipation for longer than 1 week.	Pressure on bladder from fecal impaction.	See Fecal Impaction.
• Lack of urinary control in person over age 60, plus 2 or more of following: • Inability to remember recent events. • Decline in attention to personal appearance or cleanliness. • Personality change.	• Poor nutrition. • Mental deterioration.	• See Vitamin B Deficiencies. • See Alzheimer's Disease. • See Dementia.
Lack of urinary control in child over age 3-1/2.	Several causes.	See Bed-Wetting.
• Lack of urinary control. • Chronic illness.	Several disorders.	• Call doctor now. • See Multiple Sclerosis. • See Syphilis. • See Disk, Ruptured.

*All references are to Illness section unless noted otherwise.

URINATION, PAINFUL

SYMPTOMS & FACTORS	POSSIBLE PROBLEM	WHAT TO DO*
• Painful urination. • Pain in one side of back, between waist and last rib. • Fever.	Kidney infection.	See Kidney Infection, Acute.
• Painful urination. • Frequent urination.	Bladder inflammation.	See Cystitis.
• Painful urination. • Painful blisters on genitals. • Fever.	Sexually-transmitted virus infection.	See Herpes, Genital.
• Painful urination in female. • Green-yellow or white discharge from vagina. • Itching around genitals.	Vaginal infection.	• See Vaginitis, Monilial. • See Vaginitis, Trichomonal.
• Painful urination in man. • Thick, yellow-green discharge from penis.	Sexually-transmitted infection.	• See Gonorrhea. • See Urethritis.
• Painful urination in woman. • Bad-smelling vaginal discharge. • Pain or tenderness in lower abdomen. • Fever.	Sexually-transmitted infection.	• See Gonorrhea. • See Urethritis.
• Painful urination in man. • Heavy feeling or dull pain between scrotum and anus. • Fever.	Infection of prostate gland.	See Prostatitis.
• Burning urination. • Blood in urine. • Pain in pelvic area.	Abnormal growth in bladder.	See Bladder Tumor.
• Painful urination or inability to urinate. • Forceful blow, injury or wound in lower abdomen or genitals.	Injury to genital tract.	See Genitourinary Injury.
• Discomfort on urinating. • Vaginal discharge (female). • Urethral discharge (male).	Infection.	See Chlamydia Infection.
• Discomfort with urination (male). • Painless sore or lesion on penis.	Cancer.	See Penis Cancer.

*All references are to Illness section unless noted otherwise.

URINE, ABNORMAL COLOR

SYMPTOMS & FACTORS	POSSIBLE PROBLEM	WHAT TO DO*
• Pink, red, smoky-brown or other color change in urine. • Use of new prescription drug in last 24 hours.	Side effect of drug.	Consult doctor if color change not expected.
• Dark yellow or orange urine. • Recent use of laxatives containing senna. OR • Recent consumption of rhubarb.	Effect of chemicals in these substances.	Nothing.
• Pink, red or smoky-brown urine. • Recent consumption of beets, blackberries or other red food.	Effect of natural or artificial color.	Nothing.
Pink, red or smoky-brown urine.	Disorder of urinary tract.	• Consult doctor. • See Cystitis. • See Prostate, Enlarged. • See Bladder Tumor. • See Tuberculosis. • See Urinary Calculi. • See Kidney Infection (both Acute and Chronic). • See Wilm's Tumor (children only). • See Hypernephroma. • See Glomerulonephritis.
• Clear, dark-brown urine. • Pale stool. • Yellow skin and eyes.	Liver disorder.	• Call doctor now. • See Hepatitis, Viral.
• Dark yellow or orange urine. • Fever. OR • Very hot weather. OR • Decreased fluid intake.	Concentrated urine.	• See Fever charts (in Symptoms section). • See Heatstroke or Heat Exhaustion. • See Dehydration. • Increase fluid intake.
• Dark yellow or orange urine. • Vomiting. • Diarrhea.	Concentrated urine.	• See Vomiting, Recurrent Attacks (in Symptoms section). • See Diarrhea (in Symptoms section).
Green or blue urine.	Effect of artificial color in food or drug.	Nothing.
• Colorless urine. • Excessive thirst. • Passage of large amounts of urine.	Hormone disorder.	See Diabetes Insipidus.

*All references are to Illness section unless noted otherwise.

VAGINAL BLEEDING, UNEXPECTED

SYMPTOMS & FACTORS	POSSIBLE PROBLEM	WHAT TO DO*
Vaginal bleeding during first 3 months of pregnancy.	Spontaneous abortion.	• Call doctor now. • See Miscarriage.
Vaginal bleeding during 4th to 9th month of pregnancy.	Abnormal location of placenta.	• Call doctor now. • See Placenta Previa. • See Abruptio Placenta.
• Unexpected vaginal bleeding. • Severe abdominal pain. • Pregnancy possible. OR • Current use of intrauterine contraceptive device (IUD).	Pregnancy developing outside uterus.	• Call doctor now. • See Ectopic Pregnancy.
• Unexpected vaginal bleeding in woman over age 45. • Last menstrual period more than 6 months ago.	• Hormone changes. • Tumor or cancer.	• See Menopause. • See Uterine Bleeding, Postmenopausal. • See Uterine Cancer. • See Cervix Cancer. • See Ovarian Cancer. • See Vagina or Vulva Cancer.
• Unexpected vaginal bleeding in woman over age 45. • Use of prescription drug for hormone replacement therapy.	Breakthrough bleeding.	Consult doctor.
• Unexpected vaginal bleeding. • Vaginal discharge.	• Several disorders. • Cancer.	• See Cervical Polyps. • See Cervical Erosion. • See Cervix Cancer. • See Uterine Cancer. • See Vagina or Vulva Cancer.
• Unexpected vaginal bleeding. • Pain in lower abdomen.	• Uterine fibroids. • Cancer.	• See Cervical Polyps. • See Uterine Bleeding, Dysfunctional. • See Fibroid Tumors of the Uterus. • See Ovarian Cancer. • See Uterine Malignancy.
• Unexpected vaginal bleeding. • Recent insertion of intrauterine contraceptive device (IUD).	Complications caused by IUD.	Consult doctor.
• Unexpected vaginal bleeding. • Use of oral contraceptives.	Breakthrough bleeding; common occurrence in women taking pill.	Consult doctor.
• Excessive menstrual flow. • Menstrual period lasts more than 7 days.	Menstrual irregularity.	See Menorrhagia.
• Menstrual disorders. • Course skin. • Sleepiness.	Underactive thyroid gland.	See Hypothyroidism.
• Unexpected vaginal bleeding. • Insertion of foreign object into vagina.	Vaginal injury.	Consult doctor.

*All references are to Illness section unless noted otherwise.

VAGINAL DISCHARGE, ABNORMAL

SYMPTOMS & FACTORS	POSSIBLE PROBLEM	WHAT TO DO*
• Heavy vaginal discharge. • Vaginal pain.	Irritation or infection of cervix.	See Cervicitis.
• Green-yellow, bad-smelling vaginal discharge. • No other symptoms.	Vaginal infection.	See Vaginitis, Trichomonal.
• Heavy vaginal discharge that is normal in color and consistency. • Vaginal itching or soreness.	Irritation or infection.	See Vaginal Itching (in Symptoms section).
White, curd-like vaginal discharge.	Vaginal fungus infection.	See Vaginitis, Monilial.
• Green-yellow, bad-smelling vaginal discharge. • Tampon, diaphragm or cervical cup left in vagina.	Vaginal infection.	• Remove tampon, diaphragm or cup if you can. • If not, consult doctor.
• Heavy vaginal discharge that is normal in color and consistency. • Use of oral contraceptives. OR • Possible pregnancy.	Normal occurrence caused by hormone changes.	Consult doctor to confirm pregnancy.
Heavy vaginal discharge that is normal in color and consistency during ovulation occurring during middle days between periods.	Normal occurrence.	Nothing.
• Vaginal discharge. • Reddening of vagina.	Vaginal infection.	• See Chlamydia Infection. • See Vaginitis, Bacterial. • See Vaginitis, Postmenopausal.
• Vaginal discharge, which may or may not smell bad. • Redness, itching around genital area. • Young girl (before puberty).	Infection.	See Vulvovaginitis Before Puberty.
• Red or brown vaginal discharge. • Occasional spotting of blood between menstrual periods.	Several disorders.	• See Cervical Polyps. • See Vaginal Bleeding Unexpected (in Symptoms section).
• Green-yellow, bad-smelling vaginal discharge. • Pain in lower abdomen. • Frequent or painful urination.	Infection of reproductive organs.	• See Pelvic Inflammatory Disease. • See Gonorrhea.
• Heavy, bad-smelling vaginal discharge 2 or more days after childbirth. • Fever. • Abdominal pain.	Infection of uterus.	See Puerperal Infection.

*All references are to Illness section unless noted otherwise.

VAGINAL ITCHING

SYMPTOMS & FACTORS	POSSIBLE PROBLEM	WHAT TO DO*
• Vaginal itching. • Unusual vaginal discharge.	Several disorders.	• See Vulvovaginitis Before Puberty. • See Vaginitis, Bacterial. • See Vaginitis, Postmenopausal (women over 45). • See Pruritis Vulvae. • See Vaginal Discharge, Abnormal (in Symptoms section).
• Vaginal itching. • Use of antibiotics.	Vaginal infection.	• Consult doctor. • See Vaginitis, Monilial.
• Vaginal itching. • Use of chemical spray, ointment, cream, douche or contraceptive foam.	Irritation caused by chemical or drug.	• Consult doctor. • Discontinue use of possible irritant.
Vaginal itching in woman over age 38.	Decreasing level of estrogens at menopause.	See Pruritis Vulvae.
• Vaginal itching, plus 2 or more of following: • Unexplained weight loss. • Increased hunger and thirst. • Frequent urination. • Fatigue.	Sugar in urine.	• See Diabetes Mellitus, Insulin Dependent. • See Diabetes Mellitus, Non-Insulin Dependent.

*All references are to Illness section unless noted otherwise.

VISION DISTURBANCE OR LOSS
(continued on next page)

SYMPTOMS & FACTORS	POSSIBLE PROBLEM	WHAT TO DO*
• Sensitivity to light. • Discharge from eye. • Pain in eye.	Infection.	See Conjunctivitis.
• Blurred vision. • Person over age 50.	• Clouding of eye lens. • Decreased blood supply to back of eye.	See Cataract.
• Blurred vision in past 2 days. • Eye pain.	Inflammation of iris.	See Uveitis.
• Blurred vision or sensitivity to light. • Use of prescription drug.	Adverse reaction or side effect of drug.	Consult doctor.
• Blurred vision in one eye. • Eye pain.	Excess pressure in eye.	See Glaucoma, Primary Angle Closure.
• Loss of peripheral vision in small areas. • Blurred vision on one side.	Excess pressure in eye.	See Glaucoma, Chronic Open Angle.
• Blurred or fuzzy vision. • Squinting to see objects that aren't close to you. OR • Unable to see objects that are right in front of you.	Uncorrected vision problem.	Have an eye examination.
• Flashes of light or wavy spots in vision. • Severe headache. • Nausea and vomiting.	Severe vascular headache.	See Migraine.
• Sensitivity to light. • Eye pain. • Tears.	Infection.	See Keratitis.
Uncoordinated eye movements that may cause vision problems.	Eye muscle disorder.	See Strabismus.
• Double vision. • Bulging eyes.	• Overactive thyroid gland. • Tumor. • Inflammation of tissue behind eye.	• Consult doctor. • See Hyperthyroidism. • See Exophthalmos. • See Eye Tumor.
• Vision disturbance. • Recent head injury.	Bleeding inside skull.	• Call doctor now. • See Subdural Hemorrhage & Hematoma.
Sudden, partial or total loss of vision in one or both eyes.	• Decreased blood supply to back of eye or brain. • Disorder of central nervous system.	• Call doctor now. • See Stroke. • See Transient Ischemic Attack. • See Brain Tumor. • See Multiple Sclerosis.

*All references are to Illness section unless noted otherwise.

VISION DISTURBANCE OR LOSS
(continued from previous page)

SYMPTOMS & FACTORS	POSSIBLE PROBLEM	WHAT TO DO*
• Blurred vision in one eye. • Flashing lights. • Floating spots. • No pain.	Disorder of blood vessels and structures in back of eye.	See Retinal Detachment.
• Double vision. • Drooping eyelids. • Swallowing difficulty.	Autoimmune disorder.	See Myasthenia Gravis.
• Blurred vision. • Diabetes.	Diabetic retinopathy (retina injury).	Consult doctor.
• Poor night vision. • Dry, inflamed eyes. • Rough skin. • Loss of appetite.	Lack of vitamin A.	See Vitamin A Deficiency.
• Changes in vision. • Headache; nausea; vomiting. • Seizures. • Excessive thirst.	Tumor.	See Pituitary Tumor.

*All references are to Illness section unless noted otherwise.

VOICE LOSS OR HOARSENESS

SYMPTOMS & FACTORS	POSSIBLE PROBLEM	WHAT TO DO*
Hoarseness following excessive smoking or alcohol consumption.	Inflammation of vocal cords caused by alcohol or tobacco.	• Decrease smoking or alcohol consumption. • See Laryngitis.
• Hoarseness following excessive use of voice. OR • Exposure to tobacco smoke or toxic fumes.	Inflammation of vocal cords caused by overuse or exposure.	If hoarseness doesn't disappear in a few days, consult doctor.
• Hoarseness, plus 2 or more of following: • Dry skin or hair. • Decreased tolerance for cold. • Fatigue. • Unexplained weight gain.	Underactive thyroid gland.	See Hypothyroidism.
• Voice loss or hoarseness. • Tender or hard lump in neck just below Adam's apple.	Tumor of thyroid.	See Thyroid Nodule.
Hoarseness following cold, cough or sore throat.	Inflammation of vocal cords caused by nasal drainage.	See Laryngitis.
• Hoarseness. • Recent tension or depression.	Effect of stress.	See Anxiety.
• Voice loss or hoarseness for longer than 1 week. OR • Recurrent attacks of hoarseness or voice loss in last 6 months.	• Inflammation of vocal cords. • Tumor.	• See Vocal-Cord Nodules. • See Larynx Cancer. • See Oral Cancer. • See Lung Cancer.

*All references are to Illness section unless noted otherwise.

VOMITING (INFANT 0 TO 6 MONTHS)

SYMPTOMS & FACTORS	POSSIBLE PROBLEM	WHAT TO DO*
• Vomiting. • Diarrhea.	Infection of digestive tract.	See Gastroenteritis.
• Vomiting. • Infant appears healthy. • No other symptoms.	• Single episode—no underlying disorder. • More than one episode—several disorders, such as food allergies or milk intolerance.	• Consult doctor if vomiting lasts longer than 6 hours. • Consult doctor for repeated vomiting. • See Food Allergy and Intolerance. • See Lactose Intolerance.
• Vomiting. • Recent playful bouncing. OR • Travel by airplane, boat or motor vehicle.	Disturbed equilibrium.	• Don't bounce after feedings. • See Motion Sickness.
• Vomiting. • Fever.	Infection.	See Fever (child 0 to 2 years) (in Symptoms section).
• Vomiting. • Cough or runny nose.	Virus infection.	Consult doctor if vomiting lasts longer than 6 hours.
• Vomiting. • Use of prescription drug.	Adverse reaction or side effect of drug.	Call doctor now.
• Forceful vomiting. • Possible accidental ingestion of drug, household cleaning supply or poison. OR • Recent head injury.	• Chemical irritation of stomach and toxic effect of chemical on brain. • Internal bleeding.	• Call doctor now or go to emergency room. • See Head Injury.
• Vomiting. • Fever of 101F (38.3C) rectally or higher, plus any of following: • Lethargy. • Eyes sensitive to light. • General ill appearance. • Crying with urination.	• Infection in membranes around brain. • Urinary-tract infection.	Call doctor now.
• Vomiting. • Swelling or lump in groin or testicle.	Protruding intestinal tissue.	See Hernia.
• Infant vomits forcefully after each feeding. • Infant appears healthy. • Infant is male and younger than 4 months.	Constriction in outlet to stomach.	See Pyloric Stenosis, Congenital.
• Vomiting. • Recurrent attacks of screaming or crying, as if in great pain.	Blockage in intestines.	• Call doctor now. • See Intussusception. • See Intestinal Obstruction.
• Vomiting. • Failure to gain weight. • Withdrawn affect.	Emotional deprivation from lack of touching or attention.	See Failure to Thrive.

*All references are to Illness section unless noted otherwise.

VOMITING, RECURRENT ATTACKS

SYMPTOMS & FACTORS	POSSIBLE PROBLEM	WHAT TO DO*
• Recurrent vomiting. • Burning sensation in chest or upper abdomen, especially when bending forward or lying down.	Stomach acid in esophagus.	See Gastroesophageal Reflux Disease.
• Recurrent vomiting. • Occasional pain or tenderness in upper right abdomen. • No fever.	Gallbladder disorder.	See Gallstones.
• Recurrent vomiting. • Occasional pain or tenderness in upper right abdomen. • Fever.	Gallbladder inflammation.	See Cholecystitis or Cholangitis.
• Recurrent vomiting. • Poor appetite. • Jaundice (yellow skin and eyes).	Gallbladder or liver disorder.	• See Gallstones. • See Hepatitis, Viral.
• Recurrent vomiting. • Use of prescription or nonprescription drug.	Adverse reaction or side effect of drug.	Consult doctor.
• Recurrent vomiting. • Pain or tenderness in center of upper abdomen. • Discomfort relieved by vomiting.	Peptic-ulcer disease.	See Ulcer, Peptic.
Vomiting within hours after drinking alcohol.	Stomach inflammation.	See Gastritis.
Recurrent, self-induced vomiting.	Psychological disorder.	See Bulimia.
• Vomiting. • Extreme dizziness. • Loss of balance.	Inner ear disorder.	See Labyrinthitis.
• Recurrent vomiting. • Poor appetite. • Constant pain in upper abdomen.	Tumor.	See Stomach Cancer.
• Recurrent vomiting without nausea. • Recurrent headaches, especially in morning.	• Bleeding inside skull. • Tumor.	• Consult doctor. • See Subdural Hemorrhage & Hematoma. • See Brain Tumor.
• Bloody vomit. • Bleeding from several body parts.	Blood-clotting problem.	See Disseminated Intravascular Coagulation.
• Vomiting. • Extreme abdominal pain, swelling and gas.	Disorder of the pancreas.	See Pancreatitis.

*All references are to Illness section unless noted otherwise.

VOMITING, SUDDEN ATTACK (continued on next page)

SYMPTOMS & FACTORS	POSSIBLE PROBLEM	WHAT TO DO*
• Vomiting. • Diarrhea. • Fever.	Infection of digestive tract.	See Gastroenteritis.
• Vomiting. • Feelings of nervousness and apprehension (such as before going on stage).	Emotional upset.	• Vomiting should stop when emotions calm down. • See Anxiety. • See Panic Attack.
• Vomiting. • Headache.	Headache disorder.	See Migraine.
• Vomiting. • Use of prescription or nonprescription drug.	Adverse reaction or side effect of drug.	• Consult doctor about prescription drug. • Discontinue use of nonprescription drug.
• Vomiting. • Jaundice (yellow skin or eyes).	Gallbladder or liver disorder.	• Consult doctor. • See Hepatitis, Viral. • See Gallstones.
Recent, recurrent vomiting attacks.	Several disorders.	See Vomiting, Recurrent (in Symptoms section).
• Vomiting. • Consumption of spoiled, contaminated or improperly prepared food.	Effect of toxins in food.	• See Food Poisoning. • See Salmonella Infections. • See Botulism. • See Trichinosis.
• Vomiting. • Dizziness.	Infection or disorder of inner ear.	• See Labyrinthitis. • See Meniere's Disease.
• Vomiting. • Excessive consumption of alcohol or rich food.	Stomach inflammation.	See Gastritis.
Vomiting of blood or dark "coffee ground" material.	Bleeding in stomach.	• Call doctor now. • See Ulcer, Peptic. • See Gastric Erosion.
• Vomiting. • Severe abdominal pain. • No pain relief from vomiting.	Several disorders.	• Call doctor now. • See Appendicitis.
• Vomiting. • Dizziness; headache; faintness.	Gas inhalation.	See Carbon Monoxide Poisoning.
• Vomiting. • Headache, plus any of following: • Eyes sensitive to light. • Drowsiness or confusion. • Pain when bending head forward.	Infection or bleeding in membranes around brain.	• Call doctor now. • See Meningitis, Aseptic. • See Meningitis, Bacterial. • See Subarachnoid Hemorrhage.
• Vomiting. • Headache. • Head injury in last 24 hours.	Brain injury.	• Call doctor now. • See Head Injury.

*All references are to Illness section unless noted otherwise.

VOMITING, SUDDEN ATTACK
(continued from previous page)

SYMPTOMS & FACTORS	POSSIBLE PROBLEM	WHAT TO DO*
• Vomiting. • Abdominal pain or swelling. • Inability to have bowel movement.	Blockage in intestines.	• Call doctor now. • See Intestinal Obstruction.
• Vomiting. • Eye pain. • Blurred vision.	Excess pressure inside eye.	• Call doctor now. • See Glaucoma, Primary Angle Closure.
• Vomiting and watery diarrhea. • Sudden high fever. • Rash that resembles sunburn.	Blood poisoning.	See Toxic Shock Syndrome.

*All references are to Illness section unless noted otherwise.

WEIGHT GAIN

SYMPTOMS & FACTORS	POSSIBLE PROBLEM	WHAT TO DO*
• Weight gain. • Change from active to sedentary lifestyle.	Calorie intake too high for current activity level.	Decrease food consumption and increase physical activity.
• Weight gain. • No other symptoms.	More calories consumed than burned.	See Obesity.
• Weight gain. • Depression.	Compensatory overeating.	See Depression.
• Weight gain. • Feeling of depression and tiredness. • Start of, or during, winter season.	Lack of light.	See Seasonal Affective Disorder.
• Weight gain. • Use of prescription or nonprescription drug that causes fluid retention, such as steroids, cortisone drugs, oral contraceptives or nonsteroid anti-inflammatory drugs.	Adverse reaction or side effect of drug.	Consult doctor.
• Weight gain. • Decreased tolerance for cold. • Dry skin or hair. • Fatigue. • Constipation.	Underactive thyroid gland.	See Hypothyroidism.
• Weight gain. • Recently discontinued smoking.	Normal occurrence.	Weight gain will soon stop. But be careful about what you eat. Get plenty of exercise.
• Rapid weight gain during pregnancy. • Puffiness in the face, hands and feet that is worse in the morning.	Complication of pregnancy.	See Toxemia of Pregnancy.
• Weight gain. • High blood pressure or history of heart, kidney or liver disease.	Fluid retention caused by disorder of blood vessels, heart, liver or kidney.	• See Hypertension. • See Congestive Heart Failure. • See Nephrotic Syndrome. • See Cirrhosis of the Liver.
• Weight gain with accumulation of fat over upper back and trunk. • Round face and puffy eyes.	Endocrine disorder.	See Cushing's Syndrome.
Weight gain due to fluid retention.	Several disorders.	• See Ankles, Swollen (in Symptoms section). • See Abdominal Swelling (in Symptoms section).

*All references are to Illness section unless noted otherwise.

WEIGHT GAIN, SLOW (CHILD 0 TO 5 YEARS)

SYMPTOMS & FACTORS	POSSIBLE PROBLEM	WHAT TO DO*
• Weight gain slow in young child. • Child appears healthy and content. • Birth weight low (less than 5-1/2 pounds). OR • Parent smaller than average.	Genetic causes; no underlying disorder.	Consult doctor if worried.
• Weight gain slow in breast-fed infant younger than 1 year. • Feeding schedule rigid or allows little sucking time.	Inadequate nourishment.	• Consult doctor. • Feed on demand. • Increase sucking time.
• Weight gain slow in bottle-fed infant younger than 1 year. • Too much water added to powdered formula, or water added to ready-to-feed formula.	Inadequate nourishment.	• Prepare formula according to directions. • Do not dilute ready-to-feed formula.
• Weight gain slow in bottle-fed infant younger than 1 year. • Child empties every bottle of formula.	Inadequate nourishment.	• Tell doctor at next visit. • Increase amount offered.
• Weight gain slow in young child. • Use of cortisone drugs.	Adverse reaction or side effect of drug.	Consult doctor.
• Weight gain slow in young child. • Loose, pale, bulky, bad-smelling stool.	Digestive disorder.	• See Celiac Disease. • See Lactose Intolerance.
• Weight gain slow in infant younger than 6 months. • Infant vomits after feedings.	Several disorders.	See Vomiting (Infant 0 to 6 Months) (in Symptoms section).
• Weight gain slow in young child. • Withdrawn personality. • Slow mental, physical and emotional development.	Effect of abuse or neglect.	• Consult doctor. • See Failure to Thrive.

*All references are to Illness section unless noted otherwise.

WEIGHT LOSS
(continued on next page)

SYMPTOMS & FACTORS	POSSIBLE PROBLEM	WHAT TO DO*
• Weight loss, plus 2 or more of following: • Increased hunger. • Increased thirst. • Fatigue. • Family history of diabetes. • Frequent urination. • Itching rash in genital area.	Sugar in urine.	• See Diabetes Mellitus, Insulin Dependent. • See Diabetes Mellitus, Non-Insulin Dependent.
• Weight loss, plus 2 or more of following: • Bulging eyes. • Excessive sweating. • Fatigue. • Anxiety. • Rapid heartbeat.	Overactive thyroid gland.	See Hyperthyroidism.
• Weight loss of 10 or more pounds. • Anxiety or depression.	• Effect of stress. • Psychological disorder.	• See Anxiety. • See Depression. • See Anorexia Nervosa. • See Bulimia.
• Weight loss. • Current use of prescription drug.	Adverse reaction or side effect of drug.	Consult doctor.
• Weight loss. • Recurrent diarrhea or constipation. • Recurrent pain in lower abdomen. • Black stool.	• Inflammation of intestine. • Tumor.	• See Crohn's Disease. • See Large Intestine Cancer.
• Weight loss. • Recurrent pain in upper abdomen.	• Peptic-ulcer disease. • Tumor. • Stress or emotional conflicts. • Intestinal inflammatory disorder.	• See Ulcer, Peptic. • See Stomach Cancer. • See Irritable Bowel Syndrome. • See Colitis, Ulcerative. • See Crohn's Disease.
• Weight loss, plus 2 or more of following: • Excessive sweating at night. • Fever. • Fatigue. • Persistent cough with blood in sputum.	Lung inflammation or infection.	• See Tuberculosis. • See Bronchitis, Chronic. • See Bronchiectasis.
• Weight loss. • Recurrent diarrhea. • Pale, bulky, bad-smelling stool.	Poor digestion.	See Malabsorption.
• Weight loss. • Increased physical activity.	Normal occurrence.	Consult doctor if weight loss is not expected and continues longer than 2 weeks.

*All references are to Illness section unless noted otherwise.

WEIGHT LOSS
(continued from previous page)

SYMPTOMS & FACTORS	POSSIBLE PROBLEM	WHAT TO DO*
• Weight loss. • Recurrent respiratory and skin infections.	Virus infection.	See HIV Infection and AIDS.
• Unexplained weight and appetite loss. • Abdominal discomfort. • Hard mass in upper right abdomen.	Liver tumor.	See Hepatoma.

*All references are to Illness section unless noted otherwise.

WHEEZING

SYMPTOMS & FACTORS	POSSIBLE PROBLEM	WHAT TO DO*
• Wheezing. • Fever.	Infection of bronchial tubes.	• See Bronchitis, Acute. • See Asthma. • See Bronchiolitis (young children only).
• Wheezing. • Breathing difficulty.	Spasm of bronchial tubes.	• Call doctor now. • See Asthma.
• Wheezing with a "barking" cough in an infant or young child. • Difficulty in breathing.	Bacterial or viral infection.	See Croup.
• Wheezing. • Possible inhalation of foreign object, such as peanut.	Foreign object in larynx or bronchial tubes.	Call doctor now.
• Persistent, mild wheezing. • Cough with gray or green-yellow sputum.	Chronic infection of breathing passages.	• See Bronchitis, Chronic. • See Bronchiectasis. • See Chronic Obstructive Pulmonary Disease.
• Wheezing. • Cough with frothy pink, brownish or white sputum.	Fluid in lungs.	• Call doctor now. • See Pulmonary Edema.
• Wheezing. • Breathing difficulty. • Swelling in face or hands. • Itching all over; hives.	Allergic reaction.	• Call doctor now or seek emergency help. • See Anaphylaxis.
• Symptoms similar to asthma (wheezing). • Flushed skin on the head and neck. • Diarrhea.	Tumors.	See Carcinoid Syndrome.

*All references are to Illness section unless noted otherwise.

Illness & Disorders

ABRUPTIO PLACENTA

GENERAL INFORMATION

DEFINITION—Partial separation of the placenta (after-birth) from the uterus during the last third of pregnancy.

BODY PARTS INVOLVED—Uterus.

SEX OR AGE MOST AFFECTED—Females.

SIGNS & SYMPTOMS
Small separation of the placenta:
- Vaginal bleeding.
- Mild pain or discomfort.
- Unborn child (fetus) remains healthy.

Large separation:
- Heavy vaginal bleeding.
- Severe pain in the lower abdomen.
- Hard, tender abdomen.
- Shock (rapid heartbeat, rapid breathing and dizziness).
- Fetal distress; fetal heartbeat may be inaudible.

CAUSES—Unknown.

RISK INCREASES WITH
- Women over age 35.
- Women who have had several pregnancies.
- Women who smoke.
- A direct blow to the uterus.
- High blood pressure (hypertension).
- Abuse of alcohol or drugs.
- Rectal thermometers or enema nozzles.

HOW TO PREVENT
- If pregnant, don't engage in activity more vigorous than what you were accustomed to before pregnancy.
- Avoid risk factors if possible.

WHAT TO EXPECT

DIAGNOSTIC MEASURES
- Your own observation of symptoms.
- Medical history and physical exam by a doctor.
- Laboratory studies, such as blood counts, blood-clotting tests and ultrasound examination (see Glossary) of the uterus.

APPROPRIATE HEALTH CARE
- Doctor's treatment.
- Hospitalization (except for mild cases).
- Surgery to deliver the fetus by cesarean section, or vaginal delivery (sometimes).

POSSIBLE COMPLICATIONS
- Shock or life-threatening bleeding in the mother.
- Child born brain damaged.

PROBABLE OUTCOME
- With immediate medical care, the outlook for mother and fetus is excellent.
- With delay of medical care and prolonged heavy bleeding, mother and fetus may not survive.

HOW TO TREAT

GENERAL MEASURES—Abruptio placenta is an emergency, but there is usually time to obtain advice by telephone and arrange safe transportation to the hospital. Panic is not helpful. If the placenta separation is slight, your doctor may permit you to return home for bed rest and close observation after examination.

MEDICATION—Your doctor may prescribe:
- Oxytocin to induce labor, if immediate delivery is necessary.
- Intravenous fluids.
- Blood transfusions.

ACTIVITY—Rest in bed until bleeding and other symptoms cease and your doctor approves a return to normal activity.

DIET—No special diet. Drink fluids only until your doctor determines that surgery is not likely. Solid food may cause risk if emergency surgery becomes necessary.

CALL YOUR DOCTOR IF

You have bleeding (anything more than slight spotting) during pregnancy. This is an emergency!

ACNE
(Acne Vulgaris)

 GENERAL INFORMATION

DEFINITION—A chronic inflammatory skin condition characterized by skin eruptions on the face, chest and back.

BODY PARTS INVOLVED—Skin.

SEX OR AGE MOST AFFECTED—Adolescents (more common in boys). May occur throughout life.

SIGNS & SYMPTOMS
- Blackheads (black spots the size of a pinhead).
- Whiteheads (white spots similar to blackheads).
- Pustules (small pus-filled lesions).
- Cysts (larger and firm swellings) and abscesses (swollen and inflamed areas with pus) with severe acne.
- Redness and inflammation around eruptions.

CAUSES—Oil glands in the skin become plugged for unknown reasons, but sex-hormone changes during adolescence play a role. When oil backs up, it becomes infected by bacteria normally present in glands. Contrary to myth, acne is not caused by dirt, masturbation or foods. Cleanliness can lessen it, but sexual activity has no effect on it.

RISK INCREASES WITH
- Exposure to extremely hot or cold weather.
- Stress.
- Oily skin.
- Endocrine disorders.
- Use of drugs, such as cortisone, male hormones or oral contraceptives.
- Family history of acne.
- Cosmetics (some).

HOW TO PREVENT—Cannot be prevented at present.

 WHAT TO EXPECT

DIAGNOSTIC MEASURES
- Your own observation of symptoms.
- Medical history and physical exam by a doctor.

APPROPRIATE HEALTH CARE
- Self-care after diagnosis.
- Doctor's treatment.
- Surgery (dermabrasion) to remove unsightly scars after acne heals.
- Exposure to ultraviolet light may be a recommended treatment.

POSSIBLE COMPLICATIONS
- Poor self-image and psychological distress.
- Permanent facial scars or pitting of skin.

PROBABLE OUTCOME—Most cases respond well to treatment and the condition tends to disappear after adolescence. Despite good treatment, acne will flare up from time to time.

 HOW TO TREAT

GENERAL MEASURES
- If your skin is oily, cleanse it as follows: Gently massage face with soap for 3 to 5 minutes. Don't massage sorest places. Cleanse skin gently—rough scrubbing spreads infection.
Rinse soap off for 2 to 3 minutes.
After cleansing, use an astringent, such as alcohol, to remove oil.
Use a fresh washcloth each day. Bacteria can grow in damp, wet cloths.
- Shampoo hair at least twice a week. Don't let hair hang over the face—even at night. Hair spreads oil and bacteria. Use dandruff shampoo to treat or prevent dandruff. Avoid cream rinses.
- After vigorous exercise, wash sweat and oil off as soon as possible.
- Don't squeeze, scratch, pick or rub the skin; use a comedone extractor. Acne heals better without damage to the skin. If you must squeeze pimples, blackheads or whiteheads, wash your hands first. Cleanse the area with alcohol before and after squeezing.
- Don't rest your face on your hands while reading, studying or watching TV.
- Use water-based cosmetics.

MEDICATION—Your doctor may prescribe:
- Antibiotics to fight infection.
- Cortisone injections into lesions.
- Skin lotions with drying agents.
- Isotretinoin (don't use if pregnant).
- 5% or 10% benzyl peroxide may be helpful.
Caution: If you are pregnant, don't take oral medications for acne.

ACTIVITY—No restrictions.

DIET—Foods don't cause acne, but some foods may make it worse. Keep a record of the foods you eat. To discover any food sensitivities, eliminate foods from your diet that you suspect make your acne worse. Then reintroduce them one at a time. If acne flares up 2 or 3 days after a food is eaten, leave it out of your diet. If not, you may eat it.
Acne usually improves in the summer, so some foods that cannot be eaten in the winter may be tolerated in the summer.

 CALL YOUR DOCTOR IF

- You have acne.
- New, unexplained symptoms develop. Drugs in treatment may produce side effects.

ACNE ROSACEA
(Rosacea; Adult Acne)

GENERAL INFORMATION

DEFINITION—Chronic inflammation of skin of the face. Severe nose involvement, mostly in men, is called rhinophyma.

BODY PARTS INVOLVED—Face, especially the nose, and surrounding areas.

SEX OR AGE MOST AFFECTED—Adults; it is more common in women, but more severe in men.

SIGNS & SYMPTOMS
- Flushing of the nose, cheeks and forehead that may last a few minutes or hours. In most cases, the flushing becomes permanent.
- Facial tenderness.
- Papules (small raised bumps) and pustules (small, white blisters with pus) on the affected skin (sometimes).
- Unsightly red, thickened skin (excess tissue) on the nose and cheeks. Small blood vessels are visible on the skin surface.

CAUSES
- Unknown. Some evidence suggests an underlying vascular disorder. Another factor may be a microscopic mite called Demodex folliculorum (a normal resident in human skin) that is more numerous on the skin of people with rosacea.
- The condition is worsened by stress (worry and anxiety), hot drinks, spicy foods, smoking, alcohol, exposure to temperature extremes, excessive sunlight and cosmetics or skin products containing alcohol (or other irritating ingredients).

RISK INCREASES WITH
- People who flush easily.
- Fair complexion.
- Family history of acne rosacea.
- Overuse of corticosteroid creams or ointments in treatment of other skin disorders.

HOW TO PREVENT—Avoid triggers such as hot liquids, hot or spicy foods, alcohol and stress. Extreme temperatures and sunlight may lessen occurrence.

WHAT TO EXPECT

DIAGNOSTIC MEASURES
- Your own observation of symptoms.
- Medical history and physical exam by a doctor. There is no specific test to diagnose the disorder.

APPROPRIATE HEALTH CARE
- Self-care after diagnosis.
- Doctor's treatment with medications.
- Steroid-induced rosacea is treated first by stopping the steroid drug.
- Destruction of large vessels with electric needle or a laser.
- Excess tissue removal with electric needle or a laser; or sometimes with a scalpel or rapidly rotating wire brush. The nose may be red for up to a year and then assumes a normal color.
- Psychotherapy or counseling, if disfigurement causes distress.

POSSIBLE COMPLICATIONS
- Psychological distress caused by an unsightly appearance.
- More likely to suffer from migraines.
- Autoimmune eye disorders (rare).

PROBABLE OUTCOME—Symptoms can be controlled with treatment. Acne rosacea is a disease of remissions and frequent flare-ups.

HOW TO TREAT

GENERAL MEASURES
- Seek care early if you notice evidence of acne rosacea.
- Use water-based cosmetics instead of oil-based products.
- See How to Cope With Stress in Appendix.

MEDICATION
- Your doctor may prescribe:
  Oral antibiotics, such as tetracycline or erythromycin.
  Topical antibiotics.
  Topical antiprotozoal and antibacterial medications, such as metronidazole.
  Isotretinoin (Accutane), an oral drug, may succeed where other measures fail.
- Don't use cortisone preparations, including nonprescription medicines, without doctor's approval.

ACTIVITY—No restrictions except to avoid factors that may cause a flare-up (see Causes).

DIET—No special diet. Avoid spicy foods, alcohol or anything that causes the face to flush.

CALL YOUR DOCTOR IF

You have symptoms of acne rosacea. This condition can be helped with treatment.

ADDISON'S DISEASE
(Adrenal Insufficiency)

 GENERAL INFORMATION

DEFINITION—Underactive adrenal glands. The adrenal glands secrete several hormones that are essential to a number of body functions. These hormones help to maintain body fluid balance and are involved in sugar and protein metabolism, maintenance of blood pressure and response to physical stress.

BODY PARTS INVOLVED—Adrenal glands (located over the kidneys).

SEX OR AGE MOST AFFECTED—Both sexes; all ages.

SIGNS & SYMPTOMS
Symptoms may develop slowly, including:
• Weakness and fatigue.
• Gastrointestinal disturbances (nausea, vomiting, abdominal pain, diarrhea, and appetite and weight loss).
• Low blood pressure causing faintness and dizziness.
• Brownish skin (looks suntanned) with white patches.
• Darkening of freckles, scars and breast nipples.
• Hair loss.
• Feeling cold all the time.
• Dramatic behavior or mood changes, including aggression or depression.

CAUSES
• Symptoms and signs are caused by low levels of cortisone-like hormones produced by the adrenal glands. The cause of adrenal insufficiency is usually unknown, but is sometimes a complication of tuberculosis, cancer, pituitary disease or AIDS.
• Use of cortisone drugs for other conditions. When cortisone is withdrawn, normal adrenal function sometimes does not return.

RISK INCREASES WITH
Stress; diabetes mellitus; injury to the abdomen; anticoagulant therapy; surgery.

HOW TO PREVENT—Don't discontinue use of cortisone drugs or change the dosage without consulting your doctor.

 WHAT TO EXPECT

DIAGNOSTIC MEASURES
• Your own observation of symptoms. "Before and after" pictures may emphasize the gradual skin change.
• Medical history and physical by a doctor.
• Laboratory blood counts, blood and urine measurement of adrenal hormones and a test of adrenal-gland function.

APPROPRIATE HEALTH CARE
• Doctor's treatment.
• Hospitalization for an adrenal crisis (see Possible Complications).

POSSIBLE COMPLICATIONS
• Adrenal crisis (pains, weakness, low blood pressure, high or low temperature, fainting) caused by any injury or illness.
• Increased susceptibility to infections.
• Misdiagnosis as a mental condition.

PROBABLE OUTCOME—When diagnosed in its early stages, symptoms can be controlled with hormone replacement. In advanced stages, it can be fatal without treatment.

 HOW TO TREAT

GENERAL MEASURES
• This is a lifelong condition. Learn how to care for yourself. Strict attention to medication schedules is vital.
• Learn about adrenal crisis and its relationship to body stress (infection, surgery or injury).
• Advise any doctor or dentist who treats you that you have Addison's disease.
• Wear a Medic-Alert bracelet or pendant (see Glossary).
• Stay current on immunizations, including those for influenza and pneumonia.
• If you live or travel where medical care may not be readily available, get instructions on giving yourself cortisone injections in case of emergency.

MEDICATION—Your doctor may prescribe one of several types of cortisone drugs. Follow medication schedule exactly. Never change or omit medication without your doctor's advice.

ACTIVITY—No restrictions.

DIET—Consult your doctor about diet. A diet to maintain sodium and potassium or to increase protein or carbohydrates may be required.

 CALL YOUR DOCTOR IF

• You have symptoms of Addison's disease—especially an adrenal crisis. Call immediately. Adrenal crisis is an emergency!
• The following occurs after diagnosis:
  Any signs of infection, such as fever, chills, muscle aches, headache and dizziness.
  Serious injury, such as bone fracture, dislocation or internal injuries.
• You are scheduled for elective surgery or require anesthesia for any reason.
• New, unexplained symptoms develop. Drugs used in treatment may produce side effects, such as: protruding abdomen, thin extremities, puffy face and eyes, acne, growth of facial hair.

AGRANULOCYTOSIS
(Granulocytopenia; Neutropenia)

GENERAL INFORMATION

DEFINITION—Reduction in the normal number of circulating white blood cells (granulocytes or neutrophils) in the bloodstream. These cells are the first to attack bacterial infections.

BODY PARTS INVOLVED—Blood; bone marrow.

SEX OR AGE MOST AFFECTED—Both sexes; all ages.

SIGNS & SYMPTOMS
• Fever.
• Aching.
• Sore throat.
• Ulcers (especially in the mouth and throat), which do not produce pus.
• Any sign of infection in someone who has had agranulocytosis in the past. This may signal a recurrence.

CAUSES—Increased destruction or impaired production of granulocytes (white blood cells). The most common reason for this is an adverse reaction to medications, including: anticancer drugs; anticonvulsants; antihistamines; antithyroid drugs; arsenic; chloramphenicol; Dibenzyline; gold salts; indomethacin; nitrofurantoin; nitrous oxide; phenothiazines; phenylbutazone; procainamide; sulfonamides; synthetic penicillins; and thiazide diuretics.

RISK INCREASES WITH—Genetic factors. A rare form, infantile genetic agranulocytosis, is inherited.

HOW TO PREVENT
• See your doctor if you have one infection after another (especially if you take medications).
• Prevent recurrences by avoiding any suspect medicine or drug that may have triggered agranulocytosis previously.

WHAT TO EXPECT

DIAGNOSTIC MEASURES
• Your own observation of symptoms.
• Medical history and physical exam by a doctor.
• Laboratory studies of blood and bone marrow, and cultures of blood, nose, throat and urine.

APPROPRIATE HEALTH CARE
• Doctor's treatment.
• Possible hospitalization for intensive treatment during the active phase, with strict reverse isolation techniques (see Glossary) and transfusions of white blood cells (sometimes).
• Self-care after diagnosis and hospitalization.

POSSIBLE COMPLICATIONS
• Kidney damage.
• Dangerous, sometimes fatal infections (bacterial, fungal, viral or others)—even with vigorous treatment.
• May be an early sign of leukemia or aplastic anemia.

PROBABLE OUTCOME—Depending on cause, usually curable with intensive treatment.

HOW TO TREAT

GENERAL MEASURES—Hospitalization may be necessary during the acute phase. The following may be helpful after hospitalization:
• Be extra careful about personal cleanliness.
• Keep the mouth clean by rinsing frequently with warm salt water (1 teaspoon salt to 8 oz. water) or gargling with hydrogen peroxide.
• Pay particular attention to oral hygiene. Brush teeth gently with a very soft brush, avoiding irritation of the gums.
• Avoid contact with harmful materials, such as cleaning chemicals, glue, insecticide, fertilizer and paint remover.

MEDICATION—Your doctor may:
• Prescribe intravenous and oral antibiotics if the white blood cell count is very low.
• Prescribe lithium to stimulate bone marrow to produce more granulocytes.
• Stop prescribing any drug that is suspected of causing agranulocytosis.

ACTIVITY—Rest in bed during the acute stage. Resume normal activities gradually after symptoms subside.

DIET—No restrictions.

CALL YOUR DOCTOR IF

• You have symptoms of agranulocytosis.
• The following occurs after treatment:
  Any sign of infection, especially fever.
  Swelling of the feet and ankles.
  Painful urination or decreased urine output in 1 day.
• New, unexplained symptoms develop. Drugs used in treatment may produce side effects.

ALCOHOLISM

GENERAL INFORMATION

DEFINITION—A psychological and physiological dependence on alcohol, resulting in chronic disease and disruption of interpersonal, family and work relationships.

BODY PARTS INVOLVED—Brain; central nervous system; liver; heart.

SEX OR AGE MOST AFFECTED—Both sexes, but occurs 4 times more often in men than women. The incidence of alcoholism in children is increasing.

SIGNS & SYMPTOMS
Early stages:
- Low tolerance for anxiety.
- Need for alcohol at the beginning of the day or at times of stress.
- Insomnia; nightmares.
- Habitual Monday-morning hangovers and frequent absences from work.
- Preoccupation with obtaining alcohol and hiding drinking from family and friends.
- Guilt or irritability when others suggest drinking is excessive.

Late stages:
- Frequent blackouts; memory loss.
- Delirium tremens (tremors, hallucinations, confusion, sweating, rapid heartbeat). These occur most often with alcohol withdrawal.
- Liver disease.
- Neurological impairment (numbness and tingling in hands and feet, declining sexual interest and potency, confusion, coma).
- Congestive heart failure (shortness of breath, swelling of feet).

CAUSES—Not fully understood, but include:
- Personality factors, especially dependency, anger, mania, depression or introversion.
- Family influences, especially alcoholic or divorced parents.
- Social and cultural pressure to drink.
- Body-chemistry disturbances (perhaps).

RISK INCREASES WITH
- Genetic factors. Some ethnic groups have high alcoholism rates—either for social or biological reasons.
- Use of recreational drugs.
- Crisis situations, including unemployment, frequent moves, or loss of friends or family.
- Environmental factors such as ready availability, affordability and social acceptance of alcohol in the culture group, work group or social group.

HOW TO PREVENT
- Use alcohol in moderation—if at all—to provide a healthy role model. Set limits, drink slowly, dilute drinks and don't drink alone.

- Help a spouse, friend or co-worker to admit when an alcohol problem exists and seek help.
- Learn other ways to cope with problems.

WHAT TO EXPECT

DIAGNOSTIC MEASURES
- Medical history and physical by a doctor.
- EEG (see Glossary) and laboratory studies of blood and liver function.

APPROPRIATE HEALTH CARE
- Self-care. The first and most difficult step of treatment is admitting the problem exists.
- Doctor's treatment, psychotherapy or counseling.
- May require detoxification.

POSSIBLE COMPLICATIONS
- Chronic and progressive liver disease.
- Gastric erosion, stomach inflammation.
- Neuritis, tremors, seizures, memory loss and brain impairment
- Pancreas and heart inflammation.
- Impotence and other sexual problems.
- Mental and physical damage to the fetus if a woman drinks during pregnancy (fetal alcohol syndrome).
- Loss of job, friends and breaking up of family.
- Premature death.

PROBABLE OUTCOME—With abstinence (absence of alcohol or drugs), sobriety is a way of life. The change in lifestyle is difficult and relapses occur. If you are determined to give up alcohol, you can.

HOW TO TREAT

GENERAL MEASURES
- Treatment involves short-term care that stops the drinking and long-term help to treat the problem that caused the alcoholism.
- Join a local Alcoholics Anonymous or other support group and attend regularly. Members help each other to stay away from alcohol.
- Reassess your lifestyle to identify and alter factors that encourage drinking.

MEDICATION—Your doctor may prescribe disulfiram (Antabuse), which causes several extremely unpleasant physical symptoms when alcohol is consumed.

ACTIVITY—Don't drink and drive.

DIET—Normal, well-balanced diet, vitamin supplements may be recommended.

CALL YOUR DOCTOR IF

You or a family member have symptoms of alcoholism.

ALOPECIA AREATA

GENERAL INFORMATION

DEFINITION—Sudden hair loss in circular patches on the scalp. Hair loss is not accompanied by other visible evidence of scalp disease. This is not contagious.

BODY PARTS INVOLVED—Hair; scalp; eyebrows; eyelashes; beard; genital area; underarm (sometimes).

SEX OR AGE MOST AFFECTED—Affects all ages and males more frequently than females.

SIGNS & SYMPTOMS
* Sudden hair loss in sharply defined circular patches. In rare cases, body hair loss may be total (alopecia totalis/universalis).
* No pain.
* No itch.

CAUSES
* Usually unknown, but heredity and emotional factors, such as anxiety, may contribute to hair loss. The autoimmune system may also be involved.
* May be caused by thyroiditis or pernicious anemia.

RISK INCREASES WITH
* Stress.
* Family history of alopecia areata.

HOW TO PREVENT—Cannot be prevented at present.

WHAT TO EXPECT

DIAGNOSTIC MEASURES
* Your own observation of symptoms.
* Medical history and physical exam by a doctor.

APPROPRIATE HEALTH CARE
* Self-care after diagnosis.
* Doctor's treatment.

POSSIBLE COMPLICATIONS
* Loss of all hair.
* Slow or incomplete regrowth.

PROBABLE OUTCOME—Usually curable, with spontaneous new growth, in 18 months to 3 years. Persons with a few small patches are generally cured completely. The disorder recurs in 25% of cases.

HOW TO TREAT

GENERAL MEASURES
* Consider wearing a hairpiece or wig during the acute phase.
* Continue to bathe and shampoo as usual.
* Don't tug on normal hair close to areas of hair loss.
* See Resources for Additional Information.

MEDICATION—Your doctor may prescribe:
* Topical steroids. Apply topical steroid once or twice a day unless directed otherwise. Apply immediately after bathing or shampooing for better spreading and penetration. For scalp and groin, use only low-potency steroid products without fluorine.
* Injections of steroids into affected areas and oral cortisone drugs for you to take on alternate days.
* Photochemotherapy with PUVA (see Glossary).
* A topical drug, minoxidil (a prescription drug used for hair growth), may help some patients.

ACTIVITY—No restrictions.

DIET—No special diet.

CALL YOUR DOCTOR IF

* You have symptoms of alopecia areata.
* The following occurs during treatment:
  Hair loss increases.
  Hair loss doesn't diminish in 4 weeks.
  Areas show signs of infection (redness, swelling, tenderness, warmth) after injections.

ALTITUDE ILLNESS

GENERAL INFORMATION

DEFINITION—Any of several illnesses associated with higher than usual altitudes. Illnesses are of several types, including:
- Acute mountain sickness (AMS).
- High altitude pulmonary edema (HAPE).
- High altitude cerebral edema (HACE).
- High altitude retinal hemorrhage (HARH).
- Subacute and chronic mountain sickness (CMS). This illness is a complication that represents failure to recover from AMS over a long period of time.

BODY PARTS INVOLVED—These illnesses affect most body systems, especially the brain, heart, lungs, gastrointestinal tract, circulatory system and electrolytes.

SEX AND AGE MOST AFFECTED—Young adults of both sexes.

SIGNS & SYMPTOMS
- AMS: headache, nausea, vomiting, shortness of breath, sleep disturbances.
- HAPE: shortness of breath, cough, weakness, headache, coma.
- HACE: severe headache, staggering gait, hallucinations, stupor. These indicate swelling of the brain. Death will occur with descent.
- HARH: visual disturbances, including spots before the eyes. Blood clots and bleeding into the retina occur in 50% of those who go above 17,000 feet.
- CMS: shortness of breath, fatigue, bloated face and body, congestive heart failure after years of living at high altitude (rare).

CAUSES—Insufficient oxygen at high altitudes. Following are the altitudes at which each type of illness can occur:
- AMS—7,000 to 8,000 feet or higher.
- HAPE—9,000 to 10,000 feet.
- HACE—10,000 to 12,000 feet.
- HARH—17,000 feet.

RISK INCREASES WITH
- Lack of conditioning.
- Faster and higher ascent.
- Previous episodes of altitude illness.
- Chronic illness of any sort, particularly cardiovascular and lung diseases.
- Excess alcohol consumption or use of mind-altering drugs, including narcotics and tranquilizers.

HOW TO PREVENT
- Acclimatization as you ascend; descend if troubling symptoms appear.
- Obtain maximum physical conditioning.
- Talk to your doctor about preventive drugs.

WHAT TO EXPECT

DIAGNOSTIC MEASURES
- Medical history and physical exam by a doctor.
- Laboratory blood studies and urinalysis.
- ECG (see Glossary) and chest x-rays (sometimes).

APPROPRIATE HEALTH CARE
- Self-care.
- Doctor's treatment.
- Hospitalization (severe cases).

POSSIBLE COMPLICATIONS—Respiratory distress syndrome; brain, eye, heart and lung damage.

PROBABLE OUTCOME—Complete recovery in 1-3 days.

HOW TO TREAT

GENERAL MEASURES
- In most cases, rest, mild pain relievers, avoidance of alcohol and adequate hydration will control symptoms.
- For some patients, a descent to a lower altitude will be necessary.

MEDICATION—Your doctor may prescribe:
- Pain relievers for headache.
- Antibiotics if infection is present.
- Dexamethasone or acetazolamide for more severe symptoms.
- Supplemental oxygen if required.

ACTIVITY
- If any altitude illness occurs, decrease activity to a level at which symptoms disappear.
- Resume routine activities gradually upon returning to normal altitude.

DIET—Increase fluid intake, avoid alcohol, eat small meals.

CALL YOUR DOCTOR IF

- You have symptoms of any altitude illness.
- New, unexplained symptoms develop. Drugs used in treatment may produce side effects.

ILLNESS & DISORDERS

ALZHEIMER'S DISEASE
(Presenile Dementia)

 GENERAL INFORMATION

DEFINITION—A brain disorder characterized by gradual mental deterioration. A rapidly progressive form begins in adults around ages 36 to 45. A more gradual form, with slow development of symptoms, begins around ages 65 to 70.

BODY PARTS INVOLVED—Brain.

SEX OR AGE MOST AFFECTED—Both sexes, beginning in the 40s and 50s.

SIGNS & SYMPTOMS
Early stages:
- Forgetfulness of recent events.
- Increasing difficulty performing intellectual tasks, such as accustomed work, balancing a checkbook or maintaining a household.
- Personality changes, including poor impulse control and poor judgment.

Later stages:
- Difficulty doing simple tasks, such as choosing clothing, problem solving.
- Failure to recognize familiar persons.
- Disinterest in personal hygiene or appearance.
- Difficulty feeding self.
- Belligerence and denial that anything is wrong.
- Loss of usual sexual inhibitions.
- Wandering away.
- Anxiety and insomnia.

Advanced stages:
- Complete loss of memory, speech and muscle function (including bladder and bowel control), necessitating total care and supervision.
- Extreme belligerence and hostility.

CAUSES—Irreversible damage to or loss of brain cells for unknown reasons.

RISK INCREASES WITH
- Family history of Alzheimer's disease.
- Aging.

HOW TO PREVENT—No specific preventive measures.

 WHAT TO EXPECT

DIAGNOSTIC MEASURES
- Your own observation of symptoms.
- Medical history and physical exam by a doctor.
- X-rays of the brain, including CAT scan (see Glossary) to rule out other conditions.

APPROPRIATE HEALTH CARE
- Doctor's treatment.
- Psychotherapy or counseling for family members.
- Health facility care when home care becomes impossible.

POSSIBLE COMPLICATIONS
- Decreased resistance to infections, especially pneumonia and meningitis.
- Seizures and coma (rare).

PROBABLE OUTCOME—This condition is currently considered incurable and untreatable. It is usually fatal within 5 years without skillful supportive care. Scientific research into causes and treatment continues, so there is hope for eventual treatment and cure.

 HOW TO TREAT

GENERAL MEASURES
- If a family member has this disease, don't take their hostility personally.
- If you care for a family member with the disease, try to obtain help so you can get away often. Don't feel guilty about needing a respite—even if the patient resents it.
- Join or start a support group for families of Alzheimer's victims (see Resources For Additional Information).
- Caregivers can help reduce some of the patient's behaviors by:
    Repetition: Patient with memory problem may benefit from frequent, simple reminders.
    Reassurance: A brief, firm chat with a family member may help a patient with anxiety, verbal outbursts or agitation.
    Redirection: Distract the patient who is frustrated or agitated. A short walk is helpful.

MEDICATION—Many medications are being studied. Some are useful to control symptoms such as agitation. The prescription drug, tacrine, may help some patients. Other new drugs can delay progression in patients.

ACTIVITY—As much as possible. As the condition progresses, all activity will eventually require supervision.

DIET—Regular diet. Feeding assistance will eventually be necessary.

 CALL YOUR DOCTOR IF

- You or a family member has symptoms of Alzheimer's disease.
- Signs of infection occur, such as fever, chills, muscle aches or headache.
- You care for someone with Alzheimer's disease, and you fear you are about to lose emotional control.

AMEBIASIS
(Amebic Dysentery; Entamebiasis)

 GENERAL INFORMATION

DEFINITION—Parasitic infection of the large intestine and sometimes the liver. Amebiasis is most prevalent in developing countries. In the USA, the disease is relatively rare in the general population but is concentrated in some high-risk groups. Many people, especially those who live in temperate climates, harbor the amoeba without symptoms. Symptoms occur when the parasite invades tissues of the colon. Symptoms may be very vague.

BODY PARTS INVOLVED—Intestinal tract, especially the colon; liver.

SEX OR AGE MOST AFFECTED—Both sexes; all ages.

SIGNS & SYMPTOMS
- Sometimes no symptoms are present.
- Intermittent diarrhea with bad-smelling stools. Diarrhea is often preceded by constipation in early stages.
- Gas and abdominal bloating.
- Abdominal cramps and tenderness.
- Fever.
- Mucus and blood in the stool (sometimes).
- Fatigue and muscle aches.

If the liver is involved:
- Tenderness over the liver and right side of the abdomen.
- Jaundice (sometimes).
- Chills.
- Weight loss.

CAUSES—A microscopic parasite that is spread by flies, cockroaches and direct contact with hands or food contaminated with feces. The most common sources of infection are:
- Infected food handlers.
- Faulty hotel or factory plumbing.
- Raw vegetables or fruit fertilized with human feces or washed in polluted water.

RISK INCREASES WITH
- Crowded or unsanitary living conditions.
- Travel to a foreign country.
- Combination of anal-oral sex.
- Institutional living.

HOW TO PREVENT
- Wash your hands frequently— always before eating.
- If you are in an area where food or water may be contaminated, the following measures are necessary:
  Boil drinking water for 5 minutes.
  Don't use water for any purpose that may have raw sewage.
  Don't eat unpeeled fruit or vegetables and raw fish or shellfish.

 WHAT TO EXPECT

DIAGNOSTIC MEASURES
- Your own observation of symptoms.
- Medical history and physical exam by a doctor.
- Laboratory studies of stool and blood serum; sigmoidoscopy (see Glossary); x-rays of lower bowel (barium enema).

APPROPRIATE HEALTH CARE
- Home care.
- Doctor's treatment.
- Hospitalization (severe cases only).

POSSIBLE COMPLICATIONS
- Peritonitis.
- Hepatitis or liver abscess.
- Lung abscess.
- Infection of the pericardium.
- Brain abscess.

PROBABLE OUTCOME—In most cases without complications, amebiasis is curable in 3 weeks with treatment. In the carrier state, this disease may not cause any symptoms. In severe cases, it may cause dysentery that requires hospital treatment.

 HOW TO TREAT

GENERAL MEASURES—Be extra careful about personal cleanliness. Bathe frequently and wash hands with warm water and soap after each bowel movement and before handling food.

MEDICATION—Your doctor may prescribe antiamoeba medication. Fluid replacement may be necessary to manage electrolyte imbalance due to diarrhea.

ACTIVITY—Rest in bed during an acute attack. Resume normal activities when fever disappears and diarrhea improves.

DIET—Soft diet progressing to normal diet. (See Soft Diet in Appendix.)

 CALL YOUR DOCTOR IF

- You have symptoms of amebiasis.
- The following occur during treatment:
  Abdominal cramps continue longer than 24 hours.
  Diarrhea or blood in stool increases.
  Vomiting begins.
  Pain begins over liver or jaundice occurs.
  A skin rash appears.
  Irritability or a severe headache develop.

AMENORRHEA

GENERAL INFORMATION

DEFINITION
Primary—Absence of menstruation in a young woman who is at least 16 years old or has reached age 14 with a lack of normal growth or absence of secondary sexual development.
Secondary—Cessation of menstruation in a woman who has previously menstruated.

BODY PARTS INVOLVED—Endocrine system; reproductive system.

SEX OR AGE MOST AFFECTED—Females over age 16.

SIGNS & SYMPTOMS
• Lack of menstrual periods after puberty. Most girls begin menstruating by age 14.
• Absence of menstrual periods for 3 months in a female who has menstruated at least once.

CAUSES—Usually unknown. Possibly:
• Congenital abnormalities, such as the absence or abnormal formation of female organs (vagina, uterus, ovaries).
• Intact hymen (membrane covering the vaginal opening) that has no opening to allow passage of menstrual flow.
• Disorders (tumors, infections or lack of maturation) of the endocrine system.
• Chromosome disorders.
• Emotional distress or eating disorders, including obesity, bulimia, anorexia nervosa, excessive dieting or starvation.
• Use of certain drugs, including mind-altering drugs, sedatives, hormones, oral contraceptives, anticancer drugs, barbiturates, narcotics, cortisone drugs, chlordiazepoxide and reserpine.
• Strenuous athletic activities.
Other causes of secondary amenorrhea:
• Pregnancy or breast-feeding.
• Discontinuing use of birth-control pills.
• Menopause (if woman is over 35 and not pregnant).
• Surgical removal of ovaries or uterus.
• Diabetes mellitus, tuberculosis, obesity.

RISK INCREASES WITH—See Causes.

HOW TO PREVENT
• Use drugs only if prescribed by your doctor.
• Reduce strenuous athletic activities.
• Medical treatment for underlying disorders.
• Maintain proper nutrition and body weight.

WHAT TO EXPECT

DIAGNOSTIC MEASURES
• Laboratory studies, such as a buccal smear (cells scraped from inside the cheek for chromosome studies), blood tests of hormone levels, thyroid and adrenal function tests.
• Pregnancy test and surgical diagnostic procedures, such as laparoscopy, hysteroscopy or dilatation and curettage.

APPROPRIATE HEALTH CARE
• Psychotherapy or counseling, if needed.
• Surgery (minor) to create an opening in the hymen, if necessary, or to correct abnormalities of the reproductive system (sometimes).

POSSIBLE COMPLICATIONS—Psychological distress about sexual development. May experience estrogen deficiency symptoms, such as hot flashes, vaginal dryness. May affect fertility.

PROBABLE OUTCOME
• **Primary**—The absence of menstruation is not a health risk and is usually curable with hormone treatment or removal of the underlying cause. Treatment may be delayed to age 18 unless the cause can be identified and treated.
• **Secondary**—If from pregnancy or breast-feeding, menstruation will resume when these conditions cease. If from discontinuing use of oral contraceptives, periods should begin in 2 months to 2 years. If from menopause, periods will become less frequent or may never resume. If from endocrine disorders, hormone replacement usually causes periods to resume. If from eating disorders, successful treatment of the disorder is necessary. If from diabetes or tuberculosis, menstruation may never resume. If from strenuous exercise, periods usually resume when exercise decreases.

HOW TO TREAT

GENERAL MEASURES
• Seek help in resolving emotional stress.
• Don't use mood-altering, mind-altering stimulants or sedative drugs.

MEDICATION—Your doctor may prescribe progesterone (hormone) treatment to induce bleeding. If bleeding begins when progesterone is withdrawn, the reproductive system is functioning. If progesterone withdrawal does not induce bleeding, gonad stimulants such as clomiphene or gonadotrophins may be used.

ACTIVITY
• Exercise regularly, but not to excess.
• Sleep at least 8 hours every night.

DIET—If overweight or underweight, a change in diet to correct the problem is recommended.

CALL YOUR DOCTOR IF

• You are 16 years old and have never had a period or periods have stopped for 3 months.
• Periods don't begin in 6 months, despite treatment, or new symptoms develop.

AMYOTROPHIC LATERAL SCLEROSIS
(ALS; Lou Gehrig's Disease)

 GENERAL INFORMATION

DEFINITION—A progressive breakdown of the cells of the spinal cord, resulting in gradual loss of muscle function. This is not contagious or cancerous. Symptoms may be confused with neurologic complications of Lyme Disease.

BODY PARTS INVOLVED—Central nervous system; muscle system, especially in the hands, forearms, legs, head and neck.

SEX OR AGE MOST AFFECTED—Men over age 40.

SIGNS & SYMPTOMS—Symptoms appear in the following order:
- Muscle twitching and weakness, beginning in the hands and spreading to the arms and legs. Weakness eventually affects muscles that control breathing and swallowing.
- Stiffening and spasticity of muscle groups.

CAUSES—Unknown.

RISK INCREASES WITH
- Age over 40.
- Family history of ALS.

HOW TO PREVENT—Cannot be prevented at present.

 WHAT TO EXPECT

DIAGNOSTIC MEASURES
- Your own observation of symptoms.
- Medical history and physical exam by a doctor.
- Laboratory studies, such as electromyography (see Glossary).

APPROPRIATE HEALTH CARE
- Self-care after diagnosis.
- Doctor's treatment.
- Psychotherapy or counseling to learn to cope with disability.
- Eventual hospitalization or medical facility care.

POSSIBLE COMPLICATIONS
- Pressure sores caused by immobility.
- Pneumonia caused by swallowing difficulty and choking.
- The progressive physical degeneration affects the patient's relationships, career, income, muscle coordination, sexuality and energy.

PROBABLE OUTCOME—This condition is currently considered incurable. It is usually fatal. However, pain can be relieved or controlled. Scientific research into causes and treatment continues, so there is hope for increasingly effective treatment and cure.

 HOW TO TREAT

GENERAL MEASURES
- There is no specific treatment. Supportive care is provided to control symptoms and for complicating emergencies.
- Obtain good nursing care to prevent pressure sores.
- Learn to do self-suction in order to handle increased accumulation of secretions in the lungs.
- Patients may benefit from a hospice program or local chapter of the ALS support group (see Resources for Additional Information).

MEDICATION—Your doctor may prescribe:
- Antibiotics to fight infection if pneumonia develops.
- Baclofen to help reduce spasticity.
- Antidepressant to help decrease saliva production.

ACTIVITY
- Stay as active as possible. Weakness will gradually limit capability. A rehabilitation program can help in maintaining independence as long as possible.
- Obtain equipment that will aid in mobility, such as walker or wheelchair.

DIET—If swallowing is difficult, eat soft, easy-to-swallow foods. (See Soft Diet in Appendix.)

 CALL YOUR DOCTOR IF

- You have symptoms of amyotrophic lateral sclerosis.
- Coughing, choking or fever occurs after diagnosis.

ANAL FISSURE

GENERAL INFORMATION

DEFINITION—A laceration, tear or crack in the lining of the anus.

BODY PARTS INVOLVED—Anus.

SEX OR AGE MOST AFFECTED—All ages, but most common in infants, young children and adults over 60. This affects more women than men.

SIGNS & SYMPTOMS
● Sharp pain with passage of a hard or bulky stool. The pain may last up to an hour and returns with the next bowel movement.
● Pain when sitting on a hard surface.
● Streaks of blood on the toilet paper, underwear or diaper.
● Itching around the rectum.
● Children may refuse to have a bowel movement.

CAUSES—The exact cause is unknown, but the symptoms usually occur after the stretching of the anus from a large, hard stool.

RISK INCREASES WITH
● Constipation.
● Multiple pregnancies.
● Leukemia, Crohn's disease, immunodeficiency disorders.

HOW TO PREVENT
● Avoid constipation by:
   Drinking at least 8 glasses of water daily.
   Eating a diet high in fiber.
   Using stool softeners or other laxatives, if needed.
● Don't strain at stool.
● Avoid anal intercourse.

WHAT TO EXPECT

DIAGNOSTIC MEASURES
● Your own observation of symptoms.
● Medical history and physical exam by a doctor.
● Examination of the anus and rectum with an anoscope or sigmoidoscope to rule out other causes of anal or rectal bleeding.

APPROPRIATE HEALTH CARE
● Home care.
● Doctor's treatment.
● Surgery may be necessary to remove the fissure or to alter the muscle that contracts and prevents normal healing (see Anal-Fissure Removal and Anal Sphincterectomy in Surgery section).

POSSIBLE COMPLICATIONS—Permanent scarring that prevents normal bowel movements.

PROBABLE OUTCOME—Most adults recover in 4 to 6 weeks with treatment, making surgery unnecessary. Most infants and young children recover after the stool is softened.

HOW TO TREAT

GENERAL MEASURES
● The following should be done to prevent constipation in children until the fissure heals:
   For infants: Before bedtime, fill a rubber ear syringe with plain mineral oil. Gently insert the tip and squeeze the mineral oil into the infant's rectum.
   Repeat the next morning. If no bowel movement occurs, repeat at noon. After the bowel movement, clean the anus gently with cotton and water.
   For older children: Gently squeeze 4 ounces of mineral oil into the rectum. You may use a sanitary napkin to catch oil that seeps out in the night.
● To relieve muscle spasms and pain around the anus, apply a warm towel to the area.
● Sitz baths also relieve pain. Use 8 inches of very warm water 2 or 3 times a day for 10 to 20 minutes. Be careful not to burn a young child.

MEDICATION
● For minor pain, you may use nonprescription drugs, such as acetaminophen or topical anesthetics.
● Zinc oxide ointment or petroleum jelly applied to the anal opening may help prevent the burning sensation.
● Bulk stool softeners will help to avoid the pain occurring with bowel movements.
● Lidocaine ointment may be recommended.

ACTIVITY—No restrictions. Physical activity reduces the likelihood of constipation.

DIET—Encourage a high-fiber diet and extra fluids to prevent constipation.

CALL YOUR DOCTOR IF

You or your child have symptoms of an anal fissure—especially pain—that persists despite treatment.

ANAPHYLAXIS
(Allergic Shock—Life Threatening Emergency)

GENERAL INFORMATION

DEFINITION—A life-threatening allergic response to medications and many other allergy-causing substances. Reactions that occur quickly tend to be the most severe.

BODY PARTS INVOLVED—Blood vessels throughout the body; heart; lungs; skin.

SEX OR AGE MOST AFFECTED—Both sexes; all ages.

SIGNS & SYMPTOMS—Any of the following may occur within seconds or a few minutes after exposure to a substance to which you are very allergic:
- Tingling or numbness around the mouth.
- Sneezing, coughing or wheezing.
- Swelling around face or hands.
- Itching all over, often accompanied by hives.
- Watery eyes.
- Feeling of anxiety.
- Tightness in the chest; difficulty breathing.
- Swelling or itching in the mouth or throat.
- Pounding heart, faintness, weak, rapid pulse.
- Loss of consciousness.
Not all symptoms occur. Seek immediate help for any.

CAUSES—Eating or receiving injections of something to which you are sensitive. The allergic response to neutralize or get rid of the material results in a life-threatening overreaction. Things which cause reactions most often include:
- Medication of all types, especially penicillins. Injections are riskier than oral drugs.
- Stings or bites from insects, such as bees, biting ants and some spiders.
- Injected chemicals used in some types of x-ray studies.
- Foods, especially eggs, beans, seafood, fruit.
- Vaccines; pollen.

RISK INCREASES WITH
- A previous mild allergic response to things listed above.
- History of eczema, hay fever or asthma.

HOW TO PREVENT—If you have an allergic history:
- Tell your doctor before accepting any medication. Before you are given a shot, ask what it is.
- Keep an anaphylaxis kit, such as Ana-Kit, with you at all times. Be sure your family knows how to use the kit if you have a reaction.
- Always remain in your doctor's office 15 minutes after receiving any injection. Report any symptoms immediately.
- Protect yourself from insect stings.
- People with previous severe reaction to insect stings should consider immunization (allergy shots) as a preventive measure.

WHAT TO EXPECT

DIAGNOSTIC MEASURES—Laboratory skin tests to determine sensitivities.

APPROPRIATE HEALTH CARE—Doctor's treatment. Long-term treatment involves desensitization therapy.

POSSIBLE COMPLICATIONS—Without prompt treatment, anaphylaxis causes shock, cardiac arrest and death.

PROBABLE OUTCOME—Full recovery with prompt treatment.

HOW TO TREAT

GENERAL MEASURES—If you observe signs of anaphylaxis in someone and he or she stops breathing:
- Call or have someone call 911 (emergency) or call 0 (operator) for an ambulance or medical help. (If the victim is a child, perform lifesaving measures for 1 minute before calling for emergency help.) Begin mouth-to-mouth breathing immediately. If there is no heartbeat, give external cardiac massage. Don't stop CPR (cardiopulmonary resuscitation) until help arrives.
- Be alert to the possibility of a reaction when taking any medicine and be prepared to respond quickly if symptoms occur. If you have had a previous severe allergic reaction, always carry your anaphylaxis kit (make sure the kit is not outdated).
- Wear a Medic-Alert tag (see Glossary) that indicates your allergic condition.

MEDICATION
- Epinephrine by injection is the only effective immediate treatment.
- Aminophylline, cortisone drugs or antihistamines, given after the adrenalin, help prevent the return of acute symptoms.

ACTIVITY—Resume your normal activities as soon as symptoms improve after an attack. Stay under someone's observation for 24 hours in case symptoms recur.

DIET—Avoid foods to which you are allergic.

CALL YOUR DOCTOR IF

- You have symptoms of anaphylaxis. This is an emergency!
- New, unexplained symptoms develop. Drugs used in treatment may produce side effects.

ANEMIA, APLASTIC

GENERAL INFORMATION

DEFINITION—A serious disease characterized by decreased bone-marrow production of white and red blood cells and platelets.

BODY PARTS INVOLVED—Bone marrow; lymphatic system; blood.

SEX OR AGE MOST AFFECTED—Both sexes; all ages.

SIGNS & SYMPTOMS
• Paleness.
• Weakness, tiredness, faintness and breathlessness.
• Frequent infections.
• Spontaneous bleeding from the nose, mouth, rectum, vagina, gums and other sites—including the central nervous system.
• Red dots of bleeding under the skin.
• Unexplained bruising.
• Ulcers in the mouth, throat and rectum.

CAUSES—Poor bone-marrow function. Bone marrow is often infiltrated with fat cells, which supplant areas that manufacture blood cells.
  Infections occur because of reduced white cells, which normally protect against infection.
  Half of all cases are caused by drugs, especially immunosuppressive drugs, anticancer drugs, chloramphenicol or chemicals such as benzene. Other cases probably result from immunodeficiency, severe illness or unidentifiable causes.

RISK INCREASES WITH
• Family history of aplastic anemia.
• Genetic factors, such as those associated with congenital hypoplastic anemia (see Glossary).
• Use of drugs listed as causes.
• Recent severe illness.

HOW TO PREVENT
• Avoid prolonged exposure to toxic compounds, such as benzene, that are used in many industrial chemicals.
• Don't use drugs that cause aplastic anemia if substitute drugs are available.

WHAT TO EXPECT

DIAGNOSTIC MEASURES
• Your own observation of symptoms.
• Medical history and physical exam by a doctor.
• Laboratory studies of blood and bone marrow.

APPROPRIATE HEALTH CARE
• Doctor's treatment.
• Surgery to transplant bone marrow.
• Blood transfusions if necessary.
• Hospitalization for isolation until the body can resist infection.

POSSIBLE COMPLICATIONS—Poor response to treatment, resulting in uncontrollable infections and bleeding. Complications are fatal in 50% to 70% of those with severe aplastic anemia.

PROBABLE OUTCOME—If the cause can be identified and treated successfully, the disorder is curable. Anemia caused by immuno-suppressive drugs usually improves spontaneously when drugs are withdrawn. Full recovery often requires 6 to 8 months.

HOW TO TREAT

NOTE—Follow your doctor's instructions. These instructions are supplemental.

GENERAL MEASURES
• A bone-marrow transplant requires a donor with compatible antigens. A twin, brother or sister usually makes the best donor. Donated marrow is injected gradually into the patient's veins to try to replace poorly functioning bone marrow with normal cells.
• Keep the mouth scrupulously clean to decrease the chance of infection. Brush often with a soft toothbrush. Rinse the mouth with a solution of equal parts hydrogen peroxide and water or use a medicated mouthwash, if prescribed.

MEDICATION—Your doctor may prescribe:
• Immunosuppressive drugs to prevent rejection, if a bone-marrow transplant is necessary.
• Antibiotics to prevent or treat infection.
• Medicated mouthwash to suppress fungus infections.

ACTIVITY—Resume your normal activities after treatment.

DIET—No special diet. You may need iron and vitamin supplements. Ask your doctor.

CALL YOUR DOCTOR IF

• You or a family member have symptoms of aplastic anemia.
• The following occurs after a bone-marrow transplant:
  Fever.
  Any sign of infection, such as swelling anywhere in the body. Redness, tenderness or pain may not be present.
  Skin rash.
  Jaundice (yellow skin and eyes).
  Joint pain.
  Puffy feet and ankles.
  Urinary discomfort.
  Decreased urine in 1 day.

ANEMIA DURING PREGNANCY

GENERAL INFORMATION

DEFINITION—An inadequate level of hemoglobin during pregnancy. Hemoglobin is a protein that carries oxygen to body tissues.

BODY PARTS INVOLVED—Blood cells.

SEX OR AGE MOST AFFECTED—Pregnant females.

SIGNS & SYMPTOMS
- Breathlessness.
- Tiredness, weakness or fainting.
- Paleness.

Infrequent:
- Palpitations or an abnormal awareness of the heartbeat.
- Inflamed, sore tongue.
- Nausea.
- Headache.
- Forgetfulness.
- Jaundice.
- Abdominal pain.

CAUSES
- Poor diet with inadequate iron.
- Folic-acid deficiency.
- Loss of blood from bleeding hemorrhoids or gastrointestinal bleeding.
- Excess cooking of food, which destroys available iron and other nutrients.
- Even if iron and folic-acid intake are sufficient, a pregnant woman may become anemic because pregnancy alters the digestive process. The fetus consumes some of the iron or folic acid normally available to the mother's body.

RISK INCREASES WITH
- Poor nutrition, especially multiple vitamin deficiencies.
- Smoking, which reduces absorption of important nutrients.
- Excess alcohol consumption, leading to poor nutrition.
- Medical history of any disorder that reduces absorption of nutrients.
- Use of anticonvulsant drugs.
- Previous use of oral contraceptives.

HOW TO PREVENT
- Eat foods rich in iron, such as liver, beef, whole-grain breads and cereals, eggs and dried fruit.
- Eat foods high in folic acid, such as wheat germ, beans, peanut butter, oatmeal, mushrooms, collards, broccoli, beef liver and asparagus.
- Eat foods high in vitamin C, such as citrus fruits and fresh, raw vegetables. Vitamin C makes iron absorption more efficient.
- Take prenatal vitamin and mineral supplements, if your doctor prescribes them.

WHAT TO EXPECT

DIAGNOSTIC MEASURES
- Your own observation of symptoms.
- Medical history and physical exam by a doctor.
- Laboratory blood studies of hemoglobin, iron, hematocrit and folic acid.

APPROPRIATE HEALTH CARE
- Self-care after diagnosis.
- Doctor's treatment.

POSSIBLE COMPLICATIONS
- Premature labor.
- Dangerous anemia from normal blood loss during labor, requiring blood transfusions.
- Increased susceptibility to infection after childbirth.

PROBABLE OUTCOME—Usually curable with iron and folic-acid supplements by mouth or by injection.

HOW TO TREAT

GENERAL MEASURES
- If the tongue is red and sore, rinse with warm salt water 3 or 4 times a day. Use 1 teaspoon salt to 8 oz. warm water.
- Brush teeth with a soft toothbrush.

MEDICATION—Your doctor may prescribe iron, folic acid and other supplements. For better absorption, take iron supplements 1 hour before eating or between meals. Iron will turn bowel movements black and often cause constipation.

ACTIVITY—No restrictions, except rest often until anemia disappears.

DIET—Eat well and take prescribed supplements. Increase fiber and fluid intake to prevent constipation. See How to Prevent for diet suggestions.

CALL YOUR DOCTOR IF

- You have symptoms of anemia during pregnancy.
- The following occurs during treatment:
  Diarrhea.
  Nausea.
  Abdominal pain.
  Constipation.
  Bleeding—however slight—from any source.

ILLNESS & DISORDERS

ANEMIA, FOLIC-ACID DEFICIENCY

 ## GENERAL INFORMATION

DEFINITION—Anemia caused by a deficiency of folic acid. It is often accompanied by iron-deficiency anemia.

BODY PARTS INVOLVED—Blood cells, which transport oxygen to all body parts.

SEX OR AGE MOST AFFECTED—Both sexes, but most common in women over 30.

SIGNS & SYMPTOMS
- Fatigue and weakness.
- Red, sore tongue.
- Paleness.
- Shortness of breath.
- Nausea, vomiting and diarrhea (rare).

CAUSES
- Complication of pregnancy, when the body needs 8 times more folic acid than usual.
- Inadequate intake or absorption of foods with a high folic-acid content, such as meat, poultry, fish, cheese, milk, eggs, green vegetables, yeast and mushrooms.
- Alcoholism.
- Overcooking foods, which destroys folic acid.
- Deficiency of vitamin B-12 or vitamin C.

RISK INCREASES WITH
- Adults over 60, especially those who have poor diets.
- Pregnancy.
- Illness, such as tropical sprue, psoriasis, acne rosacea, eczema or dermatitis herpetiformis.
- Fad diets or general poor nutrition, especially vitamin-C deficiency.
- Surgical removal of the stomach.
- Smoking, which decreases vitamin-C absorption. Vitamin C is necessary for folic-acid absorption.
- Use of certain drugs, such as oral contraceptives, anticonvulsants, methotrexate, triamterene or sulfasalazine.

HOW TO PREVENT
- Don't drink alcohol.
- Have regular medical checkups during pregnancy. Take prenatal vitamin supplements, if they are prescribed.
- Eat well. Include fresh vegetables, meat and other animal proteins. Avoid fad diets. Don't overcook food.
- Don't smoke. Smoking increases vitamin requirements.

 ## WHAT TO EXPECT

DIAGNOSTIC MEASURES
- Your own observation of symptoms.
- Medical history and physical exam by a doctor.
- Laboratory blood studies and possibly a Schilling test to measure vitamin B-12 levels and a therapeutic trial of vitamin B-12.

APPROPRIATE HEALTH CARE
- Self-care after diagnosis.
- Doctor's treatment.

POSSIBLE COMPLICATIONS
- Infertility.
- Increased susceptibility to infection.
- Congestive heart failure (severe cases only).

PROBABLE OUTCOME—Usually curable in 3 weeks with an adequate folic-acid intake.

 ## HOW TO TREAT

GENERAL MEASURES
- If you smoke, stop smoking.
- If you take oral contraceptives, consider using another form of contraception.

MEDICATION—Your doctor may prescribe:
- Folic-acid supplements.
- Iron supplements to take orally.

ACTIVITY—Anemia causes fatigue. Schedule regular rest periods until you are able to resume normal activity.

DIET—No special diet. Eat foods daily that are high in folic acid. The liver can store folic acid for a limited time only. Foods include asparagus spears, beef liver, broccoli spears, collards (cooked), mushrooms, oatmeal, peanut butter, red beans, wheat germ.

 ## CALL YOUR DOCTOR IF

- You have symptoms of anemia.
- Symptoms don't improve in 2 weeks, despite treatment.
- Symptoms of infection (fever, chills and muscle aches) occur during treatment.

ANEMIA, HEMOLYTIC

GENERAL INFORMATION

DEFINITION—Anemia due to the premature destruction of red blood cells (a process known as hemolysis). Bone marrow cannot produce red blood cells fast enough to compensate for those being destroyed. These anemias can be acquired (develop over time) or congenital (present at birth).

BODY PARTS INVOLVED—Blood; bone marrow; spleen.

SEX OR AGE MOST AFFECTED—Both sexes; all ages.

SIGNS & SYMPTOMS
- Fatigue.
- Shortness of breath.
- Irregular heartbeat.
- Jaundice (yellow skin and eyes, dark urine).
- Enlarged spleen.

CAUSES
- Inherited disorder, such as hereditary spherocytosis, G6PD deficiency, sickle-cell anemia or thalassemia. One inherited variety, favism, is common in Greece; hemolysis occurs after eating a type of bean.
- Antibodies produced by the body to fight infections, that for unknown reason attack red blood cells. This response is sometimes triggered by blood transfusions.
- Use of medications, including nonprescription drugs, that damage red blood cells.

RISK INCREASES WITH
- Family history of hemolytic anemia.
- Use of any medication.

HOW TO PREVENT
- Don't take any medicine that has previously triggered hemolytic anemia.
- Seek genetic counseling before having children if you have a family history of hemolytic anemia (inherited forms).
- Some types may be preventable by avoidance of the drugs or foods that precipitate hemolysis.

WHAT TO EXPECT

DIAGNOSTIC MEASURES
- Your own observation of symptoms.
- Medical history and physical exam by a doctor.
- Laboratory blood studies, including blood count, examination of bone marrow, and measurement with radioactive chromium of red cell survival.

APPROPRIATE HEALTH CARE
- Doctor's treatment.
- Hospitalization for transfusions during a hemolytic crisis.

- Surgery to remove an enlarged spleen (sometimes).
- Treatment is individualized depending on the specific hemolytic problem.

POSSIBLE COMPLICATIONS
- Excessive spleen enlargement, which increases destruction of red blood cells.
- Pain, shock and serious illness caused by hemolysis (red blood cell destruction).
- Gallstones.

PROBABLE OUTCOME
- If hemolytic anemia is acquired, it can usually be cured when the cause, such as a drug, is removed. Sometimes the spleen is removed surgically.
- If hemolytic anemia is inherited, it is currently considered incurable. However, symptoms can be relieved or controlled. Scientific research into causes and treatment continues, so there is hope for increasingly effective treatment and cure.

HOW TO TREAT

GENERAL MEASURES—If removal of the spleen is required, see Spleen Removal in Surgery section for an explanation of surgery and postoperative care.

MEDICATION—Your doctor may prescribe:
- Immunosuppressive drugs to control the antibody response.
- Medication to reduce pain. For minor discomfort, you may use nonprescription drugs such as acetaminophen.

ACTIVITY—After treatment, resume normal activities as soon as possible.

DIET—No special diet.

CALL YOUR DOCTOR IF

- You have symptoms of hemolytic anemia.
- The following occurs during treatment:
  Fever.
  Cough.
  Sore throat.
  Swollen joints.
  Muscle aches.
  Bloody urine.
  Signs of infection in any part of the body (redness, pain, swelling, fever).
- New, unexplained symptoms develop. Drugs used in treatment may produce side effects.

ANEMIA, IRON-DEFICIENCY

GENERAL INFORMATION

DEFINITION—A decreased number of circulating blood cells, or insufficient hemoglobin in the cells. Anemia is a symptom of other disorders. For proper treatment, the cause must be found.

BODY PARTS INVOLVED—Blood, which affects all body cells.

SEX OR AGE MOST AFFECTED—Both sexes; all ages.

SIGNS & SYMPTOMS—Initially, there may be no symptoms.
Signs of pronounced anemia include:
- Tiredness and weakness.
- Paleness, especially in the hands and lining of the lower eyelids.
Less common signs include:
- Tongue inflammation.
- Fainting.
- Breathlessness.
- Rapid heartbeat.
- Unusual quietness or withdrawal in a child.
- Appetite loss.
- Abdominal discomfort.
- Cravings for ice, paint or dirt.
- Susceptibility to infection.

CAUSES—Decreased absorption of iron or increased need for iron.
Causes in infants and children include:
- Poor nutrition. Between 6 months and 2 years of age, children may consume large quantities of milk, to the exclusion of iron-containing foods.
- Premature birth. Premature babies often have low stores of iron at birth.
Causes in adolescents and adults:
- Rapid growth spurts.
- Heavy menstrual bleeding.
- Pregnancy.
- Malabsorption.
- Gastrointestinal disease with bleeding, including cancer.

RISK INCREASES WITH
- Poor nutrition.
- Adults over 60.
- Recent illness, such as an ulcer, diverticulitis, colitis, hemorrhoids or gastrointestinal tumors.

HOW TO PREVENT—Maintain an adequate iron intake through a well-balanced diet or iron supplements. Provide iron-fortified formula for bottle-fed infants.

WHAT TO EXPECT

DIAGNOSTIC MEASURES
- Your own observation of symptoms.
- Medical history and physical exam by a doctor.
- Laboratory blood studies of serum iron, total iron-binding capacity and ferritin levels.

APPROPRIATE HEALTH CARE
- Doctor's treatment.
- Self-care.
- Blood transfusions in rare instances.

POSSIBLE COMPLICATIONS—Failure to diagnose a bleeding malignancy.

PROBABLE OUTCOME—Usually curable with iron supplements if the underlying cause can be identified and cured.

HOW TO TREAT

GENERAL MEASURES
- The most important part of treatment for iron-deficiency anemia is to correct the underlying cause. Iron deficiency can be treated well with iron supplements.
- Avoid risk of infections.

MEDICATION—Your doctor may prescribe iron supplements:
- Take iron on an empty stomach (at least 1/2 hour before meals) for best absorption. If it upsets your stomach, you may take it with a small amount of food (except milk).
- If you take other medications, wait at least 2 hours after taking iron before taking them. Antacids and tetracyclines especially interfere with iron absorption.
- Because liquid iron supplements may discolor the teeth, a child should drink any liquid iron preparation through a straw. Iron supplements may also cause black bowel movements, diarrhea or constipation.
- Continue iron supplements until 2 to 3 months after blood tests return to normal.
- Too much iron is dangerous. A bottle of iron tablets can poison a child. Keep iron supplements out of the reach of children.

ACTIVITY—No restrictions. You may need to pace activities until symptoms of fatigue are gone.

DIET
- Adults should limit milk to 1 pint a day. It interferes with iron absorption.
- Eat protein- and iron-containing foods, including meat, beans and leafy green vegetables.
- Increase dietary fiber to prevent constipation.

CALL YOUR DOCTOR IF

- You have symptoms of anemia.
- Nausea, vomiting, severe diarrhea or constipation occur during treatment.

ANEMIA, PERNICIOUS
(B-12 Deficiency Anemia)

 ## GENERAL INFORMATION

DEFINITION—Anemia caused by inadequate absorption of vitamin B-12. Vitamin B-12 is found only in food of animal origin, such as meat, fish and dairy products. The symptoms of pernicious anemia develop slowly and subtly and may not be recognized right away.

BODY PARTS INVOLVED—Blood, which affects all body cells; stomach.

SEX OR AGE MOST AFFECTED—Adults between ages 50 and 60. This is uncommon in children.

SIGNS & SYMPTOMS
- Weakness, especially in the arms and legs.
- Sore tongue.
- Nausea, appetite loss and weight loss.
- Bleeding gums.
- Numbness and tingling in the hands and feet.
- Difficulty maintaining proper balance.
- Pale lips, tongue and gums.
- Yellow eyes and skin.
- Shortness of breath.
- Depression.
- Confusion and dementia.
- Headache.
- Poor memory (in older persons, this may be confused with Alzheimer's disease).

CAUSES
- Absence of intrinsic factor, a chemical secreted by the stomach's membrane lining that makes absorption of vitamin B-12 possible. The reason for the absence of intrinsic factor is unknown, but it may be a genetic deficiency or autoimmune disorder.
- Decreased production of hydrochloric acid, especially following stomach surgery or in combination with the absence of intrinsic factor. Hydrochloric acid is also necessary for absorption of vitamin B-12.

RISK INCREASES WITH
- Improper diet, especially a vegetarian diet lacking vitamin B-12 and without supplements.
- Thyroid disease.
- Diabetes mellitus.
- Previous stomach surgery, stomach cancer or gastritis.
- Bulimia or anorexia nervosa.
- Family history of pernicious anemia.
- Age.
- Genetic factors. The disorder is most common in people of Northern European ancestry. It is rare in blacks and Asians.

HOW TO PREVENT—If you have had stomach surgery or gastritis, have regular vitamin B-12 injections. See Medication.

 ## WHAT TO EXPECT

DIAGNOSTIC MEASURES
- Your own observation of symptoms.
- Medical history and physical exam by a doctor.
- Laboratory blood studies.
- Radioactive studies, such as the Schilling test using radioactive vitamin B-12.
- Bone marrow test.

APPROPRIATE HEALTH CARE
- Self-care after diagnosis.
- Doctor's treatment.

POSSIBLE COMPLICATIONS
- Congestive heart failure.
- Double vision.
- Greater susceptibility to infections.
- Impotence in males.

PROBABLE OUTCOME—This condition is currently considered incurable. However, regular vitamin B-12 injections will control symptoms indefinitely and reverse complications. Some symptoms should start to disappear within a few days after treatment begins; others may take several months.

 ## HOW TO TREAT

GENERAL MEASURES—Avoid very hot water and heating pads. Your nervous system may not be able to detect dangerously high temperatures.

MEDICATION
- Your doctor will prescribe vitamin B-12 injections. The amount depends on the extent of your illness. The usual dosage is 1 injection a day for 7 days, then 1 injection a week for 1 month, then once a month for the rest of your life.
- Learn to give yourself vitamin B-12 injections, because oral supplements are inadequate. Lifetime treatment is essential. Even with treatment, your ability to absorb vitamin B-12 will not be normal.

ACTIVITY—Physical activity may need to be restricted until symptoms of weakness and balance problems disappear.

DIET
- No special diet. Raw meat and raw liver are no longer prescribed.
- Iron supplements may be necessary.

 ## CALL YOUR DOCTOR IF

- You have symptoms of pernicious anemia.
- Symptoms don't improve in 2 weeks, despite treatment.

ANEURYSM

GENERAL INFORMATION

DEFINITION—An abnormal widening of an artery A weakened artery wall is stretched as blood is pumped through it which creates an oval or egg-shaped ballooning.

BODY PARTS INVOLVED—Arteries. Aneurysms occur most often in the aorta (major artery in the chest and abdomen), arteries that supply the brain or legs, or heart wall after a heart attack.

SEX OR AGE MOST AFFECTED—Adults of both sexes.

SIGNS & SYMPTOMS—Often there are no symptoms or symptoms vary according to which artery is affected:
- Thoracic (chest) aneurysm produces a dry cough; pain in the chest, neck, back and abdomen. The pain may be sudden and sharp.
- Abdominal aneurysm produces back pain (sometimes severe), appetite and weight loss, and a pulsating mass in the abdomen.
- Aneurysm in a leg artery causes poor circulation in the leg, with weakness and pallor or swelling and bluish color. A pulsating mass may appear in the groin or behind the knee.
- Aneurysm in a brain artery produces headache (often throbbing), weakness, paralysis or numbness, pain behind the eye, vision change or partial blindness, and unequal pupils.
- Aneurysm in a heart muscle causes heartbeat irregularities and symptoms of congestive heart failure (see Illness section).

CAUSES
- Most common cause is high blood pressure which weakens an artery.
- Atherosclerosis (hardening of the arteries).
- Congenitally weak artery (especially with aneurysms in blood vessels to the brain).
- Syphilis or infection in the aorta caused by syphilis (rare).
- Injury.

RISK INCREASES WITH
Adults over 60; previous heart attack; high blood pressure; smoking; obesity; family history of aneurysms; polyarteritis nodosa (inflammation of the small and medium arteries); bacterial endocarditis (infection of the heart lining); marfan syndrome.

HOW TO PREVENT
- Don't smoke; get regular exercise; maintain adequate nutrition and a low fat diet; obtain early treatment for syphilis.
- Follow your treatment program to control high blood pressure; reduce stress.
- If you have a family history of aneurysms, ask your doctor about screening tests.

WHAT TO EXPECT

DIAGNOSTIC MEASURES
- Your own observation of symptoms.
- Medical history and exam by a doctor.
- Laboratory blood studies of clotting.
- ECG (see Glossary).
- X-rays of blood vessels (angiography).
- X-rays of the head, including CT scan or ultrasound (see Glossary for both).

APPROPRIATE HEALTH CARE
- Doctor's treatment; hospitalization.
- Surgery to replace the diseased vessel or close off the aneurysm. An aneurysm to the brain may require emergency surgery. Surgery for other types of aneurysms may be scheduled at a convenient time. (See Abdominal-Aortic Aneurysm, Removal of in Surgery section.)

POSSIBLE COMPLICATIONS
- Stroke.
- Rupture of the aneurysm. Symptoms include severe headache, severe knifelike chest, abdominal or leg pain, and loss of consciousness. If not treated, it can be fatal.

PROBABLE OUTCOME—Often curable with surgery to replace the diseased vessel with grafts (artificial vessels). Surgery on a heart aneurysm can stabilize the heartbeat and prolong life. Aneurysms sometimes recur.

HOW TO TREAT

GENERAL MEASURES—Early detection and treatment before rupture are essential. See your doctor if you have any signs of an aneurysm—especially a pulsating mass in the abdomen or leg—even if it does not cause symptoms.

MEDICATION—After surgery, your doctor may prescribe:
- Anticoagulants to prevent blood-clot formation in an aneurysm.
- Pain relievers.

ACTIVITY—Avoid heavy exertion or straining prior to surgery. After surgery, resume normal activities gradually.

DIET—Before surgery, eat a high-fiber diet. After surgery, no special diet.

CALL YOUR DOCTOR IF

- You have symptoms of an aneurysm, especially a pulsating mass in your abdomen or leg, or chest or abdominal pain. This is an emergency! Call for help and rest in bed.
- You have had a heart attack and develop heartbeat irregularity or symptoms of congestive heart failure.
- After surgery, any symptoms return.

ANGINA PECTORIS

GENERAL INFORMATION

DEFINITION—Chest pain arising from the heart—usually under the sternum (breastbone)—brought on by exercise, emotional upset or heavy meals in a person who has a heart disorder. Normally the arteries that supply blood to the heart can cope with an increased demand, but if coronary artery disease or high blood pressure is present, the flow is restricted.

BODY PARTS INVOLVED—Coronary arteries.

SEX OR AGE MOST AFFECTED—Men over age 35 and postmenopausal women.

SIGNS & SYMPTOMS—Any of the following:
- Tightness, squeezing, pressure or mild ache in the chest.
- Sudden breathing difficulty (sometimes).
- Frequent chest pain similar to indigestion.
- A choking feeling in the throat.
- Chest pain that radiates to the jaw, teeth or earlobes.
- Heaviness, numbness, tingling or ache in the arm, shoulder, elbow or hand—usually on the left side.
- Pain between the shoulder blades.

CAUSES—Insufficient blood to the heart muscle. Causes include:
- Coronary artery disease with partial blockage or spasm of arteries that supply the heart.
- Anemia.
- Overactive thyroid gland.
- Heartbeat that is too fast.
- Heart-valve disease.

RISK INCREASES WITH
- Smoking, obesity, diabetes mellitus.
- High blood pressure, high blood-cholesterol levels.
- Excess intake of fat or salt.
- Sedentary lifestyle, fatigue, overwork or stress.
- Family history of coronary artery disease.
- Exposure to cold and wind.

HOW TO PREVENT
- Obtain medical treatment for underlying causes or risks.
- Don't smoke.
- Eat a diet that is low in fat and low in salt. Lose weight if you are overweight (see Appendix for special diets).
- Avoid activities that trigger angina attacks.

WHAT TO EXPECT

DIAGNOSTIC MEASURES
- Your own observation of symptoms.
- Medical history and physical exam by a doctor.
- Laboratory studies, such as blood tests and stress tests; ECG (see Glossary); x-rays of the heart.
- Therapeutic trial of nitroglycerin.

APPROPRIATE HEALTH CARE
- Self-care after diagnosis.
- Doctor's treatment.
- Surgery to bypass severely blocked coronary arteries (sometimes).
- Balloon angioplasty (see Glossary) to open blocked coronary arteries (sometimes).

POSSIBLE COMPLICATIONS—Heart attack, congestive heart failure, potentially fatal arrhythmias.

PROBABLE OUTCOME—Minor angina can be relieved with rest and use of nitroglycerin and other drugs. Other treatment may be necessary to correct underlying diseases.

HOW TO TREAT

GENERAL MEASURES
- Reduce stress (see How to Cope with Stress in Appendix for suggestions).
- Follow suggestions under How to Prevent.
- Avoid situations that increase the heart's workload, such as anger, temperature extremes, high altitude (except in commercial airline flights) or sudden bursts of activity.

MEDICATION—Your doctor may prescribe:
- Nitroglycerin to relieve acute symptoms of angina. It does not affect symptoms of other disorders. It can work within seconds to relieve pain. Always keep it with you for immediate use.
- Other drugs for coronary disease, such as aspirin, beta-blockers or calcium antagonists may be prescribed. If they are, it is important to follow the prescribed drug regimen.

ACTIVITY
- Adjust your activities to minimize attacks.
- A regular moderate exercise routine (determined by your doctor) can help to control symptoms.

DIET—See diet suggestions under How to Prevent.

CALL YOUR DOCTOR IF

- You have symptoms of angina pectoris.
- The following occurs after diagnosis:
  An attack of chest pain continues longer than 10 to 15 minutes, despite rest and treatment with nitroglycerin.
  You wake from sleep with chest pain that does not go away with 1 nitroglycerin tablet. If these attacks continue, report them to your doctor—even if nitroglycerin relieves them.
  An attack occurs and the pain is different or more severe than usual.

ANIMAL BITES

GENERAL INFORMATION

DEFINITION—Bite wounds to humans from dogs, cats or other animals including humans.

BODY PARTS INVOLVED—Usually the hands, face or legs.

SEX OR AGE MOST AFFECTED—All ages and both sexes, but more often occurs in children and males.

SIGNS & SYMPTOMS
• Bite wounds can be tears, punctures, scratches, ripping or crush injuries.
• Dog bites usually involve the hands, face or the lower extremities.
• Cat bites usually involve the hands, followed by lower extremities, face and trunk.

CAUSES
• Bite wounds are often from a domestic pet known to the victim. Large dogs are the most common source.
• Human bites are often the result of one person striking another in the mouth with a clenched fist.

RISK INCREASES WITH—Exposure to domestic pets or wild animals. Dog bites rarely become infected. Cat bites and human bites frequently become infected.

HOW TO PREVENT
• Education on how to avoid animal bites for children as well as adults.
• Avoid stray animals.

WHAT TO EXPECT

DIAGNOSTIC MEASURES
• Your own observations.
• Doctor's examination.
• Culture of wound fluids, x-rays (if wound is near a bone or joint), exploratory surgery sometimes to determine extent of injuries.

APPROPRIATE HEALTH CARE
• Self-care.
• Doctor's treatment.
• Wound cleaning.
• Surgical closure if needed.
• Wound will usually be left open to heal to lessen risk of infection.
• Splint hand if it is injured.
• Human bite wounds on the hands should not be primarily closed due to the high risk of infection.

POSSIBLE COMPLICATIONS—Complications from bites can included infection, extensive soft tissue injuries with scarring, hemorrhage, rabies, and sometimes death.

PROBABLE OUTCOME—Wounds should steadily improve and close over by 7-10 days.

HOW TO TREAT

GENERAL MEASURES
• Elevation of the injured extremity to prevent swelling.
• Contact the local health department and consult about the prevalence of rabies in the species of animal involved.
• If possible the animal that caused the bite should be held and checked for rabies.

MEDICATION—Your doctor may prescribe:
• Preventive antibiotic treatment.
• Antitetanus injection.
• Antirabies vaccine or serum (sometimes).

ACTIVITY—No restrictions, except those caused by the injury.

DIET—No special diet.

CALL YOUR DOCTOR IF

• You or your child suffers from an animal bite.
• The bite does not begin to heal within 2-3 days.
• New or unexplained symptoms develop. Drugs used in treatment may produce side effects.

ANKYLOSING SPONDYLITIS
(Marie-Strümpell Disease)

GENERAL INFORMATION

DEFINITION—A chronic, progressive, rheumatic disease of the joints, accompanied by inflammation and stiffening. It is characterized by a "bent forward" posture caused by stiffening of the spine and support structures.

BODY PARTS INVOLVED—Sacroiliac region; hip joints; lumbar, thoracic and cervical spines.

SEX OR AGE MOST AFFECTED—Within families, males and females are affected equally. In the general population, males are affected 4-5 times more frequently than females, and onset is usually late teens or early twenties.

SIGNS & SYMPTOMS
Early stages:
- Recurrent episodes of low backache. Pain can also occur along the sciatic nerve.
- Stiffness that is worse in the morning.

Later stages:
- Progressive worsening of symptoms. Pain often spreads from the low back to the middle back or higher in the neck. Joints in the arms, legs, feet and hands are sometimes affected.
- Anemia; muscle stiffness; fatigue; weight loss; iritis (in about 25% of patients).

CAUSES—Unknown, but it may be caused by genetic changes or autoimmune disorder.

RISK INCREASES WITH—Family history of ankylosing spondylitis. Occurs more frequently in North American Indians and in white populations of North America and Western Europe.

HOW TO PREVENT—No specific preventive measures.

WHAT TO EXPECT

DIAGNOSTIC MEASURES
- Your own observation of symptoms.
- Medical history and physical exam by a doctor.
- Laboratory blood studies.
- X-rays of the spine.

APPROPRIATE HEALTH CARE
- Self-care after diagnosis.
- Doctor's treatment.
- Surgery to replace a damaged hip or to insert bone grafts in the spine (advanced stages only).

POSSIBLE COMPLICATIONS
- Congestive heart failure.
- Eye inflammation, rarely causing blindness.
- Amyloidosis.
- Heart-valve disease.
- Gastrointestinal disease.
- Lung disease.

- Nerve compression causing numbness in arms or legs.
- Permanent disability and immobilization.

PROBABLE OUTCOME—This disease is currently considered incurable. Symptoms progress unpredictably with mild or moderate flares and periods of total remission. With treatment, symptoms can be relieved or controlled and most patients can lead normal, productive lives. Occasionally, the disease is severe and incapacitating due to deformities.

HOW TO TREAT

GENERAL MEASURES
- Therapy includes exercises for breathing techniques, maintaining proper posture and building up muscle groups (to oppose the direction of possible deformities). Patient compliance with therapy is important.
- Psychological counseling may be recommended.
- Sleep on your back on a firm mattress. Use a small pillow or none at all.
- Take hot baths or use heat compresses before exercising or to relieve pain. Have regular massages, if possible.
- Additional information available from the Arthritis Foundation (800)283-7800.

MEDICATION—Your doctor may prescribe:
- Nonsteroidal anti-inflammatory drugs. Don't take narcotics for pain; they are addictive.
- Stronger pain medications and muscle relaxants for short periods of time.
- Sulfasalazine, vitamin D and immunosuppressive therapy.

ACTIVITY—Stay as active as your strength allows:
- Exercise to maintain good posture and retain as much upright carriage as possible. Back braces don't help.
- Swim regularly, if possible. Your buoyancy in water will allow you to move stiff, painful areas more easily.
- Avoid activity that puts stress on the back and avoid contact sports (too much risk of spinal injury).

DIET—No special diet.

CALL YOUR DOCTOR IF

- You or your child have symptoms of ankylosing spondylitis.
- The following occurs during treatment:
  A fever occurs. Increasing pain and disability, despite measures outlined above.

ANORECTAL ABSCESS

 GENERAL INFORMATION

DEFINITION—An abscess (collection of pus due to infection) that develops in the area around the anus and rectum. Abscesses occur more frequently in men and in people with digestive diseases. They may occur on the edge of the anal opening or deeper in the rectum.

BODY PARTS INVOLVED—Anus; rectum.

SEX OR AGE MOST AFFECTED—Both sexes; all ages.

SIGNS & SYMPTOMS
- Swelling in superficial abscesses.
- Rectal redness.
- Throbbing pain.
- Fever and other toxic symptoms with deep abscesses.
- Pain when having bowel movement.

CAUSES—Common bacteria such as staphylococci and Escherichia coli are the most common cause. Fungal infections sometimes cause abscesses.

RISK INCREASES WITH
- Digestive disease.
- Injections for internal hemorrhoids.
- Enema tip abrasions.
- Puncture wounds from eggshells or fishbones.
- Foreign objects.
- Prolapsed hemorrhoid.

HOW TO PREVENT
- Avoid constipation.
- Don't use enemas.

 WHAT TO EXPECT

DIAGNOSTIC MEASURES
- Your own observation of symptoms.
- Medical history and physical exam by a doctor.

APPROPRIATE HEALTH CARE
- Treatment involves surgery to open and drain the abscess.
- Self-care after surgery.

POSSIBLE COMPLICATIONS
- Anal fistula.
- Recurrence of abscess if underlying cause not corrected.

PROBABLE OUTCOME—Slow healing depending on extent of disease. Complete healing by 6 months if no complications.

 HOW TO TREAT

GENERAL MEASURES
- Sitz bath every 2-4 hours after surgery. Sit in a bathtub with 6-8 inches of warm water for 20 minutes.
- Heating pad, heat lamp or warm compress as needed for pain.
- Prevent constipation. Don't suppress the urge to have a bowel movement, even though you may anticipate pain. Constipation can increase pressure at the wound site.
- Follow doctor's instructions for dressing changes and keeping surgical area clean.

MEDICATION
- Antibiotics or antifungal medications may be prescribed for infection.
- Stool softening laxatives to help prevent constipation.

ACTIVITY—Return to normal activities as soon as possible after surgery.

DIET—An increase in fiber in the diet may help reduce the risk of constipation.

 CALL YOUR DOCTOR IF

- You or a family member has symptoms of anorectal abscess.
- New or unexplained symptoms develop. Drugs used in treatment may produce side effects.

ANOREXIA NERVOSA

GENERAL INFORMATION

DEFINITION—A psychological eating disorder in which a person refuses to eat adequately—in spite of hunger—and loses enough weight to become emaciated. The illness usually begins with a normal weight-loss diet. The person eats very little and refuses to stop dieting after a reasonable weight loss. The body perception is distorted; person sees self as "fat" when weight is normal or much less.

BODY PARTS INVOLVED—All body cells.

SEX OR AGE MOST AFFECTED—Female adolescents and young adults.

SIGNS & SYMPTOMS
- Weight loss of at least 15% of body weight without physical illness.
- High energy level despite body wasting.
- Intense fear of obesity.
- Depression.
- Appetite loss.
- Constipation.
- Cold intolerance.
- Refusal to maintain a minimum standard weight for age and height.
- Distorted body image. The person continues to feel fat—even when emaciated.
- Cessation of menstrual periods.

CAUSES—Unknown. Possible causes include family and internal conflicts (sexual conflicts); phobia about putting on weight; changes in fashion in USA (slimness is identified with beauty); a symptom of depression or personality disorder.

RISK INCREASES WITH
- Peer or social pressure to be thin.
- History of slight overweight.
- Perfectionistic, compulsive or overachieving personalities.
- Psychological stress.
- Athletes, ballet dancers, cheerleaders.

HOW TO PREVENT—Confront personal problems realistically. Try to correct or cope with problems with the help of counselors, therapists, family and friends. Develop a realistic attitude about weight.

WHAT TO EXPECT

DIAGNOSTIC MEASURES
- Your own observation of symptoms.
- Medical history and physical exam by a doctor.
- Laboratory blood tests for anemia and electrolyte imbalance.

APPROPRIATE HEALTH CARE
- Doctor's treatment.
- Psychotherapy or counseling for the patient and family.
- Treatment can usually be done on an outpatient basis.
- Hospitalization during crises for intravenous or tube feeding.
- Psychiatric hospitalization for at least 2 to 3 weeks (sometimes).

POSSIBLE COMPLICATIONS
- Chronic anorexia nervosa caused by patient's resistance to treatment.
- Electrolyte disturbances or irregular heartbeat. These may be life-threatening.
- Osteoporosis.
- Suicide.

PROBABLE OUTCOME—Treatable if the patient recognizes the emotional disturbance, wants help and cooperates in treatment. Without treatment, this can cause permanent disability or even death. Persons with anorexia nervosa have a high rate of attempted suicide due to low self-esteem. Therapy may continue over several years. Relapses are common, especially when stressful situations occur.

HOW TO TREAT

GENERAL MEASURES
- The goal of treatment is for the patient to establish healthy eating patterns to regain normal weight. The patient can accomplish this with behavior-modification training supervised by a qualified professional.
- See Resources for Additional Information.

MEDICATION—A variety of psychotherapy medications have some benefit but there is no one medication that is consistently useful.

ACTIVITY—No restrictions, but avoid overexertion.

DIET—A controlled refeeding program will be established. Vitamin and mineral supplements may be prescribed.

CALL YOUR DOCTOR IF

- Life-threatening symptoms occur, including: rapid, irregular heartbeat; chest pain; or loss of consciousness. Call immediately. This is an emergency!
- You have symptoms of anorexia nervosa or observe them in a family member.
- Weight loss continues, despite treatment.

ANXIETY

GENERAL INFORMATION

DEFINITION—A vague, uncomfortable feeling of fear, dread or danger from an unknown source. For some it may be a one time episode; other persons become constantly anxious about everything. A certain amount of anxiety is normal and helps improve our performance and allows people to avoid dangerous situations.

Several types of anxiety are recognized including acute situational anxiety (which is usually short-term), generalized anxiety disorder and adjustment disorder. (See also Panic Disorder, Post Traumatic Stress Disorder, Phobias, and Obsessive-Compulsive Disorder in Illness section). Generalized anxiety is defined as unrealistic or excessive anxiety for 6 months or longer. Anxiety is the most common mental health problem in the U.S.

BODY PARTS INVOLVED—Central nervous system; endocrine system.

SEX OR AGE MOST AFFECTED—Females more than males, and mainly in adults ages 20-45.

SIGNS & SYMPTOMS
- Feeling that something undesirable or harmful is about to happen (edginess and apprehension).
- Dry mouth; swallowing difficulty; hoarseness.
- Rapid breathing and heartbeat, palpitations.
- Twitching or trembling.
- Muscle tension; headaches; backache.
- Sweating.
- Difficulty in concentrating.
- Dizziness or faintness.
- Nausea; diarrhea; weight loss.
- Sleeplessness.
- Irritability.
- Fatigue.
- Nightmares.
- Memory problems.
- Sexual impotence.

CAUSES—Activation of the body's defense mechanisms for fight or flight. Excess adrenalin is discharged from the adrenal glands, and adrenalin breakdown products (catecholamines) eventually affect various parts of the body. Attempts to avoid the anxiety leads to more anxiety.

RISK INCREASES WITH
- Stress from any source (such as social or financial problems).
- Family history of anxiety.
- Fatigue or overwork.
- Recurrence of situations that have been previously stressful or harmful.
- Medical illness.
- Unrealistic perfectionism.
- Withdrawal from drugs or alcohol.

HOW TO PREVENT
- Practice relaxation techniques or meditation.
- Consider lifestyle changes to reduce stress.
See How to Cope with Stress in Appendix.

WHAT TO EXPECT

DIAGNOSTIC MEASURES
- Your own observation of symptoms.
- Medical history and physical exam by a doctor.
- Laboratory studies to rule out medical conditions that produce anxiety, such as hyperthyroidism, anemia, hypoglycemia, diabetes.

APPROPRIATE HEALTH CARE
- Self-care.
- Doctor's treatment.
- Psychotherapy or counseling.

POSSIBLE COMPLICATIONS
- Impaired social and occupational functioning.
- A sudden increase in anxiety may lead to panic and violent escape behavior.
- Dependence on drugs.
- Heart arrhythmias.

PROBABLE OUTCOME—Generalized anxiety can be controlled with treatment. Overcoming anxiety often results in a richer, more satisfying life.

HOW TO TREAT

GENERAL MEASURES
- Obtain therapy to understand the specific but unconscious threat or source of stress.
- Learn techniques, including biofeedback and relaxation therapy, to reduce muscle tension.
- Follow a regular energetic fitness routine using aerobic exercise if possible.
- See Resources for Additional Information.

MEDICATION—Your doctor may prescribe:
- Antianxiety drugs for a short-term basis.
- Antidepressants for panic-disorders.

ACTIVITY—Stay active. Physical exertion helps reduce anxiety.

DIET—No special diet. Avoid caffeine and other stimulants and alcohol.

CALL YOUR DOCTOR IF

- You have symptoms of anxiety and self-treatment has failed.
- You have a sudden feeling of panic.
- New, unexplained symptoms develop. Drugs used in treatment may produce side effects.

APPENDICITIS

GENERAL INFORMATION

DEFINITION—Inflammation of the vermiform appendix, a small intestinal pouch that extends from the cecum, the first part of the large intestine. The appendix has no known function, but it can become diseased. Appendicitis affects 1 in 500 people each year. Symptoms vary widely. Appendicitis should be considered in any person with undiagnosed abdominal pain.

BODY PARTS INVOLVED—Appendix; cecum; peritoneum (membrane covering the intestinal tract).

SEX OR AGE MOST AFFECTED—All ages, but rare in children under 2. The incidence peaks between ages 15 and 24.

SIGNS & SYMPTOMS
- Pain that begins close to the navel and migrates toward the right lower abdomen. Pain becomes persistent and well-localized. It worsens with moving, breathing deeply, coughing, sneezing, walking or being touched.
- Nausea and sometimes vomiting.
- Constipation and inability to pass gas.
- Diarrhea (occasionally).
- Low fever, beginning after other symptoms.
- Tenderness in the right lower abdomen, usually about a third of the distance from the navel to the top of the hip bone. (This description applies only if the appendix is in its normal position. In some cases, the tip of the appendix is located elsewhere, making diagnosis difficult.)
- Abdominal swelling (late stages).
- Increased white-blood-cell count.

CAUSES—Infection for unknown reason, usually with bacteria from the intestinal tract. The appendix may become obstructed from contents moving through intestinal tract, or by a constricting band of tissue. When infected, it becomes swollen, inflamed and filled with pus.

RISK INCREASES WITH
- Recent illness, especially a roundworm infestation or gastrointestinal virus infection or intra-abdominal tumors.
- Family tendency.

HOW TO PREVENT—No specific preventive measures.

WHAT TO EXPECT

DIAGNOSTIC MEASURES
- Your own observation of symptoms.
- Medical history and physical exam by a doctor.
- Laboratory blood studies. Tests usually show higher levels of white blood cells.
- Urinalysis to rule out a urinary-tract infection, which can mimic appendicitis.

APPROPRIATE HEALTH CARE
- Doctor's treatment.
- Surgery to remove the appendix. Because appendicitis can be hard to diagnose, surgery is often withheld until symptoms and signs progress enough to confirm the diagnosis.

POSSIBLE COMPLICATIONS
- Rupture of the appendix, abscess formation and peritonitis. This is more common in older persons.
- Misdiagnosis because of few or atypical symptoms—especially in the very young or very old.
- Formation of an abscess.

PROBABLE OUTCOME—Usually curable with surgery. If totally untreated, a ruptured appendix can be fatal.

HOW TO TREAT

GENERAL MEASURES
- While diagnosis is uncertain, take a rectal temperature every 2 hours. Keep a record for your doctor.
- For an explanation of surgery and postoperative care, see Appendectomy in Surgery section.

MEDICATION
- Don't take any laxatives, enemas or medicines for pain. Laxatives may cause rupture, and pain or fever reducers make diagnosis more difficult.
- Your doctor may prescribe antibiotics to reduce chance of infection, pain medicine following surgery and stool softeners to prevent constipation.
- Stool softeners to prevent constipation may be recommended.

ACTIVITY—Rest in a bed or chair until surgery.

DIET
- Don't eat or drink anything until appendicitis has been diagnosed. Anesthesia for surgery is much safer if the stomach is empty. If you are very thirsty, wash your mouth out with water.
- A liquid diet, progressing to soft diet following surgery.

CALL YOUR DOCTOR IF

- You have symptoms of appendicitis.
- The following occurs while surgery is pending:
Fever spikes of 102F (38.9C) or over.
Continued vomiting.
Increased pain in the abdomen.
Fainting.
Blood in the stool or vomit.
Dizziness or headache.

ARTHRITIS, INFECTIOUS
(Septic Arthritis)

 GENERAL INFORMATION

DEFINITION—Inflammation in a joint resulting from infection. This is one of the few forms of arthritis that is curable.

BODY PARTS INVOLVED—Any joint, but most common in larger ones, such as the hip, or those subject to trauma, such as the knee or joints in the hands.

SEX OR AGE MOST AFFECTED—Both sexes; all ages.

SIGNS & SYMPTOMS
• Chills and fever (sometimes high).
• Redness, swelling, tenderness and pain (often throbbing) in the affected joint. Pain sometimes spreads to other joints. It worsens with movement.
• Pain in the buttocks, thighs or groin (sometimes).

CAUSES—Entry into a joint by bacteria (streptococci, staphylococci, gonococci, hemophilus or tubercle bacillus) or fungi. Organisms gain entry from:
• Infection elsewhere in the body, as with gonorrhea or tuberculosis.
• Infection next to the joint, as with skin boils, cellulitis or bone infection.
• Injury to the joint, including puncture wounds and skin abrasions.

RISK INCREASES WITH
• Adults over 60.
• Illness that has lowered resistance.
• Sexually transmitted infections.
• Diabetes mellitus, rheumatoid arthritis or liver disease.
• Use of immunosuppressive drugs.
• Joint surgery or injections into joints.
• Excess alcohol consumption.
• Many sexual partners.
• Use of alcohol or mind-altering drugs, especially those that are injected.
• Poor hygiene.
• Prosthetic joint.
• The use of aspirin and other nonsteroidal anti-inflammatory drugs for other disorders may suppress signs of joint inflammation, delaying diagnosis.

HOW TO PREVENT
• Protect exposed joints, such as the knee, during activities involving injury risks.
• Obtain prompt medical treatment for infections elsewhere in the body.
• Protect yourself from sexually transmitted diseases.

 WHAT TO EXPECT

DIAGNOSTIC MEASURES
• Your own observation of symptoms.
• Medical history and exam by a doctor.
• Laboratory studies, such as blood counts, blood culture and culture of fluid from the infected joint.
• X-rays of affected joints.

APPROPRIATE HEALTH CARE
• Doctor's treatment.
• Hospitalization (frequently) for complete rest and intravenous antibiotics.
• Surgery to drain fluid or remove foreign material introduced by an injury.
• Physical therapy after recovery.

POSSIBLE COMPLICATIONS
• Misdiagnosis as gout or another noninfectious condition, delaying antibiotic treatment.
• Blood poisoning.
• Permanent joint damage.

PROBABLE OUTCOME—Usually curable with early diagnosis and treatment. Recovery takes weeks or months. Treatment delay may result in a badly damaged joint and loss of movement, requiring joint replacement.

 HOW TO TREAT

GENERAL MEASURES
• No specific instructions.
• See Resources for Additional Information.

MEDICATION—Your doctor may prescribe:
• Antibiotics (often intravenous). Don't discontinue antibiotics until your doctor recommends it. Infection may return after symptoms disappear.
• Narcotic pain medicine for a short time to relieve pain.

ACTIVITY—Splints or casts may be necessary to rest the affected joint. Movement delays healing. After cure, physical therapy is often necessary to restore joint function. Resume activities gradually as symptoms improve.

DIET—No special diet.

☎ **CALL YOUR DOCTOR IF**

• You have symptoms of joint infection. Call immediately.
• The following occurs during the illness:
  Temperature spikes to 103F (39.4C).
  Fatigue, headache, muscle aches and sweating.
• New, unexplained symptoms develop.

ARTHRITIS, JUVENILE RHEUMATOID

GENERAL INFORMATION

DEFINITION—An inflammatory disease of connective tissue—mostly joints—that affects children. May be confused with the arthritis of Lyme Disease.

BODY PARTS INVOLVED—Joints, usually knees, elbows, ankles and neck. It may also involve adjacent muscles, cartilage and membranes lining the joints.

SEX OR AGE MOST AFFECTED—Starts at 2 to 5 years and usually disappears by young adulthood. It is 4 times more frequent in girls.

SIGNS & SYMPTOMS
- Pain, swelling and stiffness in the toes, knees, ankles, elbows, shoulders or neck joints. The pain may begin suddenly or gradually, and may involve only one or many joints. The child may refuse to walk without being able to explain why.
- Daily temperature rise to about 103F (39.4C)—usually in the evening. Fever is frequently accompanied by a body rash and chills.
- Poor appetite; weight loss.
- Anemia.
- Irritability; listlessness.
- Swollen lymph glands.
- Eye pain and redness.
- Chest pain (if the disease is severe enough to affect the heart).

CAUSES—Probably caused by an autoimmune disorder, in which the body's immune system attacks its own normal tissues. The first symptoms are often associated with physical or emotional stress.

RISK INCREASES WITH—There may be an inherited tendency.

HOW TO PREVENT—Cannot be prevented at present.

WHAT TO EXPECT

DIAGNOSTIC MEASURES
- Your own observation of symptoms.
- Medical history and physical exam by a doctor.
- Laboratory blood studies, including autoimmune assays.
- X-rays of the involved joints. Changes may not appear on x-rays until the late stages.

APPROPRIATE HEALTH CARE
- Home care after diagnosis.
- Doctor's treatment.
- Psychotherapy or counseling to help the family cope with the child's long-term illness. Emotional support may be the most important factor in a child's treatment.
- Surgery to correct deformed joints (sometimes).

POSSIBLE COMPLICATIONS
- Involvement of tissues other than joints, producing uveitis (eye inflammation), an enlarged spleen, pericarditis or inflammation of the heart muscle.
- Permanent joint deformity.

PROBABLE OUTCOME
- Juvenile rheumatoid arthritis is currently considered incurable. However, in 75% to 80% of cases, the disease is in complete remission by puberty or young adulthood.
- Attacks usually last a few weeks and occur off and on throughout childhood. Symptoms can usually be controlled with treatment.
- See Resources for Additional Information.

HOW TO TREAT

GENERAL MEASURES
- Both child and parents need to be involved in therapy.
- Ongoing care will include medications, physical therapy and attention to nutrition.
- Request eye examinations at least twice a year to detect uveitis.
- Encourage the child to be as independent as possible.
- See Resources for Additional Information.

MEDICATION—Your doctor may prescribe aspirin or other nonsteroidal anti-inflammatory drugs to reduce pain and inflammation.

ACTIVITY—During an attack, keep the child in bed, except to use the bathroom, until all symptoms subside. Splints may be necessary to support and protect an inflamed joint.

After an attack passes, the child may gradually resume normal activities with rest periods during the day. The child should not become overtired and should sleep at least 10 to 12 hours each night.

Your doctor may recommend exercises when the child is well enough to do them.

DIET—Regular diet with attention to adequate nutrition.

CALL YOUR DOCTOR IF

- Your child has symptoms of juvenile rheumatoid arthritis.
- The following symptoms occur during treatment:
  Chest pain.
  Fever.
  Appetite loss.
- New, unexplained symptoms develop. Drugs used in treatment may produce side effects.

ARTHRITIS, RHEUMATOID

GENERAL INFORMATION

DEFINITION—A long-term illness characterized by joint disease that involves muscles, membrane linings of the joints and cartilage.

BODY PARTS INVOLVED—Joints, including cartilage, synovial membranes, muscles and ligaments; blood vessels; eyes.

SEX OR AGE MOST AFFECTED—3 times more common in women than men. It begins between ages 20 and 60, with a peak incidence between ages 35 and 45.

SIGNS & SYMPTOMS
• Redness, pain, warmth and tenderness in any or all active joints in the hands, wrists, elbows, shoulders, feet and ankles.
• Morning stiffness.
• Low-grade fever.
• Nodules under the skin (sometimes).
• Flareups may be triggered by emotional stress.

CAUSES—Unknown, but probably an autoimmune disease.

RISK INCREASES WITH
• Family history of rheumatoid arthritis or other autoimmune disorders.
• Genetic factors, such as autoimmune-system defects.
• Female age 20-50.
• Native American ethnicity (prevalence is higher in this group).

HOW TO PREVENT—No specific preventive measures.

WHAT TO EXPECT

DIAGNOSTIC MEASURES
• Your own observation of symptoms.
• Medical history and physical exam by a doctor, x-rays of joints.
• Laboratory blood studies to detect a rheumatoid factor.

APPROPRIATE HEALTH CARE
• Self-care after diagnosis, doctor's treatment, physical therapy.
• Surgery such as synovectomy, joint reconstruction or total joint arthroplasty may be necessary in advanced disease. (See Arthroplasty, Knee; Arthroplasty, Hip; Arthroplasty, Shoulder in Surgery section.)

POSSIBLE COMPLICATIONS
• Impaired vision.
• Permanent deformity and crippling.
• Drugs used in treatment can induce complications, such as gastric problems, and those associated with long-term steroid use.
• Moderate anemia.

PROBABLE OUTCOME—The disease may be mild or severe. It is incurable, but pain relief, prevention of disability and an active, normal lifespan are usually possible with early diagnosis. Conservative treatment relieves symptoms in 1 year in 75% of patients. About 5% to 10% are eventually disabled, despite treatment.

HOW TO TREAT

GENERAL MEASURES
• Major changes in life-style will be necessary. Try to perform as many activities of daily living as possible. Physical therapy and occupational therapy will be provided.
• Splints at night may be helpful to support and protect a joint. Ask your doctor.
• Gloves at night to retain heat.
• Relieve pain with heat, including hot soaks, heat lamps, heating pads or whirlpool treatments.
• See Resources for Additional Information.

MEDICATION—Your doctor may prescribe: nonsteroidal anti-inflammatory drugs, including aspirin and other salicylates; gold compounds; immunosuppressive drugs.
  Cortisone drugs usually relieve pain dramatically for short periods, but they are less effective for long-term use. They don't prevent progressive joint destruction, and they sometimes have hazardous side effects.
  Cortisone injections into joints can temporarily relieve pain.

ACTIVITY
• Stay in bed, except to use the bathroom, until fever and other signs of an active flare-up disappear.
• Remain active, but include daily rest periods. Sleep for 10 to 12 hours each night. Don't become overtired.
• Stand, walk and sit erectly.
• When able, exercise actively to preserve strength and joint mobility. Build up slowly to the amount suggested by your doctor and physical therapist.
• Exercise disabled joints passively to help prevent contractures.

DIET—Eat a normal, well-balanced diet. Avoid arthritis diet fads. Lose weight if you are obese (see Weight Loss Diet in Appendix). Obesity stresses the joints.

CALL YOUR DOCTOR IF

• You have symptoms of rheumatoid arthritis.
• The following occurs during treatment:
  Fever.
  Symptoms appear in unaffected joints.
• New, unexplained symptoms develop. Drugs in treatment may produce side effects.

ASBESTOSIS

GENERAL INFORMATION

DEFINITION—Inflammation of the lung due to breathing asbestos particles. It is a chronic disorder, but is not contagious. It may lead to cancer of the lung (likelihood greatly increased in cigarette smokers).

BODY PARTS INVOLVED—Lungs.

SEX OR AGE MOST AFFECTED—Men over age 40 who have been exposed to asbestos.

SIGNS & SYMPTOMS
Early symptoms:
Shortness of breath; cough that produces little or no sputum; general ill feeling.
Late symptoms:
Fitful sleep; appetite loss; chest pain; hoarseness; coughing blood; symptoms of congestive heart failure; bluish nails.

CAUSES—Many years of exposure to small particles of asbestos at work or other sources. The outer part of the lung becomes irritated by the asbestos fibers, leading to inflammation and to a thickening and scarring of the lung tissue (pulmonary fibrosis). Up to 20 years or more may elapse between exposure to asbestos and the symptoms of the disease.

RISK INCREASES WITH
• Occupations involving asbestos-related industry.
• Smoking.
• Excess alcohol consumption.

HOW TO PREVENT
• During exposure to asbestos, wear a protective mask or external-air-supplied hood.
• Follow recommended industrial procedures to suppress asbestos dust.
• Don't smoke.
• Participate in a regular physical exercise program to maintain good cardiopulmonary fitness.
• For workers in asbestos industries, regular scheduled x-rays to detect any shadow on the lungs. If so, the person should stop working with asbestos, even if there are no symptoms.

WHAT TO EXPECT

DIAGNOSTIC MEASURES
• Your own observation of symptoms.
• Medical history and physical exam by a doctor.
• X-ray of the chest.

APPROPRIATE HEALTH CARE
• Self-care after diagnosis.
• Doctor's treatment.

POSSIBLE COMPLICATIONS
• Tuberculosis (late stages of silicosis).
• Heart failure due to lung disease.
• Lung collapse.
• Pleurisy.
• Lung cancer.

PROBABLE OUTCOME—This condition is currently considered incurable. However, symptoms can be relieved or controlled. Scientific research into causes and treatment continues, so there is hope for increasingly effective treatment and cure.

HOW TO TREAT

GENERAL MEASURES—The following measures may relieve symptoms and protect against recurrent lung infections:
• Obtain medical treatment for any respiratory infection, including the common cold.
• Practice bronchial drainage. Your doctor will provide instructions.
• Chest physical therapy techniques will be provided by respiratory therapist.
• Use an ultrasonic, cool-mist humidifier to loosen bronchial secretions so they can be coughed up easily. Clean humidifier daily.
• Keep influenza and pneumococcal immunizations up to date.
• Avoid crowds and persons with infections.

MEDICATION
• Your doctor may prescribe:
Antibiotics for infections.
Bronchodilators (inhaled or oral) with inhalation therapy (supervised at first by an inhalation therapist) to open bronchial tubes to the maximum.
• For minor discomfort, you may use nonprescription drugs, such as acetaminophen or aspirin.
• Supplemental oxygen may be necessary.

ACTIVITY
• Rest in bed with infections.
• After treatment, resume normal activity as soon as symptoms improve.
• Regular exercise in whatever form tolerated is important to preserve lung capacity.

DIET—No special diet.

CALL YOUR DOCTOR IF

• You have symptoms of asbestosis.
• The following occurs during treatment:
Temperature spike of 101F (38.3C) or more.
Increased chest pain or breathlessness.
Blood in the sputum.
Continuing weight loss.
• New, unexplained symptoms develop. Drugs used in treatment may produce side effects.

ASTHMA

GENERAL INFORMATION

DEFINITION—A chronic disorder with recurrent attacks of wheezing and shortness of breath.

BODY PARTS INVOLVED—Lungs; bronchi; bronchioles.

SEX OR AGE MOST AFFECTED—It affects all ages but 50% of the cases are in children under age 10 (boys with asthma outnumber girls). In adult onset asthma, women are more often affected than men.

SIGNS & SYMPTOMS
- Chest tightness and shortness of breath.
- Wheezing upon breathing out.
- Coughing, especially at night, with little sputum.
- Rapid, shallow breathing that is easier with sitting up.
- Breathing difficulty—neck muscles tighten.

Severe symptoms of acute attack:
- Bluish skin.
- Exhaustion.
- Grunting respiration.
- Inability to speak.
- Mental changes, including restlessness or confusion.

CAUSES—Overactivity and spasm of air passages (bronchi and bronchioles), followed by swelling of the passages and thickening of lung secretions (sputum). This decreases or closes off air to the lungs. These changes are caused by:
- Allergens, such as pollen, dust, animal dander, molds and some foods.
- Lung infections such as bronchitis.
- Air irritants, such as smoke and odors.
- Exposure to occupational chemicals or other materials.
- Stresses (viral infection, exercise, emotional upset, noxious odors, tobacco smoke).

RISK INCREASES WITH
- Other allergic conditions, such as eczema or hay fever.
- Family history of asthma or allergies.
- Exposure to air pollutants; smoking.
- Use of some drugs such as aspirin.

HOW TO PREVENT
- Avoid known allergens and air pollutants.
- Take prescribed preventive medicines regularly—don't omit them when you feel well.
- Investigate and avoid triggering factors.

WHAT TO EXPECT

DIAGNOSTIC MEASURES
- Your own observation of symptoms.
- Medical history and physical exam by a doctor, chest x-rays.
- Laboratory blood studies and pulmonary-function test.
- Allergy testing, usually with skin tests.

APPROPRIATE HEALTH CARE
- Self-care after diagnosis.
- Doctor's treatment.
- Emergency-room care and hospitalization for severe attacks.
- Psychotherapy or counseling for the whole family to help cope with a chronic condition.

POSSIBLE COMPLICATIONS
- Respiratory failure.
- Pneumothorax.
- Lung infection and chronic lung problems from recurrent attacks.

PROBABLE OUTCOME—Symptoms can be controlled with treatment and strict adherence to prevention measures. Half of the affected children will outgrow asthma.

HOW TO TREAT

GENERAL MEASURES
- Eliminate allergens and irritants at home and at work, if possible. Get treatment for desensitizing to specific allergens.
- Keep regular medications with you at all times.
- Sit upright during attacks.
- Stay indoors as much as possible during high allergen times.
- See Resources for Additional Information.

MEDICATION—Your doctor may prescribe:
- Expectorants to loosen sputum.
- Bronchodilators to open air passages.
- Intravenous cortisone drugs (emergencies only) to decrease the body's allergic response.
- Cortisone drugs by nebulizer, which have fewer adverse reactions than oral forms.
- Antihistamines by nebulizer. These are preventive drugs.
- Anti-inflammatory drugs directed specifically at the lungs.

ACTIVITY—Stay active, but avoid sudden bursts of exercise. If an attack follows heavy exercise, sit and rest. Sip warm water. Treatment with bronchodilators often prevents exercise-caused asthma.

DIET—No special diet, but avoid foods to which you are sensitive. Drink plenty of fluids daily to keep secretions loose.

CALL YOUR DOCTOR IF

- You have symptoms of asthma.
- You have an asthma attack that doesn't respond to treatment. This is an emergency!
- New, unexplained symptoms develop. Drugs used in treatment may produce side effects.

ATELECTASIS

GENERAL INFORMATION

DEFINITION—Collapse of part or all of one lung, preventing normal oxygen absorption.

BODY PARTS INVOLVED—Lungs.

SEX OR AGE MOST AFFECTED—Both sexes; all ages.

SIGNS & SYMPTOMS
Sudden, major collapse:
- Chest pain.
- Shortness of breath; rapid breathing.
- Shock (severe weakness, paleness of skin, rapid heartbeat).
- Dizziness.

Gradual collapse:
- Cough.
- Fever.
- Shortness of breath.
- No other symptoms.

CAUSES—Obstruction of small or large lung air passages by:
- Thick mucus plugs from infection or other disease, including cystic fibrosis.
- Tumors in the air passages.
- Tumors or blood vessels outside the air passages, causing pressure on airways.
- Inhaled objects, such as small toys or peanuts.
- Prolonged chest or abdominal surgery with general anesthetic.
- Chest injury or fractured ribs.
- Penetrating wound.
- Enlarged lymph glands.

RISK INCREASES WITH
- Smoking.
- Illness that has lowered resistance or weakened the patient.
- Chronic obstructive lung disease, including emphysema and bronchiectasis.
- Use of drugs that depress alertness or consciousness, such as sedatives, barbiturates, tranquilizers or alcohol.

HOW TO PREVENT
- Force coughing and deep breathing every 1 to 2 hours after surgery with general anesthesia. Also change position often in bed, if possible.
- Increase fluid intake during lung illness or after surgery—by mouth or intravenously—to keep lung secretions loose.
- Keep small objects that might be inhaled away from young children (peanuts are notorious).

WHAT TO EXPECT

DIAGNOSTIC MEASURES
- Your own observation of symptoms.
- Medical history and physical exam by a doctor.

- Laboratory studies to measure oxygen and carbon dioxide in the blood.
- X-rays of the chest.

APPROPRIATE HEALTH CARE
- Doctor's treatment.
- Surgery to remove tumors.
- Bronchoscopy (see Glossary) to remove foreign objects or a mucus plug.

POSSIBLE COMPLICATIONS
- Pneumonia.
- Small lung abscess.
- Permanent lung scars and collapsed lung tissue.

PROBABLE OUTCOME
- Atelectasis is seldom life-threatening and usually resolves spontaneously.
- If atelectasis is caused by a mucus plug or inhaled foreign object, it is curable when the plug or object is removed. If it is caused by a tumor, the outcome depends on the nature of the tumor.

HOW TO TREAT

GENERAL MEASURES
- Cooperate with requests to turn, cough and breathe deeply after surgery. Hold a pillow tightly against surgical incisions during the coughing exercises.
- Stop smoking.
- Learn to perform postural drainage (see Glossary) after hospitalization. An inhalation therapist, nurse or doctor can demonstrate the technique.
- See Resources for Additional Information.

MEDICATION
- Your doctor may prescribe:
  Antibiotics to fight infection that inevitably accompanies atelectasis.
  Pain relievers for minor pain.
- Don't take sedatives. They may contribute to a recurrence.

ACTIVITY—Resume your normal activities as soon as symptoms improve.

DIET—No special diet, but drink at least 8 glasses of water or other fluid daily to thin lung secretions.

CALL YOUR DOCTOR IF

- You have symptoms of atelectasis.
- The following occurs during treatment:
  Distended abdomen.
  Sudden shortness of breath.
  Blue fingernails and lips.
  Temperature of 102F (38.9C) or higher.

ATHEROSCLEROSIS
(Hardening of the Arteries)

 GENERAL INFORMATION

DEFINITION—An extremely common form of hardening of the arteries in which plaque deposits form in the walls of the blood vessels that carry oxygen and other nutrients from the heart to other body parts. Atherosclerosis may lead to kidney damage, decreased circulation to the brain and extremities, and coronary artery disease. Atherosclerosis is a major cause of strokes and heart attacks.

BODY PARTS INVOLVED—All arterial blood vessels in the body.

SEX OR AGE MOST AFFECTED—Both sexes of adolescents and adults. Up to age 45, atherosclerosis is more common in men. After menopause, women have the same incidence.

SIGNS & SYMPTOMS—Symptoms are often absent until atherosclerosis reaches advanced stages. Symptoms depend on what part of the body has a decreased blood flow and the extent of disease. Common symptoms include:
• Muscle cramps if atherosclerosis involves vessels in the legs.
• Angina pectoris or heart attack if it involves blood vessels to the heart.
• Stroke or transient ischemic attack if it involves vessels to the neck and brain.

CAUSES—Patches of fatty tissue that damage artery walls often collect at artery junctions. At these points, the inner lining of the artery may trap fatty substances that circulate in the blood. As fatty deposits accumulate, they reduce the blood vessel's elasticity and narrow the passageway, interfering with blood flow. This process may begin in early adulthood.

RISK INCREASES WITH
• Adults over 60; stress; diabetes mellitus; high blood pressure; obesity; smoking; sedentary lifestyle.
• Poor nutrition, especially too much fat and cholesterol in the diet.
• Family history of atherosclerosis.
• High cholesterol levels (high levels of the low density lipoprotein and low levels of the high density lipoprotein).

HOW TO PREVENT
• Don't smoke.
• Follow suggestions under Diet. Children and young adults of parents with this condition may benefit from a low-fat diet. Exercise regularly.
• Reduce stress when possible (see How to Cope with Stress in Appendix).
• If you have diabetes or high blood pressure, adhere strictly to your treatment program.

 WHAT TO EXPECT

DIAGNOSTIC MEASURES
• Your own observation of symptoms.
• Medical history and exam by a doctor.
• Laboratory studies, including: ECG (see Glossary); exercise-tolerance test; blood studies of cholesterol and high-density lipoproteins (see Glossary); and blood-sugar tests; x-rays of the chest and blood vessels.

APPROPRIATE HEALTH CARE
• Self-care after diagnosis.
• Doctor's treatment.
• Psychotherapy or counseling to learn to cope with stress.
• Surgery available in some cases.

POSSIBLE COMPLICATIONS—Heart attack; stroke and/or angina pectoris; kidney disease; congestive heart failure; heartbeat irregularities; sudden death.

PROBABLE OUTCOME—This condition is currently considered incurable. However, symptoms can be controlled, and progress of the disease can be slowed with treatment. Complications can be fatal. However, in the arteries that feed the heart, aggressive treatment has been shown to actually reverse blockage.

 HOW TO TREAT

GENERAL MEASURES
• Treatment for atherosclerosis is generally directed at its complications.
• Stop smoking.
• See Resources for Additional Information.

MEDICATION
• Lowering cholesterol levels in persons with high levels can increase life expectancy. If diet and exercise fail to reduce cholesterol, your doctor may prescribe antihyperlipidemic drugs.
• Other drugs may be necessary to treat symptoms of an associated problem (high blood pressure, heartbeat irregularities).
• Some studies have indicated that aspirin and vitamin E may reduce the risk of heart attack. Follow your doctor's recommendations.

ACTIVITY— Routine exercise is recommended.

DIET— Eat a diet that is low in fat, low in salt and high in fiber (see Appendix for special diets).

 CALL YOUR DOCTOR IF

You have high risk factors for atherosclerosis and want to be in a prevention program.

ATHLETE'S FOOT
(Tinea Pedis; Ringworm of the Feet)

 GENERAL INFORMATION

DEFINITION—A common, contagious fungus infection of the skin on the feet.

BODY PARTS INVOLVED—Feet, especially the soles and skin between toes (usually 4th and 5th toes).

SEX OR AGE MOST AFFECTED—Both sexes and all ages, but most common in adolescents and adults.

SIGNS & SYMPTOMS
- Moist, soft, gray-white or red scales on feet, especially between toes.
- Dead skin between toes.
- Itching in inflamed areas.
- Damp, musty foot odor.
- Small blisters on the feet (sometimes).

CAUSES—Infection by a Trichophyton fungus.

RISK INCREASES WITH
- Infrequent washing of the feet.
- Infrequent changes of shoes or socks.
- Use of locker rooms and public showers.
- Hot, humid weather.
- People who are immunosuppressed due to illness or medications.
- Persistent moisture around the feet.

HOW TO PREVENT
- Bathe feet daily. Dry thoroughly and apply drying or dusting powder.
- Go barefoot when possible.
- Change shoes and socks daily.
- Wear socks made of cotton, wool or other natural, absorbent fibers. Avoid synthetics.

 WHAT TO EXPECT

DIAGNOSTIC MEASURES
- Your own observation of symptoms.
- Medical history and physical exam by a doctor.
- Laboratory culture and microscopic examination of scales.

APPROPRIATE HEALTH CARE
- Self-care after diagnosis.
- Doctor's treatment, if infection is severe or persistent.

POSSIBLE COMPLICATIONS
- Secondary bacterial infection in the affected area.
- Id reaction on hands and face (a rare skin rash).

PROBABLE OUTCOME—Usually curable in 3 weeks with treatment, but recurrence is common.

 HOW TO TREAT

GENERAL MEASURES
- After soaking or bathing, carefully remove scales and material between the toes daily.
- Keep affected areas cool and dry. Go barefoot or wear sandals during treatment.

MEDICATION
- Use nonprescription antifungal powders, creams or ointments after each bath.
- For severe cases, your doctor may prescribe oral or more potent topical antifungal medications.

ACTIVITY—No restrictions. Temporarily avoid activities that cause feet to sweat.

DIET—No special diet.

 CALL YOUR DOCTOR IF

- You have severe symptoms of athlete's foot that persist, despite self-treatment.
- You develop fever or the infection seems to be spreading.

ATRIAL FIBRILLATION

GENERAL INFORMATION

DEFINITION—A completely irregular heartbeat rhythm. Fibrillation means a quivering of heart-muscle fibers.

BODY PARTS INVOLVED—Heart muscles; the atrium (also called auricle), a chamber of the heart that connects to the left ventricle (main chamber); heart's electrical conduction system.

SEX OR AGE MOST AFFECTED—Adults of both sexes.

SIGNS & SYMPTOMS
- No symptoms (sometimes).
- Continuously irregular heartbeat, in which no 2 beats are of equal strength or duration.
- Weakness, dizziness or faintness (sometimes).

CAUSES
- Rheumatic heart disease caused by rheumatic fever.
- Atherosclerosis of coronary arteries, with or without a previous heart attack.
- Hyperthyroidism.
- Congestive heart failure.

RISK INCREASES WITH
- Stress.
- Heart valve disease.
- Recent heart surgery.
- Electrolyte disturbances, especially low potassium.
- Pulmonary embolism.
- Hypertension.
- Excessive use of some drugs, such as thyroid hormones, caffeine and others.
- Smoking.
- Excess alcohol consumption.
- Obesity.

HOW TO PREVENT—Avoid risk factors for atherosclerosis and coronary artery disease (both in Illness section).

WHAT TO EXPECT

DIAGNOSTIC MEASURES
- Your own observation of symptoms.
- Medical history and physical exam by a doctor.
- ECG (see Glossary).
- Blood studies to measure levels of drugs used in treatment.

APPROPRIATE HEALTH CARE
- Self-care after diagnosis.
- Doctor's treatment.
- Hospitalization (sometimes).
- Electric shock (electrocardioversion), which may restore normal rhythm.

POSSIBLE COMPLICATIONS
- Acute pulmonary edema.
- Arterial thrombosis or embolus.
- Congestive heart failure.
- Other heartbeat irregularities, triggering cardiac arrest.
- Stroke.

PROBABLE OUTCOME—A normal heartbeat rhythm can be restored with electrocardioversion in about 50% of patients. In the other 50%, some symptoms can be controlled with medication. Those whose rhythm is restored to normal have a longer life expectancy, greater strength and more energy than those who have continuing atrial fibrillation.

HOW TO TREAT

GENERAL MEASURES
- Have family members and friends learn cardiopulmonary resuscitation (CPR) in case you have cardiac arrest.
- Don't smoke, use mind-altering drugs or drink more than 1 or 2 alcoholic drinks—if any—a day.
- Learn to check your own pulse for rate (beats per minute), rhythm (regular or irregular) and strength. Call your doctor if these change.
- See How to Cope with Stress in Appendix section.
- See Resources for Additional Information.

MEDICATION—Your doctor may prescribe:
- Heart medications, such as digitalis, quinidine, calcium-channel blockers or beta-adrenergic blockers to regulate the heartbeat.
- Anticoagulants to prevent blood clot.
- Avoid nonprescription decongestants.

ACTIVITY—Resume your normal activities as soon as symptoms improve. Consult your doctor before resuming sexual relations.

DIET
- Lose weight if you are obese, but don't use appetite suppressants. These may worsen rhythm disturbances. See Weight Loss diet in Appendix section.
- The underlying heart condition may require a low-salt or low-fat diet (see diets in Appendix section) and potassium supplements.

CALL YOUR DOCTOR IF

- You have symptoms of atrial fibrillation.
- The following occurs during treatment: Change in heart rate, rhythm or strength. Chest pain, sweating and weakness. Shortness of breath and swollen feet and ankles. Pain in the calf of the leg while walking.
- New, unexplained symptoms develop. Drugs in treatment may produce side effects.

ATTENTION-DEFICIT HYPERACTIVITY DISORDER (ADHD)

GENERAL INFORMATION

DEFINITION—A pattern of behavior in children characterized by short attention spans, impulsivity, with or without hyperactivity. It is implicated in learning disorders and estimated to affect 5-10% of school-aged children.

SEX OR AGE MOST AFFECTED—Boys are affected 10 times more than girls. The symptoms may appear at ages 4 to 7 and peak between 8 and 10. However, it can be seen in adults.

SIGNS & SYMPTOMS
- Squirms in seat; fidgets with hands or feet.
- Unable to remain seated when required to do so.
- Easily distracted.
- Blurts out answers before a question is finished.
- Difficulty in waiting turn in games and lines.
- Difficulty in following instructions.
- Unable to sustain attention in work or play activities.
- Shifts from one uncompleted project to another.
- Difficulty in playing quietly.
- Talks excessively.
- Interrupts or intrudes on others.
- Doesn't appear to listen.
- Loses items necessary for tasks.
- Often engages in dangerous activities without considering consequences.

CAUSES—Unknown. Many theories proposed, but none proven or disproven. It is thought to be biologic.

RISK INCREASES WITH—Family history of the disorder.

HOW TO PREVENT—No preventive measures known.

WHAT TO EXPECT

DIAGNOSTIC MEASURES
- Care must be taken in diagnosis and no specific test is available. Many of the behavioral problems are common to all children. Usually 8 out of 14 of above symptoms and signs should be present. Formal educational and psychological assessment is necessary.
- A social history, medical history and school reports are necessary to aid in diagnosis.

APPROPRIATE HEALTH CARE
- Doctor's treatment and counseling for parents and child.
- Behavioral and cognitive therapies. These can involve the child with self-monitoring, role playing and self-recording. These therapies focus on strategies that alter the undesired behavior. A combination of these techniques and psychostimulent medications seem to have the greatest affect on controlling the symptoms.

POSSIBLE COMPLICATIONS
- Child may not grow out of difficulties. Later problems occur such as academic failure, antisocial behavior and sometimes, criminal behaviors.
- Problems carry on to adulthood with a high incidence of personality trait disorders.

PROBABLE OUTCOME—In some cases, the behavior disappears completely at puberty. In others, hyperactivity diminishes with age. However, a great number of these children grow into troubled teenagers and adults.

HOW TO TREAT

GENERAL MEASURES
- Help your child at home by providing a structured environment, well-defined behavior limits and consistent parenting techniques. Get professional assistance if help is needed.
- Stay in close contact with the child's teacher. Arrange for extra lessons or tutoring if the child needs help with school subjects.

MEDICATION—Your doctor may prescribe stimulant drugs (e.g., methylphenidate). They appear to have a calming affect on children with the disorder. These drugs have unpleasant side effects such as sleep disturbances, depression, headache, stomach ache, loss of appetite, and stunted growth.

ACTIVITY—Structure your child's activity to the extent possible.

DIET—Diets that remove all food additives, special elimination diets or megavitamin therapy have been suggested. Most medical research indicates these diets benefit very few children. Many parents however, report dramatic changes in behavior after this treatment. Some of the change may be attributed to the extra attention the child receives with the preparation of special meals.

CALL YOUR DOCTOR IF

- You believe your child has symptoms of attention deficit hyperactivity disorder.
- Symptoms don't improve, or worsen after treatment is begun.
- New, unexplained symptoms develop. Drugs used in treatment may produce side effects.

BACK PAIN
(Sciatica)

GENERAL INFORMATION

DEFINITION—Pain in the lower back usually caused by muscle strain. It is often accompanied by sciatica (pain that radiates from the back to the buttock and down into the leg). Onset of pain may be immediate or occur some hours after exertion or an injury.

SEX OR AGE MOST AFFECTED—Adults of both sexes, usually between ages 20 and 40.

SIGNS & SYMPTOMS
- Pain. It may be continuous, or only occur when you are in a certain position. The pain may be aggravated by coughing or sneezing, bending or twisting.
- Stiffness.

CAUSES
- Exertion or lifting.
- Severe blow or fall.
- Back disorders, ruptured lumbar disk.
- Infections.
- Nerve dysfunction.
- Osteoporosis, tumors.
- Spondylosis (hardening and stiffening of the spinal column).
- Congenital problem.
- Childbirth.
- Often there is no obvious cause.

RISK INCREASES WITH
- Biomechanical risk factors.
- Sedentary occupations.
- Gardening and other yard work.
- Infrequent sports and exercise participation.
- Obesity.
- Poor muscle tone, poor posture.
- Wearing high heels (women).

HOW TO PREVENT
- Exercises to strengthen lower back muscles.
- Learn how to lift heavy objects.
- Sit properly.
- Back support in bed.
- Lose weight, if obese.
- Choose proper footwear.
- Wear special back support devices.

WHAT TO EXPECT

DIAGNOSTIC MEASURES
- Your own observation of symptoms.
- Medical history and exam by a doctor.
- Laboratory blood studies to determine if there is an underlying disorder, x-rays of the spine, sometimes a CT or MRI scan (see Glossary).

APPROPRIATE HEALTH CARE
- Treatment will depend on severity of the pain and discomfort.

- Bed rest for first 24 hours. Additional bed rest will be determined by severity of the problem. Recent medical studies indicate that staying more active is better for back disorders than prolonged bed rest.
- Options are available such as surgery for damaged disk (see Disk-Removal, Ruptured in Surgery section); electrical nerve stimulation; acupuncture; orthopedic care; physical therapy; treatment by a chiropractor, physiatrist or neurologist and others.
- Massage may help. Be sure person is well-trained or massage could cause more harm than help.

POSSIBLE COMPLICATIONS—Chronic low back pain and restricted lifestyle.

PROBABLE OUTCOME—Gradual recovery, but back troubles tend to recur.

HOW TO TREAT

GENERAL MEASURES—Some self-treatment guidelines include:
- Ice pack or cold massage or heat applied to affected area with heating pad or hot water bottle.
- Use a firm mattress (place a bed board under the mattress if needed). Sleep on your back with a pillow under your knees, or sleep on your side with a pillow between your knees.
- Wear a special back support device.
- Learn stress reduction techniques, if needed.
- Take breaks if you have to stand or sit for long periods.

MEDICATION—Your doctor may prescribe:
- Mild pain medications such as aspirin or ibuprofen.
- Stronger pain medicine or a muscle relaxant for severe pain.
- Note: Medications do not hasten healing. They only help to reduce symptoms.

ACTIVITY
- Try to continue with daily work or school schedules to the extent possible. Use care in resuming normal activities.
- Avoid strenuous activity for 6 weeks.
- After healing, an exercise program will help.

DIET—No special diet. A weight reduction diet is recommended if obesity is a problem (see Weight Loss Diet in Appendix).

CALL YOUR DOCTOR IF

- You have mild, low back pain that persists for 3 or 4 days after self-treatment.
- Back pain is severe or recurrent.
- New or unexplained symptoms appear.

BALANITIS

GENERAL INFORMATION

DEFINITION—Inflammation of the penis and sometimes the foreskin as well. It is usually associated with an unretractable foreskin of an uncircumcised male.

BODY PARTS INVOLVED—Penis and foreskin.

SEX OR AGE MOST AFFECTED—Males of all ages.

SIGNS & SYMPTOMS
- Pain, redness and swelling of the head of the penis.
- Inflammation of the foreskin.
- Ulceration of the penis.
- Enlarged lymph glands in the groin.
- Chills and fever (rare).
- Discharge from the penis (rare).
- Burning on urination (rare).

CAUSES
- Infection from bacteria (Borrelia vincentii, streptococci) or fungus (Candida albicans).
- Allergy to chemicals in clothing, contraceptive cream, condom latex.
- Reaction to certain medications.
- Tight foreskin.

RISK INCREASES WITH
- Poor hygiene.
- Trauma or minor injury to the foreskin and penis.
- Presence of foreskin.
- Diabetes mellitus.
- Sexual partner affected by candidal vaginitis.

HOW TO PREVENT
- Have male infants circumcised.
- Wash daily with soap and water, especially after sexual intercourse. Cleanse under the foreskin.
- Avoid any allergens.
- Use a condom during intercourse.

WHAT TO EXPECT

DIAGNOSTIC MEASURES
- Your own observation of symptoms.
- Medical history and physical exam by a doctor.
- Laboratory culture of the discharge from the infected area.

APPROPRIATE HEALTH CARE
- Doctor's treatment.
- Surgery to circumcise the penis, if balanitis recurs frequently. See Circumcision (in Surgery section).

POSSIBLE COMPLICATIONS
- Ulceration of the penis.
- Spread of infection to deeper skin layers of the penis shaft.
- Blood poisoning.
- Urinary tract infection.

PROBABLE OUTCOME—Usually curable in 1 to 2 weeks with medical treatment.

HOW TO TREAT

GENERAL MEASURES—Use warm-water soaks to relieve pain (see Soaks in Appendix section).

MEDICATION—Your doctor may prescribe:
- Steroid creams to control swelling.
- Topical or oral antibiotics or antifungals to fight infection.
- Aspirin, acetaminophen or ibuprofen to relieve minor pain and fever.

ACTIVITY—Rest in bed if you have fever. Avoid sexual intercourse during treatment. Resume your normal activities when the infection is cured.

DIET—No special diet.

CALL YOUR DOCTOR IF

- You have symptoms of balanitis.
- Symptoms don't improve in 3 days, despite treatment.
- Balanitis recurs. You may want to consider circumcision.

ILLNESS & DISORDERS

BALDNESS, PATTERN, MALE & FEMALE

 GENERAL INFORMATION

DEFINITION—Gradual, painless hair loss that occurs in a distinctive pattern as a person ages. The earlier hair loss begins, the greater the eventual loss. Some persons have short periods of intense hair loss, followed by long, stable periods.

BODY PARTS INVOLVED—Hair; scalp.

SEX OR AGE MOST AFFECTED—In men, appears as early as the 20s; in women, rarely appears before the 50s.

SIGNS & SYMPTOMS
• In men, hair loss occurs on top of the head and in the temple areas of the scalp.
• In women, hair loss usually occurs only on top of the head.
• In both sexes, some diffuse loss may also occur.

CAUSES
• Genetic factors.
• Hormonal factors. Male hormones are an important factor in balding. Men castrated at a young age don't develop pattern baldness—regardless of genetic factors—unless they receive supplemental testosterone (a male hormone).
   Correspondingly, estrogen (a female hormone) may be protective in women, because hair loss rarely begins before menopause.

RISK INCREASES WITH—Family history of pattern baldness. Hair loss that occurs after illness, pregnancy or as an adverse reaction to drugs is a different form of baldness.

HOW TO PREVENT—Cannot be prevented at present. The drug minoxidil has been shown to slow or reverse baldness to some degree in some men. Other medical treatments are undergoing study.

 WHAT TO EXPECT

DIAGNOSTIC MEASURES
• Your own observation of symptoms.
• Medical history and physical exam by a doctor, if diagnosis is in doubt.

APPROPRIATE HEALTH CARE—Self-care.

POSSIBLE COMPLICATIONS—No medical complications, but baldness can cause emotional distress.

PROBABLE OUTCOME—Incurable at present.

 HOW TO TREAT

GENERAL MEASURES
• Don't use products that promise to cure baldness such as vitamin formulas, ointments, creams or massage oils. They are useless.
• If you cannot accept balding as part of aging, there are 2 options:
   Consider wearing a toupee or wig.
   Consider a hair-transplant operation (see Hair Transplant in Surgery section). This surgery may have complications, so discuss the advantages and disadvantages with your doctor before undergoing the procedure.

MEDICATION—Medicine is not necessary for this disorder. Drugs are now available to stimulate hair growth, but their effectiveness is frequently limited.

ACTIVITY—No restrictions.

DIET—No special diet.

 CALL YOUR DOCTOR IF

• You want a medical referral for hair transplantation.
• You suffer a sudden hair loss. This could be a medical problem.

BAROTITIS MEDIA
(Barotrauma)

GENERAL INFORMATION

DEFINITION—Damage to the middle ear caused by pressure changes.

BODY PARTS INVOLVED—Middle ear; eustachian tube; nerve endings in the ear.

SEX OR AGE MOST AFFECTED—Both sexes; all ages.

SIGNS & SYMPTOMS
- Hearing loss (to varying degrees).
- A plugged feeling in the ear.
- Severe pain.
- Dizziness.
- Ringing noises in the ear.
- Mild to severe pain in the ears, or over the cheekbones and forehead.
- Crying infants or young children.

CAUSES—Damage caused by sudden, increased pressure in the surrounding air, such as occurs in the rapid descent of an airplane or while scuba diving.

In these activities, air moves from passages in the nose into the middle ear to maintain equal pressure on both sides of the eardrum. If the tube leading from the nose to the ear (eustachian tube) doesn't function properly, pressure in the middle ear is less than outside pressure. The negative pressure in the middle ear sucks the eardrum inward. Blood and mucus may later appear in the middle ear.

This damage is more likely if you have a nose or throat infection when scuba diving or traveling by air.

RISK INCREASES WITH
- Recent respiratory-tract infection.
- Airplane flight.
- Scuba diving; sky diving.
- High altitude mountain climbers.
- High impact sports.
- Infants and young children who have difficulty in dilating the eustachian tube (by swallowing).

HOW TO PREVENT
- Don't fly or scuba-dive when you have an upper-respiratory infection. If you must fly anyway, use nonprescription decongestant tablets or sprays. Follow package instructions.
- During air travel, while ascending or descending, suck on hard candy or chew gum to force frequent swallowing. Take a moderate-size breath, hold the nose and try to force air into the eustachian tube by gently puffing out the cheeks with the mouth closed (Valsalva maneuver).
- Give an infant a bottle of water or juice while ascending or descending.

WHAT TO EXPECT

DIAGNOSTIC MEASURES
- Your own observation of symptoms.
- Medical history and physical exam by a doctor.

APPROPRIATE HEALTH CARE
- Self-care.
- In most cases, no treatment is necessary and symptoms disappear in hours or days.
- Rarely, surgery to open the eardrum and release fluid trapped in the middle ear. A plastic tube may be inserted through the surgically perforated eardrum to keep it open and equalize pressure. The tube falls out spontaneously in 9 to 12 months.

POSSIBLE COMPLICATIONS
- Permanent hearing loss.
- Ruptured ear drum.
- Middle ear infection.

PROBABLE OUTCOME—With treatment, most cases of barotitis media are reversible without permanent damage or hearing loss.

HOW TO TREAT

GENERAL MEASURES—If fluid drains from the ear, place a small piece of cotton in the outer-ear canal to absorb it.

MEDICATION
- For minor discomfort, you may use nonprescription decongestants and pain relievers, such as acetaminophen.
- Your doctor may prescribe:
  Stronger prescription decongestant nasal sprays or tablets. Use for at least 2 weeks after damage.
  Steroid nasal spray.
  Antibiotics, if infection is present.

ACTIVITY—Resume your normal activities as soon as symptoms improve.

DIET—No special diet.

CALL YOUR DOCTOR IF

- You have symptoms of barotitis media.
- The following occurs during treatment:
  Severe headache.
  Fever.
  Severe pain.
  Dizziness.
- New, unexplained symptoms develop. Drugs used in treatment may produce side effects.

BED-WETTING
(Enuresis)

GENERAL INFORMATION

DEFINITION—Involuntary urination during sleep that occurs more often than once a month in girls over 5 and in boys over 6 years of age.

BODY PARTS INVOLVED—Urinary tract.

SEX OR AGE MOST AFFECTED—Both sexes, but more common in boys. The occurrence of bed-wetting in children is: 15% at age 5; 10% at age 6; 7% at age 8; 3% at age 12; and 1% at age 18.

SIGNS & SYMPTOMS—Bed-wetting at night. This is not significant until a child is older than 6.

CAUSES—In most cases, the cause of bed-wetting is unknown. Following are the most-common causes or popular theories:
• Underlying illness, such as diabetes or a urinary-tract infection.
• A small or weak bladder that cannot hold one night's urine production.
• Psychological problems caused by stress or separation from the mother.
• Child who is a deep sleeper.

RISK INCREASES WITH
• Diabetes.
• Urinary-tract infection.
• Family history of bed-wetting (44% occurrence if one parent was bed-wetter, 77% occurrence if both parents were bed-wetters).
• First born child.

HOW TO PREVENT—No effective preventive methods known. Show your child love, support and understanding.

WHAT TO EXPECT

DIAGNOSTIC MEASURES
• Your own observation of symptoms.
• Medical history and exam by a doctor.
• Laboratory studies of urine and blood to detect diabetes or urinary-tract infection (sometimes).

APPROPRIATE HEALTH CARE
• Self-care, bladder exercise.
• Doctor's treatment.
• Psychotherapy or counseling.
• Alarms triggered by wetting.

POSSIBLE COMPLICATIONS
• Child becomes anxious and embarrassed. Psychological and emotional problems.
• Urinary tract infection.

PROBABLE OUTCOME—Bed-wetting may continue for several years. Your doctor will want to rule out urinary-tract infections and diabetes as causes. If these are eliminated and your child is normal in other respects, consider your child's bed-wetting represents a delay in maturing that will resolve with time.

HOW TO TREAT

GENERAL MEASURES
• Prepare the bed and the child:
  Protect the mattress with a heavy plastic cover. Provide the child with extra-thick underwear and pajamas. Discontinue diapers or plastic pants by age 4; they inhibit the child's motivation to improve. Put an extra pair of underwear and pajama bottoms by the bed in case the child needs them during the night.
• Don't give any liquids to the child for 2-3 hours prior to bedtime.
• Have the child urinate at bedtime.
• Awaken the child to urinate after he has been asleep for several hours. If the child is old enough, he may be able to set the alarm clock to awaken himself and empty his bladder.
• Reward the child for staying dry. Praise him, hug him and tell of his success to people who are important to him, such as brothers and sisters. Use gold stars or happy faces to mark dry nights on a calendar if the child likes it.
• Respond gently to accidents. Don't blame, criticize, restrict or punish the child who has wet the bed. This can cause him to give up or lead to emotional problems.
• Follow instructions for any bladder-stretching or stream-interruption exercises or behavior-modification devices.
• Try alarms that are triggered by wetting.
• See Resources for Additional Information.

MEDICATION—Medicine usually is not necessary for this disorder, but your doctor may prescribe antidepressant drugs or a prescription nasal spray if other methods fail and the family favors medical treatment.

ACTIVITY—No restrictions.

DIET—No special diet. Encourage your child to drink as much fluid as possible during the day. Decrease fluid intake during the 2 to 3 hours before bedtime.

CALL YOUR DOCTOR IF

• You are concerned about your child's bed-wetting, and your child is older than 6.
• The child dribbles urine, has a weak urinary stream, has pain when urinating or must strain to urinate.
• Medication is prescribed for the child, and new, unexplained symptoms develop.

BELL'S PALSY

GENERAL INFORMATION

DEFINITION—Paralysis on one side of the face. The disorder is named after the physician who first described it. The onset may be sudden or may come on over several days. In a majority of patients, there is a preceding condition such as stress, fatigue, common cold, stiff neck or shoulder on the affected side.

BODY PARTS INVOLVED—7th cranial nerve and facial muscles supplied by that nerve.

SEX OR AGE MOST AFFECTED—All ages, but most common in adults.

SIGNS & SYMPTOMS
- Sudden paralysis on one side of the face, including muscles to the eyelid.
- Pain behind the ear on the affected side.
- Flat, expressionless features on one side of the face.
- Distorted smiles and frowns.
- Changes in taste, salivation or tear formation (sometimes).

CAUSES—Unknown. The paralysis is probably caused by swelling of the facial nerve. The swelling may be caused by: a virus; an autoimmune disease; or a decrease in blood flow and pressure on the facial nerve as it passes through the temporal bone of the skull.

RISK INCREASES WITH—Exposure to cold.

HOW TO PREVENT—Cannot be prevented at present.

WHAT TO EXPECT

DIAGNOSTIC MEASURES
- Your own observation of symptoms.
- Medical history and physical exam by a doctor.
- MRI or CT scan (see Glossary for both) to rule out other causes of pressure on the facial nerve (sometimes).
- The extent of nerve involvement can be assessed by diagnostic tests such as evoked electromyography or electroneuronography (see Glossary for both).

APPROPRIATE HEALTH CARE
- Self-care after diagnosis.
- Doctor's treatment.
- Surgery (rare).

POSSIBLE COMPLICATIONS
- Eye irritation or injury because the eye does not close properly and is exposed to dust. If unprotected, the eye may develop ulcers on the cornea.
- Tooth decay and gum disease due to reduced saliva and impairment of chewing.
- Psychological and self-esteem problems.

PROBABLE OUTCOME
- Bell's palsy is distressing, but it is not dangerous. The extent of nerve damage determines the extent of recovery.
- Improvement is gradual and recovery time varies, sometimes requiring many months.
- Patients with mild facial paralysis usually recover completely within several months. Patients with severe facial paralysis recover completely in 80% to 90% of cases.
- Surgery can sometimes improve facial appearance and muscle function in patients who do not recover fully.

HOW TO TREAT

GENERAL MEASURES
- If you have pain, apply heat to the painful area twice a day. Wring out a small towel soaked in hot water and apply for 15 minutes. Cover or close the eye during heat treatments.
- If you cannot wink or close your eye well, buy a pair of wrap-around, plastic bubble goggles. Wear them to protect your eye from dirt, dust and dryness. You may buy goggles from a sporting goods store or optician.
- At night, apply an eye patch to shut the lid so the eye stays moist and protected. Occasionally, a patch will be necessary during the daytime.
- As muscle strength returns, use facial massage and exercises. Massage muscles of the forehead, cheek, lips and eyes using cream or oil. Exercise the weak muscles in front of a mirror. Open and close the eye, wink, smile and bare your teeth. Perform the massage and exercise for 15 or 20 minutes several times a day.
- Brush and floss teeth more often to keep the mouth healthy.

MEDICATION—Your doctor may prescribe:
- Methylcellulose eye drops for comfort and protection of the exposed eye.
- Cortisone drugs for 2 weeks to reduce swelling and inflammation of the affected nerve.

ACTIVITY—Maintain your normal activities. Rest does not help Bell's palsy.

DIET—A soft diet is often necessary (see Soft Diet in Appendix).

CALL YOUR DOCTOR IF

- You have symptoms of Bell's palsy.
- Your eye becomes red or irritated, despite treatment.
- You cannot prevent saliva from drooling from your mouth.
- Pain worsens.
- You have a fever.
- Symptoms recur after treatment.

BIPOLAR DISORDER
(Manic-Depressive Disorder)

 GENERAL INFORMATION

DEFINITION—A disorder that is characterized by extreme mood swings. Periods of unexplainable elation, overactivity (mania), and exaggerated euphoria alternate with deep depression. Periods of normal behavior that may last for years occur in between the mania and the depression.

SEX OR AGE MOST AFFECTED—Both sexes; all ages.

SIGNS & SYMPTOMS
- Accelerated energy levels; euphoric mood.
- Waking earlier and earlier in the morning, (some may not sleep for 3 to 4 days).
- Easily distracted and restless.
- May go on spending sprees.
- May become sexually promiscuous.
- Often irritable with attacks of rage.
- Speech becomes rapid, wild and illogical.
- May have high opinion of one's abilities and exaggerated thinking (grandiosity).
- May skip meals, lose weight, become exhausted.
- May develop delusions of grandeur or intense anger at one's ability to carry out wild schemes.

Depression may cause the following symptoms:
- May become withdrawn or have disturbed sleep.
- Low self-esteem; self-neglect; decreased sex drive; slow speech and movement.
- Increased imagined illness and worry.

CAUSES
- Unknown.
- Biologic.
- Extreme stress may trigger a sudden episode of mania or depression.

RISK INCREASES WITH—Family history of the disorder.

HOW TO PREVENT—No specific preventive measures known.

 WHAT TO EXPECT

DIAGNOSTIC MEASURES—Medical history and physical exam by a doctor or psychiatrist. Psychological testing.

APPROPRIATE HEALTH CARE
- Psychotherapy or counseling along with drug treatment achieves the best results.
- Hospitalization or inpatient care at a treatment center for severe symptoms.
- Electroconvulsive therapy (ECT) may be used for patients who fail to respond to medication.

POSSIBLE COMPLICATIONS
- Relapse, especially if medication is stopped.
- Job loss; marital problems.
- Failure to improve.
- Suicide.

PROBABLE OUTCOME—Usually curable with long-term therapy that reduces the frequency and severity of episodes.

 HOW TO TREAT

GENERAL MEASURES
- Comply with your doctor's medication regimen.
- Stay under close medical supervision to monitor effectiveness and watch for side effects.
- Psychological counseling for help in adjusting.
- Seek support groups. Contact social agencies for help. Call suicide prevention hot line if you feel suicidal.

MEDICATION—Your doctor may prescribe:
- Lithium, valproic acid or carbamazepine (Tegretol). Newer medications are also frequently effective.
- Antipsychotic medications for more severe symptoms.

ACTIVITY—No restrictions. Maintain daily activities, even if you don't feel like it.

DIET—Eat a normal well-balanced diet, even if you have no appetite. Vitamin and mineral supplements may be necessary. Your doctor may advise you to avoid caffeine, which is a stimulant.

 CALL YOUR DOCTOR IF

- You or a family member has symptoms of depression or mania.
- You feel suicidal or hopeless.

BLADDER TUMOR

 GENERAL INFORMATION

DEFINITION—Abnormal tissue growth in the bladder in which cell multiplication is uncontrolled. The tumor may be benign or malignant. If malignant, it may spread to lymph nodes, bone, liver and lungs.

BODY PARTS INVOLVED—Urinary bladder.

SEX OR AGE MOST AFFECTED—Adults over 50 of both sexes, but more common in men than women.

SIGNS & SYMPTOMS
- In early stages, there may be no symptoms.
- Blood in the urine.
- Burning on urination.
- Increased frequency of urination, but passage of only small amounts of urine.
- Pain in the pelvic area.
- Unexplained weight loss.

CAUSES—Unknown. Exposure to environmental carcinogens (cancer producing substances) is the presumed cause in some cases.

RISK INCREASES WITH
- Smoking.
- Family history of bladder tumors.
- Exposure to naphthylamines (dyes containing aniline) or chemicals used in the manufacture of rubber.
- Schistosomiasis (a parasitic disorder found in Africa, Middle East and Asian countries).

HOW TO PREVENT
- Avoid exposure to chemical or environmental hazards. Protective measures in these industries and regular screening of those who have been exposed in the past has reduced the incidence.
- Don't smoke.

 WHAT TO EXPECT

DIAGNOSTIC MEASURES
- Your own observation of symptoms.
- Medical history and physical exam by a doctor.
- Urinalysis.
- Cystoscopy (see Glossary).
- X-rays of the bladder and urinary tract.

APPROPRIATE HEALTH CARE
- Doctor's treatment.
- Surgery to remove the tumor or bladder. If the tumor is malignant, anticancer drugs may be instilled in the bladder during surgery. The operation also may include a procedure to divert the urinary stream. (See Bladder Removal in Surgery section.)
- Radiation treatment for some.

POSSIBLE COMPLICATIONS
- Infection in the bladder or kidneys. Symptoms include back pain, fever and vomiting.
- Urinary obstruction.
- Impotence for males with some surgeries. A penile implant may be considered at a later date.

PROBABLE OUTCOME—When diagnosed early, bladder cancer treatment may be successful, but recurrence is common and regular checkups are necessary. When the tumor has been present for a long time, treatment outcome is poor.

 HOW TO TREAT

GENERAL MEASURES
- If urinary diversion is necessary, special training and care instructions will be provided to you following the surgery. Your spouse or a family member should participate also.
- Seek psychological help or counselling support.
- See Resources for Additional Information.

MEDICATION—Your doctor may prescribe:
- Pain relievers.
- Oral anticancer drugs.

ACTIVITY—After surgery or other treatment, resume your normal activities as soon as feasible.

DIET—No special diet.

 CALL YOUR DOCTOR IF

- You have symptoms of a bladder tumor.
- New, unexplained symptoms develop. Drugs used in treatment may produce side effects.

ILLNESS & DISORDERS

BLASTOMYCOSIS
(North American Blastomycosis; Gilchrist's Disease)

 GENERAL INFORMATION

DEFINITION—An infectious, fungus disease that starts in the lungs. Occasionally it spreads through the bloodstream to other body parts—especially the skin. Blastomycosis is not contagious from person to person, but can be transmitted through bites from infected dogs.

BODY PARTS INVOLVED—Lungs; mouth; skin and tissue below the skin; prostate; epididymis.

SEX OR AGE MOST AFFECTED—Both sexes, but most common in men from ages 20 to 40.

SIGNS & SYMPTOMS—The following symptoms begin slowly:
• Cough, either dry and nonproductive or with sputum.
• Chest pain.
• Chills, fever and drenching sweats.
• Shortness of breath.
• If skin involved, may have lesions or abscesses.

CAUSES—Infection with the fungus, Blastomyces dermatitidis, found in wood and soil. There may be some association with beaver huts. Skin lesions occur most commonly in gardeners or farmers, but the natural source of this fungus is unknown.

RISK INCREASES WITH
• Gardening and farming, especially in Southeastern states and the Mississippi River valley of the U.S.
• Diabetes mellitus.
• Use of immunosuppressive drugs.

HOW TO PREVENT—Cannot be prevented at present.

 WHAT TO EXPECT

DIAGNOSTIC MEASURES
• Your own observation of symptoms.
• Medical history and physical exam by a doctor.
• Laboratory cultures of skin lesion, pus, sputum or blood to identify the fungus; biopsy of tissue from the skin or lungs; chest x-ray.

APPROPRIATE HEALTH CARE
• Doctor's treatment.
• Hospitalization for intensive care, if the lung infection spreads to other body parts.
• Self-care after treatment.

POSSIBLE COMPLICATIONS—Spread to other body parts, with serious illness and death. If the infection spreads, the following may appear:
• Pain in long bones.
• Skin lesions that begin as small papules (small, raised bumps on the skin) or pustules (small white blisters with pus) on exposed skin surfaces. They spread slowly. When fully developed, the lesions become crusted ulcers with sloping, reddish-purple borders.
• Swelling and painful, tender nodules in the scrotum.

PROBABLE OUTCOME—This fungus can cause severe, debilitating illness that may be fatal without treatment. With intensive treatment, it is usually curable in several weeks.

 HOW TO TREAT

GENERAL MEASURES
• Weigh daily and keep a weight chart. An unexplained weight loss might indicate the infection has spread.
• Keep follow-up appointments with the doctor. It is important to monitor the effectiveness of the treatment and watch for side effects or adverse reactions from the medications.
• Heat and elevation may be helpful for joint pain.

MEDICATION—For severe cases, your doctor may prescribe potent antifungal drugs, such as ketoconazole and amphotericin B.

ACTIVITY—Rest in bed during the acute stage. Resume activities gradually as your strength returns.

DIET—No special diet.

 CALL YOUR DOCTOR IF

• You have symptoms of blastomycosis.
• Any of the following occurs during treatment:
  Weight loss.
  Fever.
  Diarrhea that cannot be controlled with home remedies.
  Severe headache and stiff neck.
• New, unexplained symptoms develop. Drugs used in treatment may produce side effects.

BLEPHARITIS

GENERAL INFORMATION

DEFINITION—Inflammation of the eyelid edges.

BODY PARTS INVOLVED—Eyelids; eyelashes; meibomian glands (those which lubricate the lid); conjunctiva (white of the eye).

SEX OR AGE MOST AFFECTED—Adults of both sexes.

SIGNS & SYMPTOMS
- Redness and greasy scales on the eyelid edges.
- Eyelashes that fall out.
- Small ulcers on the eyelid. If the lid edges ulcerate, crusts will form. If crusts are removed, lids will bleed.
- Irritation of the eye if flakes from the lid fall into the eye.
- A feeling that something is in the eye. This includes itching, burning, redness, swelling of the lid, sensitivity to bright light and tearing.
- Discharge from the lids, which glues lashes together during sleep.
- Sensitivity to light.

CAUSES
- Bacterial infection, usually staphylococcal, of the eyelash follicles and the meibomian glands.
- Allergic reaction (less serious inflammation only).
- Body lice (rare).

RISK INCREASES WITH
- Adults over 60.
- Medical history of seborrheic dermatitis of the scalp and other body parts.
- Exposure to chemical or environmental irritants.
- Crowded or unsanitary living conditions.
- Poor nutrition.
- Immunosuppression due to illness or medication.
- Diabetes mellitus.
- Acne rosacea.

HOW TO PREVENT
- Wash hands often and dry with clean towels.
- Avoid environments that contain dust or other irritating substances.
- Use hypoallergenic eye makeup.
- Control seborrhea of the scalp with medicated shampoos.

WHAT TO EXPECT

DIAGNOSTIC MEASURES
- Your own observation of symptoms.
- Medical history and physical exam by a doctor.
- Laboratory culture of the discharge from lids (sometimes).

APPROPRIATE HEALTH CARE
- Self-care after diagnosis.
- Doctor's treatment. If blepharitis is caused by lice, your doctor will remove them with tweezers or medication.

POSSIBLE COMPLICATIONS
- Loss of eyelashes.
- Ulceration of the cornea (covering of the eye).
- Scarred eyelids.
- Stye.
- Misdirected eyelash growth.

PROBABLE OUTCOME—Blepharitis is stubbornly resistant to treatment, but it is sometimes curable in 8 to 12 months. Recurrence is common.

HOW TO TREAT

GENERAL MEASURES
- Use warm-water soaks (see Appendix) to reduce inflammation and hasten healing. Apply soaks for 20 minutes, then rest at least 1 hour. Repeat as often as needed.
- Remove scales from the lids each day.
- Don't wear eye makeup until inflammation subsides.
- Discontinue soft contact lenses until condition cleared.

MEDICATION—Your doctor may prescribe:
- Antibiotic ointment or eyedrops, which may contain cortisone drugs.
- Oral medication may be prescribed in severe cases such as with acne rosacea.

ACTIVITY—No restrictions.

DIET—No special diet.

CALL YOUR DOCTOR IF

- You have symptoms of blepharitis.
- You have pain in the eye.
- Your vision changes.
- New, unexplained symptoms develop. Drugs used in treatment may produce side effects.

BLOOD POISONING
(Septicemia; Septic Shock; Bacteremia)

 GENERAL INFORMATION

DEFINITION—Bacterial infection (or toxins from bacteria) in the blood that invade the entire body via the bloodstream.

BODY PARTS INVOLVED—Total body.

SEX OR AGE MOST AFFECTED—Both sexes; all ages.

SIGNS & SYMPTOMS
- Shaking chills.
- Rapid temperature rise.
- Rapid, pounding heartbeat.
- Warm, flushed skin.
- Confusion and other symptoms of mental impairment.
- Drop in blood pressure.
- General ill feeling.
- Hyperventilation.

CAUSES—Infection in some other body part, such as: appendix, tooth, sinus, pelvis, gallbladder or urinary tract. The source may also be a burn, infected wound or open abscess.

RISK INCREASES WITH
- Adults over 60.
- Newborns and infants.
- Illness, such as diabetes, that has lowered resistance.
- Leukemia or other cancer.
- Use of immunosuppressive drugs or self-administered, intravenous drugs.
- Use of a catheter.
- Complicated labor or delivery.
- Certain surgical procedures.

HOW TO PREVENT
- Obtain medical treatment for any infection.
- If dental procedures have produced blood poisoning in the past or you have diseased heart valves, take antibiotics before any dental treatment—including simple prophylaxis by a dentist or hygienist.
- Influenza and pneumococcal vaccinations for high-risk patients.

 WHAT TO EXPECT

DIAGNOSTIC MEASURES
- Your own observation of symptoms.
- Medical history and physical exam by a doctor.
- Laboratory studies, such as: culture of the blood to identify organisms responsible for the illness; urinalysis; blood count.

APPROPRIATE HEALTH CARE
- Doctor's treatment.
- Hospitalization with intensive care treatment for severe cases.
- Removal or drainage of source of infection.
- Mechanical ventilation for respiratory failure.
- Blood transfusions.

POSSIBLE COMPLICATIONS
- Shock, with very low blood pressure, overwhelming infection and death.
- Persistent infection of the heart valves.
- Adult respiratory distress syndrome.
- Multi-organ failure (heart, lungs, kidney, liver).

PROBABLE OUTCOME—Dependent on underlying conditions, patient's health and any delay in treatment.

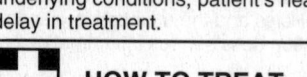 **HOW TO TREAT**

GENERAL MEASURES—This can be a frightening time for the patient's family. Intensive care units are intimidating places. Try to keep your spirits up, stay in close communications with the doctors and let them know the patient's preferences so that they can be incorporated into the clinical care.

MEDICATION—Your doctor will utilize antibiotics to fight infections.

ACTIVITY—As directed by your doctor.

DIET—May require tube or intravenous feedings.

 CALL YOUR DOCTOR IF

- You have symptoms of blood poisoning.
- The following occurs during treatment:
  Fever.
  Signs of infection (swelling, pain, redness) anywhere in your body.
- You plan elective surgery or a dental procedure after you have had an episode of blood poisoning.
- New, unexplained symptoms develop. Drugs used in treatment may produce side effects.

BLOOD-TRANSFUSION REACTION

GENERAL INFORMATION

DEFINITION—Symptoms triggered by a blood transfusion.

BODY PARTS INVOLVED—Blood; blood vessels; kidneys; heart; skin; central nervous system; lungs.

SEX OR AGE MOST AFFECTED—Both sexes. All ages.

SIGNS & SYMPTOMS
Less serious:
- Chills and fever.
- Backache or other aches and pains.
- Hives and itching.

More serious:
- Blood-cell destruction (hemolysis), causing shortness of breath, severe headache, chest or back pain and blood in the urine.

CAUSES—Transfusions of a different blood type than that of the patient. This may occur from errors in matching or from the use of incompletely matched blood in an emergency.

RISK INCREASES WITH
- Blood transfusions in emergency situations, when careful typing and matching of blood must be bypassed.
- Blood transfusions from donors who carry infections.
- Multiple blood transfusions.
- Rh negative mother.

HOW TO PREVENT
- Blood-bank and hospital personnel have safety procedures to prevent reactions except in situations that are uncontrollable (see Causes).
- Use of diphenhydramine (an antihistamine) and acetaminophen prior to transfusion may prevent minor reactions.
- Let doctor or medical personnel know of any prior history of a response to transfusions.
- If surgery is planned at least 1 month in advance, your own blood may be drawn and stored for use during surgery, if necessary. Transfusion with your own blood is least likely to produce a reaction.

WHAT TO EXPECT

DIAGNOSTIC MEASURES
- Your own observation of symptoms.
- Medical history and physical exam by a doctor.
- Laboratory blood tests to recheck compatibility and detect complications.

APPROPRIATE HEALTH CARE
- Doctor's treatment.
- Hospitalization. Patients receiving transfusions are usually in a hospital or outpatient surgical facility, and reactions can be treated when they occur.

POSSIBLE COMPLICATIONS
- Acute kidney failure.
- Anaphylaxis.
- Congestive heart failure from too rapid transfusion.

PROBABLE OUTCOME—Most reactions clear gradually after the transfusion is halted. A few reactions are fatal.

HOW TO TREAT

GENERAL MEASURES—Stay awake and alert during a blood transfusion, if possible, so you can notify medical personnel immediately if symptoms occur.

MEDICATION—Your doctor may prescribe:
- Antihistamines to decrease hives and itching.
- Cortisone drugs to decrease the likelihood of acute kidney failure.
- Antihypertensives, if blood pressure rises too high, or hypertensives, such as ephedrine or epinephrine, if blood pressure drops too low.

ACTIVITY—Resume your normal activities as soon as symptoms improve after transfusion.

DIET—No special diet.

CALL YOUR DOCTOR IF

You have symptoms of a blood-transfusion reaction during or after a transfusion. Call immediately. This is an emergency!

BOILS
(Furuncles; Carbuncles)

GENERAL INFORMATION

DEFINITION—A painful, deep, bacterial infection of a hair follicle. Boils are common and somewhat contagious. They can occur anywhere on the skin. Carbuncles are clusters of boils that occur when the infection spreads through small tunnels underneath the skin.

BODY PARTS INVOLVED—Skin on the neck, face, buttocks, and breasts; hair follicles.

SEX OR AGE MOST AFFECTED—Both sexes; all ages.

SIGNS & SYMPTOMS
- A domed nodule that is painful, tender and red and has pus on the surface. Boils can appear suddenly and ripen in 24 hours. They are usually 1-1/2cm to 3cm in diameter; some are larger.
- Fever (rare).
- Swelling of the closest lymph glands.

CAUSES—Infection, usually from Staphylococcus bacteria, that begins in the hair follicle and bores into the skin's deeper layers.

RISK INCREASES WITH
- Poor nutrition.
- Illness that has lowered resistance.
- Diabetes mellitus.
- Use of immunosuppressive drugs.

HOW TO PREVENT
- Keep the skin clean.
- If someone in the household has a boil, don't share towels or washcloths or clothing with that person.
- If you have a chronic disease (such as diabetes mellitus), be sure to follow your medical regimen.

WHAT TO EXPECT

DIAGNOSTIC MEASURES
- Your own observation of symptoms.
- Medical history and physical exam by a doctor.
- Laboratory culture of the pus (sometimes).

APPROPRIATE HEALTH CARE
- Self-care.
- Doctor's treatment, which may include incision and drainage of the boil.

POSSIBLE COMPLICATIONS
- The infection may enter the bloodstream and spread to other body parts.
- Scarring.
- Boils may recur.
- Family members may need treatment.

PROBABLE OUTCOME—Without treatment, a boil will heal in 10 to 20 days. With treatment, the boil should heal in less time, symptoms will be less severe, and new boils should not appear. The pus that drains when a boil opens spontaneously may contaminate nearby skin, causing new boils.

HOW TO TREAT

GENERAL MEASURES
- Do not burst a boil as this may spread bacteria.
- Taking showers instead of baths reduces chances of spreading infection.
- Relieve pain with gentle heat from warm-water soaks. Use 3 or 4 times daily for 20 minutes. Wash your hands carefully after touching the boil.
- Prevent the spread of boils by using clean towels only once or using paper towels and discarding them.

MEDICATION
- Your doctor may prescribe antibiotics.
- Don't use nonprescription antibiotic creams or ointments on the boil's surface. They are ineffective.

ACTIVITY—Decrease activity until the boil heals. Avoid sweating and avoid contact sports (such as wrestling) while lesions are present.

DIET—No special diet.

CALL YOUR DOCTOR IF

- You have a boil.
- The following occurs during treatment:
  Symptoms don't improve in 3 to 4 days, despite treatment.
  New boils appear.
  You have a fever.
  Other family members develop boils.
- New, unexplained symptoms develop. Drugs used in treatment may produce side effects.

BONE FRACTURE

GENERAL INFORMATION

DEFINITION—Complete or incomplete break in a bone. Following are the different types of fractures:
- Complete fracture. The broken bone is completely separated.
- Incomplete (greenstick) fracture. The broken bone is not completely separated.
- Comminuted fracture. There are more than 2 bone fragments at the fracture site.
- Open fracture (compound). The fractured bone has broken the skin.
- Closed fracture (including stress fracture). The fractured bone has not broken the skin.
- Compression fracture. The break occurs from extreme pressure on the bone.
- Impacted fracture. The broken ends have been driven into each other.
- Avulsion fracture. Force has been applied to a strong tendon, causing it to pull on and break off a portion of bone.
- Pathologic fracture. A break that occurs from minor injury in bone weakened or destroyed by disease.
- Stress fracture. A crack in a bone caused by repetitive and prolonged pressure on the bone, usually by intense exercise.

BODY PARTS INVOLVED—Bones.

SEX OR AGE MOST AFFECTED—Both sexes; all ages.

SIGNS & SYMPTOMS
- Pain and swelling at the fracture site.
- Tenderness close to the fracture.
- Paleness and deformity (sometimes).
- Loss of pulse below the fracture, usually in an extremity (this is an emergency).
- Numbness, tingling or paralysis below the fracture (rare; this is an emergency).
- Bleeding or bruising at the site.
- Weakness and inability to bear weight.

CAUSES—Injury.

RISK INCREASES WITH
- Osteoporosis.
- Tumors of the bone or bone marrow.
- Activities that carry the risk of injury.
- Reckless behavior that increases the chance of accidents.
- Older adults (they tend to fall more and bones are fragile).

HOW TO PREVENT
- Don't drink alcohol or use mind-altering drugs and drive.
- Wear protective gear for sports.
- Use your vehicle's seat belt.
- If you have osteoporosis, adhere to your treatment program and avoid situations in which injury is likely.

WHAT TO EXPECT

DIAGNOSTIC MEASURES
- Your own observation of symptoms.
- Medical history and exam by a doctor.
- Laboratory studies to determine blood loss.
- X-rays of injured parts.

APPROPRIATE HEALTH CARE
- Almost all fractures require immobilization with casts or splints.
- Hospitalization for anesthesia and treatment of severe fractures.
- Surgery, if the fracture must be repaired with rods, plates or screws (see Fracture Repair in Surgery section).
- Physical therapy for rehabilitation.

POSSIBLE COMPLICATIONS—Failure to heal (nonunion), shock from blood loss, travel of a fat embolus (clump of fat cells) from the injury site to the lungs or brain, obstruction of arteries.

PROBABLE OUTCOME
Usually curable with skillful first aid and aftercare. The broken bone should be manipulated, realigned and immobilized as soon as possible. Realignment is much more difficult after 6 hours.

HOW TO TREAT

GENERAL MEASURES—Give first aid treatment for bleeding, cover any open wounds, move patient as little as possible. Then transport to hospital or other emergency facility.

MEDICATION—Your doctor may prescribe: pain relievers, muscle relaxants.

ACTIVITY
- Immobility of a bone for a long period can cause loss of muscle bulk, stiffness in nearby joints and edema. It is important to begin to use the affected part as soon as is safely possible.
- There may be physical therapy with special exercises to maintain flexibility of the joint and strength to the muscles.
- Resume your normal activities as soon as symptoms improve.

DIET—No special diet. Take vitamin-C and zinc supplements to promote bone healing.

CALL YOUR DOCTOR IF

The following occurs after immobilization or surgery—Swelling above or below the fracture site, severe, persistent pain, blue or gray skin below the fracture site, especially under nails, numbness or loss of feeling below the fracture site. Report any of the above signs immediately.

BOTULISM

GENERAL INFORMATION

DEFINITION—A serious, noncontagious form of food poisoning caused by eating contaminated food containing a toxin that severely affects the nervous system. Two other types exist: wound botulism and infant botulism.

BODY PARTS INVOLVED—Central nervous system; muscular system.

SEX OR AGE MOST AFFECTED—All ages, but most common in adults.

SIGNS & SYMPTOMS—The following symptoms usually appear suddenly 18 to 36 hours after eating contaminated food:
- Blurred or double vision.
- Drooping eyelids.
- Dry mouth.
- Slurred speech.
- Swallowing difficulty.
- Vomiting and diarrhea.
- Weakness of the arms and legs, leading to paralysis.
- No fever.
- No disturbance of mental abilities.

The following symptoms appear in infants:
- Severe constipation.
- Feeble cry.
- Inability to suck.

CAUSES
- Infection with bacteria, Clostridium botulinum, found in contaminated or incompletely cooked, canned foods. This germ generates a powerful poison (toxin) that is absorbed from the digestive tract and spreads to the central nervous system.

  Foods likely to cause botulism include home-canned vegetables and fruits, fish, meat, under-cooked sausage, smoked meats and milk products.
- In infants under 1 year, raw honey or other uncooked foods may cause botulism.
- The bacteria also may contaminate a wound and produce the toxin.

RISK INCREASES WITH
- Infants.
- Home-canned foods. Green beans are especially susceptible to spoilage.

HOW TO PREVENT
- If a can of food is bulging, or the contents have a peculiar color or odor, don't taste it.
- Don't eat any foods not definitely known to be properly cooked and canned.
- Don't give infants honey in foods or cough suppressants.
- Boiling can prevent, but call your local home-extension service for details about canning food and cooking it safely. You may get additional information from Center for Nutrition and Dietetics National Consumer Hotline, (800) 366-1655.

- Call your local health department if you suspect botulism. The health department can notify the news media to alert others in danger and require retailers to remove contaminated food from store shelves.

WHAT TO EXPECT

DIAGNOSTIC MEASURES
- Your own observation of symptoms—especially if several persons eat the same food and become sick.
- Medical history and exam by a doctor.
- Laboratory blood tests; laboratory analysis of suspected food.

APPROPRIATE HEALTH CARE
Doctor's treatment. Hospitalization for intensive care. A respirator may be necessary.

POSSIBLE COMPLICATIONS
- Lung infections as a result of impaired swallowing and choking on food.
- Respiratory failure caused by weak breathing muscles.

PROBABLE OUTCOME—With prompt care, the outlook is good. The larger the toxin dose and the sooner symptoms begin, the more dangerous the condition. The overall death rate is 10% to 25%.

HOW TO TREAT

GENERAL MEASURES
- Induce vomiting if only a few hours have passed since the poisoned food was eaten.
- If you suspect botulism, refrigerate some of the contaminated food for laboratory testing.

MEDICATION—Botulism antitoxin injections prevent the condition from worsening. The antitoxin is available through the Center for Disease Control, Atlanta, Georgia. The antitoxin is derived from horse serum, which may be life-saving, but has serious side effects.

ACTIVITY—Bed rest is necessary during hospitalization. After treatment, resume normal activities gradually.

DIET—Intravenous fluids and foods are usually necessary during hospitalization because of swallowing difficulty. After treatment, no special diet is necessary.

CALL YOUR DOCTOR IF

- You have symptoms of botulism. Call an ambulance immediately. This is an emergency!
- Weakness, blurred vision or slurred speech occur after you return from intensive care.

BRAIN OR EPIDURAL ABSCESS

GENERAL INFORMATION

DEFINITION—A collection of pus caused by a bacterial infection in the brain or the outermost of 3 membranes that cover the brain and spinal cord.

BODY PARTS INVOLVED—Brain; meninges (membranes that cover the brain); skull.

SEX OR AGE MOST AFFECTED—All ages, but most common in young adults.

SIGNS AND SYMPTOMS—The following symptoms usually appear gradually over several hours. They resemble symptoms of a brain tumor or stroke:
- Pain in the back, if the infection is in the covering of the spinal cord.
- Headache.
- Nausea and vomiting.
- Weakness, numbness, or paralysis of one side of the body.
- Irregular gait.
- Convulsions.
- Fever.
- Confusion or delirium.
- Speaking difficulty.

CAUSES—The primary source of bacterial infection that causes a brain or epidural abscess often cannot be found. These 3 sources are the most common:
- An infection that spreads from an infected skull, such as in osteomyelitis, mastoiditis or sinusitis.
- An infection that is introduced by a skull injury.
- An infection that spreads through the bloodstream from other infected organs, such as the lungs, skin or heart valves.

RISK INCREASES WITH
- Head injury.
- Illness that has lowered resistance, especially diabetes mellitus.
- Recent infection, especially around the nose, eyes and face.
- Immunosuppressed patient due to illness (AIDS) or medications.
- Intravenous drug abuse.

HOW TO PREVENT
- Consult your doctor for treatment of any infection in your body—especially one around the nose or face (such as ear infection or dental abscess)—to prevent its spread.
- Wear protective head gear when engaging in any activity where risk of head injury is possible.

WHAT TO EXPECT

DIAGNOSTIC MEASURES
- Your own observation of symptoms.
- Medical history and physical exam by a doctor.
- Laboratory studies such as blood studies, spinal-fluid studies, CT scan (see Glossary).
- X-rays of the skull.

APPROPRIATE HEALTH CARE
- Intensive care monitoring required.
- Medical or surgical treatment will depend on location of abscess. Normally requires antibiotic therapy and surgery to drain the abscess. Other treatment may include intravenous fluids and mechanical breathing support.
- Self-care after returning home.

POSSIBLE COMPLICATIONS
- Seizures, coma and death without treatment.
- Permanent brain damage.

PROBABLE OUTCOME—Usually curable with early diagnosis and treatment.

HOW TO TREAT

GENERAL MEASURES
- The family should maintain an optimistic outlook, stay in close contact with the patient's doctor and help by making their visits with the patient brief and as supportive as possible.
- Additional information available from the Brain Research Foundation, 208 S. LaSalle Street, Suite 1426, Chicago, IL 60604, (312)782-4311.

MEDICATION—Your doctor may prescribe:
- Antibiotics for 4 to 6 weeks to fight infection.
- Anticonvulsants to prevent seizures.
- Following surgery, corticosteroids to reduce swelling (edema).

ACTIVITY—While in the hospital, you will need bed rest. After a 2- to 3-week recovery, you should be as active as your strength and feeling of well-being allow.

DIET—While hospitalized, intravenous fluids may be necessary. Following treatment, eat a normal, well-balanced diet.

CALL YOUR DOCTOR IF

- You have any symptoms of a brain or epidural abscess.
- Fever rises to 101F (38.3C) or higher.
- New, unexplained symptoms develop. Drugs used in treatment may produce side effects.

BRAIN TUMOR

GENERAL INFORMATION

DEFINITION—An abnormal growth in the brain that may be benign or malignant. A nonmalignant brain tumor may cause as much disability as a malignant tumor unless it is treated appropriately.

BODY PARTS INVOLVED—Brain; central nervous system.

SEX OR AGE MOST AFFECTED—All ages, but most common in adults between ages 20 and 60.

SIGNS & SYMPTOMS
- Headaches that worsen when lying down.
- Vomiting with nausea, or sudden vomiting without nausea.
- Vision disturbances, including double vision.
- Weakness on one side of the body.
- Lack of balance; dizziness.
- Loss of sense of smell.
- Memory loss.
- Personality changes.
- Seizures.

CAUSES—Some tumors begin in the brain (primary tumors), but most brain tumors have spread (metastasized) from other cancers—especially cancer of the breast, lungs, intestines or melanoma of the skin. Symptoms are caused by increasing pressure in the skull as the tumor enlarges.

RISK INCREASES WITH—The following risk factors are related to cancers in other body parts that spread to the brain:
- Poor nutrition, especially a low-fiber diet (intestinal cancer).
- Smoking (lung cancer).
- Excess alcohol consumption (liver cancer).
- Excess sun exposure (melanoma).
- Previous cancer at any other body site.

HOW TO PREVENT
- Practice breast self-exam, skin self-exam and testicular self-exam (see Appendix for all).
- Don't smoke.
- Eat a high-fiber diet (see Appendix).
- Protect yourself from excessive sun exposure by using sunscreens and protective clothing.

WHAT TO EXPECT

DIAGNOSTIC MEASURES
- Your own observation of symptoms.
- Medical history and physical exam by a doctor.
- Many different techniques are used to locate the site of a brain tumor: EEG, CT scan, MRI scan (see Glossary for all), x-rays of the skull, bones, lungs and gastrointestinal tract.

APPROPRIATE HEALTH CARE
- Surgery to remove the tumor, if possible.
- Radiation therapy may be given.

POSSIBLE COMPLICATIONS—Disability and death if a tumor is inoperable because of size or location.

PROBABLE OUTCOME
- Brain tumors that are not treated lead to death or permanent brain damage. Bones of the skull restrict a tumor's outward growth, so the brain is compressed as a tumor grows.
- If a tumor is discovered and treated early with surgery or radiation therapy and chemotherapy, full recovery is often possible. For an explanation of this surgery, see Craniotomy (in Surgery section).

HOW TO TREAT

GENERAL MEASURES
- The more you can learn and understand about a disease, the more you will be able to make informed decisions about where to go for your care, the treatments available, the risks involved, side effects of therapy and expected outcome.
- Additional information available from the Association for Brain Tumor Research, 2720 River, Des Plaines, IL 60018, (708)827-9910.

MEDICATION—Your doctor may prescribe:
- Cortisone drugs to diminish swelling of the brain tissue.
- Anticonvulsant drugs to control seizures.
- Pain relievers.
- Anticancer drugs.

ACTIVITY—Will depend on your symptoms.

DIET—No special diet is necessary unless recommended by your doctor.

CALL YOUR DOCTOR IF

- You have symptoms of a brain tumor.
- New, unexplained symptoms develop. Drugs used in treatment may produce side effects.

BREAST CANCER

GENERAL INFORMATION

DEFINITION—A malignant growth of breast tissue. Breast cancer spreads to nearby lymph glands, lungs, pleura, bone (especially the skull), pelvis and liver. It may affect males (rare).

BODY PARTS INVOLVED—Nipple or tissue of the breast.

SEX OR AGE MOST AFFECTED—Women; males (rare). Breast cancer is rare before age 30; the peak ages are from 45 to 65. The incidence increases after menopause.

SIGNS & SYMPTOMS—No symptoms in early stages, but pre-symptom stages may be detected by mammogram.
- Swelling or lump in the breast.
- Vague discomfort in the breast without pain.
- Retraction of the nipple.
- Distorted breast contour.
- Dimpled or pitted skin in the breast.
- Enlarged nodes under the arm (late).
- Bloody discharge from the nipple (rare).

CAUSES—Unknown.

RISK INCREASES WITH
- Family history of breast cancer (especially mother or sister).
- Women who have not had children.
- Atypical hyperplasia on previous biopsy.
- Early menstruation (before age 12); late menopause (after age 55); first pregnancy after age 30.
- Obesity; alcohol use.
- Current or previous oral contraceptive use.
- Women over 50.
- Premenopausal or postmenopausal estrogen replacement therapy.
- Previous breast, ovarian or colon cancer.

HOW TO PREVENT
- Examine breasts monthly for signs of cancer (see Breast Self-Exam in Appendix).
- Visit your doctor regularly for an examination.
- Obtain a baseline mammogram between ages 35 to 40. Have mammograms every 1 to 2 years to age 49 and annually after 50 or as recommended by your doctor.
- Eat a well-balanced diet that is low in fat.
- If you are pregnant, consider breast-feeding your baby. Women who have breast-fed have a lower incidence of breast cancer.
- A drug such as tamoxifen, may be prescribed for women at high risk for breast cancer.

WHAT TO EXPECT

DIAGNOSTIC MEASURES
- Your own observation of symptoms.
- Medical history and exam by a doctor.
- Biopsy (see Glossary), x-rays of the breast and bones.
- Laboratory blood studies of hormones.
- After diagnosis, other tests such as ultrasound, bone scan, chest x-ray, liver scan are often performed.

APPROPRIATE HEALTH CARE
- Surgery to remove the lump, or breast, lymph glands, and lymphatic channels and muscles under the breast (sometimes). See Mastectomy in the Surgery section.
- Radiation therapy, hormonal therapy or chemotherapy (sometimes).

POSSIBLE COMPLICATIONS—Spread to vital organs if not treated early, adverse reactions to anticancer drugs and radiation, postsurgical complications (infection, limited shoulder motion).

PROBABLE OUTCOME—Many breast cancers are curable if diagnosed and treated early. The 10-year survival rate is related to the stage of the disease at diagnosis.

HOW TO TREAT

GENERAL MEASURES
- The decision for treatment is very complex, and often confusing. Be sure all options are explained and that the risks and benefits of each are thoroughly understood. It is important for you to be well informed.
- Joining a support group is helpful.
- See Resources for Additional Information.

MEDICATION—Your doctor may prescribe:
- Pain relievers.
- Anticancer drugs, such as fluorouracil, cyclophosphamide, methotrexate, chlorambucil, vincristine, doxorubicin or melphalan.
- Hormones (male and/or female).
- Cortisone drugs.

ACTIVITY
- No restrictions.
- Exercise for rehabilitation following surgery will depend on how much tissue has been removed and your general physical condition.

DIET—No special diet. Keep fat intake to a minimum.

CALL YOUR DOCTOR IF

- You find a lump or change in a breast.
- The following occurs after surgery:
  Nausea or vomiting, fever, swelling in the arm.
  Pain that is not controlled by medication.
- New, unexplained symptoms develop.

BRONCHIECTASIS

GENERAL INFORMATION

DEFINITION—A lung disease in which the bronchial tubes become blocked and accumulate thick secretions. Frequent secondary infections occur. It is not contagious unless associated with tuberculosis.

BODY PARTS INVOLVED—Lungs; bronchial tubes.

SEX OR AGE MOST AFFECTED—All ages, but most common in adults.

SIGNS & SYMPTOMS
- Frequent coughing with bad-smelling, green or yellow sputum (sometimes flecked with blood).
- Repeated lung infections.
- Shortness of breath.
- General ill feeling.
- Frequent fatigue.
- Anemia (frequently).

CAUSES—Damage to the small bronchial tubes, which may develop over years. Common sources of damage include:
- Cigarette smoking.
- Repeated lung infections (pneumonia).
- Chronic bronchitis.
- Allergies; smoke or dust.
- Inhalation of a foreign object.
- Tuberculosis.
- Fungus infection.
- Cystic fibrosis.

RISK INCREASES WITH
- Smoking.
- Poor nutrition; obesity.
- Family history of tuberculosis.
- Fatigue or overwork.
- Exposure to allergens.
- Cold, humid weather.

HOW TO PREVENT
- Don't ever smoke.
- Obtain medical treatment for lung infections.
- Avoid as many risks as possible.
- Get immunization against influenza and pneumonia.
- Use a cool mist humidifier in the child's room.

WHAT TO EXPECT

DIAGNOSTIC MEASURES
- Your own observation of symptoms.
- Medical history and physical exam by a doctor. Sputum culture, x-rays of the lung, including a bronchogram (see Glossary).

APPROPRIATE HEALTH CARE
- Self-care after diagnosis.
- Doctor's treatment.
- Surgery to remove isolated areas of damaged lung tissue (rare).

POSSIBLE COMPLICATIONS
- COPD (chronic obstructive pulmonary disease).
- Repeated pneumonia.
- Destruction of lung tissue.

PROBABLE OUTCOME—With treatment, most patients with bronchiectasis can lead nearly normal lives without major disability.

HOW TO TREAT

GENERAL MEASURES
- Don't smoke.
- Learn and practice postural drainage (see Glossary) twice a day.
- Sleep with 3- to 5-inch blocks under the foot of the bed to prevent mucus from collecting in the lower lobes of the lungs.
- If you work around heavy air pollution, do everything possible to limit your exposure—including changing jobs.
- Install air conditioning with a filter and humidity control in your home.
- Avoid sudden temperature changes.
- Avoid loud talking, loud laughing, crying, exertion or sudden temperature changes, if these trigger coughing episodes.
- Keep the teeth and mouth in excellent condition.
- If you have an allergic background, avoid allergens.
- See Resources for Additional Information.

MEDICATION—Your doctor may prescribe:
- Antibiotics for 10 days every month if bacterial infections have caused bronchiectasis or triggered episodes of pneumonia or acute bronchitis.
- Bronchodilators to enlarge airways.
- Expectorants to loosen secretions.

ACTIVITY—Remain as active as possible.

DIET—Increase fluid intake. Drink a minimum of 8 glasses of fluid a day. This thins lung secretions so they can be coughed out more easily.

CALL YOUR DOCTOR IF

- You have symptoms of bronchiectasis.
- After diagnosis, you have symptoms of a respiratory infection or bronchitis.
- You have a fever.
- Blood appears in the sputum, sputum thickens despite treatment, or postural drainage reveals a change in color, amount or character of sputum.
- Chest pain increases.
- Shortness of breath occurs without coughing or when at rest.

BRONCHIOLITIS

GENERAL INFORMATION

DEFINITION—Inflammation of the bronchioles, the smallest branches of the respiratory tree. These carry air from the large bronchial tubes to microscopic air sacs in the lungs. The air sacs transfer oxygen to the bloodstream. Bronchiolitis may be confused with inhaled objects lodged in the child's lung.

BODY PARTS INVOLVED—Bronchioles.

SEX OR AGE MOST AFFECTED—Children under age 6.

SIGNS & SYMPTOMS—Sudden breathing difficulty, usually preceded by a mild common cold and cough, and characterized by the following:
• Wheezing.
• Rapid, shallow breathing (60 to 80 times a minute).
• Retractions (see-saw movements) of the chest and abdomen.
• Fever (occasionally).
• Dehydration.
• Blue skin or nails (severe cases).

CAUSES—Viral or bacterial infection, or a combination of the two. Some young children develop this disorder after every cold. Bronchiolitis is contagious and often becomes epidemic.

RISK INCREASES WITH
• Illness that has lowered resistance, especially respiratory infection.
• Family history of allergies.
• Day care environment.
• Contact with an infected person.

HOW TO PREVENT
• Observe and avoid any activities that seem to trigger attacks in the child, such as active play in cool night air.
• Decrease the child's exposure to groups of people, especially other children, to avoid colds.

WHAT TO EXPECT

DIAGNOSTIC MEASURES
• Your own observation of symptoms.
• Medical history and physical exam by a doctor.
• Laboratory blood studies.
• X-rays of the lungs.

APPROPRIATE HEALTH CARE
• Home care.
• Doctor's treatment.
• Hospitalization for intensive care and oxygen (severe cases).

POSSIBLE COMPLICATIONS—Permanent lung damage leading to chronic bronchitis, collapse of a small portion of the lung, bronchiectasis, repeated pneumonia, and rarely, chronic obstructive pulmonary disease (COPD).

PROBABLE OUTCOME—Usually curable in 7 days with treatment. Some studies indicate that infants who have 2 or more episodes of bronchiolitis before age 2 are more likely to develop allergies and asthma.

HOW TO TREAT

GENERAL MEASURES
• Keep the humidity in the child's room as high as possible. Use an ultrasonic, cool-mist humidifier. Clean humidifier daily. If you don't have a humidifier, run cold or hot water in the shower with windows and doors closed to produce a high-humidity room. Hold the child in this room for 20 minutes several times a day, especially at bedtime. If the child awakens at night with wheezing or shortness of breath, repeat the process.
• Breathing cool outside air may help.

MEDICATION—Your doctor may prescribe:
• Antibiotics to fight bacterial infections.
• Antiviral medications may help in severe cases.
• Bronchodilators (drugs that widen the airways in the lungs) may be helpful.

ACTIVITY—Have the child rest until symptoms have subsided for 48 hours. Then normal activities may be resumed gradually.

DIET—Offer the child clear fluids frequently. Give water, tea, carbonated drinks, lemonade, weak bouillon, diluted fruit juice or gelatin.

CALL YOUR DOCTOR IF

• Symptoms don't improve in 4 hours, despite treatment.
• Temperature (rectal) rises to 101F (38.3C) or higher.
• Breathing becomes more difficult.
• A cough begins that produces colored phlegm.
• The skin, lips or nails turn dark blue.
• The child becomes lethargic.

BRONCHITIS, ACUTE

GENERAL INFORMATION

DEFINITION—Inflammation of the air passages of the lungs. Acute bronchitis is of sudden onset and short duration while chronic bronchitis is persistent over a long period and recurring over several years.

BODY PARTS INVOLVED—Trachea; bronchi; bronchioles.

SEX OR AGE MOST AFFECTED—Both sexes; all ages.

SIGNS & SYMPTOMS
- Cough that produces little or no sputum initially, but does later on.
- Low fever (usually less than 101F or 38.3C).
- Burning chest discomfort or feeling of pressure behind the breastbone.
- Wheezing or uncomfortable breathing (sometimes).

CAUSES
- Infection from one of many respiratory viruses. Most cases of acute bronchitis begin with a cold virus in the nose and throat that spreads to the airways. A secondary bacterial infection is common.
- Lung inflammation from breathing air that contains irritants, such as chemical fumes (ammonia), acid fumes, dust or smoke.

RISK INCREASES WITH
- Chronic obstructive pulmonary disease (COPD), asthma, sinusitis.
- Cold, humid weather.
- Smoking; second hand smoke.
- Recent illness that has lowered resistance.
- Contact with an infected person.
- Children in day care environments.
- Immunosuppression from drugs or illness.
- Poor nutrition; elderly and very young.

HOW TO PREVENT
- Avoid exposure.
- Avoid smoking.
- Control of risk factors.

WHAT TO EXPECT

DIAGNOSTIC MEASURES
- Your own observation of symptoms.
- Medical history and physical exam by a doctor.
- Laboratory blood counts to detect complicating infections and cultures of sputum and blood to identify the bacteria.
- X-rays of the chest (for complications only).

APPROPRIATE HEALTH CARE
- Self-care, if you are in good overall health.
- Doctor's treatment, if you have chronic lung disease or complications develop.

POSSIBLE COMPLICATIONS
- Bacterial lung infection (various kinds of pneumonia).
- Chronic bronchitis from recurrent episodes of acute bronchitis.
- Pleurisy (inflammation of the lining of the lungs) (rare).

PROBABLE OUTCOME—Usually curable with treatment in 1 week. Cases with complications are usually curable in 2 weeks with medication. Cough may last several weeks after initial improvement.

HOW TO TREAT

GENERAL MEASURES
- If you are a smoker, don't smoke during your illness. This delays recovery and makes complications more likely.
- Increase air moisture. Take frequent hot showers. Use a cool-mist, ultrasonic humidifier by your bed. Clean humidifier daily.

MEDICATION
- For minor discomfort, you may use: Acetaminophen to reduce fever. Nonprescription cough suppressants. Use only if your cough is nonproductive (without sputum). It may be dangerous to stop a cough entirely—this traps excess mucus and irritants in bronchial tubes, leading to pneumonia and poor oxygen exchange in the lungs.
- Your doctor may prescribe: Antibiotics to fight bacterial infections. Expectorants to thin mucus so it can be coughed up more easily. Cough suppressants.

ACTIVITY—Rest in bed until temperature returns to normal. Then resume normal activity gradually as symptoms improve.

DIET—No special diet. Drink at least 8 to 10 glasses of fluid each day to help thin mucus secretions so they can be coughed up more easily.

CALL YOUR DOCTOR IF

- You have symptoms of bronchitis.
- The following occurs during the illness:
  High fever and chills.
  Chest pain.
  Thickened, discolored or blood-streaked sputum.
  Shortness of breath, even when the body is at rest.
  Vomiting.

BRONCHITIS, CHRONIC

GENERAL INFORMATION

DEFINITION—Chronic inflammation and degeneration of the bronchial tubes, with or without active infection. It is most commonly associated with cigarette smoking.

BODY PARTS INVOLVED—Bronchial tubes (bronchi).

SEX OR AGE MOST AFFECTED—All ages, but most common in adults, usually men.

SIGNS & SYMPTOMS
- Frequent cough or coughing spasms.
- Shortness of breath.
- Sputum that is thick and difficult to cough up. Sputum production varies according to whether infection is present.
- Barrel chest (in the late stages).

CAUSES—Repeated irritation or infection in the bronchial tubes, causing them to thicken, narrow and lose elasticity. Underlying irritants include allergens, air pollution and tobacco smoke.

RISK INCREASES WITH
- Smoking (the greatest risk factor).
- Any lung illness that has lowered resistance.
- Family history of tuberculosis or other disease of the respiratory tract.
- Exposure to air pollutants.
- Poor nutrition.
- Obesity.
- Crowded living conditions.

HOW TO PREVENT
- Don't smoke. This is the most reversible risk.
- Avoid irritating fumes in the environment.
- Obtain prompt medical treatment for respiratory infections.

WHAT TO EXPECT

DIAGNOSTIC MEASURES
- Your own observation of symptoms.
- Medical history and physical exam by a doctor.
- Laboratory studies of sputum and pulmonary function.
- X-rays of the chest.

APPROPRIATE HEALTH CARE
- Self-care after diagnosis.
- Doctor's treatment. Many lung and heart disorders cause symptoms identical to those of chronic bronchitis. Your doctor must exclude these possibilities to make a diagnosis.
- Treatment does not cure, but it can relieve symptoms and help prevent complications.

POSSIBLE COMPLICATIONS
- Recurrent pneumonia.

- Chronic obstructive pulmonary disease (COPD). COPD is incurable. It is characterized by purple lips and nails and congestive heart failure.

PROBABLE OUTCOME—Chronic bronchitis is usually curable with treatment—if you are a nonsmoker and don't have an underlying chronic disease, such as congestive heart failure, bronchiectasis or tuberculosis. Chronic bronchitis usually reduces life expectancy if you smoke and don't stop, or if you have an underlying chronic disease.

HOW TO TREAT

GENERAL MEASURES
- Stop smoking.
- If you work or live in an area with heavy air pollution, do everything you can to avoid or reduce it. Consider changing jobs and installing air-conditioning with a filter and humidity control in your home.
- Avoid sudden temperature changes or exposure to cold, wet weather.
- Avoid talking loudly, laughing loudly, crying and exertion, if these trigger coughing episodes.
- Practice bronchial drainage and deep-breathing techniques. Your physician will provide instructions.
- Sleep with 5-inch blocks under the foot of your bed.
- See Resources for Additional Information.

MEDICATION
- Don't take cough suppressants; they make chronic bronchitis worse.
- Your doctor may prescribe:
  Antibiotics to fight chronic or recurrent infection.
  Expectorants to loosen secretions.
  Bronchodilators to open bronchial tubes.
  Drugs to treat severe depression or anxiety if they occur.

ACTIVITY—No restrictions. A regular exercise routine is important as prolonged inactivity leads to excessive disability.

DIET—No special diet. Increase fluid intake to 8 to 10 glasses a day.

CALL YOUR DOCTOR IF

- You have symptoms of chronic bronchitis.
- You develop fever.
- Blood appears in the sputum.
- Chest pain increases.
- Shortness of breath occurs even when you are resting or not coughing.
- Sputum thickens despite efforts to thin it.

ILLNESS & DISORDERS

BRUCELLOSIS
(Undulant Fever; Bang's Disease)

 GENERAL INFORMATION

DEFINITION—A rare bacterial infection transmitted to humans from infected cows, pigs, sheep or goats. It is not contagious from person to person. The disease has an acute form (symptoms appear suddenly) and a chronic form (symptoms appear gradually).

BODY PARTS INVOLVED—Blood-producing organs, including bone marrow, lymph glands, liver and spleen.

SEX OR AGE MOST AFFECTED—Both sexes and all ages, but most common in men between ages 20 and 60.

SIGNS & SYMPTOMS—
Acute form:
* Chills, intermittent fever, sweating.
* Marked fatigue.
* Tenderness along the spine.
* Headache.
* Enlarged lymph glands.
Chronic form:
* Fatigue.
* Muscle pain.
* Backache.
* Constipation.
* Weight loss.
* Depression.
* Sexual impotence.
* Abscesses in the ovaries, kidney and brain (rare).

CAUSES—Infection from the bacteria, Brucella, which is transmitted to humans through unpasteurized milk or milk products (butter, cheese) or meat products.

RISK INCREASES WITH
* Pernicious anemia or previous stomach surgery. These conditions result in reduced stomach acid; stomach acid decreases the chance of infection.
* Persons with occupations involving animals, such as farmers, butchers, veterinarians or ranchers.
* Travel to some foreign countries.

HOW TO PREVENT
* Don't drink unpasteurized milk from any source.
* Use gloves and aprons when working around animals.
* Immunization of livestock.

 WHAT TO EXPECT

DIAGNOSTIC MEASURES
* Your own observation of symptoms.
* Medical history and physical exam by a doctor.
* Laboratory blood studies.

APPROPRIATE HEALTH CARE
* Doctor's treatment.
* Hospitalization.
* Self-care after treatment of the acute phase.

POSSIBLE COMPLICATIONS
* Heart, bone, brain or liver infection (rare).
* Chronic illness and disability from inadequate treatment and care.

PROBABLE OUTCOME—Usually curable in 3 to 4 weeks with treatment.

 HOW TO TREAT

GENERAL MEASURES
* It usually is not necessary to isolate the ill person.
* All family members who may have been exposed to the same infected milk products should have medical checkups and diagnostic tests.

MEDICATION—Your doctor may prescribe:
* Antibiotics to fight infection, such as tetracycline, for a minimum of 3 weeks.
* Cortisone drugs to reduce the inflammatory response in severe cases.
* Pain relievers for muscle pain.

ACTIVITY—Rest in bed until fever and other symptoms subside. Resume your normal activities gradually.

DIET—No special diet. Increase calories if weight loss has been significant.

 CALL YOUR DOCTOR IF

* You have symptoms of undulant fever.
* Fever or other symptoms recur after treatment.

BUERGER'S DISEASE
(Thromboangiitis Obliterans)

 GENERAL INFORMATION

DEFINITION—Blockage of small and medium arteries—usually in the legs and feet—from inflammation of blood vessels. This causes clot formation.

Cigarette-smoking is a very important factor in developing this disease. It is extremely rare among nonsmokers.

BODY PARTS INVOLVED—Arteries (and sometimes veins) in the extremities.

SEX OR AGE MOST AFFECTED—Both sexes, but most common in cigarette-smoking men between ages 20 and 40.

SIGNS & SYMPTOMS
• Intermittent pain in the instep or the leg when exercising. The pain improves with rest.
• Pain, blueness, heat and tingling in the legs when exposed to cold.
• Painful ulcers on the toes and fingertips (sometimes).

CAUSES—Unknown, but the disease is probably triggered by nicotine. Cigarette-smoking causes blood-vessel spasms, leading to obstruction of the essential blood vessels in the extremities.

RISK INCREASES WITH
• Collagen disease or atherosclerosis.
• Stress.
• Cold weather.
• Family history of Buerger's disease.

HOW TO PREVENT
• Don't smoke.
• Avoid exposure to the cold. This also causes blood vessels to constrict and deprives extremities of a normal blood supply.

 WHAT TO EXPECT

DIAGNOSTIC MEASURES
• Your own observation of symptoms.
• Medical history and physical exam by a doctor.
• Laboratory studies, such as ultrasound, plethysmography to help detect decreased circulation in the peripheral vessels and arteriography to locate lesions (see Glossary for all).

APPROPRIATE HEALTH CARE
• Self-care after diagnosis.
• Doctor's treatment.
• Surgery (sympathectomy) to cut sympathetic nerves to the area (sometimes).

POSSIBLE COMPLICATIONS
• Fingertip ulcerations.
• Muscle atrophy.
• Gangrene in the foot or leg caused by a loss of blood supply. This may result in amputation.

PROBABLE OUTCOME—This condition is currently considered incurable. However, symptoms can be controlled for a while, but the disease causes increasing disability—especially if amputation is necessary.

Life expectancy is reduced.
Scientific research into causes and treatment continues, so there is hope for increasingly effective treatment and cure.

 HOW TO TREAT

GENERAL MEASURES
• Other measures are rarely successful if smoking continues, so stop smoking.
• Avoid exposure to the cold. Wear warm footwear and gloves.
• Clip nails carefully to avoid injuring the skin.
• Wear well-fitting shoes and cotton or wool socks. Don't wear socks made of synthetic material.
• Insert soft padding in your shoes to protect your feet.
• Don't go barefoot outdoors.
• Counseling may be recommended to help with lifestyle changes required to cope with the restrictions of the disease.

MEDICATION—Your doctor may prescribe vasodilator drugs, but they are usually useless if you continue smoking.

ACTIVITY—Avoid cold weather, but stay active. Begin a conditioning program to become as physically fit as possible.

DIET—No special diet.

 CALL YOUR DOCTOR IF

• You have symptoms of Buerger's disease.
• Uncontrollable pain begins.
• Ulcers develop on your toes or feet.

BULIMIA NERVOSA

 GENERAL INFORMATION

DEFINITION—A psychological eating disorder characterized by abnormal perception of body image, constant craving for food and binge eating, followed by self-induced vomiting or laxative use.

BODY PARTS INVOLVED—Brain and central nervous system; kidneys; liver; endocrine system; gastrointestinal tract.

SEX OR AGE MOST AFFECTED—Adolescents or young adults, usually female.

SIGNS & SYMPTOMS—Recurrent episodes of binge eating (rapid consumption of a large amount of food in a short time, usually less than 2 hours), plus at least 3 of the following:
- Preference for high-calorie, convenience foods during a binge.
- Secretive eating during a binge. Patients are aware that the eating pattern is abnormal, and they fear being unable to stop eating.
- Termination of an eating binge with purging measures, such as laxative use or self-induced vomiting.
- Depression and guilt following an eating binge.
- Repeated attempts to lose weight with severely restrictive diets, self-induced vomiting and use of laxatives or diuretics.
- Frequent weight fluctuations greater than 10 pounds from alternately fasting and gorging.
- No underlying physical disorder.

CAUSES—Unknown. Thought to be largely emotional.

RISK INCREASES WITH
- Strict, compulsive, perfectionistic family environment.
- Anorexia nervosa.
- Depression.
- Stress, including lifestyle changes, such as moving or starting a new school or job.
- Neurotic preoccupation with being physically attractive.
- Ballet dancers, gymnasts, models, cheerleaders and athletes.

HOW TO PREVENT
- Encourage rational attitude about weight.
- Enhance self-esteem.
- Avoid overly high self-expectations.
- Avoid stress.

 WHAT TO EXPECT

DIAGNOSTIC MEASURES
- Your own observation of symptoms. Many patients are secretive, and parents may be unaware of this condition.
- Medical history and physical exam by a doctor.
- Laboratory blood studies, including measurement of electrolyte levels.

APPROPRIATE HEALTH CARE
- Doctor's treatment.
- Psychotherapy or counseling that may include hypnosis or biofeedback training.
- Treatment in an eating disorder facility (sometimes).
- Hospitalization (severe cases).

POSSIBLE COMPLICATIONS
- Fluid and electrolyte imbalance from vomiting; dental disease; stomach rupture (rare).
- Without treatment, complications can be fatal.
- Relapse.

PROBABLE OUTCOME—Outcome is variable; patients can learn to control the behavior with counseling, psychotherapy, biofeedback training and individual or group psychotherapy.

 HOW TO TREAT

GENERAL MEASURES
- Those who stay in therapy have the best chance to improve.
- See Resources for Additional Information.

MEDICATION—Antidepressants are frequently helpful in this disorder.

ACTIVITY—No restrictions.

DIET
- If hospitalization is necessary:
  Intravenous fluids may be prescribed. During recovery, vitamin and mineral supplements will be necessary until signs of deficiency disappear and normal eating patterns are established.
- For outpatient therapy:
  Supervision and regulation of eating habits. A food diary may be maintained. Feared foods will be reintroduced.

 CALL YOUR DOCTOR IF

- You have symptoms of bulimia or you suspect your child has bulimia.
- The following occurs during treatment:
  Rapid, irregular heartbeat or chest pain.
  Loss of consciousness.
  Cessation of menstrual periods.
  Repeated vomiting or diarrhea.
  Continued weight loss, despite treatment.

BUNION
(Hallux Valgus)

GENERAL INFORMATION

DEFINITION—A bony protrusion from the outside edge of the joint at the base of the big (first) toe.

BODY PARTS INVOLVED—Great (big) toe.

SEX OR AGE MOST AFFECTED—Female adolescents and adults.

SIGNS & SYMPTOMS
- An inward-turned great toe that may overlap the second—and sometimes the third—toe.
- Thickened skin over the bony protrusion at the base of the great toe.
- Fluid accumulation under the thickened skin (sometimes).
- Foot pain and stiffness.

CAUSES—Hallux valgus. The technical name for the big toe is hallux. If the big toe has grown or been forced into a position where it overlaps one or more of the other toes, that is called hallux valgus.

RISK INCREASES WITH
- Family history of foot abnormalities (inherited weakness in toe joints).
- Arthritis.
- Narrow-toed, high-heeled shoes that compress toes together.

HOW TO PREVENT
- Exercise daily to keep muscles of the feet and legs in good condition.
- Wear wide-toed shoes that fit well. Don't wear high heels or shoes without room for toes in their normal position.

WHAT TO EXPECT

DIAGNOSTIC MEASURES
- Your own observation of symptoms.
- Medical history and physical exam by a doctor.
- X-rays of the foot.

APPROPRIATE HEALTH CARE
- Self-care in the early stages. This may prevent a bunion from worsening.
- Doctor's (orthopedist's or podiatrist's) treatment. Orthotics (molded shoe inserts) will frequently reduce symptoms and delay the need for surgery.
- Surgery to remove the overgrown tissue (bunion) and correct the position of the bones (see Bunion Removal in Surgery section).

POSSIBLE COMPLICATIONS
- Infection of the bunion, especially in persons with diabetes mellitus.
- Inflammation and arthritic changes in other joints caused by walking difficulty, which places abnormal stress on the foot, hip and spine.

PROBABLE OUTCOME—Usually curable with treatment and preventive measures to guard against recurrence.

HOW TO TREAT

GENERAL MEASURES
- Before bedtime, separate the great toe from the others with a foam-rubber pad.
- Wear a thick, ring-shaped adhesive pad around and over the bunion.
- Use arch supports to relieve pressure on the bunion. These are available in shoe-repair shops.

MEDICATION—Medicine usually is not necessary for this disorder unless infection develops.

ACTIVITY—If surgery is necessary, resume your normal activities gradually afterward. Walk on your heels until the surgical site heals. Elevate the foot of the bed to reduce swelling.

DIET—No special diet.

CALL YOUR DOCTOR IF

- You have a bunion that is interfering with normal activities.
- Signs of infection, such as fever, heat, tenderness or pain, develop after treatment or surgery.

BURNS

GENERAL INFORMATION

DEFINITION—Injury to the skin, and sometimes other organs, from contact with heat, radiation, electricity or chemicals.

BODY PARTS INVOLVED—Skin; underlying tissue and respiratory system (sometimes).

SEX OR AGE MOST AFFECTED—Both sexes; all ages. The risk of damage is greatest with infants and young children.

SIGNS & SYMPTOMS—Burns are of 3 types:
* 1st-degree burns are limited to the upper skin layer. They produce redness, tenderness, pain, swelling and slight fever.
* 2nd-degree burns affect deeper skin layers. Symptoms are more severe and include blisters.
* 3rd-degree burns involve all skin layers. Skin is white (appears cooked), and there may be no pain in the initial stages.

CAUSES
* Rise in skin temperature from heat sources, such as fire, steam or electricity.
* Tissue injury caused by chemicals or radiation, including sunlight.
* Lightning strikes can cause internal burns with minimal external signs.

RISK INCREASES WITH
* Stress, carelessness, smoking in bed or excess alcohol consumption, all of which make accidents more likely.
* Occupations involving exposure to heat or radiation, such as firefighting, police work or defense-factory work.
* Faulty wiring.
* Hot water heaters set too high.

HOW TO PREVENT
* Wear sun-screen lotions outdoors.
* Fireproof your home. Install smoke alarms, plan emergency exits and have regular fire drills.
* Wear protective gear and observe safety precautions around heat or radiation.
* Don't touch uncovered electric wires.
* Teach children safety rules for matches, fires, electrical outlets and cords.
* If you have small children, put safety caps on unused outlets. Discard frayed cords.

WHAT TO EXPECT

DIAGNOSTIC MEASURES
* Your own observation of symptoms.
* Medical history and physical exam by a doctor.
* Laboratory blood and urine tests, and studies of kidney and liver function (severe burns).

APPROPRIATE HEALTH CARE
* Self-care for most 1st-degree burns.
* Doctor's treatment for more severe burns.
* Hospitalization for all large 3rd-degree burns and some 2nd-degree burns. Special burn centers exist for the worst cases.
* Surgery to graft skin over 3rd-degree burns (see Skin Graft in Surgery section).

POSSIBLE COMPLICATIONS—Infection at the burn site; pneumonia; shock due to loss of fluids and electrolytes (severe burns); permanent scars; vision impairment, if eyes are injured; tetanus and other infections.

PROBABLE OUTCOME—Most persons recover if the extent of burns (including 3rd-degree burns) is limited to 50% of the body surface. For less-severe burns, skin usually repairs itself in 1 to 3 weeks.

HOW TO TREAT

GENERAL MEASURES—For severe burns see Emergency First Aid section. For less-severe burns:
* Apply nonprescription body lotion to cool 1st-degree burns.
* Immerse small 2nd- or 3rd-degree burn areas in cold water for 10 minutes to reduce pain and swelling.
* Keep the burn area clean. Soak in a tub or use lukewarm compresses once a day. You may add 2 tablespoons of powdered detergent to the tub to help soak off crusting areas. Use plain water for compresses.
* Prop the burn area higher than the rest of the body, if possible.
* You may use dressings on the burn.

MEDICATION
* To treat minor burns, you may use nonprescription antibiotic ointments, topical anesthetics and aspirin.
* To treat severe burns, your doctor may prescribe pain relievers, antibiotics and tetanus booster shots.

ACTIVITY—Depends on location and extent of the burn. Getting a burn patient up and moving as soon as possible after treatment begins is an important part of the recovery

DIET—No special diet for minor burns. More severe burns require intravenous feeding.

CALL YOUR DOCTOR IF

* You or a family member has been burned. This can be an emergency.
* An infant has a burn, even if it seems minor.
* The following occur during treatment: No healing in 6 days; chills and fever; increased pain, redness, swelling or pus in the burn area.

BURSITIS

GENERAL INFORMATION

DEFINITION—Inflammation of bursa, a soft fluid-filled sac that serves as a cushion between tendons and bones.

BODY PARTS INVOLVED—Bursae, especially near the shoulders, elbows, knees, pelvis, hips or Achilles tendons.

SEX OR AGE MOST AFFECTED—Adults of all ages.

SIGNS & SYMPTOMS
- Pain, tenderness and limited movement in the affected area with radiation of pain into the neck, arm, fingertips.
- Severe pain with movement of the arm.
- Fever (sometimes).

CAUSES
- Injury to a joint.
- Overuse of a joint.
- Strenuous, unaccustomed exercise.
- Calcium deposits in shoulder tendons with degeneration of the tendon.
- Acute or chronic infection.
- Arthritis.
- Gout.
- Unknown (frequently).

RISK INCREASES WITH
- People who are involved in vigorous and repetitive athletic training.
- Exercise or sports participants who suddenly increase their activity levels ("weekend warriors").
- Improper or overstretching.

HOW TO PREVENT
- Avoid injuries or overuse of muscles whenever possible. Wear protective gear for contact sports.
- Appropriate warm-up and cool-down.
- Maintain a high fitness level.

WHAT TO EXPECT

DIAGNOSTIC MEASURES
- Your own observation of symptoms.
- Medical history and physical exam by a doctor.
- X-rays of the affected area.

APPROPRIATE HEALTH CARE
- Self-care after diagnosis.
- Doctor's treatment.

POSSIBLE COMPLICATIONS—Frozen joint or permanent limitation of a joint's mobility.

PROBABLE OUTCOME—This is a common—but not serious—problem. Symptoms usually subside in 7 to 14 days with treatment.

HOW TO TREAT

GENERAL MEASURES
- RICE therapy (rest, ice, compression and elevation of affected joint). See RICE therapy in Appendix.
- Apply ice packs to the affected area during a flare-up or after receiving injections in the joint.
- After the acute stage, continued ice treatment (until inflammation subsides) or heat application may be recommended. If you use heat, take hot showers, use a heat lamp, apply hot compresses or a heating pad, or rub in deep-heating ointment.
- Invasive therapy may include aspiration of the joint or surgical excision.

MEDICATION—Your doctor may prescribe:
- Nonsteroidal anti-inflammatory drugs.
- Cortisone injections into the bursa to reduce inflammation.
- Pain relievers.

ACTIVITY—Rest the inflamed area as much as possible. If you must resume normal activity immediately, wear a sling until the pain becomes more bearable. To prevent a frozen joint (especially in the shoulder), begin normal, slow joint movement as soon as possible.

DIET—No special diet.

CALL YOUR DOCTOR IF

- You have symptoms of bursitis.
- Pain increases, despite treatment.
- New, unexplained symptoms develop. Drugs used in treatment may produce side effects.

ILLNESS & DISORDERS

CALCIUM IMBALANCE
(Hypercalcemia; Hypocalcemia)

 GENERAL INFORMATION

DEFINITION—Calcium is a mineral component of blood that helps regulate the heartbeat, transmit nerve impulses, contract muscles and form bone and teeth. Too much calcium (hypercalcemia) or too little calcium (hypocalcemia) can cause serious, sometimes life-threatening medical problems.

BODY PARTS INVOLVED—Membranes of all body cells; muscles; bones; parathyroid glands and parathyroid hormones (these regulate calcium absorption and utilization).

SEX OR AGE MOST AFFECTED—Both sexes; all ages.

SIGNS & SYMPTOMS
Too little calcium:
- Muscle spasms, twitching or cramps.
- Numbness and tingling in the arms, legs, hands and feet.
- Seizures.
- Irregular heartbeat.
- High blood pressure.

Too much calcium:
- Lethargy.
- Appetite loss.
- Vomiting and diarrhea.
- Dehydration and thirst.
- Irregular heartbeat.
- Low blood pressure.
- Depression, delirium, confusion.
- Seizures or coma (worst cases only).

CAUSES
Too little calcium:
- Underactive parathyroid glands from disease or damage during neck surgery.
- Inadequate intake of calcium and vitamin D.
- Malabsorption from the gastrointestinal tract (usually for unknown reasons).
- Severe burns or infections.
- Pancreatitis.
- Kidney failure.
- Decreased blood levels of magnesium.

Too much calcium:
- Overactive parathyroid glands.
- Multiple fractures and prolonged bed rest; multiple myeloma.
- Tumors that destroy bone.

RISK INCREASES WITH
Too little calcium:
- Use of certain drugs, including thiazide diuretics and calcium-channel blockers.
- Injury, cancer or surgery of the thyroid gland or parathyroid glands.
- Excess alcohol leading to poor nutrition.

Too much calcium:
- Improper diet, especially overconsumption of milk products or antacids containing calcium.

- Repeated transfusions with citrated blood.
- Chronic kidney disease.
- Inactivity or prolonged bed rest.

HOW TO PREVENT
- Eat a normal, balanced diet.
- Don't drink more than 1 or 2 alcoholic drinks—if any—a day.
- Don't use nonprescription antacids on a regular basis.

 WHAT TO EXPECT

DIAGNOSTIC MEASURES
- Your own observation of symptoms.
- Medical history and exam by a doctor.
- Laboratory blood studies of calcium levels.
- ECG (see Glossary), x-rays of bones.

APPROPRIATE HEALTH CARE
- Doctor's treatment.
- Hospitalization.
- Self-care after hospitalization.

POSSIBLE COMPLICATIONS
- Cardiac arrest.
- Fractures of weak bones.
- Kidney stones (high calcium).
- Peptic ulcer (high calcium).

PROBABLE OUTCOME—Most cases are curable with treatment in 1 week, unless the calcium imbalance is caused by cancer.

 HOW TO TREAT

GENERAL MEASURES—The underlying cause must be corrected before you can follow a treatment program to prevent a recurrence.

MEDICATION—Your doctor may prescribe:
- Intravenous calcium gluconate or calcium carbonate for too little calcium.
- Intravenous saline solution and loop diuretics (furosemide and ethacrynic acid) for too much calcium.

ACTIVITY—After treatment, resume your normal activities as symptoms improve.

DIET
- For a mild, low calcium level, take calcium supplements and vitamin D. Increase your intake of protein, milk and milk products.
- For a mild, high calcium level, restrict consumption of dairy products and calcium-containing antacids.

 CALL YOUR DOCTOR IF

- You have symptoms of a calcium imbalance.
- Symptoms recur after treatment.

CANDIDIASIS OF SKIN
(Moniliasis)

 GENERAL INFORMATION

DEFINITION—A yeast infection in skin folds or areas of intertriginous (adjacent) skin that come in contact with each other, such as in the groin or under the breasts. This is mildly contagious from person to person and from place to place on the same person.

BODY PARTS INVOLVED—It can affect the skin of the scrotum, vagina and vaginal lips; underarm area; spaces between fingers and toes; inner thighs; under the breasts; and over the base of the spine (sacrum).

SEX OR AGE MOST AFFECTED—Both sexes; all ages.

SIGNS & SYMPTOMS—Plaques (patches or flat areas) with the following characteristics:
• Bright red patches with poorly defined borders, often 6 cm to 12 cm in diameter or larger.
• Some plaques are weeping or oozing.
• Skin appears moist or crusted.
• Itching is usually severe.
• Smaller plaques (less than 1 mm in size) sometimes surround larger plaques. They rarely form small pustules (small white blisters with pus inside).

CAUSES
• Yeast infection of the skin caused by candida fungus (usually Candida albicans). The spore form of this organism normally grows in the intestinal tract and the vagina. Skin signs do not begin until yeast changes from its spore form to another growth phase, the mycelial phase. Damaged skin, moisture and warmth are all necessary for the infection to take over.
• Inadequate immunity from the disease or immunosuppressant drugs.

RISK INCREASES WITH
• Use of oral antibiotics.
• Use of steroids (oral, injectable or topical).
• Diabetes; obesity; poor nutrition.
• Excessive sweating.
• Crowded or unsanitary living conditions.
• Use of birth control pills.
• Douching.

HOW TO PREVENT
• Take antibiotics only when prescribed.
• Avoid excessive sweets.
• Keep skin cool and dry.
• Wear cotton underwear.

 WHAT TO EXPECT

DIAGNOSTIC MEASURES
• Your own observation of symptoms.
• Laboratory study of a skin scraping or pus.

APPROPRIATE HEALTH CARE
• Treatment involves therapy for the disorder and the underlying condition that predisposes you to candidiasis.
• Self-care after surgery.

POSSIBLE COMPLICATIONS
• Secondary bacterial infections (rare).
• Id reactions (allergic response to a skin disorder) (rare).
• Blood poisoning (rare).

PROBABLE OUTCOME
• Usually curable in 2 weeks with treatment. Without treatment, healing may be slow (up to 4 to 5 years).
• Recurrence is common.

 HOW TO TREAT

GENERAL MEASURES
• Keep skin cool and dry. Expose affected areas to sunlight as much as possible.
• Wear loose cotton clothing. Avoid synthetic or wool fabrics.
• Protect skin from injury.

MEDICATION—Antifungal topical medications are usually prescribed. Gently massage a small amount into the affected area as directed. Use only enough to cover. Larger amounts don't help.

ACTIVITY—No restrictions, except to avoid heat and sweating.

DIET—No special diet. Eating yogurt, buttermilk or sour cream, or taking acidophilus tablets may help prevent yeast infections that may result as an adverse effect of the drugs.

 CALL YOUR DOCTOR IF

• You or a family member has symptoms of candidiasis.
• The following occur during treatment:
  Infection continues to spread, despite treatment.
  Signs of secondary bacterial infection develop (pain, tenderness, redness, warmth, oozing).
• New unexplained symptoms develop. Drugs used in treatment may produce side effects.

CANKER SORES
(Aphthous Ulcers)

 GENERAL INFORMATION

DEFINITION—Painful ulcers that occur in the lining of the mouth. Ulcers are not cancerous, but may be contagious. They may be confused with herpes infections.

BODY PARTS INVOLVED—Mouth and adjacent areas.

SEX OR AGE MOST AFFECTED—Both sexes, but more common in women.

SIGNS & SYMPTOMS—Mouth ulcers with the following characteristics:
• Ulcers are small, very painful, shallow and covered by a gray membrane. Borders are surrounded by an intense red halo.
• Ulcers appear on lips, gums, inner cheeks, tongue, palate and throat. 2 or 3 ulcers usually appear during an attack, but 10 to 15 ulcers are not uncommon.
• Ulcers may be so painful during first 2 or 3 days that they interfere with eating or speaking.
• Ulcers are preceded by tingling or burning for 24 hours (sometimes).

CAUSES—Unknown, but following are the most likely causes:
• Emotional or physical stress, anxiety or premenstrual tension.
• Injury to the mouth lining caused by rough dentures, hot food, toothbrushing or dental work.
• Irritation from foods, such as chocolate, citrus, acid foods (vinegar, pickles), salted nuts or potato chips.
• Virus infection.

RISK INCREASES WITH—Recent dental treatment.

HOW TO PREVENT
• Brush teeth at least twice a day and floss regularly to keep the mouth clean and healthy.
• Avoid stress if possible (see How to Cope with Stress in Appendix).
• Avoid intimate contact with infected persons.
• Observe if canker sores develop after eating specific foods. Don't eat foods that seem to trigger attacks.

 WHAT TO EXPECT

DIAGNOSTIC MEASURES
• Your own observation of symptoms.
• Medical history and physical exam by a doctor (sometimes).
• Laboratory culture of the sores to distinguish from herpes infection or detect secondary bacterial infections (sometimes).

APPROPRIATE HEALTH CARE
• Self-care.
• Doctor's treatment.

POSSIBLE COMPLICATIONS—Dehydration in severe cases where eating and drinking are limited.

PROBABLE OUTCOME—Most ulcers heal without scarring in 2 weeks. Recurrent attacks are common. They vary from a single lesion 2 or 3 times a year to an uninterrupted succession of multiple lesions.

 HOW TO TREAT

GENERAL MEASURES
• Rinse the mouth 3 or more times a day with a salt solution (1/2 teaspoon salt to 8 oz. water).
• Clean sores frequently with 2% hydrogen peroxide on a cotton applicator.
• If a canker sore is caused by a rough tooth, braces or dentures, consult your dentist. The sore won't heal until the cause is eliminated.

MEDICATION—Your doctor may prescribe:
• Topical anesthetics to relieve pain.
• Protective dental paste with a steroid derivative, such as Orabase with triamcinolone acetonide. If applied as soon as the ulcer begins, this prevents pain.
• Some new prescription medications are available that can occassionally help shorten the duration.
• Keep medicine prescribed by your doctor for the first attack. Use it immediately at the sign of a recurrent attack. The sooner treatment starts, the milder the attack.

ACTIVITY—No restrictions.

DIET—No restrictions, except to avoid foods that aggravate ulcers. Drink as many fluids and eat as well-balanced a diet as possible while healing. To minimize pain, sip liquids through straws. Foods that cause the least pain are milk, liquid gelatin, yogurt, ice cream and custard.

 CALL YOUR DOCTOR IF

• Temperature rises to 102F (38.9C) or higher.
• Ulcers don't improve in 10 days, despite treatment.
• Pain is unbearable and isn't relieved by treatment.
• A child with canker sores loses weight.

CARBON MONOXIDE POISONING

GENERAL INFORMATION

DEFINITION—Inhalation of carbon monoxide (a colorless, odorless, poisonous gas). Carbon monoxide is released by fires, combustion engines (automobiles and trucks), industrial fumes, cigarette smoke, or faulty stoves or heating systems. This is the most common form of accidental poisoning in the U.S. Initial symptoms may be similar to food poisoning, influenza or other mild gastrointestinal upsets.

BODY PARTS INVOLVED—Total body.

SEX OR AGE MOST AFFECTED—Both sexes; all ages.

SIGNS & SYMPTOMS
Mild to moderate exposure:
Headache; dizziness; nausea, vomiting; faintness.
Extensive exposure:
Severe headache; collapse; trouble breathing; slow heart rate; convulsions, coma; cherry-red skin color (rare).

CAUSES—When carbon monoxide is inhaled, it passes into the bloodstream where it interferes with the ability of the red blood cells to transport oxygen. All cells in the body need oxygen for survival.

RISK INCREASES WITH
• Faulty furnaces or heating devices; fireplace with a defective flue.
• Riding in the back of a pickup truck under a closed cover of some type.
• Poor venting (exhaust fumes escape into buildings or homes).
• Using charcoal-burning grills or Sterno heat in enclosed places.
• Using paint removers containing methylene chloride in enclosed places.
• Smoking or exposure to second-hand smoke.
• Faulty auto exhaust system.
• Winter months when heaters are in use and houses are more closed up.

HOW TO PREVENT
• Avoid risk factors where possible.
• Check furnaces, fireplaces and heaters often.
• Install a carbon monoxide alarm in your home.
• Call your local gas company if you think there may be a leak in your home.
• If the early symptoms occur only in certain places (at home, in the car, at work), but disappear once you are away, consider the possibility of a carbon monoxide problem.
• Use of fire-prevention methods in the home (smoke alarms, fire extinguishers).

WHAT TO EXPECT

DIAGNOSTIC MEASURES
• Your own observation of symptoms.
• Medical history and exam by a doctor.
• Laboratory measurements of oxygen and carbon monoxide levels.

APPROPRIATE HEALTH CARE
• Doctor's treatment.
• Hospitalization for oxygen and breathing support for more severe cases.
• Rarely, hyperbaric oxygen treatment.

POSSIBLE COMPLICATIONS
• Severe cases of poisoning can result in short-term memory problems; depression; brain, heart or lung damage; and death. Outcome is determined by the extent of the exposure.
• For pregnant women exposed to carbon monoxide poisoning, there is an increased risk of miscarriage, premature labor and death of the unborn child.

PROBABLE OUTCOME
• In mild to moderate carbon monoxide exposure with prompt diagnosis and treatment, the symptoms usually subside within minutes to a few hours.
• Long-term effects are unlikely; however, some patients experience delayed symptoms 2-4 weeks after the exposure. Symptoms of tiredness, memory problems, confusion, mood and behavior changes may occur.

HOW TO TREAT

GENERAL MEASURES
• If you suspect someone is exposed to carbon monoxide fumes (car is running or there is a fire), move them into fresh air. If the victim has stopped breathing, call 911 (emergency), then give mouth-to-mouth respiration or CPR (cardio-pulmonary resuscitation) until help arrives.
• Fresh air may be sufficient for recovery. Even so, the patient should still consult a doctor.

MEDICATION—Your doctor may prescribe:
• Supplemental oxygen.
• Anticonvulsants for seizures.

ACTIVITY—Determined by severity of symptoms.

DIET—Determined by severity of symptoms. With mild to moderate symptoms, no special diet is necessary.

CALL YOUR DOCTOR IF

• You have symptoms of carbon monoxide poisoning.
• Symptoms worsen or recur or new symptoms develop 2-4 weeks after recovery or treatment.

ILLNESS & DISORDERS

CARCINOID SYNDROME

GENERAL INFORMATION

DEFINITION—A group of symptoms caused by malignant tumors (carcinoids) in the wall of the small intestine. Carcinoids secrete serotonin, histamine, prostaglandins and hormones—powerful chemicals that cause carcinoid symptoms.

BODY PARTS INVOLVED—Primary tumors appear in the appendix, ileum, rectum, ovaries or stomach. The malignancy may spread and cause symptoms that affect the skin, blood vessels, kidney, gastrointestinal tract, liver, heart and lungs.

SEX OR AGE MOST AFFECTED—Adults of both sexes.

SIGNS & SYMPTOMS—Carcinoids are slow-growing and many persons with these tumors have no symptoms. The primary tumor may cause intestinal obstruction, characterized by painful cramps in the middle of the abdomen, vomiting, abdominal swelling and weight loss. In a few cases, carcinoid cells spread to other body parts and produce secondary, hormone-producing (serotonin) tumors. Heavy exercise, alcohol consumption, or eating bananas, tomatoes, plums, avocados, pineapple or walnuts may trigger symptoms of these secondary tumors. These symptoms include:
- Flushed skin on the head and neck that can last several hours.
- Watery eyes.
- Diarrhea with abdominal cramps.
- Respiratory symptoms similar to asthma (wheezing).
- Congestive heart failure.
- Irregular heartbeat.
- Nausea and vomiting.
- Low blood pressure.
- Unexplained weight loss.

CAUSES—Unknown.

RISK INCREASES WITH
- Adults over 60.
- Obesity.
- Smoking.
- Excess alcohol consumption.

HOW TO PREVENT—Cannot be prevented at present.

WHAT TO EXPECT

DIAGNOSTIC MEASURES
- Carcinoids may be discovered during a diagnostic test or surgery for some other disorder.
- Medical history and physical exam by a doctor.
- Laboratory urine studies for 5-hydroxyindoleacetic and serotonin level.

- Endoscopy and x-rays of the abdominal organs.
- Sigmoidoscopy and CT scan of the colon (see Glossary for both).
- Biopsy (see Glossary).

APPROPRIATE HEALTH CARE
- Self-care after diagnosis.
- Doctor's treatment. Treatment will be dependent on the extent of the disease.
- Surgical removal of the tumor if possible.

POSSIBLE COMPLICATIONS—Malignancy may spread to other body parts.

PROBABLE OUTCOME—This condition is currently considered incurable. However, symptoms can be relieved or controlled, and survival is possible for 10 to 20 years.

Scientific research into causes and treatment continues, so there is hope for increasingly effective treatment and cure.

HOW TO TREAT

GENERAL MEASURES
- The more you can learn and understand about a disease, the more you will be able to make informed decisions about where to go for your care, the treatments available, the risks involved, side effects of therapy and expected outcome.
- See Resources for Additional Information.

MEDICATION
- For minor diarrhea, you may use nonprescription drugs, such as Pepto-Bismol.
- Your doctor may prescribe:
  Anticancer drugs to kill malignant cells.
  Methyldopa to prevent formation of serotonins.
  Phenothiazines to prevent flushed skin.
  Cortisone drugs to reduce inflammation anywhere in the body.
  Bronchodilators, if asthma-like symptoms are a problem.

ACTIVITY—Resume your normal activities as soon as symptoms improve, but avoid strenuous exercise.

DIET
- Include at least 2 protein servings a day.
- Take niacin and tryptophan supplements if recommended by your doctor.
- Avoid foods that trigger symptoms of secondary tumors.
- Don't drink alcohol.

CALL YOUR DOCTOR IF

- You have symptoms of carcinoid syndrome.
- Symptoms become disabling, despite treatment.
- New, unexplained symptoms develop. Drugs used in treatment may produce side effects.

CARDIAC ARREST

 GENERAL INFORMATION

DEFINITION—Total loss of heart-pumping action. Delay of treatment for only 3 to 5 minutes may cause death or permanent brain damage.

BODY PARTS INVOLVED—Heart.

SEX OR AGE MOST AFFECTED—More common in men until age 45, then the incidence is equal in men and women.

SIGNS & SYMPTOMS
- Brief dizziness, followed by fainting and unconsciousness.
- No pulse. No breathing.
- Bluish-white skin. Dilated pupils.
- Seizures.
- Loss of bowel and bladder control (sometimes).
- Simple fainting may resemble cardiac arrest, but pulse and breathing continue.

CAUSES
- Heartbeat irregularities.
- Heart attack (myocardial infarction).
- Atherosclerotic heart disease.
- Lack of blood circulation and profound shock caused by a hemorrhage or overwhelming infection.
- Loss of oxygen from drowning, choking or anesthesia.
- Major changes in the blood's electrolyte composition, as with a potassium or fluid imbalance.
- Anaphylactic shock.
- Drug overdose.

RISK INCREASES WITH
- Stress.
- Diabetes mellitus.
- Use of drugs, such as:
  Digitalis. Even a minor excess of this powerful drug can disturb heart rhythm.
  Diuretics. These can cause low potassium in the blood.
  Adrenalin or any drug that raises blood pressure in a heart patient, including cold capsules, decongestant tablets and nasal sprays.
- Using drugs of abuse, especially cocaine and intravenous drugs.

HOW TO PREVENT
- Obtain immediate medical treatment for any conditions listed as Causes. Refer to appropriate chart in Illness section.
- If you have heart disease, learn all you can about all the drugs you take, including nonprescription drugs.
- Have family members and close friends learn CPR (cardiopulmonary resuscitation).

 WHAT TO EXPECT

DIAGNOSTIC MEASURES—Your observation of symptoms. See Signs & Symptoms. Once the patient is in the hospital, an ECG (see Glossary) will confirm the diagnosis.

APPROPRIATE HEALTH CARE—Emergency care by others present when cardiac arrest occurs.

POSSIBLE COMPLICATIONS
- Death or permanent brain damage if heart action cannot be resumed in 3 to 5 minutes.
- Mistaking a faint or other causes of unconsciousness for cardiac arrest. Check for a neck pulse before starting cardiopulmonary resuscitation (CPR).

PROBABLE OUTCOME—Bystanders skilled in recognizing cardiac arrest and performing CPR can often restore heartbeat. The final outcome, however, depends on the underlying cause of the cardiac arrest. The victim must be taken to the nearest emergency facility as soon as the heartbeat is restored. Cardiac arrest may recur.

 HOW TO TREAT

GENERAL MEASURES
- Learn CPR. Call your local Red Cross or hospital for information. You may save a life.
- If you have heart trouble, or are at risk, wear a Medic-Alert bracelet or pendant (see Glossary).

MEDICATION—Administer oxygen, if available, after CPR has restored a heartbeat. (Emergency oxygen may be available in welder's shops.)
  The doctor may later prescribe medications to treat the underlying cause of cardiac arrest.

ACTIVITY—After recovery, activities should be resumed gradually. Sexual relations may be resumed only after medical clearance from the doctor.

DIET—Don't give fluid or foods to anyone with signs of cardiac arrest. He or she could choke.

 CALL YOUR DOCTOR IF

The victim is unconscious and not breathing:
- Yell for help. Don't leave the victim.
- Call 911 (emergency) for an ambulance or medical help.
- Begin mouth-to-mouth breathing immediately.
- If there is no heartbeat, give external cardiac massage.
- Don't stop CPR until help arrives.

CARDIOMYOPATHY

 GENERAL INFORMATION

DEFINITION—An inflammatory disorder of the heart muscle. The heart muscle is weakened and cannot pump blood efficiently.

BODY PARTS INVOLVED—Heart muscle. Decreasing heart function eventually affects the lungs, liver and circulatory system.

SEX OR AGE MOST AFFECTED
- Both sexes, but more common in males.
- All ages, but most common in adults.

SIGNS & SYMPTOMS—If cardiomyopathy is extensive enough to cause congestive heart failure, the following symptoms may occur:
- Irregular or rapid heartbeat.
- Shortness of breath with activity.
- Swelling of the feet and ankles.
- Fatigue.
- Cough with frothy, bloody sputum.
- Appetite loss.
- Loss of sex drive.

CAUSES
- Virus infection.
- Late stage of coronary artery disease.
- Nutritional deficiency, especially of vitamin B-1 (thiamine).
- Mineral deficiency, especially of potassium.
- Fat tissue in the heart that replaces muscle fibers.
- Amyloid deposits (abnormal protein material deposited in tissues) due to other disorders.
- Hemochromatosis (excessive amount of iron in the liver, pancreas, skin).
- Severe anemia.
- Friedreich's ataxia (inherited nervous order disease).
- Stress.
- Unknown.

RISK INCREASES WITH
- Adults over 60.
- Obesity.
- Smoking.
- Alcoholism.
- Family history of coronary artery disease or cardiomyopathy.
- Use of certain drugs, such as alcohol, cocaine, antidepressants and antipsychotics.
- Diabetes mellitus.
- High cholesterol levels.

HOW TO PREVENT
- Drink alcohol moderately (1 or 2 drinks a day or none at all).
- Eat a well-balanced diet.
- Avoid risk factors where possible.

 WHAT TO EXPECT

DIAGNOSTIC MEASURES
- Your own observation of symptoms.
- Medical history and physical exam by a doctor.
- ECG and echocardiogram (see Glossary for both).
- X-rays of the heart and lungs, cardiac catheterization and other special tests.

APPROPRIATE HEALTH CARE
- Self-care after diagnosis.
- Doctor's treatment.
- Heart transplantation (rarely).

POSSIBLE COMPLICATIONS—Congestive heart failure.

PROBABLE OUTCOME
- If the underlying disorder can be corrected, cardiomyopathy may be curable.
- If the underlying cause can't be corrected, cardiomyopathy is incurable. Some patients are candidates for a heart transplant.

 HOW TO TREAT

GENERAL MEASURES
- Treatment goals are to ease the symptoms and to try and prevent further complications.
- Weigh daily before breakfast and record the weight. Report marked weight gain to the doctor. This may indicate excess fluid accumulation.
- Monitor blood pressure daily.
- For those with alcoholic cardiomyopathy, stopping all alcohol consumption is essential.

MEDICATION—Your doctor may prescribe:
- Digitalis to improve heart function.
- Diuretics to decrease fluid retention.
- Vitamins or potassium supplements (if the disorder is caused by a deficiency).

ACTIVITY
- Resume your normal activities gradually. There may be some limitations depending on severity of the disorder.
- Resume sexual relations when your sense of well-being allows and symptoms are controlled.

DIET
- Low-salt, low-fat diet if recommended by doctor (see Sodium Restricted Diet in Appendix).
- Weight loss diet if you are overweight.
- Stop drinking alcohol.

 CALL YOUR DOCTOR IF

- You have symptoms of cardiomyopathy or symptoms recur after treatment.
- You have chest pain.
- New, unexplained symptoms develop. Drugs used in treatment may produce side effects.

CARPAL-TUNNEL SYNDROME

GENERAL INFORMATION

DEFINITION—A nerve disorder in the hand that causes pain and loss of feeling, especially in the thumb and first 3 fingers. It is common among people using computers and word processors.

BODY PARTS INVOLVED—Median nerve at the wrist joint; blood vessels, nerves and tendons of the hand.

SEX OR AGE MOST AFFECTED—Both sexes, but most common in women between ages 29 and 62.

SIGNS & SYMPTOMS
- Tingling or numbness in part of the hand.
- Sharp pains that shoot from the wrist up the arm, especially at night.
- Burning sensations in the fingers.
- Morning stiffness or cramping of hands.
- Thumb weakness.
- Frequent dropping of objects.
- Inability to make a fist.
- Shiny, dry skin on the hand.

CAUSES—Pressure on the median nerve caused by swollen, inflamed or scarred tissue. The sources of pressure include:
- Repetitive motion injury (associated with continuous and rapid use of the fingers).
- Inflammation of the tendon sheaths (sometimes from arthritis).
- Fracture of the forearm.
- Sprain or dislocation of the wrist.

RISK INCREASES WITH
- Diabetes mellitus; hypothyroidism.
- Menopause.
- Raynaud's disease.
- Pregnancy.
- Work that requires strong hand or wrist action (computer users, some musicians, factory workers, cashiers).
- Obesity; rheumatoid arthritis; gout.
- Ganglion cyst.

HOW TO PREVENT
- Take a break at least once an hour when doing repetitive work involving hands.
- Wear a wrist brace or splint if your work involves doing repetitive work involving hands.

WHAT TO EXPECT

DIAGNOSTIC MEASURES
- Your own observation of symptoms. For a simple test, place the backs of your hands together with your fingers pointing straight down and your elbows pointing straight out to the side (wrists are at a 90° angle). If symptoms are brought on by you holding this position for one minute, you most likely have carpal-tunnel syndrome.
- Medical history and physical exam by a doctor.
- Electrophysiologic nerve tests (records electrical activity of muscles) and x-rays of the hand and wrist.

APPROPRIATE HEALTH CARE
- Self-care after diagnosis.
- Doctor's treatment.
- Surgery to free the pinched nerve. Provides almost complete relief from all symptoms in 95% of patients. Procedure may be done as an outpatient. (See Carpal-Tunnel Syndrome Repair in Surgery section.)

POSSIBLE COMPLICATIONS
- Permanent numbness and a weak thumb or fingers in the affected hand.
- Permanent paralysis of some of the hand and finger muscles.

PROBABLE OUTCOME—Usually curable—sometimes spontaneously, sometimes with surgery. Surgery usually needed if muscle wasting or nerve changes have developed. If pregnancy is the cause, the problem usually clears up after delivery.

HOW TO TREAT

GENERAL MEASURES
- Conservative treatment is usually tried first.
- Discomfort improves by shaking hands or dangling arms. If you awaken at night with pain in your hand, hang it over the side of the bed; rub or shake it.
- Wearing a splint on the affected wrist may be recommended.
- For work at a computer terminal, be sure desk, keyboard and chair are at the proper height. Take a break once an hour.

MEDICATION
- You may take aspirin or ibuprofen or naproxen to reduce pain and inflammation.
- Your doctor may prescribe:
  Anti-inflammatory drugs to reduce inflammation.
  Cortisone injections at the wrist to reduce inflammation.
  Vitamin B-6 injections.

ACTIVITY—Stay as active as your strength allows. If surgery has been necessary, allow 2 weeks for recovery. Exercises may be prescribed for the hand.

DIET—Eat a normal, well-balanced diet.

CALL YOUR DOCTOR IF

Symptoms of carpal-tunnel syndrome don't disappear in 2 weeks.

CAT-SCRATCH DISEASE

 GENERAL INFORMATION

DEFINITION—A mild infectious disease caused by a small bacteria resulting from a scratch by a cat (most often a kitten). It is not contagious from person to person. More than one family member can be infected at one time.

BODY PARTS INVOLVED—Skin; lymph glands.

SEX OR AGE MOST AFFECTED—Both sexes; all ages.

SIGNS & SYMPTOMS
- A lump, with or without pus or fluid, which starts on the scratched skin 3 to 10 days after the cat scratch.
- Swollen lymph glands near the affected area.
- Low fever of 99F to 101F (37.2C to 38.3C).
- Fatigue.
- Headache.
- Loss of appetite.
- AIDS patients may have more severe symptoms.

CAUSES—A bacterium carried on cat's claws. The infection spreads to lymph glands near the scratch by way of lymphatic vessels. Most of the animals involved are healthy.

RISK INCREASES WITH—Owning or handling cats.

HOW TO PREVENT
- Teach children to respect animals and not provoke them.
- Don't pick up strange cats.

 WHAT TO EXPECT

DIAGNOSTIC MEASURES
- Your own observation of symptoms.
- Medical history and physical exam by a doctor. Tell your doctor of any cat scratches in the previous 2 weeks.
- Skin test.

APPROPRIATE HEALTH CARE
- Self-care.
- Doctor's treatment.
- Needle aspiration (see Glossary) to drain the lymph gland, if it contains pus.

POSSIBLE COMPLICATIONS—Eye inflammation, encephalitis, hepatitis (all rare).

PROBABLE OUTCOME—Spontaneous recovery within 3 weeks.

 HOW TO TREAT

GENERAL MEASURES
- Apply heat to affected areas; use warm soaks (see Soaks in Appendix) or use heating pad.
- It is not necessary to isolate the ill person because the disease is not transmitted from person to person.
- Consult your veterinarian about the cat or kitten that caused the infection.

MEDICATION—Your doctor may prescribe antibiotics.

ACTIVITY—Rest in bed until fever subsides and energy returns. Resume your normal activities gradually.

DIET—No special diet.

 CALL YOUR DOCTOR IF

- You have symptoms of cat-scratch disease.
- A swollen lymph gland becomes painful and red. This may indicate that a doctor should open and drain the infected gland.

CATARACT

GENERAL INFORMATION

DEFINITION—A clouding of the lens of the eye. The lens is a crystal-clear, flexible structure near the front of the eyeball. It helps to keep vision in focus and screens and refracts light rays. The lens has no blood supply. It is nourished by the vitreous (watery substance that surrounds it). If hardening of the arteries prevents proper nourishment of the vitreous—as often occurs in aging—the lens loses its nourishment also. The lens may then become less transparent and flexible and form cataracts. Cataracts may form in one or both eyes. If they form in both eyes, their growth rate may be very different. Cataracts are not cancerous.

BODY PARTS INVOLVED—Lens of the eye(s).

SEX OR AGE MOST AFFECTED
• Adults over 60.
• Newborns (congenital form only).

SIGNS & SYMPTOMS
• Blurred vision that may be worse in bright light. The blurring may first become apparent to one while driving at night, when lights seem to scatter or have halos.
• Double vision (occasionally).
• Opaque, milky-white pupil (advanced stages only).

CAUSES
• Natural aging.
• Injury to the eye.
• Illnesses associated with high blood sugar, such as diabetes mellitus.
• Inflammation, such as uveitis (inflammation of the parts of the eyes that make up the iris).
• Drugs, especially cortisone and its derivatives.
• Exposure to x-rays, microwaves and infrared radiation.
• Hereditary causes, including the effect of German measles on the unborn child of a mother who contracts the disease early in pregnancy.
• Galactosemia (see Glossary) in an infant.

RISK INCREASES WITH
• Adults over 60.
• Exposure to any causes listed above.

HOW TO PREVENT
• The use of cortisone drugs or any others that affect the eye lens should be monitored carefully by a doctor.
• Eye disorders that may cause cataract formation, such as iritis and uveitis, should receive prompt medical treatment.
• Ultraviolet protecting glasses (in sunny climates) may slow progression of cataract.
• Women of child-bearing age should be vaccinated against German measles if they have not had the disease or been immunized.

WHAT TO EXPECT

DIAGNOSTIC MEASURES
• Your own observation of symptoms.
• Medical history and physical exam by a doctor.
• Eye examination with ophthalmoscopy.

APPROPRIATE HEALTH CARE
• Doctor's (ophthalmologist's) treatment.
• Surgery to remove the lens if vision deteriorates or cataract causes inflammation and pressure in the eye. Many different methods are in use today for anesthesia, hospitalization, and correction of vision after surgery. Surgery may be done on an inpatient or outpatient basis. Usually one eye is operated on at a time (if cataracts are in both eyes). (See Cataract Removal with Intraocular Lens Replacement in Surgery section.)

POSSIBLE COMPLICATIONS
• Loss of vision.
• Postoperative complications, including rupture of the eye, adhesions, infections and retinal detachment.

PROBABLE OUTCOME—Usually curable with surgery. Some cataracts never impair vision enough to require surgery. During the time cataracts are forming, frequent eyeglass changes may help vision.

HOW TO TREAT

GENERAL MEASURES
• Consider surgery when your vision problems interfere with your lifestyle: lack of confidence when driving, can't read comfortably, unable to do your best work, prevented from doing things you want to do, afraid of falling, not as independent as you want to be, just can't see well enough (even with glasses).
• For a description of cataract surgery and postoperative care, see Cataract Removal (in Surgery section). Special eyeglasses or contact lenses will be needed after surgery.

MEDICATION—Medicine usually is not necessary for this disorder.

ACTIVITY—No restrictions, except don't drive at night if your vision is poor.

DIET—No special diet.

CALL YOUR DOCTOR IF

You have symptoms of cataracts.

CELIAC DISEASE
(Gluten Enteropathy; Nontropical Sprue)

 GENERAL INFORMATION

DEFINITION—An allergic condition in the small intestine, triggered by gluten (a protein found in most grains), which prevents the intestine from absorbing nutrients. Most forms are inherited. Celiac disease is not contagious or cancerous.

BODY PARTS INVOLVED—Digestive system.

SEX OR AGE MOST AFFECTED—Usually begins during infancy or early childhood (2 weeks to 1 year). Symptoms appear when the child first begins eating food with gluten. In adults, symptoms may develop gradually over months or even years and can appear as late as age 60. It affects twice as many women as men.

SIGNS & SYMPTOMS
• Weight loss or slowed weight gain in an infant following the introduction of cereal to the diet.
• Poor appetite.
• Loose, pale, bulky, bad-smelling stools; frequent gas.
• Swollen abdomen; abdominal pain.
• General undernourished appearance.
• Mouth ulcers.
• Anemia or vitamin deficiency, with fatigue, paleness, skin rash, or bone pain.
• Mildly bowed legs in children.
• Vague tiredness, breathlessness.
• Swollen legs.
• Strange sensations in the hands and feet such as burning, prickling, tickling or tingling.

CAUSES—An inherited defect most often found in people of northwestern European ancestry.

RISK INCREASES WITH
• Family history of celiac disease.
• Pregnancy.
• Other allergies.

HOW TO PREVENT—Cannot be prevented at present.

 WHAT TO EXPECT

DIAGNOSTIC MEASURES
• Your own observation of symptoms.
• Medical history and physical exam by a doctor.
• Laboratory studies of stool and blood.
• Firm diagnosis is made by a biopsy, in which a small sample of tissue is taken from the small intestine. Three biopsies may be done, one when you are eating foods containing gluten, another when you are on a gluten-free diet, and a third when you again eat foods containing gluten.

APPROPRIATE HEALTH CARE
• Home care.
• Doctor's treatment.

 WHAT TO EXPECT

POSSIBLE COMPLICATIONS—In rare cases, gluten withdrawal does not bring immediate improvement.

PROBABLE OUTCOME—With a strict, gluten-free diet, most persons with celiac disease can expect a normal life. Improvement begins in 2 to 3 weeks.

 HOW TO TREAT

GENERAL MEASURES
• Pay careful attention to the dietary instructions provided by your doctor or dietitian.
• See Resources for Additional Information.

MEDICATION—Your doctor may prescribe:
• Iron and folic acid for anemia.
• Calcium and multiple-vitamin supplements for deficiencies.
• Oral cortisone drugs to reduce the body's inflammatory response during a severe attack.

ACTIVITY—No restrictions.

DIET—Gluten-free diet (see Gluten-Restricted diet in Appendix). It is difficult to exclude gluten from the diet completely, so be patient while becoming familiar with the diet, which a dietician can help you plan.

 CALL YOUR DOCTOR IF

• You or your child have symptoms of celiac disease.
• Symptoms don't decrease within 3 weeks after beginning a gluten-free diet.
• The child fails to regain lost weight or grow and develop as expected.
• Fever develops.

CELLULITIS
(Erysipelas)

GENERAL INFORMATION

DEFINITION—A noncontagious infection of connective tissue beneath the skin.

BODY PARTS INVOLVED—Skin anywhere on the body, but most likely on the face or lower legs. Erysipelas is the name of a severe cellulitis of the face.

SEX OR AGE MOST AFFECTED—Both sexes; all ages.

SIGNS & SYMPTOMS
- Sudden tenderness, swelling and redness in an area of the skin. The area of cellulitis is initially 5cm to 20cm in diameter and grows rapidly in the first 24 hours. A thin red line often extends from the middle of the cellulitis toward the heart. Cellulitis does not develop into a boil.
- Fever, sometimes accompanied by chills and sweats.
- General ill feeling.
- Swollen lymph glands nearest the cellulitis.

CAUSES—Infection from staphylococcus or streptococcus bacteria.

RISK INCREASES WITH
- Chronic illness, such as diabetes mellitus, or a recent infection that has lowered resistance.
- Any injury that breaks the skin.
- Poor nutrition.
- Intravenous drug use.
- Surgical wound; animal bites, burns.
- Diabetes mellitus.
- Immunosuppression due to illness or medications.
- Chronic use of antibacterial soaps that can select out resistant bacteria.

HOW TO PREVENT
- Avoid skin damage. Use protective clothing or gear if you participate in strenuous work or sports.
- Keep the skin clean.
- Avoid swimming if you have a skin lesion.

WHAT TO EXPECT

DIAGNOSTIC MEASURES
- Your own observation of symptoms.
- Medical history and physical exam by a doctor.
- Skin biopsy (sometimes).

APPROPRIATE HEALTH CARE
- Self-care after diagnosis.
- Doctor's treatment.
- If excess fluid is lost from the skin, hospitalization may be necessary to provide adequate hydration.

POSSIBLE COMPLICATIONS
- Blood poisoning, if bacteria enter the bloodstream.
- Brain infection or meningitis, if cellulitis occurs on the central part of the face.
- A recent emergence of an extremely aggressive bacteria ("flesh-eating strep") can cause rapid and extensive destruction of tissue.

PROBABLE OUTCOME—Usually curable in 7 to 10 days with treatment, unless the patient has a chronic disease or is receiving immunosuppressive treatment. In that case, cellulitis may lead to blood poisoning and become life-threatening.

HOW TO TREAT

GENERAL MEASURES
- Use warm-water soaks (see Soaks in Appendix) to hasten healing and relieve pain and inflammation.
- Elevation and restricted movement of the affected area can help reduce swelling.

MEDICATION—Your doctor may prescribe an antibiotic to fight infection. Finish the prescribed dose, even if symptoms disappear quickly.

ACTIVITY—Rest in bed until fever disappears and other symptoms improve. Resume your normal activities as soon as symptoms improve.

DIET—No special diet. Vitamin-C supplements (250mg to 500mg daily) may hasten healing.

CALL YOUR DOCTOR IF

- You have symptoms of cellulitis, especially on the face.
- The following occurs during treatment:
  Fever.
  Headache or vomiting.
  Drowsiness and lethargy.
  Blister over the area of cellulitis.
  Red streaks that continue to extend, despite treatment.
- New, unexplained symptoms develop. Drugs used in treatment may produce side effects.

CEREBRAL PALSY (CP)

 GENERAL INFORMATION

DEFINITION—A group of muscular and nervous-system disorders that begins in infancy and causes varying degrees of disability. Cerebral palsy is not inherited.

BODY PARTS INVOLVED—Central nervous system; muscular system.

SEX OR AGE MOST AFFECTED—Usually begins in infancy and remains throughout life.

SIGNS & SYMPTOMS—Number and severity of the following symptoms vary widely among children with CP:
- Early sucking difficulty with breast or bottle.
- Lack of normal muscle tone (early).
- Slow development (walking, talking).
- Unusual body postures.
- Stiffness and muscle spasms (later).
- Purposeless body movements.
- Poor coordination or balance.
- Crossed eyes.
- Deafness.
- Convulsions.
- Various degrees of mental retardation.

CAUSES—Defects in the brain and spinal column. The reason for these defects is often unknown (about 70% of the time). Known reasons include:
- Birth injury, including prolonged oxygen deprivation.
- An infection in the mother during pregnancy that spreads to the baby in the uterus; especially rubella (German measles).
- Meningitis or encephalitis during infancy or childhood.

RISK INCREASES WITH
- Prematurity.
- Excess alcohol during pregnancy.
- Seizures in the mother during pregnancy.
- Child abuse.

HOW TO PREVENT
- Arrange for good medical care during pregnancy, labor and delivery.
- Eat a well-balanced diet during pregnancy.
- Don't drink alcohol or use any drug, including nonprescription drugs, during pregnancy without consulting your doctor.
- Avoid sick people if you are pregnant.

 WHAT TO EXPECT

DIAGNOSTIC MEASURES
- Your own observation of symptoms.
- Medical history and physical exam by a doctor. A parent's intuition is often important. Obtain a second opinion, if necessary.
- Laboratory blood studies.
- EEG (see Glossary).
- Psychological tests.

APPROPRIATE HEALTH CARE
- Home care.
- Doctor's treatment.
- Psychotherapy or counseling to help the family accept the disease and help the child achieve maximum potential.
- Surgery to correct muscular-system deformities (sometimes).
- Time in an extended-care facility for children with severe CP (sometimes).

POSSIBLE COMPLICATIONS—Permanent disability and associated problems such as epilepsy, learning disabilities, mental retardation, behavioral problems, strabismus, hearing loss.

PROBABLE OUTCOME—Children vary widely in the severity of this condition. A child with CP may have high intelligence despite major muscular disability. Many children can be cared for in a loving home. Those with less-severe impairment can lead near-normal, productive lives. Children with severe impairments may require special care.

 HOW TO TREAT

GENERAL MEASURES
- Because early diagnosis is important, be sure your child has regular medical checkups. Failure to diagnose CP may deny the child opportunities for special programs .
- Maintain an optimistic outlook for yourself and your child.
- Seek help and advice from other parents whose children have cerebral palsy.
- Investigate resources in your community, including educational and physical-therapy programs and support groups. Contact the United Cerebral Palsy Foundation, 1(800)USA-1UCP.

MEDICATION—Your doctor may prescribe:
- Anticonvulsants to control seizures.
- Muscle relaxants to relieve spasms.

ACTIVITY
- Encourage your child to do as much as he or she can do.
- Physical therapy, occupational therapy, speech therapy and special equipment will help child to reach full potential within the limits set by this disorder.

DIET—No special diet. Constipation is frequent and stool softeners might be considered.

 CALL YOUR DOCTOR IF

You are concerned about your child's development or suspect CP.

CERVICAL DYSPLASIA

GENERAL INFORMATION

DEFINITION—Cervical dysplasia is the presence of abnormal cells on the lining of the cervix. It can range from mild to severe, depending on the spread of the abnormal cells. Depending on the severity, dysplasia can be considered a precancerous condition, but does not represent cancer of the cervix.

BODY PARTS INVOLVED—Cervix.

SEX OR AGE MOST AFFECTED—Females of all ages, but most common in those age 25 to 35.

SIGNS & SYMPTOMS—Usually no signs or symptoms occur. The suspected diagnosis results from a routine Pap smear evaluation.

CAUSES—There is an association with human papillomaviruses (genital warts) or similar viruses. The human papillomavirus (HPV) is usually acquired from sexual intercourse but can, in rare instances, be acquired from other skin to skin contact.

RISK INCREASES WITH
- Repeated infections.
- Smoking.
- Immunosuppression.
- Pregnancy and the immunologic changes associated with pregnancy.
- Multiple sexual partners.
- Early age of first sexual intercourse.
- Daughters of women who took DES during pregnancy.
- History of infection with the human papilloma-virus (HPV), which causes genital warts.
- Long-term oral contraceptive use.

HOW TO PREVENT
- Sexual monogamy of both partners.
- Yearly Pap smears for all women who are, or have been, sexually active, or who have reached the age of 18. Pap smears will not prevent dysplasia, but will aid in early diagnosis.
- Don't smoke.
- Use of a diaphragm by the female or a condom by the male for sexual intercourse.

WHAT TO EXPECT

DIAGNOSTIC MEASURES—To confirm the diagnosis, a colposcopy (examination of the cervix with a colposcope, a slender optical instrument with a lighted tip) is usually performed and combined with a biopsy.

APPROPRIATE HEALTH CARE—Treatment measures will vary depending on the degree and extent of the cervical dysplasia. Possibilities include cryotherapy (freezing), laser surgery, conization of the cervix, and cone biopsy. A recently developed treatment for cervical dysplasia is the loop excision electrosurgical procedure (LEEP). In LEEP, the physician uses a hand-held wire loop, activated by an electrosurgical generator, which makes a very precise and uniform cut across the cervix, in much the same way as a laser beam would.

POSSIBLE COMPLICATIONS
- Some severe dysplasia may progress to cancer of the cervix.
- Recurrence is possible, especially in the first two years following treatment. If a woman has completed childbearing, recurrent dysplasia can be treated with a hysterectomy.
- Rarely, complications can result from the treatment, such as excessive bleeding or infection.

PROBABLE OUTCOME
- With early diagnosis and treatment, the outlook is excellent.
- Spontaneous regression (reversal) occurs in a significant number of patients.

HOW TO TREAT

GENERAL MEASURES
- Follow-up Pap smears every 3 to 6 months for 1 to 2 years may be recommended to verify the success of treatment and to detect any recurrence. Thereafter, be sure to receive annual Pap smears.
- For patients with recurrent or severe dysplasia, hysterectomy may be an option.

MEDICATION
- Prescription pain medication should generally be required only for 2 to 7 days following the procedure.
- You may use nonprescription drugs, such as acetaminophen, for minor pain.

ACTIVITY
- Return to normal activities as soon as possible after surgery.
- Delay sexual relations until a follow-up medical examination determines that healing is complete.

DIET—No special diet.

CALL YOUR DOCTOR IF

- Pain, swelling, redness, drainage or bleeding increases in the surgical area.
- You develop signs of infection, including headache, muscle aches, dizziness or a general ill feeling and fever.
- Vaginal discharge increases or begins to have an unpleasant odor.

ILLNESS & DISORDERS

CERVICAL EROSION

 GENERAL INFORMATION

DEFINITION—A condition in which the lining of the uterus spreads to cover the tip of the cervix. This abnormally placed tissue is more likely to become inflamed or infected. It is not cancerous.

BODY PARTS INVOLVED—Cervix; uterus lining.

SEX OR AGE MOST AFFECTED—Adolescent and adult females.

SIGNS & SYMPTOMS
• No symptoms (usually).
• Increased mucus discharge from the vagina (sometimes).
• Unexplained vaginal bleeding (sometimes).

CAUSES—Usually unknown, but may accompany pregnancy, childbirth or the use of oral contraceptives. Some women are born with cervical erosion but have no symptoms.

RISK INCREASES WITH
• Stress.
• Repeated vaginal infections.
• Obesity.

HOW TO PREVENT—Cannot be prevented at present.

 WHAT TO EXPECT

DIAGNOSTIC MEASURES
• Medical history and physical exam—including pelvic examination—by a doctor.
• Pap smear (see Glossary).

APPROPRIATE HEALTH CARE
• Doctor's treatment.
• Treatment by local destruction of glandular tissue may involve cauterization, cryosurgery (see both in Surgery section), diathermy or laser treatment.

POSSIBLE COMPLICATIONS—None expected.

PROBABLE OUTCOME—Disorder is usually curable with treatment. Allow 3 months for the cervix to return completely to normal. Cervical erosion may recur.

 HOW TO TREAT

GENERAL MEASURES
• Don't douche unless instructed to by your doctor.
• Obtain medical treatment for any vaginal infection you may also have.

MEDICATION—Your doctor may prescribe oral antibiotics or topical antibiotics to apply to the cervix.

ACTIVITY—After treatment (except following a hysterectomy), normal activity and sexual relations may be resumed immediately.

DIET—No special diet.

 CALL YOUR DOCTOR IF

• You have symptoms of cervical erosion.
• The following occurs after treatment:
  Increased discharge.
  Pain with intercourse or bleeding afterward.
  Vaginal bleeding between periods.
• New, unexplained symptoms develop. Drugs used in treatment may produce side effects.

CERVICAL POLYPS

GENERAL INFORMATION

DEFINITION—Small, fragile, bulbous growths on stalks protruding through the cervix (lower third of the uterus) from the lining inside the uterus (endometrium). They may be single or numerous.

BODY PARTS INVOLVED—Endometrium (thin membrane lining the uterus); cervix (lower third of the uterus).

SEX OR AGE MOST AFFECTED—Women of all ages.

SIGNS & SYMPTOMS
- Unexpected spotting of blood between menstrual periods.
- Spotting of blood after sexual intercourse or bowel movements.
- Vaginal discharge.

CAUSES—Cervical polyps are caused by cervix inflammation from infection, erosion or ulceration. They frequently accompany chronic infections in the vagina or cervix, although they are not contagious. The small growths are usually benign, but in very rare cases, they represent early cancer of the cervix.

RISK INCREASES WITH
- Diabetes mellitus.
- Recurrent vaginitis or cervicitis.

HOW TO PREVENT—To prevent vaginal or cervix infections that can precede cervical polyps:
- Wear cotton underpants or pantyhose with a cotton crotch to prevent accumulation of excess heat and moisture, which can make you susceptible to vaginal and cervical infections.
- Avoid contracting sexually transmitted diseases by having your sexual partner wear a condom during intercourse.

WHAT TO EXPECT

DIAGNOSTIC MEASURES
- Your own observation of symptoms.
- Medical history and physical exam by a doctor.
- Laboratory studies, such as a Pap smear (see Glossary) and examination of the vaginal discharge.

APPROPRIATE HEALTH CARE
- Self-care after diagnosis and treatment.
- Doctor's treatment and surgery to remove cervical polyps with a wire snare, electrocautery or liquid nitrogen. This can often be done in a simple office procedure. The cervix may be cauterized after removing the polyp to prevent regrowth of the same or another polyp.
- A polyp that accompanies cervicitis (inflammation or infection of the cervix) may require more extensive surgery. See Cervicitis in Illness section.

POSSIBLE COMPLICATIONS
- Bleeding and some mild pain with removal of the polyps.
- In very rare instances, cervical polyps may become malignant.

PROBABLE OUTCOME—Usually curable with minor surgery. You may feel brief, mild pain during the procedure and have mild to moderate cramps for several hours. Spotting of blood from the vagina may occur for 1 or 2 days.

HOW TO TREAT

GENERAL MEASURES
- Don't douche unless your doctor recommends it.
- Use small sanitary pads to protect your clothing from creams or suppositories.

MEDICATION—Usually no medications are necessary for this disorder.

ACTIVITY—No restrictions. Delay sexual relations until your doctor performs a follow-up pelvic exam and determines that healing is complete.

DIET—No special diet.

CALL YOUR DOCTOR IF

- You have symptoms of cervical polyps.
- The following occur after treatment:
Discomfort persists longer than 1 week.
Symptoms recur.
Unexplained vaginal bleeding or swelling develops.
- New, unexplained symptoms develop. Drugs used in treatment may produce side effects.

CERVICAL SPONDYLOSIS

GENERAL INFORMATION

DEFINITION—Degenerative changes of bones in the neck that place pressure on nerves and muscles to the arms, legs and bladder.

BODY PARTS INVOLVED
- 7 bones of the neck.
- Disks between the bones.
- Blood vessels to the head.
- Bladder and lower legs (advanced stages).

SEX OR AGE MOST AFFECTED—Adults of both sexes. More common in males after 40, increasing after age 60.

SIGNS & SYMPTOMS—Any of the following:
- Pain in the neck, radiating to the shoulder blades, top of the shoulders, upper arms, hands or back of the head.
- Crunching sounds with movement of the neck or shoulder muscles.
- Numbness and tingling in the arms, hands and fingers; some loss of feeling in the hands; and impairment of reflexes.
- Muscle weakness and deterioration; diminished reflexes.
- Neck stiffness.
- Headache.
- Dizziness; unsteady gait.
- With advanced disease, loss of bladder control and leg weakness.

CAUSES
- Arthritis (inflammation of a joint).
- Injuries such as: automobile accidents with "whiplash" injury; athletic injuries; sudden jerks on the arms; falls.
- Osteoarthritis (wear and tear on joints that accompanies aging).
- Outgrowths of bone that sometimes occur with aging.

RISK INCREASES WITH
- Adults over 60.
- Fatigue or overwork.
- Neck injury.

HOW TO PREVENT
- Avoid sitting in cramped positions.
- Sleep without pillows. Use a soft fabric collar or towel to support the neck.
- Avoid injury. Wear protective headgear for contact sports. Use seat belts in vehicles and keep headrests at proper height.

WHAT TO EXPECT

DIAGNOSTIC MEASURES
- Your own observation of symptoms.
- Medical history and physical exam by a doctor.

- X-rays or MRI scan (see Glossary) or other diagnostic tests may be obtained to confirm the diagnosis.

APPROPRIATE HEALTH CARE
- Self-care for mild symptoms.
- Doctor's treatment for signs of nerve-root pressure (symptoms in the head, arms or bladder) or pain.
- Ultrasonic treatments may be recommended.
- Surgery (sometimes) to fuse neck bones, remove a damaged disk or enlarge the spinal-cord space.

POSSIBLE COMPLICATIONS
- Reduced neck flexibility after surgery or treatment.
- If untreated, a spastic gait may result as the disease progresses.

PROBABLE OUTCOME—Minor symptoms usually respond well to treatment and subside slowly. Severe symptoms may persist indefinitely.

HOW TO TREAT

GENERAL MEASURES
- Wear a soft fabric collar (Thomas collar) to prevent unexpected neck-muscle strain.
- Apply moist heat. Take hot showers and let the water beat on neck and shoulders for 10 to 20 minutes twice a day. Between showers, apply hot soaks to neck. Soak towel or cloth in hot water, wring out and apply.
- Improve your posture. Pull in the chin and abdomen when sitting or standing. Use a firm chair and sit with buttocks against the back.
- Sleep without a pillow. Instead, use a cervical pillow, wear a soft fabric collar, or put a small rolled towel under the neck.
- Ultrasonic treatments may be recommended.
- If numbness or pain affects the hands or arms, buy or rent a cervical-traction apparatus. To set it up, follow directions that accompany the apparatus.

MEDICATION
- For minor discomfort or disability, you may use aspirin or acetaminophen.
- For serious discomfort, your doctor may prescribe stronger pain medicine, muscle relaxants or tranquilizers.

ACTIVITY—Any activity that does not cause symptoms is recommended.

DIET—No special diet.

CALL YOUR DOCTOR IF

- You have symptoms of cervical spondylosis.
- Symptoms persist or worsen despite treatment.

CERVICITIS

GENERAL INFORMATION

DEFINITION—Inflammation or infection of the cervix. There are 2 types, and either may be contagious:
- Acute cervicitis is usually a bacterial or viral infection with specific symptoms.
- Chronic cervicitis is a long-term infection that may not have symptoms.

BODY PARTS INVOLVED—Cervix and mucous membranes covering the cervix.

SEX OR AGE MOST AFFECTED—Females of all ages after adolescence.

SIGNS & SYMPTOMS
Acute cervicitis:
- Thick, yellow vaginal discharge.
Chronic cervicitis:
- Slight—sometimes unnoticeable—vaginal discharge.
- Backache.
- Discomfort with urination.
- Discomfort with sexual intercourse.
Extensive chronic cervicitis:
- Profuse vaginal discharge.
- Bleeding between menstrual periods.
- Spotting or bleeding after sexual intercourse.

CAUSES
- Acute cervicitis is usually caused by the organisms N. gonorrhoeae or C. trachomatis. Herpes virus can also be a cause.
- Chronic cervicitis is caused by repeated episodes of acute cervicitis or one episode that is not treated long enough to heal completely.

RISK INCREASES WITH
- Multiple sexual partners.
- Diabetes mellitus.
- Acute or recurrent vaginitis.

HOW TO PREVENT
- Have an annual pelvic examination and Pap smear (see Glossary).
- Wear cotton panties or pantyhose with a cotton crotch. Avoid panties made from nonventilating materials. Synthetic materials hold in vaginal wetness and warmth, which may trigger vaginal or cervical infections.
- Avoid contracting sexually transmitted diseases by having your sexual partner wear a latex condom for intercourse.
- If cervicitis is caused by a sexually transmitted infection, your sexual partner also needs treatment.

WHAT TO EXPECT

DIAGNOSTIC MEASURES
- Your own observation of symptoms.
- Medical history and pelvic exam by a doctor.
- Laboratory studies, such as a Pap smear (see Glossary) and culture of the discharge.

APPROPRIATE HEALTH CARE
- Self-care after diagnosis.
- Doctor's treatment, including destruction of abnormal cells with silver nitrate (chemical used for cautery); cryosurgery (destruction of abnormal tissue by applying freezing temperatures, usually with liquid nitrogen); or electrocautery (destruction of tissue by heat applied with a controlled electric current).

POSSIBLE COMPLICATIONS
- Cervical polyps.
- Pelvic inflammatory disease.
- Untreated cervicitis can spread and cause endometritis (infection of the lining of the uterus) or salpingitis (infection of Fallopian tube).
- Malignant change in cervix cells (rare).

PROBABLE OUTCOME
- Mild cervicitis will heal without treatment.
- Acute cervicitis caused by venereal disease is contagious through sexual intercourse and is curable with medication.
- Most other cases of cervicitis can be cured with treatment. All women with cervicitis need regular checkups until the condition heals.

HOW TO TREAT

GENERAL MEASURES
- Use sanitary pads instead of tampons during treatment.
- Don't douche unless your doctor recommends it.

MEDICATION—Your doctor may prescribe:
- Oral antibiotics if infectious cervicitis suspected.
- Antiviral or antibiotic vaginal creams or suppositories to fight infection.

ACTIVITY—No restrictions, except to avoid sexual relations until your doctor determines that the infection has healed.

DIET—No special diet.

CALL YOUR DOCTOR IF

- You have symptoms of cervicitis.
- During treatment, discomfort persists longer than 1 week or symptoms worsen.
- Unexplained vaginal bleeding or swelling develops during or after treatment.
- New, unexplained symptoms develop. Drugs used in treatment may produce side effects.

ILLNESS & DISORDERS

CERVIX CANCER

GENERAL INFORMATION

DEFINITION—A common but treatable cancer of the female reproductive system.

BODY PARTS INVOLVED—Cervix (the lower third of the uterus, which opens into the vagina).

SEX OR AGE MOST AFFECTED—Women of all ages, but most common between ages 30 and 50.

SIGNS & SYMPTOMS
In the early, easily treatable stages:
- No symptoms.

In later stages:
- Unexplained vaginal bleeding.
- Persistent vaginal discharge.
- Pain and bleeding after intercourse.

In final stages:
- Abdominal pain.
- Leaking of feces and urine through the vagina.
- Appetite and weight loss.
- Anemia.

CAUSES—Unknown. Probably related to viral infections, including human papillomavirus.

RISK INCREASES WITH
- Early age of first intercourse.
- Multiple sex partners.
- Multiple pregnancies.
- Human papillomavirus infection (genital warts).
- Recurrent vaginal infections (bacterial or viral, including genital herpes and genital warts).
- Smoking.

HOW TO PREVENT
- Avoid the risks listed above as much as possible.
- Begin medical pelvic examinations at age 18 or at the beginning of regular sexual activity.
- Obtain regular Pap smears (see Glossary). Regular pelvic examinations and the Pap smear are very effective in detecting precancerous changes or cervical cancer in its symptom-free stage.

  Consult your doctor, Planned Parenthood or the public health department about how often to be examined. Many public agencies will perform a Pap smear at little or no cost to you.

WHAT TO EXPECT

DIAGNOSTIC MEASURES
- Your own observation of symptoms, especially unexplained vaginal bleeding.
- Medical history and physical exam by a doctor.
- Laboratory studies, such as a Pap smear and biopsy (see Glossary).
- Surgical diagnostic procedures, such as conization of the cervix (see Glossary).

APPROPRIATE HEALTH CARE
- Doctor's treatment.
- Surgery to remove the cancerous area. During early stages, this may only involve a small area of the cervix, which preserves childbearing abilities. More advanced stages may require removal of the reproductive organs and other affected tissue (see Hysterectomy in Surgery section).
- Chemotherapy and radiation therapy (advanced cancer).

POSSIBLE COMPLICATIONS—If cervical cancer is not treated early, it spreads beyond the uterus to other body parts—leading to death.

PROBABLE OUTCOME—Usually curable if diagnosed before the tumor has spread.

HOW TO TREAT

GENERAL MEASURES
- The more you can learn and understand about cervical cancer, the more you will be able to make informed decisions about where to go for your care, the treatments available, the risks involved, side effects of therapy and expected outcome.
- See Resources for Additional Information.

MEDICATION—Medicine usually is not necessary for this disorder if it is diagnosed and treated early. If radical surgery and additional treatment are required, your doctor may prescribe anticancer drugs.

ACTIVITY—No restrictions. Resume sexual activity once you have medical clearance.

DIET—No special diet.

CALL YOUR DOCTOR IF

- You have persistent vaginal bleeding or other symptoms of cervical cancer.
- You have not had a pelvic examination or Pap smear in at least 1 year.

CHALAZION

GENERAL INFORMATION

DEFINITION—A mass on the eyelid resulting from chronic inflammation of a meibomian gland (gland which lubricates the lid margins).

BODY PARTS INVOLVED—Eyelid.

SEX OR AGE MOST AFFECTED—Adults of both sexes.

SIGNS & SYMPTOMS—A painless swelling on the eyelid, which at first may resemble a sty. The eyelid may swell, and the eye may feel irritated. After a few days, these early symptoms disappear, leaving a painless, slow-growing, firm lump in the eyelid. Skin over the lump can be moved loosely.

CAUSES—Blockage of a duct leading to the surface of the eyelid from the meibomian gland. The blockage may be due to infection (usually staphylococcal) around the duct opening.

RISK INCREASES WITH—Skin conditions such as acne rosacea or seborrheic dermatitis.

HOW TO PREVENT
- If you have a tendency to get chalazions, wash eyelid area daily with water and baby shampoo applied with a cotton swab.
- At the first sign of eyelid irritation, apply warm compresses several times a day.

WHAT TO EXPECT

DIAGNOSTIC MEASURES
- Your own observation of symptoms.
- Medical history and physical exam by a doctor.
- Laboratory culture of the discharge from the chalazion (sometimes).

APPROPRIATE HEALTH CARE
- Self-care. To help the healing, gently massage the lid towards the margin. This helps to release blocked-up fluid from the gland.
- Surgical removal under local anesthesia in the doctor's office, if the chalazion does not heal spontaneously in 6 weeks, if is a large chalazion or if it becomes infected. (See Chalazion Removal in Surgery section.)

POSSIBLE COMPLICATIONS—None expected.

PROBABLE OUTCOME—A chalazion may heal spontaneously. If not, it is usually curable with surgical removal.

HOW TO TREAT

GENERAL MEASURES—Use warm-water soaks to reduce inflammation and hasten healing. Apply soaks for 20 minutes, then rest at least 1 hour. Repeat as often as needed.

MEDICATION—Your doctor may prescribe:
- Topical antibiotic ointments or creams, such as erythromycin or bacitracin. Apply a thin layer of medication to the lid edges 3 or 4 times daily. A heavy layer wastes medicine and is no more beneficial than a thin layer.
- Antibiotic eye drops to prevent the spread of infection to other parts of the eye. Oral antibiotics or antibiotic injections usually are not needed.

ACTIVITY—No restrictions.

DIET—No special diet.

CALL YOUR DOCTOR IF

- You have symptoms of a chalazion that last longer than 2 weeks.
- You have pain in the eye.
- Your vision changes.
- New, unexplained symptoms develop. Drugs used in treatment may produce side effects.

CHICKENPOX (Varicella)

GENERAL INFORMATION

DEFINITION—A very contagious, mild disease caused by the herpes zoster virus.

BODY PARTS INVOLVED—Skin and mucous membranes.

SEX OR AGE MOST AFFECTED—All ages, but most common in children.

SIGNS & SYMPTOMS—The following are usually mild in children, severe in adults:
- Fever.
- Abdominal pain or a general ill feeling that lasts 1 or 2 days.
- Skin eruptions that appear almost anywhere on the body, including the scalp, penis and inside the mouth, nose, throat or vagina. They may be scattered over large areas, and they occur least on the arms and legs. Blisters collapse within 24 hours and form scabs. New crops of blisters erupt every 3 to 4 days.
- Adults have additional symptoms that resemble influenza.

CAUSES—Infection with the herpes zoster virus. It is spread from person to person by airborne droplets or contact with a skin eruption on an infected person. Incubation after exposure is 7 to 21 days.

A newborn is protected for several months from chickenpox if the mother had the disease prior to or during pregnancy. The immunity diminishes in 4 to 12 months.

RISK INCREASES WITH
- Use of immunosuppressive drugs.
- Contact with an infected person (day care, school).

HOW TO PREVENT—A live vaccine is recommended for all children over 12 months of age who have not had chickenpox. Children taking the vaccine should not take aspirin for 6 weeks because of the possibility of Reye's syndrome.

WHAT TO EXPECT

DIAGNOSTIC MEASURES
- Your own observation of symptoms.
- Medical history and physical exam by a doctor (the observance of the skin eruptions is usually sufficient for diagnosis).

APPROPRIATE HEALTH CARE
- Self-care after diagnosis.
- Doctor's diagnosis and treatment, if complications arise.

POSSIBLE COMPLICATIONS
- Secondary bacterial infection of chickenpox blisters.
- Pneumonia.
- Viral eye infection.
- Encephalitis (rare).
- Reye's syndrome.
- Scarring, if blisters become infected (rare).
- Myocarditis.
- Arthritis (transient).

PROBABLE OUTCOME
- Spontaneous recovery. Children usually recover in 7 to 10 days. Adults take longer and are more likely to develop complications.
- After recovery, a person has lifelong immunity against a recurrence of chickenpox.
- After chickenpox runs its course, the virus sometimes remains dormant in the body. The same virus may later cause shingles.

HOW TO TREAT

GENERAL MEASURES
- Cool-water soaks (see Soaks in Appendix) or cool-water compresses to reduce itching.
- Keep the patient as quiet and cool as possible. Heat and sweat trigger itching.
- Keep the nails short to discourage scratching, which can lead to secondary infection. Have the child wear mittens if necessary.
- Notify parents of any children exposed to your child during the contagious period.

MEDICATION
- The following nonprescription medicines may decrease itching: topical anesthetics and topical antihistamines, which provide quick, short-term relief. Preparations containing lidocaine and pramoxine are least likely to cause allergic skin reactions. Lotions that contain phenol, menthol and camphor (such as calamine lotion). Follow package instructions.
- If you must reduce fever, use acetaminophen. Never use aspirin in children under age 18 as it may contribute to the development of Reye's syndrome (a form of encephalitis) when given to children during a viral illness.

ACTIVITY—Bed rest is not necessary. Allow quiet activity in a cool environment. A child may play outdoors in the shade during nice weather. Keep an ill child away from others until all blisters have crusted.

DIET—No special diet.

CALL YOUR DOCTOR IF

- You or your child have symptoms of chickenpox.
- Lethargy, headache or sensitivity to bright light develop.
- Fever rises over 103F (39.4C).
- Chickenpox lesions contain pus or otherwise appear infected.
- A cough occurs during a chickenpox infection.

CHLAMYDIA INFECTION

GENERAL INFORMATION

DEFINITION—Chlamydia are intracellular parasites that have many of the same physical characteristics of viruses. They cause inflammation of the urethra (the tube that allows urine from the bladder to pass outside the body), vagina, cervix, uterus, Fallopian tubes, anus, ovaries and epididymis. This is a common sexually transmitted disease. Chlamydia infection may also be transmitted to the eyes or lungs of a newborn infant. If chlamydia are found by microscopic exam and culture of discharge in any person who is sexually active, all sexual partners must be treated.

BODY PARTS INVOLVED—Urethra, vagina, cervix, uterus, Fallopian tubes, anus, ovaries, epididymis.

SEX OR AGE MOST AFFECTED—Both sexes, age 12 and older.

SIGNS & SYMPTOMS
- Sometimes no symptoms during early stages.
- Vaginal discharge (females).
- Urethral discharge (males).
- Anal swelling, pain or discharge.
- Reddening of the vagina or tip of the penis.
- Abdominal pain; fever, discomfort on urinating.
- Genital discomfort or pain.

CAUSES—A virus-like bacterium called Chlamydia trachomatis. Usually spread by direct contact with an infected person by vaginal or anal intercourse. Rarely, vaginal infection during birth of a newborn may infect the baby.

RISK INCREASES WITH
- Unprotected sexual activity.
- Sexual activity with multiple partners.
- Use of oral contraceptives or an intrauterine device (IUD).
- Diabetes mellitus.
- Hot weather, nonventilating clothing or any condition that increases genital moisture warmth and darkness, these foster growth of germs.

HOW TO PREVENT
- Use of latex condoms during sexual activity.
- Treatment of all sexual partners of any infected person (usually 2 weeks of an oral antibiotic such as tetracycline).

WHAT TO EXPECT

DIAGNOSTIC MEASURES
- Your own observation of symptoms.
- Medical history and physical exam by a doctor.
- Vaginal smear, rectal smear and urethral smear for laboratory analysis.
- Re-exam after completing the prescribed treatment.

APPROPRIATE HEALTH CARE
- Doctor's treatment.
- Home care after diagnosis.

POSSIBLE COMPLICATIONS
- Sterility in female.
- Infecting one's sexual partner.
- Secondary bacterial infections in pelvic organs, genitals or rectum.
- Pelvic inflammatory disease.
- Liver infection (perihepatitis)
- Reiter's syndrome.

PROBABLE OUTCOME—Complete cure with adequate antibiotic treatment.

HOW TO TREAT

GENERAL MEASURES
- Keep the genital area clean. Use plain unscented soap.
- Take showers rather than tub baths.
- Wear cotton panties or pantyhose with a cotton crotch. Avoid panties made from nonventilating materials, such as nylon.
- After urination or bowel movements, cleanse by wiping or washing from front to back (vagina to anus).
- Lose weight if you are obese.
- Avoid douches.
- If you have diabetes, adhere strictly to your treatment program.
- Avoid irritating sprays.
- Avoid pants that are tight in the crotch and thighs.
- Change tampons frequently.
- If urinating causes burning, urinate through a tubular device, such as a toilet-paper roll or plastic cup with the end cut out, or pour a cup of warm water over genital area while urinating.
- A follow-up medical examination is necessary after completing the prescribed treatment.
- Testing for other sexually transmitted diseases is recommended.

MEDICATION—Your doctor may prescribe oral antibiotics, such as tetracycline, for 2 weeks.

ACTIVITY
- Avoid overexertion, heat and excessive sweating.
- Delay sexual relations until treatment is completed and symptoms are gone.
- Allow about 3 weeks for recovery.

DIET—No special diet.

CALL YOUR DOCTOR IF

- You have symptoms of chlamydia infection.
- Symptoms persist longer than 1 week or worsen despite treatment.
- Unusual vaginal bleeding or swelling develops.

CHOLECYSTITIS OR CHOLANGITIS

GENERAL INFORMATION

DEFINITION—Infection or inflammation of the gallbladder (cholecystitis) or the ducts (cholangitis) that drain bile from the gallbladder to the small intestine. May be confused with hepatitis, pancreatitis or duodenal ulcer.

BODY PARTS INVOLVED—Gallbladder (located under the liver, in the upper right abdomen); bile ducts in the liver, leading to the gallbladder.

SEX OR AGE MOST AFFECTED
- Both sexes, but more common in women.
- Adults; rarely in children or adolescents.

SIGNS & SYMPTOMS
- Cramping pain in the upper right of the abdomen. Pain may also occur in the chest (imitating a heart attack), in the upper back or the right shoulder. These symptoms frequently follow a meal rich in fats.
- Tenderness in the upper abdomen.
- Nausea and vomiting.
- Belching.
- Slight fever. If high fever and chills occur, a bacterial infection is present.
- Jaundice (yellow skin or eyes) (sometimes).
- Pale stools (sometimes).
- Skin itching (sometimes).

CAUSES—Inflammation or bacterial infection, which are usually caused by gallstone formation and blockage of bile ducts.

RISK INCREASES WITH
- Diet that is high in fat and low in fiber.
- Chronic or acute pancreatitis.
- Coronary artery disease.
- Family history of gallbladder disease.
- Oral contraceptives.
- Rapid weight loss.
- Diabetes or cirrhosis; obesity.
- Female, middle age (40 to 50); or female with previous gallstones who takes estrogens.

HOW TO PREVENT—Avoid risk factors.

WHAT TO EXPECT

DIAGNOSTIC MEASURES
- Your own observation of symptoms.
- Medical history and exam by a doctor.
- Laboratory blood studies.
- X-rays of the gallbladder.
- Ultrasonography (see Glossary) of the gallbladder and bile ducts.
- Radioisotope studies (see Glossary) of liver and pancreas.

APPROPRIATE HEALTH CARE
- Specific treatment will depend on degree of severity, infection, size of stones, and your general health.

- Nonsurgical treatment methods include: medication to dissolve the stones or extracorporeal shock wave lithotripsy that will shatter the stones.
- Surgical treatment is usually a cholecystectomy done by laparoscopic technique or an open surgical procedure (see Surgery section for both).

POSSIBLE COMPLICATIONS
- Gallbladder rupture and peritonitis, or abscess.
- Hepatitis or cancer.
- Choledocholithiasis (stones pass from gallbladder into common bile duct obstructing flow of bile).

PROBABLE OUTCOME
- Symptoms of some mild attacks subside spontaneously in 1 to 4 days, if no complications develop.
- May require hospitalization and treatment.
- Recurrences are common. Attacks will cease with surgery to remove the gallbladder.

HOW TO TREAT

GENERAL MEASURES
- Be sure you know and understand all your treatment options.
- See Resources for Additional Information.

MEDICATION
- Don't medicate yourself with nonprescription pain relievers during an attack. These may mask symptoms of a bacterial infection—allowing it to worsen—and delay treatment.
- Your doctor may prescribe:
  Analgesics, including narcotics, to relieve pain.
  Ursodiol (brand name Actigall) to dissolve gallstones (will take about 2 years and works in 50% of patients).
  Antibiotics in acute cases.

ACTIVITY—Rest in bed until symptoms disappear or recovery from surgery is complete. While in bed, move your legs often to reduce the likelihood of deep-vein blood clotting.

DIET—Because of nausea and vomiting, intravenous fluids are usually necessary during attacks. Begin taking clear liquids or a soft diet as soon as you can tolerate solid foods.

CALL YOUR DOCTOR IF

- You have symptoms of cholecystitis or cholangitis; if accompanied by shortness of breath, sweating and nausea, call immediately!
- The following occurs during an attack:
  Fever; jaundice (yellow skin or eyes).
  Recurrent vomiting.
  Intolerable pain.

CHOLESTEROL, HIGH (Hypercholesterolemia)

GENERAL INFORMATION

DEFINITION—A total blood cholesterol level that is higher than the recommended safe range. When the blood contains too much cholesterol, the risk of heart and blood-vessel disease increases. Cholesterol is a white, fat-related (waxy) substance, manufactured by the liver, and essential for maintaining cells, making hormones and bile salts.

Total blood cholesterol is made up of LDL (low-density lipoprotein); HDL (high-density lipoprotein) and VLDL (very low density lipoprotein). Increased levels of LDL are associated with plaque deposits on artery walls that narrow them and restrict blood flow. HDL or "good cholesterol" helps prevent plaque.

SEX OR AGE MOST AFFECTED—Adults of both sexes, but more common in men.

SIGNS & SYMPTOMS—High cholesterol in itself does not produce symptoms.

CAUSES—The level of blood cholesterol is affected by diet, heredity and some diseases.

RISK INCREASES WITH
- Diet high in saturated fat.
- Hereditary factors.
- Obesity.
- Smoking.
- Sedentary life-style.
- Stress.
- Disorders such as hypothyroidism, diabetes mellitus, nephrotic syndrome, obstructive liver disease.
- Use of some drugs (progestins, anabolic steroids, diuretics, beta-blockers, some immunosuppressants).
- Alcohol excess.
- People with family members who have had a stroke or heart attack before age 50.

HOW TO PREVENT
- Low-fat diet.
- Exercise.
- Weight control.

WHAT TO EXPECT

DIAGNOSTIC MEASURES
- Medical history and exam by a doctor.
- Laboratory test to measure blood cholesterol levels. In the general population, the results usually range from 100 to 280 milligrams per deciliter (mg/dl). Readings below 200 mg/dl put you at below-average risk, borderline risk level is 200 mg/dl and high-risk level is greater than 240 mg/dl. When results are in risk ranges, further evaluation is suggested to verify the results and to determine the separate levels of LDL, HDL and triglycerides (another kind of blood fat).

APPROPRIATE HEALTH CARE
- Self-care after diagnosis.
- Doctor's treatment.

POSSIBLE COMPLICATIONS—May lead to atherosclerosis, heart disease and stroke. Smoking increases the risk.

PROBABLE OUTCOME—High cholesterol levels can usually be lowered with a change in diet and life-style modifications. When these are insufficient, medications may be prescribed.

HOW TO TREAT

GENERAL MEASURES
- The diet changes and life-style modifications do not mean you have to give up all the good things you enjoy. Moderation is important.
- Stop smoking. Consult your doctor about recommendations for a cessation program.

MEDICATION—Your doctor may prescribe: cholesterol lowering drugs if self-care measures do not reduce elevated cholesterol levels. Diet restrictions need to be continued, even if you are taking these medications.

ACTIVITY
- Regular aerobic exercise (30 minutes, 3 times a week) can help increase the level of HDL, the "good" cholesterol.
- Consult your doctor before beginning an exercise program if you have high cholesterol levels and other risk-factors for heart disease.

DIET
- Restrict your consumption of foods that contain cholesterol and saturated fats (eggs, dairy products, beef, dark meat poultry, poultry skin, and coconut and palm oils).
- Eat a low-fat, high-fiber diet (see both in Appendix).
- Begin a weight reduction diet if you are overweight (see Weight-Loss Diet in Appendix).
- Read food labels carefully. A product may have no cholesterol but still be high in fat content. Reducing your intake of both fat and cholesterol is important.
- Reduce alcohol intake.

CALL YOUR DOCTOR IF

- You want to learn your cholesterol levels.
- Self-care measures do not reduce elevated cholesterol levels.
- New or unexplained symptoms develop. Drugs used in treatment may cause side effects.

CHRONIC FATIGUE SYNDROME

GENERAL INFORMATION

DEFINITION—Chronic fatigue syndrome is characterized primarily by profound fatigue. There is usually an abrupt onset of symptoms that come and go for at least six months. It is unknown whether it represents one or many disorders. It is difficult to diagnose because there is no specific laboratory test, or a defined set of signs and symptoms. Currently, the major criteria used to define cases are: 1) persistence of relapsing fatigue that does not resolve with bed rest and is severe enough to reduce average daily activity by at least 50% for at least 6 months, and 2) other chronic clinical conditions have been satisfactorily excluded, including pre-existing psychiatric disease. Other signs and symptoms aid in the diagnosis.

BODY PARTS INVOLVED—Endocrine system, muscles, gastrointestinal system, central nervous system.

SEX OR AGE MOST AFFECTED—It is observed primarily in young adults between 20 and 40, and women outnumber the men about two to one.

SIGNS & SYMPTOMS
- Fatigue.
- Low grade fever.
- Pharyngitis.
- Painful lymph glands.
- Sore throat.
- Generalized muscle weakness.
- Muscle aches.
- Headaches.
- Sleep disturbances (hypersomnia or insomnia).
- Joint pain.
- Neuropsychological complaints (photophobia, forgetfulness, irritability, confusion, difficulty in concentrating, depression, vision changes).

CAUSES—Unknown. Immunological abnormalities may be involved. Many theories center on an infectious agent, but no such agent has been identified. Epstein-Barr virus and others have been implicated.

RISK INCREASES WITH—Unknown.

HOW TO PREVENT—Unknown.

WHAT TO EXPECT

DIAGNOSTIC MEASURES
- No specific medical test is available. The 2 major criteria mentioned in definition plus about 8 of the other signs and symptoms are necessary to establish the diagnosis.
- Medical history and social history plus physical exam by a doctor.
- Laboratory blood and urine studies as necessary to rule out other disorders.

APPROPRIATE HEALTH CARE
- Self-care after diagnosis.
- Doctor's treatment.
- Psychotherapy may be helpful for some patients.

POSSIBLE COMPLICATIONS—None specific to the disorder. Symptoms are usually most severe during the first 6 months.

POSSIBLE OUTCOME—Generally very slow improvement over months or years.

HOW TO TREAT

GENERAL MEASURES
- Basic management involves four areas:
  1) validation of the diagnosis and your education about the disorder
  2) general treatment measures
  3) treatment of specific symptoms
  4) experimental therapy
- Try to remain optimistic.
- Keep involved in life; don't isolate yourself.
- Sometimes a change of scenery can help. Take a vacation if possible.
- Be patient with family and friends and their understanding and acceptance of your disorder.
- Join a local or national support group.
- See Resources for Additional Information.

MEDICATION
- Medications must be individually tailored but may include pain medicine, local injections, antidepressants or others.
- Other experimental medication therapies are being studied.

ACTIVITY
- Rest if you feel tired.
- Exercise is important. Begin a gradual program that may be just 3-5 minutes a day to start with. Increase the activity by about 20% about every 2-3 weeks. Setbacks will occur, so don't be discouraged.

DIET—Try to maintain good nutrition, even if appetite is decreased. Eat a low-fat, high-fiber diet (see both in Appendix). Take vitamin supplements.

CALL YOUR DOCTOR IF

- You have signs and symptoms of chronic fatigue syndrome.
- Symptoms worsen after treatment is started.
- New or unexplained symptoms develop. Drugs used in treatment may cause side effects.

CHRONIC OBSTRUCTIVE PULMONARY DISEASE (COPD; Emphysema)

GENERAL INFORMATION

DEFINITION—A term used to describe chronic airway obstruction that results from emphysema, chronic bronchitis, asthma, or any combination of these disorders. The combination often involves bronchitis and emphysema.

BODY PARTS INVOLVED—Lungs.

SEX OR AGE MOST AFFECTED—More men than women are affected (until recently, men were more likely to be the heavy smokers).

SIGNS & SYMPTOMS
- Symptoms may not appear until middle-age even though COPD is thought to begin early in adult life.

Bronchitis:
- Frequent cough or coughing spasms usually with sputum.
- Shortness of breath.
- Sputum that is thick and difficult to cough up.

Emphysema:
- No symptoms in the early stages (often).
- Increasing shortness of breath over several years.
- Occasional recurrent infections of the lungs or bronchial tubes.
- Weight loss.
- Minimal wheezing or coughing; scant sputum.

CAUSES—Damage to the lung from bronchial irritation and inflammation and caused by:
- Cigarette smoking; air pollution.
- Antitrypsin deficiency (an inherited form of emphysema).
- Occupational exposure to irritants (e.g., firefighters).
- Infection, possibly (viral).

RISK INCREASES WITH
- Smoking; passive smoke (especially adults whose parents smoked).
- Severe viral pneumonia early in life.
- Aging.
- Family history of allergies, respiratory or lung disorders.

HOW TO PREVENT
Don't smoke. Also avoid secondary (or passive) smoke.

WHAT TO EXPECT

DIAGNOSTIC MEASURES
- Your own observation of symptoms.
- Medical history and exam by a doctor.
- Laboratory blood studies, pulmonary functions studies, CT scan, bronchogram (see Glossary for both) and chest x-ray.

APPROPRIATE HEALTH CARE
- Doctor's treatment.

- Overall goals of treatment are to relieve symptoms, slow the progression of the disorder and prevent complications.
- Home treatment is usually adequate, but hospitalization may be required.
- Lung transplantation is currently being evaluated.

POSSIBLE COMPLICATIONS
- Frequent infections; anxiety; depression.
- Other complications include pulmonary hypertension, cor pulmonale, secondary polycythemia, bullous lung disease and respiratory failure.

PROBABLE OUTCOME
- Gradual decline in lung function. However, treatment can reduce symptoms, help prevent infections and permit a more active life.
- Younger patients may have a fairly good prognosis; older patients have a poorer prognosis.

HOW TO TREAT

GENERAL MEASURES
- Installing air conditioning with air filters in the home may be helpful.
- Bronchial hygiene may be improved with inhalation of mist, postural drainage and chest physical therapy.
- Get pneumovax vaccine and yearly influenza vaccines.
- Join a support group.
- See Resources for Additional Information.

MEDICATION—Your doctor may prescribe:
- Bronchodilators.
- Antibiotics for infections.
- Corticosteroids may be beneficial for some.
- Drugs for anxiety or depression, but must be used with caution.
- Replacement therapy for antitrypsin deficiency.
- Supplemental oxygen for continuous use, only at night or with exercise.

ACTIVITY
- Prolonged inactivity leads to increased disability. If there is no severe heart disease, it is important to maintain regular exercise.
- Occupational therapy, vocational rehabilitation and physical therapy may be recommended.

DIET—No special diet, but good nutrition is vital to help maintain your well-being. Drink at least 8 to 10 glasses of fluid each day.

CALL YOUR DOCTOR IF

- You have symptoms of COPD.
- A fever develops or chest pain increases.
- Blood appears in the sputum or sputum thickens; vomiting occurs.
- Shortness of breath occurs even when you are resting or not coughing.

CIRRHOSIS OF THE LIVER

GENERAL INFORMATION

DEFINITION—Chronic scarring of the liver, leading to loss of normal liver function.

BODY PARTS INVOLVED—Liver and its major blood vessels.

SEX OR AGE MOST AFFECTED—Adults of both sexes, but twice as common in men.

SIGNS & SYMPTOMS
Early stages:
- Fatigue; weakness.
- Poor appetite; nausea; weight loss.
- Enlarged liver.
- Red palms.

Late stages:
- Jaundice (yellow skin and eyes).
- Dark yellow or brown urine.
- Spider blood vessels of the skin (fine vessels that spread out from a central point).
- Hair loss.
- Breast enlargement in men.
- Fluid accumulation in the abdomen and legs.
- Enlarged spleen.
- Diarrhea; stool may be black or bloody.
- Bleeding and bruising.
- Mental confusion; coma.

CAUSES—Inflammation of the liver, accompanied by destruction of liver cells, cell regeneration and scarring. These may be preceded by:
- Prolonged, excess alcohol consumption.
- Hepatitis.
- Exposure to toxic chemicals.
- Inherited causes.

RISK INCREASES WITH
- Poor nutrition.
- Hepatitis.
- Excess alcohol consumption. Individuals vary widely in the amount and duration of alcohol consumption necessary to cause cirrhosis.
- Occupational exposure to chemicals toxic to the liver.

HOW TO PREVENT
- Obtain treatment for alcoholism.
- Obtain prompt medical treatment for hepatitis.
- Survey your work environment for possible exposure to toxic chemicals.

WHAT TO EXPECT

DIAGNOSTIC MEASURES
- Your own observation of symptoms.
- Medical history and physical exam by a doctor.
- Laboratory studies, such as blood and urine tests of liver function.
- X-ray and/or biopsy of liver.

APPROPRIATE HEALTH CARE
- Treatment methods may include drug treatment, dietary restrictions, rest and other supportive measures.
- Psychotherapy or counseling (for alcoholism).
- Liver transplantation (sometimes). (See Liver Transplantation in Surgery section.)

POSSIBLE COMPLICATIONS
- Life-threatening hemorrhage, especially from the esophagus and stomach.
- Liver cancer.
- Body poisoning and coma from a buildup of ammonia and other body waste.
- Sexual impotence.

PROBABLE OUTCOME—Cirrhosis can be arrested if the underlying cause can be removed. Liver damage is irreversible, but symptoms can be relieved or controlled. A near-normal life is possible if treated early and treatment succeeds.

If the underlying cause is not removed, liver scarring will continue, resulting in death from liver failure.

HOW TO TREAT

GENERAL MEASURES
- Stop all alcohol if necessary, ask for help from family, friends and community agencies. Contact an Alcoholics Anonymous group in your community.
- Weigh daily and keep a record. Notify your doctor if there is a sudden weight gain.
- See Resources for Additional Information.

MEDICATION—Your doctor may prescribe:
- Iron supplements for anemia resulting from hemorrhage or poor nutrition.
- Diuretics to reduce fluid retention.
- Antibiotics, such as neomycin, to reduce ammonia buildup.

ACTIVITY
- Maintain as active a life as possible.
- Elevate swollen feet and legs when resting.

DIET—Eat a nutritionally balanced diet with appropriate vitamins and minerals. Eating frequent small meals may help.

CALL YOUR DOCTOR IF

- You have symptoms of cirrhosis.
- The following occurs during treatment:
  Vomiting blood or passing black stool.
  Mental confusion or coma.
  Fever or other signs of infection (redness, swelling, tenderness or pain).

CLAUDICATION

 GENERAL INFORMATION

DEFINITION—A feeling of muscle fatigue or cramp-like pain, usually in one or both legs. The discomfort occurs after minimal exercise, such as a short walk, and is normally relieved by resting. The disorder poses no immediate or even long-term danger.

BODY PARTS INVOLVED—The calf is more frequently affected, but it can occur in the thighs, buttocks, hips or feet.

SEX OR AGE MOST AFFECTED—It is more common in men than women, particularly men over age 55.

SIGNS & SYMPTOMS
- Pain, tension, weakness in the limb.
- Pain occurs while walking and pain stops when resting.
- Unable to walk distances.
- Loss of the hair on the toes.
- Lameness or limping.

CAUSES
- Blockage or narrowing of the arteries of the legs due to atherosclerosis.
- Rarer cause is spinal stenosis (pressure on nerve roots that pass into either leg).

RISK INCREASES WITH
- Smoking.
- Diabetes.
- High blood pressure.
- Obesity.
- Heart disease.
- Hyperlipidemia (fatty substances in the blood are higher than normal).

HOW TO PREVENT
- Stop smoking.
- Weight loss, if obese.
- Routine exercise program.
- Minimize the amount of saturated fats in the diet.

 WHAT TO EXPECT

DIAGNOSTIC MEASURES
- Medical history and physical exam by a doctor.
- Doppler ultrasound and arteriography (see Glossary for both) may be conducted to help rule out other disorders.

APPROPRIATE HEALTH CARE
- Self-care after diagnosis.
- Doctor's treatment.
- Balloon angioplasty for treatment in select patients.
- Various surgical procedures, depending on the site of the disease and health of patient, are available for more severe cases.

POSSIBLE COMPLICATIONS
- Pain while resting as well as when walking.
- Tissue loss and gangrene (rare).

POSSIBLE OUTCOME—Gradual improvement in ability to walk distances without pain.

 HOW TO TREAT

GENERAL MEASURES
- Routine exercise is important.
- A stop smoking program is essential. Ask your doctor for recommendations.
- Elevate head of bed with 4-6 inch blocks.
- Get treatment for control of high blood pressure if needed.

MEDICATION—Your doctor may prescribe:
- Low doses of aspirin.
- Special medication to increase blood flow.

ACTIVITY
- Daily exercise program. Walking as much as possible (up to 4-5 miles a day), resting if pain or discomfort occurs, and then walking again. Walk on level ground. Keep a log of progress in walking distances.
- Other daily activities performed as normal.

DIET
- Weight loss program if overweight.
- Low-fat diet may be helpful (see Low-fat Diet in Appendix).

 CALL YOUR DOCTOR IF

- You have symptoms of claudication.
- You experience chest pain, shortness of breath or rapid heart beat during exercise program.
- New or unexplained symptoms develop. Drugs used in treatment may cause side effects.

ILLNESS & DISORDERS

COLD, COMMON

 GENERAL INFORMATION

DEFINITION—A contagious viral infection of the upper-respiratory passages.

BODY PARTS INVOLVED—Nose; throat; sinuses; ears; eustachian tubes; trachea; larynx; bronchial tubes.

SEX OR AGE MOST AFFECTED—Both sexes; all ages.

SIGNS & SYMPTOMS
- Runny or stuffy nose. Nasal discharge is watery at first, then becomes thick and greenish yellow.
- Sore throat.
- Hoarseness.
- Cough that produces little or no sputum.
- Low fever.
- Fatigue.
- Watering eyes.
- Appetite loss.

CAUSES—Any of at least 100 viruses. Virus particles spread through the air or from person-to-person contact, especially hand-shaking.

RISK INCREASES WITH
- Winter (colds are most frequent in cold weather).
- Children attending school or day care.
- Household member who has cold.
- Crowded or unsanitary living conditions.
- Infection may be facilitated by stress, fatigue or allergic disorders.

HOW TO PREVENT
- To prevent spreading a cold to others, avoid unnecessary contact during the contagious phase (first 2 to 4 days).
- Wash hands frequently, especially after blowing your nose or before handling food.
- Avoid risks listed above if possible.
- Humidify your air.

 WHAT TO EXPECT

DIAGNOSTIC MEASURES
- Your own observation of symptoms.
- Medical history and physical exam by a doctor (sometimes).
- Laboratory throat culture to rule out bacterial infection with streptococcus or other germs (sometimes).

APPROPRIATE HEALTH CARE
- Self-care.
- Doctor's treatment (for complications only).

POSSIBLE COMPLICATIONS—Bacterial infections of the ears, throat, sinuses or lungs.

PROBABLE OUTCOME—Spontaneous recovery in 7 to 14 days.

 HOW TO TREAT

GENERAL MEASURES
- To relieve congestion, inhale steam from a pan of boiled water (after removing it from the heat); take hot showers; use salt-water drops (1/2 teaspoon salt to 1 cup of warm water).
- Use a cool-mist, ultrasonic humidifier to increase air moisture. Clean humidifier daily.
- Don't smoke if you have a cough.
- For a sore throat, drink hot liquids, use medicated throat lozenges or suck on hard candies.
- For a baby too young to blow his nose, use an infant nasal aspirator. If mucus is thick and sticky, loosen it by putting 2 or 3 drops of salt-water solution (see above) into nostrils.

  Don't insert cotton swabs into a child's nostrils. Instead, catch the discharge outside the nostril on a tissue or swab, roll it around and pull the discharge out of the nose.
- For an infant or very young child, lay the child on his stomach to sleep. This improves nasal drainage and breathing.

MEDICATION
- No medicine, including antibiotics, can cure the common cold. To relieve symptoms, you may use nonprescription drugs, such as acetaminophen, decongestants, nose drops or sprays, cough remedies and throat lozenges. Don't give a child under age 18 aspirin for cold symptoms.
- Vitamin C in large doses (up to 1000 mg a day) may shorten duration.

ACTIVITY—Bed rest is not necessary, but avoid vigorous activity. Rest often.

DIET—Drink extra fluids, including water, fruit juice, tea and carbonated drinks. Avoid milk because it may thicken secretions.

 CALL YOUR DOCTOR IF

The following occurs during the illness:
- Increased throat pain, or white or yellow spots on the tonsils or other parts of the throat.
- Coughing episodes that last longer than intervals between coughing; cough that produces thick, yellow-green or gray sputum; cough that lasts longer than 10 days; or difficult or labored breathing between coughing bouts.
- You cannot distinguish a cold from the flu.
- Fever that lasts several days; shaking chills.
- Chest pain or shortness of breath.
- Earache, headache or skin rash.
- Pain in the teeth or over the sinuses.
- Unusual lethargy or irritability.
- Delirium.
- Enlarged, tender glands in the neck.
- Dusky blue or gray lips, skin or nail beds.
- Inability to bottle-feed or breast-feed (infant).

COLIC IN INFANTS

 GENERAL INFORMATION

DEFINITION—Repeated episodes of excessive crying that cannot be explained. Crying ranges from fussiness to agonized screaming.

BODY PARTS INVOLVED—Possibly the lower intestinal tract.

SEX OR AGE MOST AFFECTED—Both sexes, but more common in boys. Colic affects infants up to 5 months old and is most common in a first child.

SIGNS & SYMPTOMS—Excessive crying with the following characteristics:
• Crying bouts usually occur in late afternoon or evening.
• Crying bouts usually begin at 2 to 4 weeks and last through 3 or 4 months.
• The infant's abdomen may rumble, and the child may draw up the legs as if in pain.
• No specific disease, such as an ear infection, hernia, allergy or urinary infection, can be discovered.

CAUSES—Unknown. Colic may be related to physical pain or emotional upset. Some likely possibilities include: hunger; insufficient sleep; milk that is too hot; overfeeding; food allergy; reactions to tension in the home; loneliness; or tiredness.

RISK INCREASES WITH—No known risk factor.

HOW TO PREVENT—No specific preventive measures. Remove any causes that can be identified.

 WHAT TO EXPECT

DIAGNOSTIC MEASURES
• Your own observation of symptoms.
• Medical history and physical exam by a doctor.

APPROPRIATE HEALTH CARE
• Home care.
• Doctor's treatment (occasionally).

POSSIBLE COMPLICATIONS—None expected.

PROBABLE OUTCOME—All babies cry, and many have fussy periods. Crying is an important activity and means of communication. Colic is a distressing, but not dangerous, condition. The symptoms can sometimes be relieved. When they can't, the colic will disappear after the 4th or 5th month.

 HOW TO TREAT

GENERAL MEASURES
• Be patient and tolerant. Since colic is not the parents' fault, do not blame yourself.
• Don't feed the baby every time he or she cries. Look for a reason, such as: a gas bubble; cramped position; too much heat or cold; soiled diaper; open diaper pin; or a desire to be cuddled.
• During an attack of gas, hold the baby securely, and gently massage the lower abdomen. Rocking may be soothing or other movement (car ride, swing or stroller).
• Offer the baby a pacifier.
• Playing music may help.
• Allow the baby to cry if you are certain everything is all right (not hungry, not soiled, no fever, no open pins) and you have done all you can. Colic is distressing, but not harmful.
• Keep the baby warm.
• Get someone to care for the baby for at least an hour or two each day. The tension can get to you and you need some relief.

MEDICATION—Medications are usually not helpful for colic. Simethicone (for gas) may be prescribed.

ACTIVITY—No restrictions.

DIET
• Cow's milk in the diet of a breast-feeding mother may cause colic. Avoid drinking it if your baby has colic.
• Interrupt bottle feedings after every ounce and burp the baby. Interrupt breast feedings every 5 minutes.
• Allow at least 20 minutes to feed the baby. Don't prop the baby for feedings.
• Nipple holes should not be too large. A vigorous baby may require blind nipples in which you can make small, homemade nipple holes.
• For formula-fed babies, try stopping the cow's milk and switching to soy-milk/hydrolyzed-protein formula.

 CALL YOUR DOCTOR IF

• The baby's rectal temperature rises to 101F (38.3C) or higher.
• You are concerned about your emotional control.

COLITIS, ULCERATIVE (Granulomatous Colitis)

GENERAL INFORMATION

DEFINITION—A serious, chronic, inflammatory disease of the colon characterized by ulceration and episodes of bloody diarrhea. The ulcerated areas are inflamed and may form abscesses in the lining of the large intestine. Ulcerative colitis may be confused with some bacterial infections of the colon.

BODY PARTS INVOLVED—Rectum; large bowel.

SEX OR AGE MOST AFFECTED—May occur at any age, but most common in women between ages 15 and 40.

SIGNS & SYMPTOMS
Early symptoms include:
- Pain in the left side of the abdomen that improves after bowel movements.
- Episodes of bloody diarrhea with mucus, alternating with symptom-free intervals.

During an acute attack:
- Increased bloody diarrhea (up to 10 to 20 bowel movements a day).
- Severe cramps and pain around the rectum.
- Sweating; dehydration.
- Nausea; appetite and weight loss.
- Bloated abdomen.
- Fever as high as 104F (40C).

CAUSES—Unknown. Genetic, infectious, immunologic and psychologic factors have all been suggested.

RISK INCREASES WITH
- Family history of ulcerative colitis.
- Stress, alcohol and certain diets seem to aggravate symptoms.

HOW TO PREVENT—No specific measures.

WHAT TO EXPECT

DIAGNOSTIC MEASURES
- Medical history and exam by a doctor.
- Laboratory stool and blood studies.
- X-ray of the colon (barium enema).
- Sigmoidoscopy (see Glossary).
- Biopsy of the colon lining.

APPROPRIATE HEALTH CARE
- Self-care after diagnosis.
- Doctor's treatment.
- Psychological counseling.
- Surgery to remove the diseased colon (sometimes). See Colostomy (in Surgery section).
- Hospitalization during worst episodes.

POSSIBLE COMPLICATIONS
- Life-threatening blood loss, ulceration through the intestinal wall or peritonitis during acute attacks.
- Malnutrition, wasting of the body or chronic disability.
- Inflammation of joints, eyes and skin.
- Colon cancer; the risk is greater in persons with ulcerative colitis.

PROBABLE OUTCOME—Often curable with counseling and medical treatment or surgery. If not curable, symptoms can be controlled with treatment.

HOW TO TREAT

GENERAL MEASURES
- To reduce cramps, apply a hot-water bottle, warm moist towels or heating pad to the abdomen or try taking a hot bath.
- Quit smoking. Ask your doctor for recommendations for cessation program.
- Try to reduce stress (see How to Cope With Stress in Appendix).
- See Resources for Additional Information.

MEDICATION
- Don't use aspirin. It increases bleeding risk.
- Your doctor may prescribe:
  Antidiarrhea medication for minor symptoms.
  Sulfa drugs, such as sulfasalazine, for moderate symptoms.
  Medicated enemas (usually with hydrocortisone).
  Cortisone drugs for severe disease.
  Immunosuppressive drugs in patients with chronic disease.

ACTIVITY—Bed rest may be necessary during acute attacks. However, resume normal activity as soon as symptoms improve.

DIET
- Vitamin and mineral supplements may be needed.
- If abdominal cramping, eat canned or cooked fruits and vegetables (skin on foods can be abrasive). Avoid raw fruits and vegetables.
- If diarrhea present, avoid roughage in diet and intestinal irritants (spicy foods, caffeine, alcohol).
- Iron replacement may be necessary.
- Avoid milk products if you have a lactose intolerance.
- Keep a food diary to discover which foods may trigger symptoms. Don't eat those foods.

CALL YOUR DOCTOR IF

- You have symptoms of ulcerative colitis.
- Fever and chills develop.
- Frequency of bowel movements or bleeding increases.
- Abdomen becomes distended.
- Jaundice (yellow eyes and skin and dark urine) develops.
- Vomiting begins or abdominal pain increases.

CONGESTIVE HEART FAILURE

GENERAL INFORMATION

DEFINITION—A complication of many serious diseases in which the heart loses its full pumping capacity. Blood backs up into other organs, especially the lungs and liver.

BODY PARTS INVOLVED—Heart; blood vessels; lungs; liver; extremities.

SEX OR AGE MOST AFFECTED—Both sexes and all ages, but more common after age 50.

SIGNS & SYMPTOMS
- Shortness of breath, especially with exertion or when lying flat in bed.
- Fatigue, weakness or faintness.
- Cough (usually with sputum).
- Swelling of the abdomen, legs and ankles.
- Rapid or irregular heartbeat.
- Low blood pressure.
- Distended neck veins.
- Enlarged liver.

CAUSES
- High blood pressure; heart-valve disease.
- Heart attack; coronary artery disease; heartbeat irregularities.
- Severe lung disease such as emphysema.
- Congenital heart disease; cardiomyopathy; hyperthyroidism.
- Severe anemia; heart tumor (rare).
- Infections complicating underlying disease.

RISK INCREASES WITH
- Infections with high fever.
- Smoking; obesity.
- Excess alcohol consumption. Alcohol depresses heart function.
- Use of certain drugs, such as beta-adrenergic blockers or excess digitalis.
- Diet that is high in fat and salt.

HOW TO PREVENT—If you have a condition that can lead to congestive heart failure, obtain medical care and adhere to your treatment program. Follow your dietary guidelines and don't drink alcohol or smoke.

WHAT TO EXPECT

DIAGNOSTIC MEASURES
- Your own observation of symptoms.
- Medical history and exam by a doctor.
- Laboratory blood studies and urinalysis.
- ECG (see Glossary).
- Heart-catheterization studies (occasionally).
- X-rays of the heart, lungs and blood vessels (angiography).
- Radioactive studies of heart muscle efficiency.
- Echocardiogram (occasionally; see Glossary).

APPROPRIATE HEALTH CARE
- Self-care after diagnosis.
- Doctor's treatment.

- Surgery on heart valves, coronary arteries or ventricular aneurysms (sometimes).
- Hospitalization (severe cases).
- Cardiac transplantation for severe cases that do not respond to medical treatment (sometimes).

POSSIBLE COMPLICATIONS
Pulmonary edema; heartbeat irregularities.

PROBABLE OUTCOME—Life expectancy is reduced, but many forms are well-controlled for a while with medication and sometimes surgery. Other forms cause chronic illness. Any infection may worsen the condition.

HOW TO TREAT

GENERAL MEASURES
- The aim of treatment is to improve the heart's pumping function usually with medications, rest, and other supportive measures.
- Weigh daily and keep a record.
- Don't smoke.
- Wear a Medic-Alert neck pendent or bracelet (see Glossary) that identifies your medical problem and the medications you take.
- See Resources for Additional Information.

MEDICATION—Your doctor may prescribe:
- Diuretics to decrease fluid retention and swelling.
- Digitalis to strengthen and regulate heartbeat.
- Antiarrhythmic drugs to stabilize heartbeat.
- "Afterload" vasodilators to reduce blood pressure, even if it's normal.
- Potassium replacements, if you take diuretics or digitalis.

ACTIVITY
In early stages, bed rest with the upper body elevated is as important as medication. Avoid unnecessary exertion (such as climbing stairs) until the condition is under control. You may need to alter your lifestyle to reduce symptoms.

DIET
- Achieve your ideal weight to reduce the heart's workload.
- Eat a low-salt, low-fat, high-fiber diet (see diets in Appendix). Don't drink alcohol.

CALL YOUR DOCTOR IF

- You have symptoms of congestive heart failure.
- The following occurs during treatment:
  Symptoms of infection, such as fever, muscle aches, headache and dizziness.
  Worsening of symptoms, especially rapid or irregular heartbeat or wheezing at night.
  Cough with increased sputum or blood.
  Weight gain of 3 or 4 pounds in 1 or 2 days.
- New, unexplained symptoms develop.

CONJUNCTIVITIS
(Pink Eye)

GENERAL INFORMATION

DEFINITION—An inflammation of the eyelid's underside and white part of the eye.

BODY PARTS INVOLVED—Eye; underside of the eyelid.

SEX OR AGE MOST AFFECTED—Both sexes and all ages, but more common in children.

SIGNS & SYMPTOMS—The following symptoms may affect one or both eyes:
- Clear, green or yellow discharge from the eye.
- After sleeping, crusts on lashes that cause eyelids to stick together.
- Eye pain.
- Swollen eyelids.
- Sensitivity to bright light.
- Redness and gritty feeling in the eye.
- Intense itching (allergic conjunctivitis only).

CAUSES
- Viral infection. Conjunctivitis may accompany colds or childhood diseases such as measles.
- Bacterial infection.
- Chemical irritation or wind, dust, smoke and other types of air pollution.
- Allergies caused by cosmetics, pollen or other allergens.
- A partially closed tear duct.
- Intense light, such as from sunlamps, snow reflection or electric arcs in welding.

RISK INCREASES WITH
- Newborns of mothers who are carriers of gonorrhea or chlamydia.
- Crowded or unsanitary living conditions.
- Exposure to others in public places, such as day care centers and public schools.

HOW TO PREVENT
- Wash hands frequently with soap and warm water.
- Avoid exposure to eye irritants.
- Newborns in hospital deliveries are routinely given antibiotic eye drops.
- Do not share eyeliners, and discard mascara after 4 to 6 months.

WHAT TO EXPECT

DIAGNOSTIC MEASURES
- Your own observation of symptoms.
- Medical history and physical exam by a doctor.
- Laboratory culture of the discharge from the eye (sometimes).

APPROPRIATE HEALTH CARE
- Self-care after diagnosis. Treatment of conjunctivitis varies with the cause.
- Doctor's treatment.
- If the infection does not improve in 2 or 3 days, it may be caused by an insensitive bacteria, virus or allergy. At this point, an ophthalmologist may need to culture the conjunctivae or make special studies to determine the cause of the conjunctivitis.

POSSIBLE COMPLICATIONS—If untreated, conjunctivitis may spread and damage the cornea permanently, impairing vision.

PROBABLE OUTCOME
- Allergic conjunctivitis can be cured if the allergen is removed. However it is likely to recur.
- Other forms are curable in 1 to 2 weeks with treatment.

HOW TO TREAT

GENERAL MEASURES
- Wash hands often with antiseptic soap, and use paper towels to dry. Don't touch eyes. Gently wipe the discharge from the eye using disposable tissues.
  Infections are frequently spread by contaminated fingers, towels, handkerchiefs or washcloths that have touched the infected eye.
- Use warm-water soaks (see Soaks in Appendix) to reduce discomfort.
- Don't use eye makeup.

MEDICATION—Your doctor may prescribe:
- Antibiotic or antiviral eye drops, sulfa eye drops, or ointment to fight infection. (Most eye care specialists believe steroid eyedrops should not be used until a diagnosis is definite. If the infection is caused by herpes simplex virus, steroids may spread it from the conjunctiva to the cornea, damaging the eye.)
- Anti-inflammatory eye drops.

ACTIVITY—Resume your normal activities as soon as symptoms improve.

DIET—No special diet.

CALL YOUR DOCTOR IF

- You have symptoms of conjunctivitis.
- The infection does not improve in 48 hours, despite treatment.
- Fever occurs.
- Pain increases.
- Vision is affected.

CONSTIPATION

GENERAL INFORMATION

DEFINITION—Difficult, uncomfortable or infrequent bowel movements that are hard and dry. In most people, constipation is harmless, but it can indicate an underlying disorder.

BODY PARTS INVOLVED—Colon.

SEX OR AGE MOST AFFECTED—Both sexes; all ages.

SIGNS & SYMPTOMS—People vary widely in bowel activity. Any of the following may be a sign of constipation:
- Infrequent bowel movements, sometimes accompanied by abdominal swelling.
- Hard feces.
- Straining during bowel movements.
- Pain or bleeding with bowel movements.
- Sensation of continuing fullness after a bowel movement.

CAUSES
- Inadequate fluid intake.
- Insufficient fiber in the diet. Fiber adds bulk, holds water and creates easily passed, soft feces.
- Inactivity; depression.
- Hypothyroidism; hypercalcemia.
- Anal fissure.
- Chronic kidney failure.
- Back pain.
- Colon or rectal cancer; irritable bowel syndrome.

RISK INCREASES WITH
- Stress.
- Illness requiring complete bed rest.
- Use of certain drugs, including: belladonna; calcium-channel blockers; beta-adrenergic blockers; tricyclic antidepressants; narcotics; atropine; or aspirin.
- Travel.
- Sedentary lifestyle.

HOW TO PREVENT
- Eat a well-balanced, high-fiber diet.
- Exercise regularly.
- Drink at least 8 glasses of water a day.

WHAT TO EXPECT

DIAGNOSTIC MEASURES
- Your own observation of symptoms. Tell your doctor of any major change in your bowel pattern that lasts longer than 1 week. It may be a sign of cancer.
- Medical history and physical exam by a doctor.
- Laboratory tests of blood and stool to detect internal bleeding.
- Sigmoidoscopy (rare; see Glossary).

APPROPRIATE HEALTH CARE
- Self-care.
- Doctor's treatment (occasionally).

POSSIBLE COMPLICATIONS—Hemorrhoids, laxative dependency, hernia from excessive straining, uterine or rectal prolapse, spastic colitis, bowel obstruction, chronic constipation.

PROBABLE OUTCOME—Usually curable with exercise, diet and adequate fluids.

HOW TO TREAT

GENERAL MEASURES
- Set aside a regular time each day for bowel movements. The best time is often within 1 hour after breakfast. Don't try to hurry. Sit at least 10 minutes, whether or not a bowel movement occurs.
- Drinking hot water, tea or coffee may help stimulate bowel.

MEDICATION—For occasional constipation, you may use mild nonprescription laxatives such as bulk-formers, lubricants, stool softeners and enemas. Don't use laxatives or enemas regularly as this can cause dependency. Avoid harsh laxatives and cathartics, such as Epsom salts. The best laxatives are bulk-formers, such as bran, psyllium, polycarbophil and methylcellulose.

ACTIVITY—Exercise and good physical fitness helps maintain healthy bowel patterns.

DIET—Drink at least 8 glasses of water each day. Include bulk foods, such as bran and raw fruits and vegetables, in your diet.

CALL YOUR DOCTOR IF

- You have constipation that persists, despite self-care—especially if the constipation represents a change in your normal bowel patterns.
- Constipation is accompanied by fever or severe abdominal pain.

ILLNESS & DISORDERS

CONVULSION, FEBRILE

GENERAL INFORMATION

DEFINITION—A seizure triggered by rapid rise in temperature and characterized by altered consciousness and uncontrolled muscle spasms.

BODY PARTS INVOLVED—Central nervous system; musculoskeletal system.

SEX OR AGE MOST AFFECTED—Infants and children.

SIGNS & SYMPTOMS—An infection with fever usually precedes the convulsions, but sometimes convulsions may be the first sign of fever. Symptoms include:
- Unconsciousness.
- Jerking or twitching of the arms, legs or face that lasts 2 to 3 minutes.
- Loss of bladder or bowel control.
- Irritability upon regaining consciousness, followed by sleep for several hours.

CAUSES—Sudden, high fever from any cause, plus an unexplained irritability of the central nervous system in some children.

RISK INCREASES WITH
- Repeated infections.
- A sister or brother who suffered febrile convulsions.

HOW TO PREVENT—When fever begins in a child who has had a febrile convulsion in the past, immediately begin measures to reduce the fever.

WHAT TO EXPECT

DIAGNOSTIC MEASURES
- Your own observation of symptoms.
- Medical history and physical exam by a doctor.
- For recurrent, frequent, febrile seizures, laboratory studies of blood and spinal fluid and electroencephalography (studying the brain by measuring electric activity ["brain waves"]).

APPROPRIATE HEALTH CARE
- Doctor's treatment for diagnosis and treatment of the underlying cause.
- Home care after the seizure has subsided and after diagnosis.

POSSIBLE COMPLICATIONS
- Body injury during a seizure.
- Brain injury with repeated seizures.
- Children with febrile seizures are at greater than average risk to develop epilepsy later in life.
- Recurrence risk is about 33%; almost all that recur do so within the one year.

PROBABLE OUTCOME
- Despite its frightening appearance, a convulsion caused solely by fever in a child is usually not serious. However, other causes should be investigated.
- Seizures do not cause retardation, developmental delays or behavioral abnormalities.
- If the first convulsion with fever occurs in a child younger than 6 months, a neurological examination and other studies may be necessary.

HOW TO TREAT

GENERAL MEASURES
- During the convulsion, move potentially dangerous objects away from the child. Lie the child on its side, be sure airway is open.
- Write down details of the convulsion, and report them to the doctor. Information should include the following:
  When did it begin?
  How soon did the seizure occur after the fever rose?
  Were the limb movements equal on both sides or was one side twitching more than the other?
  How long did the seizure last?
  Did the child sleep afterward? If so, how long?
  Did the seizure recur after a quiet interval?
- After the convulsion, try to reduce fever with a tepid sponge bath.

MEDICATION
- Your doctor may prescribe anticonvulsant drugs, such as phenobarbital, to prevent a recurrence of seizures. Some doctors recommend medication after the first convulsion; most doctors treat only if a seizure recurs. Anticonvulsant drugs are only effective if taken daily during the susceptible years (up to age 4).
- Use acetaminophen for fever.

ACTIVITY—Keep the child resting quietly in bed until fever and the underlying illness are gone. Then allow activity to return gradually to normal.

DIET—Nothing by mouth during seizure. After the seizure ends, encourage the child to drink extra liquids, including water, tea, cola and fruit juice.

CALL YOUR DOCTOR IF

- Your child has a seizure with fever. Call your doctor immediately.
- An injury occurs during a seizure.
- The underlying illness does not improve in 3 days.

COR PULMONALE
(Pulmonary Hypertension)

GENERAL INFORMATION

DEFINITION—Congestive heart failure resulting from raised blood pressure in the lungs. This is a complication of disorders that slow or block blood flow in the lungs.

BODY PARTS INVOLVED—Lungs; heart; blood vessels.

SEX OR AGE MOST AFFECTED—Both sexes and all ages, but most common in men over 40.

SIGNS & SYMPTOMS
Early stages:
- No symptoms (usually).
Later stages:
- Weakness and fatigue; fainting.
- Shortness of breath with exertion.
- Swelling of the ankles and feet caused by fluid retention.
- Distended neck veins.
- Bluish skin.
- Chest pain.
- Enlarged liver and swollen abdomen.

CAUSES
- Severe, chronic obstructive lung disease, such as emphysema, recurrent pneumonia, bronchiectasis, silicosis, lung cancer, tuberculosis or collagen diseases.
- Small blood clots that travel to the lung from another body site—usually a deep vein in the calf of the leg—and obstruct lung blood vessels.
- Primary diseases of the heart, including rheumatic heart disease and congenital heart disease.

RISK INCREASES WITH
- Prolonged bed rest for any illness. This increases the chance of blood-clot formation.
- Smoking.
- Living at high altitudes.
- Occupational exposure to lung damaging materials.
- Certain medications such as fenfluramine and dexfenfluramine.

HOW TO PREVENT
- Don't smoke.
- Obtain regular medical treatment for any underlying disorder that can be corrected with surgery or medical treatment.

WHAT TO EXPECT

DIAGNOSTIC MEASURES
- Your own observation of symptoms.
- Medical history and physical exam by a doctor.
- Laboratory studies of blood and lung function.
- X-rays of the lungs.

APPROPRIATE HEALTH CARE
- Doctor's treatment.
- You may need oxygen. An oxygen therapist can arrange for the type of oxygen that allows you to be up and about.
- Surgery to correct problems caused by congenital or acquired disorders, such as replacing damaged heart valves (sometimes).

POSSIBLE COMPLICATIONS—Irreversible congestive heart failure and death.

PROBABLE OUTCOME—This condition is currently considered incurable. Many persons live 10 or 15 years after diagnosis, but disability will slowly increase. However, symptoms can be relieved or controlled. Lung transplants may be curative.

Scientific research into causes and treatment continues, so there is hope for increasingly effective treatment and cure.

HOW TO TREAT

GENERAL MEASURES
- Avoid contact with people with infections.
- Avoid air irritants (e.g., smoke).
- Weigh daily and keep a record. Any sudden increase may indicate increased fluid retention.
- See Resources for Additional Information.

MEDICATION—Your doctor may prescribe:
- Diuretics to prevent fluid accumulation.
- Digitalis to strengthen the force of heart muscle contractions.
- Antibiotics for recurrent infections.
- Vasodilators to reduce the resistance of the blood vessels to promote improved blood flow.

ACTIVITY—No restrictions. Be as active as your condition allows, but don't overexert. Rest between activities.

DIET—Eat a diet that is moderate in salt.

CALL YOUR DOCTOR IF

- You have symptoms of cor pulmonale.
- The following occurs during treatment:
  Temperature of 101F (38.3C) or higher.
  Weight gain of 3 to 4 pounds in 1 or 2 days.
  Increased shortness of breath.
  Increased swelling of the ankles.
  Cough with sputum that is discolored or tinged with blood.

CORN OR CALLUS

GENERAL INFORMATION

DEFINITION—A corn is a thickening (bump) of the outer skin layer, usually over bony areas such as toe joints. A callus is a painless thickening of skin caused by repeated pressure or irritation.

BODY PARTS INVOLVED
- Corn: toe joints and skin between toes.
- Callus: any part of the body, especially hands, feet or knees, that endures repeated pressure or irritation.

SEX OR AGE MOST AFFECTED—All ages except infants.

SIGNS & SYMPTOMS
- Corn: a small, sometimes tender, raised bump on the side or over the joint of a toe. Corns are usually 3 mm to 10 mm in diameter and have a hard center.
- Callus: a rough, thickened area of skin that appears after repeated pressure or irritation.

CAUSES—Corns and calluses form to protect a skin area from injury caused by repeated irritation (rubbing or squeezing). Pressure causes cells in the irritated area to grow at a faster rate, leading to overgrowth.

RISK INCREASES WITH
- Shoes that fit poorly.
- Those with occupations that involve pressure on the hands or knees, such as carpenters, writers, guitar players or tile layers.

HOW TO PREVENT
- Don't wear shoes that fit poorly.
- Avoid activities that create constant pressure on specific skin areas.
- When possible, wear protective gear, such as gloves or knee pads.

WHAT TO EXPECT

DIAGNOSTIC MEASURES
- Your own observation of symptoms.
- Medical history and physical exam by a doctor of medicine or podiatrist.

APPROPRIATE HEALTH CARE
- Self-care.
- Doctor's treatment (sometimes).

POSSIBLE COMPLICATIONS—Back, hip, knee or ankle pain caused by a change in one's gait due to severe discomfort.

PROBABLE OUTCOME—Usually curable if the underlying cause can be removed. Allow 3 weeks for recovery. Recurrence is likely—even with treatment—if the cause is not removed.

HOW TO TREAT

GENERAL MEASURES
- If you have diabetes or poor circulation, consider consulting a podiatrist for treatment.
- Remove the source of pressure, if possible. Discard ill-fitting shoes.
- Use corn and callus pads to reduce pressure on irritated areas.
- Peel or rub the thickened area with a pumice stone to remove it. Don't cut it with a razor. Soak the area in warm water to soften it before peeling.
- Ask the shoe repairman to sew a metatarsal bar onto your shoe to use while a corn is healing.
- Avoid surgery. It does not remove the cause. Post-surgical scarring is painful and may complicate healing.

MEDICATION
- After peeling the upper layers of the corn once or twice a day, apply ointment. Use a nonprescription 5% or 10% salicylic ointment. Cover with adhesive tape.
- Your doctor may inject a corn or callus with cortisone medicine to suppress inflammation or pain.

ACTIVITY—Resume your normal activities as soon as symptoms improve.

DIET—No special diet.

CALL YOUR DOCTOR IF

- You have corns or calluses that persist, despite self-treatment.
- Any signs of infection, such as redness, swelling, pain, heat or tenderness, develop around a corn or callus.

CORNEAL ABRASION AND ULCER

GENERAL INFORMATION

DEFINITION—An open sore in the thin transparent layers that cover the eye.

BODY PARTS INVOLVED—Cornea (covering); conjunctiva (white of the eye); iris (colored part of the eye); and aqueous humor (fluid in the eyeball).

SEX OR AGE MOST AFFECTED—Both sexes; all ages.

SIGNS & SYMPTOMS
- Eye pain, usually severe.
- Sensitivity to bright light.
- Eyelid spasm.
- Tearing.
- Blurred vision.
- Redness in the white of the eye.

CAUSES
- Ill-fitting or prolonged use of contact lenses.
- Injury to the cornea or the embedding in the cornea of a foreign body, such as a small piece of steel, sand or glass. A bacterial infection (usually pneumococcal, streptococcal or staphylococcal) or fungal infection may follow the injury.
- Infection by the virus, herpes simplex, that produces cold sores on the mouth.
- Infections of the eyelids and conjunctiva.
- Defective closure of the lid.

The above infections are contagious from person to person or from one part of the body to another—especially finger-to-eye contact after touching cold sores on the mouth.

RISK INCREASES WITH
- Recent infection or eye injury.
- Smoking or other environmental eye irritants.
- Ill-fitting or prolonged use of contact lenses (especially soft lenses).
- Hyperthyroidism.

HOW TO PREVENT
- Wash hands frequently.
- Avoid injury. Wear safety goggles to protect eyes when exposed to flying wood shavings or splinters, or metal or stone bits.
- Don't touch your eyes if you have cold sores.
- Handle contact lenses properly.

WHAT TO EXPECT

DIAGNOSTIC MEASURES
- Your own observation of symptoms.
- Medical history and physical exam by a doctor (ophthalmologist).
- Sometimes a visual acuity test, and a laboratory culture study of corneal scraping.

APPROPRIATE HEALTH CARE
- Doctor's treatment.
- Treatment normally involves instillation of antibiotic eye drops.
- Removal of any deeply embedded foreign body using a topical anesthetic.

POSSIBLE COMPLICATIONS—Neglected corneal ulcers may penetrate the cornea, allowing infection to enter the eyeball. This can cause permanent vision loss.

PROBABLE OUTCOME—A corneal ulcer is a serious eye problem. It is usually curable in 2 to 3 weeks if treated by an ophthalmologist. If scars from previous corneal ulcers impair vision significantly, a corneal transplant (grafting a new cornea onto the eye) may make vision nearly normal.

HOW TO TREAT

GENERAL MEASURES
- Apply cool-water compresses to the eye as often as they feel good.
- Patching the eye may decrease discomfort.

MEDICATION
- Your doctor may prescribe antibiotic eye drops, ointments or oral antibiotics for bacterial infections. Your doctor will administer medication for viral and fungus infections.
- For minor pain, you may use nonprescription drugs such as acetaminophen.

ACTIVITY—After treatment, resume normal activity as soon as possible.

DIET—No special diet.

CALL YOUR DOCTOR IF

- You have symptoms of a corneal ulcer.
- The following occurs during treatment:
  Fever over 101F (38.3C).
  Pain that is not relieved by acetaminophen.
  Changed vision.
- New, unexplained symptoms develop. Drugs used in treatment may produce side effects.

CORONARY ARTERY DISEASE
(Arteriosclerotic Heart Disease)

 GENERAL INFORMATION

DEFINITION—Hardening and narrowing of the coronary arteries, which provide the blood supply to the heart. There are three main coronary arteries. When any or all become narrowed, they can no longer provide adequate oxygen for heart cells.

BODY PARTS INVOLVED—Blood vessels to the heart.

SEX OR AGE MOST AFFECTED—Adults of both sexes over age 40. Coronary artery disease is uncommon in premenopausal women.

SIGNS & SYMPTOMS
Early stages:
• No symptoms (often).
Later stages:
• Angina pectoris (burning, squeezing, heaviness or tightness in the chest that may extend to the left arm, neck, jaw or shoulder blade).
• Heart attack.

CAUSES—Often unknown, except for association with risks listed below. In addition to narrowing due to hardening of arteries, blood clots frequently form and block arteries.

RISK INCREASES WITH
• Smoking.
• Family history of coronary disease, diabetes, high blood pressure or atherosclerosis.
• Poor nutrition; too much fat in the diet.
• Previous heart attack or stroke.
• Lack of exercise; obesity; hypertension.
• Hostile or impatient personality type.
• Elevated cholesterol and/or low level of HDL (high-density lipoprotein).

HOW TO PREVENT
• Don't smoke.
• Eat a low-fat, low-salt, high-fiber diet.
• Exercise regularly; attain ideal body weight.
• One aspirin a day (consult your doctor).
• See How to Cope with Stress in Appendix.
• If you have diabetes or hypertension, adhere strictly to the treatment schedule, including diet.

 WHAT TO EXPECT

DIAGNOSTIC MEASURES
• Medical history and exam by a doctor.
• Diagnostic tests may include electrocardiogram, echocardiogram, exercise-tolerance test, thallium stress test, blood studies to measure total fat, cholesterol and lipoproteins, x-rays of the chest and coronary angiogram.

APPROPRIATE HEALTH CARE
• Self-care after diagnosis.

• Doctor's treatment.
• Surgery to bypass coronary arteries (severe cases).
• Balloon angioplasty (treatment for obstructed arteries). A small uninflated balloon is passed up the artery to the obstruction and then expanded to release the obstruction.
• Although these procedures may decrease or eliminate symptoms for a while, they do not control the underlying disease.
• Heart transplant (sometimes) for end-stage coronary artery disease.

POSSIBLE COMPLICATIONS—Life-threatening myocardial infarction (death of heart-muscle cells from inadequate blood flow).

PROBABLE OUTCOME—This condition is currently considered incurable. However, symptoms can usually be relieved or controlled. Treatment can prolong life and improve its quality. Evidence now suggests that aggressive treatment can reverse atherosclerosis to some degree. Scientific research into causes and treatment continues, so there is hope for treatment and cure.

 HOW TO TREAT

GENERAL MEASURES
• Reduce as many risk factors as possible.
• Stop smoking.
• See Resources for Additional Information.

MEDICATION—Your doctor may prescribe:
• Nitroglycerin, anticoagulants, calcium channel-blockers, ACE inhibitors or beta-adrenergic blockers for angina pectoris and blood-vessel spasms.
• Vasodilator drugs to increase the blood supply to the heart muscle. Injection of a blood clot dissolving medication (sometimes).

ACTIVITY—Engage in a program of moderate, daily physical exercise.

DIET
• Low-fat diet (see Low-Fat Diet in Appendix).
• If you are overweight, begin a moderate reducing diet and stick to it.

 CALL YOUR DOCTOR IF

• You develop deep chest discomfort (aching or pressure) with radiation to the jaw, left arm or back. Call immediately; may be an emergency!
• You sweat and feel short of breath.
• After exertion, you develop chest, neck or jaw pain that goes away with rest.
• Symptoms worsen or don't improve.
• New or unexplained symptoms develop.

COSTOCHONDRITIS
(Tietze's Syndrome)

GENERAL INFORMATION

DEFINITION—An inflammation of the cartilage of one or more ribs, most commonly the second or third ribs. The pain that results is often intensified by movements that change the position of the ribs, such as lying down, bending over, coughing or sneezing. Pain may mimic that of coronary artery disease.

BODY PARTS INVOLVED—Cartilage of one or more ribs.

SEX OR AGE MOST AFFECTED—More common in young adults, but can occur in any age group.

SIGNS & SYMPTOMS
• Pain in the chest wall, usually sharp in nature.
• Pain worsens with movement.
• Pain may occur in more than one location and may radiate into the arm.
• Tightness in the chest.
• Affected area is sensitive to the touch.

CAUSES—Inflammation of the cartilage that attaches ribs to the sternum. Cause of the inflammation is often unknown.

RISK INCREASES WITH
• Trauma, such as a severe blow to the chest.
• Unusual physical activity.
• Upper respiratory infection.

HOW TO PREVENT—Avoidance of activities that may strain or cause trauma to the rib cage.

WHAT TO EXPECT

DIAGNOSTIC MEASURES
• Your own observation of symptoms.
• Medical history and physical exam by a doctor.

APPROPRIATE HEALTH CARE—Self-care after diagnosis.

POSSIBLE COMPLICATIONS—None likely.

PROBABLE OUTCOME—Complete healing. The disorder is benign and the course is usually of a short duration.

HOW TO TREAT

GENERAL MEASURES
• Heating pad or ice massage applied to the affected area (whichever feels best).
• Avoidance of sudden movements that will intensify the pain.

MEDICATION
• You may use mild pain medications, such as aspirin or ibuprofen to help relieve discomfort.
• Your doctor may prescribe stronger pain medicines or steroid injections (rare).

ACTIVITY—As tolerated. Rest is important.

DIET—No special diet.

CALL YOUR DOCTOR IF

• You have symptoms of costochondritis.
• New or unexplained symptoms develop. Drugs used in treatment may cause side effects.

ILLNESS & DISORDERS

CROHN'S DISEASE
(Regional Ileitis; Granulomatous Ileitis or Ileocolitis)

 GENERAL INFORMATION

DEFINITION—A chronic inflammatory disease of the gastrointestinal tract. It most commonly affects the ileum (the end of the small intestine where it joins the large intestine).

BODY PARTS INVOLVED—Ileum, colon and other parts of the gastrointestinal tract; regional lymph nodes; the mesentery (outside covering of the intestines).

SEX OR AGE MOST AFFECTED—
Adolescents, young adults and after age 60.

SIGNS & SYMPTOMS
• Cramping abdominal pain—especially after eating. The pain is sometimes in the right lower abdomen, mimicking appendicitis.
• Nausea and diarrhea; general ill feeling; fever.
• Appetite and weight loss.
• Abdominal tenderness; abdominal mass that can be felt.
• Bloody stools (sometimes).
• Growth retardation in children.

CAUSES—Unknown. Can be aggravated by bacterial infection or inflammation.

RISK INCREASES WITH
• Medical history of food allergies.
• Family history of Crohn's disease.

HOW TO PREVENT—Cannot be prevented at present.

 WHAT TO EXPECT

DIAGNOSTIC MEASURES
• Your own observation of symptoms.
• Medical history and physical exam by a doctor.
• Diagnostic procedures, such as sigmoidoscopy or colonoscopy (see Glossary for both); x-rays of the colon and small intestine.

APPROPRIATE HEALTH CARE
• Self-care after diagnosis.
• Doctor's treatment.
• Surgery (see Ileostomy in Surgery section) to resect the inflamed area (sometimes), although nonsurgical treatment is preferred.

POSSIBLE COMPLICATIONS
• Intestinal obstruction.
• Bleeding and anemia.
• Fistula between the bowel and bladder.
• Perirectal abscess.
• Perforation of the inflamed bowel.
• Increased susceptibility to cancer of the ileum.
• Joint pain and inflammation; eye inflammation.
• Kidney disorders.
• Malabsorption.
• Vitamin-B-12 deficiency.

PROBABLE OUTCOME—Attacks usually begin in patients in their early 20s and may continue for years. Intervals between attacks vary from every few months to every few years. Occasionally, symptoms appear only once or twice, and the disease disappears.

If you and your doctor decide that your condition requires surgery, it can dramatically improve your condition and delay progress of the disease for many years. However, despite surgery, recurrences are quite possible.

 HOW TO TREAT

GENERAL MEASURES
• Use heat to relieve pain. Apply a heating pad or warm compresses to the abdomen. Warm water baths may help reduce discomfort. If abdominal cramps are continuous or severe, notify your doctor.
• Check your stool daily for signs of bleeding. Take any suspicious specimens to your doctor's office for analysis.
• See Resources for Additional Information.

MEDICATION—Your doctor may prescribe:
• Pain relievers.
• Antidiarrhea medication.
• Vitamin supplements.
• Anti-inflammatory drugs and immunosuppressant medication.
• Antibiotics to fight infections.
• Steroids in acute cases.

ACTIVITY
• During acute attacks, rest in bed or a chair. Get up only to go to the bathroom, to bathe or to eat.
• During periods between attacks, rest often during the day and sleep up to 10 hours a night.

DIET
• Usually no restrictions.
• Reducing the amount of fat in the diet may help.
• If you have possible food allergies, omit milk, wheat, eggs, nuts and other suspected foods. Omit each one, especially milk, for a short period, then try it again in a few weeks.
• If diarrhea is a problem, increase amount of fiber in your diet.

 CALL YOUR DOCTOR IF

• You have symptoms of Crohn's disease.
• You have black, tarry stools or blood in the stool.
• Your abdomen swells.
• Your temperature rises to 101F (38.3C) or higher.

CROUP
(Laryngotracheobronchitis)

GENERAL INFORMATION

DEFINITION—Infection, inflammation and swelling of the larynx (vocal cords) and surrounding tissue. This causes labored breathing and a characteristic "barking" noise with each inhalation or cough.

BODY PARTS INVOLVED—Larynx; throat; bronchial tubes; trachea (windpipe).

SEX OR AGE MOST AFFECTED—Children under age 6.

SIGNS & SYMPTOMS
- Hoarseness.
- Barking cough and difficult breathing, especially at night.
- Chest or throat discomfort or pain.
- Fever.

CAUSES—Contagious viral infection (influenza virus type A, other parainfluenza and influenza viruses; respiratory syncytial virus; other viruses such as adenovirus, rhinovirus, enterovirus, Coxsackievirus, ECHO virus, measles virus).

RISK INCREASES WITH
- Past history of croup.
- Frequent upper respiratory infections.

HOW TO PREVENT—No specific preventive measures.

WHAT TO EXPECT

DIAGNOSTIC MEASURES
- Your own observation of symptoms.
- Medical history and physical exam by a doctor (sometimes). There is no specific diagnostic test for croup.
- In rare instances, throat culture, neck x-ray or CT scan, and laryngoscopy (see Glossary for both).

APPROPRIATE HEALTH CARE
- Home care after diagnosis.
- Doctor's treatment.
- A child who has difficulty breathing may need to be hospitalized and may be given oxygen. Recovery usually takes 2 days.

POSSIBLE COMPLICATIONS—Complications are unlikely, but may occur depending on severity of the symptoms.

PROBABLE OUTCOME—Croup can be frightening, because attacks usually happen at night and the child has trouble breathing. In most cases, croup is not serious, and symptoms can be relieved. If attacks happen during the day and are accompanied by fever, the illness is more serious.

HOW TO TREAT

GENERAL MEASURES—Home care for a mild croup attack:
- Stay calm. Anxiety increases the child's breathing difficulty.
- Steam from a hot shower may help breathing. Hold child in your arms in the bathroom.
- Wrapping the child in a blanket and walking around outdoors occasionally helps.
- Keep the child comfortable in a semiseated position. Use TV, radio or a story for distraction so the child can relax. Crying can aggravate symptoms.
- Use a cool-mist, ultrasonic humidifier or vaporizer by the child's bed for several nights after an attack even if the child appears well. Simple croup often recurs. Clean humidifier daily.

MEDICATION—Usually no medicines are necessary for this disorder. In severe cases, your doctor may administer drugs that decrease airway obstruction or antibiotics if a bacterial infection occurs.

ACTIVITY—Decrease the child's activity and encourage rest as long as croup attacks are occurring. Don't allow the child to play outside in cool night air—this may trigger attacks (although cool air can help relieve symptoms during an attack).

DIET—Croup usually depresses appetite. Offer frequent small amounts of fluid, such as water, ginger ale, tea, juice or cola—not milk. Coughing may cause vomiting, so don't give the child solids during an attack.

CALL YOUR DOCTOR IF

- Your child is having trouble breathing and cannot swallow saliva or water. This is an emergency!
- Breathing rate increases to 80 breaths a minute.
- Breathing is labored, and retraction (the drawing in of neck and chest with each inhalation) is pronounced.
- Nails or lips become dark or blue.
- Child starts drooling or has trouble swallowing.
- You are worried.
- Mild croup symptoms don't improve with 30 to 60 minutes of cool-mist treatment.

CRYPTOCOCCOSIS
(Torulosis)

GENERAL INFORMATION

DEFINITION—A fungal disease that usually begins in the lung and may spread to other body parts. It is much more serious when there are underlying illnesses or risk factors. This condition has become more prevalent as an opportunistic disease since the onset of the AIDS epidemic.

BODY PARTS INVOLVED—Lung; central nervous system; kidney; bone; skin.

SEX OR AGE MOST AFFECTED—Most common in men between ages 40 and 60.

SIGNS & SYMPTOMS
- Severe headache.
- Stiff neck.
- Fever.
- Blurred vision.
- Mental disturbances, such as confusion, depression, agitation or inappropriate speech or dress.
- Cough; protein in the urine.

CAUSES—Infection from the fungus, cryptococcus neoformans (also called filobasidiella neoformans). The fungus is acquired by breathing air that contains spores of this organism, which comes from soil contaminated by bird droppings.
   The serious, progressive, systemic form of this fungus disease is most apt to occur in persons who are seriously ill with other diseases or who are receiving immunosuppressive treatment.

RISK INCREASES WITH
- Geographic location. The disease is most common in the southeastern U.S.
- Use of cortisone, immunosuppressive or antimetabolite drugs.
- Illness that has lowered resistance—especially Hodgkin's disease—or others, including: uremia; diabetes; chronic lung disease; tuberculosis; leukemia; or severe burns.
- Persons with HIV infection.

HOW TO PREVENT
- Obtain medical treatment for any of the serious illnesses listed as risks.
- Avoid bird roosts.

WHAT TO EXPECT

DIAGNOSTIC MEASURES
- Your own observation of symptoms.
- Medical history and physical exam by a doctor.
- Laboratory studies of cerebrospinal fluid, blood and urine.

- X-rays of the chest and bones.

APPROPRIATE HEALTH CARE
- Doctor's treatment.
- Hospitalization for intensive care in severe cases.
- Non-AIDS patients with no pulmonary disease may require no treatment.

POSSIBLE COMPLICATIONS—This fungus can cause severe, debilitating illness. In rare cases, the fungi spread from the lungs throughout the body, causing skin ulcers and bone and kidney infections.

PROBABLE OUTCOME
- Mild cases may require no treatment.
- Antifungal medicines are usually effective, but relapses occur.

HOW TO TREAT

GENERAL MEASURES
- It is usually not necessary to isolate ill persons.
- Weigh daily and keep a weight chart. An unexplained weight loss might indicate that infection has spread.

MEDICATION—Your doctor may prescribe:
- Antifungal drugs. These are effective for skin, bone or kidney involvement and are life-saving for cryptococcal meningitis.
- Life-long suppression drugs.

ACTIVITY—If you have a mild form of the disease that does not require strong antifungal medication, rest in bed until the cough and fever disappear.

DIET—No special diet.

CALL YOUR DOCTOR IF

- You have symptoms of cryptococcosis, especially a severe headache or stiff neck.
- The following occurs during treatment:
   Weight loss.
   Fever of 101F (38.3C) orally.
   Diarrhea that cannot be controlled.
   Severe headache and stiff neck.
- New, unexplained symptoms develop. Drugs used in treatment may produce side effects.

CUSHING'S SYNDROME

 GENERAL INFORMATION

DEFINITION—An endocrine disorder caused by excess corticosteroid hormones produced by the adrenal glands.

BODY PARTS INVOLVED—Adrenal gland (located over the kidney); pituitary gland (at the base of the brain).

SEX OR AGE MOST AFFECTED
- All ages, but most common in adults.
- Both sexes, but more common in women.

SIGNS & SYMPTOMS
- Round face and puffy eyes.
- Ruddy red complexion.
- Growth of facial hair in women.
- Fat accumulation over the upper back and trunk, accompanied by red "stretch marks."
- High blood pressure.
- Mental and emotional changes, including psychosis.
- Menstrual changes, including cessation of, increased or irregular periods.
- Enlarged clitoris.
- Low resistance to infection.

CAUSES—Symptoms and signs result from overproduction of the cortisone-like hormone produced by the adrenal glands. The overproduction may result from:
- A tumor in the adrenal glands.
- A pituitary tumor, causing production of excessive ACTH (adrenocorticotropic-hormone), which the pituitary gland produces to stimulate adrenal glands to secrete hormones.
- Prolonged use of cortisone drugs.

RISK INCREASES WITH—Prolonged use of ACTH for treatment of pituitary cancer.

HOW TO PREVENT—If use of ACTH or cortisone is necessary for other disorders, such as asthma, arthritis, kidney disease or Addison's disease, take the lowest dose possible for the shortest time. Consult your doctor.

 WHAT TO EXPECT

DIAGNOSTIC MEASURES
- Your own observation of symptoms. Pictures taken before symptoms begin are helpful in noting changes in appearance.
- Medical history and physical exam by a doctor.
- Laboratory blood and urine studies of white-blood-cell counts, pituitary and adrenal-gland function and hormone levels.
- X-rays of the pituitary and adrenal glands.

APPROPRIATE HEALTH CARE
- Doctor's treatment, including consultation with an endocrinologist.

- Surgery (sometimes) to remove ACTH-producing tumors from the pituitary or to remove adrenal-gland tumors.
- Hospitalization for high voltage radiation treatment of the pituitary gland (sometimes).

POSSIBLE COMPLICATIONS
- Bone fractures due to osteoporosis.
- Diabetes mellitus.
- Peptic ulcers.
- Osteoporosis.
- Pituitary tumor, if adrenal glands are removed (rare).

PROBABLE OUTCOME
- If caused by an adrenal-gland tumor, the disorder is curable with surgical removal of the tumor or glands. Lifelong, carefully monitored drug therapy is essential if the glands are removed.
- If caused by a pituitary tumor, the disorder is curable with surgical removal or radiation of the tumor, but tumors may recur.
- If caused by prolonged use of cortisone drugs or ACTH, the condition may improve if these are withdrawn gradually under medical supervision.

 HOW TO TREAT

GENERAL MEASURES
- Learn all you can about this condition and its treatment. You must often monitor your own reactions to medications. Discontinuing drugs suddenly is dangerous.
- Wear a Medic-Alert bracelet or pendant (see Glossary).
- Protect yourself from fractures. Accident proof your home. Wear seat belts in autos.

MEDICATION—Your doctor may prescribe:
- Drugs to suppress adrenal-gland function.
- Cortisone drugs, if adrenal glands must be removed surgically.
- Drugs to replace pituitary hormones (sometimes).
- Antihypertensive drugs to lower blood pressure.
- Calcium supplements to treat osteoporosis.
- Sedatives (sometimes).

ACTIVITY—No restrictions. Energy will increase once treatment begins.

DIET—Consult your doctor about possible salt restriction.

 CALL YOUR DOCTOR IF

- You have symptoms of Cushing's syndrome.
- Signs of infection occur, such as fever, chills, muscle aches, headache and dizziness.
- There are signs of steroid underdosage (fatigue, weakness, dizziness) or overdosage (swelling in hands or feet, weight gain).

CYSTIC FIBROSIS (CF)

GENERAL INFORMATION

DEFINITION—An inherited disease in which mucus-producing glands throughout the body—especially in the pancreas, intestine and lung—fail to produce normal enzymes and mucus.

BODY PARTS INVOLVED—Pancreas; lungs; sweat glands of the skin; gastrointestinal tract.

SEX OR AGE MOST AFFECTED—Children of both sexes.

SIGNS & SYMPTOMS
Newborn period:
- Thick, sticky stools (meconium), which may cause intestinal obstruction.

Later:
- Poor weight gain despite good appetite.
- Bad-smelling, large, fatty stools.
- Chronic cough.
- Frequent, severe respiratory infections with sticky, hard-to-cough-up sputum.
- Salty sweat.
- Enlarged liver and spleen.

CAUSES—Genetic factors. Many people carry the genes for cystic fibrosis, and 1 in 2000 newborns is born with it. The genes cause abnormal mucus in the respiratory and gastrointestinal tracts and sweat glands. This causes lung obstruction and infection, poor digestion and poor food absorption.

RISK INCREASES WITH—Family history of cystic fibrosis. If both parents come from families with cystic fibrosis, the chances are 1 in 4 that each child will have the disease.

HOW TO PREVENT—If you have a family history of cystic fibrosis, seek genetic counseling before starting a family. A medical test to determine if you are a carrier is available.

WHAT TO EXPECT

DIAGNOSTIC MEASURES
- Your own observation of symptoms. Sometimes a parent notes a salty taste when kissing a child.
- Medical history and exam by a doctor.
- Laboratory studies to analyze sweat, stools and digestive juices.

APPROPRIATE HEALTH CARE
- Team approach (respiratory therapist, nurse, nutritionist, physical therapist, counsellor, social worker) to help with the child's care.
- Goals of therapy are to prevent and treat respiratory failure and pulmonary complications.
- Surgery to relieve intestinal obstruction (sometimes).
- Hospitalization to control serious infections, which occur frequently.

- Lung transplants are becoming a method of treatment (see Lung Transplantation and Heart-Lung Transplantation in Surgery section).

POSSIBLE COMPLICATIONS
- Pneumonia.
- Chronic bronchitis; bronchiectasis.
- Fluid and electrolyte imbalance—especially in hot weather.
- Malnutrition.
- Nasal polyps.
- Rectal prolapse.

PROBABLE OUTCOME—This condition is currently considered incurable and is often fatal in childhood. Careful long-term care by parents and professionals can help children lead reasonably comfortable lives. Children with milder forms may live to adulthood, especially if the disorder is detected early.

Researchers have identified the gene that produces cystic fibrosis. New strategies are in development to prevent and treat this disease.

HOW TO TREAT

GENERAL MEASURES
- Learn as much as possible about this condition. Diet, medication and early recognition of infection are very important.
- You will be instructed on how to perform daily postural drainage to drain mucus from the lungs, and chest percussion to shake loose sticky mucus plugs.
- Use a cool-mist, ultrasonic humidifier in your child's room whenever he or she has respiratory symptoms. Moisture helps thin mucus so it can be coughed up more easily.
- Keep your child's immunizations, including influenza vaccines, up to date.
- Join a support group for parents of children with cystic fibrosis.
- Encourage your child to lead as normal and active a life as possible.
- See Resources for Additional Information.

MEDICATION—Your doctor may prescribe: Digestive enzymes; antibiotics when lung infections occur; enzymes by nebulizer to help loosen lung secretions; anti-inflammatory drugs.

ACTIVITY—As much as the condition permits.

DIET—Your child should eat a low-fat diet with adequate protein. Consult a dietitian for specific instructions. Vitamin and mineral supplements may be necessary. Encourage intake of liquids, which helps thin mucus.

CALL YOUR DOCTOR IF

- You suspect your child has cystic fibrosis.
- After diagnosis, your child develops fever, a worsening cough and muscle aches.

CYSTITIS
(Bladder Infection)

GENERAL INFORMATION

DEFINITION—Inflammation or infection of the urinary bladder.

BODY PARTS INVOLVED—Bladder; urethra.

SEX OR AGE MOST AFFECTED—All ages and both sexes, more common in females.

SIGNS & SYMPTOMS
- Burning and stinging on urination.
- Frequent urination, especially at night, although the urine amount may be small.
- Increased urge to urinate.
- Pain in the pubic area.
- Penile discharge.
- Low back pain.
- Blood in the urine, bad-smelling urine.
- Low fever.
- Painful sexual intercourse.
- Lack of urinary control (sometimes).
- Bed-wetting in a child.
- Irritability in an infant.

CAUSES
- Bacteria that reach the bladder from another part of the body through the bloodstream.
- Bacteria that enter the urinary tract from skin around the genitals and anal area.
- Injury to the urethra.
- Use of a urinary catheter to empty the bladder, such as following childbirth or surgery.
- Structural defect in the urinary tract.

RISK INCREASES WITH
- Increased sexual activity. In women, the cause is often aggravated by bruising of the urethra during intercourse.
- Infection in other parts of the genitourinary system.
- Illness that has lowered resistance.
- Obstruction of urine in the urinary tract in men—usually partial obstruction caused by an enlarged or inflamed prostate gland.
- Wearing poorly ventilated underpants.
- Sitting in bath water that contains bath salts or bubble bath product.
- Loss of suspension of female organs.

HOW TO PREVENT
- Women should drink a glass of water before sexual intercourse and urinate within 15 minutes after intercourse.
- Use a water-soluble lubricant, such as K-Y Lubricating Jelly, during intercourse.
- Use female-superior or lateral positions in sexual intercourse to protect the female urethra from injury.
- Take showers instead of tub baths.
- Request frequent urinalyses to monitor signs of infection.
- Avoid the use of catheters, if possible.

- Obtain prompt medical treatment for urinary-tract infections.
- Women should not douche and should clean the anal area thoroughly after bowel movements. Wipe from the front to the rear—rather than rear to front (avoids spreading fecal bacteria to genital area).
- Wear underwear and nylons that have cotton crotches.
- Avoid postponing urination.

WHAT TO EXPECT

DIAGNOSTIC MEASURES
- Your own observation of symptoms.
- Medical history and physical exam by a doctor.
- Urinalysis, careful urine collection for bacterial culture, cystoscopy (see Glossary) and ultrasound.

APPROPRIATE HEALTH CARE—Doctor's treatment with medication.

POSSIBLE COMPLICATIONS—Inadequate treatment can cause chronic urinary-tract infections, leading to kidney failure.

PROBABLE OUTCOME—Curable in 2 weeks with prompt medical treatment. Recurrence is common.

HOW TO TREAT

GENERAL MEASURES
- Warm baths help relieve discomfort.
- Women may pour a cup of warm water over genital area while urinating. It will help to relieve burning and stinging.

MEDICATION—Your doctor may prescribe:
- Antibiotics to fight infection.
- Antispasmodics to relieve pain.
- Urinary analgesics for pain (occasionally).

ACTIVITY—Avoid sexual intercourse until you have been free of symptoms for 2 weeks to allow inflammation to subside.

DIET—Drink 6 to 8 glasses of water daily. Avoid caffeine and alcohol during treatment. Drink cranberry juice to acidify urine.

CALL YOUR DOCTOR IF

- You have symptoms of cystitis.
- You have fever.
- Blood appears in the urine.
- Discomfort and other symptoms don't improve in 1 week.

DECOMPRESSION SICKNESS (Bends)

GENERAL INFORMATION

DEFINITION—A painful, sometimes life-threatening condition of blood gases that is caused by a sudden drop in environmental pressure.

BODY PARTS INVOLVED—Blood in all body parts.

SEX OR AGE MOST AFFECTED—Both sexes; all ages. Usually occurs in young males.

SIGNS & SYMPTOMS—The following may occur immediately or up to 24 hours after the pressure change:
- Mild to severe joint pain, especially in the shoulders, elbows, hips and knees.
- Chest pain; shortness of breath; a burning sensation behind the breastbone.
- Chokes (severe breathing difficulty experienced by scuba divers and others who go from high to normal air pressure too rapidly. Bubbles of nitrogen develop in the bloodstream and obstruct blood supply to vital organs, sometimes resulting in severe injury or death).
- Coughing.
- Weakness, loss of normal sensation, paralysis, loss of consciousness and coma (rare).
- Inability to speak, see or hear.
- Abdominal pain.
- Difficult urination.

CAUSES—Formation of nitrogen bubbles in the blood. Nitrogen is a normal blood component. If the pressure around the body drops rapidly—as in surfacing too quickly while scuba diving or climbing too rapidly in a nonpressurized aircraft—the nitrogen collects in bubbles in the blood vessels, blocking them and depriving the body of essential blood nutrients.

RISK INCREASES WITH
- Commercial diving or recreational scuba diving. Repeated dives in one day increase the risk.
- Some kinds of high-performance aircraft.
- Working in compression chambers; tunnel work (caisson disease).

HOW TO PREVENT
- Obtain professional instruction before scuba diving.
- Don't dive if you are not in good general health. You are at risk if you are obese or have a medical history of:
  Lung conditions, such as asthma.
  Spontaneous pneumothorax.
  Heart disease.
  Chronic sinusitis.
  Emotional instability.
  Alcoholism.

- Allow for a slow, gradual change to normal air pressure in situations listed above. (The U.S. Navy has tested and established guidelines.)
- Avoid air travel for 24 hours after diving.

WHAT TO EXPECT

DIAGNOSTIC MEASURES
- Your own observation of symptoms.
- Medical history and physical exam by a doctor.
- Laboratory blood studies, oxygen levels, EEG (see Glossary), chest x-ray, CT scan (see Glossary).

APPROPRIATE HEALTH CARE
- Self-care is impossible for this condition. If you observe someone with symptoms of decompression sickness, obtain emergency medical care immediately.
- Hospitalization in a decompression chamber to force nitrogen bubbles to dissolve into the blood.
- Treatment is best when it is accomplished early; however some patients may benefit even at 6 to 9 days after the incident. Referral is critical even if symptoms resolve since 25% of patients will relapse.

POSSIBLE COMPLICATIONS
- Permanent brain damage.
- Permanent bone destruction caused by inadequate nourishment from the blood.

PROBABLE OUTCOME—Excellent for patients who receive early treatment; in others, it depends on duration and severity of symptoms prior to treatment.

HOW TO TREAT

GENERAL MEASURES—Self-care is impossible for this condition. If you observe someone with symptoms of decompression sickness, obtain emergency medical care immediately.

MEDICATION—Medicine usually is not necessary for this disorder. Don't take pain relievers. These may further decrease normal breathing efficiency.

ACTIVITY—Resume your normal activities as soon as symptoms improve after treatment.

DIET—No special diet.

CALL YOUR DOCTOR IF

You develop any symptoms of decompression sickness within 24 hours after scuba diving or rapid ascent without pressurization.

DEHYDRATION
(Fluid & Electrolyte Loss)

 GENERAL INFORMATION

DEFINITION—Loss of water content and essential body salts (electrolytes) needed for normal body function. Necessary salts contain sodium, potassium, calcium, bicarbonate and phosphate. Dehydration is most dangerous in newborns, infants and persons over 60. Water accounts for about 60% of a man's weight and 50% of a woman's weight and needs to be kept in fairly narrow limits to maintain cells and body tissue.

BODY PARTS INVOLVED—Blood; gastrointestinal tract; kidneys.

SEX OR AGE MOST AFFECTED—Both sexes; all ages.

SIGNS & SYMPTOMS
- Dry mouth.
- Decreased or absent urination.
- Sunken eyes.
- Wrinkled skin.
- Fatigue.
- Dizziness; confusion; coma.
- Low blood pressure.
- Severe thirst.
- Increase in heart rate and breathing.

CAUSES
- Persistent vomiting or diarrhea from any cause.
- Persistent high fever.
- Heavy sweating.
- Use of drugs that deplete fluids and electrolytes, such as diuretics ("water pills").
- Overexposure to sun or heat.
- Not taking in sufficient amount of water.

RISK INCREASES WITH
- Newborns and infants.
- Adults over 60.
- Recent illness with high fever.
- Diabetes mellitus.
- Chronic kidney disease.
- Adrenal disease.
- Chronic lung disease.

HOW TO PREVENT
- Obtain medical treatment for underlying causes of dehydration.
- If you are vomiting or have diarrhea, drink enough water to keep urine consistently pale (you may not feel thirsty, but fluid intake is essential).
- If you use diuretics, weigh daily. Report to your doctor a weight loss of more than 3 pounds in 1 day or 5 pounds in 1 week.

 WHAT TO EXPECT

DIAGNOSTIC MEASURES
- Your own observation of symptoms.
- Medical history and physical exam by a doctor.
- Laboratory blood studies, including blood counts and electrolyte measurement (see Glossary).

APPROPRIATE HEALTH CARE
- Self-care.
- Doctor's treatment.
- Hospitalization for intravenous fluids (severe or prolonged illness only).

POSSIBLE COMPLICATIONS
- Depends on any serious underlying cause. Usually with mild symptoms, no complications are expected.
- Severe dehydration or electrolyte imbalance may lead to heartbeat irregularities, cardiac arrest and death.

PROBABLE OUTCOME—Curable in 24-48 hours with control of the underlying cause and replacement of necessary fluids.

 HOW TO TREAT

GENERAL MEASURES
- Weigh daily on an accurate home scale and record the weight so you can be aware of fluid loss.
- If you have vomiting or diarrhea, keep a record of the number of episodes so you can estimate your fluid loss.
- For minor dehydration, take frequent small amounts of clear liquids. Large amounts may trigger vomiting.

MEDICATION—Your doctor may prescribe intravenous fluids to replace lost water, anti-emetic drug if vomiting is severe, or drugs for the diarrhea if it is persistent.

ACTIVITY—Rest in bed until you recover.

DIET— Drink electrolyte solutions. For adults, diluting commercial solutions such as Gatorade or Recharge with an equal amount of water may be adequate. For children, use special commercial products (Pedialyte or Ricelyte). Instructions are on the labels.

 CALL YOUR DOCTOR IF

You have symptoms of dehydration.

DEMENTIA
(Senility)

GENERAL INFORMATION

DEFINITION—Mental impairment caused by a variety of diseases that produce brain deterioration.

BODY PARTS INVOLVED—Brain.

SEX OR AGE MOST AFFECTED—Adults over 60.

SIGNS & SYMPTOMS
- Forgetfulness, especially of recent events.
- Unpredictable, sometimes violent, behavior.
- Confusion.
- Loss of interest in normal activities.
- Disorientation, especially at night.
- Poor personal hygiene and appearance.
- Depression, sleep disturbances.
- Poor judgment.
- Fecal incontinence (late).

CAUSES—Degeneration and loss of the gray matter from the brain. The causes include:
- Alzheimer's disease (its underlying cause is not known).
- Inadequate blood supply to the brain due to blood clots, hypertension or atherosclerosis.
- Severe head injury or repeated head injury (e.g., boxing).
- Brain tumor.
- AIDS.
- Parkinson's disease, Huntington's disease.
- Secondary dementias caused by hypothyroidism, syphilis, normal pressure hydrocephalus, vitamin B deficiency and some medications. These may be reversible with treatment of primary disorder.

RISK INCREASES WITH
- High blood pressure or atherosclerotic disease.
- Adults over 60.

HOW TO PREVENT
- Obtain early medical treatment for underlying causes.
- Protect yourself from head injury. Wear seat belts in vehicles. Wear protective head gear for riding bicycles, motorcycles and participating in contact sports.
- To prevent atherosclerosis, don't smoke, eat a diet low in fat (see Low-fat Diet in Appendix), exercise regularly and reduce stress whenever possible.

WHAT TO EXPECT

DIAGNOSTIC MEASURES
- Your own observation of symptoms.
- Medical history and physical exam by a doctor.
- Laboratory blood studies, EEG (see Glossary); x-rays of the head (to rule out potentially reversible causes).

APPROPRIATE HEALTH CARE
- Doctor's treatment.
- Home care if symptoms are mild to moderate.
- Nursing-home care, if the disorder is too advanced for home care.
- Psychotherapy or counseling for family members.
- Occupational therapy.

POSSIBLE COMPLICATIONS—Infections, constipation, falls and injuries, and poor nutrition. These occur because the ill person cannot care for himself or herself.

PROBABLE OUTCOME—Primary dementia is currently considered incurable and progressive. Medicine may help a few to keep the condition from worsening, but it cannot restore lost brain function.

HOW TO TREAT

GENERAL MEASURES—Family members can help:
- Notice early behavior changes and seek prompt medical care.
- Provide simple reminders, such as a clock, daily calendar or name tag. Help the person with their personal hygiene.
- Minimize changes in daily routine and environment.
- Encourage social activities and contacts. Consider adult day care.
- Treat the person with respect and kindness.
- Provide a protected, nonjudgmental environment when the patient cannot provide self-care. When home care is no longer possible, find a good extended-care facility.
- Visit the patient often—even if he or she doesn't seem to recognize you.
- See Resources for Additional Information.

MEDICATION—Your doctor may prescribe medication appropriate to treat the underlying condition or drugs to treat the behavioral symptoms if other treatment has failed.

ACTIVITY—Encourage as much activity as possible. Caregivers should accident-proof the home.

DIET—Provide a well-balanced diet.

CALL YOUR DOCTOR IF

You observe symptoms of dementia in a family member.

DEPRESSION

GENERAL INFORMATION

DEFINITION—A continuing feeling of sadness, despondency or hopelessness with accompanying symptoms. Major depression occurs in about 1 in 10 Americans but there is continued improvement in treatment.

BODY PARTS INVOLVED—Nervous system.

SEX OR AGE MOST AFFECTED—Both sexes, but is more common in women; all ages.

SIGNS & SYMPTOMS
- Loss of interest in life; boredom.
- Listlessness and fatigue.
- Insomnia; excessive or disturbed sleeping.
- Social isolation; feeling not useful or needed.
- Appetite loss or overeating; constipation.
- Loss of sex drive.
- Difficulty making decisions; concentration difficulty; unexplained crying bouts.
- Intense guilt feelings over minor or imaginary misdeeds.
- Irritability; restlessness; thoughts of suicide.
- Various pains, such as headache or chest pain, without evidence of disease.

CAUSES
- A truly depressive illness has no single obvious cause. Some biological factors can play a part (physical illness, hormonal disorders, certain drugs).
- Social and psychological factors play a part.
- Inherited disorders may contribute (manic-depression runs in families).
- May relate to the number of disturbing events in a person's life at one time.

RISK INCREASES WITH
- Unexpressed anger or other emotion.
- Compulsive, rigid, perfectionist or highly dependent personalities.
- Family history of depression; alcoholism.
- Failure in occupation, marriage or other relationships; death or loss of a loved one.
- Loss of something important (job, home, etc).
- Job change or move to a new area.
- Surgery, such as mastectomy for cancer.
- Major illness or disability.
- Passing from one life stage to another, such as menopause or retirement.
- Use of some drugs, such as reserpine, beta-adrenergic blockers or benzodiazepines.
- Withdrawal from mood-altering drugs, such as narcotics, amphetamines or caffeine.
- Some diseases, including diabetes mellitus, cancer of the pancreas and hormonal abnormalities.

HOW TO PREVENT
Anticipate and prepare for major life changes. Avoid risk factors when feasible.

WHAT TO EXPECT

DIAGNOSTIC MEASURES
Medical history and physical exam by a doctor (sometimes a psychiatrist). Psychological testing.

APPROPRIATE HEALTH CARE
- Self-care for mild depression.
- Psychotherapy or counseling along with drug treatment appears to obtain the best results for more severe depression.
- Hospitalization or inpatient at treatment center may be required for severe depression.
- Rarely, electroconvulsive therapy.

POSSIBLE COMPLICATIONS
- Suicide. Warning signs include withdrawal from family and friends, neglect of personal appearance, mention of wanting "to end it all" or being "a burden to others", evidence of a suicide plan, such as buying or cleaning a gun, sudden cheerfulness after despondency.
- Failure to improve.

PROBABLE OUTCOME—Spontaneous recovery in many cases, but professional help can shorten the duration and help you learn to cope in the future. Recurrence is common. The recovery rate is high, despite one's pessimism.

HOW TO TREAT

GENERAL MEASURES
- If symptoms appear mild to moderate, try some self-care ideas: talk to friends and family; exercise regularly; eat a balanced, low-fat diet; avoid alcohol; maintain your normal routines (if overscheduling is a problem though, try to slow down); see fun movies; learn relaxation techniques and practice them; take a vacation if possible; write down your feelings in a journal or diary; try to work out interpersonal problems (it's best however, to avoid making major decisions at this time); stay as active as possible.
- Seek support groups. Contact social agencies for help. Call your local suicide-prevention hot line if you feel suicidal.

MEDICATION—Your doctor may prescribe:
- Antidepressant drugs to accompany therapy.
- Lithium for alternating mania and depression.

ACTIVITY—No restrictions. Maintain daily activities—even if you don't feel like it.

DIET—Eat a normal, well-balanced diet—even if you have no appetite. Vitamin and mineral supplements may be necessary.

CALL YOUR DOCTOR IF

- You have symptoms of depression.
- You feel suicidal or hopeless.

DERMATITIS, ATOPIC

 GENERAL INFORMATION

DEFINITION—A chronic inflammatory disease of the skin that is often associated with other allergic disorders that affect the respiratory system, such as asthma or hay fever.

BODY PARTS INVOLVED—Skin.

SEX OR AGE MOST AFFECTED—Both sexes, but symptoms may be worse in females; children most commonly affected.

SIGNS & SYMPTOMS
- Itching rash in areas where heat and moisture are retained, such as skin creases of elbows, knees, neck, face, hands, feet, groin, genitals and around the anus.
- Dry, thickened skin in affected areas.
- Uncontrolled scratching (frequently unconscious).
- Chronic fatigue from loss of sleep due to severe itching.

CAUSES—Unknown, but probably inherited and probably related to immune-system overactivity.

RISK INCREASES WITH
- Hay fever or asthma.
- Food allergy.
- Family history of atopic dermatitis or other allergic disorders.
- Stress. The rash and itching increase during stressful periods.
- Use of immunosuppressive drugs.
- Irritating clothes and chemicals.
- Excessively hot or cold climate.

HOW TO PREVENT
- Decrease stress if possible.
- Avoid agents that cause irritation (wool, perfumes, fabric softeners, harsh soaps, etc.).
- Minimize sweating.
- Lukewarm, not hot baths.
- Lubricate skin frequently.

 WHAT TO EXPECT

DIAGNOSTIC MEASURES
- Your own observation of symptoms.
- Medical history and physical exam by a doctor.

APPROPRIATE HEALTH CARE
- Self-care after diagnosis.
- Doctor's treatment with medication.

POSSIBLE COMPLICATIONS
- Secondary bacterial infection in the affected area.
- Cataracts (more common in people with atopic dermatitis).
- Decreased resistance to fungal and viral infections.
- Permanent scarring from scratching.
- Herpes simplex infections are more severe in people with atopic dermatitis.

PROBABLE OUTCOME—Unpredictable. Flare-ups and remissions may occur throughout life. It does tend to decrease or sometimes disappear with age.

 HOW TO TREAT

GENERAL MEASURES
- Effective treatment involves eliminating allergens, avoiding irritants and other precipitating factors and relieving itching and inflammation.
- Use cool-water soaks for crusting, oozing lesions. These decrease itching and remove crusts.
- Bathe in cool to warm water with cleansing agents other than soap.
- Keep fingernails short.
- Wear loose-fitting, cotton clothing (avoid wool and synthetics).
- Avoid fabric softeners and anti-static laundry products.
- Use petroleum- or lanolin-based ointments after bathing.
- Reduce stress in your life, if possible.

MEDICATION
- To relieve minor itching, use nonprescription topical steroids or coal-tar preparations.
- For severe itching, your doctor may prescribe:
  More potent topical steroids.
  Oral cortisone drugs (rarely, and for short periods only).
  Antihistamines or mild tranquilizers.
  Lubricating ointments for the hands.
  Antibiotics (sometimes) to fight secondary infections.

ACTIVITY—No restrictions except to keep cool. Avoid prolonged exposure to heat.

DIET—An allergy diet may be helpful, if food allergy is suspected. Consult your doctor.

 CALL YOUR DOCTOR IF

- You have symptoms of atopic dermatitis.
- You develop fever or uncontrolled itching during a flare-up.

DERMATITIS, CONTACT
(Housewives' Eczema)

GENERAL INFORMATION

DEFINITION—Skin inflammation caused by contact with an irritating substance. Contact dermatitis is not contagious.

BODY PARTS INVOLVED—Skin, especially of the hands, feet and groin.

SEX OR AGE MOST AFFECTED—All ages, but most common in women.

SIGNS & SYMPTOMS
- Itching, pain or discomfort (sometimes).
- Slight redness.
- Cracks and fissures in the skin.
- Bright red, weeping areas (severe cases).

CAUSES—Contact with irritants, such as sprays, acids or solvents. The irritant removes the fatty layer of skin. This causes dehydration and shrinking of surface cells. Some irritants can cause a reaction in moments, while others may take hours or days. Irritants include:
- Some metals in jewelry.
- Certain topical medications.
- Chemicals in some cosmetics.
- Chemicals, soaps, detergents, bleaches, metal cleaners, paint removers, gasoline and others.

RISK INCREASES WITH
- Constant exposure to hot water, detergents, or any irritant that changes the moisture content of skin.
- Burns from hot water or sunburn.
- Occupations or hobbies that bring you in contact with irritants.

HOW TO PREVENT
- Avoid contact with any irritant that has caused dermatitis in the past.
- Wear protective gloves and other clothing for protection from irritants.

WHAT TO EXPECT

DIAGNOSTIC MEASURES
- Your own observation of symptoms.
- Medical history and physical exam by a doctor.

APPROPRIATE HEALTH CARE
- Self-care.
- Doctor's treatment with medication.

POSSIBLE COMPLICATIONS
- Secondary bacterial infection.
- More generalized skin eruption.

PROBABLE OUTCOME—Symptoms can be controlled with treatment and avoidance of the irritant. Recurrence is common, so treatment may be necessary for years.

HOW TO TREAT

GENERAL MEASURES
- Avoid the chemical or material causing the skin eruption.
- Use bath oil or glycerin-based soap instead of soap for bathing.
- Pat skin dry rather than rubbing it.
- Reduce water temperature to lukewarm for bathing or other uses.
- Use only cream, lotion or ointment prescribed for the condition. Other commercial products may aggravate the condition. Apply ointment or cream to hands 6 or 7 times a day. For other body parts, lubricate twice a day, especially after bathing.
- Minimize the use of solvents, and wear heavy-duty, cotton-lined vinyl gloves to prevent contact with irritating substances such as: water; soap; detergent; metal scouring pads; scouring powder; paint; paint thinner; turpentine; and polish for cars, floors, shoes, furniture or metal. Dry the insides of gloves after use. Discard gloves if they develop a hole. Wear gloves when you peel or squeeze lemons, oranges, grapefruit, tomatoes or potatoes.
- Wear leather or heavy-duty fabric gloves for housework or gardening.
- Use a dishwasher (if available) to wash dishes or ask someone else to do it.
- Remove rings before doing housework or washing hands.
- Do not use fabric softeners in wash or anti-static sheets in dryer.

MEDICATION—Your doctor may prescribe topical creams, ointments or lotions. These may include steroid preparations to reduce inflammation or lubricants to preserve moisture.

ACTIVITY—Resume your normal activities gradually as irritation subsides.

DIET—No special diet.

CALL YOUR DOCTOR IF

- Severe pain develops.
- You develop fever.
- Signs of infection (swelling, tenderness, redness, warmth) develop at the site of irritation.
- Treatment does not relieve symptoms in 1 week.

ILLNESS & DISORDERS

DERMATITIS, HERPETIFORMIS

 GENERAL INFORMATION

DEFINITION—A chronic skin inflammation characterized by clusters of small itching blisters. The disorder is hereditary but not contagious or cancerous.

BODY PARTS INVOLVED—Skin of the elbows, knees, shoulders, arms, legs and over the bottom of the spine (sacrum).

SEX OR AGE MOST AFFECTED—Adolescents and adults.

SIGNS & SYMPTOMS—Lesions with the following characteristics:
• Lesions are small clusters of 5 to 20 blisters. Blisters usually measure 2mm to 6mm in diameter.
• Clusters appear on both sides of the body in the same places.
• Lesions itch, but they are not usually painful if there are no complications. May feel a burning or stinging sensation.

CAUSES—Unknown, but may be a disorder of the autoimmune system.

RISK INCREASES WITH
• Exposure to heat and humidity.
• Gluten sensitivity (protein found in wheat and other foods that cannot be digested by some persons because of genetic disease).
• Family history of dermatitis herpetiformis.

HOW TO PREVENT—Cannot be prevented at present. To prevent a recurrence of symptoms, continue to take medication as directed and prevent injury to normal skin.

 WHAT TO EXPECT

DIAGNOSTIC MEASURES
• Your own observation of symptoms.
• Medical history and physical exam by a doctor.
• Biopsy (see Glossary).

APPROPRIATE HEALTH CARE
• Self-care after diagnosis.
• Doctor's treatment with medication.

POSSIBLE COMPLICATIONS—People with dermatitis herpetiformis also may have disease of the small bowel (without symptoms), which pathologically resembles that of patients who are intolerant to gluten. The only way to diagnose this is with biopsy.

PROBABLE OUTCOME—This is a chronic disease. Treatment can control symptoms—including itching—but it will not cure the disease.

 HOW TO TREAT

GENERAL MEASURES—Soak in cool water or use cool-water compresses to reduce itching.

MEDICATION
• For itching, you may use nonprescription drugs such as:
Low-dose steroid lotion, ointment and cream. These reduce inflammation and itching in 24 to 48 hours.
Topical anesthetics and topical antihistamines. These provide quick, short-term relief. Many cause skin sensitivity, but lidocaine and pramoxine usually do not.
Lotions containing phenol, menthol and camphor (such as calamine lotion). These are soothing, but use with care. Large amounts may be absorbed through the skin into the bloodstream; they can be toxic.
• To control blistering, your doctor may prescribe two oral medications, dapsone or sulfapyridine. If either one is needed, it will be required indefinitely.

ACTIVITY—No restrictions, except avoid overheating and moisture.

DIET—Restricting gluten in your diet will reduce the amount of medicine you will need. For a gluten-free diet, see Appendix.

 CALL YOUR DOCTOR IF

• You have symptoms of dermatitis herpetiformis.
• New, unexplained symptoms develop. Drugs used in treatment may produce side effects.

DERMATITIS, SEBORRHEIC

GENERAL INFORMATION

DEFINITION—A skin condition characterized by greasy or dry, white scales. Dandruff and cradle cap are both forms of seborrheic dermatitis. This is not contagious.

BODY PARTS INVOLVED—Skin of the scalp, eyebrows, forehead, face, folds around the nose, behind ears, external ear canal or skin of the trunk, especially over the breastbone (sternum) or in skin folds.

SEX OR AGE MOST AFFECTED—Both sexes; all ages.

SIGNS & SYMPTOMS—Flaking, white scales over reddish patches on the skin. Scales anchor to hair shafts. They may itch, but they are usually painless unless complicated by infection.

CAUSES—Unknown. May be genetic and environmental factors.

RISK INCREASES WITH
* Stress and fatigue.
* Hot, humid weather or cold, dry weather.
* Infrequent shampoos.
* Oily skin.
* Other skin disorders, such as acne rosacea, acne or psoriasis.
* Obesity.
* Parkinson's disease.
* AIDS.
* Use of drying lotions that contain alcohol.

HOW TO PREVENT—Cannot be prevented. To minimize severity or frequency of flare-ups:
* Shampoo frequently.
* Dry skin folds thoroughly after bathing.
* Wear loose, ventilating clothing.

WHAT TO EXPECT

DIAGNOSTIC MEASURES
* Your own observation of symptoms.
* Medical history and physical exam by a doctor (sometimes).

APPROPRIATE HEALTH CARE
* Self-care after diagnosis.
* Doctor's treatment with medication.

POSSIBLE COMPLICATIONS
* Embarrassment and social discomfort.
* Secondary bacterial infection in affected areas.
* Reactions to topical medications used in treatment.

PROBABLE OUTCOME—This is a chronic condition, but it is often characterized by long periods of inactivity. During active phases, symptoms can be controlled with treatment. It does not cause hair loss.

HOW TO TREAT

GENERAL MEASURES
* Shampoo vigorously and as often as once a day. The shampoo you use is not as important as the way you scrub your scalp. Loosen scales with your fingernails while shampooing and scrub at least 5 minutes.
* Exposure to sunlight in moderate doses may help.

MEDICATION
* For minor dandruff, you may use nonprescription dandruff shampoos with selenium sulfide or zinc pyrithione and lubricating skin lotion.
* Your doctor may prescribe:
  For severe problems, shampoos that contain coal tar or scalp creams that contain cortisone. To apply medication to the scalp, part the hair a few strands at a time and rub the ointment or lotion vigorously into the scalp. Topical steroids for other affected parts.

ACTIVITY—No restrictions. Outdoor activities in summer may help.

DIET—No special diet. Avoid foods that seem to worsen your condition.

CALL YOUR DOCTOR IF

* You have symptoms of seborrheic dermatitis that don't respond to self-care.
* Patches of seborrheic dermatitis ooze, form crusts or drain pus.

DIABETES INSIPIDUS

GENERAL INFORMATION

DEFINITION—A rare disorder of the hormone system, centered in the pituitary gland.

BODY PARTS INVOLVED—Pituitary gland; endocrine system.

SEX OR AGE MOST AFFECTED—Both sexes; all ages.

SIGNS & SYMPTOMS
- Excessive thirst that is difficult to satisfy.
- Passage of large amounts (up to 15 quarts a day) of diluted, colorless urine.
- Dry hands.
- Constipation.

CAUSES—Deficiency of an antidiuretic hormone (ADH) normally secreted by the pituitary gland. The deficiency may result from the following:
- Head injury, with damage to the pituitary gland.
- Tumor of the pituitary gland.
- Other brain tumor that applies pressure to the pituitary gland.
- Infection in the brain, such as encephalitis or meningitis.
- Bleeding inside the skull.
- Aneurysm.
- Kidney disease.

RISK INCREASES WITH
- Preceding illness or injury in the brain.
- Atherosclerosis (hardening of the arteries).
- Family history of diabetes insipidus.

HOW TO PREVENT—No specific preventive measures.

WHAT TO EXPECT

DIAGNOSTIC MEASURES
- Your own observation of symptoms.
- Medical history and physical exam by a doctor.
- Laboratory studies, such as water-deprivation tests to determine levels of ADH.

APPROPRIATE HEALTH CARE
- Doctor's treatment.
- Treatment involves controlling fluid balance and preventing dehydration; identifying and eliminating the cause of the diabetes insipidus.
- Surgery if a tumor or aneurysm is present.

POSSIBLE COMPLICATIONS—Electrolyte imbalance, especially increased sodium or potassium deficiency. Either of these can cause heartbeat irregularity, fatigue and congestive heart failure.

PROBABLE OUTCOME
- If the disorder is caused by a tumor or aneurysm, it can be cured by surgery.
- If the disorder is caused by a head injury, spontaneous recovery is likely within a year.
- If the disorder is caused by a preceding brain infection, symptoms may persist indefinitely.

HOW TO TREAT

GENERAL MEASURES
- If brain surgery is necessary, see Craniotomy (in Surgery section) for an explanation of surgery and postoperative care.
- Check weight daily and maintain a record.

MEDICATION—Your doctor may prescribe synthetic ADH in nose drops, powder or injection form.

ACTIVITY—No restrictions.

DIET—No special diet. Drink as much water as you feel you need.

CALL YOUR DOCTOR IF

- You have symptoms of diabetes insipidus.
- Symptoms don't improve, despite treatment.
- New, unexplained symptoms develop. Drugs used in treatment may produce side effects.

DIABETES MELLITUS, INSULIN-DEPENDENT
(Type I Diabetes; IDDM)

GENERAL INFORMATION

DEFINITION—A chronic disease of metabolism characterized by the body's inability to produce enough insulin to process carbohydrates, fat and protein efficiently. Treatment requires injections of insulin. Insulin-dependent diabetes is often called ketosis-prone diabetes if it begins in adulthood and juvenile diabetes if it begins in childhood.

BODY PARTS INVOLVED
- Islet cells of the pancreas that produce insulin.
- All body cells that need insulin to convert food into chemicals the body can use.

SEX OR AGE MOST AFFECTED—Usually begins before age 30; may begin at any age.

SIGNS & SYMPTOMS
- Fatigue; excess thirst.
- Increased appetite and weight loss.
- Frequent urination.
- Itching around the genitals.
- Increased susceptibility to infections, especially urinary-tract infections and yeast infections of the skin, mouth or vagina.

CAUSES
- Too little insulin produced by the islet cells of the pancreas for unknown reasons.
- Interference with insulin use in the body cells for unknown reasons.
- Virus infection of the pancreas.

RISK INCREASES WITH
- Family history of diabetes mellitus. It often skips one generation.
- Pregnancy.

HOW TO PREVENT—Cannot be prevented.

WHAT TO EXPECT

DIAGNOSTIC MEASURES
- Your own observation of symptoms.
- Medical history and physical exam by a doctor.
- Laboratory urine and blood studies to measure glucose, cholesterol and insulin.

APPROPRIATE HEALTH CARE
- Self-care after diagnosis.
- Doctor's treatment.
- Hospitalization for severe complications.
- Surgery for treatment of some complications, such as failing eyesight, gangrene or coronary artery disease.
- Regular foot care by a podiatrist and regular eye examination by a specialist.

POSSIBLE COMPLICATIONS
- Cardiovascular disease, especially stroke, atherosclerosis and coronary artery disease.
- Kidney failure.
- Blindness.
- Peripheral vascular disease, with gangrene in legs and feet and sexual impotence in men.
- Life-threatening hypoglycemia (low blood sugar) if too much insulin is used.
- Life-threatening ketoacidosis (very high blood sugar) with breakdown of body cells.

PROBABLE OUTCOME—This disease is presently considered incurable, but symptoms and progress of the disease can be controlled with rigid adherence to treatment. Life expectancy is somewhat reduced, but many persons with diabetes have a nearly normal life span.

HOW TO TREAT

GENERAL MEASURES
- Learn all you can about controlling diabetes and recognizing signs and symptoms of ketoacidosis or hypoglycemia. Learn the techniques of home monitoring of blood sugar.
- Keep a vial of glucagon available at all times to use if hypoglycemia occurs.
- Learn to give yourself insulin injections. They will be necessary every day for life.
- Wear a Medic-Alert bracelet or pendant (see Glossary).
- Seek medical treatment for any infection.
- See Resources for Additional Information.

MEDICATION—Your doctor will prescribe insulin by injection. The dosage must be individualized and occasionally adjusted. Normal therapy is 2 or more injections per day under the skin (subcutaneous).

ACTIVITY
- No restrictions. Exercise is an important part of controlling diabetes. Consult your doctor.
- Insulin dosage may need to be adjusted according to the planned physical activity. Consult your doctor.

DIET—A special diet will be prescribed. A dietitian or nutritionist should be consulted.

CALL YOUR DOCTOR IF

- You have symptoms of diabetes mellitus.
- The following occurs during treatment:
  Inability to think clearly; weakness; sweating; paleness; rapid heartbeat; seizures; or coma (may indicate hypoglycemia).
  Fruity odor on the breath; changes in breathing pattern; or stupor (may indicate ketoacidosis)
  Several days of illness or weakness.
  Numbness, tingling or pain in the feet or hands.
  Chest pain.

DIABETES MELLITUS, NON-INSULIN-DEPENDENT (Type II Diabetes; NIDDM)

 GENERAL INFORMATION

DEFINITION—A disease of metabolism characterized by the body's inability to produce enough insulin to process carbohydrates, fat and protein efficiently. Non-insulin-dependent diabetes mellitus is most prevalent among obese adults.

BODY PARTS INVOLVED
- Islet cells of the pancreas that produce insulin.
- All body cells that need insulin to convert food into chemicals the body can use.

SEX OR AGE MOST AFFECTED—Both sexes of adults.

SIGNS & SYMPTOMS
- Fatigue.
- Excess thirst.
- Increased appetite.
- Frequent urination.
- Decreased resistance to infection, especially urinary-tract infections and yeast infections of the skin, mouth or vagina.

CAUSES
- Insufficient insulin produced by the pancreas to sustain normal function of body cells.
- Interference with insulin utilization in body cells for unknown reasons.

RISK INCREASES WITH
- Obesity in adults.
- Stress.
- Pregnancy.
- Use of certain drugs, including oral contraceptives, thiazide diuretics, cortisone or phenytoin.
- Family history of diabetes mellitus.

HOW TO PREVENT
- Control your weight to avoid becoming obese.
- Maintaining a regular exercise program may help prevent or delay NIDDM.

 WHAT TO EXPECT

DIAGNOSTIC MEASURES
- Your own observation of symptoms.
- Medical history and exam by a doctor.
- Laboratory urine and blood studies to measure glucose, cholesterol and insulin levels.

APPROPRIATE HEALTH CARE
- Self-care after diagnosis.
- Doctor's treatment.
- Surgery for treatment of some complications, such as gangrene or heart disease.

POSSIBLE COMPLICATIONS
- Cardiovascular disease, especially atherosclerosis, stroke and coronary artery disease.
- Vision impairment.
- Peripheral vascular disease, with gangrene in legs and feet and sexual impotence in men (sometimes).
- Hypoglycemia, if oral hypoglycemic medication is used (rare).

PROBABLE OUTCOME—This form of diabetes is often be controlled with weight loss. Good control decreases the chance of complications. In some cases, it progresses to insulin-dependent diabetes, a more serious form.

 HOW TO TREAT

GENERAL MEASURES
- Learn to test your blood for glucose (sugar).
- Learn all you can about controlling diabetes and recognizing signs and symptoms of complications.
- Wear a Medic-Alert pendant or bracelet (see Glossary).
- Lose weight to a normal level and maintain your ideal weight.
- Obtain prompt medical treatment for any infection or injury.
- See Resources for Additional Information.

MEDICATION—Early in the disease your doctor may prescribe oral medicines to reduce blood sugar (hypoglycemics). In later stages, insulin by injection with or without oral medication may be necessary. They can often be discontinued when body weight becomes normal.

ACTIVITY—Regular daily exercise is an important part of controlling diabetes. Consult your doctor.

DIET—A special diet will be necessary to: reduce weight; limit refined carbohydrates; balance unrefined carbohydrates, protein and fat; and increase plant fiber. Your doctor will provide instructions.

 CALL YOUR DOCTOR IF

- You have symptoms of diabetes mellitus.
- The following occurs during treatment: Inability to think clearly; weakness; sweating; paleness; rapid heartbeat; seizures; coma (may indicate hypoglycemia).
  Numbness, tingling or pain in the feet or hands.
  Infection that does not improve in 3 days.
  Chest pain.
  Worsening of original symptoms, despite adherence to treatment.

DIABETIC FOOT & SKIN PROBLEMS

GENERAL INFORMATION

DEFINITION—Infections of the skin, particularly of the feet, are more common in people with diabetes than in nondiabetics. The feet of a diabetic person are very susceptible to all forms of trauma. The common response is infection.

BODY PARTS INVOLVED—Feet and skin.

SEX OR AGE MOST AFFECTED—Both sexes; all ages.

SIGNS & SYMPTOMS
- Often there is no pain associated with infection or trauma to the foot.
- New sores or ulcers that take unusually long to heal.
- Unusual, persistent warmth or coolness.
- Numbness or muscle weakness.

CAUSES—Susceptibility to infections and other foot problems results from circulation problems, nerve damage and impaired immune system in diabetic patients.

RISK INCREASES WITH
- Ingrown toenail.
- Plantar corn or callus; blisters.
- Poor-fitting shoes.

HOW TO PREVENT
- Wash feet daily with soap and warm (not hot) water. Dry thoroughly and gently, especially between the toes. Powder the feet once a week with talcum.
- When the feet are thoroughly dry, rub lanolin into the skin of the feet to keep the skin soft and free from scales and dryness. Do not rub so vigorously that the feet become tender. Do not cut corns or calluses or try to remove them with patent or other medicines.
- Prevent calluses under the balls of the feet by exercise: curl and stretch the toes 20 times a day; finish each step that you walk on the toes (not on the balls) of the feet.
- If toenails are brittle and dry, apply lanolin generously under and about the nails for a few nights after soaking. Clean the nails carefully with clean orange-wood sticks. Cut nails carefully straight across. Do not cut on the sides of the nail or the cuticle. If you go to a podiatrist, foot specialist or chiropodist, be sure to tell this doctor that you have diabetes.
- If your toes overlap or are pushed close together, separate them with lamb's wool.
- Remove shoes for short periods when you can.
- Do not wear bedroom slippers when you should wear shoes. Slippers do not give proper support.
- Do not step on the floor or go outside with bare feet.
- Wear shoes of soft leather that fit but are not tight. Break in new shoes gradually 1 hour a day.
- Use cotton bed socks if you need extra warmth for your feet when you are in bed to sleep, but do not use hot-water bottles or electric heating pads. Don't burn the feet! Electric blankets are satisfactory.
- Do not wear garters or sit with legs crossed. Either will decrease circulation to the feet, and the circulation may already be less than normal because of the effect diabetes may have on your blood vessels.
- Wear thin socks of cotton (not wool) to prevent moisture, which stimulates germs that cause athlete's foot or other skin infections. Wear clean socks that you change at least once a day. Do not wear loose socks with raised seams.

WHAT TO EXPECT

DIAGNOSTIC MEASURES
- Your own observation of symptoms.
- Medical history and physical exam by a doctor.

APPROPRIATE HEALTH CARE
- Self-care (see How to Prevent).
- Doctor's treatment.

POSSIBLE COMPLICATIONS—Serious foot infections, gangrene and amputation.

PROBABLE OUTCOME—Using preventive measures and seeking early treatment of infections should avoid serious complications.

HOW TO TREAT

GENERAL MEASURES
- See section on prevention.
- See Resources for Additional Information.

MEDICATION—Specific drugs for infections may be prescribed.

ACTIVITY—Continue with regular activities unless foot problems interfere.

DIET—Follow prescribed diet.

CALL YOUR DOCTOR IF

- An infection on the foot does not heal.
- Feet are persistently cold.
- Corns or calluses occur despite preventive measures.
- Pain or cramps occur in the legs or feet.
- Itching.
- Its been more than a year since you had your feet inspected.

DIABETIC HYPOGLYCEMIA

 GENERAL INFORMATION

DEFINITION—Hypoglycemia means low blood sugar. When the blood sugar decreases considerably below normal, a group of symptoms develop. Hypoglycemia develops when there is too much insulin or not enough food for the condition you are in at any point in time. It is more frequent in insulin-dependent type diabetes.

BODY PARTS INVOLVED—Endocrine and metabolic.

SEX OR AGE MOST AFFECTED—Both sexes; all ages.

SIGNS & SYMPTOMS
Mild:
- Hunger; weakness; nervousness.
- Emotional ups and downs; difficulty in concentrating.
- Sweating; headache.

Moderately severe:
- Increased weakness; excessive perspiration.
- Skin cold and clammy to touch.
- Numbness about mouth and/or fingers.
- Pounding of heart.
- Loss of memory.
- Double vision.
- Staring expression.
- Difficulty in walking.
- Unawareness of surroundings.

Severe:
- Twitching of muscles; unconsciousness; convulsions.
- Passing urine unknowingly.

CAUSES
- Exercising more than usual.
- Eating meals at times other than regular hours.
- Skipping meals or eating only parts of meals.
- Loose bowel movements, diarrhea or vomiting your last meal (can also elevate blood sugar).
- Infection (can also elevate blood sugar).
- Are upset or excited (may increase blood sugar).
- Adverse reaction from other medications.
- Excessive insulin dosage.

RISK INCREASES WITH
- Presence of other disorders (such as kidney or liver disease, hypothyroidism, alcoholism, gastroenteritis, congestive heart failure).
- Elderly patient.
- "Tight control" type patient.

HOW TO PREVENT
- Maintaining a regular schedule of diet, medication and exercise.
- Regular blood-glucose testing.
- Learn to recognize the early symptoms of hypoglycemia and take prompt action. Make sure family and friends know about the symptoms so if you become disoriented or confused, they can give you something sweet.
- Always have access to a simple sugar.

 WHAT TO EXPECT

DIAGNOSTIC MEASURES
- Your own observation of symptoms.
- Medical history and exam by a doctor.

APPROPRIATE HEALTH CARE
- Doctor's treatment (sometimes).
- Hospitalization for complications or if there is any doubt about the cause.

POSSIBLE COMPLICATIONS
- Diabetic shock or seizures.
- Permanent brain damage.

PROBABLE OUTCOME—Full recovery is the usual outcome but is dependent on quickness of the diagnosis and treatment.

 HOW TO TREAT

GENERAL MEASURES
- If patient is alert to take food or drink, prompt consumption of a sugar-containing food or beverage that can be rapidly absorbed, such as unsweetened juices, Lifesaver candies, glucose tablets or syrup. If there are more than 30 minutes to the next meal, some fat or starch should also be taken (bread and butter).
- If the patient is drowsy or unconscious, glucagon should be administered. Diabetic patients and their families should have glucagon always available and know how to inject it.
- Check blood-sugar about 15-20 minutes after treatment to ensure the desired effect.
- If no glucagon is available, get the patient to the nearest emergency facility or telephone for emergency help.
- Determine the cause of the hypoglycemia. The insulin dosage may need to be adjusted.
- See Resources for Additional Information.

MEDICATION—If hospitalized, your doctor may prescribe intravenous dextrose.

ACTIVITY—Rest until symptoms resolve.

DIET—Maintain the regular diet unless eating habits are the cause of the hypoglycemia. Adjustments may need to be made.

CALL YOUR DOCTOR IF

- You have symptoms of hypoglycemia that are not controlled by simple measures.
- Attacks are recurring.
- Adjustments need to be made in insulin dosages.

DIAPER RASH

GENERAL INFORMATION

DEFINITION—A form of contact dermatitis that causes skin irritation in the diaper area of infants.

BODY PARTS INVOLVED—Skin around the genitals, rectum and abdomen in the area covered by diapers.

SEX OR AGE MOST AFFECTED—Infants and young children who wear diapers.

SIGNS & SYMPTOMS
- Moist, painful, red, spotty and itchy (sometimes) skin in the diaper area. The skin may be cracked and fissured.
- In male infants, a red, raw and occasionally bloody area may appear around the meatus (the opening at the tip of the penis).

CAUSES—Diaper rash results from skin irritation produced by substances in the urine or stool.

RISK INCREASES WITH
- Prolonged exposure to wet diapers.
- Friction from rough diapers.
- Improper laundering of diapers.
- Family history of skin allergies.
- Hot, humid weather.

HOW TO PREVENT
- Change diapers frequently.
- Don't use waterproof diapers at night.
- Keep diapers clean. After washing, rinse them twice to remove detergents and other chemicals.
- Leave diaper off for 10-30 minutes between diaper changes for air exposure.

WHAT TO EXPECT

DIAGNOSTIC MEASURES
- Your own observation of symptoms.
- Medical history and physical exam by a doctor.
- Urinalysis to rule out urinary-tract infection, which may complicate healing (sometimes).

APPROPRIATE HEALTH CARE
- Home care after diagnosis.
- Doctor's treatment, if home treatment fails to cure the rash.

POSSIBLE COMPLICATIONS—Secondary bacterial infection in the rash area.

PROBABLE OUTCOME—Usually curable with treatment. Recurrence is common.

HOW TO TREAT

GENERAL MEASURES
- Expose the diaper area to air as much as possible.
- Change diapers frequently, even at night if the rash is extensive.
- Don't use soap or boric acid to wash the rash area. Cleanse with cotton dipped in mineral oil.
- Discontinue using baby lotion, powder, ointment or baby oil unless prescribed for you.
- Don't use packaged wipes that contain alcohol. They can cause overdrying of the skin making it susceptible to irritants.
- Apply small amounts of nonprescription petroleum jelly, lanolin-based ointment or zinc oxide ointment to the rash at the earliest sign of diaper rash, and 2 or 3 times a day thereafter.
- Use boiling water to launder cloth diapers or use an antiseptic product manufactured for the purpose. Avoid fabric softeners as they may cause the rash.
- If you use disposable diapers, switching to cloth diapers for period of time may help.

MEDICATION—Your doctor may prescribe medicated anti-inflammatory ointments or creams, such as hydrocortisone, or antifungal cream such as miconazole, to apply to the skin.

ACTIVITY—No restrictions.

DIET—No special diet. Avoid foods that can make stools irritating (breads, pasta, tomatoes and acidic fruit).

CALL YOUR DOCTOR IF

- Home treatment doesn't cure the rash in 1 week.
- The following occurs during treatment:
  Fever.
  Pustules in the rash area.
  Male infant has a weak urinary stream.
  Female infant develops adhesions of the vaginal lips.

DIARRHEA, ACUTE

GENERAL INFORMATION

DEFINITION—The passage of many loose, watery or unformed bowel movements. This is a symptom, not a disease.

BODY PARTS INVOLVED—Colon; small intestine.

SEX OR AGE MOST AFFECTED—Both sexes; simple diarrhea is common among all age groups.

SIGNS & SYMPTOMS
- Cramping abdominal pain.
- Loose, watery or unformed bowel movements.
- Lack of bowel control (sometimes).
- Fever (sometimes).

CAUSES—There are many causes including infections (viral, parasitic or bacterial).

RISK INCREASES WITH
- Emotional upsets or acute stress.
- Food poisoning or food allergy.
- Infections (viral, parasitic or bacterial) or other recent illness.
- Regional enteritis.
- Malabsorption syndromes.
- Disease or tumor of the pancreas (malignant or benign).
- Diverticulitis.
- Foods, such as prunes or beans.
- Use of drugs, such as laxatives, antacids, antibiotics, quinine or anticancer drugs.
- Radiation treatments for cancer.
- Excess alcohol consumption.
- Crowded or unsanitary living conditions.
- Immunosuppression due to illness or drugs.
- Travel to foreign country.
- Ingestion of water from streams, springs or untested wells.
- Lactose or sorbitol intolerance.

HOW TO PREVENT
- If diarrhea is recurrent and a cause can be identified, treatment or avoidance of the cause should prevent recurrence.
- Everyone is likely to have bouts of diarrhea occasionally from insignificant causes that disappear and leave no lasting effects. Most cases of acute diarrhea last a short time and a search for the cause may not be necessary.
- Avoid undercooked or raw seafood, buffet or picnic foods left out several hours and food served by street vendors.
- Wash hands frequently, especially after using the toilet.

WHAT TO EXPECT

DIAGNOSTIC MEASURES
- Your own observation of symptoms.
- Medical history and exam by a doctor.

- Laboratory stool studies (for prolonged diarrhea).

APPROPRIATE HEALTH CARE
- Self-care. Diarrhea is a symptom. If possible, the underlying disorder should be treated.
- Doctor's treatment (if symptoms persist longer than 2 to 3 days).

POSSIBLE COMPLICATIONS—Dehydration if diarrhea is prolonged, especially in infants.

PROBABLE OUTCOME—Spontaneous recovery in 24 to 48 hours.

HOW TO TREAT

GENERAL MEASURES
- If you think a prescription drug is causing the diarrhea, consult with the doctor before discontinuing it.
- If cramps are present, place hot compresses, a hot-water bottle or an electric heating pad on the abdomen.
- Maintain fluid intake. Severe diarrhea may require urgent fluid and electrolyte replacement to correct dehydration.

MEDICATION—For minor discomfort, you may use nonprescription drugs such as bismuth subsalicylate (Pepto-Bismol).

ACTIVITY—Decrease activity until diarrhea stops.

DIET
- Replace lost fluids and electrolytes with a commercial rehydration product (e.g., Gatorade). There are special products for infants (Pedialyte, Ricelyte, etc.). Follow package instructions.
- After 12 hours with no diarrhea, try a diet of clear soup, salted crackers, dry toast or bread.
- Avoid alcohol, caffeine, milk and dairy products, spicy, fried and junk foods.
- Resume a normal diet 2 or 3 days after the diarrhea stops. Avoid alcohol and highly seasoned foods for several more days.

CALL YOUR DOCTOR IF

- Diarrhea lasts more than 48 hours, especially in a child.
- Mucus, blood or worms appear in the stool.
- Fever rises to 101F (38.3C) or higher.
- Severe pain develops in the abdomen or rectum.
- Dehydration develops. Signs include: dry mouth; wrinkled skin; excess thirst; little or no urination.

DIARRHEA, CHRONIC, NONSPECIFIC OF CHILDHOOD

GENERAL INFORMATION

DEFINITION—Chronic diarrhea (more than 5 watery or loose stools a day) in a healthy child.

BODY PARTS INVOLVED—Colon.

SEX OR AGE MOST AFFECTED—Young children (1-1/2 to 3-1/2 years).

SIGNS & SYMPTOMS
• Frequent, loose stools that often contain undigested vegetable fibers or mucus and occur primarily during the morning.
• Occasional irritation of the anal area caused by frequency of bowel movements.

CAUSES—Usually unknown, can be malabsorption or intolerance to specific foods or food groups.

RISK INCREASES WITH—Family history of intestinal problems.

HOW TO PREVENT—Cannot be prevented at present.

WHAT TO EXPECT

DIAGNOSTIC MEASURES
• Your own observation of symptoms.
• Medical history and physical exam by a doctor.
• Laboratory stool studies.

APPROPRIATE HEALTH CARE
• Doctor's treatment.
• Home care after diagnosis.

POSSIBLE COMPLICATIONS—Possible psychological fixation on bowel function because of excessive parental attention to bowel habits.

PROBABLE OUTCOME—Despite the chronic diarrhea, affected children develop normally and show no signs of malnutrition. The frequent stools have no special significance. Bowel movements eventually become normal, but it may take 2 to 3 years.

HOW TO TREAT

GENERAL MEASURES—Don't blame or criticize your child for this problem. Don't expect toilet training to be successful as soon as with other children. Treat your child as normal and try to ignore the problem. Avoid tension. If the child becomes anxious about diarrhea, the problem may become worse or psychological problems may arise.

MEDICATION—Medicine usually is not necessary for this disorder. Don't give your child any nonprescription antidiarrheal drugs. Side effects may be harmful.

ACTIVITY—No restrictions. Insist on full normal activity for your child's age group.

DIET
• No special diet, but vitamin and mineral supplements may be helpful.
• The child should drink at least 6 to 8 glasses of fluid each day to replace fluid lost in stools.

CALL YOUR DOCTOR IF

• Your child has chronic diarrhea or stools with mucus that haven't been diagnosed.
• There is blood in the stool.
• Your child's rectal temperature is 102F (38.9C) or higher.
• Your child becomes listless, refuses to eat or cries loudly and persistently, even when picked up.
• Your child's growth and development are not normal.

DIPHTHERIA

GENERAL INFORMATION

DEFINITION—An acute, highly contagious throat infection. Diphtheria has become less common with the widespread use of immunizations. The diphtheria vaccine is usually given with the vaccines against tetanus and pertussis (whooping cough) to infants (DTP vaccine).

BODY PARTS INVOLVED—Throat; skin; heart; central nervous system.

SEX OR AGE MOST AFFECTED—Older children (5 years and up), adolescents and adults.

SIGNS & SYMPTOMS
Early stages:
• Sore throat.
• Low fever.
• Swollen neck glands.
Late stages:
• Airway obstruction and breathing difficulty.
• Shock (low blood pressure; rapid heartbeat; paleness; cold skin; sweating; anxious appearance).

CAUSES—A bacteria, Corynebacterium diphtheriae, infects the throat and sometimes the skin. The bacteria produces poisons that spread to the heart, central nervous system and other organs.

RISK INCREASES WITH
• Adults over 60, children under 5.
• Poor nutrition.
• Outbreak in the community.
• Crowded or unsanitary living conditions.
• Lack of up-to-date immunizations.
• Alcoholism.

HOW TO PREVENT
• Immunization with diphtheria vaccine.
• Improved nutrition and standard of living.
• Notify the local health department of any case of diphtheria. Anyone having contact with the patient must be examined and treated.

WHAT TO EXPECT

DIAGNOSTIC MEASURES
• Your own observation of symptoms.
• Medical history and physical exam by a doctor.
• Laboratory studies, such as throat culture and blood counts.

APPROPRIATE HEALTH CARE
• Doctor's treatment. This is a medical emergency.
• Hospitalization and isolation of the patient until fully recovered. Protect susceptible individuals (the nonimmunized, very young or elderly) from exposure.
• Patients may require mechanical assistance in breathing.

POSSIBLE COMPLICATIONS
• Heart inflammation and heart failure.
• Suffocation.
• Nerve inflammation.
• Misdiagnosis as a less-serious infection, resulting in dangerous delay of treatment.

PROBABLE OUTCOME—Usually curable in 1 week, followed by slow recovery for several weeks. A delay in treatment may result in death or long-term heart disease.

HOW TO TREAT

GENERAL MEASURES
• Dispose of all secretions (nose and mouth) and excretions (urine and feces) in an acceptable manner. Call the local health department for instructions.
• People who have been in close contact with the patient and who have not been immunized should have throat cultures and be immunized. They should be watched closely for possible symptoms. A booster vaccine may be given for people who have been immunized.

MEDICATION—Your doctor may prescribe:
• Diphtheria antitoxin to neutralize the diphtheria toxin.
• Antibiotics to fight remaining diphtheria organisms.

ACTIVITY—Prolonged bed rest (2 to 3 months or until fully recovered), especially if the heart is involved.

DIET—Liquid to soft diet as tolerated.

CALL YOUR DOCTOR IF

• You have symptoms of diphtheria or observe them in someone else.
• Anyone in your family is exposed to diphtheria.
• Your immunizations are not current.
• The following occurs during treatment:
  Temperature spikes to 102F (38.9C).
  Increasing breathing difficulty.
  Increasing shortness of breath.
  Confusion.

DISK, RUPTURED
(Herniated Disk; Slipped Disk)

 GENERAL INFORMATION

DEFINITION—Sudden or gradual break in the supportive ligaments surrounding a spinal disk (cushions separating bony spinal vertebrae).

BODY PARTS INVOLVED—Disks of the neck or lower spine (most common sites).

SEX OR AGE MOST AFFECTED—Adults of both sexes.

SIGNS & SYMPTOMS
Lower back:
- Severe pain in the low back or back of one leg, buttock or foot (sciatica). Pain usually affects one side and worsens with movement, coughing, sneezing, lifting or straining.
- Weakness, numbness or muscular wasting of the affected leg.
Neck:
- Pain in the neck, shoulder or down one arm. Pain worsens with movement.
- Weakness, numbness or muscular wasting of the affected arm.

CAUSES—Weakening and rupture of the disk material, creating pressure on nearby spinal nerves. Rupture of the disk is caused by sudden injury or chronic stress, such as from constant lifting or obesity.

RISK INCREASES WITH
- Heavy lifting; twisting violently or jumping hard.
- Poor physical condition.
- Elderly.

HOW TO PREVENT
- Practice proper posture when lifting.
- Exercise to maintain good muscle tone.

 WHAT TO EXPECT

DIAGNOSTIC MEASURES
- Your own observation of symptoms.
- Medical history and physical exam by a doctor.
- X-rays of the neck or lower spine, including myelogram (see Glossary).
- CT scan, MRI (see Glossary for both) or diskography (dye is injected into the disk).

APPROPRIATE HEALTH CARE
- Self-care after diagnosis.
- Doctor's treatment.
- Rest at home or in the hospital (sometimes).
- Surgery to relieve nerve pressure if bed rest does not relieve symptoms.
- Rehabilitation to strengthen muscles. You may work with a physical therapist, chiropractor, osteopath, acupuncturist or others in finding the best therapy methods.

- Psychotherapy or counseling to learn coping methods for enduring pain and frustration.

POSSIBLE COMPLICATIONS
- Loss of bladder and bowel function.
- Paralysis.
- Muscle wasting and weakness.
- Disk may be prone to re-injury.

PROBABLE OUTCOME—Spontaneous recovery in many cases. At least 2 weeks in bed should be tried before considering other therapy, unless complications occur. When necessary, a ruptured disk is often curable with surgery.

 HOW TO TREAT

GENERAL MEASURES
- Apply ice packs to the painful area during the first 72 hours and occasionally thereafter, if they provide relief. Alternately, try to relieve pain with a heat lamp, hot showers or baths, compresses or a heating pad.
- Be patient about your recovery. It will take time and energy and often will mean some lifestyle changes.

MEDICATION
- For minor discomfort, you may use nonprescription drugs such as aspirin.
- Your doctor may prescribe:
  Pain relievers.
  Muscle relaxants, such as diazepam or methocarbamol.
  Nonsteroidal anti-inflammatory drugs to reduce inflammation around the rupture.
  Laxatives or stool softeners to prevent constipation.

ACTIVITY—Rest in bed during the acute phase. Resume your normal activities, including sexual relations, when symptoms improve.

DIET—No special diet. Increase consumption of dietary fiber and drink at least 8 glasses of fluid a day to prevent constipation or fecal impaction.

 CALL YOUR DOCTOR IF

- You have symptoms of a ruptured disk.
- The following occurs during treatment:
  Increased pain or weakness in the extremities.
  Loss of bladder or bowel control.
- New, unexplained symptoms develop. Drugs used in treatment may produce side effects.

ILLNESS & DISORDERS

DISLOCATION OR SUBLUXATION

GENERAL INFORMATION

DEFINITION—Dislocation is injury to a joint so that adjoining bones no longer touch each other.

Subluxation is a minor dislocation. Joint surfaces still touch, but not in normal relation to each other.

BODY PARTS INVOLVED—Bones in joints, especially the jaw, shoulder, knee and spine. Some infants are born with a hip dislocation.

SEX OR AGE MOST AFFECTED—Both sexes; all ages.

SIGNS & SYMPTOMS
- Sudden joint pain, swelling or deformity after an injury.
- Limited or absent movement around a joint.

CAUSES
- Injury that stretches or tears ligaments that surround a joint and hold the bones together.
- Shallow or abnormally formed joint surfaces (congenital).
- Rheumatoid arthritis or other diseases of ligaments and tissue around a joint.
- In small children, jerking of an arm or a leg by an adult

RISK INCREASES WITH
- Rheumatoid arthritis.
- Family history of congenital hip dislocation.
- Repeated injury to a joint.

HOW TO PREVENT
- If you are involved in heavy work or strenuous sports, learn to protect the involved joints. Use protective devices, such as wrapped elastic bandages, tape wraps, knee or shoulder pads, and special support stockings.
- Infants should be examined for congenital hip dislocation at birth and at "well-baby" checkups.

WHAT TO EXPECT

DIAGNOSTIC MEASURES
- Your own observation of symptoms.
- Medical history and physical exam by a doctor.
- X-rays of the joint and adjacent bones.

APPROPRIATE HEALTH CARE
- Self-care after diagnosis.
- Doctor's treatment. This may include manipulating the joint to reposition the bones.
- Surgery to restore the joint to its normal position (sometimes). Recurring dislocation may require surgical reconstruction or replacement of the joint.

POSSIBLE COMPLICATIONS—Damage to nearby nerves or major blood vessels, causing numbness, coldness and paleness.

PROBABLE OUTCOME—Usually curable with prompt treatment. After the dislocation has been corrected, the joint may require immobilization with a cast or sling for 2 to 8 weeks.

HOW TO TREAT

GENERAL MEASURES—Immediately after injury:
- Apply ice packs to the involved joint to prevent swelling.
- Use a splint or sling to prevent movement while transporting the injured person to the doctor.
- If your doctor puts a cast on the joint, see Care of Casts in Appendix.

MEDICATION—Your doctor may prescribe:
- General anesthesia or muscle relaxants to make joint manipulation possible.
- Acetaminophen or aspirin to relieve moderate pain.
- Narcotic pain relievers for severe pain.

ACTIVITY—Resume your normal activities gradually after treatment.

DIET—Drink only water before manipulation or surgery to correct the dislocation. Solid food makes general anesthesia more hazardous.

CALL YOUR DOCTOR IF

- You have difficulty moving a joint after injury.
- Any extremity becomes numb, pale or cold after injury. This is an emergency!
- Dislocations occur repeatedly that you can "pop" back into normal position.

DISSEMINATED INTRAVASCULAR COAGULATION
(Defibrination Syndrome; Consumption Coagulopathy; DIC)

 GENERAL INFORMATION

DEFINITION—A serious disruption of blood-clotting mechanisms, resulting in hemorrhaging or internal bleeding. This disorder is a complication of an underlying disorder.

BODY PARTS INVOLVED—Blood vessels and blood in all parts of the body.

SEX OR AGE MOST AFFECTED—Both sexes; all ages.

SIGNS & SYMPTOMS
- Bleeding and hemorrhage from any or several body parts. Bleeding may be heavy. Common signs of bleeding include:
  Bloody vomit or red or black stools.
  Vaginal bleeding.
  Red or cloudy urine.
  Unexplained bruising.
- Severe abdominal or back pain caused by bleeding into body organs.
- Convulsions (rare).
- Coma (rare).

CAUSES—Depletion of blood-clotting components, causing widespread bleeding. This condition can be the result of:
- Pregnancy abnormalities, such as placenta previa, abruptio placenta or toxemia.
- Widespread or major infection.
- Widespread cancer.
- Some kinds of surgery.
- Widespread tissue destruction, as with extensive burns.
- Poisonous snakebite.
- Transfusion of mismatched blood.

RISK INCREASES WITH
- Poor nutrition.
- Illness that has lowered resistance.

HOW TO PREVENT—Obtain prompt medical treatment for the underlying causes.

 WHAT TO EXPECT

DIAGNOSTIC MEASURES
- Your own observation of symptoms.
- Medical history and physical exam by a doctor.

APPROPRIATE HEALTH CARE
- Doctor's treatment.
- Hospitalization.
- Surgery to correct the underlying disorder (sometimes).
- Self-care after treatment.

POSSIBLE COMPLICATIONS
- Kidney failure.
- Brain damage, with seizures or coma.
- Shock; death.
- Gangrene and loss of extremities.

PROBABLE OUTCOME—If the underlying cause of DIC is treated promptly, full recovery is likely.

 HOW TO TREAT

GENERAL MEASURES
- Patients with this condition are often desperately ill and require intensive hospital care. Family members can help by maintaining a positive, hopeful attitude.
- During recovery, don't scrub or take scabs off sores. This may trigger new bleeding.

MEDICATION—Your doctor may prescribe:
- Blood transfusions or blood-component infusions.
- Heparin (an anticoagulant administered by injection).
- Antibiotics for infection.

ACTIVITY—Rest in bed until your doctor approves a return to normal activity.

DIET—Whatever type of diet is tolerated depending on patient's condition.

 CALL YOUR DOCTOR IF

- You have symptoms of DIC. This is an emergency!
- Any bleeding recurs or the abdomen swells rapidly during treatment.

ILLNESS & DISORDERS

DIVERTICULAR DISEASE
(Diverticulosis; Diverticulitis)

 GENERAL INFORMATION

DEFINITION—Diverticulosis is the presence of small, saclike swellings (diverticula) in the wall of the colon. Diverticula may be present without any symptoms. Diverticulitis is the inflammation of diverticula. It is not contagious or cancerous.

BODY PARTS INVOLVED—Left side of the large intestine.

SEX OR AGE MOST AFFECTED—Adults. Diverticula are present in 30% to 40% of persons over age 50. They increase with each decade of life.

SIGNS & SYMPTOMS
Diverticulosis symptoms:
- No symptoms (usually).
- Mild cramping or tenderness in the left side of the abdomen that is relieved by passing gas or moving bowels.
- Occasional bright red blood in the stool. noninfected diverticula sometimes bleed.
- Constipation (sometimes).

Diverticulitis symptoms:
- Intermittent cramping, abdominal pain that becomes constant. Pain may be disabling at the onset or may not become disabling for days.
- Fever or nausea.
- Tenderness over affected area of the colon.
- Diarrhea or alternating diarrhea and constipation.

CAUSES—Unknown, but the tendency is inherited. Recent evidence suggests that the highly refined, low-residue diet common in the U.S. and other developed countries may contribute to the formation of diverticula. Pressure builds up inside the sigmoid colon as a result of spasm due to lack of dietary bulk. The inner lining eventually pushes through to form the small pouches.

RISK INCREASES WITH
- Improper diet that lacks fiber.
- Family history of diverticulosis; age over 50.
- Coronary artery disease or gallbladder disease or obesity.

HOW TO PREVENT—Cannot be prevented at present, but risk can be reduced by:
- Eat a diet high in fiber; drink plenty of fluids.
- Don't strain when moving bowels.
- Maintain good cardiovascular fitness.

 WHAT TO EXPECT

DIAGNOSTIC MEASURES
- Your own observation of symptoms.
- Medical history and exam by a doctor.
- X-rays of the lower intestine (barium enema).
- Sigmoidoscopy (see Glossary).

APPROPRIATE HEALTH CARE
- Self-care after diagnosis.
- Doctor's treatment.
- Hospitalization (complications only).
- Surgery to remove part of the colon if diverticula become infected or bleed significantly. (See Sigmoid-Colon Removal in Surgery section.)

POSSIBLE COMPLICATIONS—If diverticula become infected, they may bleed profusely or perforate (erode through the intestinal wall) and cause peritonitis. Both are emergencies.

PROBABLE OUTCOME—Diverticulosis is dangerous only if diverticula become infected or bleed. Diverticulitis is curable with surgery.

 HOW TO TREAT

GENERAL MEASURES
- Treatment is usually unnecessary if there are no symptoms. For mild symptoms, a change in diet and the use of stool softeners may be sufficient. For more severe symptoms, you may require bed rest, medications and surgery.
- Try to have a bowel movement at about the same time each day. Allow at least 10 minutes, and don't strain.
- Check your stool daily for bleeding. If the stool is black, remove it from the toilet and take it to your doctor's office for analysis.
- To relieve mild pain and spasms, apply a heating pad to the abdomen.

MEDICATION—Your doctor may prescribe:
- Antibiotics, if the diverticula are infected.
- Stool-softeners or laxatives, if you are unable to eat a high-fiber diet. Don't take laxatives unless prescribed.

ACTIVITY—If you have fever or severe pain, stay in bed. Resume normal activity as soon as symptoms improve.

DIET
- Eat a well-balanced diet that is high in fiber, low in salt and low in fat (see diets in Appendix).
- Avoid foods that may constipate (bananas, applesauce, rice) and foods with small indigestible seeds that could plug the diverticula (poppy, sesame, raspberry, strawberry, etc.).

 CALL YOUR DOCTOR IF

- You have symptoms of diverticulosis or diverticulitis (e.g. blood in stool).
- Severe pain continues despite treatment.
- Fever, vomiting or abdominal swelling occurs during treatment.

DOMESTIC VIOLENCE
(Battering; Spousal Abuse)

 GENERAL INFORMATION

DEFINITION—Abuse includes different behaviors (physical, sexual, psychological and emotional forms) that are used to establish power and to control the victim, who is most frequently a woman. Often, because of shame and guilt, the victim does not report the abuse to authorities or talk about it with family or friends.

SEX OR AGE MOST AFFECTED—Both sexes, all ages, but most common in females. Over 2 million women in the U.S. are battered by a male partner each year. Some studies have shown that 1 in 4 pregnant women are battered.

SIGNS & SYMPTOMS
In victims:
- Physical injuries to the body including broken bones, bruises, burns, choking, bites and rape. Most injuries are inflicted on the head, neck, chest, breasts and abdomen. Injuries also occur on the arms which are used to deflect blows.
- Other symptoms may include chronic pelvic pain, sexual dysfunction, feelings of anxiety, sleep disorders, depression, post traumatic stress disorder (PTSD), eating disorders, psychological problems and thoughts of suicide.

In the abuser:
- Angry, suspicious, tense and moody behaviors. Sometimes the abuser can be extremely charming. They often alternate periods of abuse with periods of affection.
- May demonstrate pathological jealousy, fear of abandonment, lack of assertiveness, possessiveness and fear of dependence.
- Watches wife closely; keeps her away from her friends and sometimes her family.
- Makes threats of violence; may play with guns or knives.

CAUSES—There are a number of theories as to why domestic abuse occurs and how it evolves. Researchers are still looking for answers.

RISK INCREASES WITH
- A history of family abuse, especially during childhood of abuser or victim.
- Abusers are often men who tend to use alcohol or drugs, frequently are unemployed, and are often less educated (however, educated professional men can be abusers).
- Males who are dependent on women, have financial worries, feelings of inadequacy and have traditional attitudes, particularly about sex.
- Females lacking self-esteem or who feel dependent and useless.
- Pregnant females. Abuse is often a factor in miscarriages.

HOW TO PREVENT—Victims should seek help at the first sign of abuse and not assume that the abuser will change or the abuse will stop.

 WHAT TO EXPECT

DIAGNOSTIC MEASURES
- Your own observation of symptoms.
- Medical history and exam by a doctor.

APPROPRIATE HEALTH CARE—Doctor's treatment. Hospitalization if needed.

POSSIBLE COMPLICATIONS
- Years of emotional and physical abuse.
- Death of the abused.
- Killing of abuser.

PROBABLE OUTCOME—With the increased public awareness of the problem and availability of support systems, more people are seeking help early.

 HOW TO TREAT

GENERAL MEASURES
If you are abused:
- Protect yourself, especially the head and abdomen. Get help; if you can, get away from the abuser. Document the abuse with pictures by telling someone or by calling 911.
- Have a personal safety plan established (place to stay, money necessary to get there, survival funds, transportation, and clothing and personal essentials packed).
- Seek legal help. Police departments and prosecutory practices are rapidly improving in responding to the problems.
- Numerous agencies and shelters for helping abused women and children are available. Call your local crisis line.

Treatment steps for a victim:
Get medical help for any injuries.
Counseling is vital. The variety of treatment options will help a woman learn to cope, regain her self-confidence and the ability to function independently.

Treatment for the abuser:
Treatment is often resisted by an abuser. Educational and treatment groups have had some success for abusive men.

MEDICATION—Usually not needed, but may be prescribed for anxiety or depression.

ACTIVITY—No restrictions.

DIET—No special diet.

 CALL YOUR DOCTOR IF

You or a family member is a victim of domestic violence.

DOWN SYNDROME
(Trisomy 21)

GENERAL INFORMATION

DEFINITION—Mental retardation and abnormalities in many organs caused by a major chromosome abnormality that is congenital.

BODY PARTS INVOLVED—Central nervous system; heart; skeletal system.

SEX OR AGE MOST AFFECTED—Newborns.

SIGNS & SYMPTOMS
Shortly after birth:
- Lack of normal muscle tone. The child seems "floppy."
- Head and face abnormalities, including: a small or odd-shaped skull; slanting, almond-shaped eyes; small mouth and protruding tongue.
- Broad hands with large, unusual palm creases. The little finger curves inward (sometimes).
- Heart murmur.

Later:
- Retarded growth and development (slower than other children to walk, talk and learn).
- Mental retardation (average IQ is about 50).

CAUSES—An extra chromosome in the fertilized egg creates abnormalities as the fetus develops. In 1/3 of cases, the extra chromosome comes from the father.

RISK INCREASES WITH
- Pregnancy in females under age 16 or over 35. At age 40, incidence is 1 in 40 births.
- Family history of Down syndrome.
- Mother's exposure to drugs, radiation, chemicals or infections before pregnancy.

HOW TO PREVENT
- If you are pregnant and over age 35, or you or your partner have a family history of Down syndrome, request amniocentesis (see Glossary). This can detect whether the fetus has Down syndrome.
- If you or your partner have a family history of Down syndrome, obtain genetic counseling before starting a family.

WHAT TO EXPECT

DIAGNOSTIC MEASURES
- Parent's observation of symptoms.
- Medical history and physical exam by a doctor.
- Laboratory studies of chromosomes.

APPROPRIATE HEALTH CARE
- Doctor's treatment.
- Psychotherapy or counseling for the parents. Many parents blame themselves and need help to cope with unnecessary, harmful guilt.
- Surgery to correct congenital heart or intestinal disorders.
- Group-home care, if home care is not feasible.

POSSIBLE COMPLICATIONS
- Increased susceptibility to leukemia and thyroid disease.
- Increased susceptibility to infections.
- Congestive heart failure caused by congenital heart abnormalities.
- Alzheimer's disease in 1/3 of patients over age 35.

PROBABLE OUTCOME—Special education and training allow many children with Down syndrome to lead happy, loving and useful lives. Life expectancy is reduced—few persons with Down syndrome reach age 40.

HOW TO TREAT

GENERAL MEASURES
- Learn all you can about programs and resources in your community to help children with Down syndrome. Early intervention programs are designed to help these children develop their abilities as much as possible.
- The degree of retardation ranges from mild to severe. Children may be able to attend special education classes in regular schools and others may attend special schools for the mentally retarded.
- See Resources for Additional Information.

MEDICATION—Your doctor may prescribe antibiotics for frequent, complicating infections. There is no medication to specifically treat Down syndrome.

ACTIVITY—Encourage the child to be as active as possible in a protected environment.

DIET—No special diet. Extra patience may be necessary in feeding an infant with Down syndrome. Some have difficulty sucking or are not eager to eat.

CALL YOUR DOCTOR IF

- Your infant seems "floppy" or does not seem to be developing normally.
- A child with Down syndrome develops signs of infection (fever, warmth or pain).

DROWNING, NEAR

GENERAL INFORMATION

DEFINITION—The immediate aftereffects of prolonged submersion under water.

BODY PARTS INVOLVED—Lungs; blood; heart.

SEX OR AGE MOST AFFECTED—Both sexes; all ages.

SIGNS & SYMPTOMS
* Confusion or unconsciousness.
* Little or no breathing or heartbeat.
* Bluish-white paleness.

CAUSES—Submersion under water results in either:
* Spasm of the larynx (the tube from the throat to the lungs). After rescue, this spasm prevents oxygen from reaching the lungs.
* Water in the lungs, causing life-threatening changes in the circulating blood.

RISK INCREASES WITH
* Excess alcohol consumption.
* Accidents—especially head injury—while swimming.
* Poorly supervised children or inadequately fenced swimming pools.
* Suicidal persons.

HOW TO PREVENT
* Learn cardiopulmonary resuscitation (CPR).
* Encourage all family members—including infants—to learn to swim.
* Install a fence around your home swimming pool.
* Never swim alone.
* Don't drink alcohol and swim.

WHAT TO EXPECT

DIAGNOSTIC MEASURES
* Your own observation of symptoms.
* Medical history and physical exam by a doctor.
* Laboratory blood tests.

APPROPRIATE HEALTH CARE
* Immediate cardiopulmonary resuscitation (CPR).
* Hospitalization for observation for delayed, serious reactions.

POSSIBLE COMPLICATIONS
* Pulmonary edema (body fluid in the lungs).
* Permanent brain damage.
* Heart irregularities, including cardiac arrest and death.
* Lung infection.
* Fear of water.
* Seizures, retardation, heart and lung problems are frequent long-term complications.

PROBABLE OUTCOME—Depends on the length of time under water. With early rescue and treatment, full recovery is possible. Special body mechanisms may permit full recovery from near-drowning in icy water even after prolonged immersion.

HOW TO TREAT

GENERAL MEASURES
* If the victim is unconscious and not breathing, yell for help. Don't leave the victim.
* Call 911 (emergency) for an ambulance or medical help (if the victim is a child, give 1 minute of CPR and then call 911).
* Begin mouth-to-mouth breathing immediately.
* If there is no heartbeat, give external cardiac massage.
* Don't stop CPR until help arrives.
* The near-drowning victim should be taken to the nearest hospital for intensive care even if the victim has regained consciousness. Complications or death may occur 24 to 48 hours after the accident due to heart-rhythm disturbances.
* Remain with a recovering patient to provide support and reassurance. Near-drowning is a traumatic experience.

MEDICATION—The doctor may prescribe:
* Oxygen.
* Cortisone drugs to prevent or treat lung inflammation.
* Antibiotics to prevent lung infection.
* Bronchodilators to enable oxygen to enter the lungs.

ACTIVITY—Complete bed rest until activity is permitted by the doctor.

DIET—Intravenous nutrients, if the victim is unconscious upon hospitalization. After recovery, no special diet is necessary.

CALL YOUR DOCTOR IF

* Someone appears to have drowned. Call for emergency help immediately! See General Measures for additional emergency information.
* Signs of infection (fever, cough, muscle aches and fatigue) appear after apparent recovery.

ILLNESS & DISORDERS

DRUG ABUSE & ADDICTION

 ## GENERAL INFORMATION

DEFINITION—A compulsive and destructive use of mind-altering substances despite adverse medical, psychological and social consequences.

BODY PARTS INVOLVED—Central nervous system; liver; kidneys; blood.

SEX OR AGE MOST AFFECTED—All ages, except early childhood.

SIGNS & SYMPTOMS—Depends on the substance of abuse. Most produce:
- A temporary, pleasant mood.
- Relief from anxiety.
- False feelings of self-confidence.
- Increased sensitivity to sights and sounds (including hallucinations).
- Altered activity levels—either stupor and sleeplike states or frenzies.
- Unpleasant or painful symptoms when the abused substance is withdrawn.

CAUSES—Substances of abuse may produce addiction (a physiological need) or dependence (a psychological need). The most common substances of abuse include:
- Nicotine.
- Alcohol; caffeine.
- Marijuana or amphetamines.
- Barbiturates or cocaine.
- Opiates, including codeine, heroin, methadone, morphine and opium.
- Psychedelic drugs, including PCP ("angel dust"), mescaline and LSD.
- Volatile substances, such as glue, solvents and paints.

RISK INCREASES WITH
- Illness that requires prescription pain relievers or tranquilizers.
- Family history of drug abuse.
- Genetic factors (possibly). Some persons may be more susceptible to addiction.
- Excess alcohol consumption.
- Fatigue or overwork.
- Poverty; peer pressure.
- Psychological problems, including depression, dependency or poor self-esteem.

HOW TO PREVENT
- Don't socialize with persons who use and abuse drugs.
- Seek counseling for mental-health problems, such as depression or chronic anxiety, before they lead to drug problems.
- Develop wholesome interests and leisure activities.
- After surgery, illness or injury, discontinue the use of prescription pain relievers and tranquilizers as soon as possible. Don't use more than you need.

 ## WHAT TO EXPECT

DIAGNOSTIC MEASURES
- Your own observation of symptoms.
- Medical history and physical exam by a doctor.
- Laboratory blood tests.

APPROPRIATE HEALTH CARE
- Doctor's treatment.
- Psychotherapy or counseling.
- Hospitalization for drug-withdrawal symptoms.

POSSIBLE COMPLICATIONS
- Sexually transmitted diseases, which are more likely among addicts.
- Severe infections, such as endocarditis, hepatitis or blood poisoning, from intravenous injections with nonsterile needles.
- Malnutrition.
- Accidental injury to oneself or others while in a drug-induced state.
- Loss of job or family; incarceration.
- Irreversible damage to body organs.
- Death caused by overdose.

PROBABLE OUTCOME—Curable with strong motivation, good medical care and support from family and friends.

 ## HOW TO TREAT

GENERAL MEASURES
- Admit you have a problem.
- Seek professional help.
- Be open and honest with your family and good friends, and ask their help.
- Avoid friends who tempt you to resume your habit.
- Join self-help groups.
- See Resources for Additional Information.

MEDICATION—Your doctor may prescribe:
- Disulfiram (Antabuse) for alcoholism. This drug produces severe illness when alcohol is consumed.
- Methadone for narcotic abuse. This drug is a less-potent narcotic used to decrease the severity of physical withdrawal symptoms.

ACTIVITY—No restrictions. Exercise regularly and vigorously.

DIET—Eat a normal, well-balanced diet that is high in protein. Vitamin supplements may be necessary if you suffer from malnutrition.

 ## CALL YOUR DOCTOR IF

- You abuse or are addicted to drugs and want help.
- New, unexplained symptoms develop. Drugs in treatment may produce side effects.

DRUG HYPERSENSITIVITY

GENERAL INFORMATION

DEFINITION—A variety of allergic responses caused by medication. The reaction may be immediate—especially with a drug given intravenously—or the reaction may take a week to develop.

BODY PARTS INVOLVED—Skin; blood vessels; lungs.

SEX OR AGE MOST AFFECTED—Both sexes; all ages.

SIGNS & SYMPTOMS
- Rash, itching or hives.
- Flushed skin.
- Anxiety.
- Serum sickness (fever, rash, joint pain and nerve damage).
- Anaphylaxis (wheezing and breathing difficulty). For signs and symptoms, see Anaphylaxis (in Illness section).
- Various blood disorders, such as hemolytic anemia.
- Peripheral neuropathy (nerve damage).
- Vasculitis (blood vessel inflammation).

The following reactions to medications are usually not the result of allergy:
- Vomiting or diarrhea.
- Fever.
- Photosensitivity (a skin reaction to sunlight).

CAUSES—Medications are "foreign" materials. When injected—or less often, when taken orally—the body develops antibodies to the medication. Subsequent exposure to the medication causes an allergic reaction in the body.

RISK INCREASES WITH
- Use of almost any drugs, but especially the following:
  - Penicillin and cephalosporin antibiotics.
  - Sulfa drugs.
  - Animal serums.
  - Vaccines.
  - Local anesthetics.
  - Allergy extracts.
  - Iodine-containing compounds, such as those used in some X-rays.
- Injected medications, especially in high doses.
- Medical history of other allergies, such as hay fever, asthma or eczema.
- Current infectious illness (probably because infection increases immune-system functions).

HOW TO PREVENT
- Tell medical professionals about any drug reactions you have had.
- Learn the name of any medication you are given. If it causes a reaction, you must avoid it in the future.
- Don't take medication—including nonprescription drugs—unless necessary.

WHAT TO EXPECT

DIAGNOSTIC MEASURES
- Your own observation of symptoms.
- Medical history and physical exam by a doctor.

APPROPRIATE HEALTH CARE
- Self-care.
- Doctor's treatment.
- Discontinuing of the the offending drug. Often another drug can be substituted.

POSSIBLE COMPLICATIONS
- Death from severe anaphylaxis reactions.
- Disability for many months from serum sickness.

PROBABLE OUTCOME—Most reactions disappear once the medication is permanently discontinued.

HOW TO TREAT

GENERAL MEASURES
- Wear a Medic-Alert pendant or bracelet (see Glossary) if you have drug hypersensitivity. Even with a slight reaction the first time, subsequent exposure to the drug may initiate more severe reaction.
- Keep an anaphylaxis kit at home, on your person, nearby at work and in your car for emergency use if anyone in the family has had a severe drug reaction. Ask your doctor how to obtain one.

MEDICATION—Your doctor may prescribe:
- Cortisone drugs to decrease the inflammatory reaction.
- Antihistamines to decrease the body's allergic response.

ACTIVITY—Resume your normal activities as soon as symptoms improve.

DIET—No special diet.

CALL YOUR DOCTOR IF

You have symptoms of drug hypersensitivity or observe them in someone else.

DUMPING SYNDROME

GENERAL INFORMATION

DEFINITION—A group of symptoms that are a complication of surgical removal of all or part of the stomach. Most patients experience the problem to a minor degree for 1 to 6 months after surgery. It becomes a serious problem in 1% or 2% of patients.

The symptoms are of 2 types—early dumping syndrome and late dumping syndrome. Symptoms of the first begin a few minutes to 45 minutes after every meal. Symptoms of the second begin 2 to 3 hours after eating. Most persons experience late dumping syndrome—one person does not have both forms.

BODY PARTS INVOLVED—Gastrointestinal system; cardiovascular system.

SEX OR AGE MOST AFFECTED—Both sexes of adults following surgery on the stomach.

SIGNS & SYMPTOMS
Early dumping syndrome:
- Weakness and fainting.
- Sweating.
- Irregular or rapid heartbeat.
- Decreased blood pressure.
- Flushing of skin.
- Dizziness.
- Shortness of breath.
- Vomiting.
- Explosive diarrhea and abdominal cramps.

Late dumping syndrome:
- Sweating, anxiety and tremors.
- Exhaustion and faintness.
- Decreased blood pressure.
- Headache.

CAUSES
- Early dumping syndrome: Rapid entry of food and fluids directly into the small intestine, producing decreased blood pressure and increased blood flow to the intestines.
- Late dumping syndrome: Low blood sugar caused by excess insulin produced in response to sudden dumping of food and fluids into the intestine.

RISK INCREASES WITH—The larger the amount of stomach removed, the more severe the dumping syndrome.

HOW TO PREVENT—Some degree cannot be prevented, but recurrence and severity can be minimized with dietary changes (see Diet).

WHAT TO EXPECT

DIAGNOSTIC MEASURES
- Your own observation of symptoms.
- Medical history and physical exam by a doctor.
- Laboratory studies of blood sugar levels.

APPROPRIATE HEALTH CARE
- Self-care after diagnosis.
- Doctor's treatment.

POSSIBLE COMPLICATIONS
- Malnutrition and weight loss.
- Anxiety.

PROBABLE OUTCOME—Spontaneous recovery for most patients. Early dumping syndrome usually lasts 3 to 4 months. Late dumping syndrome usually lasts 1 year, but it may persist for many years.

HOW TO TREAT

GENERAL MEASURES
- Early syndrome: Lie down for 45 minutes until symptoms pass.
- Late syndrome: Eat small amounts of sugar candy or drink sweetened orange juice.

MEDICATION—Your doctor may prescribe:
- Anticholinergics to block the dumping-syndrome reflex.
- Pectin to reduce the severity of diarrhea.
- Vitamin and mineral supplements to compensate for poor absorption.

ACTIVITY
- Between symptoms: no restrictions.
- With symptoms: rest until they pass.

DIET
- Early dumping syndrome: Diet control is the most important treatment. Eat a diet low in sugar and other simple carbohydrates. Increase fat and protein consumption. Eat 6 small, evenly spaced meals a day. Take meals dry—without water or beverages—and drink fluids only between meals.
- Late dumping syndrome: Avoid refined sugar.

CALL YOUR DOCTOR IF

- You have symptoms of dumping syndrome not relieved by measures outlined above.
- You vomit blood, have black, tarry stools or other signs of gastrointestinal bleeding.
- New, unexplained symptoms develop. Drugs used in treatment may produce side effects.

DYSENTERY, BACILLARY
(Shigellosis)

GENERAL INFORMATION

DEFINITION—A bacterial infection of the surface layers of the intestinal tract. This is contagious with close personal contact and occurs in epidemics. It has a 1 to 4 day incubation period.

BODY PARTS INVOLVED—Lower small intestine (ileum); large intestine (colon).

SEX OR AGE MOST AFFECTED—Both sexes; all ages.

SIGNS & SYMPTOMS
- Abdominal cramps.
- Fever.
- Diarrhea (up to 20 or 30 watery bowel movements in 1 day).
- Blood, mucus or pus in the stool.
- Nausea or vomiting.
- Muscle aches or pain.
- White-blood-cell count lower than normal at the onset (sometimes).

CAUSES—Bacteria called Shigella bacillus, that invades the lining of the colon. It spreads from person to person, usually from contaminated hands to mouth, contaminated food or drinking water.

RISK INCREASES WITH
- Travel to foreign countries.
- Crowded or unsanitary living conditions.

HOW TO PREVENT
- Wash hands after bowel movements and before handling food.
- Isolate anyone with symptoms of bacillary dysentery.
- Immerse soiled clothes and bedclothes in covered buckets of soap and water until they can be boiled.

WHAT TO EXPECT

DIAGNOSTIC MEASURES
- Your own observation of symptoms.
- Medical history and physical exam by a doctor.
- Laboratory stool culture. Diagnosis is aided by knowledge of outbreaks and endemic areas.

APPROPRIATE HEALTH CARE
- Home care.
- Doctor's treatment.
- Hospitalization of persons (especially small children with dehydration) who are severely ill. Hospital care will include isolation and intravenous fluid supplements.

POSSIBLE COMPLICATIONS
- Dangerous dehydration, especially in children.
- In rare cases, the bacteria may enter the bloodstream from the digestive tract and infect other body organs, such as kidneys, gallbladder, liver or heart and joints. This may cause shock and death.

PROBABLE OUTCOME—Usually curable in 7 days with treatment. Most Shigella infections are mild and don't require drastic treatment. However, in a severe attack, excessive dehydration can be fatal (especially in infants and young children) if treatment is unsuccessful.

HOW TO TREAT

GENERAL MEASURES
- Isolate the patient from others.
- Use a heating pad or hot-water bottle on the abdomen to relieve pain.
- Maintain fluid intake.

MEDICATION
- Your doctor may prescribe antibiotics.
- Don't use paregoric preparations or other antidiarrhea drugs unless your doctor prescribes them. These may prolong the illness. If used, discontinue them as soon as possible.

ACTIVITY—Bed rest is necessary, except for trips to the bathroom, until fever, diarrhea and other symptoms have been gone for at least 3 days. The legs should be exercised regularly in bed.

DIET—Liquid (use commercial rehydration products) or soft diet until diarrhea stops, then return to normal diet.

CALL YOUR DOCTOR IF

- You or your child have symptoms of bacillary dysentery.
- The following occurs during treatment:
  Fever of 102F (38.9C) or more.
  Sore throat, headache or earache.
  Shortness of breath or severe cough.
  Traces of blood in the sputum.
  Severe abdominal pain or abdominal swelling.
  Rectal bleeding.
  Pain in the calf or leg.
  Swollen joints.
  Signs of dehydration (lethargy, sunken eyes, rapid weight loss or dry skin) appear.

DYSHIDROSIS

GENERAL INFORMATION

DEFINITION—A skin condition, characterized by small blisters on the hands or feet—apparently related to stress.

BODY PARTS INVOLVED—Tips and sides of the fingers, toes, palms and soles.

SEX OR AGE MOST AFFECTED—Both sexes and all ages, but most common in men between ages 20 and 50.

SIGNS & SYMPTOMS—Small blisters with the following characteristics:
- Blisters are very small (1mm or less in diameter). They appear on the tips and sides of fingers, toes, palms and soles.
- Blisters are opaque and deep-seated; they are either flush with the skin or slightly elevated. They don't break easily. Eventually, small blisters come together and form large blisters.
- Blisters may itch, cause pain or produce no symptoms. They worsen after contact with soap, water or irritating substances.

CAUSES—Unknown, but they are probably related to periods of anxiety, stress and frustration in ambitious people who internalize their emotions. Persons with dyshidrosis have difficulty relaxing—even during nonstressful periods.

This problem is not caused by sweat retention, as was once believed. Excessive sweating is often associated with it.

RISK INCREASES WITH
- Stress and internalized frustration or irritation.
- Obsessive-compulsive personalities.

HOW TO PREVENT—Follow instructions under General Measures. These are helpful in preventing recurrences, as well as in treating active episodes.

WHAT TO EXPECT

DIAGNOSTIC MEASURES
- Your own observation of symptoms.
- Medical history and physical exam by a doctor.

APPROPRIATE HEALTH CARE
- Self-care after diagnosis.
- Doctor's treatment.
- Psychotherapy or counseling to learn to cope with stress more effectively.

POSSIBLE COMPLICATIONS—Secondary bacterial infection (sometimes).

PROBABLE OUTCOME
- Symptoms can be controlled with treatment, but recurrence is common. Often heals spontaneously.

- Persons with mild problems have occasional attacks, and the skin returns to normal between episodes.
- Persons with severe problems sometimes have persistent peeling and fissuring of the involved skin.

HOW TO TREAT

GENERAL MEASURES—Keep heat and moisture away from the affected areas whenever possible:
- Wear cotton socks and leather-soled shoes. Don't wear tennis shoes or other footwear made of man-made materials.
- Remove shoes and socks frequently to allow sweat to evaporate.
- Wear heavy-duty, cotton-lined vinyl gloves to prevent contact with irritating substances, such as: water; soap; detergent; metal scrubbing pads; scouring powder; and other chemicals. Dry insides of gloves after use. Discard gloves if they develop a hole. Wear gloves when you peel or squeeze acid fruits and vegetables.
- Wear leather or heavy-duty fabric gloves for housework or gardening.
- Use a dishwashing machine to wash dishes if possible. If not, ask someone else to wash them.
- Avoid contact with irritating chemicals, such as: paint; paint thinner; and polish for cars, floors, shoes, furniture and metal.
- Remove rings before doing housework or washing hands.
- Use lukewarm water and very little mild soap to shower or bathe.

MEDICATION—You may use nonprescription topical steroid preparations to reduce inflammation and decrease itching. Apply once or twice a day after bathing, unless directed otherwise. If these are not effective, your doctor may prescribe stronger steroid preparations.

ACTIVITY—Avoid activities or environments that lead to stress or excessive sweating. Sweating does not cause the disorder but may aggravate it.

DIET—No special diet.

CALL YOUR DOCTOR IF

- You have symptoms of dyshidrosis.
- Signs of infection (swelling, redness, tenderness or warmth) appear around blisters.
- Symptoms don't improve after 1 week, despite treatment.
- Improvement begins and then symptoms recur.

DYSMENORRHEA
(Menstrual Cramps)

 GENERAL INFORMATION

DEFINITION—Severe, painful cramps during menstruation. Primary dysmenorrhea means pain has recurred regularly since periods began. Secondary dysmenorrhea means pain began years after periods started. Women with dysmenorrhea are generally fertile. Severity of symptoms varies greatly from woman to woman, and from one time to the next in the same woman. Dysmenorrhea usually is less severe after a woman has a baby.

BODY PARTS INVOLVED—Female reproductive system, especially the uterus.

SEX OR AGE MOST AFFECTED—Women of childbearing age.

SIGNS & SYMPTOMS
- Cramping and sometimes sharp pains in the lower abdomen, lower back and thighs.
- Nausea and vomiting (sometimes).
- Diarrhea (occasionally); urinary frequency.
- Sweating; lack of energy.
- Irritability; nervousness; depression.

CAUSES
- Strong or prolonged contractions of the muscular wall of the uterus. These may be caused by concentration of prostaglandins (hormones manufactured by the body). Research shows that women with dysmenorrhea produce and excrete more prostaglandins than those who don't have as much discomfort.
- Dilation of the cervix to allow passage of blood clots from the uterus to the vagina.
- Other causes include pelvic infections; endometriosis, especially if dysmenorrhea begins after age 20; benign tumors of the uterus.

RISK INCREASES WITH
- Use of caffeine.
- Stress. The degree of dysmenorrhea may vary according to physical or mental health. While emotional or psychological factors don't cause the pain, they can worsen pain or cause less responsiveness to treatment.
- Family history of dysmenorrhea.
- Lack of exercise; poor diet.

HOW TO PREVENT
- Take female hormones that prevent ovulation, such as oral contraceptives.
- Treatment of the underlying cause.

 WHAT TO EXPECT

DIAGNOSTIC MEASURES
Medical history and physical exam, including a pelvic examination, by a doctor.

APPROPRIATE HEALTH CARE
- Self-care after diagnosis.

- Doctor's treatment.
- Initial treatment aims are to relieve pain. Long term goals of treatment involve treating any underlying cause with medication, counseling or possibly surgery.
- Transcutaneous electrical nerve stimulator (TENS) treatment may help relieve pain.
- Psychotherapy or counseling, if dysmenorrhea is stress-related. Hypnosis therapy may help.
- Treatment for the cause for secondary dysmenorrhea.

POSSIBLE COMPLICATIONS—Severe pain that regularly interferes with normal activity.

PROBABLE OUTCOME—Symptoms can be controlled with treatment.

 HOW TO TREAT

GENERAL MEASURES
- Heat helps relieve pain. Use a heating pad or hot-water bottle on the abdomen or back, or take hot baths. Sit in a tub of hot water for 10 to 15 minutes as often as necessary.
- Keep yourself warm. Women in cold environments seem to suffer more severe symptoms.
- See How to Cope with Stress in Appendix for suggestions to reduce stress.

MEDICATION
- For minor discomfort, you may use nonprescription drugs such as aspirin or ibuprofen.
- Your doctor may prescribe:
  Antiprostaglandins, including nonsteroidal, anti-inflammatory drugs.
  Oral contraceptives, which prohibit ovulation.

ACTIVITY
- No restrictions. When resting in bed, elevate your feet or bend your knees; lie on your side.
- Regular, vigorous exercise reduces discomfort of future periods.

DIET
- No special diet. Your doctor may prescribe vitamin-B supplements. These help relieve symptoms in some persons.
- Some herbal teas can relieve symptoms.
- Drink lots of nonalcoholic fluids.

 CALL YOUR DOCTOR IF

- You have symptoms of dysmenorrhea you cannot control by yourself.
- Your bleeding is excessive (you saturate more than one pad or tampon each hour).
- You develop signs of infection, such as fever, a general ill feeling, headache, dizziness or muscle aches.
- New, unexplained symptoms develop.

DYSPAREUNIA

GENERAL INFORMATION

DEFINITION—Recurrent and persistent genital pain for a woman during sexual intercourse.

BODY PARTS INVOLVED—Vaginal muscles; hymen (sometimes); uterus (sometimes); brain.

SEX OR AGE MOST AFFECTED—Sexually active females of all ages.

SIGNS & SYMPTOMS—Pain in the genital area during sexual activity, including foreplay, intercourse or attempted intercourse. Pain may be mild or severe, and it may vary with different intercourse positions.

CAUSES
Physical causes include:
- Infection of the genitals, including herpes and others involving the vagina, cervix, Fallopian tubes or ovaries.
- Pressure against the vaginal wall caused by scarring from operations or radiation treatment.
- A tight episiotomy scar from vaginal repair after childbirth.
- A fibroid or other uterine tumor.
- Endometriosis.
- A hymen that is torn or thicker than normal.
- A bruised opening to the urethra.
- Inadequate vaginal or condom lubrication.
- Allergic reactions to diaphragms, condoms or contraceptive foams and jellies.
- Dryness and thinness of the vaginal wall after menopause.
- Pelvic inflammatory disease.

Psychological causes include:
- Fear of pregnancy.
- Fear of injury to the unborn child during pregnancy.
- Lack of sexual arousal and vaginal lubrication caused by inadequate sexual foreplay, aversion to a sexual partner, fatigue or anxiety.
- Lack of sexual experience or information.
- Past sexual injury or psychological trauma.
- Temporary lack of desire for sexual partner.

RISK INCREASES WITH
- Stress, recent illness.
- Fatigue or overwork.
- Alcohol consumption.

HOW TO PREVENT
- Obtain medical treatment if you have symptoms of infection of the reproductive organs.
- Discontinue use of contraceptive foams or jellies that produce allergic reactions.
- Obtain professional counseling to resolve feelings about past sexual trauma.
- Discuss the lack of sexual arousal with your partner, including ways to improve foreplay. Enlist your partner's support and patience to overcome the problem. Use a lubricant, if necessary.

WHAT TO EXPECT

DIAGNOSTIC MEASURES
- Your own observation of symptoms.
- Medical history and exam by a doctor.
- Laboratory studies, such as a Pap smear (see Glossary) and culture of any vaginal discharge.

APPROPRIATE HEALTH CARE
- Appropriate treatment will be directed to physical causes or psychological causes.
- Correction of any underlying disease, injury or structural defect.
- Treatment for psychological causes will vary depending on the needs of the patient. It can involve education about contraception, counseling to uncover hidden conflicts, sensate focus exercises and teaching of appropriate foreplay techniques.

POSSIBLE COMPLICATIONS—Damage to personal relationships, permanent inability to enjoy sexual experiences and loss of self-esteem.

PROBABLE OUTCOME—Depends on the cause. Medical disorders are usually curable with treatment. Psychological problems can often be cured with therapy, and interpersonal problems can improve with communication and patience.

HOW TO TREAT

GENERAL MEASURES
- Sitz baths frequently relieve tenderness. Sit in a tub of hot water for 10 to 15 minutes. Repeat baths as often as 3 or 4 times a day.
- Use a nonprescription lubricant, such as baby oil or K-Y Lubricating Jelly, during sexual intercourse.
- Your doctor may provide instructions for exercises or techniques to dilate the vagina.
- Try different positions for sexual intercourse to discover new ones that might reduce penile penetration and be pain-free.

MEDICATION—Your doctor may prescribe antibiotic, antiviral, or antifungal medications for underlying infection.

ACTIVITY—No restrictions.

DIET—No special diet.

CALL YOUR DOCTOR IF

- You have symptoms of dyspareunia.
- Pain worsens, despite treatment.
- Symptoms don't disappear after 3 months of treatment.

DYSPHAGIA

GENERAL INFORMATION

DEFINITION—Difficulty or pain in swallowing. It is a fairly common symptom with a wide variety of causes that can be benign or possibly malignant. Chances of a serious disorder are slight, but if it is a serious disorder, early diagnosis is essential.

BODY PARTS INVOLVED—Pharynx; esophagus.

SEX OR AGE MOST AFFECTED—Both sexes; all ages.

SIGNS & SYMPTOMS
- Pain associated with swallowing.
- The feeling that food "gets stuck" on the way down.
- The swallowing difficulty may progress over several weeks.
- Choking.
- Pressure sensation in mid chest.

CAUSES
- Foreign object lodging at back of throat.
- A scratch in the throat lining caused by a foreign object.
- Insufficient production of saliva.
- Esophageal spasm.
- Tumors (benign or cancer).
- Stricture (narrowing of the passage).
- Inflammation (esophagitis).
- In children, may be caused by malformation, delayed maturation, cerebral palsy, muscular dystrophy.
- Hernia of part of the esophagus through a weak area in the surrounding muscle.
- Nervous system disorder (stroke, myasthenia gravis).
- Outside pressure on the esophagus possibly caused by a goiter or aortic aneurysm.

RISK INCREASES WITH
- Older adults.
- Smoking.
- Some medications.
- Long history of esophageal reflux.

HOW TO PREVENT—No specific preventive measures.

WHAT TO EXPECT

DIAGNOSTIC MEASURES
- Your own observation of symptoms.
- Medical history and physical exam by a doctor.
- Test may include endoscopy, esophageal manometry, barium x-ray examination, CT scan of the chest (see Glossary for all).

APPROPRIATE HEALTH CARE
- Self-care.
- Doctor's treatment.
- Hospitalization may be required for severe disorders.
- Surgery may be needed for some benign or malignant disorders.

POSSIBLE COMPLICATIONS—Complications will depend on underlying disorder (may include aspiration, esophageal "asthma," pneumonia, Barrett's esophagus).

PROBABLE OUTCOME—Outcome will vary depending on the cause.

HOW TO TREAT

GENERAL MEASURES—Specific recommendations will need to be based on the cause of the dysphagia. Some patients may need to learn how to chew food differently or have speech therapy that will teach them swallowing techniques.

MEDICATION—Medication will depend upon the cause. If a drug is causing the problem, your doctor may discontinue it, reduce the dosage or substitute a different drug.

ACTIVITY—Usually no restrictions apply, but will be determined by diagnosis and treatment.

DIET—Can range from normal to total intravenous feeding depending on degree of obstruction.

CALL YOUR DOCTOR IF

- You develop difficulty or pain while swallowing. Do not delay calling as this is a major symptom of what could be a malignant disorder. Early diagnosis is essential.
- New or unexplained symptoms develop. Drugs used in treatment may cause side effects.

ILLNESS & DISORDERS

DYSPLASTIC NEVI

GENERAL INFORMATION

DEFINITION—Nevi are skin lesions that often begin to grow in childhood (occasionally, they are congenital) and have appeared on the skin by early adult life. The most common types are freckles and common moles. Dysplastic nevi are a type that may continue to appear even after age 35. They are more suspect as precursors of melanomas (a serious type of skin cancer). Dysplastic nevus syndrome refers to the presence of multiple dysplastic nevi and melanoma in 2 or more first-degree family members.

BODY PARTS INVOLVED—Skin.

SEX OR AGE MOST AFFECTED—Both sexes; late teens and adults.

SIGNS & SYMPTOMS—Lesions with the following characteristics:
- Borders are irregular and ill-defined.
- Have both flat and elevated areas.
- Measure 5-15mm in diameter (larger than common moles).
- Color ranges from tan to dark brown on a pink background.
- May appear anywhere on the body, but most frequently found on the back, chest, buttocks, breast and scalp. They are found in sun-exposed as well as sun-protected areas.
- Persons with dysplastic nevi may have about 100 lesions (most individuals have up to 15-20 common moles).

CAUSES—May be inherited or appear sporadically. Sunlight damage may play a part in distribution patterns of the nevi, but sun damage is not absolutely necessary, as the nevi appear on buttocks and female breasts, which are usually always covered.

RISK INCREASES WITH
- Family history of dysplastic nevi, melanomas or other skin cancers.
- Persons of northern European background (Celtic) with light colored hair and freckles.

HOW TO PREVENT
- Routine use of sunscreens. Use one with SPF of 15 or higher and that protects against ultraviolet A and ultraviolet B (most sunscreens protect against ultraviolet B only).
- If you have a family history of dysplastic nevi or skin cancer, get regular physical examinations to detect any new lesions or changes in existing ones. These may be as often as every 3 months for high-risk individuals. Also perform routine, self-examinations of your skin (see Skin Self Examination in Appendix) to determine any changes in individual lesions. Have a family member help check the areas of your body that are difficult for you to see.

WHAT TO EXPECT

DIAGNOSTIC MEASURES
- Your own observation of symptoms.
- Medical history and physical exam by a doctor.
- Skin biopsy (see Glossary) of suspicious lesions.

APPROPRIATE HEALTH CARE
- Treatment may involve excision of suspicious lesions (those that have changed grossly), or excision of all lesions (even if there have been no changes in appearance).
- Color photographs may be taken of your body, so that on subsequent office visits, any changes can be verified.

POSSIBLE COMPLICATIONS—Melanoma, a possibly fatal form of skin cancer.

PROBABLE OUTCOME—The prognosis is good for those patients who have early diagnosis and treatment.

HOW TO TREAT

GENERAL MEASURES—Follow your doctor's instructions. Compliance with your medical treatment plan is essential for the best outcome.

MEDICATION—No medication is necessary for this disorder.

ACTIVITY—Be sure to use sunscreens and protective clothing for any exposure to the sun. Avoid sun exposure between 10 a.m. and 3 p.m. if possible.

DIET—No special diet.

CALL YOUR DOCTOR IF

- You have skin lesions (moles) that have changed in appearance.
- New lesions appear after treatment.

DYSTHYMIA
(Low-Grade Depression)

 GENERAL INFORMATION

DEFINITION—A chronic depressive mood (or irritability in children and adolescents) with symptoms that are milder but longer-lasting than a major depressive episode. The onset of dysthymia is often unnoticed and many people are not aware of the change in their lives. Symptoms may begin in childhood or in adolescence and continue over years or decades.

BODY PARTS INVOLVED—Nervous system.

SEX OR AGE MOST AFFECTED—Both sexes; late teens, young to middle-age adults.

SIGNS & SYMPTOMS—Several of the following signs and symptoms have been going on for most of the day, for most days, for two years or more (one year for children or teens) and with no more than two months being symptom free:
- Poor appetite or eating too much.
- Sleep problems (too much or too little).
- Lack of energy; feel tired all the time.
- Preoccupied with failure, inadequacy and negative thoughts (hopelessness).
- Feelings of self-pity; pessimistic attitude.
- Lack of productivity at home and work.
- Trouble with concentration and making decisions.
- Lack of interest or enjoyment in pleasurable activities or social activities.
- Irritability.
- Crying for no reason.
- Over critical or complaining
- Skeptical.

CAUSES—Probably due to a combination of genetic factors, development factors and psychosocial factors (job loss, divorce).

RISK INCREASES WITH
- Family history of depressive illnesses.
- Alcohol dependency or abuse. It may be a contributor to the depression, or depression gives people a reason to start drinking.

HOW TO PREVENT—No specific preventive measures. Anticipate and prepare for major life changes where possible.

 WHAT TO EXPECT

DIAGNOSTIC MEASURES
- Your own observation of symptoms.
- Medical history and physical exam by a doctor.

APPROPRIATE HEALTH CARE
- Doctor's treatment.
- Psychotherapy or counseling (may be combined with antidepressant medications). Several techniques are effective in treating dysthymia such as cognitive-behavior therapy (focuses on changing negative thought patterns into positive ones), interpersonal therapy (focuses on building better relationships) and cultural analysis (deals with the role of society in contributing to low self-esteem and powerless feelings).
- Vocational counseling for some patients to be sure their work suits their temperament.

POSSIBLE COMPLICATIONS
- Chronic course; major depression.
- Alcohol abuse or dependency.

PROBABLE OUTCOME—The majority of people can be helped with treatment. It may take several months before symptoms show improvement. Sometimes, it's not until they are treated and feeling better that people realize how depressed they were.

 HOW TO TREAT

GENERAL MEASURES
- Join a support group. They help many people with the sharing of problems and fostering friendships.
- Avoid alcohol. If you need help with stopping, ask your doctor or contact an Alcoholics Anonymous group in your community.
- Reduce emotional stress in your life (see How to Cope with Stress in Appendix).
- See Resources for Additional Information.

MEDICATION—Your doctor may prescribe antidepressants such as fluoxetine. The medication may be needed for several months or several years. If one medication doesn't work, it's likely that another will.

ACTIVITY—No restrictions. A routine physical exercise program is recommended.

DIET—Eat a nutritionally-balanced diet to help maintain optimum health.

 CALL YOUR DOCTOR IF

- You have symptoms of dysthymia.
- Symptoms worsen or don't improve despite treatment.
- You have thoughts of death or suicide.

EAR INFECTION, MIDDLE (Otitis Media)

GENERAL INFORMATION

DEFINITION—Infection in the middle ear. This is not contagious from person to person, but the preceding respiratory infection causing it may be infectious.

BODY PARTS INVOLVED—Middle-ear space where nerves and small bones connect to the eardrum on one side and the eustachian tube on the other side.

SEX OR AGE MOST AFFECTED—All ages, but most common in infants and children ages 3 months to 5 years.

SIGNS & SYMPTOMS
- Irritability.
- Earache; feeling of fullness in the ear; hearing loss.
- Fever.
- Discharge or leakage from the ear.
- Diarrhea, vomiting (sometimes).
- Pulling at the ear (small children).

CAUSES
- Viral or bacterial infection that spreads to the middle ear by way of the eustachian tube. These are usually upper-respiratory virus infections in the nose or throat.
- Sinus and eustachian-tube blockage caused by nasal allergies or enlarged adenoids.
- A ruptured eardrum.

RISK INCREASES WITH
- Recent illness, such as a respiratory infection, that has lowered resistance.
- Crowded or unsanitary living conditions.
- Genetic factors. Some American Indians, especially the Navajo, seem more susceptible.
- Cold climate.
- Change in altitude, such as flying or driving up mountains.
- Family history of ear infections.
- Day care.
- Smoking in household.

HOW TO PREVENT
- Bottle- or breast-feed an infant in a sitting position with head up, never lying down.
- Breast-feeding decreases chances of child having ear infections.
- No smoking in the household.

WHAT TO EXPECT

DIAGNOSTIC MEASURES
- Your own observation of symptoms.
- Medical history and exam by a doctor.
- Fluid from the ear may be cultured.

APPROPRIATE HEALTH CARE
- Doctor's treatment.
- Home care after diagnosis.

- Surgery to insert plastic tubes through the eardrum to drain pus or fluid from the middle ear (rare).
- If the eardrum is bulging, a small cut, or myringotomy, (see Glossary) may be made in it to relieve pressure and pain.

POSSIBLE COMPLICATIONS
- May recur.
- Chronic otitis media (pus comes from perforation in eardrum).
- Hearing impairment usually temporary, but sometimes permanent leading to delay of normal language development in children.
- Enlarged adenoids in children from repeated middle-ear infections, causing chronic middle-ear infections.
- Rarely, mastoiditis (infection of the mastoid, the bony area just behind the ear).
- Meningitis (rare).

PROBABLE OUTCOME—Symptoms usually improve in 2 to 3 days.

HOW TO TREAT

GENERAL MEASURES
- Apply heat to the area around the ears to relieve pain.
- Swimming should be avoided until infection clears.

MEDICATION
- Use ear drops to relieve pain. You may use nonprescription drops or those prescribed for a previous infection. They will not cure the infection.
- Use nonprescription drugs, such as acetaminophen, to reduce pain and fever.
- Your doctor may prescribe antibiotics if the infection appears to be bacterial rather than viral. Finish the medication. The infection may remain active for several days after symptoms disappear.

ACTIVITY—Rest in bed or reduce activity until fever and pain subside.

DIET—No special diet.

CALL YOUR DOCTOR IF

- You or your child have symptoms of a middle-ear infection.
- The following occurs during treatment:
  Fever.
  Severe headache.
  Earache that persists longer than 2 days, despite treatment.
  Swelling around the ear.
  Convulsions.
  Twitching of the face muscles.
  Dizziness.

EAR INFECTION, OUTER
(Otitis Externa; Swimmer's Ear)

GENERAL INFORMATION

DEFINITION—Inflammation or infection of the ear canal that extends from the eardrum to the outside.

BODY PARTS INVOLVED—Skin of the ear canal.

SEX OR AGE MOST AFFECTED—Both sexes; all ages.

SIGNS & SYMPTOMS
- Ear pain that worsens when the earlobe is pulled.
- Slight fever (sometimes).
- Discharge of pus from the ear.
- Itching in the ear.
- Temporary loss of hearing on the affected side.

CAUSES
- Bacterial or fungal infection of the delicate skin lining of the ear canal.
- Injury to the ear canal.

RISK INCREASES WITH
- Swimming in dirty, polluted water.
- Excessive swimming in chlorinated pools. Chlorinated water dries out the ear canal, allowing bacteria or fungi to enter the skin.
- Excess moisture from any cause.
- Irritation from swabs; metal objects, such as bobby pins; or ear plugs, especially if they are left in a long time.
- Inadequate production of protective ear wax (cerumen).
- Previous ear infections.
- Skin allergies.
- Diabetes mellitus or other disorders that predispose to infection.
- Use of hair spray or hair dye that may enter the ear canal.

HOW TO PREVENT
- Don't clean your ears with any object or chemical.
- After you have had otitis externa, keep the prescription ear drops on hand. If the ear canals get wet for any reason, such as swimming or shampooing, put drops in both ears at bedtime.

WHAT TO EXPECT

DIAGNOSTIC MEASURES
- Your own observation of symptoms.
- Medical history and physical exam by a doctor.
- Laboratory culture of ear fluid (sometimes).

APPROPRIATE HEALTH CARE
- Self-care after diagnosis.
- Doctor's treatment. Severe cases may require treatment by an ear, nose and throat specialist.

POSSIBLE COMPLICATIONS
- Severe pain.
- Chronic inflammation that is difficult to cure.
- A boil in the ear canal.
- Cellulitis (deep-tissue infection).

PROBABLE OUTCOME—Usually curable with treatment in 7 to 10 days.

HOW TO TREAT

GENERAL MEASURES
- Warm compress over the ear may help relieve the pain.
- Keep the infected ear dry. Wear ear plugs or shower cap for showering.

MEDICATION
- You may use nonprescription drugs, such as acetaminophen or aspirin, for minor pain.
- Your doctor may prescribe:
  Ear drops that contain antibiotics and cortisone drugs to control inflammation and fight infection.
  Topical creams or ointments for fungal or bacterial infections.
  Oral antibiotics for severe infection.

ACTIVITY—Resume your normal activities as soon as symptoms improve. Avoid getting water in the ears for 3 weeks after all symptoms disappear. Any moisture—even from showering or washing hair—can trigger a recurrence.

DIET—No special diet.

CALL YOUR DOCTOR IF

- You have symptoms of otitis externa.
- The following occurs during treatment:
  Pain persists, despite treatment.
  You feel your ears need cleaning. Remember that a small amount of ear wax helps protect against infection.

EARDRUM, RUPTURED
(Tympanic Membrane Perforation)

 GENERAL INFORMATION

DEFINITION—A perforation of the thin membrane (tympanic membrane) that separates the inner ear from the outer ear.

BODY PARTS INVOLVED—Eardrum (tympanic membrane); middle ear.

SEX OR AGE MOST AFFECTED—Both sexes; all ages.

SIGNS & SYMPTOMS
- Sudden pain in the ear.
- Partial hearing loss.
- Bleeding or discharge from the ear. The discharge may resemble pus within 24 to 48 hours after rupture.
- Ringing in the ear.
- Dizziness.

CAUSES
- Perforation of the eardrum when a sharp object is inserted in the ear, such as: a cotton swab to clean the ear or relieve an itch; an unseen twig on a tree; hot slag from an industrial site.
- Sudden inward pressure in the ear, such as with: a slap; a swimming or diving accident; a nearby explosion.
- Sudden outward pressure or suction, such as with a kiss over the ear.
- Severe middle-ear infection.

RISK INCREASES WITH
- Recent middle-ear infection.
- Head injury.

HOW TO PREVENT
- Don't put any object into the ear canal.
- Avoid injuries that may cause a rupture (see Causes).
- Obtain prompt medical treatment for middle-ear infections.

 WHAT TO EXPECT

DIAGNOSTIC MEASURES
- Your own observation of symptoms.
- Medical history and physical exam by a doctor. When the eardrum ruptures, contents of the middle ear (primarily bones) can be seen with a special instrument called an otoscope. A healthy eardrum is almost transparent.
- Culture of the fluid from the ear (sometimes).

APPROPRIATE HEALTH CARE
- Self-care. Treatment involves medication to prevent infection and supportive care for pain.
- Doctor's treatment.
- Microsurgery to repair the perforation (rare).

POSSIBLE COMPLICATIONS
- Ear infection.
- Meningitis; mastoiditis.
- Significant blood loss (rare).
- Some permanent hearing loss (rare).

PROBABLE OUTCOME
- The eardrum will usually repair itself in a week or two (but may take up to 2 months) and normal hearing is restored. If it becomes infected, the infection is curable with treatment.
- If the perforation does not heal, minor surgery is needed.

 HOW TO TREAT

GENERAL MEASURES
- Don't blow your nose, if possible. If you must, blow gently.
- Don't use cotton swabs except to clean the out ear.
- Keep the ear canal dry. Don't swim, take showers or get caught in the rain. Insert a wisp of cotton in the ear canal to keep moisture out of it when bathing.

MEDICATION—Your doctor may prescribe:
- Antibiotics to prevent or treat infections.
- Pain relievers. For minor pain, you may use nonprescription drugs such as acetaminophen.

ACTIVITY—Resume your normal activities as soon as symptoms improve.

DIET—No special diet.

 CALL YOUR DOCTOR IF

- You have symptoms of a ruptured eardrum, especially a pus-like discharge.
- The following occurs during treatment:
  Fever.
  Pain that persists, despite treatment.
  Dizziness that continues longer than 12 to 24 hours.
- New, unexplained symptoms develop. Drugs used in treatment may produce side effects.

EARWAX BLOCKAGE
(Cerumen Impaction)

 GENERAL INFORMATION

DEFINITION—Overproduction of earwax (cerumen), causing blockage of the external ear canal. Wax is produced by the ear to protect the canal leading from the eardrum to the outside. The amount of wax produced varies from person to person. Some produce so little wax that it never accumulates. Others produce enough to block the canal every few months.

BODY PARTS INVOLVED—External ear canal on one or both sides.

SEX OR AGE MOST AFFECTED—Both sexes; all ages.

SIGNS & SYMPTOMS
- Decreased hearing.
- Ear pain.
- Plugged feeling in the ear.
- Ringing in the ear.

CAUSES—Overproduction of wax by glands in the external-ear canal.

RISK INCREASES WITH
- Exposure to dust or debris.
- Family history of overproduction of earwax.
- Water in the ear can cause the wax to swell.
- Use of cotton swabs in an attempt to clean the ear canal.

HOW TO PREVENT
- Avoid areas where the air is dusty or filled with debris. This stimulates overproduction of earwax. Consider wearing earplugs if you must be in this type of environment.
- Monthly use of 1-2 drops of glycerin in the ear may soften the wax and prevent recurrent blockage.

 WHAT TO EXPECT

DIAGNOSTIC MEASURES
- Your own observation of symptoms.
- Medical history and physical exam by a doctor.

APPROPRIATE HEALTH CARE
- Self-care. Sometimes wax can be removed easily at home with ear drops and irrigation of the ear canal.
- Doctor's treatment if the wax is difficult to remove.

POSSIBLE COMPLICATIONS
- Ear infection.
- Eardrum damage.

PROBABLE OUTCOME—Earwax can be removed, but stubborn cases require patience.

 HOW TO TREAT

GENERAL MEASURES—To remove earwax at home:
- Buy nonprescription wax-softening ear drops.
- Lie down with the affected ear toward the ceiling.
- Pull the top of the ear gently up and back toward the back of the head.
- Instill the ear drops; use the amount given in the package directions.
- Leave the drops in the ear for 20 minutes. Continue to lie down, if possible. Plug the ear with cotton.
- Sit up, leaning a little toward the affected side.
- Use a soft rubber bulb syringe to irrigate the ear canal gently with plain warm water or equal parts warm water and hydrogen peroxide.
- Repeat irrigations until the ear feels clear. If the ear doesn't clear, consult your doctor.
- Don't try to remove wax with a stick or cotton swab. You may damage the eardrum or cause infection in the ear canal. Caution—if you have a perforated eardrum, don't try to remove wax, see your doctor.

MEDICATION—For minor pain, you may use nonprescription drugs such as acetaminophen.

ACTIVITY—No restrictions.

DIET—No special diet.

 CALL YOUR DOCTOR IF

- You have symptoms of an earwax blockage that does not clear, despite treatment.
- A child younger than 4 has an earwax blockage.
- Fever and ear pain accompany an earwax blockage. Do not irrigate the ear in this case.

ILLNESS & DISORDERS

ECTOPIC PREGNANCY

 GENERAL INFORMATION

DEFINITION—A pregnancy that develops outside the uterus. The most common site is in one of the narrow tubes that connect each ovary to the uterus (Fallopian tube). Other sites include the ovary or outside the reproductive organs in the abdominal cavity or the cervix. About 1 in 100 pregnancies is ectopic.

BODY PARTS INVOLVED—Female reproductive system; abdominal cavity.

SEX OR AGE MOST AFFECTED—Females of childbearing age.

SIGNS & SYMPTOMS
Early stages:
• Missed menstrual period or a heavy, painful period.
• Unexplained vaginal spotting or bleeding.
• Lower abdominal pain and cramps.
• Pain in the shoulder (rare).
Late stages:
• Sudden, sharp, severe abdominal pain caused by rupture of the Fallopian tube.
• Dizziness, fainting and shock (paleness, rapid heartbeat, drop in blood pressure and cold sweats). These may precede or accompany pain (sometimes).

CAUSES—An egg from the ovary is fertilized and becomes implanted outside the uterus—usually in the Fallopian tube. As the fertilized egg enlarges, the Fallopian tube stretches and ruptures, causing life-threatening internal bleeding.

RISK INCREASES WITH
• Use of an intrauterine device (IUD) for contraception.
• Previous pelvic infections.
• Adhesions (bands of scar tissue) from previous abdominal surgery.
• Previous tubal pregnancy.
• Previous tubal or uterine surgery.
• History of endometritis.

HOW TO PREVENT
• Use a contraceptive method other than IUD.
• Obtain prompt treatment for pelvic infection.

 WHAT TO EXPECT

DIAGNOSTIC MEASURES
• Your own observation of symptoms.
• Medical history and exam by a doctor.
• Laboratory studies, such as a pregnancy test and blood count.
• Surgical diagnostic procedures, such as laparoscopy and culdocentesis, D & C (dilatation and curettage) and exploratory laparotomy (see Glossary for all).
• Ultrasound to outline the fetus (see Glossary).

APPROPRIATE HEALTH CARE
• Doctor's treatment.
• Surgery to remove the developing fetus, the placenta and any damaged tissue. If the Fallopian tube cannot be repaired, it is removed. Future normal pregnancy is possible with one Fallopian tube.

POSSIBLE COMPLICATIONS
• Infection.
• Diminished fertility.
• Loss of reproductive organs after complicated surgery.
• Shock and death from internal bleeding.

PROBABLE OUTCOME—An ectopic pregnancy cannot progress to full term or produce a viable fetus. Rupture of an ectopic pregnancy is an emergency requiring immediate hospitalization and surgery. Full recovery is likely with early diagnosis and surgery. Subsequent pregnancies are usually normal.

 HOW TO TREAT

GENERAL MEASURES—After surgery:
• You may wash normally over the stitches in your incision.
• Use heat to relieve pain. Apply a heating pad or hot-water bottle to the abdomen or back. Hot baths also relieve discomfort and relax muscles. Sit in a tub of hot water for 10 to 15 minutes. Repeat as often as needed.

MEDICATION—Medicine usually is not necessary for this disorder.

ACTIVITY—Resume your normal activities, including sexual relations, as soon as possible. Frequent, satisfying sexual activity helps you feel closer to your mate and promotes healing.
   Attempt sexual intercourse soon, but provide adequate lubrication. Spend extra time touching, conversing intimately and caressing. During early encounters, the woman must decide how much penile penetration and vigorous thrusting is comfortable.

DIET—No special diet.

 CALL YOUR DOCTOR IF

• You have symptoms of ectopic pregnancy, especially a rupture. Call immediately. This is an emergency!
• The following occurs after surgery:
  Excessive vaginal bleeding (soaking a pad or tampon every hour).
  Signs of infection, such as fever, chills, headache, dizziness or muscle aches.
  Increased urinary frequency that lasts longer than 1 month. This may be a sign of bladder irritation or infection resulting from surgery.

ECZEMA
(Infantile Eczema; Neurodermatitis)

 GENERAL INFORMATION

DEFINITION—A chronic allergic skin disorder.

BODY PARTS INVOLVED—Skin, especially of the hands, scalp, face, back of the neck or skin creases of elbows and knees.
- Atopic eczema occurs in people who have a tendency toward allergy and is common in babies.
- Nummular eczema occurs in adults and the cause is unknown.
- Hand eczema usually results from irritation by a substance.

SEX OR AGE MOST AFFECTED—May begin between 1 month and 1 year. It usually subsides somewhat by age 3, but it may flare again at any age.

SIGNS & SYMPTOMS—Skin affected by eczema has the following characteristics:
- Itching (sometimes severe).
- Small blisters with oozing.
- Thickening and scaling from chronic inflammation.

CAUSES
- Often occurs for no known reason.
An allergic reaction to a wide variety of things, including:
- Foods, such as eggs, wheat, milk or seafood.
- Wool clothing.
- Skin lotions and ointments.
- Soaps, detergents, cleansers.
- Plants, tanning agents used for shoe leather, dyes, topical medications.

RISK INCREASES WITH
- Stress.
- Medical history of other allergic conditions, such as hay fever, asthma or sensitivity to certain drugs.
- Clothing made of synthetic fabric, which traps perspiration.
- Weather extremes, including humidity, severe cold and severe heat (especially with increased sweating).

HOW TO PREVENT
- Avoiding risk factors.
- Wearing cotton-lined rubber gloves for household tasks.

 WHAT TO EXPECT

DIAGNOSTIC MEASURES
- Your own observation of symptoms.
- Medical history and exam by a doctor.
- Laboratory studies, such as blood and skin tests to identify allergies.

APPROPRIATE HEALTH CARE
- Home care.
- Doctor's treatment.

POSSIBLE COMPLICATIONS—Bacterial infections caused by injury to the skin.

PROBABLE OUTCOME—Variable. Some children outgrow eczema. Others are resistant to treatment, and eczema may persist through puberty. However, symptoms can usually be controlled with treatment.
  Skin irritation from any other cause can trigger a flare-up or aggravate existing eczema.

 HOW TO TREAT

GENERAL MEASURES
- Wear loose, cotton clothing to help absorb perspiration.
- Minimize stress whenever possible.
- Keep fingernails short and put soft gloves on at night to minimize scratching. Scratching worsens eczema.
- Bathe less frequently to avoid excessive skin dryness. Soap and water may trigger flare-ups. When bathing, use special nonfat soaps and tepid water. Use no soap on inflamed areas.
- Lubricate the skin after bathing.
- Avoid extreme temperature changes.
- Avoid anything that has previously worsened the condition.

MEDICATION—Your doctor may prescribe:
- Ointments containing coal tar or cortisone drugs to decrease inflammation. These may help more if used at night under occlusive plastic wrap. Ask your doctor.
- Antihistamines to decrease itching.
- Antibiotics for complicating infections, if they occur.
- Sedatives or tranquilizers (rarely).

ACTIVITY—No restrictions. Sometimes being exposed to sunlight helps heal the rash. Take care not to get burned.

DIET—No special diet. Eliminate any foods known to cause flare-ups of eczema.

 CALL YOUR DOCTOR IF

- You have symptoms of eczema that don't clear up with self-care.
- New, unexplained symptoms develop. Drugs used in treatment may produce side effects.

ELECTRIC SHOCK

GENERAL INFORMATION

DEFINITION—Injury caused by electricity passing through the body.

BODY PARTS INVOLVED—Total body.

SEX OR AGE MOST AFFECTED—Both sexes; all ages.

SIGNS & SYMPTOMS—Depends on where the current enters the body and the kind of electrical current. Following are the most common:
- Burns at areas of contact. The burns are often deep.
- Heart damage, including cardiac arrest.
- Severe muscle spasms that may cause fractures.
- Breathing paralysis.

CAUSES—Contact with electricity from downed power lines, exposed appliance wires, faulty electrical equipment, lightning strikes or other electrical sources.

RISK INCREASES WITH
- Standing on wet ground or under a tree during an electrical storm.
- Mishandling of electrical equipment.
- Occupations that involve electrical machinery or lines.

HOW TO PREVENT
- Inspect your house, especially the kitchen, bathroom and workshop, for hazards. Use grounded plugs wherever possible.
- Don't use hair dryers or radios in the bathroom where they can fall into a tub or sink.
- Use safety plugs in empty electrical outlets to prevent children from inserting metal objects.
- Don't try to repair electrical equipment unless you know how.
- Wear protective gloves and clothing for work that involves exposure to electricity.
- Replace worn cords or wiring at home or work.
- Use ground fault electrical interrupters when possible.
- Go indoors during electrical storms. Lightning may strike several miles away from actual rainfall.

WHAT TO EXPECT

DIAGNOSTIC MEASURES—Diagnosis is usually obvious from the circumstances.

APPROPRIATE HEALTH CARE
- Self-care after diagnosis (minor burns only).
- Emergency cardiopulmonary resuscitation (CPR) at the time of injury, if the victim is unconscious and not breathing.
- Doctor's treatment.
- Hospitalization for moderate to severe injuries.

POSSIBLE COMPLICATIONS
- Pneumonia.
- Permanent brain damage.
- Severe burns of the skin and underlying muscle.
- Death from heart damage.

PROBABLE OUTCOME—Depends on the extent of injury. Full recovery is likely if major brain or heart damage does not occur.

HOW TO TREAT

GENERAL MEASURES
- If the victim is touching live electrical wires, shut off the power or remove the wires with a nonmetal object before giving aid. Don't electrocute yourself trying to help someone else.
- If the victim is unconscious and not breathing:
  Yell for help. Don't leave the victim.
  Call O (operator) or 911 (emergency) for an ambulance or medical help. Begin mouth-to-mouth breathing immediately.
  If there is no heartbeat, give external cardiac massage.
  Don't stop cardiopulmonary resuscitation (CPR) until help arrives.
- If multiple persons are struck, give CPR first to victims who are not moving (those moving are likely to recover).

MEDICATION—Medicine usually is not necessary for electric shock.

ACTIVITY—No restrictions, if the shock is mild. If the shock is severe, the victim may resume activities gradually as injuries heal.

DIET—No special diet following electric shock.

CALL YOUR DOCTOR IF

- You or someone around you receives an electric shock severe enough to cause injury.
- The following occurs during convalescence:
  Irregular heartbeat.
  Fever.
  Cough with sputum.

ENCEPHALITIS, VIRAL

GENERAL INFORMATION

DEFINITION—An acute inflammation involving the brain caused by a viral infection. The viral infection may cause encephalitis as a primary disorder or as a secondary complication following viral disorders such as measles, chickenpox, rubella, vaccinia and other less known viruses or a smallpox vaccination.

BODY PARTS INVOLVED—Brain; sometimes meninges (membranes that cover the brain).

SEX OR AGE MOST AFFECTED—Both sexes; all ages.

SIGNS & SYMPTOMS
Mild cases:
- No symptoms (sometimes).
- Fever.
- General ill feeling.

Severe cases:
- Vomiting.
- Headache.
- Stiff neck.
- Pupils of different size.
- Unconsciousness.
- Personality changes.
- Seizures.
- Occasional weakness or paralysis of an arm or leg.
- Double vision.
- Speech impairment.
- Hearing loss.
- Drowsiness that progresses to coma.

CAUSES
- Viruses that cause other illnesses, including: polio; herpes; measles; mumps; chickenpox; infectious mononucleosis; infectious hepatitis; German measles; smallpox; Coxsackie virus; echovirus diseases; and Eastern & Western equine virus.
- Viruses carried by mosquitoes or other insects.
- Lead poisoning.
- Vaccine reactions.
- Leukemia.

RISK INCREASES WITH
- Newborns and infants.
- Adults over 60.
- Illness that has lowered resistance.
- Crowded or unsanitary living conditions.
- HIV or AIDS.

HOW TO PREVENT
- Avoid contact with anyone who has encephalitis.
- Consult your doctor for treatment of any infection in your body—especially those mentioned as causes—to attempt to prevent the spread of infection.
- Use insect repellent and mosquito netting if you travel to an area of risk.

WHAT TO EXPECT

DIAGNOSTIC MEASURES
- Your own observation of symptoms.
- Medical history and physical exam by a doctor.
- Laboratory studies of blood and cerebrospinal fluid, skull x-ray, electroencephalography (studying the brain by measuring electric activity ["brain waves"]).

APPROPRIATE HEALTH CARE
- Doctor's treatment.
- Hospitalization, care in an intensive care unit (worst cases only).
- Self-care after diagnosis or hospitalization.

POSSIBLE COMPLICATIONS—A very small percentage of patients suffer permanent brain damage that impairs mental or muscle functions.

PROBABLE OUTCOME—Mild viral encephalitis is common and may go unnoticed. Severe cases usually require hospitalization.

Complications and fatalities from encephalitis are most common in infants and the elderly. People in other age groups usually recover completely. Unless the attack is severe, you can expect full recovery within 2 to 3 weeks.

HOW TO TREAT

GENERAL MEASURES
- Susceptible individuals should avoid contact with the patient.
- The illness can be frightening, both to the patient and to the family. Most hospitals have social workers who are there for your support.

MEDICATION—Your doctor may prescribe:
- Acetaminophen for headache and fever.
- Antiviral drugs, such as acyclovir or amantadine.
- Cortisone drugs to suppress inflammation (rare).
- Drugs to control seizures if needed.

ACTIVITY—You will need bed rest in a darkened room. After a 2- to 3-week recovery, you should be as active as your strength and feeling of well-being allow.

DIET—No special diet.

CALL YOUR DOCTOR IF

- You have any symptoms of encephalitis.
- Fever.
- New, unexplained symptoms develop. Drugs used in treatment may produce side effects.

ENCOPRESIS

GENERAL INFORMATION

DEFINITION—Lack of bowel control in a child who has previously been toilet-trained and does not have diarrhea or constipation. A child cannot be expected to have complete bowel control until at least 2-1/2 years of age.

BODY PARTS INVOLVED—Bowels.

SEX OR AGE MOST AFFECTED—Both sexes of children over age 2-1/2.

SIGNS & SYMPTOMS
• Bowel movements in underwear.
• Mass in left lower abdomen (sometimes).

CAUSES
• Physical or emotional crisis in the child's life, such as birth of a sibling or recent illness with diarrhea.
• Resistance to using the toilet because of too much pressure to do so.
• If the problem is long-term, the original cause may be forgotten and the behavior may persist as a habit.
• Less frequently, might be due to impairment in the child's nervous system.
• Painful bowel movements.
• Resistance to using toilet facilities at school, on camping trips, or outdoor toilets.
• Dietary problems that cause constipation.

RISK INCREASES WITH
• Stress.
• Recent illness that brought the child increased attention.
• Child abuse.

HOW TO PREVENT
• Don't lavish attention on a child for being ill.
• Avoid undue emphasis on toilet-training. Approach it calmly with realistic expectations. Don't shame or blame the child for accidents.
• Be sensitive to stressful situations your child faces. Talk together about the child's feelings.
• Protect your child against physical and sexual abuse.
• Maintain good diet and nutrition for your child.

WHAT TO EXPECT

DIAGNOSTIC MEASURES
• Your own observation of symptoms.
• Medical history and physical exam by a doctor, if necessary.

APPROPRIATE HEALTH CARE
• Home care.
• Doctor's treatment, if home care fails.
• Psychotherapy or counseling (sometimes).

POSSIBLE COMPLICATIONS
• Anal fissure.
• Skin rash in rectal area.
• Stool impaction.

PROBABLE OUTCOME—Usually curable, unless there is a serious underlying physical problem.

HOW TO TREAT

GENERAL MEASURES
• Let your child decide when it is time to go to the bathroom. Don't remind him or make him sit on the toilet against his will. This fosters a negative attitude.
• Praise your child for having bowel movements in the toilet—he deserves positive reinforcement for success. Other family members may also praise the child.
• Provide a prearranged reward if the child stays clean all day. The favorite reward of many children is 30 minutes of free time with either parent, doing whatever the child chooses. Incentives build motivation to succeed.
• Respond gently to accidents. When the child is soiled, he should clean himself and change into clean underwear. For younger children (under age 5), the parent will probably have to do this.
• Don't blame, criticize, restrict or punish the child for accidents. This may cause him to give up, as well as lead to secondary emotional problems.
• Don't allow siblings or others to tease the child.
• Never put the child back in diapers.
• Ask for the school's cooperation. The child needs quick access to the bathroom at school, especially if he is shy or new at school. Remind him that there should be nothing embarrassing about leaving the classroom to go to the bathroom.

MEDICATION
• Stool softeners and bulk producers may be helpful.
• Enemas or suppositories may be necessary if there is an impaction. Ask your doctor before giving any to your child.

ACTIVITY—No restrictions.

DIET
• Avoid excessive milk, bananas, apples and gelatin.
• Increase fiber in the child's diet.

CALL YOUR DOCTOR IF

Your child has encopresis and it persists longer than 2 months, despite your efforts.

ENDOCARDITIS
(Bacterial Endocarditis; Infective Endocarditis)

 GENERAL INFORMATION

DEFINITION—A noncontagious infection of the valves or lining of the heart.

BODY PARTS INVOLVED—Heart muscle; heart valves; endocardium (lining of the heart chambers and valves).

SEX OR AGE MOST AFFECTED—Both sexes; all ages.

SIGNS & SYMPTOMS
Early symptoms:
- Fatigue and weakness.
- Intermittent fever, chills and excessive sweating, especially at night.
- Weight loss.
- Vague aches and pains.
- Heart murmur.

Late symptoms:
- Severe chills and high fever.
- Shortness of breath on exertion.
- Swelling of the feet, legs and abdomen.
- Rapid or irregular heartbeat.

CAUSES—Bacteria or fungi that enter the blood and infect the valves and heart lining of persons with damaged hearts (see risks below). Bacteria or fungi further damage the heart valves, muscles and linings.

RISK INCREASES WITH
Risk of heart-valve damage increases with:
- Rheumatic fever.
- Congenital heart disease.

Risk of endocarditis following heart-valve damage increases with:
- Pregnancy.
- Injections of contaminated materials into the bloodstream, such as with self-administered intravenous drugs.
- Use of immunosuppressive drugs.
- Artificial heart valves.

HOW TO PREVENT—If you have heart-valve damage or a heart murmur:
- Request antibiotics prior to medical procedures that may introduce bacteria into the blood. These include dental work, childbirth and surgery of the urinary or gastrointestinal tract.
- Consult your doctor before becoming pregnant.
- Don't use illicit drugs like heroin or cocaine.

 WHAT TO EXPECT

DIAGNOSTIC MEASURES
- Medical history and physical exam by a doctor.
- Your own observation of symptoms.
- Laboratory blood counts and blood cultures.

- ECG (see Glossary).
- X-rays of the heart and lungs, including echocardiogram (see Glossary).

APPROPRIATE HEALTH CARE
- Doctor's treatment.
- Hospitalization.
- Self-care after the acute illness.
- Surgery to replace infected valve in some patients.

POSSIBLE COMPLICATIONS
- Blood clots that may travel to the brain, kidneys or abdominal organs, causing infections, abscesses or stroke.
- Heart-rhythm disturbances (atrial fibrillation is most common).

PROBABLE OUTCOME—Usually curable with early diagnosis and treatment, but recovery may take weeks. If treatment is delayed, heart function deteriorates, resulting in congestive heart failure and possible death.

 HOW TO TREAT

GENERAL MEASURES
- If you have damaged heart valves, tell any doctor or dentist who treats you.
- Once you have had endocarditis, stay under a doctor's care to prevent a relapse.
- Ongoing dental hygiene is important to prevent infection.
- Wear a medical alert type bracelet or neck tag that indicates your medical problem. Carry a wallet card listing the antibiotic regimens needed for medical and dental procedures.

MEDICATION—Your doctor may prescribe antibiotics for many weeks to fight infection. Antibiotic treatment is often intravenous.

ACTIVITY—Rest in bed until you are fully recovered. While in bed, flex your legs often to prevent clots from forming in deep veins. Resume your normal activities, including sexual relations, when strength allows.

DIET—No special diet.

 CALL YOUR DOCTOR IF

- You have symptoms of endocarditis.
- The following occurs during or after treatment:
  Weight gain without diet changes.
  Blood in the urine.
  Chest pain.
  Sudden weakness or numbness in muscles of the face, trunk or limbs.

ILLNESS & DISORDERS

ENDOMETRIAL HYPERPLASIA
(Adenomatous Hyperplasia of the Uterus)

 GENERAL INFORMATION

DEFINITION—An overgrowth of tissue in the endometrium (inner lining of the uterus). This is not cancerous.

BODY PARTS INVOLVED—Endometrium.

SEX OR AGE MOST AFFECTED—Women over age 35.

SIGNS & SYMPTOMS
- Bleeding between normal menstrual periods.
- Heavy menstrual flow (saturating a tampon or pad once every hour).
- Bleeding after menopause.
- Vaginal discharge.

CAUSES—Excessive estrogen, a female hormone. This is caused internally or from the use of hormone-containing medications. Endometrial hyperplasia rarely occurs in women who have a normal menstrual cycle.

RISK INCREASES WITH
- Use of oral contraceptives or estrogen replacement therapy after menopause.
- Obesity in post menopausal women.
- Late menopause (over age 55).

HOW TO PREVENT—No specific preventive measures.

 WHAT TO EXPECT

DIAGNOSTIC MEASURES
- Your own observation of symptoms.
- Medical history and physical exam by a doctor.
- Laboratory tests, such as blood tests of hormone levels and Pap smear (see Glossary).

APPROPRIATE HEALTH CARE
- Doctor's treatment.
- D & C (see Dilatation and Curettage of the Uterus in Surgery section) to obtain tissue for microscopic examination to rule out malignancy.
- Hysterectomy (see in Surgery section) sometimes.

POSSIBLE COMPLICATIONS
- Perforation of the uterus and peritonitis as a complication of surgery (rare).
- Excessive, uncontrollable bleeding.

PROBABLE OUTCOME—Often curable with D & C or hysterectomy. If a woman chooses not to have surgery, hormone therapy usually controls symptoms. In most cases, hormonal treatment with a progesterone will reverse the hyperplasia caused by the excess estrogen.

 HOW TO TREAT

GENERAL MEASURES
- Try to reduce psychological stress that can complicate your illness and delay your recovery. If you can't resolve the stress, ask for help from family, friends or competent counselors.
- Use heat to relieve pain. Place a heating pad or hot-water bottle on your abdomen or back.
- Take frequent hot baths to relax muscles and relieve discomfort. Sit in a tub of hot water for 10 to 15 minutes.
- Don't douche unless your doctor recommends it.
- For an explanation of surgery and postoperative care, see Hysterectomy in Surgery section.

MEDICATION
- If the D & C does not relieve symptoms and you don't want a hysterectomy (or you are a poor surgical risk), you will probably be prescribed progesterone, a female hormone.
- Avoid aspirin; it may increase bleeding.

ACTIVITY—No restrictions unless you have surgery. Then resume your activities gradually. Ask your doctor about resuming sexual relations following surgery or D & C. Don't hesitate to discuss this—it is an important part of your life.

DIET—No special diet.

 CALL YOUR DOCTOR IF

- You have symptoms of endometrial hyperplasia.
- The following symptoms occur during hormone treatment or after surgery or D & C:
  Excessive bleeding (saturating more than 1 pad or tampon every hour).
  Signs of infection, such as fever, general ill feeling, headache, dizziness or muscle aches.
- New, unexplained symptoms develop. Hormones used in treatment may produce side effects

ENDOMETRIOSIS

GENERAL INFORMATION

DEFINITION—A disorder in which tissue resembling the inner lining of the uterus (endometrium) appears at unusual locations in the lower abdomen. This tissue may be found: on the ovary surfaces; behind the uterus, low in the pelvic cavity; on the intestinal wall; and rarely, at other sites far away.

BODY PARTS INVOLVED—Uterus; ovaries; Fallopian tubes; outer layer of the intestines.

SEX OR AGE MOST AFFECTED—Females between puberty and menopause, but most common between ages 20 and 30.

SIGNS & SYMPTOMS—The following symptoms may begin abruptly or develop over many years:
- Increased pelvic pain during menstrual periods, especially the last days.
- Pain with sexual intercourse.
- Blood in the urine; premenstrual spotting.
- Back pain.
- Pain with intestinal contractions.
- Blood in the stool (sometimes).

CAUSES—Unknown, but the following theory is most accepted among doctors:

Normally during ovulation, the uterus lining thickens to prepare for implantation of a fertilized egg. If this does not occur, the lining tissue peels away from the uterus and is expelled in the menstrual flow. In some cases, this material builds up and passes backward out of the Fallopian tubes into the pelvic cavity. Here it floats freely and attaches itself to other tissues.

The transplanted tissue reacts each month as if it were still in the uterus, thickening and peeling away. New bits of peeled-off tissue create new implants. The growing endometrial tissue between pelvic organs may cause them to adhere together, producing pain and other symptoms.

RISK INCREASES WITH
- Adult women who don't become pregnant.
- Family history of endometriosis.

HOW TO PREVENT—Having children while you are young. Pregnancy permanently cures some people with endometriosis.

WHAT TO EXPECT

DIAGNOSTIC MEASURES
- Your own observation of symptoms.
- Medical history and exam by a doctor.
- Laboratory blood studies.
- Surgical diagnostic procedures, such as laparoscopy (see Glossary).
- X-rays of the lower intestines (barium enema).

APPROPRIATE HEALTH CARE
- Self-care after diagnosis.
- Doctor's treatment. Diagnosing the disorder may be difficult, requiring repeated examinations or surgical diagnostic procedures.
- Surgery to remove implants, or a hysterectomy (see in Surgery section) to remove the uterus, Fallopian tubes and ovaries in women who don't want to become pregnant.

POSSIBLE COMPLICATIONS
- Sterility from tissue implants that constrict the Fallopian tubes.
- Disabling, but never life-threatening, pain.
- Adhesions of pelvic organs.
- Bowel or bladder problems.

PROBABLE OUTCOME—Without treatment, endometriosis becomes increasingly severe. It subsides after menopause when estrogen production decreases.

Symptoms can be relieved with medication, and it is sometimes curable with surgery.

HOW TO TREAT

GENERAL MEASURES
- If you want children, consider pregnancy as soon as possible. Pregnancy often cures the disorder. Delaying pregnancy may cause infertility.
- Use sanitary napkins instead of tampons. Tampons may make backward menstrual flow more likely.
- Use heat to relieve pain. Place a heating pad or hot-water bottle on your abdomen or back, or take hot baths to relax muscles and relieve discomfort.
- See Resources for Additional Information.

MEDICATION
- You may use nonprescription drugs, such as acetaminophen, to relieve minor pain.
- Your doctor may prescribe: danazol, gonadotropin-releasing hormones, oral contraceptives or progestogens that are commonly used drugs for treating endometriosis by suppressing ovarian function.

ACTIVITY—No restrictions.

DIET—No special diet.

CALL YOUR DOCTOR IF

- You have symptoms of endometriosis.
- The following occurs during treatment:
  Intolerable pain.
  Unusual or excessive vaginal bleeding.
- New, unexplained symptoms develop. Drugs used in treatment may produce side effects.
- Symptoms recur after treatment.

ENTROPION & ECTROPION

 GENERAL INFORMATION

DEFINITION
- Entropion is a disorder of the eyelid (usually the lower) in which it curls inward toward the eye.
- Ectropion is when the eyelid turns outward (inside out).

BODY PARTS INVOLVED—Eyelids.

SEX OR AGE MOST AFFECTED—Adults over 40.

SIGNS & SYMPTOMS
- Inflammation of the eye (swelling, redness, pain and excessive tears) caused when the inward-turning eyelid and lashes rub against the cornea.
- Turning out of the eyelid (usually the lower), causing an unattractive facial appearance.

CAUSES—Several different factors may cause entropion:
- Relaxation of the eyelid's supporting tissue, coupled with the inward pull of the eyelid muscles.
- Chronic eye inflammation (including allergy), creating scar tissue in the eyelid.
- Weakening of the muscles and tissues that normally support the lid against the eye.
- Paralysis of the nerve that supplies the eyelid muscles.
- Contraction of scar tissue (from burns, wounds or surgery) near the eye.

RISK INCREASES WITH—Aging.

HOW TO PREVENT—Obtain prompt medical attention for any eye infection.

 WHAT TO EXPECT

DIAGNOSTIC MEASURES
- Your own observation of symptoms.
- Medical history and physical exam by a doctor.

APPROPRIATE HEALTH CARE
- Self-care after diagnosis.
- Doctor's treatment. Your doctor may attach a small strip of adhesive tape to the lower lid as a temporary measure before surgery.
- Minor surgery (usually) to correct the condition. (See Entropion and Ectropion Repair in Surgery section.)

POSSIBLE COMPLICATIONS
- Ulceration of the cornea from eyelash and eyelid irritation.
- Cornea damage caused by dryness.

PROBABLE OUTCOME—Usually curable with surgery.

 HOW TO TREAT

GENERAL MEASURES
- Apply warm compresses to the eyelids several times a day to relieve inflammation and discomfort. To prepare compresses:
  Pour warm water in a clean bowl.
  Soak a clean cloth in the water. Wring it out almost dry.
  Apply the warm, moist cloth to the closed eye for 10 to 15 minutes.
  Remoisten the cloth frequently.
- Wear protective glasses or goggles if you are exposed to wind or pollutants.

MEDICATION—Your doctor may prescribe:
- Artificial tears until surgery can be performed.
- Antibiotics if infection is present.

ACTIVITY—No restrictions.

DIET—No special diet.

☎ **CALL YOUR DOCTOR IF**

- You have symptoms of entropion or ectropion.
- The following occurs after surgery:
  Eye pain, redness and photosensitivity.
  Your vision changes in any way.

EPIDIDYMITIS

GENERAL INFORMATION

DEFINITION—An inflammation and infection of the epididymis, an oblong structure attached to the upper part of each testis.

BODY PARTS INVOLVED—Epididymis.

SEX OR AGE MOST AFFECTED—Males between puberty and old age.

SIGNS & SYMPTOMS
- Enlarged, hardened, painful testicle.
- Fever.
- Acute urethritis (often).
- Rapid onset of pain, heat and swelling at the back of one testicle (sometimes both).

CAUSES—Usually a complication of a bacterial infection elsewhere in the body, such as: gonococcal infection of the urethra; prostate infection; or bladder or kidney infection.

Epididymitis may also complicate an infection of the scrotum or be caused by scrotal injury.

RISK INCREASES WITH
- Recent illness, especially acute or chronic prostatitis, urethritis or urinary-tract infection.
- Urethral stricture.
- Indwelling urethral catheter.

HOW TO PREVENT
- Use condoms during intercourse to protect from venereal disease. Don't engage in sexual activity with persons who have venereal disease.
- Avoid urethral catheters if possible.

WHAT TO EXPECT

DIAGNOSTIC MEASURES
- Your own observation of symptoms.
- Medical history and physical exam by a doctor.
- Laboratory studies, such as urinalysis and culture of prostate secretions, to identify the cause.

APPROPRIATE HEALTH CARE
- Self-care after diagnosis.
- Doctor's treatment.
- An exploratory operation to make a firm diagnosis and save the testicle (rare).
- Surgical procedure may be necessary for severe cases not responding to antibiotics (rare).

POSSIBLE COMPLICATIONS
- Constipation (sometimes) because bowel movements aggravate pain.
- Sterility or narrowing and blockage of the urethra if the epididymitis involves both testicles. This requires surgery.

PROBABLE OUTCOME—Usually curable with treatment. Pain usually resolves in 1-3 days, but complete healing may take weeks or months.

HOW TO TREAT

GENERAL MEASURES
- Support the weight of the scrotum and tender testicles. Roll a soft bath towel and place it between the legs under the inflamed area.
- Apply an ice bag to the inflamed parts to help reduce swelling and relieve pain. Don't use heat.
- Wear an athletic supporter or two pairs of athletic briefs when you resume normal activity.

MEDICATION—Your doctor may prescribe:
- Antibiotics to fight infection.
- Ibuprofen or acetaminophen for mild pain; or stronger pain drugs for moderate to severe pain.
- Stool softeners.

ACTIVITY—Rest in bed until fever, pain and swelling improve. Don't engage in sexual intercourse Wait at least 1 month after all symptoms disappear before resuming sexual relations.

DIET
- Don't drink alcohol, tea, coffee or carbonated beverages. These irritate the urinary system.
- Eat natural laxative foods, such as prunes, fresh fruit, whole-grain cereals and nuts, to prevent constipation.

CALL YOUR DOCTOR IF

- You have symptoms of epididymitis.
- Pain is not relieved by measures outlined above.
- You develop fever.
- You become constipated.
- Symptoms don't improve within 4 days after treatment begins.

EPIGLOTTITIS, ACUTE

GENERAL INFORMATION

DEFINITION—A sudden, life-threatening childhood infection of the epiglottis (a small flap of tissue in the back of the throat that guards the airway entrance to the lung). Epiglottitis is contagious and is often confused with croup, which is less serious.

BODY PARTS INVOLVED—Epiglottis and surrounding tissue.

SEX OR AGE MOST AFFECTED—Children (2 to 12 years).

SIGNS & SYMPTOMS
- Muffled voice or cry (in croup it is more hoarse).
- Minimal cough (in croup it is a barking cough).
- Sore throat.
- Fever.
- Hoarseness.
- Drooling caused by difficulty swallowing saliva.
- Increasing breathing difficulty.
- Noisy, high-pitched, squeaky inhalations.
- Purple skin and nails.
- Odd head posture. The child tilts the neck back and leans forward with the tongue stuck out and the nostrils flared, trying to inhale more air.

CAUSES—Infection of the epiglottis by a bacteria (usually hemophilus influenza, pneumococcus or streptococcus). The swollen epiglottis blocks the trachea (the main lung airway).

RISK INCREASES WITH
- Illness that has lowered resistance.
- Crowded or unsanitary living conditions.

HOW TO PREVENT
- If your child has had epiglottitis previously, treat all respiratory infections early and with medical supervision.
- Immunize children against hemophilus influenza.

WHAT TO EXPECT

DIAGNOSTIC MEASURES
- Your own observation of symptoms.
- Medical history and physical exam by a doctor.
- Laboratory blood culture, throat culture and others that are performed under special controls to prevent complications.

APPROPRIATE HEALTH CARE
- Doctor's treatment.
- Hospitalization for oxygen and other intensive care.
- Surgery to make an opening in the windpipe (trachea) or to place a tube in the trachea to permit breathing. Usually the tube is withdrawn or the opening is closed in 4 to 7 days.

POSSIBLE COMPLICATIONS—Without treatment, complete airway obstruction and death within hours.

PROBABLE OUTCOME—Full recovery with prompt diagnosis and treatment.

HOW TO TREAT

GENERAL MEASURES
- Caution—Never attempt to look at back of child's throat if you suspect epiglottitis.
- Have the child sit up rather than lie down.
- Keep the child calm and still until reaching the hospital. Panic increases breathing difficulty.
- After hospitalization, use a cool-mist ultrasonic humidifier at night in the child's room for 2 to 3 weeks. Clean humidifier daily.

MEDICATION
- Your doctor may prescribe antibiotics to control infection. Continue for a minimum of 10 days.
- Corticosteroids to reduce inflammation.

ACTIVITY—Bed rest is necessary until all symptoms disappear. Activities may then be resumed gradually.

DIET—Fluids only (usually intravenous) until the child can swallow. After hospitalization, encourage extra fluids and provide a normal diet.

CALL YOUR DOCTOR IF

- Your child has symptoms of epiglottitis, especially signs of breathing difficulty. This is an emergency!
- Your child has had epiglottitis in the past, and symptoms of respiratory infection appear.

ERYTHEMA MULTIFORME

GENERAL INFORMATION

DEFINITION—An acute inflammatory disorder of the skin and mucous membranes (thin moist tissues that line body cavities). In the majority of cases, it is a self-limited, benign disorder, but can be potentially severe. The severe form of the disorder is known as Stevens-Johnson syndrome or erythema multiforme major; the less severe form is referred to as erythema multiforme minor.

BODY PARTS INVOLVED—Skin and mucous membranes.

SEX OR AGE MOST AFFECTED—Men more than women; adults age 20-40; rare under age 3 or over age 50.

SIGNS & SYMPTOMS
- Rash spots that are red and symmetrical in shape, frequently appearing as concentric rings like bull's-eyes.
- Rash usually appears on palms, soles, other areas of arms and legs, may spread to face and rest of the body.
- Rash is itchy, sometimes painful or has burning sensation.
- Rash develops into blisters, hives or becomes ulcerated.
- In the major form, the mucous membranes of the mouth, eyes and genitals become inflamed.
- Fever; headache; sore throat; diarrhea.

CAUSES
- In 50% of the cases, the cause is unknown.
- Viral infections, particularly the herpes simplex virus.
- Bacterial or protozoan infections.
- Collagen vascular disease.
- Medications, such as: sulfonamides, penicillins, anticonvulsants, salicylates, barbiturates. The reaction to the drug may not occur until 7-14 days after first using it.
- Malignancy; pregnancy; radiation therapy; premenstrual hormone changes.

RISK INCREASES WITH
- Previous history of erythema multiforme.
- Taking medications that may cause the disorder.

HOW TO PREVENT
- Avoiding suspected causes where feasible.
- Prompt treatment of any illness or infection that may cause erythema multiforme.
- Prevention of herpes simplex virus outbreaks by avoiding sun exposure and reducing stress.

WHAT TO EXPECT

DIAGNOSTIC MEASURES
- Medical history and exam by a doctor.
- Skin biopsy (see Glossary).

APPROPRIATE HEALTH CARE
- Self-care after diagnosis for mild cases.
- Doctor's treatment.

- If there is extensive, advanced skin damage present, hospitalization in a special burn unit for treatment may be required.

POSSIBLE COMPLICATIONS
- Progression from the minor form to the major form of erythema multiforme.
- Eyes may develop corneal ulcerations, iritis or other serious problems.
- Recurrence of the disorder.
- Serious illness or even death may may result due to shock or inflammation spreading throughout the body.

PROBABLE OUTCOME—Rash evolves over 1-2 weeks and usually clears up in 2-3 weeks, but may take 5-6 weeks.

HOW TO TREAT

GENERAL MEASURES
- Bed rest, if fever is present.
- Discontinuing any implicated medication.
- Wet dressings and soaks or lotions to soothe the skin.
- Bathing in lukewarm to cool water three times a day for 30 minutes.
- Careful monitoring of any eye involvement to prevent complications.
- If mouth sores are present, good oral hygiene is important to reduce possibility of infection and to relieve discomfort.

MEDICATION—Your doctor may prescribe:
- Corticosteroids to reduce inflammation and irritation.
- Acyclovir may be prescribed to treat viral infection such as herpes simplex virus.
- Antibacterial medications, if secondary infection present.
- Topical medications or mouthwashes if mouth sores are present, .
- Eyewashes or other topical medications if eyes are involved.
- Pain medications, sedatives or antihistamines to help provide relief of symptoms.

ACTIVITY—As tolerated by your symptoms.

DIET
- Usually no special diet is necessary.
- If mouth sores are present, a soft or liquid diet may be better tolerated.
- Increased fluid intake sometimes helpful.
- Intravenous fluids may be required in hospitalized patient.

CALL YOUR DOCTOR IF

- You or a family member has signs or symptoms of erythema multiforme.
- Symptoms worsen during treatment. Complications can be potentially severe.
- New or unexplained symptoms develop.

ERYTHEMA NODOSUM

GENERAL INFORMATION

DEFINITION—An inflammatory disease of the skin and tissue under the skin, characterized primarily by painful red nodules on the legs. It is not contagious.

BODY PARTS INVOLVED—Skin of the legs, especially areas over the large bone in the lower leg. The disease occasionally involves the arms or other areas.

SEX OR AGE MOST AFFECTED—Both sexes and all ages, but more likely in females (ages 12 to 40).

SIGNS & SYMPTOMS—Nodules with the following characteristics:
- Nodules are red, painful or tender, and warm.
- Nodules are large (4cm to 10cm). Usually no more than 6 nodules appear at one time.
- Nodules usually occur on the front of the lower legs. They appear on one side and then the other.
- Nodules usually appear suddenly. They are often accompanied by fever and swollen, red, tender ankles and knees.
- Nodules change color from pink to red to blue to brown over 7 to 10 days.

CAUSES—Sometimes unknown. Known causes include:
- Use of drugs, such as birth-control pills (especially those high in estrogen), sulfonamides, iodides and bromides.
- Preceding infection, including: streptococcus (most common), coccidioidomycosis, histoplasmosis, sarcoidosis, blastomycosis, tuberculosis and Yersinia infections (see Glossary).
- Autoimmune disease.
- Chronic bowel inflammation.
- Dysproteinemia (see Glossary).
- Consumption of foods with food dyes or preservatives.
- Cancer.

RISK INCREASES WITH
- Pregnancy.
- Those listed in causes.

HOW TO PREVENT—Remove or treat the cause, if it can be identified.

WHAT TO EXPECT

DIAGNOSTIC MEASURES
- Medical history and physical exam by a doctor.
- Laboratory studies, such as antistreptococcal titre or sedimentation rate.
- X-rays of the chest to detect sarcoidosis or tuberculosis.

APPROPRIATE HEALTH CARE
- Doctor's treatment.
- Self-care after diagnosis.

POSSIBLE COMPLICATIONS
- None expected from erythema nodosum.
- Other complications can arise depending on the cause.

PROBABLE OUTCOME—Individual nodules diminish in size and tenderness and heal in 10 to 20 days. However, others may begin. The disease may last several months. Once it disappears, erythema nodosum probably will not return. Treatment hastens recovery.

HOW TO TREAT

GENERAL MEASURES
- Elevate the legs whenever possible.
- Use elastic wrap or support stockings.
- Use wrapped or immersion soaks (see Appendix) to hasten healing and relieve discomfort. Warm-water soaks are usually more soothing for pain or inflammation. Cool-water soaks feel better for itching.

MEDICATION
- For minor discomfort, you may use nonprescription drugs such as acetaminophen.
- Your doctor may prescribe aspirin, a nonsteroidal anti-inflammatory drug or cortisone drugs to reduce inflammation. (Topical medications usually do not help.)

ACTIVITY—Rest in bed as much as possible with the legs elevated. Overexertion will cause lesions to recur. When symptoms subside, resume normal activity slowly. Allow 3 weeks for recovery.

DIET—No special diet.

CALL YOUR DOCTOR IF

- You have symptoms of erythema nodosum.
- The following occurs during treatment: Symptoms don't improve after 3 days of treatment.
  Fever.
- Any new symptoms arise that you think may be due to the disorder or the medications prescribed.

ESOPHAGEAL STRICTURE OR CORROSIVE ESOPHAGITIS

 GENERAL INFORMATION

DEFINITION
- Esophageal stricture is narrowing of the esophagus (the tube connecting the mouth to the stomach) caused by inflammation. The narrowing interferes with swallowing.
- Corrosive esophagitis is narrowing of the esophagus caused by chemical damage.

BODY PARTS INVOLVED—Esophagus.

SEX OR AGE MOST AFFECTED—Both sexes; all ages.

SIGNS & SYMPTOMS
- Sudden or gradual decrease in the ability to swallow. Gradual swallowing difficulty affects solid foods first, then liquids.
- Pain in the mouth and chest after eating.
- Increased salivation.
- Rapid breathing.
- Vomiting, sometimes with mucus or blood. Cancer of the esophagus often causes similar symptoms.

CAUSES—Scarring of the esophagus following inflammation or damage caused by:
- Chronic heartburn or hiatal hernia.
- Prolonged use of feeding tubes.
- Accidental swallowing of lye or other corrosive chemicals by a child. This is an emergency!
- Deliberate swallowing of lye or other corrosive chemicals by a suicidal person.
- Bulimia.
- Radiation therapy to throat, neck or chest.

RISK INCREASES WITH—Careless storage of corrosive chemicals, such as lye, kerosene, harsh detergent or bleach.

HOW TO PREVENT
- Store all chemicals out of the reach of young children.
- Avoid prolonged use of feeding tubes.

 WHAT TO EXPECT

DIAGNOSTIC MEASURES
- Your own observation of symptoms.
- Medical history and physical exam by a doctor.
- Surgical diagnostic procedures such as endoscopy (see Glossary). A small amount of tissue will be removed for biopsy to make sure the stricture is benign.
- X-rays of the esophagus (barium swallow).

APPROPRIATE HEALTH CARE
- Doctor's treatment.
- Hospitalization for supportive care and intravenous nutrition (sometimes).
- Surgery to remove stricture if other measures fail (rare).
- Periodic dilatation of esophagus.

POSSIBLE COMPLICATIONS
- Malnutrition from inability to eat normally.
- Perforation of the damaged esophagus. This may be life-threatening.

PROBABLE OUTCOME—Usually curable with treatment. Normal swallowing can be maintained with regular treatment to stretch the stricture.

 HOW TO TREAT

GENERAL MEASURES—The stricture must be stretched regularly, about once a month for some people and for others, every 4 to 6 months. There are several methods available and your doctor will provide information about the options. The techniques require an experienced operator. Don't be hesitant to inquire about the experience of the person scheduled to perform the procedure on you. The stricture will eventually return if regular treatments are not continued.

MEDICATION—Your doctor may prescribe:
- Cortisone drugs to reduce inflammation and diminish the possibility of scarring.
- Antibiotics to prevent infection.

ACTIVITY—Resume normal activities gradually.

DIET
- Eat a soft or liquid diet (see both in Appendix) after treatment until normal swallowing is possible. Avoid spicy foods that irritate the esophagus.
- Don't drink alcohol.

 CALL YOUR DOCTOR IF

- You have symptoms of esophageal stricture or corrosive esophagitis.
- The following occurs during treatment:
  Chest pain.
  Fever.
  Inability to speak.
  Feeling of air bubbles under the skin of the chest.

ESOPHAGUS, CANCER OF

GENERAL INFORMATION

DEFINITION—A new growth of tissue in the esophagus (tube connecting the mouth to the stomach) in which cells multiply in an uncontrolled fashion. Cancer that begins in the esophagus (primary) usually occurs in the lower third of the esophagus where it passes through the chest.

BODY PARTS INVOLVED—Esophagus.

SEX OR AGE MOST AFFECTED
• Adults (age 50 and over).
• Both sexes, but more likely in men.

SIGNS & SYMPTOMS
• Swallowing difficulty or pain.
• Rapid weight loss.
• Regurgitation of bloody mucus.

CAUSES—Unknown. Most esophagus cancers are primary (begin there), but some spread from other body parts (secondary). It is not inherited.

RISK INCREASES WITH
• Smoking.
• Excess alcohol consumption.
• Previous head and neck tumors.
• Celiac disease.
• Hiatal hernia.
• Strictures.
• Iron deficiency.
• Chronic gastric reflux.

HOW TO PREVENT
• Don't smoke.
• Don't drink more than 1 or 2 alcoholic drinks—if any—a day.
• Obtain medical treatment for any gastrointestinal disorder that lasts longer than 5 days.

WHAT TO EXPECT

DIAGNOSTIC MEASURES
• Your own observation of symptoms.
• Medical history and physical exam by a doctor.
• Biopsy, CT scan, esophagoscopy (see Glossary for all).
• X-ray of the upper-intestinal tract.

APPROPRIATE HEALTH CARE
• Doctor's treatment.
• Surgery, radiation, chemotherapy or a combination of these.

POSSIBLE COMPLICATIONS—If treatment doesn't begin immediately, esophagus cancer spreads rapidly to the lungs and liver.

PROBABLE OUTCOME—This condition is currently considered incurable. Early diagnosis and aggressive treatment offer the only chance of survival. In any case, symptoms can be relieved or controlled.

Medical literature cites a few instances of unexplained recovery. Scientific research into causes and treatment continues, so there is hope for increasingly effective treatment and cure.

HOW TO TREAT

GENERAL MEASURES
• The more you can learn and understand about esophageal cancer, the more you will be able to make informed decisions about where to go for your care, the treatments available, the risks involved, side effects of therapy and expected outcome.
• Esophageal dilation therapy may help if swallowing is a problem. Ask your doctor.
• See Resources for Additional Information.

MEDICATION—Your doctor may prescribe:
• Analgesics or narcotics to relieve pain.
• Tranquilizers to reduce anxiety.
• Anticancer drugs (sometimes).
• Anticholinergics or calcium-channel blockers for esophageal spasms.

ACTIVITY—Remain as active as possible.

DIET
• Soft to liquid diet if necessary (see both in Appendix). Avoid chocolates, alcohol and fats.
• Prior to surgery, special nutritional support may be required (feeding tube with formula diet).

CALL YOUR DOCTOR IF

• You have symptoms of cancer of the esophagus, especially difficulty swallowing.
• Pain becomes intolerable despite treatment.
• New, unexplained symptoms develop. Drugs used in treatment may produce side effects.

EXOPHTHALMOS (Proptosis)

GENERAL INFORMATION

DEFINITION—A protrusion or bulging of one or both eyes.

BODY PARTS INVOLVED—Eyes.

SEX OR AGE MOST AFFECTED—Both sexes; all ages.

SIGNS & SYMPTOMS
- Bulging eyes, which creates a staring or frightened look.
- Double vision.
- Pain (sometimes).
- Infrequent blinking (sometimes).

CAUSES—Swelling of tissue behind the eye. Swelling may be caused by:
- Overactive thyroid gland (most common cause).
- Infection or tumor in the supportive tissues behind the eye.
- Aneurysm, blood clot or hemorrhage in the veins or arteries behind the eye.
- Injury to the eye or face.
- Congenital deformity of the head.

RISK INCREASES WITH—Unknown.

HOW TO PREVENT—Obtain prompt medical treatment for the underlying disorder.

WHAT TO EXPECT

DIAGNOSTIC MEASURES
- Your own observation of symptoms.
- Medical history and physical exam by a doctor.
- Biopsy (see Glossary) of tissue behind the eyes.
- Blood tests for thyroid function.
- Radioactive studies for thyroid function.
- X-rays of the head.
- CT scan (see Glossary).

APPROPRIATE HEALTH CARE
- Doctor's treatment.
- Surgery to:
  Remove a tumor, blood clot or aneurysm.
  Return the eyes to their normal position, if necessary, after the underlying cause is corrected.
  Correct congenital abnormalities.

POSSIBLE COMPLICATIONS—Injury to the eye and impaired vision.

PROBABLE OUTCOME—Spontaneous recovery in most cases after the underlying cause is treated. If not, surgery can often correct any remaining protrusion.

HOW TO TREAT

GENERAL MEASURES
- If the disorder is caused by injury, see a doctor immediately.
- If your vision is affected, don't drive or engage in dangerous activity.
- If eyelids don't blink properly, wear goggles to protect them from wind or dust.

MEDICATION
- If the lids don't blink properly, you should use nonprescription, lubricating eye drops.
- Your doctor may prescribe drugs to treat the underlying cause, such as:
  Antithyroid drugs for hyperthyroidism.
  Antibiotics to fight infection.
  Cortisone drugs to reduce inflammation.

ACTIVITY—No restrictions.

DIET—No special diet.

CALL YOUR DOCTOR IF

- You have symptoms of exophthalmos.
- Symptoms don't improve within 5 days after treatment begins.
- New, unexplained symptoms develop. Drugs used in treatment may produce side effects.

ILLNESS & DISORDERS

EXTRADURAL HEMORRHAGE
(Epidural Hemorrhage)

 GENERAL INFORMATION

DEFINITION—Bleeding between the skull and the outermost of 3 membranes that cover the brain (meninges). May be confused with meningitis. A hematoma (collection of clotted blood) forms and rapidly enlarges, increasing pressure within the skull and causing symptoms.

BODY PARTS INVOLVED—Skull; meninges; brain.

SEX OR AGE MOST AFFECTED—Both sexes; all ages.

SIGNS & SYMPTOMS—These symptoms develop within 24 to 96 hours after a head injury:
• Headache that steadily worsens.
• Drowsiness or unconsciousness.
• Nausea or vomiting.
• Inability to move arms and legs.
• Change in the size of eye pupils.

CAUSES—Head injury.

RISK INCREASES WITH
• Use of anticoagulant drugs.
• Bleeding disorders, such as hemophilia, ITT or aplastic anemia.
• Injuries. These occur more often after excess alcohol consumption or use of mind-altering drugs.

HOW TO PREVENT—Avoid head injury in the following ways:
• Use seat belts in cars.
• Wear protective head gear during contact sports or while riding a bicycle or motorcycle.
• Don't drink alcohol or use mind-altering drugs and drive.
• Seek medical advice for even a moderate blow to the head.

 WHAT TO EXPECT

DIAGNOSTIC MEASURES
• Your own observation of symptoms.
• Medical history and physical exam by a doctor.
• Laboratory studies of blood and cerebrospinal fluid.
• Hospital diagnostic tests, such as x-rays of the head, arteriography, radioscopic scan and CT scan (see Glossary for all).

APPROPRIATE HEALTH CARE
• Doctor's treatment.
• Extradural hemorrhage is an emergency that requires rapid treatment to prevent permanent brain damage or death. Surgical treatment consists of drilling a hole in the skull, draining the blood clot and clipping the ruptured blood vessel.
• Home-care after surgery.

POSSIBLE COMPLICATIONS—Fatal compression of the brain if bleeding lasts longer than 24 hours.

PROBABLE OUTCOME—Quick diagnosis and prompt surgery usually bring complete recovery.

 HOW TO TREAT

GENERAL MEASURES
• The family should maintain an optimistic outlook, stay in close contact with the patient's doctor and help by making their visits with the patient brief and as supportive as possible.
• See Resources for Additional Information.

MEDICATION—Your doctor may prescribe cortisone drugs to reduce swelling inside the skull.

ACTIVITY—Stay as active as your strength allows. Work and exercise moderately. Rest when you tire. If speech or muscle control has been damaged, you may need physical therapy or speech therapy.

DIET—Eat a normal, well-balanced diet. Vitamin and mineral supplements should not be necessary unless you cannot eat normally.

 CALL YOUR DOCTOR IF

• You have had a head injury—even if it seems minor—and you develop any symptoms of extradural hemorrhage.
• The following occurs during treatment:
  Fever.
  Surgical wound becomes red, swollen or tender.
  Headache worsens.

EYE CONTUSION OR LACERATION

GENERAL INFORMATION

DEFINITION—Eye injury, including blunt injury (contusion) or cut (laceration).

BODY PARTS INVOLVED—Eyeball; eyelid; bones around the eyeball (eye socket); muscles attached to the eyeball.

SEX OR AGE MOST AFFECTED—Both sexes; all ages.

SIGNS & SYMPTOMS
- Swelling, redness, tenderness, pain, bleeding or bruising ("black eye") in or around the eye.
- Change in ability to see clearly.

CAUSES—A blunt or sharp blow or cut to the eye or surrounding structures.

RISK INCREASES WITH
- Eye injuries often occur in fights. Fights are more likely with alcohol consumption or in hostile environments that foster aggression.
- Occupations that expose the eye to injury, such as carpentry or steel-construction work.
- Using rotary lawn mower.
- BB gun or slingshot usage.
- Participation in sports such as basketball, football, hockey, etc.

HOW TO PREVENT—Always wear protective eye coverings, if possible, for any exposure to eye injury risks.

WHAT TO EXPECT

DIAGNOSTIC MEASURES
- Your own observation of symptoms.
- Medical history and physical exam by a doctor.
- X-rays of bone surrounding the eye.

APPROPRIATE HEALTH CARE
- Doctor's treatment, which may include suturing a laceration.
- For a major laceration, repair should be done by an eye surgeon.
- For trauma to the eyeball, emergency treatment by a specialist is necessary.
- Self-care after treatment.

POSSIBLE COMPLICATIONS
- Permanent vision loss.
- Infection.
- Cataract.

PROBABLE OUTCOME—Usually curable with treatment to prevent infection and suture of lacerations in and around the eye. Allow 2 weeks for complete healing.

HOW TO TREAT

GENERAL MEASURES
- For a lid contusion (black eye) during the first 24 hours, use ice packs to reduce swelling. The next day, prepare a hot compress by folding a clean cloth in several layers. Dip in hot water, wring out slightly and apply to the eye. Dip the compress often to keep it moist. Apply the compress for an hour, rest an hour and repeat.
- Protect eyes from bright light or sunlight by wearing dark glasses temporarily.
- Sleep with the head elevated with 2 pillows until symptoms subside.

MEDICATION—Your doctor may prescribe:
- Antibiotic eye drops or ointments to prevent infection.
- Pain relievers.
- Eye drops to dilate the eye pupil and rest the eye muscles (sometimes).

ACTIVITY—Resume normal activities gradually after treatment.

DIET—No special diet.

CALL YOUR DOCTOR IF

- You have a cut or other eye injury.
- The following occurs after eye injury:
  Fever.
  Severe eye pain that persists, despite treatment.
  Vision changes.

ILLNESS & DISORDERS

EYE, FOREIGN BODY IN

GENERAL INFORMATION

DEFINITION—Embedding of a small speck of metal, wood, stone, sand, paint or other foreign material in the eye.

BODY PARTS INVOLVED—Eye, usually the conjunctiva (outer eye covering).

SEX OR AGE MOST AFFECTED—Both sexes; all ages.

SIGNS & SYMPTOMS
• Severe pain, irritation and redness in the eye.
• Foreign body visible with the naked eye (usually). Sometimes the foreign body is very small, trapped under the eyelid and invisible except with medical examination.
• Scratchy feeling with blinking.

CAUSES—Accident.

RISK INCREASES WITH
• Windy weather.
• Occupations or activity, such as carpentry or grinding, in which fine particles of wood or other materials fly loose in the air.

HOW TO PREVENT—Wear protective eye coverings if your occupation or hobby involves the risk of eye injury.

WHAT TO EXPECT

DIAGNOSTIC MEASURES
• Your own observation of symptoms.
• Medical history and physical exam by a doctor. This may include staining the eye with a harmless substance (fluorescein dye) to outline the object and examine the eye through a magnifying lens.

APPROPRIATE HEALTH CARE
• Doctor's treatment.
• The procedure to remove the object will be determined by its size and location within the eye.
• An eye patch will be applied to keep the eye closed.
• Follow-up examination should be done in 1 to 2 days.
• Self-care after removal of the particle.

POSSIBLE COMPLICATIONS
• Infection, especially if the foreign body is not removed completely.
• Severe, permanent vision damage caused by penetration of deeper eye layers.

PROBABLE OUTCOME—Most objects can be removed simply under local anesthesia in a doctor's office or emergency room.

HOW TO TREAT

GENERAL MEASURES
• Ask someone else to drive you to the doctor's office. Don't try to drive yourself.
• Don't rub the eye.
• Keep the eye closed, if possible, until you are examined.
• Wear an eye patch to keep the eye closed, or dark glasses, for 24 hours after removal to protect your eye from bright light.

MEDICATION—Your doctor may prescribe:
• Antibiotic eye drops or ointment to prevent infection.
• Pain relievers.
• Local anesthetic eye drops.

ACTIVITY—Resume your normal activities gradually after removal of the foreign body and the patch, if one is applied.

DIET—No special diet.

CALL YOUR DOCTOR IF

• You have a foreign body in the eye.
• The following occurs after removal:
  Pain increases or does not disappear in 2 days.
  You develop a fever.
  Your vision changes.

EYE TUMOR

GENERAL INFORMATION

DEFINITION—A growth in the eye in which cell multiplication is uncontrolled and progressive. Eye tumors are of 3 types: retinoblastoma, malignant melanoma or secondary tumors that have spread from other parts of the body.

BODY PARTS INVOLVED—Usually one eye. Retinoblastoma invades both eyes in 25% of cases.

SEX OR AGE MOST AFFECTED
• Melanoma: Adults over 60.
• Retinoblastoma: Young children between ages 1 and 5.
• Secondary tumors: All ages.

SIGNS & SYMPTOMS—The following are characteristic of all 3 types:
• Possibly no signs in the early stages except occasionally a whitish light reflection in pupil.
• Gradual loss of vision.
• Bulging eyes (sometimes).
Retinoblastoma may have the following additional signs:
• Crossed eyes.
• A tumor that is visible through the pupil.

CAUSES
• Melanoma and secondary tumors: Unknown.
• Retinoblastoma: Inherited tendency.

RISK INCREASES WITH—Family history of retinoblastoma. The genetic trait is dominant, but it does not affect all children.

HOW TO PREVENT—Cannot be prevented at present. If the family has a history of retinoblastoma, obtain genetic counseling before having children.

WHAT TO EXPECT

DIAGNOSTIC MEASURES
• Your own observation of symptoms.
• Medical history and physical exam by a doctor.
• Echography (see Glossary).
• Fluorescein dye tests (see Glossary) to outline blood vessels in the eye.
• X-rays of the skull.

APPROPRIATE HEALTH CARE—One of the following:
• Surgery to remove the tumor.
• Radiation therapy.
• Cryotherapy (see Glossary).
• Treatment with laser beams.

POSSIBLE COMPLICATIONS
• Spread to other parts of the body.
• Partial or complete loss of vision.

PROBABLE OUTCOME—Some eye tumors are curable in 6 months with medical treatment.
Other eye tumors are considered incurable. A fatal spread to other body parts usually occurs rapidly. However, medical literature cites a few instances of unexplained recovery. Scientific research into causes and treatment continues, so there is hope for increasingly effective treatment and cure.

HOW TO TREAT

GENERAL MEASURES
• The more you can learn and understand about this disorder, the more you will be able to make informed decisions about where to go for your care, the treatments available, the risks involved, side effects of therapy and expected outcome.
• See Resources for Additional Information.

MEDICATION—Your doctor may prescribe:
• Pain relievers.
• Anticancer drugs.

ACTIVITY—After treatment, resume your normal activities as soon as possible.

DIET—No special diet.

CALL YOUR DOCTOR IF

• You have symptoms of an eye tumor.
• Pain becomes intolerable during treatment.
• New, unexplained symptoms develop that may indicate the malignancy has spread to other body parts.

FAILURE TO THRIVE

 GENERAL INFORMATION

DEFINITION—Failure of infants or children to grow and develop normally. This term is used until a specific diagnosis can be established.

BODY PARTS INVOLVED—All.

SEX OR AGE MOST AFFECTED—Children under 5, usually infants, ages 3-6 months.

SIGNS & SYMPTOMS
- Height, weight and head circumference do not progress normally, as measured on doctors' growth charts.
- Physical skills are often slow to develop. Such skills include turning over in bed, sitting, standing and walking.
- Mental and social skills are often delayed. These skills include talking, social interaction, self-feeding, toilet training.
- Normal growth and development vary widely. The rate of change—as measured at regular medical checkups—is more significant.

CAUSES
- In some of these children, the cause is organic, usually gastrointestinal problems or neurological problems.
- In most of the children, the cause is environmental, such as incorrect feeding.

RISK INCREASES WITH
- Malnutrition; parental inexperience; a negative emotional environment (neglect, abuse or rejection).
- Chronic disease (e.g., kidney failure).
- Fetal Alcohol Syndrome.
- Genetic disorders, such as Down syndrome or cystic fibrosis.
- Endocrine diseases, including disorders of the thyroid, pituitary, adrenal, pancreas and sexual glands.
- Poverty.
- Parents who were raised in a negative emotional environment or are poorly educated.
- Crowded or unsanitary living conditions.
- Premature or sick newborn.
- Infant with physical deformity.

HOW TO PREVENT
- Arrange for parenting classes if you are an expectant mother or father.
- Take your child regularly to the doctor for "well-baby" checkups.
- Provide a stable home life with caring parents.
- Read books on parenting.

 WHAT TO EXPECT

DIAGNOSTIC MEASURES
- Your own observation of symptoms.
- Medical history and exam by a doctor.

- Diagnostic tests: Repeated measurements of height, weight and head circumference; psychological tests, such as the Denver Developmental test, which measures growth and development; laboratory blood tests, including hormone studies; x-rays of the wrists (bone age), which measure body growth.

APPROPRIATE HEALTH CARE
- Doctor's treatment.
- Psychotherapy or counseling, if parents have emotional problems that prevent a healthy relationship with the child.
- Hospitalization (short-term), if complicated diagnostic procedures are necessary or food intake must be verified.

POSSIBLE COMPLICATIONS
- Permanent mental, emotional or physical disability.
- Child remains small and developmentally slow.
- If proper care is not provided in the home, foster care may be necessary.

PROBABLE OUTCOME
- If failure to thrive is caused by parental inexperience or psychological problems, recovery is possible with education and counseling for the parents.
- If failure to thrive is caused by an underlying physical illness or disorder, including malnutrition, recovery depends on whether the condition can be corrected.

 HOW TO TREAT

GENERAL MEASURES
- Read books and pamphlets on child-rearing or attend parenting classes.
- Ask a visiting nurse for guidance.
- Provide as much love and support as possible for your child. Examine your feelings and behavior toward your child. If you don't think they are what they should be, arrange for psychological counseling.

MEDICATION—If an underlying disorder is causing failure to thrive, your doctor may prescribe medication to treat the condition.

ACTIVITY—No restrictions.

DIET
- Provide your child with an adequate, well-balanced diet.
- If malnutrition is causing failure to thrive, your doctor may prescribe a special diet.

 CALL YOUR DOCTOR IF

You are concerned that your child is not developing properly.

FAINTING
(Syncope)

GENERAL INFORMATION

DEFINITION—Sudden, temporary loss of consciousness due to insufficient oxygen reaching the brain.

BODY PARTS INVOLVED—Circulatory system (heart and blood vessels); brain.

SEX OR AGE MOST AFFECTED—Both sexes; all ages.

SIGNS & SYMPTOMS
- Sudden lightheadedness.
- General weakness, then falling.
- Blurred vision (sometimes).
- Nausea (sometimes).
- Paleness and sweating.
- Rapid heartbeat and rapid breathing. If heartbeat or breathing is not present, this may be cardiac arrest rather than fainting.

CAUSES—A sudden decrease in blood flow to the brain. This may result from:
- Heartbeat abnormalities—too fast, too slow or irregular.
- Prolonged straining, such as from severe coughing or attempted bowel movements when constipated.
- Sudden emotional stress.
- Heart diseases that limit the amount of blood the heart pumps.
- Getting out of bed or a chair suddenly (orthostatic hypotension).
- Acute pain.
- Epilepsy.
- Heart attack (rare).

RISK INCREASES WITH
- Stress.
- Heart disease.
- Some drugs such as alcohol.
- Use of certain drugs, such as heart medications that slow the heartbeat. These include digitalis, beta-adrenergic blockers and other antihypertensive drugs.
- Hot, humid weather; dehydration.
- Elderly.
- Diabetes mellitus.

HOW TO PREVENT
- Avoid sudden changes in physical activity.
- If fainting episodes are caused by medication, consult your doctor about changing drugs.

WHAT TO EXPECT

DIAGNOSTIC MEASURES
- Observation of symptoms by those nearby.
- Medical history and exam by a doctor.
- Diagnostic tests for an underlying cause may include CT scan or MRI of the head and an EEG (see Glossary for all).

APPROPRIATE HEALTH CARE
- Care from bystanders.
- Self-care after regaining consciousness.
- Doctor's treatment, if fainting is caused by other conditions (see Causes).

POSSIBLE COMPLICATIONS
- Injury while fainting.
- Mistaking cardiac arrest for fainting.

PROBABLE OUTCOME—People recover from a simple faint in 1 or 2 minutes.

HOW TO TREAT

GENERAL MEASURES
- If someone faints, check for breathing and a neck pulse. If neither is present:
  Dial 911 (emergency) for an ambulance or medical help. (If the victim is a child, perform 1 minute of lifesaving procedures first, then call 911).
  Then give first aid immediately.
  Begin cardiac massage and mouth-to-mouth breathing (CPR). Don't stop until help arrives.
- If someone faints, is breathing and has a pulse, leave the person on the ground and elevate both legs. This helps return blood to the heart. Person should remain lying down for 10-15 minutes.
- If you feel faint, sit down immediately and bend over, or lie down.
- If you are subject to frequent fainting spells, avoid activities in which fainting may endanger your life, such as climbing to high places, driving vehicles or operating dangerous machinery.

MEDICATION—Medication usually is not necessary for fainting. Medication may be necessary for underlying disorders.

ACTIVITY—Resume your normal activities as soon as you regain consciousness.

DIET—No special diet unless fainting episodes are caused by low blood sugar. If so, eat 5 or 6 small meals a day. The meals should be high in protein, high in complex carbohydrates and low in simple carbohydrates (sugar). Drink adequate fluids and avoid alcohol.

CALL YOUR DOCTOR IF

- An unconscious person has no pulse and is not breathing. Give CPR first.
- Someone faints and does not regain consciousness quickly.
- Fainting is a symptom of another condition (see Causes).

FECAL IMPACTION

 ## GENERAL INFORMATION

DEFINITION—A severe form of acute constipation in which a large mass of feces cannot be passed. Fecal impaction is not a serious condition, but it complicates other illnesses.

BODY PARTS INVOLVED—Lower colon; rectum.

SEX OR AGE MOST AFFECTED—Both sexes; all ages.

SIGNS & SYMPTOMS
- Absence of normal bowel movements.
- Sense of fullness in the rectum, but inability to pass stool.
- Lack of urinary control.
- A firm mass in the lower left abdomen (sometimes).
- Pain or cramps (sometimes). Impaction often develops slowly without discomfort.
- Thin, watery discharge from the rectum.
- Nausea, vomiting, loss of appetite (rare).

CAUSES
- Rectal disorders that make normal bowel movements uncomfortable, such as painful hemorrhoids or anal fissure.
- Rectal or colon tumors.
- Barium that is swallowed for x-rays of the intestinal tract.
- Loss of nerve supply to the colon or rectum, as with a spinal-cord injury.
- Insufficient fiber and liquid in the diet.

RISK INCREASES WITH
- Bed rest for any condition, such as a recent heart attack, surgery or fracture.
- Back disorders with nerve pressure.
- Decreased fluid and fiber intake.
- Chronic or long-term use of laxatives.
- Use of some drugs, such as narcotic pain killers, antiparkinsonism drugs, atropine, phenothiazines or tricyclic antidepressants.

HOW TO PREVENT
- If confined to bed, drink extra fluids and increase consumption of dietary fiber.
- If simple constipation develops, use a mild laxative, such as milk of magnesia, a stool softener or an enema.
- Set aside a regular time each day for bowel movement (within an hour after breakfast is best). Don't try to hurry. Sit at least 10 minutes.

 ## WHAT TO EXPECT

DIAGNOSTIC MEASURES
- Your own observation of symptoms.
- Medical history and physical exam, including a rectal exam, by a doctor.

APPROPRIATE HEALTH CARE
- Self-care.
- Doctor's treatment to remove feces by enema or manually.

POSSIBLE COMPLICATIONS
- Persons who have had a recent (within 1 week) heart attack may suffer fatal rupture of the heart muscle while straining to pass a fecal impaction.
- Rectal prolapse (protrusion outside the body).
- Aggravation of hemorrhoids.

PROBABLE OUTCOME—Usually curable with treatment, but recurrence is common unless the underlying cause is removed.

 ## HOW TO TREAT

GENERAL MEASURES
- If your doctor prescribes it, use an oil-retention enema before and after manual removal of the impaction. Follow instructions on the package.
- See Constipation (in Illness section) for suggestions to improve bowel habits.

MEDICATION
- After removal of the impaction, your doctor may prescribe laxatives or stool softeners.
- Clomiphene citrate may be prescribed, but its effectiveness is questionable.

ACTIVITY—No restrictions. Be as active as possible. Good physical fitness improves bowel function.

DIET
- Eat a normal, well-balanced diet high in fiber (see Appendix).
- Drink at least 8 glasses of fluid each day.

 ## CALL YOUR DOCTOR IF

- You have symptoms of a fecal impaction.
- Your normal bowel pattern changes.
- You cannot pass feces while under treatment for other conditions.

FERTILITY PROBLEMS IN MEN

GENERAL INFORMATION

DEFINITION—The inability to impregnate a female after 1 year of sexual activity without contraception. Infertility occurs in 10% of all couples. Fertility depends on the production of normal quantities of healthy sperm, ability to achieve an erection and to ejaculate sperm into the vagina during sexual intercourse.

BODY PARTS INVOLVED—Genitals; endocrine system; brain.

SEX OR AGE MOST AFFECTED—Males after puberty.

SIGNS & SYMPTOMS—Inability to impregnate a fertile woman.

CAUSES—Infertility is caused by an absence of sperm, defective sperm or insufficient sperm in ejaculation. Reasons include:
- Anatomical abnormalities of the penis or testicles, including undescended testicles.
- Excessive alcohol intake.
- Urinary-tract infection.
- Hormone disturbance.
- Mumps.
- Use of some drugs, such as antihypertensives, cytotoxic drugs, male hormones and MAO inhibitors.
- Sexually transmitted diseases.
- Injury to the genitals; ejaculatory dysfunction.
- Varicose veins in the testicles.
- Psychological reasons, such as fear of infertility.
- Overheating of the testicles caused by vigorous, repetitive exercise or underwear that is too tight and holds the testicles too close to the body.
- Intercourse problems, e.g., premature withdrawal, poor timing with menses, too infrequent.

RISK INCREASES WITH
- Diabetes mellitus.
- Poor nutrition.
- Family history of Klinefelter's syndrome (see Glossary).
- Smoking (men who smoke produce fewer and less healthy sperm).
- Hot tub use.

HOW TO PREVENT—No specific preventive measures except to avoid risk factors or causes.

WHAT TO EXPECT

DIAGNOSTIC MEASURES
- Your own observation of symptoms.
- Medical history and exam by a doctor.
- Blood studies of hormones; semen analysis.
- Testicular biopsy.
- Special tests of sperm function and quality.

APPROPRIATE HEALTH CARE
- Self-care after diagnosis.
- Doctor's treatment.
- A variety of treatments are available such as devices that lower scrotal temperatures, intrauterine insemination of concentrated washed sperm and in-vitro fertilization.
- Psychotherapy or counseling for sexual therapy techniques, marital problems or alcoholism.
- Surgery to correct anatomical abnormalities of the reproductive system.

POSSIBLE COMPLICATIONS—Psychological distress caused by feelings of guilt, inadequacy and loss of self-esteem.

PROBABLE OUTCOME—Many fertility problems are minor and reversible. Approach treatment with optimism.

HOW TO TREAT

GENERAL MEASURES
- Heat may decrease sperm production in the testicles. To prevent this: Don't wear tight underwear or athletic supporters that hold the testicles too close to the body, don't take hot baths or extended hot showers, avoid long bicycle rides.
- Have sexual intercourse during the time your partner is ovulating. Don't ejaculate for 3 days prior. Intercourse should occur every 36 hours during the fertile period.
- Don't smoke; avoid alcohol or use in moderation.
- Don't use commercial sexual lubricants (they may kill sperm).
- See Resources for Additional Information.

MEDICATION—Your doctor may prescribe medications for any underlying problem discovered during medical testing.

ACTIVITY—Work and exercise moderately. Overexercising can be a factor in infertility. Rest when you tire.

DIET—Eat a normal, well-balanced diet.

CALL YOUR DOCTOR IF

- You want help for infertility.
- Conception doesn't occur within 6 months, despite recommendations and treatment.
- New, unexplained symptoms develop. Drugs used in treatment may produce side effects.

FERTILITY PROBLEMS IN WOMEN

GENERAL INFORMATION

DEFINITION—The inability to become pregnant after 1 year of sexual activity without contraception. Infertility occurs in 10% of all couples.

BODY PARTS INVOLVED—Genitals; endocrine system; brain.

SEX OR AGE MOST AFFECTED—Females between puberty and menopause.

SIGNS & SYMPTOMS—Inability to conceive.

CAUSES
- Minor anatomic abnormalities of the reproductive system.
- Emotional stress.
- Repeated weight-gain/weight-loss cycles.
- Hormone dysfunction, especially thyroid disorders.
- Vaginitis; ovarian cysts; endometriosis; tumors.
- Disorders of the cervix, such as infection, laceration from previous childbirth or narrowing of the cervical opening for any reason.
- Amenorrhea (lack of menstrual periods) caused by strenuous exercise programs or nutritional disorders (bulimia or anorexia nervosa).
- Chemical changes in the cervical mucus.
- The use of some medications, including oral contraceptives. Many women cannot conceive for many months after discontinuing use.
- Disorders probably not related to infertility include: a tilted uterus; small fibroid tumors of the uterus; or inability to achieve orgasm.

RISK INCREASES WITH
- Stress.
- Marital discord and infrequent sexual intercourse.
- Abuse of drugs, like heroin.

HOW TO PREVENT
- Obtain treatment for any treatable disorder that causes infertility.
- Avoid preventable causes of infertility, especially poor nutrition.

WHAT TO EXPECT

DIAGNOSTIC MEASURES
- Your own observation of symptoms.
- Medical history and physical exam by a doctor.
- Laboratory studies, such as: blood studies; Rubin's insufflation tests (see Glossary); culdoscopy (see Glossary); and studies of mucus of the cervix.
- Surgical diagnostic procedures such as laparoscopy (see Glossary).

APPROPRIATE HEALTH CARE
- Self-care after diagnosis.
- Doctor's treatment.
- Psychotherapy or counseling, if marital problems exist.
- Surgery to correct anatomical abnormalities of the reproductive system.
- In-vitro fertilization; eggs from the female are harvested, impregnated with sperm from the male and implanted in the uterus.

POSSIBLE COMPLICATIONS—Psychological distress, including feelings of guilt, inadequacy and loss of self-esteem.

PROBABLE OUTCOME
- Many fertility problems are minor and reversible. Approach treatment with optimism.
- Research is offering new options to couples.

HOW TO TREAT

GENERAL MEASURES
- Keep a basal body-temperature chart to become familiar with your ovulation pattern. Ask your doctor for instructions.
- Have intercourse just before ovulation, which can be determined from the chart.
- Don't use a lubricant during sexual relations. Lubricants may interfere with sperm mobility.
- Your partner should withdraw his penis quickly from your vagina after ejaculation. If left in, it reduces the number of sperm that can swim toward the egg.
- After your partner's ejaculation, place pillows under your buttocks to provide an easier downhill swim for the sperm.
- Avoid physical exhaustion prior to intercourse.
- Maintain a positive attitude. Worry and tension contribute to infertility.
- See Resources for Additional Information.

MEDICATION—Your doctor may prescribe:
- Hormones for a hormone imbalance.
- Clomiphene, a gonad stimulant.
Recognize that fertility drugs may cause multiple births.

ACTIVITY—Work and exercise moderately. Overexercising may contribute to infertility.

DIET—Eat a normal, well-balanced diet. If you are overweight, try to achieve your ideal weight (see Weight-Loss diet in Appendix).

CALL YOUR DOCTOR IF

- You want help for infertility.
- Conception doesn't occur within 6 months, despite recommendations and treatment.
- New, unexplained symptoms develop. Hormones used in treatment may produce side effects.

FETAL ALCOHOL SYNDROME (FAS)

GENERAL INFORMATION

DEFINITION—A combination of irreversible birth abnormalities resulting from alcohol abuse by the mother during pregnancy. Fetal alcohol syndrome has been reported in babies of women who drank 2 mixed drinks or 2-3 bottles of beer or glasses of wine a day. Lesser degrees of alcohol abuse can result in less severe birth defects (fetal alcohol effect). No safe level of alcohol consumption is known.

SEX OR AGE MOST AFFECTED—Newborns.

SIGNS & SYMPTOMS
Newborn behaviors:
- Poor sucking ability; poor sleeping habits.
- Irritability; effects of alcohol withdrawal.

Possible physical abnormalities:
- Small head; small eyes; unusually short.
- Epicanthic folds (vertical folds of skin extending from upper eyelid to the side of nose).
- Small jaw; protruding forehead.
- Cleft palate.
- Small brain; heart defects.
- Hip dislocation; other joint deformities.

Later:
- Mental retardation; severe growth retardation.
- Poor coordination; learning disabilities.
- Speech and language difficulties; minimal brain dysfunction; hyperactivity; other behavioral problems.

Adolescence to adulthood:
- Maladaptive behaviors (social withdrawal, failure to consider consequence of actions, inappropriate emotional responses, excessive unhappiness, conduct problems).

CAUSES—Chronic (and probably binge-type) alcohol consumption during pregnancy. Alcohol intake can affect the unborn child during the first trimester by interfering with organ development, in the second trimester with mental retardation and the third trimester, retardation of fetal growth.

RISK INCREASES WITH
- The greater the alcohol consumption, the greater the risk for severe birth defects.
- Pregnant women not receiving prenatal health care.

HOW TO PREVENT
- Pregnant women (or those likely to become pregnant) should not drink any alcoholic drinks or abuse drugs. There is insufficient evidence that indicates an occasional glass of wine or beer is dangerous, but complete abstinence is recommended.
- If you are concerned about your alcohol consumption, seek help from your doctor, Alcoholics Anonymous or other support groups.
- Get early and continuing prenatal care.

WHAT TO EXPECT

DIAGNOSTIC MEASURES
- There is no diagnostic test that can determine an infant born with fetal alcohol syndrome. Some defects will be apparent at the time of birth; other defects will show up later.
- The diagnosis is difficult to confirm once the child is older. The mother may not remember if she drank during pregnancy or how much she drank. The child's academic performance may be blamed on behavior problems.

APPROPRIATE HEALTH CARE
- For the pregnant woman—Get prenatal care.
- For the child—Early diagnosis and recognition of a child at risk. A referral to medical professionals who can start immediately on special programs designed to enhance motor skills, improve communication skills and develop social interactions.

POSSIBLE COMPLICATIONS—The defects are generally irreversible. The complications may be mild or severe and include one or several of the problems listed in Signs and Symptoms.

PROBABLE OUTCOME—Since the effects of fetal alcohol syndrome can vary a great deal, the outcome is unpredictable.

HOW TO TREAT

GENERAL MEASURES
- If you are pregnant and continuing to drink alcohol, call your doctor and discuss.
- If you know a family member or friend who is pregnant and continues to drink alcohol, talk to her about your concern and the risk she is taking with her unborn child.
- If you are the parent of a child with fetal alcohol syndrome, get the appropriate help needed for the child's development. Get help for yourself if the alcohol problem is continuing or if you need other psychological support.

MEDICATION—Medicine is usually not necessary for this disorder.

ACTIVITY—No restrictions.

DIET—No special diet.

CALL YOUR DOCTOR IF

- You are pregnant or think you might be pregnant and have not had a check-up.
- You are concerned about your newborn's behavior, physical development or appearance.

FEVER OF UNKNOWN ORIGIN

 GENERAL INFORMATION

DEFINITION—Prolonged temperature above 101F (38.3C) on at least four occasions over a 14 day period for which no cause is evident and illness of 14 days duration without an obvious cause.

BODY PARTS INVOLVED—Any body organs or system may be the source of a fever-producing condition.

SEX OR AGE MOST AFFECTED—Both sexes; all ages.

SIGNS & SYMPTOMS—Fever (measured rectally) for at least 2 weeks. Fever may be intermittent.

CAUSES
In infants and children:
- Infections.
- Collagen or autoimmune diseases.
- Tumors and cancer, especially leukemia.
In adults:
- Infections.
- Collagen or autoimmune diseases.
- Tumors and cancer, especially kidney cancer and leukemia.
- Self-induced in some psychologically unstable persons.
- Medications can cause fever as an adverse reaction.

RISK INCREASES WITH
- Poor nutrition.
- Illness that has lowered resistance.
- Chemical or environmental exposure to polluted water or air.
- Travel in areas with unsanitary conditions.
- Exposure to others with contagious diseases.
- Elderly person.
- People in AIDS risk group.
- Drug abuse.

HOW TO PREVENT—No specific preventive measures.

 WHAT TO EXPECT

DIAGNOSTIC MEASURES
- Your own observation of symptoms.
- Accurate daily temperature chart.
- Medical history and physical exam by a doctor.
- Because fever may be the first evidence of a serious condition (in its early stages), thorough diagnostic testing may be recommended. This may include laboratory studies, such as blood studies and a urine culture, x-rays of the chest, CT scan, ultrasound, echocardiogram (see Glossary for all), thyroid studies, liver function tests, HIV antibody test and others.

APPROPRIATE HEALTH CARE
- Self-care after diagnosis.
- Doctor's treatment.

POSSIBLE COMPLICATIONS—Depends on the underlying condition causing fever.

PROBABLE OUTCOME—Spontaneous recovery in about 10% of cases. In other cases, the outcome depends on successful detection and treatment of the underlying disorder.

 HOW TO TREAT

GENERAL MEASURES
- Until the fever's cause has been diagnosed, keep a daily temperature chart. Rectal temperatures are most accurate.
- Treatment will be determined by underlying cause that is found.

MEDICATION
- For minor discomfort, you may use nonprescription drugs such as acetaminophen. Until the underlying cause is determined, your doctor may withhold prescription drugs to avoid masking symptoms of the underlying disorder.
- Occasionally, in critically ill patients awaiting results of laboratory studies, the doctor may recommend a therapeutic trial of antibiotics or other drugs.

ACTIVITY—As tolerated. Encourage bed rest.

DIET—No special diet.

 CALL YOUR DOCTOR IF

- You have unexplained fever that lasts longer than 24 hours.
- New symptoms develop. They may provide a clue about the underlying cause of the fever.

FIBROCYSTIC BREAST DISEASE
(Chronic Cystic Mastitis; Benign Breast Lesions)

GENERAL INFORMATION

DEFINITION—A disorder of the female breast characterized by nonmalignant lumps. This condition is quite prevalent in women. The majority of these benign lesions are not associated with an increased risk of breast cancer.

BODY PARTS INVOLVED—Breasts.

SEX OR AGE MOST AFFECTED—Females from puberty to old age. This condition affects about 50-80% of women to some degree. It usually disappears after menopause unless estrogen-replacement therapy is used.

SIGNS & SYMPTOMS—Lumps in the breasts with the following characteristics:
- Lumps are usually on both sides. Solitary lumps may occur, but multiple lumps are common.
- Lumps offer resistance when pressed with fingertips; they may be tender.
- Lumps may be accompanied by generalized breast pain, especially before menstrual periods.
- Lumps often enlarge before menstrual periods and shrink afterward.
- Lumps come in different sizes. When the lumps are relatively large and near the surface, they can be moved freely within the breast.
- Nipple discharge.

CAUSES—Unknown, but probably related to estrogen and other hormones produced by the ovaries and possibly to dietary fat intake. Family history of cysts is common.

RISK INCREASES WITH
- Unknown.
- Some studies indicate that drinking coffee and smoking cigarettes are associated with a higher incidence and greater extent of fibrocystic breasts. Other studies have failed to show them as risk factors.

HOW TO PREVENT
- Until research is conclusive, avoid smoking and drinking coffee.
- Monthly breast self-examination to check breasts for lumps and changes in lumps after diagnosis. Report any changes to your doctor.
- Routine mammogram studies as recommended for your age group.

WHAT TO EXPECT

DIAGNOSTIC MEASURES
- Your own observation of symptoms.
- Medical history and physical exam by a doctor.

- Diagnostic tests including mammogram, ultrasound (useful for distinguishing cystic from solid lesion) and surgical diagnostic procedures such as biopsy or cyst aspiration (sometimes). (See Breast Biopsy by Incision and Breast Biopsy by Needle Aspiration in Surgery section.)

APPROPRIATE HEALTH CARE
- Monthly breast self-examination (see Appendix).
- Doctor's supervision.

POSSIBLE COMPLICATIONS—Some lumps appear benign but are cancerous. Diagnostic studies, including biopsy, are often necessary to rule out malignancy.

PROBABLE OUTCOME—Women with fibrocystic breast disease continue to have breast lumps that appear and dissolve; some remain permanently. The disorder is presently incurable, but normally does not jeopardize health.

HOW TO TREAT

GENERAL MEASURES
- Examine breasts carefully each month prior to or at the onset of menstruation. Report changes in lumps that have been diagnosed previously.
- Visit your doctor regularly (usually twice a year) for a breast exam or other studies, especially if you have a family history of cancer.

MEDICATION—Your doctor may prescribe:
- For pain, spironolactone and vitamin B-6 or iodine (kelp tablets).
- For severe disease, danazol or bromocriptine.
- Vitamin E (there is some evidence that it is beneficial).
- A mild diuretic for 7 to 10 days before menses may help some patients.

ACTIVITY—No restrictions. Regular exercise is important, but avoid activities that may cause trauma to the breasts.

DIET
- No special diet, but avoid smoking, caffeine, chocolate and other sweets, cola drinks.
- Control your weight (see Weight-Loss Diet in Appendix).

CALL YOUR DOCTOR IF

- You have undiagnosed lumps in the breast.
- You detect a change in a lump or new lumps appear.
- Nipple discharge appears.
- You have not had a breast exam in 2 years.
- New, unexplained symptoms develop. Hormones used in treatment may produce side effects.

FIBROID TUMORS OF THE UTERUS
(Myomas; Leiomyomas)

 GENERAL INFORMATION

DEFINITION—An abnormal, benign (noncancerous) growth of cells in the muscular wall of the uterus (myometrium). It is a common disorder in women. The term "fibroids" is misleading. The cells are not fibrous; they are composed of abnormal muscle cells. They can grow to the size of a cantaloupe.

BODY PARTS INVOLVED—Uterus; cervix (sometimes).

SEX OR AGE MOST AFFECTED—Fibroids affect 20% to 40% of all women over 35. They don't develop after menopause.

SIGNS & SYMPTOMS
- No symptoms (often).
- More frequent menstruation, frequently associated with large clots and discomfort.
- Increased menstrual flow and discomfort.
- Bleeding between periods.
- Painful sexual intercourse or bleeding after intercourse.
- Anemia (weakness, fatigue and paleness).
- Feelings of pressure on the urinary bladder or rectum.
- Increased vaginal discharge (rare).

CAUSES—Exact cause is unknown. Estrogen is required for their stimulation and growth, as they are rare in prepubertal girls or menopausal women.

RISK INCREASES WITH
- Use of oral contraceptives.
- Genetic factors. Fibroid tumors are 3 to 5 times more common in black women than Caucasian women.

HOW TO PREVENT—Cannot be prevented at present, but avoiding the use of oral contraceptives decreases risk of developing fibroids.

 WHAT TO EXPECT

DIAGNOSTIC MEASURES
- Your own observation of symptoms.
- Medical history and exam by a doctor.
- Laboratory studies, such as ultrasound, laparoscopy or hysterogram (see Glossary).

APPROPRIATE HEALTH CARE
- Self-care after diagnosis.
- Doctor's treatment.
- For minimal symptoms, no treatment may be needed and you will be re-examined in 3-6 months.
- Surgery may be recommended for certain situations and different surgical options are possible, depending on whether or not reproductivity is desired.

POSSIBLE COMPLICATIONS
- Complications can occur in pregnancy such as spontaneous abortion and premature labor.
- Fibroids may return following surgery to remove them.
- Malignant change in the fibroid tumor (occurs in less than 0.5%). This rare complication is usually signaled by very rapid growth.
- Fibroids are sometimes associated with decreased fertility.

PROBABLE OUTCOME—If surgery is not necessary prior to menopause, these tumors usually decrease in size without treatment after menopause.

Fibroids can often be removed surgically without removing the entire uterus. The ability to conceive continues as long as the uterus remains.

 HOW TO TREAT

GENERAL MEASURES
- Be sure you understand all the options concerning treatment and you decide with your doctor what you want to do.
- For minimal symptoms, no treatment may be needed and you will be re-examined in 3-6 months.
- Record dates of bleeding and number of pads used each day.

MEDICATION
- If you have a small fibroid, don't take contraceptive pills with a high estrogen content. Estrogen may cause fibroids to enlarge. Consider other forms of contraception, such as a diaphragm, cervical cap, IUD, condom or contraceptive foam, sponge or jelly.
- Danazol to stem heavy menstrual bleeding.
- Your doctor may prescribe:
  Iron supplements if you are anemic from excessive blood loss.
  A gonadotropin releasing hormone. It will induce an abrupt, artificial menopause that will stop the bleeding and reduce the size of the fibroid. Do not use for longer than 6 months.

ACTIVITY—No restrictions unless surgery performed. Then you may need bed rest for a period of time, some restricted activity and no sexual intercourse for approximately one month.

DIET—No special diet.

 CALL YOUR DOCTOR IF

- You have symptoms of a fibroid tumor.
- A fibroid tumor has been diagnosed, and symptoms become more severe.
- You saturate a pad or tampon more often than once an hour.

FIBROSITIS
(Fibromyositis; Fibromyalgia)

GENERAL INFORMATION

DEFINITION—Inflammation or pain of muscles, muscle sheaths and connective-tissue layers of tendons, muscles, bones and joints.

BODY PARTS INVOLVED—Muscular areas of the low back, neck, shoulder, chest, arms, hips and thighs.

SEX OR AGE MOST AFFECTED—Adults (usually begins between ages 30 and 60) and in women more often than men (ratio of 5 to 1).

SIGNS & SYMPTOMS
- Stiffness and weakness.
- Sudden, painful muscle spasms ("charley horse") that worsen with activity.
- Nodules or localized areas that are tender to the touch (trigger points).
- Painful muscle areas.
- Fatigue.
- Difficulty remaining asleep.

CAUSES—Unknown. Possibly an imbalance in brain chemicals or an autoimmune disorder. Until recently, this was thought to be a psychological disorder, but this is no longer the wide-spread belief. Research continues into the cause.

RISK INCREASES WITH
- Stress.
- Sleep disturbances.
- Muscle injury.
- Exposure to dampness or cold.
- Medical history of disorders that produce joint inflammation, such as rheumatoid arthritis or polyarteritis.
- Viral infections.
- Poor nutrition.
- Fatigue or overwork.

HOW TO PREVENT
- Avoid risk factors when possible.
- Get adequate sleep.
- General conditioning exercises.

WHAT TO EXPECT

DIAGNOSTIC MEASURES
- Your own observation of symptoms.
- Medical history and physical exam by a doctor.
- Laboratory blood studies to measure inflammation and tests to rule out rheumatoid arthritis or polymyalgia. There is no specific test for fibromyositis.

APPROPRIATE HEALTH CARE
- Self-care after diagnosis.
- Doctor's treatment.

POSSIBLE COMPLICATIONS
- Muscle atrophy, disability.
- Abuse of pain-killing medications.

PROBABLE OUTCOME—Spontaneous recovery in some persons. Other persons may have flare-ups and remissions indefinitely. The disease is uncomfortable, but not life-threatening. Symptoms can be controlled with treatment.

HOW TO TREAT

GENERAL MEASURES
- Heat relieves pain. Take hot showers, and let the water beat on painful areas. Use heat lamps, electric heating pads, whirlpool or plain tub baths and hot compresses.
- Have someone gently massage painful areas.
- Regular rest patterns may be helpful.
- Eliminate unnecessary stress in your life (see How to Cope with Stress in Appendix).
- Learn relaxation techniques.
- Biofeedback is helpful for some patients who use it to relax contracted muscles.
- Maintain your social life and contact with friends, even though the pain may be distracting at times.
- Surface electrical stimulation (TENS units) may be helpful.

MEDICATION
- For minor discomfort, you may use nonprescription drugs such as aspirin, acetaminophen or ibuprofen.
- Your doctor may prescribe:
  Cortisone injections into "trigger points."
  Nonsteroidal anti-inflammatory drugs.
  Antidepressants in low dosages and for short periods.

ACTIVITY
- Stay as active as possible, even when you are in pain. Stretching exercises may be helpful.
- General conditioning exercises are helpful.

DIET—No special diet, but avoid substances that interfere with sleep, such as caffeine and alcohol.

CALL YOUR DOCTOR IF

- You have symptoms of fibrositis that last more than 2 or 3 days.
- New, unexplained symptoms develop. Drugs used in treatment may produce side effects.

FIFTH DISEASE
(Erythema Infectiosum)

 GENERAL INFORMATION

DEFINITION—An infectious, mild, viral illness that occurs in localized outbreaks (often during the winter and spring months). The name comes from its position on a list developed in the early 1900s of childhood diseases.

SEX OR AGE MOST AFFECTED—Children and adolescents ages 5-14; rare in infants and adults.

SIGNS & SYMPTOMS
- Widespread rash—called "slapped cheeks appearance" because it starts as a rash on the cheeks. The rash then spreads to the trunk, buttocks and limbs, usually in a lacy pattern.
- Low-grade fever (sometimes).
- Slight tiredness or fatigue.
- Mild joint pain or swelling (in adults).
- Sometimes no symptoms are apparent (about 20% of patients).

CAUSES—A virus called human parvovirus B-19 spread by airborne particles. The incubation period is 4-14 days. Once the rash appears, the child is no linger infectious.

RISK INCREASES WITH—School and day care attendance.

HOW TO PREVENT—No preventive measures. Outbreaks can last for months, so keeping a child out of a school or day care where the infection has occurred will accomplish little. Infection provides future immunity.

 WHAT TO EXPECT

DIAGNOSTIC MEASURES
- Your own observation of the symptoms.
- Awareness of an outbreak in the school or community.
- Medical history and physical exam by a doctor (sometimes).

APPROPRIATE HEALTH CARE—Self-care after diagnosis.

POSSIBLE COMPLICATIONS
- None expected in the general population. In rare instances (patients with other disorders such as sickle cell anemia or the immunocompromised), fifth disease can cause a serious anemic reaction.
- In pregnant women there is a small risk of miscarriage if the woman is infected during the first 20 weeks of pregnancy. There is no evidence that fifth disease causes birth defects.

PROBABLE OUTCOME—Complete recovery. The rash usually clears in 10 days to 2 weeks.

 HOW TO TREAT

GENERAL MEASURES
- Use cool soaks if the rash itches.
- External factors such as sun exposure, bathing, excitement or exercise can cause the rash to redden or reappear weeks after the initial infection. This is no cause for concern.

MEDICATION
- There are no medicines for treating fifth disease. You may use acetaminophen for fever. Don't give a child younger than 18 aspirin for fever.
- If the rash itches, use plain calamine lotion.

ACTIVITY—Extra rest during symptomatic period.

DIET—No special diet. Drink plenty of fluids.

 CALL YOUR DOCTOR IF

- If you or your child has symptoms of fifth disease and you are concerned.
- Symptoms don't improve or worsen after self-care treatment.
- You are pregnant and have been exposed to fifth disease.

FOLLICULITIS

GENERAL INFORMATION

DEFINITION—Inflammation and infection of one or more hair follicles of the skin. This is contagious. It often spreads from one family member to another.

BODY PARTS INVOLVED—Skin anywhere on the body, but usually the exposed areas of arms, legs and beard area of the face.

SEX OR AGE MOST AFFECTED—Both sexes; all ages.

SIGNS & SYMPTOMS—Pustules (small white blisters with pus inside) with the following characteristics:
- Pustules are yellow-white and surrounded by narrow red rings.
- Pustules are 1mm to 2mm in size; there may be few or many.
- Pustules discharge a blood-stained pus made from dead cells.
- Some pustules are pierced by hair; others may be adjacent to hair follicles.

CAUSES
- Infection of the hair follicles with Staphylococcus bacteria or a fungus usually after minor skin injury. Infection spreads to other parts of the body by fingernails, frequently from Staphylococcus in the nose.
- Infection with Pseudomonas bacteria following the use of contaminated hot tubs or spas. This is rare but increasing.

RISK INCREASES WITH
- Abrasion, injury or surgical wound.
- Recent illness such as a nose infection.
- Diabetes.
- Eczema or dermatitis.
- Crowded or unsanitary living conditions.
- Inflammation or chronic skin abrasion (tight clothing or chronic rubbing).
- Hot tub exposure.

HOW TO PREVENT
- Keep skin clean. Scrub skin twice daily with an antibacterial soap. Use separate towels and washcloths.
- Avoid hot, humid environments, which foster bacterial growth.
- Treat family members who may be source of infection.

WHAT TO EXPECT

DIAGNOSTIC MEASURES
- Your own observation of symptoms.
- Medical history and physical exam by a doctor.
- Laboratory culture of the discharge from the pustule (rare).

APPROPRIATE HEALTH CARE
- Self-care after diagnosis.
- Doctor's treatment.

POSSIBLE COMPLICATIONS
- Boils (furuncles) or deep skin infections may develop (rare).
- This infection may enter the bloodstream and spread to other body parts.

PROBABLE OUTCOME— Without treatment, an individual pustule heals in 7 days but as some heal, new ones may appear. Treatment may shorten the course of the infection. Healing should be complete in 2 weeks, but may sometimes recur.

HOW TO TREAT

GENERAL MEASURES
- Don't scratch pustules. The germs that cause them can be transferred from under the fingernails to other parts of the body.
- Use warm-water soaks (see Soaks in Appendix) to relieve itching and hasten healing.
- Clean area with antibacterial soap.
- Avoid use of oils on the skin.
- If you shave, use a new blades each time.
- Shampoo daily if lesions are on scalp.

MEDICATION
- If there are only a few pustules, you may use nonprescription topical antibiotics, such as bacitracin, Mycitracin or neomycin. Apply and gently massage a small amount into the affected areas 3 or 4 times a day. Use only the small amount needed to cover—larger quantities don't help.
- Your doctor may prescribe antibiotics or antifungal medication.

ACTIVITY—No restrictions.

DIET—No special diet.

CALL YOUR DOCTOR IF

- The pustules spread, despite treatment.
- Symptoms of folliculitis recur after treatment.

FOOD ALLERGY & INTOLERANCE

 ## GENERAL INFORMATION

DEFINITION—Food allergy is an overreaction of the immune system to certain foods or substances that are otherwise harmless. These adverse reactions may be inborn or an acquired biochemical defect. Symptoms may occur within minutes or up to two hours after ingesting the food. In some instances, the symptoms may not appear until a day or two later.

Food intolerance is mainly from an unknown cause, but may be due to irritants, toxins or food additives. More people have food intolerances than true food allergies. With intolerance, a person may consume small amounts of the offending substance without symptoms, such as milk intolerance.

BODY PARTS INVOLVED—Skin, lungs, gastrointestinal, central nervous system.

SEX OR AGE MOST AFFECTED—Males more often than females; all ages; food allergies are more common in children.

SIGNS & SYMPTOMS
- Diarrhea or abdominal pain (common).
- Flatulence and bloating (common).
- Skin rash; hives; itching.
- Swelling of hands and feet or face and lips.
- Hay fever; cough or wheezing.
- Nausea and vomiting.
- Asthma.
- Migraine headache.
- Fainting or near-fainting.

CAUSES—Any food or swallowed substance can cause allergic reactions. Foods most often involved are cow's milk, egg whites, wheat, soybeans, peanut, fish, tree nuts (walnut and pecan), shellfish, melons, sesame seeds, sunflower seeds, chocolate.

RISK INCREASES WITH
- People who have other allergy problems.
- Having family members with a history of food allergy.

HOW TO PREVENT
- Identify responsible foods and avoid them. Keep a food diary.
- Breast-fed infants who are started on solid foods late tend to have fewer allergies.

 ## WHAT TO EXPECT

DIAGNOSTIC MEASURES
- Your own observation of symptoms.
- Medical history and exam by a doctor.
- Elimination diets for both diagnosis and treatment.
- Skin tests may help identify the offending food, but frequently give results indicating that you are allergic to certain foods when you aren't.

APPROPRIATE HEALTH CARE
- Self-care.
- Doctor's treatment (severe reactions).

POSSIBLE COMPLICATIONS
- Anaphylaxis (difficulty in breathing, heart irregularities, blood pressure drop).
- Hive-like reaction.
- Bronchial asthma.
- Bowel inflammation.
- Eczema-like lesions.

PROBABLE OUTCOME
- Infants will usually outgrow food hypersensitivity by 2-4 years of age.
- Adults with food hypersensitivity (particularly to milk, fish, shellfish or nuts) are more likely to maintain their allergy for many years.

 ## HOW TO TREAT

GENERAL MEASURES
- Eliminate the suspected foods from your diet for two weeks (or until all symptoms disappear) and then begin eating the foods again one by one to see if the symptoms return. Keep a diary and note the foods and any symptoms you feel.
- Patients with a severe allergy hypersensitivity to a food should be extra cautious in their avoidance of that food.
- Carry a kit with an adrenaline-containing syringe in case the offending food is eaten accidentally and a subsequent immediate reaction develops.
- Many fruit sensitive people may also have a reaction to latex (widely used in surgical gloves and medical devices as well as balloons, condoms, etc.) Advise any doctor or dentist about this reaction before any invasive medical procedure.
- Wear a Medic-Alert bracelet or pendant (see Glossary) that indicates your particular allergy.
- See Resources for Additional Information.

MEDICATION—No medication is available to treat food allergy, but medications may be prescribed to relieve some of the symptoms.

ACTIVITY—No restrictions.

DIET
- Avoidance of the offending food, or limiting yourself to small amounts of it. Read food labels.
- Maintain a nutritionally balanced diet.
- Ask your doctor about a more advanced elimination diet if symptoms don't improve.

 ## CALL YOUR DOCTOR IF

Someone appears to have a severe reaction after eating. Call for emergency help immediately.

FOOD POISONING

GENERAL INFORMATION

DEFINITION—A term commonly used to describe illnesses suspected of being caused by food contaminated with bacteria. It can affect several members of a household, multiple customers who dined at a particular restaurant, nursing home patients, or children in day care facility. In some cases, symptoms can begin within 1 hour of eating the contaminated foods, others may take 8-16 hours and some may not begin for 3-5 days. Symptoms similar to those caused by food poisoning can also be caused by viral gastroenteritis, emotional stress, food allergy, drugs, hepatitis, appendicitis or other disorders.

BODY PARTS INVOLVED—Gastrointestinal.

SEX OR AGE MOST AFFECTED—Both sexes; all ages.

SIGNS & SYMPTOMS
- Nausea and vomiting.
- Abdominal cramps or pain.
- Diarrhea (sometimes bloody).
- Fever.
- In severe cases, shock and collapse.

CAUSES—Bacterial organisms such as Salmonella, staphylococci, clostridia, Escherichia coli, Bacillus cereus and others. Botulism is a rare, life-threatening form of food poisoning.

RISK INCREASES WITH
- Eating food that is improperly prepared or stored.
- Lack of good hygiene when preparing food.
- Drinking water or eating raw foods when traveling in a foreign country.

HOW TO PREVENT
- Avoid raw seafood or meat.
- Don't consume raw or undercooked eggs.
- Avoid unpasteurized dairy products.
- Keep picnic foods cool, especially those made with mayonnaise.
- Proper cooking and storage of foods. Keeping food preparation areas, cutting boards and cooking utensils clean.
- Throwing out food items that are old, have an "off" smell, or those in bulging tin cans.
- Attention to handwashing before preparing food.

WHAT TO EXPECT

DIAGNOSTIC MEASURES
- Your own observation of symptoms.
- Medical history and exam by a doctor.
- Stool culture (sometimes).

APPROPRIATE HEALTH CARE
- Self-care.
- Doctor's treatment (sometimes).

POSSIBLE COMPLICATIONS
- Shock and collapse.
- Respiratory problems.
- Hospitalization may be required for a very young patient or an elderly debilitated patient.

PROBABLE OUTCOME—Most food poisoning is not serious and recovery generally occurs within 3 days.

HOW TO TREAT

GENERAL MEASURES
- Replacement of fluids and electrolytes is the most important aspect of treatment.
- If several persons are affected, local health departments should be contacted so they can interview patients and food handlers and take samples of suspected contaminated food.

MEDICATION
- Medications usually not prescribed for this disorder. You may take take acetaminophen for fever.
- If symptoms are severe (protracted vomiting, painful abdominal cramps) and the causative agent is known, antibiotics may be prescribed.

ACTIVITY—Bed rest during acute phase. Convenient access to a bathroom or bedpan is important.

DIET
- Liquid diet using commercial rehydration preparations, clear broth or bouillon. Use salt and sugar in liquids to replace what was lost. Try to take small sips even if vomiting continues. This will help with volume replacement and oral rehydration.
- Progress to soft, bland diet. Return to regular diet gradually.

CALL YOUR DOCTOR IF

- You or a family member has signs or symptoms of food poisoning and symptoms continue after self-care.
- Symptoms worsen after treatment begins. Hospitalization may be required to prevent dehydration.

ILLNESS & DISORDERS

FROSTBITE

GENERAL INFORMATION

DEFINITION—Temporary or permanent tissue damage from exposure to subfreezing temperature.

BODY PARTS INVOLVED—Arms and legs (especially fingers and toes); face (especially nose and ears).

SEX OR AGE MOST AFFECTED—Both sexes; all ages.

SIGNS & SYMPTOMS
During exposure:
- Gradual numbness, hardness and paleness in the affected area.
- Whiteness or yellowness of the skin.

Upon rewarming:
- Pain and tingling or burning (sometimes severe) in the affected area, with color change from white to red, then purple.
- Blisters (severe cases).
- Shivering.
- Slurred speech.
- Memory loss.

CAUSES—Blood flow to the outer area of the body decreases when exposed to cold (the body tries to protect vital, internal organs). As a result, skin tissue freezes and dies because of the lack of a warm blood supply.

RISK INCREASES WITH
- Diabetes mellitus.
- Blood-vessel disease such as Raynaud's phenomena.
- Peripheral neuropathy.
- Smoking.
- Excess alcohol consumption.
- Windy weather, which increases the chill factor.
- Elderly.

HOW TO PREVENT
- Anticipate sudden temperature changes and carry a jacket, gloves, socks, hat and scarf.
- Don't drink or smoke prior to anticipated exposure.

WHAT TO EXPECT

DIAGNOSTIC MEASURES
- Your own observation of symptoms.
- Medical history and exam by a doctor.
- X-rays of damaged areas.

APPROPRIATE HEALTH CARE
- Doctor's treatment.
- Hospitalization (sometimes).
- Cautious rewarming; continuous temperature monitoring.
- Surgery to remove permanently damaged (gangrenous) tissue (sometimes).

POSSIBLE COMPLICATIONS
- Gangrene.
- Amputation of dead or infected tissue, especially fingers, toes, nose or ears, following severe exposure.
- Cardiac arrest, if frostbite is accompanied by total body hypothermia.

PROBABLE OUTCOME—For mild cases, full recovery is possible with treatment. You may be sensitive to cold and experience burning and tingling. Healing process may take 6 to 12 months. Severe cases often require amputation of the affected part.

HOW TO TREAT

GENERAL MEASURES—The following instructions apply to emergency care until medical care is available:
- Upon reaching shelter, remove clothing from the frostbitten parts.
- Never massage damaged tissue.
- Immerse the affected parts in warm water (about 100F or 37.8C). Use a thermometer, if available. Higher temperatures may cause further injury. Pat the skin dry.
- Drink warm fluids with a high sugar content.
- Don't smoke.
- After rewarming, cover the affected areas with soft cloth bandages.
- Don't use affected limbs until you have medical care (if feet are involved, don't walk).
- Maintain skin-to-skin contact with any companion.

MEDICATION
- Your doctor may prescribe:
  Warm intravenous fluids and heated oxygen.
  Analgesics, including narcotics, to relieve severe pain.
  Antibiotics to fight infection.
  Antitetanus toxoid.
- You may use nonprescription drugs, such as acetaminophen, for minor pain.

ACTIVITY—Physical therapy may be required after healing progresses sufficiently.

DIET—Whatever is tolerated. Warm fluids to start with.

CALL YOUR DOCTOR IF

- You have symptoms of frostbite or observe them in someone else.
- The following occurs during treatment:
  Increased pain, swelling, redness or drainage at the site of injury.
  Fever, muscle aches, dizziness or a general ill feeling.
- New, unexplained symptoms develop. Drugs used in treatment may produce side effects.

GALLSTONES
(Cholelithiasis)

GENERAL INFORMATION

DEFINITION—Stones in the gallbladder (the organ under the liver that stores bile). Most gallstones are composed primarily of cholesterol, others contain bile pigment or calcium. They are not cancerous.

BODY PARTS INVOLVED—Gallbladder; bile ducts.

SEX OR AGE MOST AFFECTED—Adolescents and adults of both sexes, but more common in women. 10% of the U.S. population—and 20% of those over 40—have gallstones.

SIGNS & SYMPTOMS
- Colicky (severe, spasmodic) pain in the upper right abdomen or between the shoulder blades.
- Nausea and vomiting.
- Bloating or belching.
- Intolerance for fatty foods (indigestion, bloating and belching).
- Jaundice.
- No symptoms in about 40% of cases.

CAUSES
- Failure of the gallbladder to empty competently.
- Alterations in bile mucus.
- Increased bilirubin concentration in bile. (Bilirubin is a yellowish, red-blood-cell waste product in bile that the blood carries to the liver. It contributes to urine's yellowish color and can cause jaundice if it builds up in the blood.)
- Infection in the tubes that carry bile out of the liver.

RISK INCREASES WITH
- Recent illness, such as coronary artery disease, cirrhosis of the liver or disorder of the small intestine.
- Family history of gallstones.
- Genetic factors. Some ethnic groups are more susceptible.
- Obesity.
- Excess alcohol consumption.
- Oral contraceptives and estrogen replacement therapy.
- High fat, low fiber diet.
- Rapid weight loss.
- Women who have had many children.
- Smoking.

HOW TO PREVENT—Avoid risk factors where possible.

WHAT TO EXPECT

DIAGNOSTIC MEASURES
- Your own observation of symptoms.
- Medical history and physical exam by a doctor.
- Laboratory studies, such as: blood count; blood chemistry; CT scan; cholecystography and ultrasound (see Glossary for all).

APPROPRIATE HEALTH CARE
- Self-care.
- Doctor's treatment.
- Surgery to remove the gallbladder and stones in the bile ducts may be needed for patients with severe symptoms. Laparoscopic cholecystectomy is usually the preferred procedure (see Gallbladder Removal in Surgery section).
- Shockwave (lithotripsy) treatment to break up (shatter) the stones may be recommended in some cases.

POSSIBLE COMPLICATIONS—Infection or rupture of the gallbladder.

PROBABLE OUTCOME—Many persons with gallstones have no symptoms. For those who do, the disorder is curable with surgery.

HOW TO TREAT

GENERAL MEASURES
- If you know you have gallstones and experience pain in the upper right abdomen, apply heat to the area. If pain worsens or continues more than 3 hours, call your doctor.
- See Resources for Additional Information.

MEDICATION
- For minor discomfort, you may use nonprescription drugs such as acetaminophen.
- Oral medication to try to dissolve stones. This treatment is used for certain types of stones and can take up to two years.

ACTIVITY—No restrictions, except to rest during attacks of gallbladder colic.

DIET
- During an attack, sip water occasionally, but don't eat.
- Eat a low-fat diet (see Low-Fat Diet in Appendix). Fatty meals may bring on mild attacks.
- If you are overweight, begin a weight reduction program (see Weight-Loss Diet in Appendix).

CALL YOUR DOCTOR IF

- You have symptoms of gallstones.
- Fever rises to 101F (38.3C).
- Pain occurs that lasts for more than 3 hours.

GANGRENE

GENERAL INFORMATION

DEFINITION—Dead tissue. Gangrene develops when a wound becomes infected or tissue is destroyed by an accident. It can involve any body part, but the most common sites are toes, feet, legs, fingers, hands and arms. There are two types, dry gangrene where there is no bacterial infection and wet gangrene when a wound becomes infected with bacteria. The term gas gangrene pertains to a form of wet gangrene.

BODY PARTS INVOLVED—Any body part, but the most common sites are toes, feet, legs, fingers, hands and arms. The most dangerous sites are abdominal organs.

SEX OR AGE MOST AFFECTED—Both sexes; all ages.

SIGNS & SYMPTOMS
- Black skin with dead underlying muscle and bone.
- Crepitation of the skin. This feels like pressing on air bubbles under the skin.
- Swelling.
- Severe abdominal pain.
- Pain or loss of sensation in affected area.
- Bad-smelling discharge from ulcers in dead tissues.
- Moderate fever up to 101F (38.3C).

CAUSES—Gangrene occurs when blood flow to a body part is blocked or severely reduced. The following may interrupt blood flow and cause gangrene:
- Infection with clostridia perfringens germs.
- Tissue injury caused by accidents, surgery or deep puncture wounds.
- Crushing injury that cuts off blood supply.
- Blood clot in artery or hardening of arteries.
- Prolonged frostbite.
- Ruptured appendix or gallbladder.
- Herniated bowel.
- Burning by heat or acid.

RISK INCREASES WITH
- Diabetes mellitus.
- Smoking, which impairs blood circulation.
- Excess alcohol consumption, which interferes with blood-vessel function.
- Poor blood circulation; older age.
- Raynaud's phenomenon; Buerger's disease.

HOW TO PREVENT
- If you have diabetes, adhere closely to your treatment program to control diabetes. Examine your feet often for signs of unhealthy tissue. Keep your nails trimmed. Wear comfortable, well-fitting shoes.
- Burned skin requires careful, antiseptic handling to avoid infection.
- Handle frostbitten skin with great care.

- Consult your doctor for signs of infection (warmth, swelling, redness, pain or tenderness) in a skin injury.
- Avoid trauma.
- Don't smoke.

WHAT TO EXPECT

DIAGNOSTIC MEASURES
- Medical history and exam by a doctor.
- Cultures from the gangrene site or blood.
- X-rays of any suspicious area to detect gas in tissues.

APPROPRIATE HEALTH CARE
- Doctor's treatment and hospitalization.
- Surgery to remove dead tissue, sometimes by amputation; surgery for abdominal organs.
- Physical therapy, if amputation is necessary.

POSSIBLE COMPLICATIONS
- Blood poisoning or shock.
- DIC (disseminated intravascular coagulation), a blood-clotting disorder.
- Limb amputation to prevent death.
- Death, if not diagnosed in abdominal organs.

PROBABLE OUTCOME—Usually curable in the early stages with antibiotic treatment and surgery to remove dead tissue. Without treatment, gangrene may lead to fatal infection.

HOW TO TREAT

GENERAL MEASURES—The family should maintain an optimistic outlook, stay in close contact with the patient's doctor and help by making their visits with the patient as supportive as possible.

MEDICATION—Your doctor may prescribe:
- Antibiotics—usually intravenously in the early stages—to fight infection.
- Pain relievers.
- Anticoagulants to prevent blood clotting.

ACTIVITY
- Rest in bed until gangrene stops progressing and healing begins. Then resume activity gradually.
- Physical therapy, if amputation is necessary.

DIET
- Eat a high-protein, high-calorie diet while your body is repairing damaged tissue.
- Take vitamin and mineral supplements, including zinc. Ask your doctor for advice.
- Drink adequate fluids (6 to 8 glasses daily).

CALL YOUR DOCTOR IF

- You have symptoms of gangrene.
- You have persistent pain, despite treatment.
- Fever develops during convalescence.

GASTRIC EROSION

 GENERAL INFORMATION

DEFINITION—A slight break (ulceration) in the innermost layer (mucosa) of the stomach's lining. If an ulceration extends deeper than this layer, it is called a gastric ulcer. Erosions are not contagious or cancerous.

BODY PARTS INVOLVED—Stomach.

SEX OR AGE MOST AFFECTED—All ages, but most common in men.

SIGNS & SYMPTOMS
- Often there are no symptoms.
- Vomiting blood. Blood may be bright red or resemble black coffee grounds.
- Blood in stool. Blood will appear black or tarry.

CAUSES—Probably caused by drugs that irritate the stomach lining. Most likely drugs are: alcohol; caffeine; tobacco; aspirin; nonsteroidal anti-inflammatory drugs used to treat arthritis and gout; and cortisone drugs used to treat asthma, Addison's disease or other conditions.

RISK INCREASES WITH
- Stress.
- Use of any oral medication.
- Serious illness.
- Growth of a specific bacteria, Helicobacter pylori, in the stomach.

HOW TO PREVENT
- Don't take medicines without enteric (protective) coatings if possible.
- Don't drink alcohol if you have had gastric erosion. It may trigger bleeding.

 WHAT TO EXPECT

DIAGNOSTIC MEASURES
- Your own observation of symptoms.
- Medical history and physical exam by a doctor.
- Laboratory studies of stool and blood tests for anemia.
- X-rays of the upper digestive tract.

APPROPRIATE HEALTH CARE
- Self-care after diagnosis.
- Doctor's treatment.

POSSIBLE COMPLICATIONS—Bleeding is an uncommon but dangerous complication, especially in the elderly. Another major complication is perforation, in which the erosion penetrates the stomach wall. Surgery is necessary to correct either complication. It involves little risk except for those over 70 years of age.

PROBABLE OUTCOME—Curable in 2 weeks with treatment if the cause is eliminated. Recurrence is common.

 HOW TO TREAT

GENERAL MEASURES
- Check your stool every day for signs of bleeding. If the stool is black, remove a stool portion from the toilet bowl and take it to your doctor's office for examination.
- Avoid stressful situations (see How to Cope with Stress in Appendix).
- Don't smoke or drink alcoholic beverages.

MEDICATION
- Your doctor may prescribe:
  H-2 blockers to reduce production of stomach acid.
  Ulcer-healing drugs such as cimetidine, ranitidine or famotidine.
- For minor pain, you may use nonprescription antacids.

ACTIVITY—Resume normal activities as soon as symptoms improve.

DIET—Avoid hot and spicy foods. Eat small frequent meals for 2 weeks. Don't drink alcohol.

 CALL YOUR DOCTOR IF

- You have signs of bleeding described in Signs & Symptoms.
- You develop diarrhea. This may represent an adverse reaction to drugs used in treatment. The prescription may need adjustment.
- You have severe pain that is not relieved by treatment.
- You are unusually weak, pale or lightheaded.
- Symptoms of gastric erosion recur after treatment.

GASTRITIS

GENERAL INFORMATION

DEFINITION—Mild irritation, inflammation, erosion or infection of the stomach lining. The illness may be acute, occurring as a sudden attack, or chronic, developing gradually over a long period of time. Gastritis is part of a spectrum of diseases that include erosion and gastric ulcer.

BODY PARTS INVOLVED—Stomach.

SEX OR AGE MOST AFFECTED—Both sexes; all ages.

SIGNS & SYMPTOMS
- Abdominal pain and cramps.
- Vomiting (occasionally).
- Appetite loss.
- Fever (rare).
- Weakness.
- Swollen abdomen.
- Sharp, dull or annoying pain in the chest.
- Acid taste in the mouth.
- Mild nausea and diarrhea (rare).
- Belching or gas.

CAUSES
- Excess stomach acid caused by heavy drinking, smoking or overeating (especially foods you don't digest easily).
- Virus infection. This form may be contagious.
- Adverse reaction to alcohol, caffeine or drugs.
- Unknown (sometimes).

RISK INCREASES WITH
- Stress, including surgery and hospitalization for other problems.
- Improper diet.
- Illness that has lowered resistance.
- Smoking.
- Use of drugs, such as aspirin, nonsteroidal anti-inflammatories, cortisone, caffeine and many more.
- Excess alcohol consumption.
- Fatigue or overwork.
- The presence of a bacteria, Helicobacter pylori, in the stomach.

HOW TO PREVENT
- Eat and drink moderately.
- Don't skip meals or eat irregularly.
- Avoid foods you find hard to digest.
- Don't smoke.
- Discuss with your doctor all medicines you take. Avoid medicines that irritate your stomach, if possible.

WHAT TO EXPECT

DIAGNOSTIC MEASURES
- Your own observation of symptoms.
- Medical history and physical exam by a doctor.
- Diagnosis is made by examining the stomach through a gastroscope (a viewing tube passed down the esophagus to the stomach). A small amount of tissue may be removed for a biopsy (see Glossary).

APPROPRIATE HEALTH CARE
- Self-care.
- Doctor's treatment.
- Hospitalization may be required if excessive bleeding occurs.

POSSIBLE COMPLICATIONS—Bleeding is an uncommon but dangerous complication, especially in the elderly.

PROBABLE OUTCOME—Usually curable in several days if the cause is eliminated.

HOW TO TREAT

GENERAL MEASURES
- Consider lifestyle changes if they are contributing to symptoms.
- Stop smoking. Consult your doctor about recommendations for a cessation program.

MEDICATION
- For minor discomfort, you may use nonprescription antacids or H-2 blockers such as cimetidine, famotidine, etc. Don't use aspirin.
- Your doctor may prescribe additional medication such as ulcer-healing drugs, depending on the cause of your gastritis.

ACTIVITY—Resume normal activities as soon as symptoms improve.

DIET—Don't eat solid food on the first day of the attack. Drink liquids frequently, preferably milk or water. Resume a normal diet slowly, but avoid hot and spicy foods until symptoms disappear.

CALL YOUR DOCTOR IF

- You vomit blood.
- Bowel movements become black or tarry.
- Pain becomes severe.
- Signs of dehydration, such as a dry mouth, wrinkled skin, excess thirst or decreased urination, develop.

GASTROENTERITIS
("Stomach Flu"; "Intestinal Flu")

 GENERAL INFORMATION

DEFINITION—Irritation and infection of the digestive tract that can often cause sudden and sometimes violent upsets. Gastroenteritis is a generic term and often is used when there is a nonspecific, uncertain or unknown cause. Infectious causes can be spread by contact with an infected person or consumption of contaminated food or water.

BODY PARTS INVOLVED—Stomach; small intestine; colon.

SEX OR AGE MOST AFFECTED—All ages, but most severe in young children (1 to 5 years) and adults over 60.

SIGNS & SYMPTOMS
• Nausea; vomiting.
• Diarrhea that ranges from 2 or 3 loose stools to many watery stools.
• Abdominal cramps, pain or tenderness.
• Appetite loss; fever; weakness.
• Headache; loss of appetite.

CAUSES
• A viral infection is the most common cause. Types includes Norwalk virus (second only to the common cold in prevalence of viral infections), rotavirus (causes about 50% of diarrheal illnesses among infants and children), adenovirus and enterovirus.
• Bacterial or parasitic infection.
• Food poisoning (see in Illness section).
• Food allergy (see in Illness section).
• Excess alcohol consumption.
• Use of drugs, such as aspirin, nonsteroidal anti-inflammatories, antibiotics, harsh laxatives, cortisone or caffeine.

RISK INCREASES WITH
• Adults over 60.
• Newborns and infants.
• Travel to foreign countries.

HOW TO PREVENT
• There are no specific preventive measures. If you or someone around you has symptoms of gastroenteritis, be extra careful about personal hygiene. Wash hands frequently.
• Medical researchers are experimenting with various vaccines that may be effective against some viruses.

 WHAT TO EXPECT

DIAGNOSTIC MEASURES
• Medical history and exam by a doctor.
• Laboratory studies, such as blood counts and stool studies (sometimes.)

APPROPRIATE HEALTH CARE
• Self-care.
• Doctor's treatment (sometimes).
• Hospitalization, if dehydration is severe.

POSSIBLE COMPLICATIONS—Serious dehydration that requires intravenous fluids.

PROBABLE OUTCOME—Vomiting and diarrhea usually disappear in 2 to 5 days, but adults may feel weak, fatigued and depressed for about 1 week.

 HOW TO TREAT

GENERAL MEASURES
• It is not necessary to isolate persons with gastroenteritis.
• Supportive care is the most important aspect of treatment (rest, fluids, close proximity to bathroom or bedpan).
• Consult your doctor if you are a breast-feeding mother and your infant has gastroenteritis.

MEDICATION—Medicine is usually not necessary. If gastroenteritis is severe or prolonged, your doctor may prescribe antinausea and antidiarrhea medication. Antibiotics do not help.

ACTIVITY—Rest in bed until nausea, vomiting, diarrhea and fever are gone.

DIET
• Suck ice chips or drink small amounts of clear fluids frequently.
• Replace lost fluids and electrolytes with commercial products such as Pedialyte or Ricelyte for infants and children; diluted rehydration fluids (Gatorade) for adults.
• After diarrhea and vomiting stop, drink small amounts of clear liquids, such as tea, "flat" ginger ale or lemon-lime soda, broth and gelatin.
• If you tolerate liquids for 12 hours, eat small amounts of soft foods, such as cooked cereal, rice, eggs, custard, baked potato and yogurt.
• If you tolerate soft food for 2 or 3 days, gradually return to a normal diet.

 CALL YOUR DOCTOR IF

• Symptoms of gastroenteritis persist longer than 2 to 3 days.
• The following occurs during treatment:
Mucus or blood in the stool.
Fever of 101F (38.3C) or higher.
Abdominal swelling.
Severe pain in the abdomen or rectum, especially pain that begins in the center and moves to the lower right side.
• Signs of dehydration develop.

ILLNESS & DISORDERS

GASTROESOPHAGEAL REFLUX DISEASE
(Heartburn; GERD)

 GENERAL INFORMATION

DEFINITION—A reflux (backward or return flow) of fluid of gastric or intestinal contents into the esophagus. Normally, the esophagus transports food from the pharynx to the stomach by coordinated contractions. Heartburn (pyrosis) is a symptom of this disorder, not a disease, and has nothing to do with the heart.

BODY PARTS INVOLVED—Gastrointestinal.

SEX OR AGE MOST AFFECTED—All ages, but most common in adults over 60.

SIGNS & SYMPTOMS—The following signs may range from mild to severe, infrequent or chronic, and are often worse at night:
• Regurgitation of stomach contents into the mouth, producing an acid taste; belching.
• Sensations of heaviness, warmth, burning or uncomfortable feeling in the chest.
• Swallowing difficulty.
• Mild abdominal pain or vomiting (rarely).

CAUSES—The lower esophageal sphincter that closes off the upper stomach becomes lax, allowing stomach juices to enter the esophagus and irritate its lining. Causes may include:
• Hiatal hernia (part of stomach protrudes into the chest).
• Pregnancy.
• Scleroderma.
• Ulcer or tumor of the esophagus.
• Delayed gastric emptying.

RISK INCREASES WITH
• Stress; improper diet; overeating, hurried eating, improper chewing.
• Obesity.
• Smoking.
• Excess alcohol consumption.
• Naps after meals; squatting, bending or lifting with a full stomach.
• Use of some medications that can lower the pressure of the lower esophageal sphincter.
• Chest trauma.
• Consumption of coffee.

HOW TO PREVENT
Preventing gastroesophageal reflux disease:
• No specific measures.
Preventing symptoms:
• Avoid smoking.
• Don't bend over, lie down or exercise immediately after eating.
• Don't wear tight, restrictive clothing.
• Elevate the head of the bed 4 to 6 inches with blocks.
• Follow instructions under Diet.
• Lose weight if you are overweight.
• Talk to your doctor about any drugs you take that could cause the problem.

 WHAT TO EXPECT

DIAGNOSTIC MEASURES
• Medical history and exam by a doctor.
• Sometimes tests are done to rule out other disorders. Blood studies, ECG to exclude chance of heart disease; endoscopy, biopsy (see Glossary for all), x-rays of the upper digestive tract.

APPROPRIATE HEALTH CARE
• Self-care; doctor's treatment.
• Antireflux surgery for severe cases.

POSSIBLE COMPLICATIONS—Peptic or gastric ulcer. Stomach acids can damage the esophagus.

PROBABLE OUTCOME—Symptoms can be controlled but recurrence is common.

 HOW TO TREAT

GENERAL MEASURES—The symptoms usually begin within about an hour after eating and may continue for several hours. Usually no medical care is necessary. Self-treatment with antacids and taking preventive measures should control the symptoms.

MEDICATION
• For minor discomfort, you may use nonprescription liquid antacids. These coat the inside of the esophagus and neutralize stomach acid. Pregnant women should not take any drugs without doctor's approval.
• You may use H-2 blockers such as cimetidine, famotidine, ranitidine, etc. Your doctor may prescribe a proton pump inhibitor, such as lansporazole, omeprazole, or pantoprazole.
• Avoid aspirin and other nonsteroidal anti-inflammatory drugs. They irritate stomach lining.

ACTIVITY—Resume normal activities as soon as symptoms subside.

DIET
• Avoid foods and beverages that stimulate heavy stomach-acid secretion, such as spicy dishes, coffee, citrus fruit juice, alcohol, chocolate or peppermint, and reduce your consumption of high-fat foods.
• Eat small, frequent meals, 4 or 5 a day.
• Don't eat close to bedtime.
• Lose weight, if you are overweight (see Weight-Loss Diet in Appendix).

 CALL YOUR DOCTOR IF

• Swallowing becomes more difficult.
• You regurgitate blood.
• Symptoms continue despite self-care.

GENITOURINARY INJURY
(Bladder Injury; Kidney Injury; Urethra Injury; Ureter Injury; Penis or Testis Injury)

 GENERAL INFORMATION

DEFINITION—Injury to a part of the genitourinary tract that may result from a variety of causes.

BODY PARTS INVOLVED—Kidney (organ that filters the blood and excretes waste products); bladder (the organ that stores urine); ureter (two tubes that carry urine from the kidneys to the bladder); urethra (the tube through which urine travels from the bladder to the outside); penis; scrotum.

SEX OR AGE MOST AFFECTED—Both sexes; all ages.

SIGNS & SYMPTOMS
- Severe abdominal pain.
- Shock (sweating; faintness; nausea; panting; rapid pulse; pale, cold, moist skin).
- Painful urination or inability to urinate.
- Pain or tenderness in the back, just below the ribs on the injured side.
- Fever (sometimes).
- Blood in the urine.
If you have severe pain with large amounts of blood in your urine, one or both kidneys may be seriously injured.

CAUSES—Forceful or penetrating blow or wound to lower abdomen (gunshot or stab wounds, pelvic surgery, pelvic fracture, straddle injuries, kicks, penis amputation).

RISK INCREASES WITH
- Excess alcohol consumption.
- Hazardous occupations.
- Motor vehicle accidents.
- Sexually abused children.
- Medical treatments including surgery, shock waves, laser therapy, instrument use, radiation.
- Physical combat or physical violence.
- Penile rings.
- Excessive trauma during intercourse or other sexual activity.

HOW TO PREVENT
- Protect yourself from injury whenever possible.
- Buckle your automobile seat belt to minimize internal injury in case of accident.
- Don't drink and drive.
- Avoid alcohol or limit amount you consume.

 WHAT TO EXPECT

DIAGNOSTIC MEASURES
- Your own observation of symptoms.
- Medical history and physical exam by a doctor.
- Laboratory urine studies.
- X-rays of the urinary tract, intravenous urography, cystography (see Glossary for both).

APPROPRIATE HEALTH CARE
- Doctor's treatment.
- Hospitalization; emergency care.
- Surgery to repair any wounds, control bleeding and repair damage to the organs involved. A temporary catheter may be necessary for urinary drainage while the body heals.
- Injury to external male genitalia may require skin grafts.
- An amputated penis may be re-implanted using microsurgical techniques.

POSSIBLE COMPLICATIONS
- Internal bleeding.
- Urine leakage into the abdomen, causing abdominal inflammation or infection.
- Recurrent infections from scars in the urethra that narrow the urinary passage.
- Scarring and narrowing of the injured ureter.
- Atrophy of testes following a rupture injury.

PROBABLE OUTCOME—A genitourinary tract injury usually requires emergency treatment. Most cases heal with bed rest, time, supportive treatment or surgery.

 HOW TO TREAT

GENERAL MEASURES—No specific instructions except those under other headings.

MEDICATION—Your doctor may prescribe:
- Antibiotics to prevent infection.
- Pain medicine as required.
- Anticholinergics for spasms.

ACTIVITY—Stay as active as your strength allows. Allow 1 month for recovery. Don't return to work or resume sexual relations until healing is complete.

DIET
- No special diet.
- Drink 6 to 8 glasses of fluid daily.
- Don't drink alcohol.

 CALL YOUR DOCTOR IF

- You have any symptoms of genitourinary injury.
- During or after treatment, you develop fever and chills.
- New, unexplained symptoms develop. Drugs used in treatment may produce side effects.

GIARDIASIS

GENERAL INFORMATION

DEFINITION—Bowel infection caused by a parasite found in contaminated water. It is becoming increasingly common among day care and preschool children.

BODY PARTS INVOLVED—Gastrointestinal tract, especially the small bowel.

SEX OR AGE MOST AFFECTED—All ages, but most common in children.

SIGNS & SYMPTOMS
- Often no symptoms are present.
- Sudden diarrhea and abdominal cramping. Some persons have only mild diarrhea and indigestion.
- Loose, bulky, bad-smelling stools.
- Slight fever (uncommon).
- Weight loss.
- Occasionally persistent symptoms over weeks and months.

CAUSES—Infestation by a microscopic parasite, giardia lamblia. Giardia parasites enter the body through food or water and multiply in the small intestine. Local inflammation, causing diarrhea and other symptoms, occurs in 1 to 3 weeks.

RISK INCREASES WITH
- Crowded or unsanitary living conditions, especially a substandard water supply and poor sanitation system.
- Drinking stream water while camping.
- Previous stomach surgery. Stomach acid normally provides some protection against this infection.
- Oral-anal sexual practices.
- Day care centers; preschools.
- Institutional living.

HOW TO PREVENT
- Boil water that is not known to be safe or treat it with commercial chemical purifiers.
- Avoid uncooked foods that may have been rinsed in contaminated water.
- Wash hands often, especially before meals, to avoid catching infection from other persons.
- Isolate children until infection has cleared.

WHAT TO EXPECT

DIAGNOSTIC MEASURES
- Your own observation of symptoms.
- Medical history and physical exam by a doctor. Tell your doctor if you have been traveling or camping in the previous month.
- Laboratory stool studies to detect parasites. May need to be repeated if early studies are negative. Antibody tests may soon be available.
- Since stool examinations are frequently false-positive, your doctor may treat on the basis of clinical history and examination.

APPROPRIATE HEALTH CARE
- Home-care.
- Doctor's treatment.
- Hospitalization may be required for patients with severe diarrhea to replace lost fluids.

POSSIBLE COMPLICATIONS
- Malabsorption and weight loss.
- Dehydration.

PROBABLE OUTCOME—Spontaneous recovery in about 1 month for most persons. Medication hastens recovery.

HOW TO TREAT

GENERAL MEASURES
- Prevention is the best treatment. Be cautious when away from normal water supplies.
- Practice careful personal hygiene if you have diarrhea or are around those who do.

MEDICATION
- Don't use nonprescription drugs for gastrointestinal problems. These can mask symptoms.
- Your doctor may prescribe an antiparasitic drug such as quinacrine or metronidazole. Alcohol interacts with metronidazole to cause abdominal cramps and nausea, so don't drink alcohol during treatment.

ACTIVITY—No restrictions.

DIET—Maintain an adequate fluid intake (at least 8 glasses of water or liquid a day).

☎ CALL YOUR DOCTOR IF

- You have symptoms of giardiasis.
- New, unexplained symptoms develop. Drugs used in treatment may produce side effects.

GILBERT'S SYNDROME
(Hyperbilirubinemia)

 GENERAL INFORMATION

DEFINITION—Increased blood levels of bilirubin (a yellow chemical byproduct of red-blood-cell breakdown). This is not a disease; rather it is a normal variant and is usually an incidental finding of routine testing.

BODY PARTS INVOLVED—Blood.

SEX OR AGE MOST AFFECTED—Both sexes and all ages, but most common in men between ages 20 and 45.

SIGNS & SYMPTOMS
- Usually there are no symptoms.
- Rarely, a slight jaundice (yellow skin and eyes), tiredness, appetite loss or upper abdominal pain may occur.

CAUSES—The liver is inefficient in changing bilirubin to bile, leaving above-normal levels of bilirubin in the blood. If blood levels are high enough, jaundice may appear. Any liver abnormality associated with this disorder is minor.

RISK INCREASES WITH—None known; sufferers are otherwise healthy.

HOW TO PREVENT—No specific preventive measures.

 WHAT TO EXPECT

DIAGNOSTIC MEASURES
- Your own observation of symptoms (sometimes). The minor jaundice may be unnoticeable.
- Medical history and physical exam by a doctor.
- Laboratory blood studies of bilirubin and liver function.

APPROPRIATE HEALTH CARE—None necessary.

POSSIBLE COMPLICATIONS—No known complications.

PROBABLE OUTCOME—The condition is harmless.

 HOW TO TREAT

GENERAL MEASURES—If you or others notice a yellowing of your eyes or skin—it may seem like a good suntan—see your doctor for a diagnosis. Some more serious conditions also begin with mild jaundice.

MEDICATION—Medicine is not necessary for this disorder.

ACTIVITY—No restrictions.

DIET—No special diet.

 CALL YOUR DOCTOR IF

You or anyone else thinks your skin looks a bit yellow.

ILLNESS & DISORDERS

GINGIVITIS

 GENERAL INFORMATION

DEFINITION—Inflammation or infection of the gums.

BODY PARTS INVOLVED—Gum tissue around teeth.

SEX OR AGE MOST AFFECTED—All ages, but most common in adults.

SIGNS & SYMPTOMS
- Gums that are swollen, tender, red and soft around the teeth.
- Gums that bleed easily.
- Bad breath.
- Fever (rarely).
- No pain.

CAUSES
- Poor nutrition, especially vitamin deficiencies that cause diseases such as scurvy or pellagra.
- Plaque (food particles, germs and mucus at the base of the teeth).
- Blood disorders, including leukemia.
- Adverse reactions to drugs, such as anticonvulsants (primarily phenytoin and barbiturates).
- Exposure to lead and bismuth.

RISK INCREASES WITH
- Diabetes.
- Poor nutrition, especially vitamin deficiency.
- Infections.
- Pregnancy.
- Poor dental hygiene.

HOW TO PREVENT
- Practice good oral hygiene (see General Measures) to prevent plaque formation.
- Have regular dental checkups twice a year.
- Eat a well-balanced diet. Take vitamin supplements if you cannot eat well-balanced meals.

 WHAT TO EXPECT

DIAGNOSTIC MEASURES
- Your own observation of symptoms.
- Medical history and physical exam by a doctor or dentist.
- Laboratory culture of the plaque to identify the bacteria responsible for the infection.

APPROPRIATE HEALTH CARE
- Self-care after diagnosis.
- Doctor's or dentist's treatment.
- Surgery to remove infected gum tissue, if other treatment fails.

POSSIBLE COMPLICATIONS
- Extensive involvement may require gum surgery.

- Untreated gingivitis may lead to periodontitis, an advanced stage of gum disease that can lead to bone loss and loosening of teeth.
- Acute necrotizing gingivitis (trench mouth) that can causes destruction of gum tissue. Treatment is with antibiotics.

PROBABLE OUTCOME—Prognosis is generally favorable with appropriate treatment.

 HOW TO TREAT

GENERAL MEASURES
- Brush your teeth properly. Scrub clear, sticky plaque off the teeth daily with a soft toothbrush. Place the brush at the gum line and gently rotate it, pointing bristles toward the gum. Brush one section of teeth at a time. A soft brush is less likely to damage teeth and gums than a hard brush.
- Floss your teeth at least once a day. Use waxed or unwaxed dental floss. Wind most of it around the middle finger of each hand. Use index fingers as guides to force the floss between the teeth gently. Gently clean adjacent tooth surfaces with a back-and-forth, sawing motion at the gum line. Floss between all lower teeth. Loosen floss and place it on the tops of the thumbs. Floss between all upper teeth, using the thumbs as guides.
- Use a fluoride toothpaste.
- Make regular appointments with your dentist for cleaning and treatment of cavities.
- Avoid smoking.

MEDICATION—Your doctor or dentist may prescribe:
- Antibiotics to fight infection.
- Fluoride mouthwash.
- Vitamins, if you have a deficiency.

ACTIVITY—No restrictions.

DIET—No special diet. Avoid candy, sweet drinks or sweet snacks. Sugar stimulates the production of acid, which attacks normal teeth. The best desserts are fruit and cheese rather than ice cream or other high-sugar desserts.

 CALL YOUR DOCTOR OR DENTIST IF

- You have symptoms of gingivitis.
- The following occurs during treatment:
  Bleeding increases.
  Pain becomes intolerable.
  Temperature rises to 101F (38.3C) or higher.
  Neck or face becomes swollen.
  Swallowing becomes difficult.
- New, unexplained symptoms develop. Drugs used in treatment may produce side effects.

GLAUCOMA, CHRONIC OPEN-ANGLE
(Open-Angle Glaucoma)

 GENERAL INFORMATION

DEFINITION—A condition of the eye in which the fluid that normally drains into and out of the eye is gradually obstructed. This causes loss of vision. Chronic glaucoma—unlike acute glaucoma—usually causes no pain.

BODY PARTS INVOLVED—Eye.

SEX OR AGE MOST AFFECTED—Adults of both sexes over 40.

SIGNS & SYMPTOMS
Early stages:
• Loss of peripheral vision in small areas.
• Blurred vision on one side toward the nose.
Advanced stages:
• Larger areas of vision loss, usually in both eyes.
• Hard eyeball.
• Halos around lights.
• Blind spots.
• Poor night vision.

CAUSES—Symptoms are caused by pressure in the eyeball that damages fibers in the optic nerve.
  Glaucoma is probably hereditary, but it may be suspected in any person who requires frequent lens changes, has mild headaches or vague visual disturbances, sees halos around electric lights, or whose vision does not adapt well from light to dark.

RISK INCREASES WITH
• Adults over 60.
• Family history of acute or chronic glaucoma.
• Diabetes mellitus.

HOW TO PREVENT
• Make sure that tension in the eyeball is measured with every eye examination (at least once a year after age 40).
• Tell your doctor of any changes in your ability to see.

 WHAT TO EXPECT

DIAGNOSTIC MEASURES
• Your own observation of symptoms.
• Medical history and physical exam by a doctor.
• Laboratory studies such as tonometry (measurement of pressure within the eyeball).

APPROPRIATE HEALTH CARE
• Self-care after diagnosis.
• Doctor's treatment.
• Laser surgery can be performed if eyedrops do not control the disease.

POSSIBLE COMPLICATIONS—Loss of vision before other symptoms begin.

PROBABLE OUTCOME—Symptoms can usually be controlled with treatment. Glaucoma treatment is lifelong. Vision is usually not impaired permanently if glaucoma is treated.

 HOW TO TREAT

GENERAL MEASURES
• Avoid emotional upheavals and fatigue, which increase pressure in the eye.
• Don't smoke. Tobacco constricts blood vessels, restricting the blood supply to the eye.
• See Resources for Additional Information.
• Periodic eye exams are necessary to recheck pressure and change medications if required.

MEDICATION—Your doctor may prescribe:
• Eye medications to lower pressure inside the eye will be prescribed. Follow the instructions and schedule carefully, even if symptoms subside.
• Diuretics to reduce excess fluid.

ACTIVITY—No restrictions.

DIET—No special diet.

 CALL YOUR DOCTOR IF

• You have symptoms of chronic glaucoma.
• Medicine in the eye becomes intolerable.
• Any sign of eye infection, such as fever, develops.
• Pain begins in the eye.
• Redness occurs in the eye.
• Vision changes suddenly.
• Patients should be aware that many medications increase ocular pressure, exacerbating the disease. These drugs include cold and allergy pills, antihistamines, tranquilizers, cortisones and several remedies for stomach and intestinal problems.

ILLNESS & DISORDERS

GLAUCOMA, PRIMARY ANGLE-CLOSURE (Acute Glaucoma; Narrow-Angle Glaucoma; Closed-Angle Glaucoma)

GENERAL INFORMATION

DEFINITION—A condition of the eye in which the fluid that normally drains into and out of the eye is gradually obstructed and the pressure of the fluid becomes abnormally high. This causes damage to the optic nerve and loss of vision. Angle-closure glaucoma can occur in subacute, acute (which is an emergency) and chronic forms.

BODY PARTS INVOLVED—Eye.

SEX OR AGE MOST AFFECTED—Adults ages 55-70, women more than men.

SIGNS & SYMPTOMS
Acute:
- Severe, throbbing eye pain and headache.
- Redness in the eye.
- Blurred vision or halos around lights.
- Tender, firm eyeball.
- Dilated, fixed pupil.
- Swollen upper eyelid.
- Vomiting and weakness (due to severe eye pain).
Subacute:
- Symptoms may be mild and intermittent. They may occur while watching TV or movies in a dark room and be relieved by sleep or rest.
- Dull ache in or around one eye.
- Mildly blurred vision.
Chronic:
- May be no symptoms.
- Symptoms may be similar to subacute form.

CAUSES—Precise cause is unknown.

RISK INCREASES WITH
- Adults over 60.
- Family history of glaucoma or farsightedness.
- Use of certain medications with cholinergic inhibition.
- Cataracts.

HOW TO PREVENT—Consult your doctor regularly for checkups to detect glaucoma before symptoms begin. If you are over 40, have pressure inside the eye checked at least once a year. The test is simple and painless.

WHAT TO EXPECT

DIAGNOSTIC MEASURES
- Your own observation of symptoms.
- Medical history and physical exam by a doctor.
- Laboratory studies such as tonometry (measurement of pressure within the eyeball).

APPROPRIATE HEALTH CARE
- Doctor's treatment.
- Hospitalization for the acute form during the attack. Various treatments (pills, liquids, intravenous fluids) are given to try and reduce the very high eye pressure.
- Surgery (iridectomy with laser beam) to prevent further attacks if other treatment is unsuccessful. A small opening is made in the periphery of the iris so that the aqueous humor (fluid in the eye) can drain. This may control the attack, but medications may still be necessary to control the pressure.

POSSIBLE COMPLICATIONS—Total blindness in the affected eye, if treatment is delayed or unsuccessful.

PROBABLE OUTCOME—Symptoms can be controlled if treatment begins quickly.

HOW TO TREAT

GENERAL MEASURES
- Avoid emotional upset, which raises pressure in the eye.
- Don't smoke. Tobacco constricts blood vessels, reducing the blood supply to the eye.
- Follow your doctor's instructions.
- See Resources for Additional Information.

MEDICATION—Your doctor may prescribe:
- Eye drops to lower pressure inside the eye. Follow the instructions and schedule carefully, even if symptoms subside or the eye drops are occasionally uncomfortable.
- Diuretics to decrease fluid pressure in the eye.
- Pain relievers.

ACTIVITY—After treatment, resume your normal activities gradually—but avoid fatigue. Resume sexual relations when eye pressure is under control.

DIET—No special diet.

CALL YOUR DOCTOR IF

- You have symptoms of glaucoma. Acute glaucoma is an emergency!
- New, unexplained symptoms develop. Drugs used in treatment may produce side effects.

GLOMERULONEPHRITIS
(Post-Infectious, Acute or Chronic Glomerulonephritis)

GENERAL INFORMATION

DEFINITION—Inflammation of the glomeruli (small, round filters in the kidney). Damaged glomeruli cannot effectively filter waste products from the bloodstream and serious kidney complications may result.

BODY PARTS INVOLVED—Kidneys.

SEX OR AGE MOST AFFECTED—All ages, but most common in children (2 to 12 years).

SIGNS & SYMPTOMS—Mild glomerulonephritis produces no symptoms. Diagnosis is possible only with urine studies. Severe glomerulonephritis produces the following:
- Smoky or slightly red urine.
- General ill feeling; drowsiness.
- Nausea or vomiting; headaches.
- Fever (sometimes).
- Appetite loss; decreased urination.
- Fluid accumulation in the body, especially puffy eyes and ankles.
- Shortness of breath; high blood pressure.
- Protein in the urine.
- Disturbed vision.

CAUSES
- Acute glomerulonephritis follows a streptococcal infection. The most common infection sites are the throat and skin. Kidney symptoms usually begin 2 or 3 weeks after the strep infection.
- Chronic glomerulonephritis is rare and may have different causes than acute glomerulonephritis.

RISK INCREASES WITH
- Exposure to people in public places where streptococcal infections can be transmitted.
- Streptococcal infection (scarlet fever or erysipelas).

HOW TO PREVENT
- Consult your doctor about antibiotic treatment of any infection that may be strep.
- Avoid exposure to people with strep infection.

WHAT TO EXPECT

DIAGNOSTIC MEASURES
- Your own observation of symptoms.
- Medical history and exam by a doctor.
- Laboratory studies, such as: blood counts; repeated urinalyses to determine the presence of protein or other abnormal elements; streptococcal antibody titer (a sophisticated blood study).
- Kidney-function tests.

APPROPRIATE HEALTH CARE
- Doctor's treatment.
- Hospitalization (severe cases).

POSSIBLE COMPLICATIONS
- Chronic glomerulonephritis in which the disease tends to progress slowly so that there may be no symptoms until kidneys can no longer function (may be 20-30 years).
- Kidney failure, which may require dialysis or kidney transplant.

PROBABLE OUTCOME—Symptoms subside in 2 weeks to several months. 90% of children recover without complications. Adults recover also—but more slowly.

HOW TO TREAT

GENERAL MEASURES
- Record temperature 3 times a day.
- Collect and record the amount of urine passed in each 24-hour period. Some of this collection will be analyzed in the doctor's office.
- See Resources for Additional Information.

MEDICATION—Your doctor may prescribe:
- Cortisone or cytotoxic drugs, if the illness is severe.
- Diuretics to increase urination.
- Antihypertensives, if high blood pressure accompanies the illness.
- Iron and vitamin supplements, if anemia develops.

ACTIVITY—Stay in bed, except to go to the bathroom, until all signs of illness have passed. Bed rest ensures an adequate blood flow to the kidney; blood flow is best when lying down. Resume normal activities after recovery.

DIET
- As long as your kidneys function properly, you may eat a normal, well-balanced diet. Greatly decrease the sodium in your diet.
- In severe cases, fluids may need to be restricted, and sodium and protein intake forbidden for a time.

CALL YOUR DOCTOR IF

- You have symptoms of glomerulonephritis.
- The following occur during treatment:
  Severe headache or convulsion.
  Failure to pass at least 22 ounces of urine in a 24-hour period.
  Fever or skin rash.
  Increased fluid retention.
  Increased nausea, vomiting or diarrhea.

GONORRHEA

GENERAL INFORMATION

DEFINITION—An infectious disease of the reproductive organs that is sexually transmitted (venereal disease). Symptoms usually develop within 2 days to 3 weeks of exposure.

BODY PARTS INVOLVED
- Males—urethra.
- Females—urethra; reproductive system.
- Both sexes—rectum; throat; joints; eyes (sometimes).

SEX OR AGE MOST AFFECTED—Both sexes and all ages—even young children—of persons who have sexual contact with infected persons. The peak incidence is between ages 20 and 30.

SIGNS & SYMPTOMS
- Burning urination.
- Thick green-yellow discharge from the penis or vagina.
- Little or no fever.
- Pain or tenderness with sexual intercourse (sometimes).
- Rectal discomfort and discharge (sometimes).
- Joint pain.
- Rash, especially on palms.
- Mild sore throat (sometimes). Females often have few or no symptoms. Males usually have more pronounced symptoms.

CAUSES—Infection from gonococcus bacteria that grow well on delicate, moist tissue. The bacteria is transmitted sexually, but some cases are of unknown origin. Sexual activity involving the rectum or mouth may transmit infection to those areas if either partner is infected.

RISK INCREASES WITH
- Many sexual partners, whether heterosexual or homosexual; prostitution.
- Child sexual abuse.
- Infant who passes through the infected birth canal of the mother.

HOW TO PREVENT
- Avoid sexual partners whose health practices and status are uncertain.
- Use a latex condom during sexual intercourse.
- This condition must be reported to the local health department to prevent its spread. It sometimes occurs simultaneously with syphilis. Your cooperation is important, and your confidentiality will be maintained.

WHAT TO EXPECT

DIAGNOSTIC MEASURES
- Your own observation of symptoms.
- Medical history and exam by a doctor.
- Blood studies.

- Laboratory culture and microscopic analysis of the discharge from the reproductive organs, rectum or throat.
- Patients should be tested for other sexually transmitted diseases.

APPROPRIATE HEALTH CARE
- Doctor's treatment.
- Hospitalization for complications.

POSSIBLE COMPLICATIONS
- Gonococcal eye infection. This may cause blindness in children.
- Blood poisoning (gonococcal septicemia).
- Infectious arthritis.
- Pelvic inflammatory disease in females.
- Epididymitis.
- Endocarditis.
- Sexual impotence in men, if untreated (sometimes).
- Infertility in women.

PROBABLE OUTCOME—Usually curable in 1 to 2 weeks with treatment.

HOW TO TREAT

GENERAL MEASURES
- Use separate linens and disposable eating utensils during treatment.
- Wash hands frequently—especially after urination and bowel movements.
- Don't touch eyes with hands.
- Inform all sexual contacts so they can seek treatment.
- See Resources for Additional Information.

MEDICATION
- Your doctor will usually prescribe injectable and oral antibiotics to fight the infection.
- You may take nonprescription drugs, such as acetaminophen or aspirin, to reduce discomfort—but not in place of antibiotics. Home remedies or folk-medicine treatments are ineffective.

ACTIVITY—No restrictions, except don't resume sexual activity until a follow-up culture shows the infection is cured. Treatment failures and resistance to antibiotics can occur.

DIET—No special diet. Reduce consumption of caffeine and alcohol during treatment. These irritate the urethra.

CALL YOUR DOCTOR IF

- You have symptoms of gonorrhea.
- You develop chills, fever, abdominal pain, swelling of the testicles, genital sores or joint pain—either before or during treatment.
- New, unexplained symptoms develop.
- If you learn that a sex partner has been infected

GOUT

GENERAL INFORMATION

DEFINITION—Recurrent attacks of joint inflammation caused by deposits of uric-acid crystals in the joints, especially the base of the big toe. Gout is a form of arthritis.

BODY PARTS INVOLVED—Joints: base of the big toe; may also involve the elbow, knee, hand, foot, ankle, arm or shoulder.

SEX OR AGE MOST AFFECTED—Adults of both sexes, but 20 times more frequent in men than women.

SIGNS & SYMPTOMS
- Sudden onset of severe pain in the inflamed joint, usually at the base of the big toe or larger joints.
- Involved joints are red, hot, swollen and very tender. Skin over the joint is red and shiny.
- Fever (sometimes).

CAUSES—A high level of uric acid in the blood due to increased production of uric acid or decreased elimination of uric acid by the kidneys. Not all people with excess uric acid levels develop gout.

RISK INCREASES WITH
- Use of diuretic drugs (water pills) such as furosemide and hydrochlorothiazide.
- Use of some antibiotics.
- Some blood diseases, such as polycythemia and leukemia.
- Men over 60.
- Family history of gout.
- Obesity.
- Many disorders including thyroid problems, kidney disease, anemia, hyperlipidemia, high blood pressure, diabetes and vascular disease.
- Trauma, surgery, radiation treatment.
- Eating large amounts of anchovies, sardines, sweetbreads, kidney or liver.
- Chemotherapy may raise uric acid levels.

HOW TO PREVENT—Avoidance of risk factors where possible.

WHAT TO EXPECT

DIAGNOSTIC MEASURES
- Your own observation of symptoms.
- Medical history and physical exam by a doctor.
- Laboratory studies such as blood levels of uric acid and studies of the fluid in the joint; x-ray (usually normal in the first year of the disease); bone scan (sometimes).
- Therapeutic trial with antigout medications.

APPROPRIATE HEALTH CARE
- Self-care after diagnosis.
- Doctor's treatment.

POSSIBLE COMPLICATIONS—If untreated, may cause:
- Crippled, deformed joints.
- Kidney stones.
- Inflammation of bones, ligaments and tendons.

PROBABLE OUTCOME—The first attack may last a few days, but recurrent attacks are common without treatment to reduce the uric-acid level in the blood. Symptoms can be eliminated with treatment.

HOW TO TREAT

GENERAL MEASURES
- Use warm or cold compresses on painful joints.
- Keep the weight of bedclothes off any painful joint by making a frame that raises sheets off the feet.

MEDICATION—Your doctor may prescribe:
- Nonsteroidal anti-inflammatory drugs to control inflammation in the painful joints.
- Prescription medications such as colchicine, indomethacin or prednisolone to control the pain of the acute attack.
- For some patients, lifelong medication, such as allopurinol to decrease uric-acid production or probenecid to increase the kidneys' excretion of uric acid. These medications have significant side effects and adverse reactions. Obtain as much information as possible regarding their use.

ACTIVITY—Acute attacks will end sooner with complete rest.

DIET
- Don't eat liver, sweetbreads, kidney or sardines.
- Drink 10 to 12 glasses of water daily.
- Don't drink alcoholic beverages, especially beer or red wine (they can worsen or trigger an attack).
- If you are overweight, begin a medically approved weight loss diet. Do not go on a crash diet, as quick weight loss may bring on gout

CALL YOUR DOCTOR IF

- You have symptoms of gout.
- The following occurs during treatment:
  Fever of 101F (38.3C) or higher.
  Skin rash, sore throat, red tongue or bleeding gums.
  Marked swelling of feet or abrupt weight increase.
  Diarrhea or vomiting.
- Symptoms are not relieved in 3 days despite treatment.
- New, unexplained symptoms develop.

GRANULOMA ANNULARE

 GENERAL INFORMATION

DEFINITION—A chronic benign skin disorder characterized by lesions that appear in the shape of a ring. This is not malignant or contagious.

BODY PARTS INVOLVED—Skin on the bottoms of feet and backs of fingers, hands, arms, elbows, legs and knees.

SEX OR AGE MOST AFFECTED—All ages, but most common in children (4 to 12 years).

SIGNS & SYMPTOMS—Papules (small, raised bumps on the skin) with the following characteristics:
- Papules have a domed or slightly flat shape, 3mm to 6mm in diameter.
- Papules are nonscaling.
- Papules are pink or violet. Those on the lower extremities are darker than ones on other parts of the body.
- Papules don't itch or hurt.
- Multiple papules cluster in a ring. Ring diameters range from 1cm to 10cm. Papules around the ring border are close but don't grow completely together. This gives the border a beaded appearance. The ring's center is often darker than the edge. Ringed lesions change in size and shape over a period of several weeks to 6 months.

CAUSES—Unknown.

RISK INCREASES WITH
- Diabetes mellitus.
- Positive family history of granuloma annulare.

HOW TO PREVENT—Avoid injury to the skin. Protect skin from sunburn with sunscreen or clothing.

 WHAT TO EXPECT

DIAGNOSTIC MEASURES
- Your own observation of symptoms.
- Medical history and physical exam by a doctor.
- Biopsy (see Glossary) to confirm diagnosis (sometimes).

APPROPRIATE HEALTH CARE
- Self-care after diagnosis.
- Doctor's treatment.

POSSIBLE COMPLICATIONS—Recurrences of the disorder.

PROBABLE OUTCOME—Spontaneous recovery within 2 years, but therapy may hasten recovery.

 HOW TO TREAT

GENERAL MEASURES
- Protect involved areas from injury.
- No treatment is usually necessary.

MEDICATION—Your doctor may prescribe topical steroids with occlusion to hasten healing. To use steroids:
- Gently rub a small amount of the steroid drug into the affected area.
- Reapply a small amount.
- Cover the affected area with clear kitchen plastic wrap. If skin becomes dry and itchy, provide additional moisture by covering the affected area with a damp, clean cloth before applying plastic. You may also soak the affected area briefly in water after applying medicine.
- Reapply medicine every time you change the plastic dressing.

ACTIVITY—No restrictions.

DIET—No special diet.

 CALL YOUR DOCTOR IF

- You have symptoms of granuloma annulare.
- Lesions ulcerate.
- New lesions occur during treatment.
- Signs of infection, such as redness, swelling, pain or tenderness, develop around the lesions.
- You become sensitive to the occlusive plastic dressing.
- New, unexplained symptoms develop. Steroid drugs used in treatment may produce side effects.

GRANULOMA INGUINALE
(Donovanosis)

GENERAL INFORMATION

DEFINITION—A sexually transmitted disease generally affecting people living in tropical climates. It is becoming more common in the U.S., especially in the South and Southwest. Incubation period is 8 to 12 weeks.

BODY PARTS INVOLVED—Genitals.

SEX OR AGE MOST AFFECTED—Both sexes; all ages.

SIGNS & SYMPTOMS
- Formation of a nonpainful lesion (cyst, papule, or nodule) in the genital area that does not readily heal. This lesion ulcerates (becomes open and runny) and may spread so that it involves most of the vulva, and sometimes the buttocks and lower abdomen.
- Marked discomfort occurs if the ulceration spreads to the urethra or anal area. Walking, sitting and sexual intercourse become painful.
- Vaginal discharge that has an unpleasant odor.
- For men, sites of infection include the penis, scrotum, groin and thighs.

CAUSES—An organism, Calymmatobacterium granulomatis (also called Donovania granulomatis or Donovanosis), that is spread via sexual intercourse with an infected person.

RISK INCREASES WITH
- Multiple sexual partners.
- Unprotected intercourse.
- Infection with other sexually transmitted diseases.

HOW TO PREVENT
- Maintain a mutually monogamous sexual relationship.
- Have the male partner use a latex condom during sexual activity.
- Cleansing of the genital area before and after sex. Douching is usually not effective.
- If there has been good possibility of exposure, seek medical care immediately. Early treatment may prevent painful symptoms from developing.

WHAT TO EXPECT

DIAGNOSTIC MEASURES
- Diagnosis is confirmed with laboratory studies of scrapings or biopsies of the lesions.
- Testing (screening) for other sexually transmitted diseases is often recommended.

APPROPRIATE HEALTH CARE—Doctor's treatment.

POSSIBLE COMPLICATIONS
- Secondary bacterial infection.
- Relapse may occur if treatment is stopped too soon.
- Scars may form where infection occurred.
- Surgical intervention may be required in cases where the infection has caused advanced tissue destruction.

PROBABLE OUTCOME—With treatment, healing should begin within a week, but complete resolution will take up to 3 weeks.

HOW TO TREAT

GENERAL MEASURES
- Sitz baths frequently relieve discomfort caused by the lesions. Sit in a tub of hot water for 10 to 15 minutes. Repeat baths as often as 3 or 4 times a day.
- Sexual partners should be examined and, if necessary, treated for infection.
- A follow-up medical examination after treatment is important to verify that healing is complete.

MEDICATION—An antibiotic, such as tetracycline, will be prescribed. Take all the medication as prescribed, even if symptoms subside. Antibiotics may reduce the effectiveness of oral contraceptives. If you are currently using oral contraceptives for birth control, discuss this with your doctor.

ACTIVITY—Avoid sexual intercourse during the active phase of the infection.

DIET—No special diet. If taking tetracycline, avoid dairy products within 3 hours of taking the medicine.

CALL YOUR DOCTOR IF

- You or a family member has symptoms of granuloma inguinale.
- Symptoms worsen despite treatment.
- New, unexplained symptoms develop. Drugs used in treatment may produce side effects.

GRANULOMA, PYOGENIC

 GENERAL INFORMATION

DEFINITION—Skin lesions composed of small blood vessels. These are not contagious or cancerous.

BODY PARTS INVOLVED—Skin anywhere on the body, but most commonly on the face and shoulder.

SEX OR AGE MOST AFFECTED
• Children of both sexes (ages 5 to 15).
• Pregnant women.

SIGNS & SYMPTOMS—Papules (small, raised bumps on the skin) with the following characteristics:
• Papules appear first as pinhead-sized but grow rapidly within weeks to full size (2mm to 20mm).
• Papules bleed easily when injured.
• Papules don't hurt or itch.

CAUSES—Unknown. Pyogenic refers to an infectious process, but these lesions are misnamed. Because they frequently appear in late childhood or pregnancy, hormonal changes may be a factor in their development.

RISK INCREASES WITH
• Pregnancy.
• Recent injury (sometimes lesions develop at the injured site).

HOW TO PREVENT—Cannot be prevented at present.

 WHAT TO EXPECT

DIAGNOSTIC MEASURES
• Your own observation of symptoms.
• Because pyogenic granuloma resembles melanoma (skin cancer), medical diagnosis is important.
• Medical history and physical exam by a doctor.
• Biopsy (see Glossary).

APPROPRIATE HEALTH CARE
• Doctor's treatment.
• Lesions can be removed by surgical excision, electrocoagulation or cryosurgery.
• Self-care after surgery.

POSSIBLE COMPLICATIONS—None expected.

PROBABLE OUTCOME—Spontaneous recovery, usually within 2 to 6 months. Recurrence is common.

 HOW TO TREAT

GENERAL MEASURES—After surgery:
• Apply rubbing alcohol to the scab twice a day.
• Apply an adhesive bandage to the scab during the day. Leave it uncovered at night.
• Wash the wound as usual. Dry gently and completely after bathing or swimming.

MEDICATION
• For minor pain, you may use nonprescription drugs, such as acetaminophen or aspirin.
• If the scab cracks or oozes, apply a nonprescription antibiotic ointment several times a day.

ACTIVITY—No restrictions except to avoid trauma to lesion while it is healing.

DIET—No special diet.

 CALL YOUR DOCTOR IF

• You have symptoms of pyogenic granuloma.
• The wound bleeds after surgery, and bleeding cannot be stopped by applying pressure for 10 minutes.
• The wound shows signs of infection, such as redness, swelling, pain or increased tenderness.

GRIEF
(Bereavement)

GENERAL INFORMATION

DEFINITION—The emotional reaction following the death of a loved one, loss of a body part or function, or other significant loss. Grieving people gradually adjust to their loss and begin to make positive plans for the future. There are no guidelines for the normal duration of grieving. Occassionally, grief is so intense or prolonged that professional help is needed.

SEX OR AGE MOST AFFECTED—Both sexes; all ages.

SIGNS & SYMPTOMS
Recognized expressions of grief:
- Feelings of sadness, numbness, pain, anger, despair, guilt (these feelings can come and go for months and may be overwhelming at times).
- Sudden crying spells.
- Hallucinations (such as a sense of having seen or heard the dead person).
- Anxiety and depression.
- Unwillingness to accept the loss; for example, maintaining the dead person's room.
- Insomnia; nervousness and hyperactivity.
- Gastrointestinal problems.
- Tiredness, agitation, tearfulness.
- Increased intake of alcohol, tranquilizers and other drugs is common (but may cause problems).

CAUSES—Grief follows a loss.

RISK INCREASES WITH— An existing emotional problem, such as depression; social isolation; strong feelings of guilt or anger due to one's relationship with the dead person

HOW TO PREVENT—Grieving should not be prevented or denied. It is a normal expected response to a loss and should be encouraged by open expression of feeling and social recognition of the loss.

WHAT TO EXPECT

DIAGNOSTIC MEASURES
- Your own observation of symptoms.
- Examination by a doctor or counselor.

APPROPRIATE HEALTH CARE—Counseling to deal with loss.

POSSIBLE COMPLICATIONS
- Difficulty maintaining relationships and jobs.
- Excess use of alcohol or tranquilizer drugs.

- The following grieving expressions may require medical help:
  Panic attacks.
  Excessive feelings of guilt, bitterness or remorse.
  Chronic anxiety and depression.
  Prolonged grief (usually more than 2 years). A person may build a life around the grief and never accept the loss.
  Talk about or threats of suicide.

PROBABLE OUTCOME—With time, grief lessens and adjustment begins. The feelings of grief may return unpredictably and will probably recur occasionally for years.

HOW TO TREAT

GENERAL MEASURES
- Hold a memorial service or funeral for the loved one.
- Express your feelings following the loss. Don't keep them bottled up. Look to family and friends for help and support.
- Join a grief support group.
- Don't expect your feelings of grief to follow any pattern or particular timetable.
- Slowly begin to rebuild your life. Meet new people and interest yourself in new activities.
- Avoid the overuse of alcohol or medications to suppress the emotion you are feeling.
- Seek professional counseling or psychotherapy if you or your family think it is needed. Therapy can help bring about a healthy resolution of grief.

MEDICATION—Your doctor may prescribe medications, such as sedatives or antidepressants, for a short time. In most cases, drugs are not needed.

ACTIVITY—Normally, no restrictions unless directed by your doctor.

DIET—Eat a normal, well balanced diet to maintain optimum health.

CALL YOUR DOCTOR IF

- You or a family member has symptoms or intense grief.
- You want information about grief support groups.

GUILLAIN-BARRÉ SYNDROME
(Infectious Polyneuropathy; Acute Idiopathic Polyneuritis)

GENERAL INFORMATION

DEFINITION—A rare, inflammatory condition involving the central nervous system that causes rapid weakness and loss of sensation.

BODY PARTS INVOLVED—Central nervous system.

SEX OR AGE MOST AFFECTED—All ages, but most common between 30 and 50.

SIGNS & SYMPTOMS
Early stages:
- Muscle weakness that usually starts in the legs and ascends to arms and face. The weakness spreads within 72 hours; it may create life-threatening breathing difficulty.
- Shock (weakness; faintness; cold hands and feet; rapid heartbeat; sweating).

Later stages:
- Complete paralysis (sometimes) for weeks or months.

CAUSES—Unknown, but may be an autoimmune disorder. It sometimes follows an immunization or minor surgery.

RISK INCREASES WITH
- Recent surgery.
- Recent immunization.
- Recent illness, such as a minor respiratory infection, gastroenteritis, Hodgkin's disease or lupus erythematosus.

HOW TO PREVENT—Cannot be prevented at present.

WHAT TO EXPECT

DIAGNOSTIC MEASURES
- Your own observation of symptoms.
- Medical history and physical exam by a doctor.
- Spinal fluid analysis and electromyography (see Glossary).

APPROPRIATE HEALTH CARE
- Doctor's treatment.
- Hospitalization in an intensive care unit so condition can be closely monitored.
- A respirator may be necessary if muscles of respiration become greatly weakened.
- Plasmapheresis in severe cases (blood plasma is withdrawn from the patient, treated to remove antibodies and replaced).

POSSIBLE COMPLICATIONS
- Paralysis of eyelid muscles, resulting in eye damage.
- Thrombophlebitis.
- Pneumonia.
- Respiratory failure.
- Pressure sores, if the person is immobilized.
- Constipation or fecal impaction.
- Chronic nerve difficulty.

PROBABLE OUTCOME—Complete recovery without residual effects in most cases. Some persons recover in 15 to 20 days, others require a year or more. Many mechanical devices can aid mobility until the person recovers. Adults recover better than children.

HOW TO TREAT

GENERAL MEASURES
- The family should maintain an optimistic outlook, stay in close contact with the patient's doctor and help by making their visits with the patient brief and as supportive as possible.
- Additional information available from the Guillain-Barré Foundation at (215)667-0131.

MEDICATION—Your doctor may prescribe:
- Laxatives to prevent constipation.
- Cortisone drugs, although they are not always effective.

ACTIVITY
- Remain as active as muscle strength permits. Have a family member or physical therapist passively move and stretch muscles.
- Ongoing physical therapy as your recovery progresses.

DIET—No special diet. Drink at least 8 glasses of fluid a day to prevent constipation.

CALL YOUR DOCTOR IF

- You have symptoms of Guillain-Barré syndrome.
- The following occurs during treatment:
  Fever.
  Breathing difficulty.
  Sores on the skin.
  Vision changes.
  Swollen or tender calves.
  Constipation.
- New, unexplained symptoms develop. Drugs used in treatment may produce side effects.

HAND, FOOT & MOUTH DISEASE

 GENERAL INFORMATION

DEFINITION—A common infectious, viral infection that begins in the throat.

BODY PARTS INVOLVED—Throat; tonsils; skin; gastrointestinal tract; central nervous system.

SEX OR AGE MOST AFFECTED—Infants and young children (2 weeks to 3 years).

SIGNS & SYMPTOMS
- Sudden fever.
- Sore throat with blisters and ulcers in the mouth and throat lining.
- Headache.
- Rash with blisters on the hands, feet and groin.
- Appetite loss.
- Abdominal pain (sometimes).

CAUSES—Infection from the coxsackievirus A-16, which is transmitted from person to person.

RISK INCREASES WITH—Summer and fall seasons.

HOW TO PREVENT—Prevent exposure of infants and young children to anyone with a respiratory illness.

 WHAT TO EXPECT

DIAGNOSTIC MEASURES
- Your own observation of symptoms.
- Medical history and physical exam by a doctor.

APPROPRIATE HEALTH CARE
- Home care.
- Doctor's treatment.

POSSIBLE COMPLICATIONS—None expected.

PROBABLE OUTCOME—Spontaneous recovery in 4 to 5 days

 HOW TO TREAT

GENERAL MEASURES
- The disorder has a mild course and the child can be cared for at home.
- Dip a cotton applicator in 2% hydrogen peroxide and apply to the blisters in the mouth.
- Rinse the mouth with salt water (1/2 teaspoon salt to 1 cup water) after eating, if the child is old enough to rinse without swallowing.
- Boil eating utensils and other items that touch the mouth or saliva—or use disposable utensils—to avoid transmitting the disease.
- Boil bottle nipples separately for 20 minutes before sterilizing formula in the bottles.

MEDICATION—To reduce high fever, you may use nonprescription drugs such as acetaminophen. Do not use aspirin. Antibiotics are not effective against this disease.

ACTIVITY—Keep the child in bed until fever and other symptoms disappear. Normal activities may be resumed gradually.

DIET—Encourage the child to increase fluid intake, including milk, liquid gelatin, ice cream, custard or drinks made with syrup of wild cherry (available from your druggist). If drinking is painful, older children may use a straw.

 CALL YOUR DOCTOR IF

- Your child has symptoms of hand, foot and mouth disease.
- Symptoms worsen or do not improve.

ILLNESS & DISORDERS

HANTAVIRUS
(Hantaviral Pulmonary Syndrome)

 GENERAL INFORMATION

DEFINITION—A group of viruses (named after the Hantaan River in Korea) spread by rodents. The viruses are responsible for widespread illness in Europe and Asia. New strains have recently been identified in the U.S. To date, the majority of patients reside in the Four Corner region of New Mexico, Arizona, Colorado and Utah. The disorder begins with mild symptoms, but can quickly give rise to acute respiratory failure.

BODY PARTS INVOLVED—Respiratory system.

SEX OR AGE MOST AFFECTED—Both sexes; all ages.

SIGNS & SYMPTOMS
Early symptoms (flu-like):
- Chills.
- Fever.
- Muscle aches.
- Cough.
- Listlessness; tiredness.

Later symptoms:
- Extreme difficulty in breathing (the virus causes capillaries in the lungs to leak blood).

CAUSES—Exact mode of transmission is still to be determined. In the U.S., the virus is found mainly in deer mice and is probably spread to humans who breath in air that has been contaminated by the urine, feces or saliva of the mouse. It is not spread by person-to-person contact. Incubation time is 1-5 weeks. Deer mice live in rural areas of many states in the U.S. and Canada. Studies are ongoing to see if other rodents harbor the virus and if any animals that prey on rodents may carry it. There is no indication that Norway rats, common to urban areas, or house mice harbor the virus.

RISK INCREASES WITH—No known specific risk factors. Some environmental factors are involved that allow a population of rodents (like deer mice) to increase. A decline in their population should lessen the risk for contacting the virus.

HOW TO PREVENT
- Avoid contact with deer mice by keeping them out of your home. Contact your county or state health department or an exterminator for information about removing them.
- Research on possible vaccines is underway.

 WHAT TO EXPECT

DIAGNOSTIC MEASURES
- Your own observation of symptoms.
- Medical history and physical exam by a doctor.
- Laboratory blood and urine studies. Quick, specific diagnostic tests are under development.

APPROPRIATE HEALTH CARE—Hospitalization for supportive care and assisted breathing. There is no specific treatment for the disease.

POSSIBLE COMPLICATIONS—The disorder is fatal to about 60% of those infected due to respiratory failure or blood loss.

PROBABLE OUTCOME—Outcome is variable. To date, there are no effective treatment procedures to stop the infection once it sets in.

 HOW TO TREAT

GENERAL MEASURES—The family should maintain an optimistic outlook, stay in close contact with the patient's doctor and help by making their visits with the patient brief and as supportive as possible.

MEDICATION—Your doctor may prescribe medications as needed to help control the bleeding and improve lung function.

ACTIVITY—Bed rest for acute illness; resume normal activities gradually.

DIET—May require intravenous feeding while hospitalized, then progress slowly to regular diet with recovery.

 CALL YOUR DOCTOR IF

You have symptoms of Hantavirus, especially if you live in an area, or traveled to an area, where the virus is present.

HAY FEVER (Seasonal Allergic Rhinitis)

 GENERAL INFORMATION

DEFINITION—An allergic response to airborne allergens that affects the eyes and upper respiratory tract. The name is confusing since hay does not cause an allergic reaction and there is no fever. Attacks flare up in pollen season and disappear when it is over.

BODY PARTS INVOLVED—Nose; eyes; sinuses; throat; mouth; lungs.

SEX OR AGE MOST AFFECTED—Both sexes; all ages.

SIGNS & SYMPTOMS
- Itching, watery eyes.
- Frequent sneezing; stuffy nose with a clear discharge; itching in the roof of the mouth.
- Wheezing (sometimes); burning in the throat.

CAUSES
- The body's immune system produces allergic antibodies that release a chemical called histamine, which produces swelling and irritation in sensitive areas (nose, sinuses, eyes).
- Airborne allergens causing an allergic sensitivity include:
  Pollen from weeds, flowers, grasses, trees.
  Mold and dust
  Mites.
  Tobacco smoke and other air pollutants.

RISK INCREASES WITH
- Medical history of allergic reactions, such as eczema or asthma.
- Smoking.
- Spring and autumn (pollen in air).
- Family history of allergies.
- Immunosuppression (due to drugs or illness).

HOW TO PREVENT—Follow suggestions in General Measures.

 WHAT TO EXPECT

DIAGNOSTIC MEASURES
- Your own observation of symptoms.
- Medical history and exam by a doctor.
- Laboratory tests such as a blood count and allergy skin tests may be recommended, but are usually not required for diagnosis.

APPROPRIATE HEALTH CARE
- Self-care.
- Doctor's treatment.

POSSIBLE COMPLICATIONS
- Sleeping difficulty and chronic fatigue.
- Susceptibility to other respiratory infections.
- Ear infections.

PROBABLE OUTCOME—Symptoms can be controlled with treatment, but the condition persists over a lifetime. It is usually more troublesome than disabling.

 HOW TO TREAT

GENERAL MEASURES—Eliminate as many allergens in your environment as possible. Prepare your bedroom as follows:
- Empty the room of furniture, rugs or carpet, and drapes or curtains.
- Clean the walls, woodwork and floors with a damp mop. Wax the floor.
- Cover the box springs, mattress and pillows with plastic covers.
- Use only rugs that can be washed weekly.
- Use bedclothes that can be washed often, such as cotton sheets, washable mattress pads and synthetic fiber blankets. Don't use chenille bedspreads, quilts or comforters.
- Use wood or plastic chairs.
- Use plastic curtains, if possible. Dust daily.
- Use a vacuum cleaner, damp rags, and a damp or oiled mop to clean the bedroom thoroughly once a week.

Other preventive measures:
- Keep windows and doors closed as much as possible.
- Don't handle objects that are very dusty, such as books or stored clothing.
- Don't keep stuffed animals or toys around.
- Remove all pets (except fish) from the house.
- Wear a filter face mask during exposure to allergens, including during housecleaning.
- Install an air-purification unit in your home's heating and air-conditioning system.
- Drive an air-conditioned car.
- Have someone else mow the lawn.

MEDICATION—To reduce the body's allergic response, your doctor may prescribe:
- Antihistamines; decongestants; cortisone eye drops or nasal spray; cortisone tablets (severe cases only); cromolyn nasal spray; cromolyn nose drops. These medications relieve symptoms, but they don't cure hay fever.
- Desensitization injections for known allergens for severe or year-round cases. Once allergens are known (through skin or blood tests), small amounts are injected periodically. This helps block the immune system from releasing the histamine. This process may take months or years for effective results.

ACTIVITY—No restrictions.

DIET—Avoid foods that cause allergies.

 CALL YOUR DOCTOR IF

- Signs of infection, such as fever, headache, muscle aches, or thick, discolored nasal discharge, appear. A sinus infection may be complicating the allergy.
- New, unexplained symptoms develop.

HEAD INJURY

GENERAL INFORMATION

DEFINITION—Injury to the head, with or without unconsciousness or other visible signs. Head wounds may be "open" or "closed" depending on the nature of the injury.

BODY PARTS INVOLVED—Head.

SEX OR AGE MOST AFFECTED—Both sexes; all ages, but most frequent in young males.

SIGNS & SYMPTOMS—Depends on the extent of injury. The presence or absence of swelling at the injury site is not related to the seriousness of injury. Signs and symptoms include any or all of the following:
- Drowsiness or confusion.
- Vomiting and nausea.
- Blurred vision; pupils of different size.
- Loss of consciousness—either temporarily or for long periods.
- Amnesia or memory lapses.
- Irritability; headache.
- Bleeding of the scalp, if the skin is broken.

CAUSES—Injury. The worst injuries usually result from motor-vehicle accidents.

RISK INCREASES WITH
- Excess alcohol consumption.
- Contact sports, especially football or boxing.
- Seizure disorders.
- Falls.
- Bicycle or motorcycle riding without a helmet.

HOW TO PREVENT
- Don't drink or use mind-altering drugs and drive.
- Wear protective headgear for contact sports and cycling.
- Use your auto seat belt always. Place young children in safety car seats.
- Don't leave small children unattended in high chair, stroller, buggy or walker.
- Make sure ladders are in good condition.
- Make your home as safe as possible.

WHAT TO EXPECT

DIAGNOSTIC MEASURES
- Your own observation of symptoms.
- Medical history and exam by a doctor.
- Laboratory studies of blood and cerebrospinal fluid.
- X-rays of the skull and neck.
- CT scan (see Glossary) of the head.

APPROPRIATE HEALTH CARE
- Home care.
- Doctor's treatment.
- Hospitalization for observation, if signs and symptoms are severe.
- Emergency surgery to relieve skull pressure.

POSSIBLE COMPLICATIONS
- Bleeding under the skull (subdural hemorrhage and hematoma).
- Bleeding into the brain.
- Permanent disability or death.

PROBABLE OUTCOME—Usually curable with early recognition of danger signs and medical treatment. Patient is normally able to return home after recovery; some may require time in a rehabilitation facility.

HOW TO TREAT

GENERAL MEASURES
- The extent of injury can be determined only with careful examination and observation. After a doctor's examination, the injured person may be sent home, but a responsible person must stay with the person and watch for serious symptoms. The first 24 hours after injury are critical, although serious after-effects can appear later (up to 6 months after the injury).
- If you are watching the patient, awaken him or her every 2 hours for 24 hours or as recommended. Report to the doctor immediately if you can't awaken or arouse the person. Report also any of the following:
  Vomiting.
  Inability to move arms and legs equally well on both sides.
  Temperature above 100F (37.8C).
  Stiff neck.
  Pupils of unequal size or shape.
  Convulsions.
  Noticeable restlessness.
  Severe headache that persists longer than 4 hours after injury.
  Confusion or disorientation.
- See Resources for Additional Information.

MEDICATION
- Don't give any medicine—including nonprescription acetaminophen or aspirin—until the diagnosis is certain.
- Your doctor may prescribe anticonvulsants.

ACTIVITY—The patient should rest in bed until the doctor determines the danger is over. Normal activity may then be resumed as symptoms improve.

DIET—Full liquid diet (see Appendix) until the danger passes.

CALL YOUR DOCTOR IF

- You or a family member has symptoms of a head injury or observe them in someone else.
- After an injury, you observe any of the symptoms discussed in General Measures.

HEADACHE, CLUSTER

 GENERAL INFORMATION

DEFINITION—A very severe headache that typically causes pain on one side of the head, behind or around one eye. The headaches tend to recur at the same time each day for several days or weeks.

BODY PARTS INVOLVED—Central nervous system.

SEX OR AGE MOST AFFECTED— Approximately 90% of those affected are males. Onset is around age 30 in men, later in women.

SIGNS & SYMPTOMS
- Sudden onset of headache often at night while sleeping.
- Headache reaches crescendo within 15 minutes and lasts about 2 hours
- Pain is unilateral around the eye.
- Severe, piercing or boring pain.
- Teary eyes.
- Infected conjunctiva.
- Swollen and droopy eyelid.
- Nasal congestion and runny nose.
- Slow heartbeat.
- Nausea.
- Perspiration.
- Restless, active, violent (sometimes).
- Episodes of headache occur at same time on consecutive days, with clusters of these days, separated by attack-free weeks or months.

CAUSES—Actual cause is unknown. Some indication that a neurological disturbance of the body's circadian rhythm (biologic clock) may contribute to cluster headache.

RISK INCREASES WITH
- Male, age over 30.
- Possible relationship to previous head injury or surgery.
- Significantly higher incidence of peptic ulcer, coronary artery disease (males).
- Prior history of migraine frequent (significant in females).

HOW TO PREVENT—Since the cause is unknown, no specific measures to prevent the first episode.

 WHAT TO EXPECT

DIAGNOSTIC MEASURES
- Your own observation of symptoms.
- Medical history and physical exam by a doctor.
- Diagnosis is usually determined by the patient's history of the headache patterns and symptoms.

APPROPRIATE HEALTH CARE
- Self-care after diagnosis.
- Doctor's treatment.
- Consider surgical treatments to trigeminal nerve if drug therapy is ineffective (rare).

POSSIBLE COMPLICATIONS
- Self-injury during attack.
- Side effects of drugs.

PROBABLE OUTCOME
- No cure is available, but treatment can help control the pain and shorten the cluster period.
- Prolonged remissions.

 HOW TO TREAT

GENERAL MEASURES
- Therapy may involve medications and lifestyle changes.
- During cluster periods, avoid bright light or glare, alcohol, excessive anger, stressful activity or excitement. These will precipitate attacks.
- Avoid smoking; tobacco may make cluster unresponsive to drug treatment.
- See Resources for Additional Information.

MEDICATION—Your doctor may prescribe:
- Sumatriptan (the brand name is Imitrex) subcutaneous (self-injected under the skin) may help during an acute attack. Follow all prescription instructions carefully.
- Ergotamine aerosol to be used during an attack and also as a preventive. Follow prescription instructions carefully, especially if you take more than one medication.
- Oxygen therapy for at home use.
- Caffeine containing medications (oral and suppository) can help during acute attack.
- Local anesthetic, such as lidocaine.
- Phenylephrine for nasal stuffiness.
- Other medications that are available that can help suppress headaches during a cluster period (prednisone, lithium, ergotamine, verapamil, indomethacin and methysergide).

ACTIVITY
- Avoid any activities that could cause you to injure yourself during attacks.
- Vigorous physical activity at first symptoms may abort attack.

DIET
- During clusters, avoid alcohol as it can precipitate attack.
- Rarely, specific foods (chocolate, eggs, dairy products) trigger attacks.

 CALL YOUR DOCTOR IF

- You have symptoms of cluster headache.
- Attacks continue after treatment is started.

HEADACHE, TENSION (Stress Headache)

GENERAL INFORMATION

DEFINITION—Tension headaches are the most common type of headache. These headaches can occur infrequently, such as one brought on by a stressful event, or they can occur on a chronic basis (15 or more times a month for 6 months). Symptoms may be mild to severe.

BODY PARTS INVOLVED—Sensory nerves in the skin, scalp, blood vessels and muscles of the head.

SEX OR AGE MOST AFFECTED—Both sexes; all ages.

SIGNS & SYMPTOMS—Any of the following:
- Dull, aching feeling on both sides of the head.
- Tight muscles in the neck or scalp.
- Not preceded by warnings (aura, prodrome).
- Feelings of fatigue, weakness.
- If severe, nausea, light and sound sensitivity.
- Often present when you wake up.

CAUSES
- Tension, producing strain on muscles of the neck, scalp, face and jaw.
- Clenching or grinding of the teeth.
- Sleep disturbances; anxiety or depression.
- Excessive eating or drinking.
- Physically exhausting work.
- Eye strain, including sun glare.
- Use of drugs or alcohol; low blood sugar.
- Hormone changes during the menstrual cycle.
- Allergic reactions.

RISK INCREASES WITH
- Stress, either mental or physical.
- Environments that are noisy, stuffy, hot, poorly lit or have irritating odors.
- Exposure to or consumption of nitrites, sulfites, monosodium glutamate or other food additives.
- Maintaining a sitting position for long periods.

HOW TO PREVENT
- Get enough sleep—an average of 8 hours for men and 7 hours for women.
- Don't skip meals; don't overeat; don't smoke.
- Exercise regularly to improve circulation.
- Drink alcohol moderately—no more than 1 or 2 drinks a day, if at all.
- Don't use mood-altering, mind-altering, stimulant or sedative drugs.
- Avoid foods that contain nitrites or other additives to which you are sensitive.

WHAT TO EXPECT

DIAGNOSTIC MEASURES
- Medical history and exam by a doctor.
- Diagnostic tests are usually not needed, but may be indicated if a serious underlying cause is suspected.

APPROPRIATE HEALTH CARE
- Self-care.
- Doctor's treatment, if headache persists.
- Biofeedback training relaxation therapy, hypnotherapy are sometimes useful.

POSSIBLE COMPLICATIONS—None expected for most tension headaches. Rebound headaches can occur from long-term use of analgesics.

PROBABLE OUTCOME—Most tension can be relieved (see How to Treat).

HOW TO TREAT

GENERAL MEASURES
- If possible, take a break.
- Massage shoulders, neck, jaw and scalp.
- Take a hot bath or long shower.
- Lie down. Place a warm or cold cloth (or ice packs), whichever feels better, over the aching area.
- For jobs requiring long hours of sitting, be sure to get up and move around at least hourly.
- Identify your headache triggers: keep a record of the time and duration of each headache, what foods or drinks you consumed in the previous 12 hours; list any physical, emotional or personal factors that occurred prior.
- See Resources for Additional Information.

MEDICATION
- You may take acetaminophen or aspirin to relieve pain.
- Your doctor may prescribe:
  Nonsteroidal anti-inflammatory medications. Antianxiety drugs if anxiety is a problem; antidepressants if headaches are chronic. Stronger pain medicines; muscle relaxants.

ACTIVITY—Participate in a regular physical fitness program. Focus on exercises that help muscles in the back, shoulders and neck.

DIET
- Most persons feel better if they don't eat, unless the headache is from low blood sugar.
- Don't drink alcohol.

CALL YOUR DOCTOR IF

You have a headache and any of the following:
- Fever; recent head injury.
- Drowsiness; nausea or vomiting.
- Pain in one eye; blurred vision; vision disturbances and vomiting prior to the headache; high blood pressure.
- Pain and tenderness around the eyes and cheekbones that worsens when you lean forward.
- Persistent headache pain for longer than 24 hours without other symptoms.
- You suspect a drug caused the headache.

HEARING IMPAIRMENT OR LOSS (Deafness)

GENERAL INFORMATION

DEFINITION—Decreased ability or complete inability to hear. Classifications include:
• Conductive loss, in which mechanical problems keep the sound from reaching the middle ear.
• Sensorineural loss, in which the 8th cranial nerve (the acoustic nerve) is damaged—often due to excess noise over a period of time.
• Mixed loss, involving both conductive and sensorineural disabilities.

BODY PARTS INVOLVED—Middle-ear bones that conduct sound; branches of the 8th cranial nerve that transmit sound to the brain.

SEX OR AGE MOST AFFECTED—Both sexes; all ages.

SIGNS & SYMPTOMS
In an infant:
• Lack of response to environmental sounds—especially startling sounds.
• Older infant (5-10 months) doesn't turn head to side where sound originates.
In older persons:
• Difficulty in discriminating (listening selectively) to environmental sounds.
• Ringing in the ears, dizziness, pain.
• Turning up the volume of the radio or TV.
• Frequently asking people to repeat speech.

CAUSES
• Impacted earwax or fluid behind the eardrum.
• Congenital, transmitted as a dominant or recessive genetic trait.
• Chronic middle-ear infections or spread of infection to the inner ear.
• Blood-vessel disorders, including hypertension.
• Head injury or other trauma; brain tumor.
• Blood clot that travels to the acoustic nerve.
• Multiple sclerosis.
• Blood-coagulation disorders.
• Pressure changes due to flying or diving.
• Prolonged exposure to sound levels of 85 decibels or above.
• Aging. Most persons over 65 have some hearing loss of high-pitched tones.

RISK INCREASES WITH
• Family history of congenital or acquired deafness.
• Use of drugs, such as nonsteroidal anti-inflammatories, cisplatin, erythromycins, gentamycin, streptomycin, tobramycin, quinine, furosemide, ethacrynic acid or heavy doses of aspirin and others.
• Persons with occupations or hobbies involving high noise levels.

HOW TO PREVENT
• Avoid prolonged use or overdosage of drugs that cause hearing loss.
• Obtain medical treatment for underlying disorders that cause hearing loss, particularly ear infections, allergic and respiratory problems.
• Avoid prolonged exposure to loud noise. If exposure is unavoidable, protect your ears with ear plugs or ear muffs.

WHAT TO EXPECT

DIAGNOSTIC MEASURES
• Medical history and exam by a doctor.
• Audiometry (test of hearing ability) and hearing tests performed with a tuning fork (Rinne test) will be used to diagnose hearing disorders.

APPROPRIATE HEALTH CARE
• Doctor's treatment.
• Earwax removal or eardrum puncture repair may resolve hearing problem.
• If related to medications, changes in dosage or discontinuation may help.
• Treatment for other underlying causes.
• Surgery for conductive-type deafness (sometimes).
• Speech therapy and rehabilitation, if needed.

POSSIBLE COMPLICATIONS
• Permanent deafness.
• Delayed language development in a child.
• Emotional impact of deafness.

PROBABLE OUTCOME—Some conductive hearing loss is curable with surgery. Hearing loss caused by prolonged exposure to loud noise sometimes disappears when the noise is eliminated. Other types of hearing loss are usually permanent.

HOW TO TREAT

GENERAL MEASURES
• If hearing loss is permanent and disabling: Learn sign-language and lip-reading skills. Wear a hearing aid, if one is prescribed. Speech therapy and rehabilitation, if needed. Special phone equipment is available. Resist the temptation to withdraw socially because of your hearing difficulty. Isolation will increase your communication problems and frustration, and make adjustment more difficult.
• See Resources for Additional Information.

MEDICATION—Medicine usually is not needed.

ACTIVITY—No restrictions.

DIET—No special diet.

CALL YOUR DOCTOR IF

• Your child shows signs of hearing impairment.
• You suspect you have a hearing loss.

HEART ATTACK
(Myocardial Infarction)

GENERAL INFORMATION

DEFINITION—Death of heart-muscle cells from reduced or obstructed blood flow through the coronary arteries.

BODY PARTS INVOLVED—Coronary arteries; heart muscle; platelets and clotting factors circulating in the blood.

SEX OR AGE MOST AFFECTED—Adults over 40. This is more common in men, but the incidence is rising for women.

SIGNS & SYMPTOMS
- Chest pain or "heavy, squeezing or crushing" feeling in the chest.
- Pain that radiates from the midchest over the breast bone to the jaw, neck, either arm, the area between the shoulder blades or upper abdomen (sometimes).
- Feeling of impending doom.
- Shortness of breath; dizziness; weakness.
- Nausea and vomiting; sweating.

CAUSES—Partial or complete blockage of coronary arteries by a blood clot, spasm or contracture; or a severe disruption in the heart's rhythm.

RISK INCREASES WITH
- Smoking; obesity; stress.
- High blood-cholesterol levels or low HDL cholesterol.
- High blood pressure; sedentary lifestyle.
- Diet that is high in fat, refined sugar and salt.
- Diabetes mellitus.
- Family history of coronary artery disease.
- Exercise in heat or cold and wind.

HOW TO PREVENT
- Follow suggestions for prevention of Atherosclerosis (in Illness section). Ask your doctor about taking one aspirin daily.
- Avoid risk factors where possible.

WHAT TO EXPECT

DIAGNOSTIC MEASURES
- Medical history and exam by a doctor.
- Diagnostic tests may include ECG, radioactive technetium 99 scan, angiography (see Glossary) and measurement of enzymes released into blood from damaged heart muscle.

APPROPRIATE HEALTH CARE
- Hospitalization for oxygen and medications.
- Electrical stimulation to start the heart may be necessary.
- Surgery (pacemaker insertion, balloon angioplasty or coronary artery bypass graft. See Surgery section).

POSSIBLE COMPLICATIONS
- Irregular heart rhythms; shock; pericarditis; congestive heart failure.
- Pleural effusion (see Glossary).
- Deep-vein thrombosis; pulmonary embolism; rupture of the heart septum or wall.
- Ventricular aneurysm (see Glossary).
- Risk of future heart attacks.

PROBABLE OUTCOME—With immediate emergency care and hospitalization in a coronary-care unit, most persons recover from a first heart attack. Treatment delay is often fatal. Survivors should allow 4 to 8 weeks for recovery. Repeat heart attacks are common.

HOW TO TREAT

GENERAL MEASURES
- The family should maintain an optimistic outlook and be as supportive as possible.
- See Resources for Additional Information.

MEDICATION—Your doctor may prescribe:
- Drugs that quickly dissolve the blood clots (must be given within 1-3 hours of attack).
- Pain relievers.
- Antiarrhythmic and anti-anginal drugs, such as beta-adrenergic blockers or calcium-channel blockers, to stabilize an irregular heartbeat.
- Anticoagulants to prevent blood clots.
- Nitroglycerin to widen arteries and increase blood supply to the heart.
- Digitalis to strengthen heart muscle contractions and stabilize the heartbeat.

ACTIVITY
- Resume your normal activities gradually during recovery. Consult your doctor before resuming sexual relations.
- Enroll in a cardiac rehabilitation program.

DIET
- Eat a low-fat, low-salt, high-fiber diet (see Appendix for all).
- Maintain ideal weight.

CALL YOUR DOCTOR IF

- You have symptoms of a heart attack. This is a life-threatening emergency!
- The following occurs during recovery:
  Chest pain that is not relieved by prescribed medication.
  Shortness of breath or cough while at rest.
  Nausea, vomiting or diarrhea; fever.
  Bleeding from the gums or other sites.
  Palpitations or skip beats.

HEART BLOCK
(Atrioventricular Block)

GENERAL INFORMATION

DEFINITION—A persistent disruption (either mild or major) in transmission of electrical signals between the heart's upper and lower chambers. Contractions of the atria (upper heart chambers) lose synchronization with those of the ventricles (lower heart chambers). The heartbeat is no longer regulated normally to quicken under exertion or stress and slow down at other times.

BODY PARTS INVOLVED—Heart's electrical-transmission system that coordinates contractions of heart-muscle cells. The heart's natural pacemaker initiates the electrical system.

SEX OR AGE MOST AFFECTED—All ages, but most common in men over 40 and women after menopause.

SIGNS & SYMPTOMS
- No symptoms (sometimes) for less-severe forms.
- Slow, irregular heartbeat.
- Sudden loss of consciousness.
- Convulsions (sometimes).
- Attacks of dizziness, weakness or confusion.

CAUSES
- Coronary artery disease, a sign of atherosclerosis (hardening of the arteries).
- Congenital heart abnormalities.
- Excessive digitalis and some other medications.
- Some heart blocks are seen in well-trained athletes.

RISK INCREASES WITH
- Adults over 60.
- Stress.
- Improper diet that is high in fat and salt.
- Obesity.
- Smoking.
- Diabetes mellitus.
- Heart disease, including atherosclerosis, congestive heart failure or heart-valve disease.
- High blood pressure.
- Previous electrolyte imbalance.
- Use of some drugs, such as digitalis, quinidine or beta-adrenergic blockers.

HOW TO PREVENT
- Obtain medical treatment for any underlying disease.
- Don't smoke.
- Exercise regularly.
- Eat a diet that is low in fat and low in salt (see Appendix for both).

WHAT TO EXPECT

DIAGNOSTIC MEASURES
- Your own observation of symptoms.
- Medical history and physical exam by a doctor.
- ECG (see Glossary). The ECG provides information about the degree of heart block (1st, 2nd or 3rd) and will help determine what treatment, if any, is appropriate.

APPROPRIATE HEALTH CARE
- Self-care after diagnosis. Some heart blocks require no treatment.
- Doctor's treatment.
- Surgery to implant an artificial pacemaker (sometimes). It provides a regular, mild electric stimulus that maintains a normal heartbeat.

POSSIBLE COMPLICATIONS—Uncontrolled slow, rapid or irregular heartbeat and cardiac arrest.

PROBABLE OUTCOME
- Heart blocks that do not bring on symptoms usually require no treatment.
- More serious heart blocks can be controlled with surgery to implant a pacemaker.

HOW TO TREAT

GENERAL MEASURES
- Wear a Medic-Alert bracelet or pendant (see Glossary) in case you suddenly lose consciousness.
- Don't smoke.
- See Resources for Additional Information.

MEDICATION
- Your doctor may prescribe atropine for short-term therapy.
- Don't take medications to relieve allergy or nasal congestion. They can worsen symptoms.

ACTIVITY—Don't think of yourself as an invalid. Unless your doctor advises against it, mild exercise is helpful and not to be feared. Begin a regular exercise program—walking is ideal.

DIET
- Lose weight if you are overweight (see Weight-Loss Diet in Appendix).
- Avoid excessive use of alcoholic beverages. Alcohol depresses the heartbeat.

CALL YOUR DOCTOR IF

- You have symptoms of heart block, especially an episode with loss of consciousness.
- After diagnosis, stress increases in your life.

HEART MURMURS

GENERAL INFORMATION

DEFINITION—Heart murmurs are not a disease or illness. They involve the sounds, as heard through a stethoscope, of blood flowing through the heart. With murmurs, there is an extra sound (sometimes described as "swishing") in addition to the normal sounds (described as "lub-dup") of the heartbeat. Most heart murmurs are harmless or "innocent" and are detected at a routine physical or well-baby examination. Murmurs are heard in many healthy people.

BODY PARTS INVOLVED—Heart.

SEX OR AGE MOST AFFECTED—All ages, both sexes; more often heard in children and teenagers.

SIGNS & SYMPTOMS—People with heart murmurs have no symptoms, unless associated with other disorders.

CAUSES—The stethoscope picks up sounds made when the ventricles of the heart contract and the 4 heart valves snap shut. Most extra sounds caused by turbulent blood flow are known as murmurs. What causes innocent type heart murmurs is unknown.

RISK INCREASES WITH
- Congenital heart defects.
- Rheumatic fever.
- Myocarditis.
- Children with anemia.
- Pregnancy.

HOW TO PREVENT—There are no preventive measures.

WHAT TO EXPECT

DIAGNOSTIC MEASURES
- Heart murmurs are detected by a medical professional listening to the heart sounds through a stethoscope. By listening to these sounds, a trained person can judge by their quality, intensity, location and timing that the murmur is insignificant (most cases).
- In a few cases, the sounds that are heard may indicate a need for more testing in order to determine the cause. Chest x-ray, ECG and echocardiography (see Glossary for both) may be done for further study.

APPROPRIATE HEALTH CARE—No medical treatment is necessary for an innocent heart murmur.

POSSIBLE COMPLICATIONS
- None expected with innocent heart murmurs.
- If there is any underlying organic heart problem, it can usually be corrected surgically.

PROBABLE OUTCOME—Most innocent heart murmurs detected (particularly in children) disappear or become undetectable over time. People with these murmurs live a completely normal life.

HOW TO TREAT

GENERAL MEASURES—If your child has an innocent type heart murmur, treat him or her like any other healthy child. Parents sometimes become concerned about the idea of a heart murmur and become over-protective. This can cause problems for the child's emotional well-being.

MEDICATION—No medication is necessary.

ACTIVITY—Do not limit activity.

DIET—No special diet.

CALL YOUR DOCTOR IF

You need further assurance about heart murmurs.

HEART RHYTHM IRREGULARITY
(Arrhythmia)

GENERAL INFORMATION

DEFINITION—Abnormalities in the rhythm of the heartbeat. The heart may beat too slowly (bradycardia) or too rapidly (tachycardia) and the condition may be benign or serious.

BODY PARTS INVOLVED—Heart; nerves that transmit impulses to coordinate heart muscle contractions. Most people have some irregular beats.

SEX OR AGE MOST AFFECTED—All ages, but most likely over age 65.

SIGNS & SYMPTOMS
- Awareness of one's own heartbeat (palpitations), including whether it skips, is always fast, slow, irregular, or suddenly changes rhythm.
- Shortness of breath.
- Sudden faintness or weakness.
- No symptoms (frequently).

CAUSES
- Heart diseases, such as: rheumatic fever; congenital heart disease; cardiomyopathy; previous heart attack; or heart muscle inflammation.
- Endocrine disorders, especially thyroid and adrenal-gland diseases.
- Fluid and electrolyte imbalance, especially too little or too much potassium.
- Side effects of certain drugs, especially digitalis, beta-adrenergic blockers, stimulants and diuretics.
- Overdose of certain drugs, including antidepressants, marijuana and cocaine.
- Postoperative effects following chest or heart surgery.

RISK INCREASES WITH
- Stress; chronic kidney disease; hypertension; smoking.
- Use of certain drugs, such as caffeine, alcohol, amphetamines and many nonprescription cough and cold remedies.
- Fatigue, overwork or sleep deprivation.

HOW TO PREVENT—If you have any disorders listed as causes or risks, follow your treatment program carefully to control the disease. If medication is part of your treatment, consult your doctor about having blood levels monitored and electrolytes measured periodically.

WHAT TO EXPECT

DIAGNOSTIC MEASURES
- Medical history and exam by a doctor.
- Laboratory blood studies.

- ECG and sometimes, a 24-hour Holter monitor (see Glossary for both).
- Radioactive technetium 99 scan, angiography (see Glossary), and measurement of enzymes released into blood from damaged heart muscle.

APPROPRIATE HEALTH CARE
- Frequently no treatment is necessary.
- Medication.
- DC cardioversion (see Glossary).
- Surgery to correct some heart problems.

POSSIBLE COMPLICATIONS
- Fainting; congestive heart failure.
- A few arrhythmias are fatal unless cardiopulmonary resuscitation (CPR) is performed immediately.
- Death from prolonged (more than 3 to 6 minutes) cardiac arrest.

PROBABLE OUTCOME
- Very occasionally irregular heartbeats are harmless and require no treatment.
- Most other rhythm disturbances can be controlled with treatment.

HOW TO TREAT

GENERAL MEASURES
- Consider lifestyle changes. Ask for professional help if needed.
- Stop smoking.
- Take a course to learn CPR, especially if someone in your home or neighborhood has heart disease.
- Wear a Medic-Alert bracelet or pendant (see Glossary) showing the name of your condition.
- See Resources for Additional Information.

MEDICATION—Your doctor may prescribe antiarrhythmic medications. You may need to try several to find the most effective one. Certain arrhythmias (atrial fibrillation) will require anticoagulant medicine.

ACTIVITY—Resume most normal activities as soon as symptoms improve. Consult your doctor about an exercise program.

DIET
- Some heart medicines require extra potassium, found mostly in citrus fruits, bananas, dried apricots or peaches, raisins, lentils and whole-grain cereals. Ask your doctor if you need to eat more of these.
- Avoid caffeine-containing beverages, such as coffee, tea, cola or chocolate. Avoid alcohol.

CALL YOUR DOCTOR IF

- You have symptoms of heart rhythm irregularity.
- New, unexplained symptoms develop.

HEART VALVE DISEASE
(Valvular Heart Disease)

 GENERAL INFORMATION

DEFINITION—A complication of diseases that distort or destroy valves of the heart. The heart has 4 valves. The mitral and tricuspid valves (main heart valves) control blood flow into the ventricles. The aortic and pulmonic valves control blood flow out of the heart. The correct functioning of the valves is vital to the efficiency of the heart as a pump.

BODY PARTS INVOLVED—Heart valves (aortic, mitral, tricuspid and pulmonic valves).

SEX OR AGE MOST AFFECTED—Both sexes; all ages.

SIGNS & SYMPTOMS
- No symptoms (sometimes).
- Fatigue and weakness.
- Dizziness or fainting.
- Chest pain.
- Shortness of breath.
- Lung congestion.
- Heart rhythm irregularities.
- Heart murmurs (abnormal heart sounds heard by the doctor through a stethoscope).
- Abnormal blood pressure (high or low).

CAUSES—Heart valve disease can be either narrowed valves, which obstruct blood flow (stenosis), or widened or scarred valves, which allow blood to leak backward into the heart (insufficiency). The disorder may be inherited or caused by any of the following:
- Rheumatic fever.
- A complication of strep throat.
- Atherosclerosis.
- High blood pressure.
- Congenital heart defects.
- Endocarditis and intravenous drug abuse.
- Syphilis (rare).
- Self-injected intravenous drugs are a major risk.

RISK INCREASES WITH
- Persons over 60.
- Family history of heart valve disease.
- Pregnancy.
- Fatigue or overwork.
- Marfan's syndrome.

HOW TO PREVENT
- Obtain medical treatment for diseases that cause heart valve damage, such as high blood pressure, endocarditis and syphilis.
- Take antibiotics for streptococcal infections to prevent rheumatic fever.
- If you have a family history of congenital heart disease, obtain genetic counseling before starting a family.

 WHAT TO EXPECT

DIAGNOSTIC MEASURES
- Medical history and exam by a doctor.
- Laboratory blood tests.
- ECG, echocardiogram (see Glossary).
- Heart catheterization (see Glossary).
- Angiography (see Glossary).

APPROPRIATE HEALTH CARE
- Doctor's treatment.
- Hospitalization.
- Surgery may be recommended to correct a heart valve defect or remove a diseased or damaged valve and replace it by a mechanical one (a valve made from human or bovine tissue, or a human valve from a deceased person). (See Heart Valve Replacement in Surgery section.)

POSSIBLE COMPLICATIONS
- Infection of the valves.
- Congestive heart failure.

PROBABLE OUTCOME—Depends on the underlying condition. Many complications of valvular disease can be controlled with medication or cured with surgery.

 HOW TO TREAT

GENERAL MEASURES
- Tell any doctor, dentist or anesthesiologist who treats you that you have heart valve disease. Remind those involved, even if you think they know your medical history.
- See Resources for Additional Information.

MEDICATION—Your doctor may prescribe:
- Antibiotics to treat or prevent bacterial infection of abnormal heart valves.
- Antiarrhythmic drugs to stabilize heartbeat irregularities.
- Digitalis medication to strengthen or regulate the heartbeat.
- Anticoagulants after surgery in some cases.

ACTIVITY—As much as can be tolerated. No restrictions are necessary with some forms of heart valve disease.

DIET—Eat a low-fat, low-salt diet (see Appendix for both).

 CALL YOUR DOCTOR IF

- You have symptoms of heart valve disease.
- During treatment, you develop signs of infection, such as fever, chills, muscle aches, headache, fatigue and a general ill feeling.

HEARTBEAT, RAPID
(Tachycardia; Paroxysmal Tachycardia)

 GENERAL INFORMATION

DEFINITION—Heartbeat that is much more rapid than usual and is not caused by overexertion. Tachycardia ranges from 150 to 300 beats per minute. A person with no heart disease may exercise and raise the heartbeat to 160 or more. This is normal and is not a medical problem. Types of tachycardia include atrial fibrillation, sinus tachycardia, supraventricular tachycardia and ventricular tachycardia.

BODY PARTS INVOLVED—Heart muscle; electrical system of the heart.

SEX OR AGE MOST AFFECTED—Both sexes; all ages.

SIGNS & SYMPTOMS
- Heart pounding or palpitations. The pulse at the wrist or neck will be 100 to 180 beats per minute, which is much faster than normal.
- Faintness or a feeling of impending death.
- Chest pain.
- Involuntary cough.
- Breathlessness.

CAUSES—Unknown. This usually occurs in young persons with no evidence of disease, but it may also occur in older patients who have coronary artery disease.

RISK INCREASES WITH
- Heart disease.
- Fever.
- Hyperthyroidism.
- Stress; anxiety.
- Smoking.
- Use of some drugs, such as caffeine, cocaine, ephedrine or other sympathomimetic drugs.

HOW TO PREVENT
- Don't smoke.
- Reduce stress, if possible (see How to Cope with Stress in Appendix).
- Avoid decongestants, appetite suppressants, excessive coffee, cola and other stimulants with or without caffeine, cocaine, amphetamines.

 WHAT TO EXPECT

DIAGNOSTIC MEASURES
- Your own observation of symptoms.
- Medical history and physical exam by a doctor.
- ECG (see Glossary).
- Holter monitor (see glossary).

APPROPRIATE HEALTH CARE
- Sometimes no treatment.
- Doctor's treatment.
- Self-care after diagnosis.
- Hospitalization if the attack persists, despite treatment.
- DC electrocardioversion, a controlled electric shock (rarely necessary).

POSSIBLE COMPLICATIONS—Uninterrupted tachycardia can lead to life-threatening congestive heart failure, heart attack or cardiac arrest.

PROBABLE OUTCOME—Most arrhythmias are temporary and benign. Rapid heartbeat can usually be controlled with treatment.

 HOW TO TREAT

GENERAL MEASURES
- The following sometimes reduce heartbeat:
  Hold your breath briefly.
  Pinch the skin on your arm enough to cause pain.
  Bathe your face in cold water, submerge your head briefly in a sink of cool water or take a cool shower and let the water beat on your head.
  Hold your nostrils closed and blow gently through the nose, making the eardrums pop.
  Massage the carotid area in the neck, if you have been taught to do this safely. Ask your doctor for instructions.
- See Resources for Additional Information.

MEDICATION—For repeated attacks, your doctor may prescribe medication to control heart rhythm. These include: digitalis; quinidine; calcium-channel blockers; procainamide; and beta-adrenergic blockers.

ACTIVITY
- Lie down during an attack until your heartbeat returns to normal, then resume your activities.
- Exercise regularly with your doctor's approval. Physical fitness helps prevent tachycardia.

DIET—No special diet.

 CALL YOUR DOCTOR IF

- You have an episode of rapid, irregular heartbeat that does not end in 4 or 5 minutes.
- You develop shortness of breath.
- You have chest pain.

ILLNESS & DISORDERS

HEATSTROKE OR HEAT EXHAUSTION
(Sunstroke; Heat Prostration)

GENERAL INFORMATION

DEFINITION—Illness caused by prolonged exposure to hot temperatures, limited fluid intake or failure of temperature regulation mechanisms in the brain.

BODY PARTS INVOLVED—Total body.

SEX OR AGE MOST AFFECTED—All ages, but most common in the elderly.

SIGNS & SYMPTOMS
Heat exhaustion:
- Dizziness, fatigue, faintness, headache.
- Skin that is pale and clammy.
- Pulse rapid and weak.
- Breathing is fast and shallow.
- Muscle cramps.
- Intense thirst.

Heatstroke:
- Often preceded by heat exhaustion and its symptoms.
- Skin that is hot, dry and flushed.
- No sweating.
- High body temperature.
- Rapid heartbeat.
- Confusion.
- Loss of consciousness.

CAUSES
- Heat exhaustion is caused by insufficient water intake, insufficient salt intake and a deficiency in the production of sweat. (Sweat evaporation is what helps to cool the body.)
- Heat stroke is caused by overexposure to extreme heat and a breakdown in the body's heat-regulating mechanisms. The body becomes overheated to a dangerous degree (body temperature can reach 107F).

RISK INCREASES WITH
- General effects of aging.
- Alcohol or other drug abuse.
- Chronic illness, such as diabetes or blood-vessel disease.
- Recent illness involving fluid loss from vomiting or diarrhea.
- Hot, humid weather.
- Working in a hot environment.
- Loss of body fluids from sweating and failure to drink enough replacement fluid.
- Heavy, restrictive clothing.
- Severe fever.

HOW TO PREVENT
- Wear light, loose-fitting clothing in hot weather.
- Drink water often, don't wait until thirsty.
- Drink extra water if you sweat heavily. If urine output decreases, increase your water intake.

- If you become overheated, improve your ventilation. Open a window or use a fan or air conditioner. This promotes sweat evaporation, which cools the skin.
- Acclimate yourself to hot weather.

WHAT TO EXPECT

DIAGNOSTIC MEASURES
- Your own observation of symptoms.
- Medical history and physical exam by a doctor.
- Laboratory studies of blood and urine to measure electrolyte levels.

APPROPRIATE HEALTH CARE
- Self-care after diagnosis (mild cases).
- Doctor's treatment.
- Hospitalization to lower body temperature and provide intravenous replacement fluids.

POSSIBLE COMPLICATIONS
- Can involve any major organ system (heart, lungs, kidneys, brain).
- Related to duration and intensity of heat, and to speed and effectiveness of treatment.

PROBABLE OUTCOME—Prompt treatment usually brings full recovery in 1 to 2 days.

HOW TO TREAT

GENERAL MEASURES
- If someone with symptoms is very hot and not sweating:
  Cool the person rapidly. Use a cold-water bath or wrap in wet sheets.
  Arrange for transportation to the nearest hospital. This is an emergency!
- If someone is faint but sweating:
  Give the person liquids (water, soft drinks or fruit juice). Don't give salt pills.
  Arrange for transportation to the hospital, except in mild cases. Call your doctor for advice.

MEDICATION—Medicine usually is not necessary for these disorders.

ACTIVITY—Activity may be resumed as soon as symptoms improve. Rest with legs elevated while symptoms are present.

DIET—No special diet.

CALL YOUR DOCTOR IF

You have symptoms of heatstroke or heat exhaustion or observe them in someone else. Call immediately! These conditions may be serious or fatal.

HEEL SPUR
(Calcaneal Spur)

GENERAL INFORMATION

DEFINITION—A hard, bony growth in the tissue of the heel that causes pain and difficulty walking.

BODY PARTS INVOLVED—Heel, including the calcaneus (the major bone in the heel).

SEX OR AGE MOST AFFECTED—Adults. The condition is fairly common among runners and other athletes.

SIGNS & SYMPTOMS
- No symptoms sometimes.
- Pain and tenderness in the sole of the foot, under the heel bone. Pain occurs after resting or after rising in the morning.

CAUSES—Stress or injury to the heel tissues, which causes inflammation and calcification of ligaments in the foot.

RISK INCREASES WITH
- Running or jogging. The condition is less likely with vigorous walking.
- Prolonged standing.
- Obesity.

HOW TO PREVENT
- Avoid activities that put constant strain on the foot. Switch to swimming or cycling.
- Wear a shoe with a rubber or felt heel cushion.

WHAT TO EXPECT

DIAGNOSTIC MEASURES
- Your own observation of symptoms.
- Medical history and physical exam by a doctor.
- X-rays of the heel.

APPROPRIATE HEALTH CARE
- Self-care after diagnosis.
- Doctor's treatment.
- Surgery to remove the spur if other treatments fail (rare). (See Heel-Spur Removal in Surgery section.)

POSSIBLE COMPLICATIONS—Lower-back or knee disorders caused by constant limping.

PROBABLE OUTCOME—Usually curable with conservative treatment. If not, heel spurs are curable with surgery.

HOW TO TREAT

GENERAL MEASURES
- Place a heel cup or felt insert in the shoe to relieve pressure on the heel.
- Get advice from your doctor or a podiatrist (see Glossary) about custom made shoe inserts to correct structural foot problems.
- For acute pain, use a cold compress or ice pack 3-4 times a day for 10-15 minutes each time.

MEDICATION
- To relieve minor pain and inflammation, you may use nonprescription drugs, such as ibuprofen or aspirin.
- Your doctor may inject steroids into the inflamed area to reduce inflammation.

ACTIVITY—Stay off your feet as much as possible, especially at the beginning of treatment.

DIET—No special diet, unless you are overweight. If so, lose weight to reduce stress on the foot.

CALL YOUR DOCTOR IF

- You have symptoms of a heel spur.
- Pain or disability persists, despite treatment.

ILLNESS & DISORDERS

HEMOPHILIA

GENERAL INFORMATION

DEFINITION—An inherited deficiency of a blood-clotting factor that results in episodes of dangerous bleeding. Blood normally contains multiple factors that enable clotting to occur. The factors are designated I through XIII. In hemophilia A, the clotting factor VIII is deficient. Factors I-VII function properly, but the clotting process is then interrupted. Hemophilia B occurs less often and is caused by a deficiency of factor IX.

BODY PARTS INVOLVED—All body parts.

SEX OR AGE MOST AFFECTED—Affects 1 in 10,000 males, and appears early in childhood. Rarely in a female when her mother is a carrier and her father is hemophiliac.

SIGNS & SYMPTOMS
- Painful, swollen joints or swelling in the leg or arm (especially the knee or elbow) when bleeding occurs.
- Frequent bruises.
- Excessive bleeding from minor cuts.
- Spontaneous nosebleeds.
- Blood in the urine.

CAUSES—The deficiency of a coagulation factor (X-linked recessive gene) is passed by an affected male to all of his daughters, but to none of his sons. These females become carriers of the condition. Some of the sons of female carriers may be affected, and some of the daughters of female carriers may themselves become carriers.

RISK INCREASES WITH—Positive family history of hemophilia.

HOW TO PREVENT—Cannot be prevented at present. If your family has a history of hemophilia, obtain genetic counseling before having children.

WHAT TO EXPECT

DIAGNOSTIC MEASURES
- Your own observation of symptoms.
- Medical history and physical exam by a doctor.
- Hemophilia is diagnosed by blood-clotting tests that reveal factor VIII (or IX) activity is abnormally low.

APPROPRIATE HEALTH CARE
- Doctor's treatment. Doctor should be a qualified hematologist (blood specialist).
- Hospitalization or care in an outpatient facility for transfusions of plasma and various blood factors.
- Self-care.

POSSIBLE COMPLICATIONS
- Dangerous bleeding episodes requiring emergency treatment.
- Permanent joint disability caused by persistent bleeding.
- Risk of contacting HIV/AIDS or hepatitis through donated blood problems is lessened with genetically engineered factor VIII product.

PROBABLE OUTCOME—This condition is currently considered incurable, but not fatal. If bleeding can be controlled, patients can expect a nearly normal life span.

Scientific research into causes and treatment continues, so there is hope for increasingly effective treatment and cure.

HOW TO TREAT

GENERAL MEASURES
- Learn the signs and symptoms of bleeding episodes to watch for.
- Bleeding episodes can usually be controlled with home care by self-administered replacement therapy.
- For possible emergency situations, wear a bracelet or pendant that identifies you as a person who has hemophilia.
- See Resources for Additional Information.

MEDICATION
- Your doctor may prescribe:
  Medication to reduce joint pain.
  Transfusions of plasma or clotting factors.
- Don't take aspirin. It may increase bleeding.

ACTIVITY—Avoid activities that can cause injury, such as contact sports. Swim, bicycle or walk instead. Otherwise, no restrictions.

DIET—No special diet.

CALL YOUR DOCTOR IF

- You have symptoms of hemophilia.
- The following occurs after diagnosis:
  Injury with swelling. This may indicate bleeding under the skin.
  Bleeding that isn't quickly controlled.
  Tender, painful, swollen joint.

HEMORRHOIDS (Piles)

GENERAL INFORMATION

DEFINITION—Dilated (varicose) veins of the rectum or anus. Hemorrhoids may be located at the beginning of the anal canal (internal hemorrhoids), or at the anal opening (external hemorrhoids). Hemorrhoids may be present for years, but go undetected until bleeding occurs.

BODY PARTS INVOLVED—Veins under the rectal or anal membrane.

SEX OR AGE MOST AFFECTED—Adults of both sexes.

SIGNS & SYMPTOMS
- Rectal bleeding. Bright-red blood may appear as streaks on toilet paper adhering to fecal residue, or it may be a slow trickle for a short while following bowel movements. It almost always colors the toilet water.
- Pain, itching or mucus discharge after bowel movements. Straining during bowel movements increases pain.
- A lump that can be felt in the anus.
- A sensation that the rectum has not emptied completely after a bowel movement (large hemorrhoids only).

CAUSES—Repeated pressure in the anal or rectal veins.

RISK INCREASES WITH
- Diet that lacks fiber; constipation.
- Prolonged sitting (especially truck drivers and pilots) or prolonged standing.
- Obesity.
- Pregnancy.
- Constipation.
- Loss of muscle tone due to older age, rectal surgery or episiotomy.
- Liver disease.
- Anal intercourse.
- Colon malignancy.
- Portal hypertension.

HOW TO PREVENT
- Don't try to hurry bowel movements, but avoid straining and prolonged sitting on the toilet.
- Lose weight if you are overweight.
- Include plenty of fiber in your diet.
- Drink 8-10 glasses of water a day.
- Exercise regularly.

WHAT TO EXPECT

DIAGNOSTIC MEASURES
- Your own observation of symptoms.
- Medical history and exam by a doctor.
- Anoscopy or proctoscopy (see Glossary).

APPROPRIATE HEALTH CARE
- Self-care.
- Doctor's treatment.

- Surgery may be required in stubborn cases. Procedures include ligation (tying off hemorrhoid with a rubber band to strangulate it); sclerotherapy (injection of chemical to induce scarring); cryosurgery (freezing the hemorrhoid with liquid nitrogen); coagulation (by infrared light or laser) or hemorrhoidectomy (surgical removal). (See Hemorrhoid Banding and Hemorrhoid Removal in Surgery section.)

POSSIBLE COMPLICATIONS
- Iron-deficiency anemia if blood loss is significant.
- Severe pain caused by a blood clot in a hemorrhoid.
- Infection or ulceration of a hemorrhoid.

PROBABLE OUTCOME—Hemorrhoids usually clear up with proper care, but symptoms may flare up after a bout of constipation. Stubborn cases may require surgery.

HOW TO TREAT

GENERAL MEASURES
- Never strain to push stool out.
- Lift feet on a low footstool to aid bowel movement.
- Clean the anal area gently with soft, moist paper after each bowel movement.
- To relieve pain, sit in 8 to 10 inches of hot water for 10 to 20 minutes several times a day.
- To reduce pain and swelling of a blood clot or protruding hemorrhoid, stay in bed for 1 day and apply ice packs to the anal area.

MEDICATION
- For minor pain, itching or to reduce swelling, you may use nonprescription drugs that are formulated to relieve symptoms of hemorrhoids.
- Your doctor may prescribe a stool softener or bulk laxative, such as psyllium seed.

ACTIVITY—No restrictions. Bowel function improves with good physical conditioning.

DIET
- To prevent constipation, eat a well-balanced diet that contains many high-fiber foods such as fresh fruit, bran muffins, beans, vegetables and whole-grain cereals.
- Drink 8-10 glasses of fluid daily.
- Weight loss diet if overweight.

CALL YOUR DOCTOR IF

- A hard lump develops where a hemorrhoid has been.
- Hemorrhoids cause severe pain that isn't relieved by treatment above.
- Rectal bleeding is excessive (more than a trace or streak on toilet paper or stool).

HEPATITIS, VIRAL

 GENERAL INFORMATION

DEFINITION—Inflammation of the liver caused by a virus. Hepatitis has several forms. The most common are type A (infectious hepatitis) and type B (serum hepatitis). Other types include hepatitis C, D, E and G.

BODY PARTS INVOLVED—Liver.

SEX OR AGE MOST AFFECTED—Both sexes; all ages.

SIGNS & SYMPTOMS
Early stages:
• Flulike symptoms, such as fever, fatigue, nausea, vomiting, diarrhea and loss of appetite.
Several days later:
• Jaundice (yellow eyes and skin) caused by a buildup of bile in the blood.
• Dark urine from bile spilling into the urine.
• Light, "clay-colored" or whitish stools.

CAUSES
• Types A and E: The virus usually enters the body through water or food, especially raw shellfish, that has been contaminated by sewage (fecal-oral contact). This type can occur in epidemics.
• Type B: Usually sexually transmitted (contact with body fluids of an infected person), through blood transfusions contaminated with the virus, or from injections with nonsterile needles or syringes. An infected mother can pass it to her newborn. Some cases appear sporadically.
• Type C: Usually transmitted through intravenous drug use, blood transfusions and other exposures from contaminated blood or its products. In 40% of the cases, mode of transmission is unknown.
• Type D: Always associated with an infection of hepatitis type B.

RISK INCREASES WITH
• Travel to areas with poor sanitation.
• Oral-anal sexual practices.
• Use of intravenous, mind-altering drugs.
• Alcoholism; blood transfusions.
• Hospital workers; day-care centers or residential programs; kidney-dialysis treatment; poor nutrition; illness that has lowered resistance.

HOW TO PREVENT
• If you are exposed to someone with hepatitis, consult your doctor about receiving gamma-globulin injections to prevent or decrease risk.
• If you are in a high-risk group, such as hospital workers, dentists, dental workers, male homosexuals, sexually promiscuous men and women, or intravenous drug abusers, consider vaccination for Type-B hepatitis. Vaccines are under development for other forms.
• Routine hepatitis B vaccination for all newborn infants.

 WHAT TO EXPECT

DIAGNOSTIC MEASURES
• Medical history and exam by a doctor.
• Laboratory blood tests to identify infection, liver function studies, liver biopsy in severe or chronic cases.

APPROPRIATE HEALTH CARE
• Doctor's treatment.
• Hospitalization in severe cases.

POSSIBLE COMPLICATIONS
• Liver failure, cirrhosis of the liver, liver cancer, even death.
• Chronic hepatitis. These patients are carriers and potentially infectious to household and sexual contacts. These people may look and feel well and not know they are infected.

PROBABLE OUTCOME—Jaundice and other symptoms peak and then gradually disappear over 3 to 16 weeks. Most people in good general health recover fully in 1 to 4 months. A small percentage proceed to chronic hepatitis. Recovery from viral hepatitis usually provides permanent immunity against it.

 HOW TO TREAT

GENERAL MEASURES
• Most persons with hepatitis can be cared for at home without undue risk. Strict isolation is not necessary, but the ill person should have separate eating and drinking utensils, or use disposable ones.
• If you have hepatitis or are caring for someone with it, wash your hands carefully.

MEDICATION—There are few specific medicines to treat hepatitis. Cortisone drugs may be prescribed for severe cases to reduce liver inflammation. Chronic hepatitis B or C may be treated with alpha-interferon.

ACTIVITY—Bed rest is not usually necessary, but extreme exertion or exercise as well as contact sports should be avoided.

DIET—Despite poor appetite, small well-balanced meals help promote recovery. At least 8 glasses of water are necessary each day. Don't drink alcohol.

 CALL YOUR DOCTOR IF

• You have symptoms of hepatitis, or have been exposed to someone who has it.
• The following occurs during treatment:
Increasing loss of appetite.
Excessive drowsiness or mental confusion.
Vomiting, diarrhea or abdominal pain.
Deepening jaundice; skin rash or itching.

HEPATOMA
(Malignant Liver Tumor; Hepatocellular Carcinoma)

GENERAL INFORMATION

DEFINITION—A malignant tumor that begins in the liver (primary), as opposed to cancer that has spread from another site. Hepatoma is usually associated with an underlying liver disease such as cirrhosis of the liver.

BODY PARTS INVOLVED—Liver.

SEX OR AGE MOST AFFECTED—Adults of both sexes, but more common in men.

SIGNS & SYMPTOMS
- Hard mass in the right upper abdomen.
- Unexplained weight loss and appetite loss.
- Jaundice (yellow skin and eyes; rare).
- Abdominal discomfort that resembles a pulled muscle.
- Low blood sugar (weakness, sweating, hunger, tremor and headache).
- Fever.
- Fluid in the abdomen; enlarged spleen.
- Bleeding tendency in the gastrointestinal tract and other sites.

CAUSES
- Pre-existing cirrhosis of the liver. 50% of persons with hepatoma have cirrhosis.
- Possible slow virus.
- Hepatitis type B or type C infection.

RISK INCREASES WITH
- Medical history of hepatitis; alcoholism.
- Birth control pills.
- Anabolic steroids used by some athletes to build muscles.
- Geographic locations. This is especially common in South Africa and Southeast Asia.

HOW TO PREVENT
- Don't drink more than 1 or 2 alcoholic drinks—if any—a day.
- Immunization against hepatitis B may be helpful.
- Regular screening laboratory tests in high-risk individuals (those with cirrhosis or chronic active hepatitis).

WHAT TO EXPECT

DIAGNOSTIC MEASURES
- Your own observation of symptoms.
- Medical history and physical exam by a doctor.
- Laboratory blood studies of liver function and hepatitis B antigen.
- CT scan (see Glossary) of the liver, and ultrasound.
- X-rays of the abdomen, including angiography (see Glossary) of liver blood vessels.
- Liver biopsy (see Glossary).

APPROPRIATE HEALTH CARE
- Doctor's treatment.
- Surgery to remove the tumor, if possible. Only 25% can be removed successfully. Liver transplantation has been successful in a few patients (see Liver Transplantation in Surgery section).
- Psychotherapy or counseling to help in coping with incurable illness.

POSSIBLE COMPLICATIONS
- Liver failure.
- Spread (metastases) to other organs, especially the lungs, adrenal glands and bones.

PROBABLE OUTCOME—This condition is currently considered incurable. Only a small number of patients survive 5 years following surgery. However, symptoms can be relieved or controlled, and medical literature cites a few instances of unexplained recovery.

Scientific research into causes and treatment continues, so there is hope for increasingly effective treatment and cure.

HOW TO TREAT

GENERAL MEASURES
- The more you can learn and understand about this disorder, the more you will be able to make informed decisions about where to go for your care, the treatments available, the risks involved, side effects of therapy and expected outcome.
- See Resources for Additional Information.

MEDICATION
- For minor discomfort, you may use nonprescription drugs such as acetaminophen. Your doctor may prescribe pain relievers, if necessary.
- Anticancer drugs have produced disappointing results so far.

ACTIVITY—Stay as active as your strength allows.

DIET—No special diet. Don't drink alcohol.

CALL YOUR DOCTOR IF

- You have symptoms of hepatoma.
- You develop signs of bleeding, especially from the gastrointestinal tract. Signs include bloody vomit or vomit that contains black material resembling coffee grounds, blood in the stool or black, tarry stools.

HERNIA

GENERAL INFORMATION

DEFINITION—Protrusion of an internal organ through a weakness or abnormal opening in the muscle around it. The most common types include:
- Inguinal hernia and femoral hernia (both involve connective tissue in the groin).
- Incisional hernia (involves muscles at the site of previous surgery).
- Umbilical hernia (in newborns, involves muscles around the navel).
- Epigastric hernia (occurs in the upper abdomen, between breastbone and navel).
- Periumbilical hernia (develops around the navel, more common in women).

BODY PARTS INVOLVED—Muscles.

SEX OR AGE MOST AFFECTED—Both sexes; all ages.

SIGNS & SYMPTOMS
- A swelling that usually returns to normal position with gentle pressure or by lying down.
- Mild discomfort or pain at the site of the lump (sometimes).
- Scrotal swelling, with or without pain.
- Constipation, indigestion.
- Vomiting (rare, dangerous).

CAUSES—Weakness in connective tissue or a muscle wall. This may be present at birth or acquired later in life. Incisional hernias result from previous surgery.

RISK INCREASES WITH
- Premature infants.
- Adults over 60.
- Chronic cough.
- Obesity.
- Pregnancy.
- Straining, as with chronic constipation.

HOW TO PREVENT
- Most hernias cannot be avoided, but maintaining proper weight and regular exercise to keep muscles toned may prevent some types of hernias.
- Seek medical help if constipation is a problem.
- If chronic cough is present, seek appropriate medical care.

WHAT TO EXPECT

DIAGNOSTIC MEASURES
- Your own observation of symptoms.
- Medical history and physical exam by a doctor.
- Laboratory blood studies.
- X-rays of the abdomen.

APPROPRIATE HEALTH CARE
- Doctor's treatment.
- Surgery to repair the opening caused by weakened muscle or connective tissue. The surgery can normally be done as an outpatient. (See 3 topics on Hernia Repair in Surgery section.)

POSSIBLE COMPLICATIONS—If the hernia becomes strangulated (loses its blood supply), the protruding part may cause intestinal obstruction with fever, severe pain, vomiting and shock.

PROBABLE OUTCOME—Umbilical hernias usually heal spontaneously by age 4 and rarely require surgery. Other hernias are usually curable with surgery.

HOW TO TREAT

GENERAL MEASURES
- For an explanation of surgery and postoperative care, see Hernia (in Surgery section).
- If hernia is causing only mild discomfort and can readily be pushed back, a supportive garment or truss may be recommended.

MEDICATION—For minor discomfort, you may use nonprescription drugs such as acetaminophen.

ACTIVITY
- Avoid heavy lifting either before or after surgery.
- Speed of recovery will depend on general heath and type of hernia repaired. Light activities can usually be resumed in a few days.
- Don't return to exercise program until you have medical approval.

DIET
- Adjust diet to avoid constipation.
- Maintain ideal weight.

CALL YOUR DOCTOR IF

You have symptoms of a hernia. If you have fever or severe pain, call immediately!

HERPANGINA

GENERAL INFORMATION

DEFINITION—A viral inflammation of the mouth and throat. It may be confused with canker sores, strep throat or herpes.

BODY PARTS INVOLVED—Soft palate (back of the mouth and tonsil area).

SEX OR AGE MOST AFFECTED—Young children (1 to 10 years).

SIGNS & SYMPTOMS
- Fever.
- Sudden sore throat, with redness, inflammation and painful swallowing.
- General ill feeling.
- Vomiting and abdominal pain (sometimes).
- Tiny blisters (vesicles) in the affected areas. The blisters become small ulcers.

CAUSES—Infection from a virus (coxsackievirus) that is spread from person to person. Incubation period is usually from 2-7 days.

RISK INCREASES WITH—Summer and early fall seasons.

HOW TO PREVENT
- Cannot be prevented at present, but wash hands carefully to prevent its spread.
- Avoid close personal contact such as kissing or sharing food.

WHAT TO EXPECT

DIAGNOSTIC MEASURES
- Your own observation of symptoms.
- Medical history and physical exam by a doctor.

APPROPRIATE HEALTH CARE—Home care. Usually no treatment is necessary other than simple painkillers.

POSSIBLE COMPLICATIONS—Febrile convulsions.

PROBABLE OUTCOME—Spontaneous recovery in a few days to a week.

HOW TO TREAT

GENERAL MEASURES
- Careful handwashing and sanitary disposal of excretions is important.
- Try to reduce high fever which might cause dehydration. Use tepid sponge baths.

MEDICATION—Medicine usually is not necessary for this disorder. You may use nonprescription drugs, such as acetaminophen, to relieve pain and fever. Don't give aspirin to children under age 18.

ACTIVITY—Bed rest is necessary until the fever and sore throat disappear.

DIET—No special diet. Encourage extra fluids, such as water, fruit ices, ice chips or cool-gelatin solutions. Avoid acid fruit juices, which irritate inflamed tissues.

CALL YOUR DOCTOR IF

Your child has symptoms of herpangina.

ILLNESS & DISORDERS

HERPES, GENITAL

GENERAL INFORMATION

DEFINITION—A virus infection of the genitals transmitted by sexual relations (intercourse or oral sex).

BODY PARTS INVOLVED—Penis; vagina; cervix; thighs; buttocks (sometimes).

SEX OR AGE MOST AFFECTED—Both sexes and all ages of sexually active persons.

SIGNS & SYMPTOMS
- Painful blisters, preceded by itching and irritation, on the vaginal lips or penis. In women, the blisters may extend into the vagina to the cervix and urethra. After a few days, the blisters rupture and leave painful, shallow ulcers which last 1 to 3 weeks.
- Difficult, painful urination.
- Enlarged lymph glands (sometimes).
- Fever and a general ill feeling (sometimes).

CAUSES
- Herpes type 2 virus (HSV-2). (Herpes type 1 virus causes common cold sores, which appear around the mouth.)
- Genital herpes is transmitted by a sexual partner who has active herpes lesions. Lesions may be on the genitals, hands, lips or mouth (including type 1 virus).

RISK INCREASES WITH
- Serious illness that has lowered resistance.
- Use of immunosuppressive or anticancer drugs.
- Stress may lead to diminished efficiency of the immune responses that usually suppress growth of the virus.
- Other "triggers" that can cause a recurrence include genital trauma, menstruation, sunbathing and infection of some other type.

HOW TO PREVENT
- Avoid sexual intercourse if either partner has blisters or sores.
- Use a latex condom during intercourse if either sex partner has inactive genital herpes.
- Avoid oral sex with a partner who has cold sores on the mouth.
- If you are pregnant, tell your doctor if you have had herpes or any genital lesions in the past. Precautions should be taken to prevent infection of the baby.

WHAT TO EXPECT

DIAGNOSTIC MEASURES
- Your own observation of symptoms.
- Medical history and exam by a doctor.
- Laboratory study of fluid from the lesion (sometimes).

APPROPRIATE HEALTH CARE
- Self-care after diagnosis.

- Doctor's treatment.

POSSIBLE COMPLICATIONS
- Generalized disease and death in persons who must take anticancer drugs or immunosuppressive drugs.
- Transmittal of life-threatening systemic herpes to a newborn infant from an infected mother.
- Secondary bacterial infection.
- Genital herpes may increase the risk of cervical cancer.

PROBABLE OUTCOME—Genital herpes is currently considered incurable, but symptoms can be relieved with treatment.

During symptom-free periods, the virus returns to its dormant state. Symptoms recur when the virus is reactivated. Recurrent symptoms are not new infections.

The discomfort varies from person to person and from time to time in the same person. The first herpes infection is often much more uncomfortable than following ones.

HOW TO TREAT

GENERAL MEASURES
- Women should wear cotton underpants or pantyhose with a cotton crotch.
- To reduce pain during urination, women may urinate in a shower or through a tubular device, such as a toilet-paper roll or plastic cup with the end cut out or pour a cup of warm water over genitals while urinating.
- Warm baths with a tablespoon of salt added can ease discomfort.
- Women should have an annual Pap smear and physical examination to rule out any complications.

MEDICATION
- Your doctor may prescribe acyclovir (an antiviral medication) in oral form for treatment of initial episodes and management of recurrent genital herpes. For some patients, it may be prescribed for prevention purposes. A topical form of acyclovir is available but is not as effective.
- You may use mild painkillers, such as acetaminophen.

ACTIVITY
- Avoid intercourse until symptoms disappear.
- Appropriate rest if symptoms are present.

DIET—No special diet.

CALL YOUR DOCTOR IF

- Symptoms don't improve in 1 week, despite treatment.
- Unusual vaginal bleeding or swelling occurs.
- Fever returns during treatment or you become generally ill.

HERPES SIMPLEX (Cold Sores; Fever Blisters)

GENERAL INFORMATION

DEFINITION—A common, contagious virus (herpes simplex or HSV-1) infection. Cold sores are sometimes confused with impetigo.

BODY PARTS INVOLVED—Lip; gums and mouth; cornea (rare); genitals (occasionally).

SEX OR AGE MOST AFFECTED—Both sexes. Most persons have their first infection before age 5.

SIGNS & SYMPTOMS
- Eruptions of very small, painful blisters—usually around the mouth, but sometimes on the genitals. The blisters are grouped together and each surrounded by a red ring. They fill with fluid, then dry up and disappear.
- If the eye is infected: Eye pain and redness; feeling that something is in the eye; sensitivity to light; and tearing.

CAUSES—Infection with a herpes virus that invades the skin, often remaining for months or years before causing active inflammation. Most persons develop antibodies that control the virus unless risk factors develop. The virus is transmitted by person-to-person contact or by contact with saliva, stools, urine or discharge from an infected eye. The blisters and ulcers of herpes simplex are contagious until they heal, both in the first and in succeeding flare-ups.

RISK INCREASES WITH
- Newborns; children who have eczema.
- Physical or emotional stress.
- Illness that has lowered resistance, including a cold, minor gastrointestinal upset or fever.
- Excess sun exposure.
- Menstrual periods.
- Dental treatment that stretches the mouth.
- Use of immunosuppressive drugs.

HOW TO PREVENT
- Avoid physical contact with others who have active lesions.
- Wash your hands often during a flare-up.

WHAT TO EXPECT

DIAGNOSTIC MEASURES
- Medical history and exam by a doctor.
- Laboratory virus cultures (rare).

APPROPRIATE HEALTH CARE
- Self-care after diagnosis.
- Doctor's treatment, especially if the eye is affected.

POSSIBLE COMPLICATIONS
- Permanent vision impairment, if herpes eye infections are untreated.
- Severe infection in patients with eczema.
- Meningitis or encephalitis (rare).

PROBABLE OUTCOME—Spontaneous recovery in a few days to a week, occasionally longer. Recurrence is common. The virus remains in the body for life, but it is usually dormant. Research continues in developing a vaccine.

HOW TO TREAT

GENERAL MEASURES
- Drink cool liquids or suck frozen juice bars to reduce discomfort.
- Apply an ice cube for 1 hour during the first 24 hours after a lesion appears. This may make it heal more quickly.
- Don't rub or scratch an infected eye.
- To prevent flare-ups, use zinc oxide or sunscreen on your lips when outdoors.

MEDICATION
- Use aspirin or ibuprofen to relieve minor pain and reduce inflammation. Don't use aspirin for children and adolescents under 18. The use of aspirin during some viral illnesses may lead to Reye's syndrome, a form of encephalitis.
- Use nonprescription cold sore remedies. They may help the discomfort, but don't prevent flare-ups or hasten healing.
- Don't try to treat an infected eye—especially with cortisone ointments or drops—without consulting your doctor. Cortisone promotes growth of the herpes virus in the cornea.
- Your doctor may prescribe:
  Antiviral topical or oral medication.
  Antibiotic ointment if lesions become infected with bacteria.
  Anticancer topical medication for eye infections.

ACTIVITY
- No restrictions, except to avoid close contact—especially kissing or oral sex—until lesions heal.
- Avoid newborns or patients who are taking immunosuppressant drugs.

DIET—No special diet.

CALL YOUR DOCTOR IF

The following occurs with a cold sore:
- Signs of secondary bacterial infection, such as fever, pus instead of clear fluid in the lesions, headache and muscle aches.
- Eruption of lesions on the genitals similar to those around the mouth.
- New, unexplained symptoms.

HERPES ZOSTER (Shingles)

GENERAL INFORMATION

DEFINITION—A painful viral infection of the central nervous system.

BODY PARTS INVOLVED—Sensory nerves of the skin on one side of the body.

SEX OR AGE MOST AFFECTED—All ages, but most common in adults over 50.

SIGNS & SYMPTOMS
- Painful red blisters anywhere on the body. Blisters appear 4 to 5 days after early symptoms begin. The blisters appear on a broad streak of reddened skin along sensory-nerve routes to a particular area of skin. They occur most often on the chest, and spread only on one side of the body.
- Mild chills and fever.
- General ill feeling.
- Mild nausea, abdominal cramps or diarrhea.
- Chest pain, face pain, or burning pain in the skin of the abdomen, depending on the affected area.

CAUSES—Herpes zoster is caused by the varicella-zoster virus, the same virus that causes chickenpox. It may lie dormant in the spinal cord until triggered by risk factors.

RISK INCREASES WITH
- Adults over 50.
- Stress.
- Hodgkin's disease.
- Illness that has lowered resistance.
- Use of immunosuppressive or anticancer drugs.
- Spinal surgery or radiation.
- Leukemia or lymphoma.

PREVENTIVE MEASURES—Cannot be prevented at present. Varicella vaccines under investigation have not eliminated zoster. With rare exceptions, one attack of zoster confers lifelong immunity.

WHAT TO EXPECT

DIAGNOSTIC MEASURES
- Your own observation of symptoms.
- Medical history and physical exam by a doctor.
- Diagnosis is usually not possible until rash appears. Before then, the symptoms may mimic appendicitis, pleurisy or other conditions. Diagnostic tests may include laboratory blood tests and culture of fluid from blister, and skin biopsy (rare).

APPROPRIATE MEDICAL CARE
- Self-care after diagnosis.
- Doctor's treatment.

POSSIBLE COMPLICATIONS
- Secondary infection in the blisters.
- Chronic pain, especially in the elderly, that persists for months or years in the sensory nerves where the blisters have been.
- Corneal ulceration.
- Central nervous system infection.
- Direct contact with herpes zoster can give a susceptible person chickenpox.

PROBABLE OUTCOME—The rash usually clears in 14 to 21 days. The nerve pain may last for another month or longer. One attack usually provides immunity against herpes zoster, but a few persons have had more than one attack.

HOW TO TREAT

GENERAL MEASURES
- Primary goal of treatment is to relieve the itching and pain as much as possible, usually with topical and oral medications. The nerve pain (post-herpetic neuralgia) that lingers after the skin clears is the most difficult to treat. There are no therapies to prevent it.
- When bathing, wash blisters gently.
- Don't bandage the sores.
- Apply cool, moist compresses if this decreases the pain.
- Soak in a tub of water to which cornstarch or colloidal oatmeal (Aveeno) has been added.
- Other pain remedies have been advocated, but none has been shown to be consistently effective. These include skin stimulation by intermittent rubbing, use of alternating electrical currents passed through the skin, local heat, cold spraying, and surgical cutting of nerves.

MEDICATION
- Use calamine lotion for the blisters.
- For minor discomfort, you may use nonprescription drugs such as acetaminophen.
- Your doctor may prescribe:
  Stronger pain relievers if needed.
  Tranquilizers for a short time.
  Cortisone drugs to relieve pain in severe cases.
  An antiviral drug.
  Injections of nerve block in severe cases.

ACTIVITY—No restrictions. Avoid chilling drafts.

DIET—No special diet. Maintain a nutritious diet. Use supplemental vitamins if recommended.

CALL YOUR DOCTOR IF

- You or a family member has symptoms of herpes zoster.
- Pain is intolerable, despite treatment.
- New, unexplained symptoms develop.

HERPETIC WHITLOW

GENERAL INFORMATION

DEFINITION—An inflammation of skin folds around the fingernails caused by a contagious herpes virus.

BODY PARTS INVOLVED—Fingernail or toenail bed.

SEX OR AGE MOST AFFECTED—All ages, but most common in adults.

SIGNS & SYMPTOMS
- Sudden pain around the nail.
- Redness, swelling and warmth around the nail.
- Swelling of the lymph glands nearby, such as in the elbow or armpit.
- Groupings of tiny blisters that are barely visible around the nail.

CAUSES—Herpes virus hominus, Type 1 or Type 2. Herpetic whitlow is often transmitted to the fingers from cold sores (herpes simplex) on the mouth.

RISK INCREASES WITH
- Occupational exposure to constant wetness, such as with dishwashers or maintenance personnel.
- Occupational exposure to herpes infection, such as with nurses, dentists or dental assistants who provide mouth care.

HOW TO PREVENT
- Avoid exposure to people who have active herpes infections.
- Keep hands warm and dry.

WHAT TO EXPECT

DIAGNOSTIC MEASURES
- Your own observation of symptoms.
- Medical history and physical exam by a doctor.
- Laboratory culture of discharge from the infected area.

APPROPRIATE HEALTH CARE
- Self-care after diagnosis.
- Doctor's treatment.

POSSIBLE COMPLICATIONS—Spread of herpes infection to other body parts, such as the lips or genitals.

PROBABLE OUTCOME—The first episode is usually curable in 2 months with treatment. However, recurrent attacks are common.

HOW TO TREAT

GENERAL MEASURES
- Protect your hands to prevent further injury or spread of the infection to others. Wear heavy-duty vinyl gloves to avoid contact with irritating substances, such as water, soap, detergent, metal scrubbing pads, scouring pads, scouring powder and other chemicals.
- Don't touch other persons until inflammation clears.

MEDICATION—Your doctor may prescribe:
- Topical steroid preparations to reduce inflammation. They include creams, ointments and lotions. Apply the topical steroid only once or twice a day unless directed otherwise. Apply immediately after bathing for better spreading and penetration.
- Oral antiviral medications.

ACTIVITY—No restrictions.

DIET—No special diet.

CALL YOUR DOCTOR IF

- You have symptoms of herpetic whitlow.
- Temperature rises over 101F (38.3C).
- Symptoms don't improve in 3 days, despite treatment.
- Herpes lesions appear elsewhere on the body.

ILLNESS & DISORDERS

HIATAL HERNIA

GENERAL INFORMATION

DEFINITION—A weakness or stretching of the hiatus (an opening for the esophagus) located in the diaphragm (the broad, thin muscle separating the chest cavity and abdominal cavity). When this opening becomes weakened, gastric (stomach) acid flows backward from the stomach into the esophagus, irritating the esophagus. The stomach may even protrude into the lower chest.

BODY PARTS INVOLVED—Esophagus; stomach; diaphragm.

SEX OR AGE MOST AFFECTED—All ages, but most common in adults over 50.

SIGNS & SYMPTOMS—The following symptoms usually develop within 1 hour or more after eating:
• Heartburn (a burning sensation in the area of the heart and behind the breastbone). May be confused with heart attack symptoms.
• Belching.
• Swallowing difficulty (rare).

CAUSES—Underlying cause is unknown.

RISK INCREASES WITH
• Congenital weakness in the muscular ring of the diaphragm through which the esophagus passes and empties into the stomach.
• Abdominal injury, causing tremendous pressure that tears a hole in some part of the diaphragm.
• Chronic constipation and straining during bowel movements.
• Obesity; pregnancy; smoking.
• Constant straining or lifting with tightening of the abdominal muscles.
• Age over 50.

HOW TO PREVENT—No specific preventive measures.

WHAT TO EXPECT

DIAGNOSTIC MEASURES
• Medical history and exam by a doctor.
• For diagnosis, an esophagogastroscopy (passage of a viewing tube down the throat into the esophagus) may be performed. If cancer is suspected, a small amount of tissue may be removed for a biopsy. Manometry (pressure measurement) may be performed to confirm the reduced pressure at the esophagogastric junction.

APPROPRIATE HEALTH CARE
• Doctor's treatment.
• Surgery to close the weakness in the diaphragm and keep the stomach in its natural place (rare). (See Hernia, Repair, Hiatal in Surgery section.)

POSSIBLE COMPLICATIONS
• Bleeding from the esophagus. This can be excessive, leading to shock.
• Misdiagnosis as a heart attack.

PROBABLE OUTCOME—Symptoms can usually be controlled. If symptoms cannot be controlled and it appears that irritation of the esophagus is causing scarring and ulceration, the condition can be corrected with surgery.

HOW TO TREAT

GENERAL MEASURES
• The primary goals of treatment are to relieve symptoms and to manage and prevent complications. Medical therapy is used first.
• Raise the head of your bed 4 to 6 inches. This allows gravity to keep stomach acid away from the hernia.
• Don't smoke.
• Don't wear tight pantyhose, girdles, belts or pants.
• Don't strain during bowel movements, urination or lifting.

MEDICATION—Your doctor may prescribe:
• Antacids. These are most effective for some persons when they take them 1 hour before meals and at bedtime. Others find them more helpful 1 to 2 hours after meals and at bedtime. Try both ways to find the best schedule for you.
• H-2 blockers or other acid blocking agents.
• Drugs which hasten gastric emptying.

ACTIVITY—Don't bend over or lie down immediately after a meal.

DIET
• Avoid large meals. Eat 4 or 5 small meals a day instead. Don't eat anything for at least 2 hours before bedtime.
• Lose weight, if you are overweight. Frequently symptoms may disappear below a specific weight. (See Weight-Loss Diet in Appendix.)
• Avoid alcoholic beverages, caffeine-containing beverages (coffee, tea, cocoa, cola drinks) and any other food, juice or spice that aggravates symptoms. Eat slowly.

CALL YOUR DOCTOR IF

• You have symptoms of a hiatal hernia, especially the sensation that food stops beneath the breastbone. Call immediately if pain is accompanied by shortness of breath, sweating or nausea.
• You vomit blood or have recurrent vomiting.
• Temperature rises over 100F (37.8C).
• Symptoms don't improve with treatment in 1 month.

HICCUP
(Hiccough; Singultus)

GENERAL INFORMATION

DEFINITION—Repeated, involuntary spasmodic contractions of the diaphragm. Hiccups are a symptom, not a disease. Hiccups involve the diaphragm (large, thin muscle which separates the chest from the abdomen) and phrenic nerve (nerve that connects the diaphragm to the brain). Almost everybody gets hiccups, even a fetus in a mother's womb.

BODY PARTS INVOLVED
- Diaphragm (big muscle which separates the chest from the abdomen).
- Phrenic nerve (nerve that connects the diaphragm to the brain).

SEX OR AGE MOST AFFECTED—Both sexes, but more common in men.

SIGNS & SYMPTOMS—A sharp, quick sound produced from the mouth by a spasm of the diaphragm. The spasm closes muscles in the back of the throat during inhalation.

CAUSES—Irritation of nerves from the brain that control breathing muscles, especially the diaphragm. The cause of short hiccup episodes is usually unknown. Prolonged or recurrent hiccup episodes may be caused by:
- Swallowing hot or irritating substances.
- Diseases of the pleura (thin membrane layers that cover the lung).
- Pneumonia.
- Uremia.
- Alcoholism.
- Use of certain prescription or nonprescription drugs.
- Disorders of the stomach, esophagus, bowel or pancreas.
- Pregnancy.
- Bladder irritation.
- Hepatitis.
- Spread of cancer from another part of the body to the liver or part of the pleura.
- Recent surgery, especially abdominal surgery.
- Emotional causes.

RISK INCREASES WITH
- Illness that has diminished health.
- Recent abdominal surgery.
- Use of drugs, especially those that irritate the stomach.
- Full stomach.
- Laughter or intense emotions.
- Changes in temperature.
- Alcohol consumption.

HOW TO PREVENT—Cannot be prevented at present.

WHAT TO EXPECT

DIAGNOSTIC MEASURES
- Your own observation of symptoms.
- Medical history and physical exam by a doctor (sometimes).

APPROPRIATE HEALTH CARE
- Self-care.
- Doctor's treatment (prolonged hiccups).
- Surgery to cut phrenic nerve (severe, prolonged cases only).

POSSIBLE COMPLICATIONS—None unless hiccups are prolonged, which may indicate serious disease.

PROBABLE OUTCOME—Short hiccup episodes usually don't indicate disease. They will subside on their own or often with the treatment discussed below. Continued hiccups can be debilitating and require medical attention to determine the cause.

HOW TO TREAT

GENERAL MEASURES—These instructions are for short hiccup episodes. Prolonged hiccups require medical care. Try one or more methods to see which works best for you.
- Hold your breath and count to 10.
- Breathe into a paper bag and rebreathe air in the bag. Don't use a plastic bag because it may cling to nostrils.
- Insert your thumb between your teeth and upper lip; press the upper lip with your index finger just below the right nostril.
- Press a forefinger into each ear for about 20 seconds.
- Drink a glass of water rapidly.
- Swallow dry bread or crushed ice.
- Pull gently on the tongue.
- Close eyelids and apply gentle pressure to the eyeballs.
- Swallow a teaspoon of dry sugar.

MEDICATION—Usually no medications are needed for this disorder.

ACTIVITY—No restrictions.

DIET—No special diet.

CALL YOUR DOCTOR IF

- Hiccups persist longer than 8 hours.
- You suspect a prescription drug may be causing hiccups.

HIDRADENITIS SUPPURATIVA

GENERAL INFORMATION

DEFINITION—A skin disorder characterized by nodules in the armpit.

BODY PARTS INVOLVED—Armpits. It appears rarely on buttocks, groin or under breasts.

SEX OR AGE MOST AFFECTED—Both sexes, but more common in females (13 to 16 years).

SIGNS & SYMPTOMS—Nodules with the following characteristics:
- Nodules are firm, tender and domed.
- Nodules are 1cm to 3cm in diameter.
- Larger nodules soften in the center and become painful. When pressed, they feel like an overfilled inner tube.
- Nodules open and drain pus spontaneously.
- Individual nodules (with or without drainage) heal slowly over 10 to 30 days.
- Nodules leave scars.
- Severity of the disorder varies from a few lesions per year to a constant succession of lesions that form as old ones heal. Lesions frequently recur at the same site.

CAUSES—Hormonal influences that activate the apocrine glands under the arms. Secretions in these glands enlarge the gland. The outlets become blocked, probably by heat, sweat or incomplete gland development. The secretions that are dammed in the glands force sweat and bacteria into surrounding tissue, which becomes infected.

RISK INCREASES WITH
- Obesity.
- Exposure to environmental heat and moisture.
- Genetic factors. This disorder is most common in black females.

HOW TO PREVENT—No specific preventive measures.

WHAT TO EXPECT

DIAGNOSTIC MEASURES
- Your own observation of symptoms.
- Medical history and physical exam by a doctor.
- Laboratory culture of the discharge from the draining abscess.

APPROPRIATE HEALTH CARE
- Self-care after diagnosis.
- Doctor's treatment.
- Surgery to open and drain abscesses or to remove involved skin (severe cases only).

POSSIBLE COMPLICATIONS—Scarring.

PROBABLE OUTCOME—This disorder may last many years—from puberty through the following 10 to 20 years. Symptoms can be controlled with treatment.

HOW TO TREAT

GENERAL MEASURES
- Don't use commercial underarm deodorants.
- Minimize heat and sweating.
- Avoid constrictive clothing and clothing made of synthetic fibers.
- Lose weight, if you are overweight.
- Wash with antibacterial soaps.
- Use soaks (see Soaks in Appendix) to relieve itching and hasten healing. Warm-water soaks are usually more soothing for pain or inflammation. Cool-water soaks feel better for itching.

MEDICATION
- Your doctor may prescribe:
  Injection of cortisone drugs directly into the lesions.
  Antibiotics to fight infection.
  Hormones to help subdue inflammation.
  Isotretinoin (has been effective in some patients). This is a potent drug and must be given under doctor's supervision.
- For minor discomfort, you may use nonprescription drugs such as acetaminophen.

ACTIVITY—Restrict your activity in hot weather and avoid hot jobs if possible. Swimming is excellent.

DIET—No special diet unless you need to lose weight. Obesity is a main risk factor for this disorder. See Weight-Loss Diet in Appendix.

CALL YOUR DOCTOR IF

- You have symptoms of hidradenitis suppurativa.
- Lesions don't improve after 5 days of treatment.
- Your temperature rises to 101F (38.3C).
- Lesions appear that become soft and seem to have pus, but don't drain spontaneously.
- New, unexplained symptoms develop. Drugs used in treatment may produce side effects.

HIP DISLOCATION, CONGENITAL

 GENERAL INFORMATION

DEFINITION—A disorder in which the head of the thigh bone doesn't fit properly into, or is outside of, the hip socket.

BODY PARTS INVOLVED—One or both hip joints.

SEX OR AGE MOST AFFECTED—About 1 of every 60 newborns has a possible hip dislocation. About 85% are girls.

SIGNS & SYMPTOMS—The earliest symptom may be a clicking sound in a newborn when the legs are pulled apart. However, this symptom is not always present.

After the newborn period, partial dislocation may become full dislocation. Then the thigh bone (femur) rides up behind or to the side of its hip socket. The limb will appear shorter than its mate. Skin folds of the buttocks will not be symmetrical; the side with the dislocated hip will have more creases than the other.

When the child is old enough to walk, he or she may limp or favor one side.

CAUSES—Unknown. Congenital hip dislocations seem more common after breech deliveries than following head-first or Cesarean deliveries. Theories about the reasons include: hormonal changes in the mother during pregnancy; abnormal fetal position in the uterus; or birth injury.

RISK INCREASES WITH
• Family history of hip dislocation.
• Breech birth.
• Position of unborn child in the uterus (possibly).

HOW TO PREVENT—Cannot be prevented at present.

 WHAT TO EXPECT

DIAGNOSTIC MEASURES
• Your own observation of symptoms.
• Medical history and physical exam by a doctor.
• Ultrasound (see Glossary) and/or x-rays of the hip.

APPROPRIATE HEALTH CARE
• Home care after diagnosis.
• Doctor's treatment.
• Surgery (rare).

POSSIBLE COMPLICATIONS—Late detection and treatment can lead to permanent crippling.

PROBABLE OUTCOME—If congenital hip dislocation is detected early, it can often be cured. Surgery is used only when conservative treatment fails or the disorder has not been discovered until late in childhood.

 HOW TO TREAT

GENERAL MEASURES
• To correct the dislocation, the head of the thigh bone must be returned to its socket in the pelvic bone and held firmly in place.

For mild forms, use triple diapers to immobilize the child and arrange for frequent medical exams.

For more severe forms, splints, casts or traction are used to immobilize the ball and socket until it heals. Plaster casts may be necessary for several months. They must be replaced every 1-1/2 to 2 months.
• While an infant or young child is immobilized, he or she will require more physical care than normal. Soiled diapers, especially, should not be left on the child for any length of time.
• During the first few days that the child is in a cast, splints, or traction, stay as close by as possible to give reassurance and love.
• Remove braces or splints for bathing but replace them immediately afterward.
• Turn the child in bed at least every 2 hours during the day and every 4 hours at night.

MEDICATION—Medicine usually is not necessary for this disorder.

ACTIVITY
• If traction is required, the child must stay in bed until the dislocation is corrected.
• If a cast or splints are used and the child's condition allows it, put the child on the floor for short play periods—either alone or with other children. Car rides are acceptable.

DIET—No special diet.

 CALL YOUR DOCTOR IF

• Your child has signs of a congenital hip dislocation.
• The following occurs during treatment:
Rectal temperature rises to 101F (38.3C) or higher, which may indicate infection of the skin or urinary tract.
The cast, bar or other immobilization device does not seem to hold the hip in position.
A dent appears in the cast, which might cause a pressure sore.
The child shows signs of severe pain.
Color or mobility of the child's legs and feet change.
The child loses appetite.

ILLNESS & DISORDERS

HIP FRACTURE (Femoral Neck Fracture)

GENERAL INFORMATION

DEFINITION—A complete or partial break in the femur, the major bone in the hip joint. More than 200,000 hip fractures occur every year, and about 50% of those occur in people age 80 or over.

BODY PARTS INVOLVED—Femur, including muscles and tendons that attach the head of the femur to the acetabulum (hip socket in the bony pelvis).

SEX OR AGE MOST AFFECTED
• Breaks from common injuries affect both sexes and all ages.
• Spontaneous breaks or breaks from minor injuries affect mostly older people.

SIGNS & SYMPTOMS
• Intolerable pain when trying to walk.
• Swelling, tenderness and bruising in the hip.
• Deformed hip appearance.
• Shock from internal bleeding.

CAUSES
• Injury, especially falls and auto accidents.
• Spontaneous in pathologic conditions.

RISK INCREASES WITH
• Osteoporosis, especially postmenopausal osteoporosis.
• Bone cancer.
• Multiple medications which reduce alertness.
• Osteogenesis imperfecta (inherited condition in which bones are brittle and easily broken).
• Calcium imbalance.
• Poor nutrition, especially insufficient calcium and protein.
• Brain disorders.
• Activities that increase the risk of injury.

HOW TO PREVENT
• Ensure an adequate calcium intake (1000 mg to 1500 mg a day) with milk and milk products or calcium supplements.
• Protect against falls, especially in the home.
• Women should consider taking estrogen after menopause. Consult your doctor.
• Use cane or walker if you feel unsteady.
• Obtain bone density study at or shortly after menopause to evaluate risk of osteoporosis.

WHAT TO EXPECT

DIAGNOSTIC MEASURES
• Your own observation of symptoms.
• Medical history and exam by a doctor.
• X-rays of the hip.

APPROPRIATE HEALTH CARE
• Doctor's treatment.
• Surgery is the recommended treatment. (See Hip Nailing for Hip fracture in Surgery section.)

• Traction may rarely be used.
• Physical therapy and rehabilitation.

POSSIBLE COMPLICATIONS
• Surgical-wound infection.
• Nerve and blood-vessel damage at the fracture site.
• Osteoarthritis.
• Inadequate blood supply to the injured area, causing tissue death of the bone.
• Poor healing (nonunion) of the fracture.
• Blood clots due to bed confinement.
• Following surgery, older persons sometimes have a period of mental deterioration which usually subsides.

PROBABLE OUTCOME—In most patients, the condition is curable with surgery and rehabilitation.

HOW TO TREAT

GENERAL MEASURES
• After surgery, you will be up as soon as possible (usually the next day).
• Occasionally, the complications after the first surgery may require the need for further surgery, such as hip joint replacement.

MEDICATION—Your doctor may prescribe:
• Pain relievers as needed.
• Antibiotics to fight infection, if necessary.
• Stool softeners to prevent constipation.
• Estrogen replacement or other medication to build bone density and calcium supplements to help retard more bone loss.

ACTIVITY
• After awakening from anesthesia, move the unaffected leg often to decrease the possibility of deep-vein blood clots.
• Physical therapy and rehabilitation will be started as soon as you are able. You will start by using a walker with someone nearby.
• Eventually develop a weight-bearing exercise program to help increase bone density and decrease risk of subsequent fracture.

DIET—Clear liquids for the 1st day after surgery, then no special diet. Ask your doctor if you should take calcium supplements.

CALL YOUR DOCTOR IF

• You have symptoms of a hip fracture. Call immediately if you have numbness or loss of feeling below the fracture site. This is an emergency!
• The following occurs after surgery:
Swelling above or below the fracture site.
Chills, fever, muscle aches or headache.
Increased pain, swelling, redness or discharge at the surgical site.
Constipation.

HIRSUTISM

GENERAL INFORMATION

DEFINITION—Excessive growth of hair on the face and body of a woman, in places where hair growth is ordinarily absent. It usually occurs gradually over an extended period of time.

BODY PARTS INVOLVED—Endocrine system.

SEX OR AGE MOST AFFECTED—Post-pubescent females.

SIGNS & SYMPTOMS
- Hair thickens and darkens and grows in a male pattern (beard, moustache, chest).
- Irregular or no menstruation.
- Acne.
- Sometimes accompanied by deepening of the voice, increased muscle mass and enlargement of the clitoris. When these symptoms occur, the complex is known as "virilization".
- Infertility problems (sometimes).

CAUSES
- Usually due to excessive production of androgens (male hormones) from the ovary or adrenal gland caused by some conditions, such as polycystic ovarian syndrome or congenital adrenal hyperplasia.
- Adrenal or ovarian tumor (uncommon).
- Hormonal imbalance can be induced by significant stress.
- Idiopathic (no apparent cause).

RISK INCREASES WITH
- Family history of hirsutism.
- Dark-haired individuals, especially those of Hispanic, African-American, Mediterranean, or Indian ancestry.
- Use of male hormones (androgens) or corticosteroid medications, birth control pills, hormones and some antihypertensive drugs.
- Stress.
- Menopause or anovulation (failure to ovulate).

HOW TO PREVENT—No specific preventive measures.

WHAT TO EXPECT

DIAGNOSTIC MEASURES
- A physical examination, laboratory studies, and possibly, some imaging studies (CT scan or MRI) will aid in diagnosing any underlying cause.

APPROPRIATE HEALTH CARE
- The specific type of treatment will depend on the cause of the hirsutism. A mild case of hirsutism with no menstrual irregularities may require no treatment. For others, treatment sometimes depends on the patient's desire for future childbearing.
- Ovarian or adrenal tumors should be surgically removed.
- Self-care after surgery.

POSSIBLE COMPLICATIONS
- Poor self image; may feel unattractive and find social interaction with other people difficult.
- Infertility.
- Abnormal uterine bleeding and anemia.
- Increased risk of diabetes mellitus if the cause of hirsutism is polycystic ovarian disease.
- May be unresponsive to initial treatment.

PROBABLE OUTCOME—Diagnosis and treatment of any underlying cause can frequently halt further hair growth. Response to treatment may take 6 to 12 months.

HOW TO TREAT

GENERAL MEASURES—Cosmetic treatment choices for removing excess hair include: shaving, plucking, bleaching, waxing or laser treatment. Chemical depilatories may also be used, but are not always effective on thick or coarse hair. Shaving and plucking can cause infection or scarring. Electrolysis will remove hair permanently, but should be done by a licensed professional. Laser treatment can be effective depending on hair and skin color, but is expensive and temporary.

MEDICATION
- There are no medicines specifically approved for the purpose of treating hirsutism. However, medicines that may be recommended for hirsutism caused by excess androgen production include dexamethasone, oral contraceptives, leuprolide, spirinolactone (a mild diuretic), and other antiandrogens. They vary in effectiveness, and take 3 to 6 months for results. They may help decrease new hair growth, but will usually not change the amount of hair you already have.
- If skin becomes irritated from shaving, use nonprescription 1% hydrocortisone cream.
- Depilatories or creams to remove hair are often recommended.

ACTIVITY—Usually, no restrictions.

DIET
- No special diet.
- If overweight, a weight loss diet is recommended.

CALL YOUR DOCTOR IF

- You or a family member has symptoms of hirsutism.
- New, unexplained symptoms develop. Drugs used in treatment may produce side effects.
- You become pregnant. Some medicines used to treat hirsutism will need to be discontinued.

HISTOPLASMOSIS

GENERAL INFORMATION

DEFINITION—A fungus infection confined mostly to people who live in eastern and midwestern parts of the U.S. Most cases are minor and go undiagnosed.

BODY PARTS INVOLVED—Lungs; central nervous system; gastrointestinal system.

SEX OR AGE MOST AFFECTED—Both sexes; all ages.

SIGNS & SYMPTOMS
- Frequently no symptoms are present.
- Persistent cough and other symptoms similar to a cold.
- Loss of appetite, diarrhea and weight loss.
- Fever; headache.
- Irritability.
- Paleness.
- Abdominal swelling.
- Breathing difficulty (rare).

CAUSES—Infection by the fungus, Histoplasma capsulatum. People become infected by breathing dust that contains fungus spores. The fungus is found in soil contaminated by feces of birds and bats that carry the fungus. Contaminated soil is most often in pigeon lofts, barns, chicken houses, damp areas under bridges, along streams and in caves.

RISK INCREASES WITH
- Recent severe illness, especially uremia, diabetes mellitus, chronic lung disease, cancer or severe burns.
- Geographic location. The disease occurs most often in the western Appalachian slopes and the Mississippi, Missouri and Ohio River valleys. Millions of people living in these areas have been infected, but never experience symptoms or they are so mild, they go unrecognized.
- Use of immunosuppressive, anticancer or cortisone drugs.

HOW TO PREVENT—Avoid areas where the soil is likely to be infected with histoplasma spores.

WHAT TO EXPECT

DIAGNOSTIC MEASURES
- Your own observation of symptoms.
- Medical history and physical exam by a doctor.
- Laboratory studies, such as a sputum culture, blood studies, skin tests and chest x-ray.

APPROPRIATE HEALTH CARE
- Self-care after diagnosis.
- Doctor's treatment.
- Hospitalization for complications.

POSSIBLE COMPLICATIONS
- Spread of infection to the heart, spleen, adrenal glands and meninges (membranes that cover the brain). This is rare, but it can be fatal.
- Histoplasmosis often recurs in AIDS patients.

PROBABLE OUTCOME
- Mild cases usually resolve spontaneously. Most people only feel tired or "bad" for several weeks.
- Severe cases are treatable with antifungal drugs.

HOW TO TREAT

GENERAL MEASURES
- Isolation is not necessary. The disease is not transmitted from person to person.
- Use a cool-mist or ultrasonic humidifier with distilled water and no medicine in it to increase air moisture. This helps thin lung secretions so they can be coughed up more easily. Clean humidifier daily.
- Don't smoke.
- Use warm compresses or a heating pad on the chest to relieve pain.
- Weigh daily and keep a record.

MEDICATION
- For mild cases, no medicine is usually necessary.
- For severe cases, your doctor may prescribe antifungal drugs (some must be given intravenously in a hospital).
- For AIDS patients with histoplasmosis, chronic therapy with antifungal medication will be necessary.
- You may use nonprescription drugs, such as acetaminophen or aspirin, to relieve pain.

ACTIVITY—Stay in bed until fever, pain and shortness of breath disappear for at least 48 hours. Then resume your normal activities gradually. Many people are fatigued and weak after recovery. Don't expect too much too soon.

DIET—No special diet.

CALL YOUR DOCTOR IF

- You have symptoms of histoplasmosis.
- The following occurs during treatment:
  Weight loss continues.
  Fever rises to 101F (38.3C) orally.
  Diarrhea is uncontrollable.
  Severe headache and stiff neck begin.

HIV INFECTION & AIDS
(Human Immunodeficiency Virus; Acquired Immunodeficiency Syndrome)

GENERAL INFORMATION

DEFINITION—A major failure of the body's immune system (immunodeficiency). This decreases the body's ability to fight infection and suppress multiplication of abnormal cells, such as cancer. It affects the immune system, including special blood cells (lymphocytes) and cells of the organs (bone marrow, spleen, liver and lymph glands). These cells manufacture antibodies to protect against disease and cancer. AIDS is a secondary immunodeficiency syndrome resulting from HIV infection.

BODY PARTS INVOLVED—Lungs; central nervous system; gastrointestinal system.

SEX OR AGE MOST AFFECTED—Both sexes; all ages; most common in young males ages 25-44.

SIGNS & SYMPTOMS
- Initial HIV infection may produce no symptoms.
- Fatigue; unexplained weight loss; mouth sores.
- Night sweats; fever; diarrhea.
- Recurrent respiratory and skin infections.
- Swollen lymph glands throughout the body.
- Genital changes; enlarged spleen.

CAUSES
- HIV is a virus that invades and destroys cells of the immune system, resulting in lowered resistance to infections and some cancers.
- The virus is transmitted by:
  Sexual contact among infected persons.
  Using contaminated needles for IV drug use.
  Transfusions of blood or blood products from a person with acquired immune deficiency syndrome (rare).
  Children born to an HIV infected mother.
  Note: Usual nonsexual contact does not transmit the disease.

RISK INCREASES WITH
- Multiple male-to-male sexual partners or male-to-female sexual partners (less likely).
- Exposure of hospital workers and laboratory technicians to blood, feces and urine of HIV positive patients. Greatest risk is with an accidental needle injury.
- Infants born to mothers with HIV infection.
- Intravenous drug abuse.

HOW TO PREVENT
- Avoid sexual contact with affected persons or known intravenous drug users.
- Sexual activity should be restricted to partners whose sexual histories are known.
- Use condoms for vaginal and anal intercourse.
- The risk of oral sex is not fully known. Ejaculation into the mouth should be avoided.
- Avoid intravenous self-administered drugs. Do not share unsterilized needles.
- Avoid unscreened blood products.
- Infected people or those in risk groups are not to donate blood, sperm, organs or tissue.

WHAT TO EXPECT

DIAGNOSTIC MEASURES—Laboratory studies of blood cells and HIV antibody test (may not become positive for 6 months after contact).

APPROPRIATE HEALTH CARE–Ultra-close medical monitoring is important.

POSSIBLE COMPLICATIONS
Serious infection; cancer; death.

PROBABLE OUTCOME—This condition is currently considered incurable. However, symptoms can be relieved or controlled and scientific research into causes and treatment continues. AIDS may not develop for years following a positive HIV test. Once ill, survival averages 2-1/2 years, but may vary.

HOW TO TREAT

GENERAL MEASURES
- Early diagnosis is helpful. If you are at risk, get a medical evaluation even if you feel well.
- Contact AIDS support groups.
- Avoid exposure to infections.
- See Resources for Additional Information.

MEDICATION
- Antiretroviral drugs (didanisone, stavudine, zalcitabine, etc.) and protease inhibitor drugs are used to treat HIV infection and AIDS and may slow the progression. In an HIV infected pregnant woman these drugs reduce the risk of HIV infection in the newborn.
- Research continues into new drugs and vaccines against HIV.

ACTIVITY
- No restrictions on normal activity.
- Get adequate rest, and exercise.

DIET
- Maintain good nutrition. Malabsorption, altered metabolism and weight loss are common; take vitamin supplements.
- Avoid raw eggs, unpasteurized milk or other potentially contaminated foods.

CALL YOUR DOCTOR IF

- Infection occurs after diagnosis. Symptoms include fever, cough, diarrhea.
- New symptoms develop.

HIVES
(Urticaria; Giant Urticaria)

GENERAL INFORMATION

DEFINITION—An allergic disorder characterized by skin changes with raised areas, redness and itching.

BODY PARTS INVOLVED—Skin anywhere, including the scalp, lips, palms and soles.

SEX OR AGE MOST AFFECTED—Both sexes; all ages.

SIGNS & SYMPTOMS—Itchy skin papules (small, raised bumps) with the following characteristics:
- They swell and produce pink or red lesions called wheals. Wheals have clearly defined edges and flat tops. They measure 1cm to 5cm in diameter.
- Wheals join together quickly and form large, flat plaques (larger areas of raised, skin-colored lesions).
- Wheals and plaques change shape, resolve and reappear in minutes or hours. This rapid change is unique to hives.

CAUSES—Release of histamines, sometimes for unknown reason. Following are the most common causes:
- Medications. Nearly every drug causes hives in some persons.
- Insect bites; viral infections; autoimmune disease; dysproteinemias.
- Exposure to cold, heat, water or sunlight.
- Cancer, especially leukemia.
- Exposure to animals, especially cats.
- Eating eggs, fruits, nuts and shellfish. Other foods sometimes cause hives in infants, but not in adults.
- Food dyes and preservatives (possibly).
- Infection (bacterial, viral, fungal).

RISK INCREASES WITH
- Stress.
- Other allergies or a family history of allergies.

HOW TO PREVENT
- If you have had hives and identified the cause, avoid the source.
- Keep an anaphylaxis kit if you experience severe reactions.

WHAT TO EXPECT

DIAGNOSTIC MEASURES
- Your own observation of symptoms.
- Medical history and exam by a doctor.
- Diagnostic tests may include laboratory blood studies, urinalysis, erythrocyte sedimentation rate and chest x-ray to rule out inflammatory infection.

APPROPRIATE HEALTH CARE
- Self-care after diagnosis.
- Doctor's treatment.
- Emergency-room care for life-threatening reactions.
- Allergy skin tests and injections.

POSSIBLE COMPLICATIONS
- Swelling of the larynx and inability to breathe.
- Hives may be the first sign of life-threatening anaphylaxis. If so, it will be followed by itching, runny nose, wheezing, paleness, cold sweats and low blood pressure. Without prompt treatment, coma and cardiac arrest can occur.

PROBABLE OUTCOME—Unpredictable, depending on the cause. If a medication or acute viral infection is responsible, hives usually disappear within hours or days. Some cases become chronic and last for months or years. Most eventually go into spontaneous remission—even if the cause is not identified.

HOW TO TREAT

GENERAL MEASURES
- Don't take drugs (including aspirin, laxatives, sedatives, vitamins, antacids, pain killers or cough syrups) not prescribed for you.
- Don't wear tight underwear or foundation garments. Any skin irritation may trigger new outbreaks.
- Don't take hot baths or showers.
- Apply cold-water compresses or soaks (see Soaks in Appendix) to relieve itching.

MEDICATION—Your doctor may prescribe:
- Antihistamines, ephedrine, terbutaline or cortisone drugs to relieve itching and rash.
- Sedatives or tranquilizers for anxiety.
- Epinephrine by injection for severe symptoms.

ACTIVITY—Decrease activities until several days after hives disappear. Avoid getting hot, sweaty or excited.

DIET
- If foods are suspected as a cause, keep a food diary to help identify the offending food.
- Avoid alcohol and coffee or other caffeine-containing beverages.

CALL YOUR DOCTOR IF

- The following occurs during an episode of hives:
  Swollen lips.
  Shortness of breath or wheezing.
  A tight or constricted feeling in the throat.
  This is an emergency!
- New, unexplained symptoms develop. Drugs used in treatment may produce side effects.

HODGKIN'S DISEASE

GENERAL INFORMATION

DEFINITION—Malignant tumor of the lymph glands. This is a form of lymphoma.

BODY PARTS INVOLVED
- Lymphocytes (white blood cells).
- Lymph glands (glands which check infection and produce immune substances).
- Spleen (a large lymph gland).

SEX OR AGE MOST AFFECTED—All ages, but most common in young adults and older persons. Hodgkin's disease is rare in children under 10.

SIGNS & SYMPTOMS
- Itching all over the body.
- Swollen, nontender, rubbery, distinct lymph glands anywhere in the body—but most commonly in the armpit or groin.
- Intermittent fever and night sweats.
- Pain in the diseased area after drinking alcohol.
- Weight loss.
- Jaundice (yellow skin and eyes).
- General ill feeling.
- Anemia.
- Bleeding from the gastrointestinal tract.

CAUSES—Unknown, but research suggests a virus infection may be a factor.

RISK INCREASES WITH—Immunodeficiency (acquired or inherited).

HOW TO PREVENT—No specific preventive measures.

WHAT TO EXPECT

DIAGNOSTIC MEASURES
- Your own observation of symptoms.
- Medical history and physical exam by a doctor.
- Laboratory studies of blood and bone marrow.
- Lymphangiogram (see Glossary).
- Biopsy (see Glossary) of lymph node.
- CT scan (see Glossary) of chest and abdomen, and chest x-ray.

APPROPRIATE HEALTH CARE
- Doctor's treatment.
- Hospitalization for short periods to confirm diagnosis and for treatment.
- Surgery to discover the extent of disease.
- Radiation therapy.

POSSIBLE COMPLICATIONS
- Spread of malignancy to other parts of the body.
- Sterility in males from treatment.
- Heart or lung disorders, anemia, hypothyroidism and infections.

PROBABLE OUTCOME—Usually curable with radiation therapy and anticancer drugs if diagnosed and treated early. With treatment, the 10-year survival rate is about 80%. The potential for cure varies according to the cell type discovered from biopsy of the lymph node.

HOW TO TREAT

GENERAL MEASURES
- Try to remain optimistic about your treatment and chances for cure. A good mental attitude is a powerful ally.
- Good oral hygiene is important to prevent mouthsores, if receiving chemotherapy.
- Males receiving therapy may want to consider sperm-banking in case of sterility.
- See Resources for Additional Information.

MEDICATION—Your doctor may prescribe anticancer drugs. Medication may cause side effects or adverse reactions in some people. New symptoms may be caused by the medicine, original disorder or a new illness. Side effects caused by medicine usually disappear when the body adjusts to the drug or when the drug is discontinued.

ACTIVITY—Remain as active as your strength allows.

DIET—No special diet.

CALL YOUR DOCTOR IF

- You have symptoms of Hodgkin's disease.
- The following occurs during treatment:
  Fever.
  Signs of infection (redness, swelling, pain or tenderness) anywhere in the body.
  Swelling of the feet and ankles.
  Discomfort when urinating or decreased urination in 1 day.
- You think your medicine is causing symptoms.

HYPERALDOSTERONISM
(Aldosteronism)

GENERAL INFORMATION

DEFINITION—An endocrine disease caused by overproduction of aldosterone, a hormone manufactured by the adrenal gland. Excess aldosterone causes the kidneys to absorb too much sodium and water and eliminate too much potassium.

BODY PARTS INVOLVED—Adrenal glands, which are attached at the upper part of the kidneys; kidneys; fluids and electrolytes in the bloodstream and body cells.

SEX OR AGE MOST AFFECTED
- Both sexes, but more common in females.
- All ages, but most common in adults between ages 30 and 50.

SIGNS & SYMPTOMS
- Fatigue and weakness.
- Temporary paralysis (sometimes).
- Tingling sensations in the arms, legs, hands and feet.
- Urinary frequency, especially at night.
- Thirst.
- Severe muscle spasms.
- Vision disturbances.

The following are apparent with diagnostic tests:
- Low blood levels of potassium.
- High blood levels of sodium.
- High blood pressure.

CAUSES—Increased adrenal secretion of aldosterone. This is caused by:
- A tumor of the adrenal gland.
- High blood pressure or kidney disease, causing increased production in the kidneys of a hormone (renin) that controls aldosterone levels.

RISK INCREASES WITH
- Diet that contains large amounts of black licorice.
- Kidney disease.
- Congestive heart failure.
- Cirrhosis of the liver.
- Use of oral contraceptives.
- Use of diuretic drugs that cause potassium loss.
- Pregnancy.

HOW TO PREVENT—If you have kidney disease or high blood pressure, remain under a doctor's care and adhere strictly to your treatment program—even if you have no symptoms.

WHAT TO EXPECT

DIAGNOSTIC MEASURES
- Your own observation of symptoms.
- Medical history and physical exam by a doctor.
- Laboratory blood studies of electrolyte levels.
- CT scan (see Glossary) of the kidneys and adrenal glands.

APPROPRIATE HEALTH CARE
- Self-care after diagnosis.
- Doctor's treatment.
- Hospitalization and surgery to remove adrenal gland (adrenalectomy) in some patients.

POSSIBLE COMPLICATIONS
- Congestive heart failure.
- Atherosclerosis.
- Kidney failure.

PROBABLE OUTCOME—If the disorder is caused by an adrenal tumor, it is usually curable with surgery. If it is caused by kidney disease or high blood pressure, medical treatment for these disorders will control symptoms of hyperaldosteronism.

HOW TO TREAT

GENERAL MEASURES
- Weigh daily and keep a record. Report a gain of 3 or more pounds in a 24-hour period.
- Wear a Medic-Alert bracelet or pendant (see Glossary) to identify your medical condition and any medications you take.

MEDICATION—Your doctor may prescribe:
- Spironolactone to decrease the aldosterone effect. This drug may cause breast enlargement and sexual impotence in men. Other drug options are amiloride and triamterene.
- High-blood pressure medication.

ACTIVITY—No restrictions, if surgery is not necessary. If it is, resume your normal activities gradually.

DIET—Eat a diet that is low in sodium and high in potassium. Foods rich in potassium include dried apricots and peaches, raisins, citrus fruits, lentils and whole-grain cereals. Don't eat black licorice.

CALL YOUR DOCTOR IF

- You have symptoms of hyperaldosteronism.
- New, unexplained symptoms develop. Drugs used in treatment may produce side effects.

HYPEREMESIS GRAVIDARUM

GENERAL INFORMATION

DEFINITION—Severe nausea and vomiting in a pregnant woman, causing dehydration and drastic changes in body chemistry. This is different and much more serious than morning sickness during pregnancy.

BODY PARTS INVOLVED—Gastrointestinal tract; vomiting center in the brain.

SEX OR AGE MOST AFFECTED—Pregnant females.

SIGNS & SYMPTOMS
- Severe nausea.
- Vomiting, first of mucus, then of bile and finally of blood.
- Dehydration.
- Failure to gain weight, or weight loss to less than prepregnancy weight.
- Pale, waxy, dry and sometimes yellow skin.
- Rapid heartbeat.
- Headache, confusion or lethargy.

CAUSES—Unknown. The most common theories include:
- Multiple pregnancy (more than one fetus), producing high levels of a hormone, human chorionic gonadotrophin.
- Inflammation of the pancreas.
- Bile-duct disease.
- Psychological factors, such as depression or a poor response to stress.

RISK INCREASES WITH
- Younger maternal age; first pregnancy.
- Maternal overweight.
- Single marital status.
- Emotional stress.
- Caucasian women.

HOW TO PREVENT
- Don't use any drugs, including nonprescription drugs or alcohol, during pregnancy without consulting your doctor.
- Maintain an adequate diet during all stages of pregnancy.

WHAT TO EXPECT

DIAGNOSTIC MEASURES
- Your own observation of symptoms.
- Medical history and exam by a doctor.
- Diagnostic tests may be conducted to rule out other disorders of the liver, kidney, pancreas, intestine and gastrointestinal tract.

APPROPRIATE HEALTH CARE
- Self-care after diagnosis.
- Doctor's treatment.
- Hospitalization to replace fluid and electrolytes intravenously, if needed.
- Repeated eye exams are necessary to prevent possible hemorrhagic retinitis.

POSSIBLE COMPLICATIONS
- Severe dehydration.
- Poor fetal growth and outcome (rare).

PROBABLE OUTCOME—Usually curable with treatment.

HOW TO TREAT

GENERAL MEASURES
- Reduce stress whenever possible (see How to Cope with Stress in Appendix).
- Weigh daily and report any unusual changes to the doctor.

MEDICATION
- Your doctor may prescribe:
  Intravenous fluid and electrolyte replacement if your condition is serious.
  Therapeutic trial of vitamin B-6.
- If other drugs are prescribed for you, carefully follow instructions on the label.
- Don't use any medicine, including nonprescription medicine to prevent vomiting, without telling your doctor.

ACTIVITY
- Stay in bed until symptoms disappear.
- After recovery, stay as active as your strength allows. Work and exercise moderately. Rest often.

DIET—If the condition has not reached the point to warrant hospitalization for intravenous fluids, follow these instructions:
- If you feel nauseated in the morning, eat dry toast or saltine crackers before you get out of bed.
- Eat small, frequent meals.
- Don't eat fried foods; they increase nausea.
- Sit upright for 45 minutes after eating.
- Obtain additional dietary instructions from your doctor or nutritionist.
If intravenous fluids are necessary, you will probably progress from them to a clear liquid diet, full liquid diet and then regular diet with small, frequent meals.

CALL YOUR DOCTOR IF

- You have symptoms of hyperemesis gravidarum.
- Nausea, vomiting or continued weight loss despite treatment.

ILLNESS & DISORDERS

HYPERHIDROSIS

GENERAL INFORMATION

DEFINITION—Excessive sweating. Sweating is a normal body function that helps maintain even body temperature. Excess sweat serves no purpose and often creates social embarrassment because of odor or stained clothes. In extreme cases, excess sweat can ruin clothes and shoes.

BODY PARTS INVOLVED—Skin, especially of the underarms, palms and soles.

SEX OR AGE MOST AFFECTED—Both sexes and all ages, except young children.

SIGNS & SYMPTOMS
- Heavy perspiration from underarm area, soles and palms—and to a lesser degree, from other body parts.
- Unpleasant odor, which is caused by bacteria in sweat.

CAUSES
- Genetic factors may contribute to development of hyperhidrosis.
- Stress or chronic anxiety.
- Fever and infection.
- Malignancy, such as lymphoma.
- Hyperthyroidism.
- Heart attack.
- Menopause (hormonal changes).
- Some drugs and medicines, such as narcotics.
- Withdrawal from addicting drugs.
- Obesity.
- Unknown in some cases.

RISK INCREASES WITH
- Stress.
- Strenuous activity.
- Hot weather.
- Family history of hyperhidrosis.

HOW TO PREVENT—Avoiding the causes where possible; treatment of any underlying condition contributing to hyperhidrosis.

WHAT TO EXPECT

DIAGNOSTIC MEASURES
- Your own observation of symptoms.
- Medical history and physical exam by a doctor.

APPROPRIATE HEALTH CARE
- Self-care.
- Doctor's treatment for underlying conditions, or if self-care is unsuccessful.
- Psychotherapy or counseling, if stress is a major factor.
- Surgery to remove sweat glands or sever nerves to major sweat areas (rare).

POSSIBLE COMPLICATIONS
- Psychological distress caused by social embarrassment.
- Rashes from deodorants or antiperspirants.
- Dehydration if water intake is insufficient to replace water lost in sweat.

PROBABLE OUTCOME—Symptoms can be controlled with treatment.

HOW TO TREAT

GENERAL MEASURES
- Bathe frequently.
- Change clothes frequently.
- Wear loose-fitting clothes of natural fibers, such as cotton.
- Use underarm sweat shields.
- Use antiperspirants and deodorants.
- Use drying powders.
- Wear cotton socks.
- Wear leather shoes or sandals. Don't use man-made materials.
- Electrical devices (iontophoresis) temporarily reduce sweating of palms, armpit or feet. Ask your doctor.
- Shave underarm hair.

MEDICATION
- Your doctor may prescribe special solutions to reduce sweating, such as topical applications of aluminum chloride. Beta-adrenergic blockers may occasionally help.
- Tranquilizers or anticholinergics to reduce activity of the central nervous system. Don't use if you have glaucoma or prostate disease.

ACTIVITY—No restrictions.

DIET
- No special diet. Drink at least 8 glasses of water a day—more in hot weather.
- Control your weight. See Weight-Loss Diet in Appendix).
- Don't drink alcohol.

CALL YOUR DOCTOR IF

- Excessive sweating is causing you problems at work or in social situations.
- Excessive sweating is accompanied by other symptoms (unexplained weight loss, cough, bulging eyes, rapid heartbeat).

HYPERLIPIDEMIA, TYPES I, II, III, IV, V
(Hyperlipoproteinemia; Dyslipidemia)

GENERAL INFORMATION

DEFINITION—Above-normal levels of fat in the blood. The types of hyperlipidemia (I, II, III, IV, V) are defined according to the levels of fatty substances in the blood, and how much above normal these levels are.

BODY PARTS INVOLVED—Blood and arteries.

SEX OR AGE MOST AFFECTED—All ages, but most common in adults. Different types appear at different ages.

SIGNS & SYMPTOMS
- Usually none.
- Yellowish nodules of fat in the skin beneath eyes, elbows and knees, and in tendons.
- Enlarged spleen and liver (some types).
- Whitish ring around the eye pupil (some types).

CAUSES
- The blood contains a variety of fats (lipids) joined to blood proteins, forming lipoproteins. They provide energy and are "building blocks" for some tissues and hormones. Lipoproteins include cholesterol and triglycerides. The cholesterol is made of fractions called high density lipoprotein (HDL), low density lipoprotein (LDL), and very low density lipoprotein (VLDL). The LDL will deposit onto artery walls (if it is excessive), causing atherosclerosis. The HDL is protective, by helping to prevent deposit of LDL.
- Each type of hyperlipidemia may be inherited, or secondary to some other disorder.

RISK INCREASES WITH
- Improper diet that is high in fat and cholesterol.
- Family history of hyperlipidemia.
- Use of oral contraceptives or estrogen.
- Diabetes mellitus.
- Hypothyroidism.
- Nephrosis.
- Alcoholism.

HOW TO PREVENT
- Eat a diet that is low in fat.
- Lose weight if you are overweight.
- Regular aerobic exercise.
- If you have diabetes, adhere closely to your treatment program.
- Get a medical test to check your blood level of cholesterol and its fractions.

WHAT TO EXPECT

DIAGNOSTIC MEASURES
- Medical history and exam by a doctor.
- Laboratory blood studies to measure blood lipids.

APPROPRIATE HEALTH CARE
- Self-care after diagnosis.
- Doctor's treatment.

POSSIBLE COMPLICATIONS
- Atherosclerosis. This is a major cause of heart disease (coronary artery disease), strokes, kidney failure and poor circulation.
- Acute pancreatitis.

PROBABLE OUTCOME—Usually treatable or controllable with lifelong dietary control and medication.

HOW TO TREAT

GENERAL MEASURES
- For some, an altered diet, weight loss and exercise may be sufficient for treatment, others may require medications to reduce blood lipids.
- Stress increases the risk of heart disease, a major complication of hyperlipidemia. Look for ways to reduce stress in your life. Learn relaxation methods. See How to Cope with Stress in Appendix.
- Stop smoking. Smoking accelerates the deposit of fats onto blood vessels.

MEDICATION
- Your doctor may prescribe:
  Medications to control blood lipids. Several drugs are available with variable and unpredictable results.
  Medications to treat underlying diseases, such as diabetes or thyroid conditions.
- Don't take oral contraceptives. Use other forms of birth control.

ACTIVITY
- No restrictions unless tendons are weakened by fat deposits or you have coronary artery disease.
- A regular exercise program is helpful for reducing weight, controlling stress, and raising HDL levels to help in increasing the body's ability to clear fat from the blood after meals. Consult your doctor.

DIET
- Eat a diet that is low in fat; lose weight if you are overweight (see both diets in Appendix).
- Don't drink alcohol.
- Evidence suggests 1 glass of red wine or purple grape juice daily may help raise HDL and lower risk.

CALL YOUR DOCTOR IF

- You have symptoms or a family history of hyperlipidemia.
- New, unexplained symptoms develop. Drugs used in treatment may produce side effects.

HYPERNEPHROMA
(Kidney Tumor)

GENERAL INFORMATION

DEFINITION—A form of kidney cancer with uncontrolled growth of malignant cells in the kidney.

BODY PARTS INVOLVED—Kidney.

SEX OR AGE MOST AFFECTED—Men over age 40.

SIGNS & SYMPTOMS
- Firm mass in an enlarged abdomen.
- Appetite and weight loss.
- Persistent low-grade fever.
- Vomiting.
- Mild abdominal pain.
- Red or smoky urine caused by bleeding from the tumor.

If the tumor grows large enough to cause kidney failure, symptoms include:
- Increasing fatigue and weakness.
- Headache
- Bad breath.
- Nausea, vomiting or diarrhea.
- Shortness of breath.
- Chest pain.
- Itching skin.

CAUSES—Unknown.

RISK INCREASES WITH
- Multiple congenital abnormalities.
- Smoking.

HOW TO PREVENT
- Cannot be prevented at present. If you are a woman of childbearing age with a family history of kidney tumors, seek genetic counseling before becoming pregnant.
- If kidney tumors run in your family, get medical advice about tests. Even if you feel well and don't have the disease, get regular checkups.

WHAT TO EXPECT

DIAGNOSTIC MEASURES
- Your own observation of symptoms.
- Medical history and physical exam by a doctor.
- Laboratory blood and urine studies of kidney function and to detect blood in the urine.
- CT scan, ultrasound, MRI and venography (see Glossary for all).

APPROPRIATE HEALTH CARE
- Doctor's treatment.
- Treatment consists of removal of the kidney (or partial removal in some patients) and regional lymph nodes. This may be followed by radiation therapy, chemotherapy and immunotherapy.

POSSIBLE COMPLICATIONS
- Spread to other organs, especially the liver, lungs, brain and bones, before discovery of the primary tumor.
- Softening of the bones (osteoporosis or osteomalacia).
- Increased susceptibility to urinary-tract infections.

PROBABLE OUTCOME—Usually curable with surgery, if the tumor is detected before it spreads to other body parts.

HOW TO TREAT

GENERAL MEASURES
- The more you can learn and understand about this disorder, the more you will be able to make informed decisions about where to go for your care, the treatments available, the risks involved, side effects of therapy and expected outcome.
- See Resources for Additional Information.

MEDICATION—Your doctor may prescribe anticancer drugs.

ACTIVITY
- Follow medical advice about returning to normal activities after surgery.
- Take short, frequent rests during the day. Otherwise, stay as active as your strength allows.

DIET
- Eat a low-protein diet. Because of dietary restrictions, multiple-vitamin and mineral supplements may be necessary.
- Increase fluid intake to several pints a day.

CALL YOUR DOCTOR IF

- You have symptoms of hypernephroma.
- The following occurs during treatment:
  Fever rises to 101F (38.3C) or higher.
  Urination decreases.
- New, unexplained symptoms develop. Anticancer drugs used in treatment may produce side effects.
- Symptoms recur after treatment.

HYPERPARATHYROIDISM

GENERAL INFORMATION

DEFINITION—Excess parathyroid hormone circulating in the blood. The excess amounts increase blood levels of calcium (hypercalcemia) and decrease blood levels of phosphorous (hypophosphatemia).

BODY PARTS INVOLVED—Parathyroid glands (4 pea-sized glands located on the back and side of the thyroid gland); teeth; blood, which affects all body tissues—especially the heart, blood vessels, bones, kidneys, gastrointestinal tract, central nervous system and skin.

SEX OR AGE MOST AFFECTED—Both sexes and all ages, but most common in women between ages 30 and 50.

SIGNS & SYMPTOMS—Often none; may be discovered as part of routine blood screening. When there are symptoms, they may include:
- Severe flank pain caused by kidney stones.
- Chronic low-back pain caused by bone softening.
- Easy bone fractures caused by decreased calcium in the bones.
- Upper abdominal pain caused by a peptic ulcer or pancreatitis.
- Depression.

CAUSES
- Benign tumors of the parathyroid glands.
- Sometimes caused by enlargement of the glands; the cause for this is unknown.

RISK INCREASES WITH
- Recent illness, especially endocrine disorders.
- Medical history of rickets or vitamin-D deficiency.
- Kidney failure.
- Use of laxatives.
- Use of digitalis.
- Female over age 50.

HOW TO PREVENT—No specific preventive measures.

WHAT TO EXPECT

DIAGNOSTIC MEASURES
- Your own observation of symptoms.
- Medical history and physical exam by a doctor.
- Laboratory studies of blood and urine.
- X-rays of bones; CT or MRI scan and ultrasound (see Glossary for all).

APPROPRIATE HEALTH CARE
- Doctor's treatment.
- Surgery to remove all abnormal parathyroid tissue usually cures the condition. Normally the remaining parathyroid tissue is sufficient to produce enough hormone. If it isn't, you may require treatment for underactive parathyroid (hypoparathyroidism).
- Sometimes, in mild cases, therapies other than surgery may be recommended. They consist of forcing fluids, limiting dietary intake of calcium, or forced diuresis to get rid of excess calcium.
- Treatment may be necessary to correct any underlying disorder causing the hyperparathyroidism.

POSSIBLE COMPLICATIONS
- Cataracts.
- Kidney damage.
- Peptic ulcer.
- Pancreatitis.
- Psychosis.
- Hypoparathyroidism caused by removal of too much parathyroid tissue during surgery.
- Hypothyroidism if the thyroid gland is injured inadvertently during surgery on the parathyroid glands.

PROBABLE OUTCOME—Curable with surgery.

HOW TO TREAT

GENERAL MEASURES—Sometimes, in mild cases, therapies other than surgery may be recommended. They consist of forcing fluids, limiting dietary intake of calcium, or forced diuresis to get rid of excess calcium.

MEDICATION
- Your doctor may prescribe:
  Diuretics to force sodium and calcium excretion.
  Vitamin D.
  Estrogen for postmenopausal women.
- Don't take antacids that contain calcium.

ACTIVITY—Follow medical advice about returning to normal activities following surgery.

DIET
- Drink extra water to prevent kidney stones.
- Limit calcium-containing foods, such as milk and cheese.
- Avoid highly seasoned or spicy foods, especially if you have an ulcer.

CALL YOUR DOCTOR IF

- You have symptoms of hyperparathyroidism.
- The following occurs during treatment:
  Muscle cramps, numbness or weakness.
  Breathing difficulty.
  Persistent heartburn or pain in the upper abdomen.
  Drastic mood or behavior changes.

HYPERTENSION
(High Blood Pressure)

 GENERAL INFORMATION

DEFINITION—Blood is forced through the arteries under systolic pressure; when the heart rests between beats, a diastolic pressure remains. Blood pressure is a measure of these two pressures. Normal pressure is considered 120/80. Blood pressure normally goes up as a result of stress or physical activity, but a person with hypertension has high blood pressure at rest. The diagnosis of hypertension is made when the readings are consistently high. Hypertension is sometimes called "the silent killer" because it often has no early symptoms.

BODY PARTS INVOLVED—Heart; blood vessels; kidneys and eyes (advanced stages).

SEX OR AGE MOST AFFECTED—All ages, but most common in adults.

SIGNS & SYMPTOMS—Usually no symptoms unless disease is severe. Following are symptoms of a hypertensive crisis:
- Headache; drowsiness; confusion.
- Numbness and tingling in the hands and feet.
- Coughing blood; nosebleeds.
- Severe shortness of breath.

CAUSES—Usually unknown. A small number of cases result from:
- Chronic kidney disease.
- Severe narrowing of the aorta (major artery of the heart).
- Disorders of some endocrine glands.
- Hardening of the arteries.

RISK INCREASES WITH
- Adults over 60; sedentary lifestyle.
- Obesity; smoking; stress; alcoholism.
- Diet that is high in salt or saturated fat.
- Genetic factors. Hypertension is most common among blacks.
- Family history of hypertension, stroke, heart attack or kidney failure.
- Use of contraceptive pills, steroids and some appetite suppressants or decongestants.

HOW TO PREVENT—Essential hypertension (from unknown causes) cannot be prevented at present. If you have a family history of hypertension, obtain frequent blood-pressure checks. If hypertension is detected early, treatment that includes diet, exercise, stress management and medication can usually prevent complications.

 WHAT TO EXPECT

DIAGNOSTIC MEASURES
- Medical history and exam by a doctor.
- Laboratory studies such as blood studies of kidney function, urinalysis and ECG (see Glossary).
- X-rays of the chest and kidneys.

APPROPRIATE HEALTH CARE
- Self-care after diagnosis.
- Doctor's treatment.
- Overall treatment goals will be individualized and may involve weight loss; smoking cessation; exercise program; reduction in alcohol consumption; and lifestyle changes to reduce stress.

POSSIBLE COMPLICATIONS
- Stroke; heart attack; kidney failure.
- Congestive heart failure and pulmonary edema.

PROBABLE OUTCOME
- With treatment, complications are preventable (except for possible side effects of drugs). Life expectancy is near normal.
- Without treatment, life expectancy is reduced because of likelihood of heart attack or stroke.

 HOW TO TREAT

GENERAL MEASURES
- Consider lifestyle changes and practice relaxation techniques to reduce stress (see How to Cope with Stress in Appendix).
- Learn to take your own blood pressure. Your doctor or nurse can teach you.
- See Resources for Additional Information.

MEDICATION
- Antihypertensive medications can reduce blood pressure if more conservative measures don't work.
- Don't take nonprescription cold and sinus remedies. These contain drugs, such as ephedrine and pseudoephedrine, that raise blood pressure.

ACTIVITY—Normal activity with exercise program at least 3 times a week. This helps reduce stress and maintain normal body weight; it may lower blood pressure. Seek medical advice (your doctor or an exercise physiologist) about an exercise prescription.

DIET—Low-salt diet and reducing diet if overweight (see both in Appendix).

 CALL YOUR DOCTOR IF

- You have symptoms of a hypertensive crisis.
- Chest pain occurs. This may be an emergency. Seek help immediately!
- Symptoms of high-blood pressure continue despite treatment.
- New, unexplained symptoms develop.

HYPERTHYROIDISM
(Thyrotoxicosis; Toxic Goiter; Graves' Disease)

GENERAL INFORMATION

DEFINITION—Overactivity of the thyroid, an endocrine gland that regulates all body functions. The most common form of hyperthyroidism is called Graves' disease.

BODY PARTS INVOLVED—Thyroid gland and most other body organs, especially the endocrine system, which includes the pituitary gland, parathyroid glands, pancreas, adrenal glands, and ovaries or testicles.

SEX OR AGE MOST AFFECTED—Adults between ages 20 and 50, mostly women.

SIGNS & SYMPTOMS
- Hyperactivity.
- Feeling warm or hot all the time.
- Tremors.
- Sweating.
- Itching skin.
- Pounding, rapid, irregular heartbeat.
- Weight loss, despite overeating. Older persons may gain weight.
- Marked anxiety and restlessness.
- Sleeplessness.
- Fatigue and weakness.
- Protruding eyes (exophthalmos) and double vision (sometimes).
- Diarrhea (sometimes).
- Hair loss (sometimes).
- Goiter (enlarged thyroid) (sometimes).

CAUSES
- Autoimmune disorder (body develops antibodies that stimulate excessive amounts of thyroid hormone).
- Thyroid nodules or tumors.
- Thyroiditis (inflammation of thyroid gland).

RISK INCREASES WITH
- Family history of hyperthyroidism.
- Stress.
- Female gender.
- Other autoimmune disorders.

HOW TO PREVENT—No specific preventive measures.

WHAT TO EXPECT

DIAGNOSTIC MEASURES
- Your own observation of symptoms.
- Medical history and physical exam by a doctor.
- Laboratory blood studies.
- ECG (see Glossary).
- Radioactive studies such as I-131 uptake (see Glossary).

APPROPRIATE HEALTH CARE
- Self-care after diagnosis.
- Doctor's treatment.
- Appropriate treatment will depend on the size of the goiter, the causes, your age and how long surgery may be delayed (if you are a candidate for it).
- Medication controls the problem in most patients.
- Surgery to remove part of the thyroid (see Thyroid-Gland Removal in Surgery section) if needed.

POSSIBLE COMPLICATIONS
- Congestive heart failure.
- "Thyroid storm"—a sudden worsening of all symptoms. This is a life-threatening emergency.
- Misdiagnosis as a psychiatric anxiety reaction.

PROBABLE OUTCOME—Usually curable with medication or surgery. Allow 6 months of treatment for the condition to stabilize. Some forms may return to normal without treatment.

HOW TO TREAT

GENERAL MEASURES
- Since this condition develops gradually, symptoms may be difficult to recognize. If family and friends mention changes in your behavior or appearance, consult your doctor.
- It is important for your doctor to monitor the treatment. Be sure to keep follow-up appointments.

MEDICATION—Your doctor may prescribe:
- Antithyroid drugs to depress thyroid activity.
- Beta-adrenergic blockers to decrease a rapid heartbeat.
- Radioactive iodine, which selectively destroys thyroid cells.

ACTIVITY—Limit activity as much as possible until the disorder is controlled. Modify activities according to disease severity.

DIET
- Eat a diet high in protein to replace tissue lost from thyroid overactivity.
- Weight loss diet if you are overweight (see Weight-Loss Diet in Appendix).

CALL YOUR DOCTOR IF

- You have symptoms of hyperthyroidism.
- Symptoms worsen suddenly, especially after surgery.
- New, unexplained symptoms develop. Drugs used in treatment may produce side effects.

HYPOCHONDRIASIS

 GENERAL INFORMATION

DEFINITION—A person's conviction that he or she has a serious or fatal disease, despite evidence to the contrary from medical examinations and tests. The person becomes quite informed and knowledgeable about illnesses, diagnosis and treatment, usually as a result of multiple medical evaluations and numerous contacts with health care professionals.

BODY PARTS INVOLVED—Brain.

SEX OR AGE MOST AFFECTED—Both sexes; all ages.

SIGNS & SYMPTOMS—Anxiety and persistent reports of symptoms involving any body part. Concern about heart disease or cancer is common. Symptoms may change, but the person's belief that a serious condition exists does not. Frequently reported symptoms include insomnia, sexual dysfunction and gastrointestinal discomfort, such as bloating, belching and cramps. Symptom complaints may shift and change and be very specific to general to vague.

CAUSES—Possibly a complication of other psychological disorders, but the cause is uncertain. It is more common in people who had a true organic illness in childhood or were closely involved with a sick relative.

RISK INCREASES WITH—Unknown.

HOW TO PREVENT—No specific measures known. In childhood, don't reward illness by giving a child special privileges and undue attention for being sick. Provide adequate love and support during healthy periods.

 WHAT TO EXPECT

DIAGNOSTIC MEASURES
• Medical history and physical exam by a doctor. The diagnosis is difficult.
• Medical testing as needed to rule out an organic disease.
• Psychological evaluation.

APPROPRIATE HEALTH CARE
• Doctor's treatment.
• Psychotherapy or counseling with the patient and the family. It is very difficult for persons with hypochondriasis to accept the conclusion that their health problem is not a serious organic illness.
• Regular follow-up visits with the doctor can help the patient deal with the symptoms.

POSSIBLE COMPLICATIONS
• Wasting money on unnecessary—and sometimes dangerous—medical care.
• Insisting on unnecessary surgical procedures or medications.

PROBABLE OUTCOME—Generally resistant to treatment. Most patients maintain a lifelong belief that they have a serious disease and they change doctors frequently.

 HOW TO TREAT

GENERAL MEASURES
• For family members—Persons with hypochondriasis are often difficult to live with because of their constant worry and demands for attention. Realize that the person really suffers and try to be supportive. Reward positive behavior that is not related to physical complaints. Don't encourage the "sick role."
• For patients—Try to focus on other aspects or problems in life, rather than on these symptoms. Make an effort to avoid going to different doctors continuously and getting repeat medical tests.

MEDICATION—Medicine usually is not necessary for this disorder. Your doctor may prescribe mild tranquilizers for a short time.

ACTIVITY—No restrictions.

DIET—No special diet. Avoid alcohol.

 CALL YOUR DOCTOR IF

• You have symptoms of hypochondriasis and want professional help to overcome the problem.
• New, unexplained symptoms develop. Tranquilizers used in treatment may produce side effects or dependence.

HYPOGLYCEMIA, FUNCTIONAL

 ## GENERAL INFORMATION

DEFINITION—Low blood sugar caused by excessive production of insulin by the pancreas. This is not a disease. Often misdiagnosed when based on symptoms alone. It is not a common medical condition (except in diabetic patients) as many would believe.

BODY PARTS INVOLVED—Pancreas.

SEX OR AGE MOST AFFECTED—Both sexes; all ages.

SIGNS & SYMPTOMS—The following vary greatly among people in frequency and severity:
- Weakness or faintness.
- Sweating.
- Excessive hunger.
- Nervousness and trembling hands.
- Headache.
- Confusion.
- Personality changes.
- Seizures (rare).
- Heartbeat irregularities (rare).
- Loss of consciousness (rare).

CAUSES
- Functional hypoglycemia probably results when the pancreas produces too much insulin in response to sugars and other carbohydrates, heavy exercise, pregnancy or unknown causes.
- The following drugs decrease blood-sugar levels in some persons: tobacco, caffeine, alcohol, aspirin, sulfonurea medications, phenformin, haloperidol, propoxyphene, chlorpromazine, propanolol, pentamidine, disopyramide.
- Tumor in the pancreas (rare).
- Chronic renal failure.

RISK INCREASES WITH
- Stress.
- Improper diet.
- Smoking.
- Use of drugs, such as those listed above.
- Fatigue or overwork.

HOW TO PREVENT
- Follow instructions under diet. Don't skip meals.
- Avoid stress.
- Don't smoke.
- Don't drink alcohol.
- Recognize early symptoms and take corrective action.

 ## WHAT TO EXPECT

DIAGNOSTIC MEASURES—Laboratory studies may be recommended, such as blood sugar and glucose tolerance tests.

APPROPRIATE HEALTH CARE
- Doctor's treatment.
- Self-care after diagnosis.

POSSIBLE COMPLICATIONS—Possibility of an attack while you are swimming, operating machinery, or driving a motor vehicle.

PROBABLE OUTCOME—Symptoms can be controlled with treatment.

 ## HOW TO TREAT

GENERAL MEASURES
- Comply with your doctor's advice.
- Consider lifestyle changes.
- Psychotherapy or counseling for help in coping with stress.

MEDICATION—Medicine is usually not necessary for this disorder.

ACTIVITY—No restrictions.

DIET—Eat 5 or 6 small meals a day that are low in simple carbohydrates, moderate in fats and high in protein. Don't skip meals. Between-meal snacks should include protein, such as chicken, eggs, cheese, nuts or skim milk rather than carbohydrates. Avoid highly concentrated sweets such as candy.

 ## CALL YOUR DOCTOR IF

You or a family member has symptoms of functional hypoglycemia.

HYPOPARATHYROIDISM

GENERAL INFORMATION

DEFINITION—Decreased production of hormones by the parathyroid glands (which lie behind the thyroid glands in the neck), causing a low level of calcium in the blood. The parathyroid hormone along with vitamin D and calcitonin (a hormone produced by the thyroid gland) regulates the calcium level in the body.

BODY PARTS INVOLVED—Parathyroid glands (4 pea-sized glands located on the back and side of the thyroid gland); teeth; blood, which affects all body tissues, especially the heart, blood vessels, bones, kidneys, gastrointestinal tract, central nervous system and skin.

SEX OR AGE MOST AFFECTED—Both sexes; all ages.

SIGNS & SYMPTOMS
Acute phase:
- Tetany (painful cramplike spasms of the face, hands, arms and sometimes feet).
- Tingling and numbness in feet or hands.

Chronic phase:
- Scaling skin.
- Splitting nails.
- Poor tooth development.
- Seizures.
- Mental retardation in children.
- Psychosis in adults.

CAUSES
- Complication of surgery on the parathyroid glands, the thyroid glands or other neck tissues.
- Genetic autoimmune disorder (possibly).
- Radiation of the thyroid gland.
- Hemochromatosis (see Glossary).
- No apparent reason (sometimes).
- Occasionally the parathyroids are absent from birth.

RISK INCREASES WITH—Neck surgery or trauma.

HOW TO PREVENT—No specific preventive measures.

WHAT TO EXPECT

DIAGNOSTIC MEASURES
- Your own observation of symptoms.
- Medical history and physical exam by a doctor.
- Laboratory blood and urine studies.
- ECG (see Glossary).
- X-rays of bones to detect increased bone density.

APPROPRIATE HEALTH CARE
- Doctor's treatment during the acute stage.
- Self-care after diagnosis during the chronic stage.
- Hospitalization for severe muscle spasms.

POSSIBLE COMPLICATIONS
- Cataracts.
- Brain damage.
- Heartbeat abnormalities and congestive heart failure.
- Difficulty breathing.
- Malformation of teeth.
- Seizures.

PROBABLE OUTCOME—This condition is currently considered incurable. It requires lifelong replacement therapy to control symptoms. Without treatment, it is fatal.
  Scientific research into causes and treatment continues, so there is hope for increasingly effective treatment and cure.

HOW TO TREAT

GENERAL MEASURES
- If you are suffering an acute attack of tetany (see Symptoms) you may need hospitalization for calcium injections to provide quick relief.
- For self-care, if muscle cramps start, place a paper bag over your mouth. Blow into it and rebreathe your breath. This will raise carbon-dioxide levels in the blood and decrease muscle spasms.
- Apply lubricating creams or ointments to dry, scaling skin.
- Keep nails trimmed to prevent splitting.
- Get periodic laboratory tests to check calcium levels in your blood. It is important to remember to have these tests on time.

MEDICATION—Your doctor may prescribe:
- Vitamin D and calcium supplements in high doses. A lifelong course of these medications is necessary.
- Intravenous calcium supplements during hospitalization for severe muscle spasms.
- Sedatives and anticonvulsants for frequent muscle spasms.

ACTIVITY—No restrictions.

DIET—High calcium, low-phosphorous diet. Your doctor or dietitian will provide specific instructions.

CALL YOUR DOCTOR IF

- You have unexplained muscle spasms of the hands, feet or throat, or numbness or tingling in the hands or feet.
- Muscle spasms don't decrease in 1 week, despite treatment.

HYPOTHERMIA

GENERAL INFORMATION

DEFINITION—A fall in body temperature to below 95F (35C). It can affect all ages; however most victims are elderly people who are unable to keep warm in winter. Sometimes body temperature is deliberately reduced during some surgical procedures.

BODY PARTS INVOLVED—All major organ systems, including decreased blood flow through the kidneys and brain.

SEX OR AGE MOST AFFECTED—All ages, but most common in adults over 60.

SIGNS & SYMPTOMS
Early symptoms:
- Poor muscle coordination.
- Mental confusion.
- Shivering and low body temperature (95F to 98F or 35C to 36.7C) rectally.
- Slow pulse.
- Weakness, drowsiness.

Late symptoms:
- Rigid muscles.
- Temperature drop to 77F to 84F (25C to 28.9C).
- Purple fingers, toes and nail beds.
- Loss of consciousness.

CAUSES—Prolonged exposure to cold temperatures, especially outdoors with a high wind-chill factor; cold-water near drowning; also can occur with exposure to near normal temperatures if person is ill or debilitated.

RISK INCREASES WITH
- Adults over 60 or infants.
- Thin or wet clothing.
- Slender body size. Slender persons lose heat more rapidly than obese persons.
- Smoking, which decreases circulation.
- Excess alcohol consumption.
- Mental impairment.
- Chronic disease, such as heart failure, pulmonary disorders.

HOW TO PREVENT
- Obtain warm housing and adequate clothing before winter.
- In cold weather, wear windproof clothing in many layers, including a scarf, hat and mittens.
- In rain, change to dry clothing quickly.
- Keep moving to generate body heat.
- Don't leave your home during a severe winter storm.
- Don't skate or fish on ice unless you have determined the ice is safe. Supervise children.
- If camping, walking or hiking in cold climate, carry emergency provisions for use if stranded.
- Persons who are unable to care for themselves fully, such as the elderly, mentally impaired or alcoholic, should be visited or supervised during cold weather.

WHAT TO EXPECT

DIAGNOSTIC MEASURES
- Your own observation of symptoms.
- Medical history and exam by a doctor.
- Laboratory studies, such as kidney-function studies.

APPROPRIATE HEALTH CARE
- Doctor's treatment.
- Hospitalization. Arrange transportation to the nearest emergency center immediately.

POSSIBLE COMPLICATIONS
- Shock.
- Pneumonia.
- Kidney failure.
- Frostbite; gangrene.
- Death.

PROBABLE OUTCOME—Sometimes fatal, depending on the length and amount of temperature loss. Chances of survival are excellent if the patient is conscious on arrival at the emergency center. Some children have been successfully revived despite immersion in ice water for an hour or more.

HOW TO TREAT

GENERAL MEASURES—The following may be helpful while waiting for emergency help:
- Note: Victim may be confused and resist helpful measures.
- Place the person in bed and cover with a blanket or electric blanket at normal body temperature.
- A warm (not hot) bath may be helpful—but call the nearest emergency center for advice.
- If the person is outdoors, cover with blankets or shield from the wind.
- If possible, warm victim with direct body heat (skin to skin contact).

MEDICATION—The doctor may prescribe medicine to support blood pressure if the person's condition is critical.

ACTIVITY—After treatment, normal activity should be resumed gradually.

DIET—Don't give alcohol to a person with hypothermia. It is of no help and may be harmful. Warm fluids may be given if patient is able to swallow.

CALL YOUR DOCTOR IF

You observe symptoms of hypothermia in someone.

HYPOTHYROIDISM

 GENERAL INFORMATION

DEFINITION—Underactive thyroid gland which causes an underproduction of thyroid hormone. The thyroid is a small butterfly-shaped gland in the neck. Virtually all metabolic processes are affected by the thyroid hormone.

BODY PARTS INVOLVED—Thyroid gland (located in the neck below the Adam's apple); endocrine system.

SEX OR AGE MOST AFFECTED—Both sexes of adults, but more common in women.

SIGNS & SYMPTOMS—It is unlikely one person will have all the following symptoms, but most will have several:
- Decreased tolerance for cold.
- Decreased sweating.
- Decreased appetite.
- Constipation.
- Chest pain.
- Coarse or slow-growing hair.
- Slow, rapid or irregular heartbeat.
- Weight gain or extreme thinness.
- Placidity or nervousness.
- Sleepiness or insomnia.
- Mental impairment, including depression, psychosis or poor memory.
- Fluid retention, especially around the eyes.
- Dull facial expression and droopy eyelids.
- Coarse skin.
- Decreased tolerance for medication.
- Decreased sex drive and infertility.
- Menstrual disorders.
- Anemia.
- Numbness and tingling of the hands and feet.
- Deepened or hoarse voice.

CAUSES—Sometimes unknown. Following are the most common causes:
- Autoimmune disease, in which the body's immune system functions abnormally and attacks the thyroid gland.
- Radioactive iodine treatment.
- Surgery for hyperthyroidism.
- Iodine deficiency in the diet.
- Decreased activity of the pituitary gland, which secretes a thyroid-stimulating hormone.
- Use of drugs, such as lithium, that may depress thyroid function.

RISK INCREASES WITH
- Adults over 60.
- Obesity.
- Surgery for hyperthyroidism.
- X-ray treatments.

HOW TO PREVENT
- No known measures to prevent primary hypothyroidism.
- Take replacement thyroid for life after thyroid surgery or destruction of the thyroid gland by radiation treatment.

 WHAT TO EXPECT

DIAGNOSTIC MEASURES
- Your own observation of symptoms.
- Medical history and physical exam by a doctor.
- Laboratory blood studies of thyroid hormones. Lab studies can confirm the diagnosis of hypothyroidism, but they cannot indicate how much replacement therapy is needed.

APPROPRIATE HEALTH CARE
- Self-care after diagnosis.
- Doctor's treatment.
- You may require hospitalization if complicating emergencies occur, such as myxedema coma (extremely rare in warm climates, more common in cold climates).

POSSIBLE COMPLICATIONS
- Myxedema coma, a life-threatening complication of hypothyroidism.
- Increased susceptibility to infection.
- Adrenal crisis with vigorous treatment of hypothyroidism.
- Infertility.
- Overtreatment over long periods can lead to bone demineralization.

PROBABLE OUTCOME—Usually curable with careful thyroid-replacement therapy.

 HOW TO TREAT

GENERAL MEASURES— The goal of treatment is to provide the body with enough thyroid substance for efficient body function. Medical evaluation may be necessary for several months to establish the correct dose of thyroid replacement.

MEDICATION—Your doctor will prescribe thyroid-replacement hormones. Dosage requirements will depend on age, weight, sex, capacity of thyroid function, other drugs you take and intestinal function.

ACTIVITY—No restrictions. Stay as active as possible.

DIET—No special diet for hypothyroidism. Avoid constipation by eating a high-fiber diet. Weight loss diet recommended if you are overweight (see both diets in Appendix).

 CALL YOUR DOCTOR IF

- You have symptoms of hypothyroidism.
- Symptoms don't improve within 3 weeks after treatment begins.
- New, unexplained symptoms develop. Drugs used in treatment may produce side effects.
- Coma or seizures occur. Get emergency help immediately!

ID REACTION
(Autoeczematization; Autosensitization)

 GENERAL INFORMATION

DEFINITION—An allergic response to a skin disorder of the feet, groin or other area, producing an itching rash somewhere else in the body.

BODY PARTS INVOLVED
- Parts with the original disorder: groin, ears, hands, feet.
- Parts with the allergic response: hands, feet, arms, legs or trunk.

SEX OR AGE MOST AFFECTED—Both sexes; all ages.

SIGNS & SYMPTOMS
- Itching (often severe).
- Vesicles (fluid-filled, small blisters) of varying size on the skin.

CAUSES—Unknown. An id reaction may be a disorder of the body's immunological response to the original ailment. They occur most often with some forms of dermatitis, outer-ear infections and eczema of the hand or foot.

RISK INCREASES WITH
- Recent skin rash anywhere.
- Stress.
- Medical history of allergies.

HOW TO PREVENT—Treat all skin disorders thoroughly until they disappear.

 WHAT TO EXPECT

DIAGNOSTIC MEASURES
- Your own observation of symptoms.
- Medical history and physical exam by a doctor.
- Laboratory culture of the original skin disorder.

APPROPRIATE HEALTH CARE
- Doctor's treatment.
- Self-care after diagnosis.

POSSIBLE COMPLICATIONS—Adverse reaction to medication used in treatment.

PROBABLE OUTCOME—Usually curable in 2 weeks. Recurrence is rapid if treatment is discontinued before the id reaction and original disorder are completely gone.

 HOW TO TREAT

GENERAL MEASURES
- Treat the original skin disorder until it heals completely to prevent a recurrence of the id reaction.
- Id reaction does not respond well to simple measures such as soaks.
- Minimize stress, if possible.

MEDICATION—Your doctor may prescribe topical or oral cortisone drugs. Oral steroids quickly control the id reaction but slow the healing of the underlying disorder.

ACTIVITY—No restrictions.

DIET—No special diet.

 CALL YOUR DOCTOR IF

- You have symptoms of an id reaction.
- The following occurs during treatment:
  Fever higher than 101F (38.3C).
  Heat, redness, pain or tenderness in any of the lesions. This indicates infection.
- New, unexplained symptoms develop. Drugs used in treatment may produce side effects.

ILLNESS & DISORDERS

IDIOPATHIC HYPERTROPHIC SUBAORTIC STENOSIS (IHSS)

GENERAL INFORMATION

DEFINITION—A chronic heart condition that produces an enlarged heart muscle, restricting the amount of blood the heart pumps. Cardiac output may be low, normal or high depending on whether stenosis is obstructive or nonobstructive. If output is normal, IHSS could go undetected for years.

BODY PARTS INVOLVED—Heart.

SEX OR AGE MOST AFFECTED—Both sexes; all ages.

SIGNS & SYMPTOMS
- Chest pain (angina pectoris).
- Heart-rhythm irregularity.
- Fainting.
- Shortness of breath.
- Swollen feet and ankles.
- Distended neck veins.
- Heart failure.
- Heart murmur.

CAUSES—Thickening of the left chamber (ventricle) of the heart for unknown reason. This obstructs the flow of blood, and the heart may be unable to pump enough blood during exertion. In some cases, this condition is inherited as a dominant genetic trait.

RISK INCREASES WITH—Family history of IHSS.

HOW TO PREVENT—If you have a family history of IHSS, obtain genetic counseling before starting a family.

WHAT TO EXPECT

DIAGNOSTIC MEASURES
- Your own observation of symptoms.
- Medical history and physical exam by a doctor.
- Laboratory studies, such as cardiac catheterization to measure blood flow through heart chambers.
- X-rays of the heart.
- EKG and echocardiogram (see Glossary for both) of the heart.

APPROPRIATE HEALTH CARE
- Doctor's treatment, including consultation with a cardiologist.
- Surgery to reduce the obstruction, if medication does not control the problem.
- DC electrocardioversion (electric shock to the heart) for treatment of life-threatening heartbeat irregularities and to improve heart output.

POSSIBLE COMPLICATIONS
- Heartbeat irregularity.
- Bacterial infection of the heart valve.
- Sudden death.

PROBABLE OUTCOME—Usually curable with medication or surgery.

HOW TO TREAT

GENERAL MEASURES
- Treatment goals are to relax the ventricle and relieve outflow obstruction. First therapy is usually with medications.
- Stay under close medical supervision.
- Psychological counseling for help in adjusting to emotional effects of chronic illness.

MEDICATION—Your doctor may prescribe:
- Beta-adrenergic blockers (usually propranolol) or calcium-channel blockers to prevent heartbeat irregularities.
- Don't use nitroglycerin for angina pain. It dilates arteries, which may be harmful.

ACTIVITY
- Instructions will be provided about how much physical activity is ideal. Your ability to increase activity is dependent on your response to therapy. Don't regard yourself as an invalid.
- Strenuous activities and sports are to be avoided because of high risk of sudden death.

DIET—Usually no special diet. A low-salt diet may be recommended, if you have fluid accumulation (a possible sign of congestive heart failure).

CALL YOUR DOCTOR IF

- You have symptoms of IHSS, or symptoms worsen during treatment.
- New, unexplained symptoms develop. Drugs used in treatment may produce side effects.

IMMUNODEFICIENCY DISEASE

GENERAL INFORMATION

DEFINITION—Defects in the body's immune system. A healthy immune system protects the body against germs (bacteria, viruses and fungi), cancer (partial protection) and any foreign material that enters the body. When the system fails, the body becomes susceptible to infection and cancer.

Similar, but entirely different disorders are caused by acquired immune deficiency syndrome (AIDS). Also different is the immunosuppression some people develop due to potent drugs used to treat several disorders.

BODY PARTS INVOLVED—Immune system (blood, bone marrow, lymph tissue, liver, spleen and thymus gland).

SEX OR AGE MOST AFFECTED—Both sexes; all ages.

SIGNS & SYMPTOMS—Recurrent, severe infections and illnesses. The most common include:
- Ear or respiratory infections, such as otitis media and pneumonia.
- Yeast infections, especially candidiasis.
- Cancer, especially leukemia and lymphoma.
- Bleeding disorders.
- Eczema.
- Meningitis or encephalitis.

CAUSES
- Congenital defects that involve an incomplete or absent immune system.
- Surgical removal of the spleen before age 2.
- Use of immunosuppressive drugs.
- Radiation treatment.
- Some cancers, such as Hodgkin's disease.
- Hypogammaglobulinemia (see Glossary).
- Some viral infections.

RISK INCREASES WITH
- Family history of immunodeficiency disease.
- Poor nutrition.
- Blood transfusions; intravenous drug use.
- Male homosexual activity and/or multiple sexual partners.

HOW TO PREVENT—No preventive measures known. If you have a family history of immunodeficiency disease, seek genetic counseling before starting a family. Prenatal amniotic fluid culture analysis may identify some of these disorders.

WHAT TO EXPECT

DIAGNOSTIC MEASURES
- Your own observation of symptoms, especially repeated infections in children.
- Medical history and physical exam by a doctor.
- Laboratory blood studies of antibodies, microscopic examination of blood and tissue cells and skin tests.
- Chest x-rays of the thymus gland.
- Radioactive studies of immune function.

APPROPRIATE HEALTH CARE
- Doctor's treatment.
- Surgery to transplant bone marrow or the thymus gland (occasionally).
- Hospitalization for treatment of serious infection.

POSSIBLE COMPLICATIONS
- Uncontrolled bacterial, viral or fungal infections that don't respond to treatment.
- Cancer.
- Infectious arthritis.

PROBABLE OUTCOME—Severe forms of immunodeficiency are usually fatal. Minor forms can be treated successfully.

HOW TO TREAT

GENERAL MEASURES
- Treatment will depend on the complexity of the immune deficiency. Basically, goals are to maintain optimal health, prevent emotional problems and manage infections.
- Avoid exposure to persons with contagious illnesses.
- Don't take any type of vaccine without medical advice.
- See Resources for Additional Information.

MEDICATION—Your doctor may prescribe:
- Antibiotics to fight infections.
- Injections of antibodies.
- Transfusions of blood components.
- Injections of gamma globulin (sometimes).

ACTIVITY—Bed rest is usually necessary during acute illnesses. Otherwise, there are no restrictions on activity.

DIET—No special diet.

CALL YOUR DOCTOR IF

- You have symptoms of immunodeficiency disease.
- After diagnosis, you have signs of infection, such as: chills; fever; muscle aches; headache; dizziness; and cough with thick, discolored or blood-streaked sputum.

IMPETIGO
(Pyoderma)

 GENERAL INFORMATION

DEFINITION—A contagious, common bacterial skin infection that affects the superficial layers of the skin.

BODY PARTS INVOLVED—Skin of the face, arms and legs.

SEX OR AGE MOST AFFECTED—All ages, but most common in infants and children.

SIGNS & SYMPTOMS
- A red rash with many small blisters. Some blisters contain pus, and yellow crusts form when they break. The blisters don't hurt, but they may itch.
- Slight fever (sometimes).

CAUSES—Staphylococcal or streptococcal (or combination) bacteria growing in the upper skin layers.

RISK INCREASES WITH
- Skin that is sensitive to sun and irritants, such as soap and makeup.
- Poor nutrition.
- Illness that has lowered resistance.
- Warm, moist weather.
- Crowded or unsanitary living conditions.
- Poor hygiene.

HOW TO PREVENT—Pay close attention to family hygiene, particularly hand washing.

 WHAT TO EXPECT

DIAGNOSTIC MEASURES
- Your own observation of symptoms.
- Medical history and physical exam by a doctor.
- Laboratory skin culture to identify the germ causing the infection.

APPROPRIATE HEALTH CARE
- Home care after diagnosis.
- Doctor's treatment.

POSSIBLE COMPLICATIONS
- A baby can be quite ill if the impetigo spreads all over.
- Penetration of the infection to deeper skin layers (ecthyma or cellulitis). This may cause scarring. Treatment is the same as for impetigo.
- Acute glomerulonephritis (a kidney disorder).

PROBABLE OUTCOME—Rarely becomes serious and is curable in 7-10 days with treatment.

 HOW TO TREAT

GENERAL MEASURES
- Keep fingernails short. Don't scratch impetigo blisters.
- If there is an outbreak in the family, urge all members to use antibacterial soap.
- Use separate towels for each family member, or substitute paper towels temporarily.
- Scrub lesions with gauze and antiseptic soap. Break any pustules. Remove all crusts and expose and cleanse all lesions. If crusts are difficult to remove, soak them in warm soapy water and scrub gently.
- Cover impetigo sores with gauze and tape to keep hands away from them.
- Treat new lesions the same way, even if you are not sure they are impetigo.
- Separate and boil bed linen, if possible, and towels, clothes and other items that have touched sores.
- Men should shave around sores on the face, not over them. Use an aerosol shaving cream and change razor blades each day. Don't use a shaving brush—it may harbor germs.

MEDICATION
- Your doctor may prescribe oral antibiotics to avoid complications. Take antibiotics for 10 days even if symptoms disappear.
- You may use antibiotic ointments.

ACTIVITY—No restrictions.

DIET—No special diet.

 CALL YOUR DOCTOR IF

- You or your child have symptoms of impetigo.
- A fever occurs.
- The sores continue to spread or don't begin to heal in 3 days, despite treatment.

IMPOTENCE, MALE SEXUAL
(Erectile Dysfunction)

 GENERAL INFORMATION

DEFINITION—A consistent inability to achieve or maintain an erection of the penis necessary to have sexual intercourse. (The occasional periods of impotence that occur in just about all adult males is not considered dysfunctional.)

Impotence is not inevitable with aging. The capacity for erection is retained, though a man may need more stimulation to achieve erection. Sometimes, erections may be less firm or full.

BODY PARTS INVOLVED—Male reproductive system; central nervous system.

SEX OR AGE MOST AFFECTED—Male adolescents and adults, but most common in men over 45.

SIGNS & SYMPTOMS
- Inability to achieve an erection.
- Inability to maintain an erection for the normal duration of intercourse (erection may be too weak, too brief or too painful).

CAUSES
Physical causes include:
- Diabetes mellitus.
- Atherosclerosis (hardening of the arteries).
- Medications (antihypertensive, antipsychotics, antihistamines, anti-ulcer drugs, sedatives).
- Central nervous system disorders, such as spinal injury, multiple sclerosis, stroke or syphilis.
- Endocrine disorders that involve the pituitary, thyroid, adrenal or sexual glands.
- Alcoholism; drug abuse.
- Decreased circulation to the penis.
- Hormone imbalance (rare).
- Surgery (prostate, back or genital surgery).
- Peyronie's disease, a condition where scar tissue causes painful or curved erections.
Psychological causes include:
- A poor relationship with the sexual partner.
- Psychological disorders, including depression, anxiety, stress and psychosis; guilt feelings.
- Lack of sexual information, including an understanding of the emotional aspects of sexuality and information about female anatomy.
Situational or environmental causes:
- Presence of visitors in the home.
- Rushed or routine lovemaking.
- Smoking; exposure to toxic chemicals.

RISK INCREASES WITH
- Problems listed in Causes.
- Recent illness that has lowered strength.
- Recent major surgery, especially cardiovascular or prostate surgery.

HOW TO PREVENT
- Maintain good communication with partner.
- Don't drink more than 1 or 2 alcoholic drinks—if any—a day. Don't use other drugs that can be abused.
- If you have diabetes, adhere to treatment.
- Maintain overall good health.
- If any new medication is prescribed, ask your doctor if it can cause erection problems.

 WHAT TO EXPECT

DIAGNOSTIC MEASURES
- Medical history and exam by a doctor.
- Medical tests as needed for diagnosis of any underlying disorder. Diagnosis at a special diagnostic center to measure erections.

APPROPRIATE HEALTH CARE
- Self-care after diagnosis.
- Doctor's treatment.
- Psychotherapy or counseling (alone or with your partner) from a qualified, sex therapist.
- If medication is the cause, a change in medication or in dosage may help.
- Self-administered penile injection therapy may be prescribed.
- Use of vacuum erectile device may be recommended for some patients.
- Surgery to implant an inflatable or noninflatable penile prosthesis (sometimes).

POSSIBLE COMPLICATIONS
- Depression and loss of self-esteem.
- Marital problems or breakdown of close personal relationships.

PROBABLE OUTCOME—Spontaneous recovery or recovery after brief counseling in many cases with psychological origins. For other cases with physical origins, treatment and improvement in the underlying disorder may improve sexual performance.

 HOW TO TREAT

GENERAL MEASURES
- Don't be hesitant about discussing the problem, exploring your needs and asking for help. Your partner's understanding is critical.
- See Resources for Additional Information.

MEDICATION—Medication can be very effective for many kinds of impotence.

ACTIVITY—No restrictions. Resume sexual relations when potency returns or surgery heals.

DIET—Eat a well-balanced diet.

 CALL YOUR DOCTOR IF

You have symptoms of impotence, especially if you take medications or have disorders listed as causes.

ILLNESS & DISORDERS

INCONTINENCE

 GENERAL INFORMATION

DEFINITION—An involuntary loss of bladder control. There are several types:
- Stress: An involuntary loss of urine that accompanies any action that suddenly increases pressure in the abdomen.
- Urge: Inability to control the bladder once the urge to urinate occurs. It may occur alone or sometimes with stress incontinence.
- Functional: Incontinence that occurs infrequently (transient) or there is failure to comprehend the need to urinate (functional).

BODY PARTS INVOLVED—Kidneys and urinary system.

SEX OR AGE MOST AFFECTED—Older adults of both sexes.

SIGNS & SYMPTOMS
- Unintentional loss of urine with lifting, sneezing, singing, coughing, laughing, crying or straining to have a bowel movement.
- Involuntary loss of urine almost immediately after feeling a slight urge to urinate. The volume of lost urine may range from a few drops to complete bladder emptying.
- Forgetting to urinate.
- Urinating at inappropriate times or places.
- Occasional problems in getting from bed to toilet in time.

CAUSES
- Females—shortening of the urethra and loss of the normal muscular support for the bladder and floor of the pelvis. These changes occur during pregnancy and after childbirth, particularly repeated childbirth. They may also occur as a natural consequence of aging.
- Males—damage to the sphincter mechanism.
- Overactive muscles that cause bladder to contract and empty.
- Stone, cancer, or obstruction in urinary tract.
- Dementia; depression; mobility disorders.

RISK INCREASES WITH
- Repeated childbirth.
- Adults over 60; obesity; diabetes.
- Chronic lung disease with a cough.
- Surgery, cancer or radiation damage to the sphincter mechanism in males.
- Central nervous system disorders (stroke, Parkinson's); spinal cord injury.
- Surgery that may traumatize the urethra.
- Injury of the urethra; urinary tract infection.
- Females—estrogen deficiency.
- General debilitated condition.

PREVENTIVE MEASURES
- Maintain good nutrition; exercise regularly.
- Regular physical exams.
- Don't hold urine. Go when you feel the need.

 WHAT TO EXPECT

DIAGNOSTIC MEASURES—Medical history and exam by a doctor. Medical tests to determine underlying causes.

APPROPRIATE HEALTH CARE
- Self-care; doctor's treatment.
- Treatment for any infections or tumors.
- Biofeedback, electrical stimulation or special weights for pelvic muscle strengthening.
- A pessary (support device) made of rubber or other material to fit inside the vagina to support the uterus and lower bladder muscles.
- Surgery to tighten relaxed or damaged muscles that support the bladder.
- External catheters for some impaired men.

POSSIBLE COMPLICATIONS
- Urinary-tract infections; kidney failure.
- Social isolation due to embarrassment.
- Loss of urinary control. This requires surgery.

PROBABLE OUTCOME—Most people with incontinence can be helped and even chronic cases can often be cured.

 HOW TO TREAT

GENERAL MEASURES
- Practice good genital hygiene.
- May require caregiver assistance.
- Absorbent pads or diapers may be worn. For mild incontinence, sanitary pads or panty liners may be sufficient.
- Get a portable urinal or bedside commode.
- Plan a schedule for emptying the bladder.
- Keep a daily diary of fluid intake and urination.
- See Resources for Additional Information.

MEDICATION—Your doctor may prescribe:
- Antibiotics for any urinary-tract infection.
- Sympathomimetic (alpha-adrenergic) drug therapy, which helps urethral muscles.
- Anticholinergic drugs.
- Estrogen therapy.

ACTIVITY—No restrictions.

DIET
- Lose weight if you are overweight (see Weight-Loss Diet in Appendix).
- Decrease amount of caffeine and alcohol.
- Avoid high volume of fluid intake in situations where access to bathroom facilities is limited.

 CALL YOUR DOCTOR IF

Any sign of infection develops, such as fever, pain on urination, frequent urination or a general ill feeling.

INDIGESTION
(Dyspepsia; Nonulcer Dyspepsia)

GENERAL INFORMATION

DEFINITION—Vague chest or abdominal discomfort —with no apparent organic cause—that occurs during or soon after eating or drinking. Symptoms may persist for months.

BODY PARTS INVOLVED—Stomach; esophagus; small intestine.

SEX OR AGE MOST AFFECTED—Both sexes; all ages.

SIGNS & SYMPTOMS
- Mild nausea; rarely, vomiting.
- Heartburn.
- Upper abdominal pain; gas or belching.
- Bloated or full feeling.
- Acid taste.
- Borborygmus ("growling stomach").

CAUSES—Exact cause is unknown. Symptoms seem related to eating, drinking, or swallowing air while talking or chewing gum. They occur most often with: emotional upset while eating; excessive smoking; constipation; eating improperly cooked food; eating food with a high fat content; poor digestion of gas-forming foods such as beans, cucumbers, cabbage, turnips and onions; food allergy; or excess alcohol.
  Persistent symptoms can indicate disease in the digestive tract or other body parts. Occasionally, symptoms occur in patients with no apparent disease. This indicates an abnormal function in a normal part of the body.

RISK INCREASES WITH
- Other functional disorders.
- Excess alcohol consumption.
- Use of drugs that may irritate the stomach.
- Anxiety, stress or depression.

HOW TO PREVENT—Follow suggestions in General Measures.

WHAT TO EXPECT

DIAGNOSTIC MEASURES
- Medical history and exam by a doctor.
- If symptoms are persistent or severe, x-rays of the upper digestive tract, endoscopy and gastroscopy (see Glossary for both) to rule out ulcers or stomach inflammation.

APPROPRIATE HEALTH CARE
- Self-care.
- Doctor's care (severe, recurrent indigestion only).

POSSIBLE COMPLICATIONS—Indigestion may mimic signs of a heart attack or serious disease of the esophagus or stomach, causing the serious disorder to be ignored.

PROBABLE OUTCOME—Symptoms can be controlled with treatment but recurrence is likely.

HOW TO TREAT

GENERAL MEASURES—Treatment and prevention are similar:
- Allow time for leisurely meals. Chew food carefully and thoroughly. Avoid conflicts during meals.
- Don't smoke immediately before a meal.
- Avoid excitement or exercise immediately after a meal.
- Avoid situations than make you swallow air, such as chewing gum.
- Avoid tight clothing.
- Learn relaxation techniques.
- Reduce stress (see How to Cope with Stress in Appendix).
- Observe episodes of indigestion for changes in symptoms. If character, timing, frequency or severity changes, a more serious disorder may be responsible. These include heartburn from irritation of the lower esophagus, gallbladder disease, ulcers or stomach cancer.

MEDICATION
- For minor discomfort, you may use nonprescription antacids or H2 blockers.
- For serious discomfort, your doctor may prescribe acid suppressants, antispasmodics or tranquilizers to relieve tension.
- Avoid aspirin and nonsteroidal anti-inflammatory drugs.

ACTIVITY—No restrictions. A routine exercise program is important to maintain fitness.

DIET
- No special diet. Avoid foods—especially those listed under causes—if they cause discomfort.
- Keep a food diary. Write down what you eat or drink and when symptoms occur. This will help you identify any offending foods or liquids.

CALL YOUR DOCTOR IF

- The pattern of indigestion symptoms changes markedly.
- You develop the following:
  Vomiting, weight loss or appetite loss.
  Black, tarry stool or vomiting of blood.
  Fever.
  Severe pain in the upper right abdomen.
  Discomfort that continues unrelated to meals, eating or chewing gum.
- Indigestion is accompanied by:
  Shortness of breath.
  Sweating.
  Pain radiating to the jaw, neck or arm.

INFLUENZA (Flu; Grippe)

GENERAL INFORMATION

DEFINITION—A common, contagious respiratory infection caused by a virus. Incubation after exposure is 24 to 48 hours. There are three main types of influenza (A, B, C), but they have the ability to mutate into different forms. Outbreaks of different forms occur almost every winter with varying severity.

BODY PARTS INVOLVED—Upper-respiratory system.

SEX OR AGE MOST AFFECTED—Both sexes; all ages except infants.

SIGNS & SYMPTOMS
- Chills and moderate to high fever.
- Muscle aches, including backache.
- Cough, usually with little or no sputum.
- Sore throat; hoarseness; runny nose; headache; fatigue.

CAUSES—Infection by viruses of the myxovirus class. The viruses spread by personal contact or indirect contact (such as use of a contaminated drinking glass).

RISK INCREASES WITH
- Stress; excessive fatigue; poor nutrition.
- Recent illness that has lowered resistance.
- Chronic lung or heart disease.
- Pregnancy (3rd trimester).
- Students; people in semi-closed environments.
- Immunosuppression from drugs or illness.
- Crowded places during an epidemic.

HOW TO PREVENT
- Avoid risks listed above if possible.
- Have a yearly influenza vaccine injection if you are over age 65, have chronic heart or lung disease (no matter what age), live in close institutional quarters (nursing home, dorms, military base) or you are a health care worker. The vaccine only protects against two or three specific strains of influenza A.
- Avoid unnecessary contact with persons who have upper-respiratory infections.
- Use of drug (amantadine or rimantadine) for high-risk persons that have not been vaccinated.
- Avoid crowds during flu season.

WHAT TO EXPECT

DIAGNOSTIC MEASURES
- Medical history and exam by a doctor.
- Laboratory studies, such as blood tests and sputum culture, x-rays of the chest (only for complications).

APPROPRIATE HEALTH CARE
- Self-care after diagnosis.
- Doctor's treatment.

POSSIBLE COMPLICATIONS—Bacterial infections, including middle-ear infection, bronchitis or pneumonia. These can be especially dangerous for chronically ill persons or those over age 65.

PROBABLE OUTCOME—Spontaneous recovery in 7 to 14 days if no complications occur. If complications arise, treatment with antibiotics is usually necessary and recovery may take 3 to 6 weeks.

HOW TO TREAT

GENERAL MEASURES
- To relieve nasal congestion, use salt-water drops (1 teaspoon of salt to 1 quart of water).
- To relieve a sore throat, gargle often with warm or cold, double-strength tea.
- Use an ultrasonic cool-mist humidifier to increase air moisture. This thins lung secretions so they can be coughed up more easily. Don't put medicine in the humidifier; it does not help.
- To avoid spreading germs to others, wash your hands frequently.
- Use warm compresses or heating pad for aching muscles.
- Use a sponge bath to reduce a fever.

MEDICATION
- For minor discomfort, you may use nonprescription drugs, such as acetaminophen, cough syrups, nasal sprays or decongestants.
- Don't give aspirin to a person younger than 18. Some research shows a link between the use of aspirin in children during a virus illness and the development of Reye's syndrome.
- Your doctor may prescribe an antiviral drug for seriously ill persons or for those at greatest risk.

ACTIVITY—Rest is the best medicine. If you are in good general health, rest aids recovery.

DIET
- Appetite is usually lacking. You may just want liquids at first, then progress to small meals of bland starchy foods (dry toast, rice, pudding, cooked cereal, baked potatoes)
- Drink at least 8 glasses of water a day (especially if you have a high fever). Extra fluids, including fruit juice, tea and noncarbonated drinks, also help thin lung secretions.

CALL YOUR DOCTOR IF

- You have symptoms of influenza.
- The following occurs during treatment: Increased fever or cough; blood in the sputum; earache.
  Shortness of breath or chest pain; thick discharge from the nose, sinuses or ears.
  Sinus pain; neck pain or stiffness.
- New, unexplained symptoms develop.

INSECT BITES & STINGS

GENERAL INFORMATION

DEFINITION—Skin eruptions and other symptoms caused by insect bites or stings. The victim often doesn't remember being bitten or stung.

BODY PARTS INVOLVED
- Skin on any part of the body.
- Lymph glands in the neck, armpit, groin or elbow.

SEX OR AGE MOST AFFECTED—Both sexes; all ages.

SIGNS & SYMPTOMS
Skin reactions:
- Red lumps in the skin. The lumps usually appear within minutes after the bite or sting, but some don't appear for 6 to 12 hours.
- A toxic reaction with pain, such as from bee stings.
- A toxic reaction with itching due to the body's release of histamine at the bite site, such as from mosquitoes.
Systemic reactions:
- Nausea or vomiting; headache; fever; dizziness; lightheadedness; swelling; convulsions.
Allergic reactions:
- Itching eyes; facial flushing; dry cough; wheezing; chest/throat constriction.

CAUSES—Bites or stings from mosquitoes, fleas, chiggers, bedbugs, ants, spiders, bees, scorpions and other insects.

RISK INCREASES WITH
- Areas with heavy insect infestations.
- Warm weather in spring and summer.
- Lack of protective measures.
- Perfumes, colognes.
- Previous sensitization.

HOW TO PREVENT
- After identifying the cause, remove it if possible. Treat animals for fleas and exterminate the house or kennel.
- If you cannot avoid exposure, apply insect repellents with diethyltoluamide (DEET).
- Wear protective clothing (long sleeves and long pants in areas of risk, gloves for yardwork).

WHAT TO EXPECT

DIAGNOSTIC MEASURES
Medical history and physical exam by a doctor (sometimes).

APPROPRIATE HEALTH CARE
- Self-care.
- Doctor's treatment (sometimes).

POSSIBLE COMPLICATIONS
- Secondary bacterial infection at the site of the bite. This may cause swollen lymph glands in the neck, armpit, groin or elbow.

- Anaphylaxis (for hypersensitive persons). See Anaphylaxis in Illness section.
- Scarring.

PROBABLE OUTCOME—Most troublesome symptoms disappear in 2 to 3 days, but scratching may prolong symptoms for several weeks. Treatment helps but it doesn't cure quickly.

HOW TO TREAT

GENERAL MEASURES
- Give first-aid and emergency services in severe reactions.
- Insect bites or stings:
  For bee, wasp, yellow-jacket or hornet stings, remove stinger. (Scrape it out. Don't use tweezers.) Wash the area, then rub a paste of meat tenderizer and water into the site.
  For fleas, gnats and mosquitoes, wash the area with soap and water, apply cool compress.
  For ant bites rub bite with ammonia; repeat as often as necessary.
  For spider or scorpion bites, capture the insect if possible, wash the wound, apply ice pack and seek medical attention.
  For ticks and mites, apply a petroleum product until the animal withdraws or pick it off with sterilized tweezers. Wash wound with soap and water.
- If you have had anaphylaxis (severe allergic reaction) following an insect bite, carry an anaphylaxis kit to treat it in the future.

MEDICATION—For minor discomfort, you may use:
- Nonprescription oral antihistamines to decrease itching.
- Nonprescription topical steroid preparations to reduce inflammation and decrease itching. Use according to label directions. For face and groin, use only low-potency steroid products without fluorine.

ACTIVITY—No restrictions.

DIET—No special diet.

CALL YOUR DOCTOR IF

- You have symptoms of anaphylaxis. This is an emergency!
- Self-care does not relieve symptoms, or symptoms don't improve after 2 to 3 days of medical treatment.
- A bitten area becomes red, swollen, warm and tender, indicating infection.
- Temperature rises to 101F (38.3C).

ILLNESS & DISORDERS

INSOMNIA (Sleep Disorder)

 GENERAL INFORMATION

DEFINITION—Sleep disturbance that includes difficulty in falling asleep, remaining asleep, intermittent wakefulness, early morning awakening or a combination of these. Insomnia affects all age groups but is more common in the elderly. Insomnia may be transient due to a life crisis or lifestyle change; or chronic, due to medical or psychological problems or drug intake.

BODY PARTS INVOLVED—Nervous.

SEX OR AGE MOST AFFECTED—Both sexes; all ages.

SIGNS & SYMPTOMS
* Restlessness when trying to fall asleep.
* Brief sleep followed by wakefulness.
* Normal sleep until very early in the morning (3 a.m. or 4 a.m.), then wakefulness (often with frightening thoughts).
* Periods of sleeplessness, alternating with periods of excessive sleep or sleepiness at inconvenient times.

CAUSES
* Depression. This is usually characterized by early-morning wakefulness.
* Overactivity of the thyroid gland.
* Anxiety caused by stress.
* Sexual problems, such as impotence or lack of a sex partner.
* Daytime napping.
* Noisy environment (including a snoring partner).
* Allergies and early-morning wheezing.
* Heart or lung conditions that cause shortness of breath when lying down.
* Painful disorders, such as a fibromyositis or arthritis.
* Urinary or gastrointestinal problems that require urination or bowel movements during the night.
* Consumption of stimulants, such as caffeine.
* Use of some medications, including dextroamphetamines, cortisone drugs or decongestants.
* Erratic work hours.
* New environment or location; jet lag after travel; lack of physical exercise.
* Alcoholism; drug abuse, including overuse of sleep-inducing drugs; withdrawal from addictive substances.

RISK INCREASES WITH—Stress, obesity, smoking.

HOW TO PREVENT
Establish a lifestyle that fosters healthy sleep patterns.

 WHAT TO EXPECT

DIAGNOSTIC MEASURES
* Medical history and exam by a doctor.
* Laboratory thyroid studies, EEG (see Glossary).
* Tests in a sleep-study laboratory (sometimes).

APPROPRIATE HEALTH CARE
* Self-care after diagnosis.
* Doctor's treatment; psychotherapy or counseling, if the cause is psychological.

POSSIBLE COMPLICATIONS
* Transient insomnia becomes chronic.
* Increased daytime sleepiness that can affect all aspects of your life.

PROBABLE OUTCOME—Most persons can establish good sleep patterns if the underlying cause of insomnia is treated or eliminated.

 HOW TO TREAT

GENERAL MEASURES
* Seek ways to minimize stress. Learn and practice relaxation techniques.
* Don't use stimulants close to bedtime.
* Treat any underlying or medical cause.
* Relax in a warm bath before bedtime.
* Don't turn your bedroom into an office or a den. Create a comfortable sleep setting.
* Turn off your mind. Focus on peaceful and relaxing thoughts. Play soft music or relaxation tapes. Set a rigid sleep schedule.
* Use mechanical aids such as ear plugs, eye shades or electric blanket.

MEDICATION—Your doctor may prescribe sleep-inducing drugs for a short time if:
* Temporary insomnia is interfering with your daily activities.
* You have a medical disorder that regularly disturbs sleep.
* You need to establish regular sleep patterns. Long-term use of sleep inducers may be counter-productive or addictive.

ACTIVITY
Exercise regularly to create healthy fatigue, but not within 2 hours of going to bed.

DIET
* No special diet, but don't eat within 3 hours of bedtime if indigestion has previously disturbed your sleep. Drinking warm milk before bedtime helps some. Limit caffeine consumption.

 CALL YOUR DOCTOR IF

* You have insomnia and self-help methods are ineffective.
* New, unexplained symptoms develop.

INTERSTITIAL CYSTITIS

GENERAL INFORMATION

DEFINITION—A chronic inflammation of the interstitium (the area between the bladder lining and the bladder muscle).

BODY PARTS INVOLVED—Bladder.

SEX OR AGE MOST AFFECTED—The average age of onset is 40, but it affects all ages, women more commonly than men.

SIGNS & SYMPTOMS
- Pelvic pain and pressure.
- Urgent need to urinate (sometimes 60 to 80 times a day in severe cases).
- Sensation of incomplete emptying of the bladder.
- Frequent, excessive need to urinate at night (nocturia).
- Pain during sexual intercourse.
- Burning when urinating.
- Vaginal and rectal pain (sometimes).

CAUSES—Exact cause is unknown. Studies suggest that it is a syndrome of bladder inflammation possibly initiated by bacterial infection, autoimmune process (misdirected immune response in which the body's defenses become self destructive) or contact irritants. It is probably not an infectious disease.

RISK INCREASES WITH
- A history of sensitivities or allergies to medications, food, or other substances; hay fever or asthma.
- Rheumatoid arthritis.
- Previous hysterectomy.

HOW TO PREVENT—No known preventive measures.

WHAT TO EXPECT

DIAGNOSTIC MEASURES
- Initial diagnostic tests will include urine studies (which are usually normal) and a pelvic examination. Conditions that have similar symptoms (bladder infection, kidney problems, vaginal infections, endometriosis, and sexually transmitted diseases) will need to be excluded.
- If other tests are negative, a cystoscopy (use of a small lighted telescope to view the inside of the bladder) is often recommended. A biopsy is taken at this time to rule out a malignancy. As an added benefit, cystoscopy often helps relieve symptoms. It involves distention of the bladder by filling it with water, thereby stretching the bladder and increasing its capacity.

APPROPRIATE HEALTH CARE—There is no consistently effective treatment for the disorder. Options include various oral medications, medication instilled into the bladder, special routines for stretching the bladder, diet changes, bladder retraining, relaxation training, and transcutaneous electrical nerve stimulation (TENS).
- Surgical measures are rarely used (only as a last resort when other methods of treatment have failed and quality of life warrants drastic steps).

POSSIBLE COMPLICATIONS—Unrelieved symptoms that come and go and may vary in intensity from mild to severe.

PROBABLE OUTCOME
- Treatments are available that may control or minimize the symptoms, but do not cure the disorder. Medical studies are ongoing to help determine the cause, more beneficial treatments and a possible cure.
- The disorder may have flare-ups and remissions.

HOW TO TREAT

GENERAL MEASURES—Counseling, biofeedback or self-hypnosis, or self-relaxation therapy is recommended to help manage the stress, anger, anxiety and, sometimes, depression that accompanies disorders of chronic pain.

MEDICATION
- Antihistamines, anticholinergics, nonsteroidal anti-inflammatory drugs (NSAIDs), and antidepressants all have limited success with decreasing the symptoms.
- Sodium pentosanpolysulfate has demonstrated effectiveness in relieving symptoms for some patients.
- DMSO (dimethyl sulfoxide) or other medications may be instilled (placed directly) into the bladder. The DMSO is left in for about 15 minutes and then expelled. The treatment is repeated every 2 weeks or until symptoms are relieved. DMSO use produces a garlic-like smell to the skin and breath lasting up to 72 hours.

ACTIVITY—No restrictions other than those caused by the symptoms.

DIET
- Elimination of caffeinated beverages, alcohol, artificial sweeteners, spicy foods, brewer's yeast, citrus fruits and tomatoes in the diet may help relieve symptoms.
- A bland diet helps some patients.

CALL YOUR DOCTOR IF

- You or a family member has symptoms of interstitial cystitis.
- Intolerable pain occurs during treatment.
- New, unexplained symptoms develop. Drugs used in treatment may produce side effects.
- Symptoms recur after treatment.

INTESTINAL OBSTRUCTION

GENERAL INFORMATION

DEFINITION—Partial or complete blockage of the intestines.

BODY PARTS INVOLVED—Small and large bowel.

SEX OR AGE MOST AFFECTED—Both sexes; all ages.

SIGNS & SYMPTOMS
- Cramping abdominal pain.
- Nausea and vomiting. In the advanced stages, vomit resembles feces.
- Weakness, dizziness or fainting.
- Little or no urine due to fluid loss.
- Failure to pass stools or gas.
- Audible noises from the abdomen in early stages; later, no sounds are audible.
- Abdominal bloating, swelling and gas.
- Fever (sometimes).
- Diarrhea (partial obstruction only).
- Rectal bleeding (sometimes).

CAUSES
- Paralytic ileus. Peristalsis (normal muscle contraction of the intestine) stops for unknown reasons.
- Adhesions (constricting bands of fibrous tissue that result from previous surgery).
- Intestinal hernias.
- Intestinal inflammation or tumors—either benign or cancerous.
- Tumors in adjacent organs that cause pressure on the intestines.
- Foreign objects inside the intestines (swallowed objects or parasites such as worms).
- Twisted bowel (volvulus, see Glossary).
- Severe constipation (fecal impaction).

RISK INCREASES WITH—Previous abdominal surgery.

HOW TO PREVENT
- Eat a diet high in fiber and drink at least 6 to 8 glasses of liquid a day to avoid constipation or fecal impaction.
- Obtain prompt medical treatment for repair of hernias.
- See your doctor if your bowel habits change significantly for longer than 7 days. This may be an early symptom of bowel cancer.

WHAT TO EXPECT

DIAGNOSTIC MEASURES
- Your own observation of symptoms.
- Medical history and physical exam by a doctor.
- Laboratory blood studies to measure fluids and electrolytes and to detect bleeding or infection.
- X-rays of the intestinal tract and abdomen (upper and lower GI series).

APPROPRIATE HEALTH CARE
- Doctor's treatment.
- Surgery to remove the obstruction (usually).
- Hospitalization for diagnosis and replacement of lost fluids prior to surgery.

POSSIBLE COMPLICATIONS
- Dehydration and shock.
- Bowel gangrene.
- Peritonitis.

PROBABLE OUTCOME—Surgery can usually correct the obstruction, but it may not correct the underlying cause, such as cancer. Without treatment, complications can be fatal.

HOW TO TREAT

GENERAL MEASURES—Intestinal obstruction usually develops rapidly into an emergency. Home remedies are of no value and some—such as enemas or laxatives—may be harmful.

MEDICATION—Medication is not helpful for intestinal obstruction. However, your doctor may prescribe medication appropriate for the underlying disorder.

ACTIVITY—Rest in bed until the obstruction is corrected. If surgery is necessary, resume normal activities gradually.

DIET—Don't eat or drink anything until the obstruction is corrected. You will probably receive intravenous nourishment until then.

CALL YOUR DOCTOR IF

- Your bowel habits change.
- You have early symptoms of intestinal obstruction.

INTUSSUSCEPTION

 GENERAL INFORMATION

DEFINITION—An intestinal obstruction in which the bowel telescopes (folds into itself) forming a tube within a tube.

BODY PARTS INVOLVED—Intestine, usually the large intestine.

SEX OR AGE MOST AFFECTED—All ages, but most common in infants and children between 2 months and 6 years. It is more common in boys.

SIGNS & SYMPTOMS
Early stages:
• Cramping abdominal pain. Infants cry out, bring the legs up to the abdomen and become pale and sweaty during an attack.
• Vomiting.
Later stages:
• Rectal bleeding. This may be dark red material that resembles jelly.
• Swollen abdomen.
• Mass in the abdomen that can be felt.
• Weakness and lethargy.
• Shock.

CAUSES—Unknown factors cause a loop of bowel to turn in on itself. This blocks the bowel's blood supply, causing gangrene and peritonitis. The disorder may be caused by a virus infection but that is unproven.

RISK INCREASES WITH
• Family history of intussusception.
• The seasons (for unknown reasons). It is most common in late spring, early summer and midwinter.
• Leukemia, lymphoma, or cystic fibrosis.
• Recent upper respiratory infection.
• Recent operation (1-24 days previously).

HOW TO PREVENT—Observe your child carefully if symptoms develop. Prevent complications by seeking medical treatment during early stages. No other specific preventive measures.

 WHAT TO EXPECT

DIAGNOSTIC MEASURES
• Your own observation of symptoms.
• Medical history and physical exam by a doctor.
• Laboratory blood tests.
• X-rays of the abdomen and intestinal tract (barium enema, see Glossary). The radiologist may manipulate the barium, which may clear the obstruction.

APPROPRIATE HEALTH CARE
• Doctor's treatment.
• Surgery to correct the problem by pushing out the telescoped portion of the intestine. Occasionally a segment of the bowel must be cut out.
• Home care during convalescence.

POSSIBLE COMPLICATIONS
• Dehydration and shock.
• Intestinal perforation and peritonitis.
• Postsurgical infection.

PROBABLE OUTCOME—Spontaneous recovery in 24 hours (sometimes). If not, this is curable with early diagnosis and surgery or barium treatment. Without treatment, complications are life-threatening. The disorder sometimes recurs.

 HOW TO TREAT

GENERAL MEASURES—Observe your child carefully if symptoms develop. Prevent complications by seeking medical treatment during early stages.

MEDICATION—Medicine usually is not necessary for this disorder unless infection develops. Then your doctor may prescribe antibiotics.
  Don't use home remedies or nonprescription drugs, such as laxatives, for this condition. They may be dangerous.

ACTIVITY—The child should rest in bed until the obstruction is cleared. Activities may then be resumed gradually.

DIET—Don't feed a child with signs of intestinal obstruction. Intravenous fluids are necessary until the obstruction is removed. No special diet is required afterward.

 CALL YOUR DOCTOR IF

Your child has signs or symptoms of intestinal obstruction. This condition changes quickly from a curable one to a life-threatening one.

ILLNESS & DISORDERS

IRITIS

 GENERAL INFORMATION

DEFINITION—Inflammation of the tissues that support the iris (the ring of colored tissue around the pupil of the eye). May sometimes be confused with pink eye (conjunctivitis).

BODY PARTS INVOLVED—Eye.

SEX OR AGE MOST AFFECTED—Both sexes; all ages.

SIGNS & SYMPTOMS
Acute iritis of sudden onset:
- Severe eye pain.
- Photophobia (sensitivity to light).
- Eye redness.
- Smaller pupil in the affected eye (sometimes).
- Tears.
- Blurred vision.

Iritis of gradual onset:
- Eye pain.
- Photophobia.
- Floating spots in the field of vision.
- Blurred vision.

CAUSES
- Infection that spreads to the eye from other body parts. Common causes include:
  Toxoplasmosis.
  Tuberculosis.
  Histoplasmosis.
  Syphilis.
  Sarcoidosis.
  Viruses.
- Injury to the eye.
- Autoimmune reaction (possibly).
- Unknown in many cases.

RISK INCREASES WITH
- Rheumatoid arthritis.
- Ulcerative colitis.
- Viral, bacterial, fungal or parasitic infection.
- Other eye disease.

HOW TO PREVENT—No specific preventive measures known.

 WHAT TO EXPECT

DIAGNOSTIC MEASURES—Special eye exam will confirm the diagnosis.

APPROPRIATE HEALTH CARE—Treatment for any underlying condition.

POSSIBLE COMPLICATIONS
- Glaucoma.
- Cataracts.
- Permanent or partial vision loss.

PROBABLE OUTCOME—Vision can usually be preserved with prompt treatment. Usually dependent on the underlying condition.

 HOW TO TREAT

GENERAL MEASURES—Wear dark glasses, even indoors, until treatment is complete.

MEDICATION—Your doctor may prescribe:
- Eye drops (mydriatics) that dilate the pupil and prevent scarring. You may need to use the eyedrops for a long time.
- Oral cortisone drugs or cortisone eye drops to reduce inflammation.

ACTIVITY—Rest in bed until symptoms subside.

DIET—Eat a normal well-balanced diet.

 CALL YOUR DOCTOR IF

- You or a family member has symptoms of iritis, either sudden or gradual. Call immediately.
- Vision changes in any way.
- New, unexplained symptoms develop. Drugs used in treatment may produce side effects.

IRRITABLE BOWEL SYNDROME
(Spastic Colon or Colitis; Mucous Colitis)

GENERAL INFORMATION

DEFINITION—An irritative and inflammatory disorder of the intestine. It is not contagious, inherited or cancerous.

BODY PARTS INVOLVED—Small and large intestines.

SEX OR AGE MOST AFFECTED—Often begins in adolescents or young adults; twice as likely to affect women as men.

SIGNS & SYMPTOMS—The following symptoms usually begin in early adult life. Episodes may last for days, weeks or months.
* Mucous with or around the stool.
* Cramp-like pain in the middle or to one side of the lower abdomen. Pain is usually relieved with bowel movements.
* Nausea; bloating and gas; headache; rectal pain; backache.
* Occasional appetite loss that may lead to weight loss.
* Diarrhea or constipation, usually alternating; fatigue; depression; anxiety; concentration difficulty.

CAUSES
* Unknown. May be related to stress and emotional conflict that results in anxiety, anger, guilt or depression. Situations that often precede an attack include: obsessive worry about everyday problems; marital tension; fear of, or actual loss of a loved one.
* Increased activity of the colon with hyper secretion.
* Low residue diet.
* Symptoms may also be triggered by eating, though no specific food has been identified as responsible.

RISK INCREASES WITH
* Stress; improper diet; smoking; excess alcohol consumption; use of drugs.
* Fatigue or overwork; poor physical fitness.
* Family history of similar bowel problems.

HOW TO PREVENT—Reduce stress or try to modify your response to it (see How to Cope with Stress in Appendix) and pay attention to good diet habits.

WHAT TO EXPECT

DIAGNOSTIC MEASURES
* Medical history and exam by a doctor.
* Laboratory studies, including stool studies, to exclude other disorders such as lactose intolerance, ulcers, parasites, enzyme deficiency and ulcerative colitis.
* X-ray of the colon (barium enema).
* Sigmoidoscopy (see Glossary).

APPROPRIATE HEALTH CARE
* Self-care.
* Doctor's treatment.

POSSIBLE COMPLICATIONS—Psychological fixation on bowel function, leading to psychologic disability.

PROBABLE OUTCOME—The condition is usually recurrent throughout life. Symptoms decrease or may disappear for periods of time. It is not life-threatening and doesn't progress to cancer or inflammatory disease.

HOW TO TREAT

GENERAL MEASURES
* Warm heat to the abdomen (compresses, hot-water bottle or heating pad) may help ease discomfort.
* Reduce stress in your life. Try techniques that can help you relax (meditation, self-hypnosis or biofeedback). Keep a stress diary so you know who or what may bring on symptoms.
* Quit smoking. Nicotine may contribute to the problem.

MEDICATION—Medication may help but it will not cure this disorder. Your doctor may prescribe:
* Antispasmodics to relieve severe abdominal cramps.
* Short-term tranquilizers to reduce anxiety.
* Other drugs including bulk-producing agents, constipating agents, anticholinergics, antiflatulents and lactose for milk intolerance.

ACTIVITY—No restrictions. Good physical fitness improves bowel function and helps reduce stress.

DIET
* Increase fiber in the diet to promote good bowel function (see High Fiber Diet in Appendix). Add fiber to your diet slowly to give the body time to adjust.
* Don't eat foods or drinks that aggravate symptoms. Coffee or milk may be a major cause of symptoms in some people. Keep a food diary so you can find out which foods aggravate symptoms.
* Avoid gas-producing and spicy foods.
* Avoid large meals, but eat regularly.
* Limit alcohol consumption.

CALL YOUR DOCTOR IF

* Fever develops.
* Stool is black or tarry-looking.
* You begin vomiting.
* Unexplained weight loss of 5 pounds or more occurs.
* Symptoms don't improve despite treatment.

JET LAG

 GENERAL INFORMATION

DEFINITION—Jet lag results from east-west travel between different time zones. (North-south travel does not cause jet lag.) The degree of severity depends on the number of time zones crossed and the direction traveled. Most people find traveling eastward and adapting to a shorter work day is more difficult than traveling westward and adapting to a longer work day.

SEX OR AGE MOST AFFECTED—Both sexes; all ages.

SIGNS & SYMPTOMS
- Extreme fatigue.
- Sleep disturbances.
- Loss of concentration.
- Malaise.
- Disorientation.
- Sluggishness.
- Stomach upset.
- Loss of appetite.
- Swollen feet.

CAUSES—Disturbance in the body's physiological processes that control not only sleep and wakefulness, but also alertness, hunger, digestion, urine production, temperature and hormone secretion.

RISK INCREASES WITH—Frequent travel in short periods of time.

HOW TO PREVENT
- Don't drink alcohol.
- No other specific preventive measures have been shown to be of particular value.

 WHAT TO EXPECT

DIAGNOSTIC MEASURES—Your own observation of symptoms.

APPROPRIATE HEALTH CARE—No medical care is necessary for typical mild cases of jet lag. For severe cases doctor's treatment may be necessary.

POSSIBLE COMPLICATIONS
- Motor vehicle or other accident or injury due to exhaustion.
- Job problems due to lack of concentration.

PROBABLE OUTCOME—Symptoms usually resolve themselves after a short period of time in the same geographic location.

 HOW TO TREAT

GENERAL MEASURES
- Plan destination activities to accomodate for time differences.
- Spend some time every day in natural sunlight.
- Adjust your bed and mealtimes to the new timetable as soon as possible
- Set your watch to local time as soon as possible after takeoff.

MEDICATION
- Your doctor may prescribe short-acting benzodiazepines for sleep in transit.
- The hormone melatonin has been used for this condition, but long-term data are lacking.

ACTIVITY—Don't operate motor vehicles or swim alone if you feel tired.

DIET
- Eat a normal well-balanced diet, even if you have no appetite.
- Stay clear of alcoholic drinks.

 CALL YOUR DOCTOR IF

You or a family member has symptoms of jet lag and they don't subside after one week.

KAPOSI'S SARCOMA

GENERAL INFORMATION

DEFINITION—A form of skin cancer that is found most often in patients with acquired immunodeficiency syndrome (AIDS). It is an aggressive disorder and the skin tumors soon become widespread. A second form of Kaposi's sarcoma is associated with immunosuppressive medications, and another form, referred to as classic, is usually found in elderly men of Mediterranean ancestry.

BODY PARTS INVOLVED—Skin.

SEX OR AGE MOST AFFECTED—Adult males.

SIGNS & SYMPTOMS
- Skin lesions (blue-red nodules) on the face, arms and trunk.
- Lesions may also be found in mucous membranes, lymph nodes and respiratory and gastrointestinal tracts.
- Lesions in the mouth may interfere with eating or swallowing.
- Lesions on the feet may interfere with walking.
- Swelling (edema) face and lower extremities.
- Breathing difficulty due to lesions in the lungs.

CAUSES—Unknown transmission agent. Researchers have tentatively identified a type of herpes virus that causes Kaposi's sarcoma.

RISK INCREASES WITH
- HIV (human immunodeficiency virus) infection.
- Taking immunosuppressant medications.

HOW TO PREVENT—No preventive measures for Kaposi's sarcoma; safe sex practices help prevent HIV infection.

WHAT TO EXPECT

DIAGNOSTIC MEASURES
- Your own observation of symptoms.
- Medical history and physical exam by a doctor.
- Skin biopsy (see Glossary).
- Other tests to determine if tumors have spread to lungs or liver.

APPROPRIATE HEALTH CARE
- Doctor's treatment.
- Discontinuing or reducing dosage if the disorder is related to immunosuppressant drugs.
- Freezing (cryotherapy) of superficial lesions.
- Low-dose radiation therapy, if disease is not too widespread.
- Surgical excision in some patients.

POSSIBLE COMPLICATIONS
- Spreading of lesions.
- Other infections.

PROBABLE OUTCOME—Generally poor for AIDS-related disease.

HOW TO TREAT

GENERAL MEASURES
- Primary goals of treatment are to relieve symptoms and improve cosmetic appearance.
- Good cosmetic results can improve your appearance as well as improve your overall outlook.

MEDICATION—Your doctor may prescribe:
- Injections into the lesions with anticancer medications.
- One or more oral anticancer drugs (may be necessary for patients with advanced, widespread disease).

ACTIVITY—As tolerated.

DIET—No special diet.

CALL YOUR DOCTOR IF

- You or a household member develop symptoms of Kaposi's sarcoma.
- New or unexplained symptoms develop. Drugs used in treatment may cause side effects.

KELOIDS

GENERAL INFORMATION

DEFINITION—An overgrowth of fibrous tissue (scar) on the skin. They usually arise in an area of injury (such as after a burn or from severe acne), but sometimes arise from a very minor scratch. Keloids are more frequent in black people than in white people.

BODY PARTS INVOLVED—Anywhere on the skin, but most commonly appear on the breastbone, upper back and shoulder.

SEX OR AGE MOST AFFECTED—Both sexes; all ages.

SIGNS & SYMPTOMS
- Firm, raised, hard scars that are slightly pink.
- Scars may itch, cause pain or be tender to the touch.
- Scars may continue to grow and develop claw-like projections over a period of time.

CAUSES—Keloids occur due to a defective healing process in which an excess of collagen forms at the site of a healing scar.

RISK INCREASES WITH
- Family history of keloids.
- Dark skin pigment.
- Surgical wound.
- Acne.
- Burn injury.
- Ear piercing.
- Vaccination.
- Insect bite.
- Folliculitis barbae (inflammation of a hair follicle).

HOW TO PREVENT
- Avoidance of trauma to the skin.
- Compressive pressure dressings for high-risk patients (burns).
- For patients with known tendency to keloid formation, elective surgery should be avoided. If a procedure is necessary, special precautions should be implemented.

WHAT TO EXPECT

DIAGNOSTIC MEASURES
- Your own observation of symptoms.
- Medical history and physical exam by a doctor.

APPROPRIATE HEALTH CARE
- Patients often want scars removed for cosmetic and functional reasons including itching, swelling and restrictions of movement.
- Injections (may be combined with surgical removal of the excess tissue) for some patients.
- Cryosurgery (see Glossary) using nitrous oxide and liquid nitrogen. Treatment may be repeated (every 30-60 days) until no further improvement is observed.
- Other experimental therapies with drugs, lasers, topical medications are currently undergoing study.

POSSIBLE COMPLICATIONS—Recurrence, despite adequate treatment.

PROBABLE OUTCOME—Scars gradually diminish following treatment. Keloids are generally considered harmless and noncancerous.

HOW TO TREAT

GENERAL MEASURES—There is no self-treatment for keloids. Follow doctor's instructions for follow-up measures after treatment.

MEDICATION—Injection of corticosteroid drugs directly into the keloid. May be repeated every three to four weeks until desired degree of flattening and softening has been achieved.

ACTIVITY—No restrictions.

DIET—No special diet.

CALL YOUR DOCTOR IF

You have signs of keloids.

KERATITIS

GENERAL INFORMATION

DEFINITION—Inflammation of the cornea (the clear central portion of the eye that covers the pupil).

BODY PARTS INVOLVED—Eye.

SEX OR AGE MOST AFFECTED—Both sexes; all ages.

SIGNS & SYMPTOMS
- Eye pain.
- Photophobia (sensitivity to light).
- Tears.

CAUSES
- Bacterial, viral or fungal infections. The most common is herpes simplex virus, Type I.
- Drying of the eye caused by an eyelid disorder or insufficient tear formation.
- Foreign object in the eye.
- Intense light, such as from welding arcs or the reflection of intense sunlight from snow or water. (Symptoms may not appear for 24 hours after exposure.)
- Vitamin-A deficiency (rare in normal diet).
- Allergy or sensitivity to eye cosmetics, air pollution, airborne particles (pollen, dust, mold or yeasts) and other allergens.

RISK INCREASES WITH
- Poor nutrition, especially insufficient vitamin A.
- Illness that has lowered resistance.
- Crowded or unsanitary living conditions.
- Viral infections elsewhere in the body, especially cold sores or genital herpes.

HOW TO PREVENT
- Wear protective glasses if your work involves eye hazards.
- Eat a well-balanced diet that contains sufficient vitamin A or take multiple-vitamin supplements containing vitamin A.

WHAT TO EXPECT

DIAGNOSTIC MEASURES
- Your own observation of symptoms.
- Medical history and physical exam by a doctor.
- Special eye exam confirms keratitis. A vision test may be performed also.

APPROPRIATE HEALTH CARE
- Doctor's (ophthalmologist's) treatment.
- Treatment usually involves eye medication.
- Surgery to replace the cornea (severe cases only).

POSSIBLE COMPLICATIONS
- Glaucoma.
- Ulceration of the cornea.
- Permanent scarring in the eye.
- Vision loss.

PROBABLE OUTCOME—Depends on the cause. With early treatment, most types of keratitis are curable.

HOW TO TREAT

GENERAL MEASURES—A temporary eye patch is often necessary. It may limit your ability to take care of yourself.

MEDICATION
- Your doctor may prescribe:
Antibiotic or antiviral eye drops and ointments.
Artificial tears.
- Don't treat any eye inflammation without consulting your doctor. Don't use nonprescription eye drops containing topical corticosteroids. These may worsen the condition or cause eyeball perforation.

ACTIVITY—Eye patching will restrict activity. Resume your normal activities gradually.

DIET—No special diet.

CALL YOUR DOCTOR IF

- You have symptoms of keratitis.
- Your vision diminishes in any way.

KERATOSES, SEBORRHEIC

GENERAL INFORMATION

DEFINITION—A noncontagious, inflammatory, scaling disease of the skin.

BODY PARTS INVOLVED—Chest; back; face; arms.

SEX OR AGE MOST AFFECTED—Adults of both sexes. By age 60, almost everyone has a few seborrheic keratoses.

SIGNS & SYMPTOMS—Papules (small, raised bumps) with the following characteristics:
• Papules are flat-topped with well-defined borders.
• Young papules are relatively flat and light brown. More-advanced papules are dark brown or black.
• Papules are wider than tall and they appear "stuck on."
• Papules measure 5mm to 20mm in diameter. They are distributed on the chest, back, face and arms.
• Papules don't itch or hurt.
• There may be only 1 or 2 papules, or there may be up to 100.

CAUSES—Unknown.

RISK INCREASES WITH
• Aging.
• Family history of the disorder.
• Excessive sun exposure or other skin injury.

HOW TO PREVENT—No specific preventive measures.

WHAT TO EXPECT

DIAGNOSTIC MEASURES
• Your own observation of symptoms.
• Medical history and physical exam by a doctor.
• Biopsy (see Glossary).

APPROPRIATE HEALTH CARE
• Self-care.
• Removal of lesions if they are unsightly, are irritated by clothing or interfere with grooming. Removal methods include cryosurgery, chemocautery, light electrosurgery or shave biopsy (see Glossary for all).

POSSIBLE COMPLICATIONS—Seborrheic keratoses on the eyelid borders may require special treatment.

PROBABLE OUTCOME—The number of lesions increases with time. Each lesion is permanent unless removed. Seborrheic keratoses are harmless and require no treatment, but most people want them removed (especially if they are unsightly or irritated by clothing).

HOW TO TREAT

GENERAL MEASURES—After removal, a blister (sometimes with blood) will develop at the treatment site. The top of the blister will come off spontaneously in about 2 weeks. You should have little or no scarring. Wash and use make-up or cosmetics as usual. If clothing irritates the blister, cover it with a small adhesive bandage.

MEDICATION—Medicine usually is not necessary for this disorder.

ACTIVITY—No restrictions.

DIET—No special diet.

CALL YOUR DOCTOR IF

• You have symptoms of seborrheic keratoses.
• You want unsightly seborrheic keratoses removed.
• Treated areas become infected, as evidenced by pain, tenderness, redness, swelling or heat.
• Any lesion changes color or bleeds.

KERATOSIS, ACTINIC

GENERAL INFORMATION

DEFINITION—A small area of sun-damaged skin that is precancerous.

BODY PARTS INVOLVED—Skin of exposed areas, especially the scalp, face, ears, lips, arms and hands.

SEX OR AGE MOST AFFECTED—Adults.

SIGNS & SYMPTOMS—Brownish or reddish scaly patches on exposed areas of skin. The patches are painless.

CAUSES—Prolonged exposure to the sun's radiation (may develop years after the person's most intense sun-exposure).

RISK INCREASES WITH
- Outdoor occupations such as farming.
- Outdoor sports.
- Light complexioned persons who tan poorly.
- Immunosuppression due to illness or medication.

HOW TO PREVENT—Protect yourself against direct sun exposure. When outdoors, wear a hat and protective clothing. Use sunscreen lotions and creams with rating of 15 or more.

WHAT TO EXPECT

DIAGNOSTIC MEASURES
- Your own observation of symptoms.
- Medical history and physical exam by a doctor.

APPROPRIATE HEALTH CARE
- Self-care after diagnosis.
- Doctor's treatment.

POSSIBLE COMPLICATIONS
- Skin damage.
- Skin cancer (squamous-cell carcinoma).

PROBABLE OUTCOME—An individual keratosis will disappear with treatment, but new lesions are likely to recur. If neglected, actinic keratosis can lead to skin cancer.

HOW TO TREAT

GENERAL MEASURES—After diagnosis:
- Minimize direct sun exposure.
- See your doctor for checkups every 6 months to ensure early detection and treatment of skin cancers.

MEDICATION—Your doctor may use:
- Liquid nitrogen to freeze the affected tissue.
- Applications of 5-fluorouracil to the affected area. This causes uncomfortable inflammation, but it is very effective.
- Vitamin A, which is still experimental.

ACTIVITY—No restrictions.

DIET—No special diet.

CALL YOUR DOCTOR IF

You have signs of actinic keratosis. Even though this causes no symptoms, it is precancerous.

ILLNESS & DISORDERS

KERATOSIS PILARIS

GENERAL INFORMATION

DEFINITION—A common skin disorder in which the openings of the hair follicles become filled with hard plugs. These are not contagious.

BODY PARTS INVOLVED—Skin on the backs of upper arms, fronts of thighs or buttocks.

SEX OR AGE MOST AFFECTED—Children and young adults.

SIGNS & SYMPTOMS—Papules (small, raised bumps) with the following characteristics:
- Papules are small, firm and white, with a dry "sandpaper" feeling.
- Papules are clustered. Each one is about 1mm in size.
- Papules are at the openings of hair follicles. They can be scooped out with the fingernails.
- When scooped out, a papule usually contains a coiled hair inside of white, semisolid material.
- Papules don't itch or hurt.

CAUSES—Unknown, but it may be hereditary. These commonly occur in association with allergic dermatitis and several types of ichthyosis, both of which have strong hereditary links.
  Lesions that are similar—possibly identical—to those of keratosis pilaris appear in persons with vitamin-A deficiency.

RISK INCREASES WITH
- History of skin allergies.
- Family history of keratosis pilaris.
- Poor nutrition, especially vitamin-A deficiency.

HOW TO PREVENT—Cannot be prevented at present.

WHAT TO EXPECT

DIAGNOSTIC MEASURES
- Your own observation of symptoms.
- Medical history and physical exam by a doctor.
- Biopsy (see Glossary).

APPROPRIATE HEALTH CARE—Self-care. Treatment is usually unnecessary and if done, often unsatisfactory.

POSSIBLE COMPLICATIONS—Secondary infection of papules.

PROBABLE OUTCOME—Keratosis pilaris is a chronic, harmless skin problem with no permanent cure. Individual papules may come and go over a matter of weeks. All gradually disappear by age 30.

HOW TO TREAT

GENERAL MEASURES
- Take long soaking tub baths.
- Use mild, unscented soap.
- Scrub gently with a stiff brush to remove the plugs in the follicles temporarily.
- Apply lubricating ointments or creams to the affected areas 6 or 7 times a day. The most useful time is immediately after bathing when lubrication helps the skin retain moisture.

MEDICATION—Apply lubricating ointments or creams to the affected areas 6 or 7 times a day. The most useful time is immediately after bathing when lubrication helps the skin retain moisture.

ACTIVITY—No restrictions.

DIET—No special diet.

CALL YOUR DOCTOR IF

Signs of infection develop around the keratoses pilaris. Signs include pain or tenderness, redness, swelling and fever of 101F (38.3C) or higher.

KIDNEY INFECTION, ACUTE
(Pyelonephritis, Acute)

 GENERAL INFORMATION

DEFINITION—A noncontagious bacterial infection of the kidneys (kidneys filter waste material from the bloodstream and produce urine).

BODY PARTS INVOLVED—Kidneys; urinary tract.

SEX OR AGE MOST AFFECTED—Both sexes, but more common in females of all ages. Acute kidney infections in males of any age may indicate a serious underlying disease, such as a tumor, obstruction or prostate disorder.

SIGNS & SYMPTOMS—Sudden onset of:
- Fever and shaking chills.
- Burning, frequent urination.
- Cloudy urine or blood in the urine.
- Aching (sometimes severe) in one or both sides of the lower back.
- Abdominal pain.
- Marked fatigue.
Note: Young children and the elderly may not have typical symptoms or signs.

CAUSES—Bacteria (most commonly Escherichia coli) invade one or both kidneys. The infection may begin in the bladder. The most common sources of bacterial infection are:
- Vigorous sexual activity in women, which allows bacteria to enter the urethra and bladder.
- Infections elsewhere in the body that travel to the kidneys through the bloodstream or lymph glands.
- Blockage or abnormality of the urinary system, caused by stones, obstructions, bladder dysfunction from nerve diseases, tumors or congenital abnormalities.
- Catheters, tubes or surgical procedures used for other medical conditions.

RISK INCREASES WITH
- Diabetes mellitus.
- Chronic urinary-bladder infection or tumor.
- Infrequent emptying of urinary bladder.
- Paralysis from spinal-cord injury or tumor.
- Pregnancy.

HOW TO PREVENT—No specific preventive measures for males. For females:
- After bowel movements, always wipe from the vaginal area toward the rectum.
- Avoid prolonged moistness around the urethra, such as that caused by nylon underpants or wet swim suits.
- Avoid sexual positions that irritate or hurt the urethra or bladder.
- Urinate within 15 minutes after sexual intercourse.
- Don't hold urine; when you have the urge to void, do so.

 WHAT TO EXPECT

DIAGNOSTIC MEASURES
- Your own observation of symptoms.
- Medical history and physical exam by a doctor.
- Urinalysis and urine culture; cystoscopy, ultrasound, intravenous pyelogram (IVP) (see Glossary for all). Other special tests may be recommended.

APPROPRIATE HEALTH CARE
- Self-care after diagnosis.
- Doctor's treatment.

POSSIBLE COMPLICATIONS
- Chronic kidney infection.
- High blood pressure (hypertension).

PROBABLE OUTCOME—Usually curable in 10 to 14 days with treatment. Make a return doctor visit to assure complete cure.

 HOW TO TREAT

GENERAL MEASURES
- Avoid long periods without urinating (such as on a trip).
- Treatment for men may take longer in order to prevent a relapse.
- See Resources for Additional Information.

MEDICATION—Your doctor may prescribe:
- Oral antibiotics. Take all the antibiotics prescribed, even if symptoms disappear.
- Antibiotics (intravenous or by injection), if oral antibiotics don't cure the infection.
- Urinary analgesics to relieve pain.

ACTIVITY—Rest in bed until high fever and discomfort subside. Don't resume sexual relations until fever or urinary symptoms have cleared.

DIET—No special diet. Drink at least 2 quarts of liquid daily; include cranberry juice or vitamin C to acidify the urine.

 CALL YOUR DOCTOR IF

- You have symptoms of a kidney infection.
- The following occurs during treatment:
  Symptoms and fever persist after 48 hours of antibiotic treatment. Occasionally a different antibiotic is needed.
  Symptoms return (especially if accompanied by fever) after antibiotic treatment.
- New, unexplained symptoms develop. Drugs used in treatment may produce side effects.

KIDNEY INFECTION, CHRONIC
(Pyelonephritis, Chronic)

GENERAL INFORMATION

DEFINITION—Infection of the kidneys that develops slowly and lasts for months or years. It leads to scarring and eventual loss of kidney function. Kidneys filter waste material from the bloodstream and produce urine.

BODY PARTS INVOLVED—Kidneys.

SEX OR AGE MOST AFFECTED—Adults of both sexes, but more common in women.

SIGNS & SYMPTOMS—Usually no signs or symptoms, unlike acute kidney infection. The following occur if chronic kidney failure develops:
- Anemia.
- Weakness.
- Loss of appetite.
- Hypertension.
- Pain in one or both sides of the lower back.
- Blood in the urine.

CAUSES
- Frequent, acute bacterial kidney infections.
- Untreated lower urinary tract infections.

RISK INCREASES WITH
- History of diabetes mellitus.
- Urinary obstruction, such as stones or tumors.
- Long-term use of catheters.

HOW TO PREVENT
- Obtain prompt medical treatment for acute kidney infections, including 2 or more weeks of antibiotic treatment. Don't discontinue prescribed medication even if symptoms disappear after a few days of treatment.
- Obtain treatment for any abnormality of the urinary tract that causes infection.

WHAT TO EXPECT

DIAGNOSTIC MEASURES
- Medical history and physical exam by a doctor.
- Urinalysis and urine culture; cystoscopy, ultrasound, intravenous pyelogram (IVP) (see Glossary for all). Other special tests may be recommended.

APPROPRIATE HEALTH CARE
- Self-care after diagnosis.
- Doctor's treatment.
- Surgery to relieve obstruction in the urinary tract, if one exists.

POSSIBLE COMPLICATIONS
- Kidney-caused hypertension.
- Chronic kidney failure.

PROBABLE OUTCOME
- Symptoms can be controlled with treatment. If only one kidney is chronically infected and antibiotic treatment is unsuccessful, surgical removal of the affected kidney may prevent complications.
- If chronic kidney failure develops in both kidneys, a kidney transplant or kidney dialysis can be life-saving.

HOW TO TREAT

GENERAL MEASURES
- Follow your treatment plan carefully. This may not be easy for an illness that causes few symptoms in the early stages.
- See Resources for Additional Information.

MEDICATION—Your doctor may prescribe:
- Antibiotics for months or years.
- Drugs to keep the urine slightly acid.

ACTIVITY—No restrictions.

DIET—No special diet. Drink 2 quarts of liquid daily; include cranberry juice to acidify the urine.

CALL YOUR DOCTOR IF

- You have symptoms of chronic kidney infection.
- You have symptoms of an acute kidney infection, such as: urgent, frequent or burning urination; fever and chills; fatigue; cloudy urine.

KIDNEY, POLYCYSTIC

GENERAL INFORMATION

DEFINITION—An inherited kidney disorder in which cysts develop in the kidneys. The cysts enlarge the kidney and reduce its function. This is not cancerous. Most cases show no symptoms until adulthood. Then symptoms progress slowly for up to 20 years. It is the most common hereditary disease in the U.S.

BODY PARTS INVOLVED—Kidneys.

SEX OR AGE MOST AFFECTED—Both sexes; all ages.

SIGNS & SYMPTOMS
Early stages:
- Blood in the urine that may be visible only by microscopic examination.
- Repeated kidney infections.
- A mass in the abdomen.
- Hypertension.
- No symptoms (frequently) until the cysts replace so much normal kidney structure that kidney failure occurs.
Symptoms of kidney failure are:
- Pain in the lower back.
- Frequent urination.
- Increasing fatigue and weakness.
- Headache.
- Bad breath.
- Nausea, vomiting or diarrhea.
- Fluid retention, especially swelling around the ankles or eyes.
- Shortness of breath.
- Chest pain.
- Itching skin.
- Cessation of menstruation in women of childbearing age.

CAUSES—This disease is inherited; the cause is unknown.

RISK INCREASES WITH—Family history of polycystic disease.

HOW TO PREVENT—Cannot be prevented at present. If polycystic kidney disease runs in your family, consult your doctor for tests to discover if you have kidney cysts. Even if you feel well and don't have the disease, get regular checkups. If you have a family history of polycystic kidney, seek genetic counseling before starting a family.

WHAT TO EXPECT

DIAGNOSTIC MEASURES
- Your own observation of symptoms.
- Medical history and physical exam by a doctor.

- Diagnostic tests may include laboratory studies of blood, serum creatinine, renal concentration ability; CT scan and ultrasound (see Glossary for both).

APPROPRIATE HEALTH CARE
- Self-care after diagnosis.
- Doctor's treatment.
- Home dialysis or hospitalization for dialysis (rare).
- Surgery to perform a kidney transplant (rare).

POSSIBLE COMPLICATIONS
- Progression to kidney failure.
- Kidney stones.
- Infection or rupture of cysts.

PROBABLE OUTCOME—Polycystic kidney disease is currently considered incurable. Medical care may slow the progressive kidney damage by treating complications as they arise.
  Scientific research into causes and treatment continues. This offers hope for increasingly effective treatment and eventual cure.

HOW TO TREAT

GENERAL MEASURES
- Treatment is aimed at preventing complications and preserving renal function.
- Prompt treatment of any infection is important.
- See Resources for Additional Information.

MEDICATION
- Without complications, medicine usually is not necessary for this disorder. If necessary, your doctor may prescribe antibiotics for infection or antihypertensives to control high blood pressure.
- Most drugs are excreted by the kidney. If you have chronic kidney failure and take prescription drugs, the dose may need adjustment because of this disorder.

ACTIVITY—Take short, frequent rest periods during the day. Otherwise, stay as active as your strength allows.

DIET
- Eat a low-salt, low-protein diet (ask your doctor).
- Drink at least 8 glasses of fluid every day.
- Iron and multiple-vitamin supplements may be necessary to ensure good nutrition because of the dietary restrictions. Calcium and vitamin D supplements may be recommended to prevent softening of the bones (osteoporosis).

CALL YOUR DOCTOR IF

- You have symptoms of polycystic kidney.
- You have symptoms of kidney failure.
- You have fever or other signs of infection.
- Urination decreases.

LABYRINTHITIS

 GENERAL INFORMATION

DEFINITION—Inflammation of the semicircular canals in the inner ear.

BODY PARTS INVOLVED—Semicircular canals of the inner ear. The fluid-filled canals help maintain balance.

SEX OR AGE MOST AFFECTED—Adults.

SIGNS & SYMPTOMS
- Vertigo (sensation that you or your surroundings are spinning around).
- Extreme dizziness, especially with head movement, that begins gradually and peaks in 48 hours.
- Involuntary eye movement.
- Nausea and vomiting (sometimes).
- Loss of balance, especially falling toward the affected side.
- Temporary hearing loss (sometimes).
- Ringing in the ear (tinnitus).

CAUSES
- Virus infection (usually) in the inner ear.
- Bacterial infection in the inner ear (sometimes due to cholesteatoma, an infected collection of debris in the middle ear).
- Head injury.

RISK INCREASES WITH
- Spread of a chronic middle-ear infection.
- Ingestion of toxic drugs.
- Stress.
- Recent viral illness, especially respiratory infection.
- Allergy or family history of allergies.
- Smoking.
- Excess alcohol consumption.
- Use of some prescription or nonprescription drugs, especially aspirin.
- Cardiovascular or cerebrovascular disease.

HOW TO PREVENT
- Obtain prompt medical treatment for ear infections.
- Don't take medication that has produced dizziness without consulting your doctor.

 WHAT TO EXPECT

DIAGNOSTIC MEASURES
- Your own observation of symptoms.
- Medical history and physical exam by a doctor.
- Diagnostic tests may include hearing studies, culture of any purulent drainage, other studies as needed to determine any underlying disorder.

APPROPRIATE HEALTH CARE
- Self-care after diagnosis.
- Doctor's treatment.
- Surgical removal of cholesteatoma (an infected collection of debris in the middle ear) and drainage of infected areas may be necessary if conservative measures fail.

POSSIBLE COMPLICATIONS—Permanent hearing loss on the affected side (rare).

PROBABLE OUTCOME—Recovery—either spontaneous or with treatment—in 1 to 6 weeks.

 HOW TO TREAT

GENERAL MEASURES—This disorder can be frightening and debilitating but complete recovery is usual.

MEDICATION—Your doctor may prescribe:
- Antinausea medications may be prescribed (oral or suppositories).
- Tranquilizers to reduce dizziness (rarely).
- Diuretics to decrease fluid accumulation in the inner ear.
- Antibiotics if bacterial infection present.
- Antihistamines to relieve symptoms.

ACTIVITY—Keep the head as still as possible. Rest in bed until dizziness subsides. Then resume your normal activities gradually. Avoid hazardous activities, such as driving, climbing or working around dangerous machinery, until 1 week after symptoms disappear.

DIET—No special diet, but decreasing salt and fluid intake may help.

 CALL YOUR DOCTOR IF

- You have symptoms of labyrinthitis.
- The following occurs during treatment:
  Decreased hearing in either ear.
  Persistent vomiting.
  Convulsions.
  Fainting.
  Fever of 101F (38.3C) or higher.
- New, unexplained symptoms develop. Drugs used in treatment may produce side effects.

LACTOSE INTOLERANCE
(Milk Intolerance; Lactase Deficiency)

 GENERAL INFORMATION

DEFINITION—Difficulty digesting cow's milk. Lactose is the primary sugar in milk. Lactose intolerance occurs—with varying severity—in 75% of the black population, 90% of Orientals or American Indians, and less than 20% of Caucasians of northwest European origin. It is not contagious or cancerous.

BODY PARTS INVOLVED—Digestive system.

SEX OR AGE MOST AFFECTED—Both sexes; all ages.

SIGNS & SYMPTOMS
In children:
- Foamy diarrhea with diaper rash.
- Vomiting (sometimes).
- Slow weight gain, growth and development.
In adults:
- Rumbling abdominal sounds, abdominal cramps and diarrhea.
- Gas and bloating.
- Nausea.
- Mucous with or around stool.

CAUSES—Deficiency or absence of the enzyme lactase. Lactase is necessary to digest all milk except mother's milk. Without it, sugars in milk absorb fluid and cause diarrhea. Although some infants are born with the disorder, lactose intolerance usually develops in adulthood.
   Temporary lactose intolerance can occur in an infant after a severe bout of gastroenteritis that damages the intestinal lining.

RISK INCREASES WITH—Family history of enzyme-lactase deficiency.

HOW TO PREVENT—Cannot be prevented at present. If you are pregnant and there is a history of lactose intolerance in your family, consider breast-feeding your baby. If not, you may need an alternate nonmilk formula.

 WHAT TO EXPECT

DIAGNOSTIC MEASURES
- Your own observation of symptoms.
- Medical history and physical exam by a doctor.
- Laboratory studies, such as a stool exam and lactose-tolerance test.

APPROPRIATE HEALTH CARE
- Self-care after diagnosis.
- Doctor's treatment.

POSSIBLE COMPLICATIONS—Calcium deficiency (rare).

PROBABLE OUTCOME—This condition is currently considered incurable. However, symptoms can be relieved or controlled with a diet free of milk and milk products. Symptoms worsen at times for unexplained reasons.

 HOW TO TREAT

GENERAL MEASURES—Symptoms can be controlled by diet restrictions or use of lactase products.

MEDICATION
- A supplement to digest milk. The enzyme lactase is available without a prescription to be added to milk and milk products and products are available that have the enzyme added already.
- Calcium supplements may be recommended.

ACTIVITY—No restrictions.

DIET
- If the condition is present at birth, an infant formula that contains little or no lactose, such as a soybean-based formula, will be recommended.
- If the lactose intolerance is temporary and caused by gastroenteritis, the substitute formula should be necessary for a short time only. Cow's milk can be introduced again later.
- Older persons with lactose intolerance should reduce or restrict milk and milk products, such as cheese and ice cream. Some patients tolerate whole milk or chocolate milk better than skim.
- Yogurt and fermented products such as hard cheese are better tolerated than milk.
- Read labels on food products. Milk-sugar is used in many and may cause symptoms.

 CALL YOUR DOCTOR IF

- You or your child have symptoms of lactose intolerance.
- Temperature rises to 101F (38.3C) or higher.
- Your infant fails to gain weight.
- Your infant refuses food or formula.
- Vomiting or diarrhea reappears in a child who has previously had a temporary intolerance to milk or milk products.
- A milk-free diet doesn't relieve symptoms.

LARGE-INTESTINE CANCER
(Colon Cancer; Colorectal Cancer)

GENERAL INFORMATION

DEFINITION—Uncontrolled growth of malignant cells in the rectum or colon (large intestine). It is the second most common cancer site (following lung) in the U.S.

BODY PARTS INVOLVED—Large intestine, including the cecum, ascending colon, transverse colon, descending colon and sigmoid colon; rectum (50% of all colorectal cancers occur here).

SEX OR AGE MOST AFFECTED—Adults over 40.

SIGNS & SYMPTOMS
- No symptoms in the early stages (frequently).
- Bloody or black, tarry stools.
- Cramping abdominal pain.
- Feeling of fullness.
- Change in bowel habits, such as diarrhea, constipation or narrow caliber stools.
- Unexplained weight loss.
- Pain in the rectum.
- Anemia.
- Loss of bowel control (sometimes).

CAUSES—Unknown. Both genetic and environmental factors may contribute.

RISK INCREASES WITH
- Adults over 60.
- Ulcerative colitis and some other chronic disorders of the gastrointestinal tract.
- Improper diet that is low in fiber and high in fat.
- Previous rectal polyps.
- Family history of rectal polyps or colorectal cancer.

HOW TO PREVENT
- Eat a diet that is high in fiber and low in fat.
- If you fall into a high-risk group, have annual physical examinations and request rectal and colon exams.
- If you have any of the risk factors listed above, buy from your pharmacy a detection kit for blood in the stool. Check for bleeding every 2 months. Simple-to-use home test kits are available.

WHAT TO EXPECT

DIAGNOSTIC MEASURES
- Your own observation of symptoms.
- Medical history and physical exam by a doctor.
- Laboratory blood studies.
- Sigmoidoscopy; colonoscopy (see Glossary for both).
- X-rays of the colon (barium enema) and kidney (intravenous pyelogram).
- CT scan, and ultrasound (see Glossary for both).

APPROPRIATE HEALTH CARE
- Doctor's treatment.
- Surgery to remove the tumor. It is sometimes necessary to divert the bowel through a surgical opening in the abdomen (see Colostomy in Surgery section). If you have a colostomy, you will require special instructions for care of the opening.
- Radiation treatment before and after surgery.

POSSIBLE COMPLICATIONS
- Spread to other body parts and death.
- Complications of surgery (infection, pneumonia, abscess).

PROBABLE OUTCOME—Overall outlook is variable depending on the stage the disease has reached when it is discovered. More than 50% of patients survive 5 years after surgery. The earlier the tumor is detected, the greater the chances for full recovery following treatment.

HOW TO TREAT

GENERAL MEASURES
- The more you can learn and understand about this disorder, the more you will be able to make informed decisions about where to go for your care, the treatments available, the risks involved, side effects of therapy and expected outcome.
- See Resources for Additional Information.

MEDICATION—Your doctor may prescribe:
- Pain relievers.
- Medicine to regulate bowel movements.
- Anticancer drugs, although they are usually not very effective.

ACTIVITY
- Avoid sports or activities that might injure the stoma (surgical bowel opening).
- Resume your normal activities, including sexual relations, as soon as possible after surgery. A colostomy should not prevent intercourse.

DIET—Eat a low-fat, high-fiber diet (see both in Appendix). Avoiding gas-producing foods may help symptoms (cabbage, beans, onions).

CALL YOUR DOCTOR IF

- You have symptoms of cancer of the large intestine, especially rectal bleeding or a significant change in bowel habits that lasts longer than 7 days.
- You develop anemia (fatigue, paleness and rapid heartbeat).

LARGE-INTESTINE POLYP

GENERAL INFORMATION

DEFINITION—A growth shaped like a grape on a stalk or lying flat against the inner lining of the large intestine. Polyps occur singly or in groups.

BODY PARTS INVOLVED—Large intestine, most often in the rectum and sigmoid colon.

SEX OR AGE MOST AFFECTED—Adults of both sexes.

SIGNS & SYMPTOMS
- No symptoms (usually).
- Rectal bleeding (sometimes).
- Mucus discharge from the rectum (sometimes).
- Cramps or abdominal pain.

CAUSES—Unknown.

RISK INCREASES WITH—Family history of intestinal polyps.

HOW TO PREVENT—If you have had polyps in the past, you should have regular sigmoidoscopic (see Glossary) examinations—at least once a year or more, depending on your doctor's recommendation.

WHAT TO EXPECT

DIAGNOSTIC MEASURES
- Your own observation of symptoms.
- Medical history and physical exam by a doctor.
- Laboratory studies of blood and stool.
- Sigmoidoscopy; colonoscopy (see Glossary).

APPROPRIATE HEALTH CARE
- Doctor's treatment.
- Surgery to remove a polyp is usually done with insertion of a proctoscope or sigmoidoscope in the anus. Polyps are snipped off or destroyed by electric cauterization. If a pathologist's report indicates the polyp is malignant, total excision of the polyp and surrounding tissue is necessary.
- For multiple polyps, a portion of the colon may be removed through an abdominal incision (see Laparotomy in Surgery section).

POSSIBLE COMPLICATIONS—Malignant change in about 1% of polyps.

PROBABLE OUTCOME—Usually curable with surgery, although polyps may recur.

HOW TO TREAT

GENERAL MEASURES—Follow your doctor's instructions for self-care after any surgical procedure.

MEDICATION—Medicine usually is not necessary for this disorder.

ACTIVITY—No restrictions.

DIET—Eat a diet that is high in fiber and low in fat (see both in Appendix).

CALL YOUR DOCTOR IF

- You have bleeding or mucus discharge from the rectum.
- Other members of your family have polyps or colorectal cancer. You should have periodic examinations.
- The following occurs after surgery:
  Increased rectal bleeding.
  Fever, chills or aches. This may indicate an infection at the surgical site.

ILLNESS & DISORDERS

LARVA MIGRANS, CUTANEOUS
(Creeping Eruptions)

GENERAL INFORMATION

DEFINITION—Skin infestation of hookworm or roundworm larvae. These parasites usually infect dogs and cats.

BODY PARTS INVOLVED—Skin areas that come in contact with the ground, usually feet, legs or buttocks.

SEX OR AGE MOST AFFECTED—Both sexes; all ages.

SIGNS & SYMPTOMS—Skin rash or small blister, progressing to thin, raised lines on the skin leading from the parasite's entry point. The random lines create tunnel-like lesions that lengthen up to 1cm a day. Most persons have several tracks simultaneously, each of different length and pattern.

CAUSES—Infestation by larvae of hookworms and roundworms found in the intestinal tracts of dogs and cats.

RISK INCREASES WITH
• Play in warm, moist sand in which cats or dogs have defecated.
• Work that requires crawling in confined spaces and contact with infected soil, as when plumbers work under houses.

HOW TO PREVENT
• Handle cat litter carefully. Avoid touching soil.
• Don't work or play in soil used by cats and dogs for elimination.
• Have pets treated for worms.

WHAT TO EXPECT

DIAGNOSTIC MEASURES
• Your own observation of symptoms.
• Medical history and physical exam by a doctor.

APPROPRIATE HEALTH CARE
• Home care after diagnosis.
• Doctor's treatment.

POSSIBLE COMPLICATIONS—Secondary bacterial infection of affected skin.

PROBABLE OUTCOME—Usually curable in 1 to 2 weeks with treatment.

HOW TO TREAT

GENERAL MEASURES—No measures other than medication treatment.

MEDICATION—Your doctor may prescribe:
• Topical thiabendazole for local application in a 2% solution with dimethyl sulfoxide (DMSO). Follow instructions carefully. Apply it to the end of the track (farthest from the point of entry).
• Oral thiabendazole for serious infestations by many larvae. This form causes adverse reactions and side effects.

ACTIVITY—No restrictions.

DIET—No special diet.

CALL YOUR DOCTOR IF

• You have symptoms of larva migrans.
• Skin lesions develop pus, indicating secondary infection.
• You take oral thiabendazole and new, unexplained symptoms develop.

LARYNGITIS

GENERAL INFORMATION

DEFINITION—A minor inflammation of the larynx (voice box) and surrounding tissues, causing temporary hoarseness. It is more common during epidemics of seasonal virus infections (late fall, winter, early spring).

BODY PARTS INVOLVED—Larynx (voice box); the upper part of the neck, behind the Adam's apple.

SEX OR AGE MOST AFFECTED—Both sexes; all ages.

SIGNS & SYMPTOMS
- Hoarseness or loss of voice.
- Sore throat; tickling in the back of the throat.
- Sensation of a lump in the throat.
- Slight fever (sometimes).
- Swallowing difficulty (rare).
- Tiredness.

CAUSES—Inflammation of the vocal cords and surrounding area caused by:
- Viruses (common).
- Bacteria (rare).
- Allergies.
- Excessive use of the voice.
- Electrolyte-balance disturbances, especially low potassium, that cause muscle weakness (sometimes).
- Tumors (rare).

RISK INCREASES WITH
- Exposure to irritants distributed by air-conditioning systems, such as mold, pollen and pollutants.
- Extremely cold weather.
- Smoking.
- Excess alcohol consumption.
- Recent respiratory illness, such as bronchitis or pneumonia.

HOW TO PREVENT
- Avoid yelling or straining your voice.
- Treat respiratory infections carefully.

WHAT TO EXPECT

DIAGNOSTIC MEASURES
- Your own observation of symptoms.
- Medical history and physical exam by a doctor. Treatment by an ear, nose and throat specialist might be helpful for persistent cases.

APPROPRIATE HEALTH CARE
- Self-care after diagnosis.
- Doctor's treatment.

POSSIBLE COMPLICATIONS—Chronic hoarseness.

PROBABLE OUTCOME—Spontaneous recovery for viral laryngitis in 10 to 14 days. Bacterial infections are usually curable in 7 to 10 days with antibiotic treatment.

HOW TO TREAT

GENERAL MEASURES
- Don't use your voice (even whispering may strain vocal cords). For most cases, resting the voice for a few days is all that is needed.
- Use a cool-mist, ultrasonic humidifier to increase air moisture and ease the constricted feeling in the throat. Clean humidifier daily.
- Hot, steamy showers also help.
- Avoid smoking and secondary cigarette smoke.
- Don't gargle or use mouthwashes (many contain alcohol, which is irritating).

MEDICATION—For minor discomfort, you may use nonprescription drugs, such as acetaminophen, aspirin or cough syrup.

ACTIVITY—Avoid extreme exertion or high intensity sports.

DIET—No special diet.

CALL YOUR DOCTOR IF

- You have hoarseness or other symptoms of laryngitis that last longer than 2 weeks. Though rare, it could be an early sign of cancer.
- You feel very ill, have a high fever or breathing difficulty. If these symptoms develop in a child, call your doctor immediately.

LARYNX CANCER
(Laryngeal Cancer)

GENERAL INFORMATION

DEFINITION—Uncontrolled growth of malignant cells in the vocal cords and surrounding tissues.

BODY PARTS INVOLVED—Larynx (back of the throat and "voice box").

SEX OR AGE MOST AFFECTED—Both sexes of adults over age 40, but more common in men.

SIGNS & SYMPTOMS
- Hoarseness that does not disappear after resting the voice.
- "Lump-in-the-throat" feeling.
- Painful or difficult swallowing.
- Hard, swollen lymph glands in the neck.
- Weight loss.
- Tenderness in the neck.
- Chronic cough.

CAUSES—Smoking or alcohol abuse.

RISK INCREASES WITH
- Heavy smoking.
- Excess alcohol consumption.
- Vocal-cord polyps.
- Chronic vocal-cord inflammation from any cause.

HOW TO PREVENT
- Stop smoking.
- Don't drink more than 1 or 2 alcoholic drinks—if any—a day.
- Don't abuse your voice.

WHAT TO EXPECT

DIAGNOSTIC MEASURES
- Your own observation of symptoms. Be alert to hoarseness that persists beyond 2 weeks.
- Medical history and physical exam by a doctor.
- Biopsy (see Laryngeal Biopsy in Surgery section) of the vocal cords or other affected tissue.
- CT scan or MRI (see Glossary for both), bone scan, x-ray of chest to determine if cancer has spread.

APPROPRIATE HEALTH CARE
- Doctor's treatment (usually ear, nose and throat specialist).
- If diagnosed early, radiation therapy or laser cordectomy (excision of vocal cord) may be done on an outpatient basis.
- Advanced disease requires surgery to remove cancer and involved tissue (see Laryngectomy in Surgery section) and postoperative radiation therapy.
- Speech therapy to learn to speak without vocal cords, if surgery is necessary.

POSSIBLE COMPLICATIONS
- Frequent complications arise from treatments (radiation and surgical procedures) that affect the voice, swallowing and digestion.
- Life-threatening spread to other body parts.

PROBABLE OUTCOME—Often curable with early diagnosis and treatment. In the late stages, this condition is currently considered incurable. However, symptoms can be relieved or controlled.

Scientific research into causes and treatment continues, so there is hope for increasingly effective treatment and cure.

HOW TO TREAT

GENERAL MEASURES
- Early diagnosis and treatment—as with other cancers—are the best hope for complete cure.
- If your vocal cords are removed, join a support group for persons like you who have faced the same situation. This helps minimize stress and adjustment.
- See Resources for Additional Information.

MEDICATION—Medicine usually is not necessary for this disorder. Anticancer drugs are not often prescribed; radiation therapy is used instead.

ACTIVITY—Resume your normal activities gradually after treatment or surgery.

DIET—No special diet, unless surgery is performed. In that case, a liquid diet (see Appendix) is necessary until the affected area heals.

CALL YOUR DOCTOR IF

You have symptoms of larynx cancer.

LEAD POISONING

GENERAL INFORMATION

DEFINITION—A high body level of lead, an element with no known biological value. Lead is found everywhere (in the air, such as from exhaust fumes, on the ground, in the home and in objects). A little bit of lead finds its way into everyone and usually causes no problems. Too much lead in the body can cause serious consequences. It affects almost every body organ, especially the kidneys and the central nervous system.

BODY PARTS INVOLVED—Gastrointestinal; nervous.

SEX OR AGE MOST AFFECTED—Both sexes; all ages, most common in young children.

SIGNS & SYMPTOMS
- Often no symptoms are apparent or they may be delayed.

Mild to moderate levels of lead:
- Paleness, fatigue, lethargy.
- Behavioral changes (e.g., irritability).
- Abdominal discomfort.
- Difficulty concentrating; headache; tremor.
- Vomiting; weight loss; sleep disorders.

Severe lead poisoning:
- Metallic taste; constipation; severe abdominal cramps; rigidity of the abdominal wall.
- Muscular weakness or paralysis.
- Cerebral type or lead encephalopathy (more common in children)—seizures, coma, long-term sequelae including neurologic defects, retarded mental development, chronic hyperactivity.

CAUSES—Inhalation of lead dust or fumes, or ingestion of lead. The body excretes lead very slowly, so it accumulates in the body tissues, particularly the bones.

RISK INCREASES WITH
- Children are at increased risk because of incomplete development of the blood-brain barrier before age 3 years allowing more lead into the central nervous system.
- Common childhood behaviors such as frequent hand-to-mouth activity and pica (see Pica in Illness section) greatly increase the risk of ingesting lead.
- Residence or frequent visitor in deteriorating, pre-1980 housing with leaded-paint surfaces. Children may lick or eat the old paint.
- Lead dissolved in water from lead or lead-soldered plumbing.
- Lead glazed ceramics, especially with acidic food or drink; crayons made outside U.S.
- Food stored in inverted plastic bread bags printed with colored ink.
- Soil/dust near lead industries.
- Hobbies such as glazed pottery making, lead soldering, painting, preparing lead shot, stained-glass making, car or boat repair, etc.

- Occupational exposure—plumbers, pipe fitters, lead miners, auto repairers.

HOW TO PREVENT
- Screening of blood-lead levels in all children at 9-12 months and again at age 2.
- If ceramic tableware is purchased outside the U.S., have it tested for lead release at a commercial laboratory when you return, or use it for decorative purposes only.
- Routine blood-lead testing for workers who are exposed to lead.

WHAT TO EXPECT

DIAGNOSTIC MEASURES
- Medical history and exam by a doctor.
- Diagnostic tests may include blood and urine studies to measure lead levels, and x-rays of the bones and abdomen to reveal lead deposits.

APPROPRIATE HEALTH CARE—Treatment involves the avoidance of further exposure to the lead, and for some patients, medical therapy that will help the body excrete the lead.

POSSIBLE COMPLICATIONS
- Long-term lead exposure may cause chronic renal failure, gout, lead line (blue-black) on gingival tissue.
- High blood pressure; miscarriages (possibly).
- If brain damage occurs, permanent problems (mental retardation, seizure disorder, blindness, muscle weakness) may occur.
- Coma, death.

PROBABLE OUTCOME—Symptomatic lead poisoning without any apparent brain damage generally improves with treatment, but subtle central nervous system toxicity may be long lasting or permanent.

HOW TO TREAT

GENERAL MEASURES
- If the source is in the home, the patient must reside elsewhere until the source is eliminated.
- See Resources for Additional Information.

MEDICATION—Chelating agents to help the body excrete the lead at a faster rate may be prescribed.

ACTIVITY—No restrictions.

DIET—Consume adequate calcium and iron. Eat a low fat diet to reduce absorption of lead.

CALL YOUR DOCTOR IF

- You have symptoms of lead poisoning.
- Symptoms worsen or don't improve after treatment.

LEGG-CALVÉ PERTHES DISEASE
(Slipped Femoral Epiphysis; Coxa Plana)

 GENERAL INFORMATION

DEFINITION—Gradual weakening of the head of the thigh bone where it meets the pelvis.

BODY PARTS INVOLVED—Either leg at the hip joint (occasionally both).

SEX OR AGE MOST AFFECTED—Older children (4 to 12 years) of both sexes, but more common in boys.

SIGNS & SYMPTOMS
* Pain and stiffness in the hip and thigh. Sometimes both sides are involved.
* Pain in the leg—often the knee—even though the disorder is in the hip.
* Limping.
* Difference in leg length.
* Symptoms usually have a gradual onset.

CAUSES—Unknown. Injury is usually not a factor.

RISK INCREASES WITH
* Use of cortisone drugs for other disorders.
* Overweight.
* Periods of rapid growth.
* Increased incidence in children with low birth weight and delayed development.

HOW TO PREVENT—No specific preventive measures.

 WHAT TO EXPECT

DIAGNOSTIC MEASURES
* Your own observation of symptoms, especially a limp or knee pain in your child.
* Medical history and physical exam by a doctor.
* X-ray of the hip, MRI and bone scan (see Glossary for all).

APPROPRIATE HEALTH CARE
* Doctor's treatment, including consultation with an orthopedist.
* Surgery to reinforce the bone's attachment to the joint and prevent further deformity (sometimes).
* Hospitalization (sometimes) for traction (a steady pull on the leg).

POSSIBLE COMPLICATIONS
* Bone infection.
* Permanent damage to the thigh bone and hip joint.
* Misdiagnosis for hypothyroidism or sickle cell anemia.

PROBABLE OUTCOME—Often curable in 3 to 4 years with early treatment. Delayed treatment may cause permanent bone injury and require surgery to replace the hip.

 HOW TO TREAT

GENERAL MEASURES
* Youngsters often have difficulty accepting the need for bed rest, casts, braces or other treatment. Enlist the help of your doctor, a counselor, school nurse or other significant persons, if necessary, to discuss the situation with your child.
* Help your child find activities and interests that don't involve athletics.
* Use heat to relieve pain. Warm compresses, heating pads, whirlpool baths, heat lamps, diathermy and ultrasound are effective.

MEDICATION—For minor discomfort, you may use nonprescription drugs, such as aspirin, acetaminophen or ibuprofen.

ACTIVITY—Bed rest may be necessary for 6 months to 1 year until the condition improves or until after surgery. When the bones can bear weight, crutches, braces or casts are usually necessary. After that, activities may be resumed gradually.

DIET—No special diet, unless the child is overweight.

 CALL YOUR DOCTOR IF

* Your child has hip pain, knee pain, stiffness or a limp.
* The following occurs during treatment:
Symptoms don't improve in 4 weeks, despite treatment.
Pain increases.
Temperature rises to 101F (38.3C).

LEGIONNAIRE'S DISEASE
(Legionella Pneumophilia Bronchopneumonia)

 GENERAL INFORMATION

DEFINITION—A form of lung infection (bronchopneumonia) named after an epidemic that affected 182 people attending an American Legion convention in 1976.

BODY PARTS INVOLVED—Bronchial tubes; lungs.

SEX OR AGE MOST AFFECTED—Both sexes, but more common in men over age 40.

SIGNS & SYMPTOMS
- General ill feeling.
- Headache.
- Chills and fever up to 105F (40.6C).
- Muscle aches.
- Cough without sputum that progresses to one with gray or blood-streaked sputum.
- Nausea, vomiting, diarrhea.
- Disorientation.

CAUSES—Infection from bacteria (Legionella pneumophilia) that is not contagious between persons. The germ is transmitted through the air, and the incubation period after exposure is 2 to 10 days.

In the 1976 epidemic, the germ was transmitted through the cooling and evaporating elements of a large, central air-conditioning system. The bacteria are also found in excavation sites and newly plowed soil.

RISK INCREASES WITH
- Chronic, debilitating illness including diabetes mellitus, chronic kidney failure or emphysema.
- Smoking. This increases the risk 3 to 4 times.
- Excess alcohol consumption.
- Use of immunosuppressive drugs, including cortisone and anticancer drugs.

HOW TO PREVENT
- Have cooling and heating systems cleaned and inspected regularly. Change filters often.
- Don't smoke.
- Don't drink more than 1 or 2 alcoholic drinks—if any—a day.

 WHAT TO EXPECT

DIAGNOSTIC MEASURES
- Your own observation of symptoms.
- Medical history and physical exam by a doctor.
- Laboratory blood studies and culture of sputum, bronchoscopy (see Surgery section).

APPROPRIATE HEALTH CARE
- Doctor's treatment.
- Hospitalization for intensive care and oxygen (severe cases).
- Self-care for mild cases or during convalescence after hospitalization.

POSSIBLE COMPLICATIONS
- Shock or delirium.
- Congestive heart failure.
- Kidney failure.
- Heart-rhythm disturbances.

PROBABLE OUTCOME—Usually curable with prompt diagnosis and treatment. If untreated, 15% of cases are fatal.

 HOW TO TREAT

GENERAL MEASURES—The following apply to mild cases or to care after hospitalization:
- Use a cool-mist ultrasonic humidifier to increase air moisture and thin lung secretions so they can be coughed up more easily. Clean humidifier daily.
- Use warm compresses or a heating pad on the chest to relieve chest pain.
- Practice deep-breathing exercises as often as your strength allows.
- Avoid loud talking, laughing or singing. They may trigger excessive coughing.
- Keep warm. If you become chilled, the infection can become more severe.

MEDICATION
- Your doctor may prescribe antibiotics. Be sure to finish all prescribed medication.
- If the cough is painful and doesn't produce sputum, you may use nonprescription medicine to suppress it. If the cough produces sputum, don't suppress it.
- You may take aspirin or acetaminophen to reduce fever.

ACTIVITY—Rest in bed until completely well. Allow 2 to 4 weeks for recovery.

DIET—No special diet. Maintain adequate fluid by drinking 6-8 glasses daily.

 CALL YOUR DOCTOR IF

- You have symptoms of Legionnaire's disease.
- The following occurs during or after treatment:
  Temperature spike to 102F (38.9C).
  Severe chest pain, despite treatment.
  Increased shortness of breath.
  Dark or bluish nails, lips or skin.
  Blood in the sputum.
- New, unexplained symptoms develop. Drugs used in treatment may produce side effects.

LEUKEMIA, ACUTE

GENERAL INFORMATION

DEFINITION—A cancer of the white blood cells in bone marrow or tissues that are part of the lymphatic system (lymph glands, spleen, liver). These excess cells accumulate and spill into the bloodstream, eventually involving other tissues.

Common forms of leukemia include: acute lymphocytic leukemia (ALL), especially prevalent in children; acute myelogenous leukemia (AML); and acute nonlymphocytic leukemia (ANLL). Acute leukemia is the most common form of cancer in children.

BODY PARTS INVOLVED—Bone marrow and lymph tissue in early stages. The disease eventually affects all body tissues.

SEX OR AGE MOST AFFECTED
- Both sexes, but more common in males.
- All ages. Acute lymphocytic leukemia has a peak incidence between ages 2 and 5.

SIGNS & SYMPTOMS
- Low fever; tiredness; anemia.
- Increasing paleness; general ill feeling.
- Easy bruising and spontaneous bleeding (nosebleeds, bleeding from the gums or prolonged menstruation).
- Enlarged spleen and abdominal pain.
- Susceptibility to infection, especially pneumonia.
- Mouth infections with ulcers and sores.
- Headache and lethargy, if meninges (brain membranes) are affected.

CAUSES—Precise cause unknown, but there are many suspected, predisposing factors.

RISK INCREASES WITH
- Family history of leukemia.
- Excess exposure to x-rays.
- Congenital disorders, especially Down syndrome.
- Identical twins.
- Exposure to benzenes and other toxic industrial chemicals; use of cytotoxic drugs.
- Immunosuppression due to illness or medications.
- Smoking.

HOW TO PREVENT—Cannot be prevented. If you have a family history of leukemia, seek genetic counseling before starting a family.

WHAT TO EXPECT

DIAGNOSTIC MEASURES
- Medical history and exam by a doctor.
- Laboratory studies of blood, bone marrow and cerebrospinal fluid
- Chest x-ray, CT scan, ultrasound (see Glossary for both) and spinal tap.

APPROPRIATE HEALTH CARE
- Treatment steps include transfusions of blood and platelets, anticancer drugs to kill the leukemic cells, followed by radiation therapy.
- Bone marrow transplant may be considered in patients if leukemia relapses after the first remission.

POSSIBLE COMPLICATIONS
- Hemorrhage.
- Death from destruction of the body's defenses against infection.

PROBABLE OUTCOME—Treatment brings remission in 90% of patients and cure in 30% for some forms of leukemia—especially in children.

HOW TO TREAT

GENERAL MEASURES
- Remission occurs when there is no evidence of leukemic cells in the blood or bone marrow.
- Patient should avoid ill persons and crowds to prevent dangerous exposure to infection.
- Mouth care is important. Rinse the mouth often with a warm salt-water solution to decrease mouth ulcers. Use 1 tablespoon salt in 8 oz. water. Use a soft toothbrush to prevent gum abrasion.
- See Resources for Additional Information.

MEDICATION—Your doctor may prescribe:
- Blood transfusions.
- Anticancer drugs; cortisone drugs.
- Pain relievers. Don't take aspirin or any product containing aspirin. Aspirin increases the likelihood of bleeding.
- Antibiotics to fight infection.
- Uricosuric drugs to increase excretion of uric acid that may accumulate as a side effect of anticancer drugs.

ACTIVITY—No restrictions during remissions. Bed rest is usually necessary during active phases.

DIET—Drink extra fluids. Adults should drink 8 to 10 glasses of fluid daily and children should drink 4 to 6 glasses of fluid. During chemotherapy, eat and drink high-calorie foods and beverages, such as milkshakes or eggnog.

CALL YOUR DOCTOR IF

- You or your child have symptoms of leukemia.
- The following occurs during active stages or remissions:
  Fever, chills, cough or sore throat.
  Abnormal bleeding. Apply pressure and ice while awaiting your doctor's return call.
  Constipation.

LEUKEMIA, CHRONIC LYMPHOCYTIC

 GENERAL INFORMATION

DEFINITION—A very slow-growing cancer of the blood-forming organs of older persons. About 1/3 of leukemia victims have this form. It is often discovered in a routine blood test for unrelated purposes.

BODY PARTS INVOLVED—Blood-forming organs: bone marrow; lymph glands; liver; spleen.

SEX OR AGE MOST AFFECTED—Both sexes, but more common in men over 50.

SIGNS & SYMPTOMS
In early stages, the following appear gradually:
- Fatigue and general weakness.
- Mild to moderate anemia.
- Firm, enlarged lymph nodes.
- Unexplained weight loss.
- Enlarged liver and spleen.
- Susceptibility to infection.
- Skin nodules (sometimes).

In late stages:
- Inability to resist bacterial, viral or fungal infections.
- Incapacitating weakness.

CAUSES—Unknown. Diagnostic tests show a proliferation of lymphocytes (a type of white blood cell). Unlike some forms of leukemia, excess exposure to radiation does not seem to be a factor in chronic lymphocytic leukemia.

RISK INCREASES WITH—Adults over 60.

HOW TO PREVENT—No specific preventive measures.

 WHAT TO EXPECT

DIAGNOSTIC MEASURES
- Your own observation of symptoms.
- Medical history and physical exam by a doctor.
- Laboratory studies of blood, bone marrow and cerebrospinal fluid; chest x-ray, CT scan, ultrasound (see Glossary for both) and spinal tap.
- The severity of the disease can be determined by the enlargement of the liver and spleen, anemia and the lack of platelet cells in the blood.

APPROPRIATE HEALTH CARE
- Self-care after diagnosis.
- Doctor's treatment.
- Sometimes, if it is a mild case, no treatment is needed.
- Treatment may include giving the patient anticancer drugs, followed by radiation therapy, and sometimes transfusions of blood and platelets.

POSSIBLE COMPLICATIONS
- Bleeding.
- Severe anemia.
- Infections.
- Gout.

PROBABLE OUTCOME—This condition is currently considered incurable. However, symptoms can be relieved or controlled. Many patients live for years with few or no symptoms, and medical literature cites a few instances of unexplained recovery.

Scientific research into causes and treatment continues, so there is hope for increasingly effective treatment and cure.

 HOW TO TREAT

GENERAL MEASURES
- Patient should avoid ill persons and crowds to prevent dangerous exposure to infection.
- Mouth care is important. Rinse the mouth often with a warm salt-water solution to decrease mouth ulcers. Use 1 tablespoon salt in 8 oz. water. Use a soft toothbrush to prevent gum abrasion.
- See Resources for Additional Information.

MEDICATION—Many persons with this disorder require little treatment. Treatment plans are highly individualized.
- Your doctor may prescribe:
  Anticancer medications, including cortisone drugs.
  Antigout drugs.
- Don't take aspirin or any product containing aspirin. Aspirin increases the likelihood of bleeding.

ACTIVITY—No restrictions.

DIET—No special diet. Eat as heartily as possible.

 CALL YOUR DOCTOR IF

- You have symptoms of chronic lymphocytic leukemia.
- The following occurs after diagnosis and treatment:
  Recurrence or worsening of symptoms.
  Signs of infection, such as fever and chills.
  Black, tarry stools, bleeding gums or nosebleed.

LEUKOPLAKIA

 GENERAL INFORMATION

DEFINITION—A thickened area in the delicate lining of the mouth or tongue. This is not contagious, but it may be premalignant.

BODY PARTS INVOLVED—Inside of cheek; floor of mouth; tongue; palate; roof of mouth.

SEX OR AGE MOST AFFECTED—All ages, but most common in adults over 60.

SIGNS & SYMPTOMS
- Sensitivity to hot and spicy food.
- A small white patch in the mouth. The patch feels firm, rough and stiff.
- No symptoms in the early stages.

CAUSES—Some are unknown; others include:
- Deficiency of vitamins A or B.
- Deficiency of male or female hormones.
- Syphilis.
- Chronic irritation in the mouth. The irritation may be from jagged teeth, ill-fitting dentures, hot or spicy food, excess alcohol consumption or nicotine.

RISK INCREASES WITH
- Use of tobacco products, including cigarettes, chewing tobacco, snuff, pipe or cigars.
- Dentures.
- Repeated or chronic trauma to oral regions (biting inside of cheek or lip).
- Alcohol consumption.

HOW TO PREVENT
- Don't smoke or use tobacco products.
- Inspect the mouth regularly if you wear dentures or smoke.
- Decrease consumption of hot or highly seasoned foods if suspicious lesions develop.
- Avoid alcohol.

 WHAT TO EXPECT

DIAGNOSTIC MEASURES
- Your own observation of symptoms.
- Medical history and physical exam by a doctor or dentist.
- Biopsy (see Glossary).

APPROPRIATE HEALTH CARE
- Doctor's treatment.
- Surgery to remove the lesions.
- Patches may be surgically removed (cryosurgery) using a local anesthetic.

POSSIBLE COMPLICATIONS
- The lesion may become cancerous if untreated (about 5% of patients).
- New lesions may develop after treatment.

PROBABLE OUTCOME—Sometimes curable with removal of the source of irritation (such as tobacco) or with surgery.

 HOW TO TREAT

GENERAL MEASURES
- Any recognizable irritation should be corrected or removed. Eliminate tobacco and alcohol (including alcoholic mouthwashes). Lesions may clear up after these factors are removed.
- Following surgery or biopsy:
  If bleeding occurs, press cotton gauze gently for 5 minutes against the operation site.
  24 hours after the operation, rinse the mouth with a warm salt-water solution. Use 1/2 teaspoon salt in 8 oz. warm water. Repeat every 1 or 2 hours.
  Brush and floss teeth often and use antiseptic mouthwash during the healing process. A clean mouth heals faster.

MEDICATION
- For minor pain, you may use nonprescription drugs such as acetaminophen.
- Your doctor may prescribe topical or oral forms of vitamin A (sometimes).

ACTIVITY—No restrictions.

DIET—Liquid or soft diet for 24 hours; then no special diet.

 CALL YOUR DOCTOR IF

- You have symptoms of leukoplakia.
- The following occurs after surgery:
  Bleeding after 12 hours or more.
  Severe pain.

LICE
(Pediculosis; Head Lice; Body Lice; "Crabs")

 GENERAL INFORMATION

DEFINITION—Skin inflammation caused by tiny parasites (lice) that live on the body or in clothing.

BODY PARTS INVOLVED—Hairy areas anywhere, especially the scalp, eyebrows or genital area; skin, especially areas in which clothing is in close contact with skin, such as the shoulders, waist, genital area or buttocks.

SEX OR AGE MOST AFFECTED—Both sexes; all ages.

SIGNS & SYMPTOMS
- Itching and scratching, sometimes intense and usually in hair-covered areas.
- Eggs ("nits") on hair shafts.
- Scalp inflammation and matted hair.
- Enlarged lymph glands at the back of the scalp or in the groin (sometimes).
- Red bite marks and hives.

CAUSES—Tiny (3mm to 4mm) parasites that bite through skin to obtain nourishment (blood). The bites cause itching and inflammation. Some lice live on skin, although they are difficult to see. Others live in clothing near skin. Eggs (nits) adhere to hairs.

RISK INCREASES WITH
- Crowded living conditions.
- Family history of lice.
- Sexual intercourse with an infected person.
- Contact with infected object such as combs, hats, clothing, or with infected person.

HOW TO PREVENT
- Bathe and shampoo often.
- Avoid wearing the same clothing more than a day or two; change bed linens often.
- Don't share combs, brushes or hats with others.

 WHAT TO EXPECT

DIAGNOSTIC MEASURES
- Your own observation of symptoms. You may see nits (like tiny footballs) on the side of hairs.
- Medical history and exam by a doctor.

APPROPRIATE HEALTH CARE
- Self-care after diagnosis.
- Doctor's treatment.

POSSIBLE COMPLICATIONS—Infection at the site of deep scratching.

PROBABLE OUTCOME—Usually curable with medicated creams, lotions and shampoos. Allow 5 days after treatment for symptoms to disappear. Lice often recur.

 HOW TO TREAT

GENERAL MEASURES—The following measures apply to all members of the household and to any sexual partners:
- Use the prescribed medicated shampoo, cream or lotion.
- Machine-wash all clothing and linen in hot water. Dry in the dryer's hot-air cycle. Iron the clothing and linen, if possible. Washing removes the lice, and ironing destroys nits.
- If you don't have a washing machine, iron the clothes and linen, or seal for 10 days in a plastic bag to kill lice and nits.
- Dry-clean nonwashable items or seal in a plastic bag for 10 days.
- Boil articles such as combs, curlers, hairbrushes and barrettes.
- Spray (with Lysol or similar product) all furniture that comes in contact with infected body areas.
- See Resources for Additional Information.

MEDICATION—Your doctor may prescribe anti-lice (pediculicide) cream, lotion or shampoo. Apply creams or lotions to infected body parts according to instructions. To use the shampoo:
- Wet the hair. Apply 1 tablespoon of shampoo. Lather for 4 minutes, working the lather well into the scalp.
- If shampoo gets in eyes, wash out right away.
- Rinse hair thoroughly and towel dry. Don't use this towel again without laundering.
- Comb the hair with a fine comb dipped in hot vinegar to remove the lice. The comb must run through the hair repeatedly from the scalp outward until the hair is completely free of nits.
- A single application of shampoo is effective in more than 90% of cases. Don't use more frequently than recommended, because the shampoo may cause skin irritation or be absorbed into the body. A repeat application may be necessary in 10 to 14 days.
- If the lice infect eyelashes, they must be removed carefully by the doctor. The prescribed medications should not go into the eye or on the eyelashes. You may apply petroleum jelly to the eyelashes for 7 or 8 days after removal.

ACTIVITY—No restrictions.

DIET—No special diet.

 CALL YOUR DOCTOR IF

You, your sexual partner or anyone in your household have symptoms of lice, or symptoms recur after treatment.

ILLNESS & DISORDERS

LICHEN PLANUS

 GENERAL INFORMATION

DEFINITION—A chronic skin eruption that is not cancerous or contagious.

BODY PARTS INVOLVED
- Skin of the legs, trunk, arms, wrists, scalp or penis.
- Lining of the mouth or vagina.
- Toenails and fingernails (around or partially under the nailbed).

SEX OR AGE MOST AFFECTED—All ages, but most common in adults over 40.

SIGNS & SYMPTOMS
- Small, slightly raised bumps that itch. The bumps are purplish with a whitish surface.
- An irregular whitish line inside the mouth or vagina.
- Sudden hair loss in patches on the head.

CAUSES—Unknown, but may be caused by a virus. In a few cases, lichen planus may be an adverse reaction to certain drugs.

RISK INCREASES WITH
- Stress.
- Fatigue or overwork.
- Exposure to drugs or chemicals.

HOW TO PREVENT—Cannot be prevented at present.

 WHAT TO EXPECT

DIAGNOSTIC MEASURES
- Your own observation of symptoms.
- Medical history and physical exam by a doctor.
- Biopsy of questionable papules (raised bumps).

APPROPRIATE HEALTH CARE
- Self-care after diagnosis.
- Doctor's treatment.

POSSIBLE COMPLICATIONS
- Hair loss.
- Nail destruction.
- Chronic disease where new lesions appear as old lesions resolve.

PROBABLE OUTCOME—Symptoms can be controlled with treatment, but the disorder lasts months or years. Be patient and persist with your treatment, even if results are disappointing or slow.

 HOW TO TREAT

GENERAL MEASURES
- Goal of treatment is to relieve the symptoms, particularly, the itching.
- Use cool-water soaks to relieve itching.
- Reducing stress in your life may help prevent recurrences. Learn relaxation techniques or obtain counseling if necessary.
- If lichen planus is related to a medication, get medical advice about changing dosage or a substitute drug.

MEDICATION—Your doctor may prescribe:
- Antihistamines for their sedative effect to control itching.
- Cortisone creams or ointments to reduce inflammation and decrease itching. Use only once or twice a day unless directed otherwise. Apply immediately after bathing for better spreading and penetration. For the face and groin, use only low-potency steroid products without fluorine.
- Cortisone tablets for severe cases.

ACTIVITY—No restrictions.

DIET—No special diet.

 CALL YOUR DOCTOR IF

- You have symptoms of lichen planus.
- New, unexplained symptoms develop. Drugs used in treatment may produce side effects.

LIPOMAS

GENERAL INFORMATION

DEFINITION—Benign tumors of fat cells.

BODY PARTS INVOLVED—Trunk; neck; back; upper thighs; arms.

SEX OR AGE MOST AFFECTED—Both sexes of persons from puberty to old age.

SIGNS & SYMPTOMS—Nodules that grow under the skin (subcutaneous) with the following characteristics:
• Nodules are dome-shaped and about 2cm to 10cm in diameter. Some grow larger.
• Nodules feel "doughy," smooth and easily movable.
• Skin over the nodule is normal in appearance.
• The nodules usually cause no symptoms such as itching or pain.

CAUSES—Unknown, but the tendency is probably inherited. Minor injury may trigger growth.

RISK INCREASES WITH—Family history of lipomas.

HOW TO PREVENT—Cannot be prevented at present. If you are obese, you can reduce the size of lipomas by losing weight.

WHAT TO EXPECT

DIAGNOSTIC MEASURES
• Your own observation of symptoms.
• Medical history and physical exam by a doctor.

APPROPRIATE HEALTH CARE
• Doctor's treatment.
• No treatment is needed for lesions that are stable in size.
• Surgical removal (if recommended) is usually done in a doctor's office. Lipomas can be surgically excised or removed by liposuction. (See Lipoma Removal in Surgery section.)

POSSIBLE COMPLICATIONS—Large lipomas may interfere with muscle function.

PROBABLE OUTCOME—These tumors are benign and require no treatment, but they may be removed if they are unsightly or interfere with muscle function.

HOW TO TREAT

GENERAL MEASURES—After surgical removal:
• Apply rubbing alcohol to the scab twice a day.
• Apply an adhesive bandage to the scab during the day. Leave it uncovered at night.
• Wash the wound as usual. Dry gently and completely after bathing or swimming.
• If the scab cracks or oozes, apply nonprescription antibiotic ointment several times a day.

MEDICATION—Medication usually is not necessary for this disorder.

ACTIVITY—After surgical removal, resume your normal activities gradually. Allow 1 month for complete healing.

DIET—No special diet.

CALL YOUR DOCTOR IF

The following occurs after surgery:
• Fever.
• Bleeding that does not respond to moderate pressure.
• Signs of infection (warmth, swelling or redness) at the surgical site.

ILLNESS & DISORDERS

LIVER CANCER

GENERAL INFORMATION

DEFINITION—Uncontrolled growth of malignant cells in the liver. Liver cancer may be primary—resulting from abnormal liver or bile-duct cells—or it may result from spread of cancer from another site (metastases). The most common sources are cancers of the rectum, colon, lung, breast, pancreas, esophagus or skin (melanoma).

BODY PARTS INVOLVED—Liver; bile ducts.

SEX OR AGE MOST AFFECTED—All ages, but most common in men over 60.

SIGNS & SYMPTOMS
- Loss of appetite and weight loss.
- Tender mass in the right upper abdomen.
- Pain in the upper abdomen.
- Low fever, usually less than 101F (38.3C).
- Yellow eyes and skin (sometimes).
- Swollen abdomen from fluid retention (sometimes).
- Lethargy.

CAUSES—Unknown. It occurs most often in population groups with a high incidence of viral hepatitis and other chronic liver diseases.

RISK INCREASES WITH
- Primary liver disease, such as cirrhosis of the liver.
- Use of anabolic steroids.
- Excess alcohol consumption.
- Previous hepatitis B infection.
- Chronic use of oral contraceptives.
- Hemochromatosis.
- Metabolic disorders.
- Gallstones, choledochal cysts, clonorchiasis (infection with a liver fluke commonly found in the Far East).

HOW TO PREVENT
- Hepatitis B vaccination and prevention education for high-risk individuals.
- Cancer screening and early diagnosis for high-risk individuals (laboratory test called alpha-fetoprotein or AFP).

WHAT TO EXPECT

DIAGNOSTIC MEASURES
- Your own observation of symptoms.
- Medical history and physical exam by a doctor.
- A variety of diagnostic tests may be used to confirm diagnosis including blood studies, liver biopsy, x-ray, ultrasound, CT scan, MRI, arteriography, angiography and radioactive studies (see Glossary for all).

APPROPRIATE HEALTH CARE
- Self-care after diagnosis.
- Doctor's treatment.
- Anticancer drugs and radiation therapy are often used. They may afford some relief but won't cure (palliative).
- Surgery to remove the tumor may be recommended, depending on type and spread of the disease.
- Liver transplant may be considered for some patients.

POSSIBLE COMPLICATIONS
- Sodium retention, leading to life-threatening fluid accumulation in the abdomen and lower body parts.
- Kidney failure.
- Spread of cancer to other organs.
- Death from loss of liver function.

PROBABLE OUTCOME—This condition is currently considered incurable and fatal within a short time. However, pain can be controlled. Treatment is usually attempted, although it is not likely to be successful.

Scientific research into causes and treatment continues, so there is hope for increasingly effective treatment and cure.

HOW TO TREAT

GENERAL MEASURES
- Patient care should involve comprehensive supportive care and emotional support.
- The more you can learn and understand about this disorder, the more you will be able to make informed decisions about where to go for your care, the treatments available, the risks involved, side effects of therapy and expected outcome.
- See Resources for Additional Information.

MEDICATION—Your doctor may prescribe:
- Anticancer drugs.
- Pain relievers.

ACTIVITY
- No restrictions. Stay as active as your strength allows.
- Hospice care, as an outpatient or inpatient, may be recommended as disease progresses.

DIET—High-calorie, low-protein diet.

CALL YOUR DOCTOR IF

- You have symptoms of liver cancer, especially unexplained weight loss, low fever or a mass in the abdomen.
- You develop a swollen abdomen during treatment.
- New, unexplained symptoms develop. Drugs used in treatment may produce side effects.

LUNG ABSCESS

GENERAL INFORMATION

DEFINITION—An infected area of lung tissue, surrounded by lung inflammation. The infected lung tissue dies and is replaced with pus. The infection is not contagious from person to person.

BODY PARTS INVOLVED—Lung.

SEX OR AGE MOST AFFECTED—Both sexes; all ages.

SIGNS & SYMPTOMS
- Cough with sputum. The sputum is pus-like, often blood-streaked and sometimes smells bad.
- Bad breath.
- Sweating.
- Fever to 101F (38.3C) or higher.
- Chills.
- Weight loss.
- Chest pain (sometimes).

CAUSES—Usually a complication of pneumonia. A lung abscess sometimes occurs when an unconscious or sedated person inhales infected material from the upper-breathing passages. The patient may be unconscious from a head injury, an anesthetic (including dental anesthesia), intoxicated from alcohol or heavily sedated. Lung abscesses are generally caused by virulent bacteria, such as klebsiella, Pseudomonas, staphylococcus or beta-hemolytic streptococcus.

RISK INCREASES WITH
- Recent illness, especially pneumonia that has been slow to heal.
- Alcoholism.
- Periodontal disease.
- Recent general anesthesia or injury causing unconsciousness.

HOW TO PREVENT
- Obtain prompt medical treatment for respiratory infections, especially pneumonia.
- Keep the teeth and mouth in good condition to prevent oral infections that could result in a lung abscess.

WHAT TO EXPECT

DIAGNOSTIC MEASURES
- Your own observation of symptoms.
- Medical history and physical exam by a doctor.
- Laboratory blood tests and a culture of pus from the abscess to determine what antibiotic to use.
- X-rays of the lung, lung scan, bronchoscopy (see Surgery section).

APPROPRIATE HEALTH CARE
- Doctor's treatment.
- Surgery (sometimes) to aspirate pus from the abscess or to remove the abscess and part of the lung, if the abscess does not heal.
- Self-care during convalescence.

POSSIBLE COMPLICATIONS
- Chronic abscess, leading to weight loss, anemia, bronchiectasis or chronic lung disease, if the abscess does not respond well to antibiotic treatment.
- Rupture of the abscess, causing empyema or massive bleeding in the lung.
- Spread of infection to other body parts, especially the brain.

PROBABLE OUTCOME—Usually curable with prolonged antibiotic treatment (up to 6 months).

HOW TO TREAT

GENERAL MEASURES
- Don't smoke.
- Practice deep-breathing exercises as often as possible.
- Learn postural drainage to help rid the lung of bronchial secretions. Lie on the bed on your stomach with your head and chest hanging over the edge. Force yourself to cough. Continue until you cannot raise any more sputum. Practice this twice a day for 5 to 10 minutes.

MEDICATION—Your doctor may prescribe antibiotics for prolonged periods to fight infection and prevent a recurrence.

ACTIVITY—Reduced activity until x-ray shows evidence of clearing.

DIET—No special diet. Increase your fluid intake to a minimum of 1 glass of fluid at least 8 times a day. By drinking extra liquids, the body is forced to eliminate part of the fluid through the lungs. This makes thick lung secretions thinner, so they can be coughed up more easily.

CALL YOUR DOCTOR IF
- You have symptoms of a lung abscess.
- The following occurs during treatment:
  Fever rises to 101F (38.3C) or higher.
  Sputum thickens, despite treatment.
  Postural drainage reveals a change in color, amount or consistency of the sputum.
- Symptoms of a lung infection recur after treatment, especially a sputum-producing cough, fever or general ill feeling.

LUNG CANCER
(Bronchogenic Carcinoma)

GENERAL INFORMATION

DEFINITION—Malignant tissue growth in the lung. It is related almost exclusively to cigarette smoking.

BODY PARTS INVOLVED—Bronchial tubes and lungs. Cancer spreads to the larynx, liver, brain, bones and kidneys.

SEX OR AGE MOST AFFECTED—Adults of both sexes between ages 40 and 70.

SIGNS & SYMPTOMS
- Persistent cough.
- Sputum that may contain blood.
- Wheezing.
- Chest pain.
- Fatigue and weakness.
- Weight loss.
- Shoulder, arm or bone pain.
- Sometimes, no symptoms.

CAUSES
- Cigarette smoking.
- Air pollution.
- Unknown (some forms).
- Asbestos exposure.
- Spread of cancer from somewhere else in the body.
- Chronic interstitial pneumonitis.
- Radon gas.

RISK INCREASES WITH
- Adults over 60.
- Smoking. A smoker is 22 times more likely to develop lung cancer than a nonsmoker.
- Environmental exposure to asbestos, uranium ore, nickel, chromates, bischloromethyl ether or air pollution.

HOW TO PREVENT
- Avoid pollutants. Wear a protective mask if you work with pollutants.
- Don't smoke. Because tumors don't develop for a long time, smokers can quit at any time and greatly reduce the risk of developing lung cancer.
- Obtain regular health checkups that may include a chest x-ray if you are a heavy smoker.
- Check your house for radon gas.

WHAT TO EXPECT

DIAGNOSTIC MEASURES
- Your own observation of symptoms.
- Medical history and physical exam by a doctor.
- Laboratory studies of cells in sputum and pleural fluid.
- X-rays of lungs, CT scan (see Glossary) and pulmonary function studies.

APPROPRIATE HEALTH CARE
- Doctor's care.
- Surgery for diagnosis (bronchoscopy), biopsy (see Glossary) or removal of cancerous lung tissue.
- Treatment steps will be determined by the extent of the spread of the disease.
- Surgery to remove all of the lung (pneumonectomy) or part of the lung (lobectomy) may be recommended if cancer is at an early stage. (See Lung Resection in Surgery section.)
- Radiation treatment and anticancer drugs to stop the spread of the tumor or destroy cancerous cells may be recommended.

POSSIBLE COMPLICATIONS
- Destructive spread to other body parts, including the brain.
- Lung collapse; fluid on the lung.

PROBABLE OUTCOME—Without surgery, this condition is currently considered incurable. Only 25% of tumors can be removed surgically. The survival rate to 5 years is less than 10%. Lung cancer causes more deaths than any other form of cancer and the incidence is increasing, especially among women.

HOW TO TREAT

GENERAL MEASURES
- The more you can learn and understand about this disorder, the more you will be able to make informed decisions about where to go for your care, the treatments available, the risks involved, side effects of therapy and outcome.
- See Resources for Additional Information.

MEDICATION
- For minor pain, you may use nonprescription drugs such as acetaminophen or aspirin.
- Your doctor may prescribe:
  Medication to reduce pain, nausea or anxiety.
  Anticancer drugs.

ACTIVITY—Remain as active as possible. If surgery performed, follow medical advice about resuming activities.

DIET—No special diet.

CALL YOUR DOCTOR IF

- The following occurs after surgery or during drug treatment:
  Intolerable pain.
  Nausea or vomiting.
  Sleeplessness.
- New, unexplained symptoms develop. Drugs used in treatment may produce side effects.

LUPUS ERYTHEMATOSUS, DISCOID (DLE)

GENERAL INFORMATION

DEFINITION—A chronic skin disorder. Localized DLE, the more common form, involves the skin on the face, scalp, ears and neck. Generalized DLE involves the skin on the arms and chest. DLE is different from systemic lupus erythematosus, a connective-tissue disease that affects many different organs. Discoid lupus progresses to systemic lupus in about 1 in 20 persons.

BODY PARTS INVOLVED—Skin.

SEX OR AGE MOST AFFECTED—Adults of both sexes. The peak incidence occurs in women in their late 20s.

SIGNS & SYMPTOMS—Plaques (red, raised skin lesions) with the following characteristics:
• Plaques are 1cm to 4cm in diameter and have clearly defined borders.
• They may appear anywhere on the face, but the cheeks and jawline are the most common sites. Some people describe them as "butterfly" lesions when two lesions of unequal size appear on both sides of the nose.
• Lesions sometimes appear on the scalp with localized patches of hair loss.
• Lesions scar as they heal.

CAUSES—Unknown, but probably an autoimmune disorder.

RISK INCREASES WITH—Exposure to sunlight.

HOW TO PREVENT—No specific preventive measures. Protection from sunlight decreases the severity.

WHAT TO EXPECT

DIAGNOSTIC MEASURES
• Your own observation of symptoms.
• Medical history and physical exam by a doctor.
• Laboratory blood studies and biopsy of skin lesions to rule out systemic lupus erythematosus.

APPROPRIATE HEALTH CARE
• Self-care after diagnosis.
• Doctor's treatment.

POSSIBLE COMPLICATIONS
• Extensive scarring of the face.
• Systemic lupus erythematosus (1-5% of patients).

PROBABLE OUTCOME—This disorder is characterized by remissions and flare-ups. It runs its course in 10 to 20 years. 95% of patients (those who don't progress to systemic lupus) live a normal life-span.

HOW TO TREAT

GENERAL MEASURES
• Don't go outdoors between 10 a.m. and 2 p.m., when the sun's ultraviolet light is strongest. If you can't avoid exposure to bright sunlight, wear protective clothing and maximum-protection sunscreen products. Avoid fluorescent lighting, if possible.
• See your doctor for regular checkups, even when in remission.
• See Resources for Additional Information.

MEDICATION—Your doctor may prescribe:
• Injections of triamcinolone into lesions or hydroxychloroquine by mouth to shrink lesions.
• Topical steroids (occasionally) to decrease redness of lesions.

ACTIVITY—No restrictions.

DIET—No special diet.

CALL YOUR DOCTOR IF

• You have symptoms of discoid lupus erythematosus.
• The following occurs during treatment:
  Lesions on the hands.
  Swelling, redness, pain in joints.

LUPUS ERYTHEMATOSUS, SYSTEMIC (SLE)

GENERAL INFORMATION

DEFINITION—An inflammatory disease of connective tissue. Lupus is not inherited or cancerous.

BODY PARTS INVOLVED—Connective tissue (collagen). Many body systems are affected, including joints, skin, kidneys, brain, heart and lungs.

SEX OR AGE MOST AFFECTED—All ages and both sexes, but 90% of cases occur in women between ages 30 and 50.

SIGNS & SYMPTOMS—Lupus symptoms frequently flare up and then subside. Episodes generally include fever and fatigue, plus any 4 of the following:
- Rash, usually on the cheeks.
- Ulcers in the mouth.
- Red palms and hands.
- Joint pain with redness, swelling and tenderness—but no deformity.
- Swelling of the face and legs.
- Shortness of breath; rapid or irregular heartbeat; chest pain; hair loss.
- Swelling of the lymph glands.
- Protein in the urine; anemia.
- Increased sensitivity to the sun.
- Mental changes, including psychosis.

CAUSES—Unknown, but lupus is probably an autoimmune disorder. In an autoimmune disorder, the body's immune system functions abnormally and attacks its own normal tissue.

RISK INCREASES WITH
- Stress.
- Use of drugs, such as hydralazine, procainamide, methyldopa and chlorpromazine.
- Genetic factors. The incidence is higher among blacks, Hispanics, Native Americans and Asians.

HOW TO PREVENT—Cannot be prevented at present.

WHAT TO EXPECT

DIAGNOSTIC MEASURES
- Medical history and exam by a doctor.
- Patients with vague, recurrent symptoms may require long-term observation before a final diagnosis can be made. Laboratory studies of antinuclear antibodies, blood count and sedimentation rate aid in the diagnosis.

APPROPRIATE HEALTH CARE
- Self-care after diagnosis.
- Doctor's treatment.

POSSIBLE COMPLICATIONS
- Bacterial or viral pneumonia.
- Impaired kidney function.
- Pericarditis.
- Seizures.
- Hypertension.
- SLE is sometimes associated with other autoimmune disorders such as arthritis, diabetes, hypothyroidism.

PROBABLE OUTCOME—Lupus is currently considered incurable. The disease is characterized by remissions and relapses. The prognosis is variable depending on the organs involved and the extent of the inflammation. Symptoms can be relieved or controlled for many years. Medical literature cites instances of unexplained recovery.

HOW TO TREAT

GENERAL MEASURES
- Obtain prompt medical treatment for any infection.
- Sunlight sensitivity may occur in some patients. If so, avoid exposure or use protection of hats, sunglasses, sunscreens, long sleeved clothing.
- Apply heat or ice to relieve joint pain.
- Control the stress in your life.
- Don't take any immunizations or drugs without consulting your doctor. Immunizations and some drugs may cause relapses or worsen current symptoms.
- Don't become pregnant without consulting your doctor. Pregnancy may overload the kidneys and cause death.

MEDICATION—Your doctor may prescribe immunosuppressive, steroid and nonsteroidal anti-inflammatory drugs or anti-malarial drugs. These relieve symptoms but don't cure the disease.

ACTIVITY
- Remain as active as possible; however extra rest may be needed.
- Active exercises are encouraged to retain full range-of-motion. Physical therapy may be recommended.

DIET—If your kidneys or heart are affected, restrict your salt intake. Otherwise, no special diet is necessary.

CALL YOUR DOCTOR IF

- You have symptoms of systemic lupus erythematosus.
- Any of the following occurs after diagnosis: Fever of 101F (38.3C) or higher, blood in the urine, shortness of breath, chest pain, bloody stool, severe abdominal pain, any illness with fever.
- New, unexplained symptoms develop. Drugs used in treatment may produce side effects.

LYME DISEASE
(Lyme Arthritis)

GENERAL INFORMATION

DEFINITION—An inflammatory disorder characterized by a skin rash, followed in weeks to months by symptoms in the central nervous system, cardiovascular system and joints. The majority who get Lyme disease do not become seriously ill. It can be a self-limited illness that goes away without treatment.

Named for Lyme, Connecticut, where it was first described, it's often confused with juvenile rheumatoid arthritis of children.

BODY PARTS INVOLVED—Skin of the thighs, buttocks or underarms; central nervous system; heart and blood vessels; large joints, especially in the knee.

SEX OR AGE MOST AFFECTED—Both sexes; all ages.

SIGNS & SYMPTOMS
First stage:
• A red papule (small, raised bump) on the skin of the thighs, buttocks or armpits that grows as large as 50cm, usually with clearing of the center area. They may be multiple.
Later stages—any or some of the following:
• Muscle aches and pains.
• Fatigue and lethargy.
• Chills and fever.
• Stiff neck with headache.
• Backache.
• Nausea and vomiting.
• Sore throat.
• Enlargement of the spleen and lymph glands.
• Migrating joint pain, eventually accompanied by redness and warmth.
• Enlarged heart and heart rhythm disturbances.

CAUSES—Infection with a spirochete (term for organism or germ), Borrelia burgdorferi, transmitted by a deer tick bite. Many patients report a tick bite at the site of the lesion 3 days to 4 weeks prior to the rash.

RISK INCREASES WITH—Areas where ticks are numerous, such as long grass or brush.

HOW TO PREVENT
• Wear protective clothing with tight collars and cuffs.
• Use effective insect repellents, such as DEET, in areas with ticks.
• Have dogs and cats wear tick-repellant collars.
• Careful skin inspection; removal of any ticks.

WHAT TO EXPECT

DIAGNOSTIC MEASURES
• Your own observation of symptoms.
• Medical history and physical exam by a doctor.
• Laboratory blood studies and sometimes a skin biopsy (see Glossary).

APPROPRIATE HEALTH CARE
• Self-care after diagnosis during treatment and convalescence.
• Doctor's treatment.

POSSIBLE COMPLICATIONS
• Congestive heart failure.
• Permanent joint deformity.
• Permanent brain damage (rare).
• Nerve disorder (peripheral neuropathy).

PROBABLE OUTCOME—The skin rash is curable in some patients in 10 days with treatment, and this may prevent development of other symptoms. If not, symptoms in the joints, central nervous system and cardiovascular system usually subside slowly over 2 to 3 years. Symptoms often recur after several years—without another tick bite.

HOW TO TREAT

GENERAL MEASURES
• Early treatment is important to prevent progression.
• Use crutches to keep weight off affected joints, if necessary.
• Heat relieves joint pain. Take hot baths or use heating pads, heat lamps or whirlpool treatments.
• See Resources for Additional Information.

MEDICATION—Your doctor may prescribe:
• An oral antibiotic for 14-21 days for early stage of the disease.
• Intravenous antibiotics for late stages.
• Nonsteroidal anti-inflammatory drugs.
• Cortisone drugs to reduce the inflammatory response in the heart or central nervous system.

ACTIVITY—Rest in bed until symptoms of active inflammation subside. Then resume normal activities gradually.

DIET—No special diet.

CALL YOUR DOCTOR IF

• You have symptoms of Lyme disease.
• New, unexplained symptoms develop. Drugs used in treatment may produce side effects.

ILLNESS & DISORDERS

LYMPHOGRANULOMA VENEREUM
(LGV; Lymphogranuloma Inguinale)

 GENERAL INFORMATION

DEFINITION—A contagious venereal disease that involves the genitals and lymph glands. This disease is found mostly in tropical and subtropical areas. It is rare in North America.

BODY PARTS INVOLVED—Genitals; lymph glands.

SEX OR AGE MOST AFFECTED—Both sexes of adults, but most common in men aged 20 to 40.

SIGNS & SYMPTOMS—The following begin 1 to 4 weeks after exposure and progress in order:
- A painless blister on the genitals that ulcerates and heals quickly.
- Enlarged lymph glands in the groin that form large, red, tender masses.
- Multiple areas of deep infection that discharge thick pus and blood-stained material.

Other symptoms include:
- Fever.
- Muscle aches and pain, including backache.
- Headaches.
- Joint pain.
- Appetite loss.
- Vomiting.

CAUSES—The bacterium, Chlamydia, which is transmitted by sexual activity. Incubation period is about 3-12 days.

RISK INCREASES WITH
- Travel to a country with a tropical or subtropical climate.
- Anal intercourse.
- Unprotected sexual activity with new partners.

HOW TO PREVENT
- Use condoms during sexual intercourse with new partners.
- Don't engage in sexual activity with an infected person.

 WHAT TO EXPECT

DIAGNOSTIC MEASURES
- Your own observation of symptoms.
- Medical history and physical exam by a doctor.
- Laboratory studies, such as a blood study to rule out syphilis, culture of the discharge from lesions and Frei test (see Glossary) and antibody tests for the chlamydia organism.

APPROPRIATE HEALTH CARE
- Doctor's treatment.
- Surgery to drain affected lymph glands or remove abscesses and fistulas.

POSSIBLE COMPLICATIONS
- Chronic infection.
- Interference with bowel and bladder function.
- Impotence (sometimes).

PROBABLE OUTCOME—Usually curable in 6 months if treatment is successful. If not, the disorder is incurable, although it does not reduce life expectancy.

 HOW TO TREAT

GENERAL MEASURES
- Your sexual contacts should be examined also.
- Heat applied to affected area may help discomfort.

MEDICATION
- For minor discomfort, you may use nonprescription drugs such as acetaminophen.
- Your doctor may prescribe:
  Antibiotics to fight infection, taken for 21 days.
  Pain relievers.

ACTIVITY—After treatment, resume normal activity as soon as symptoms improve. Don't resume sexual relations until completely healed.

DIET—No special diet.

 CALL YOUR DOCTOR IF

- You have symptoms of lymphogranuloma venereum.
- The following occurs during treatment:
  Fever spikes to 101F (38.3C) or higher.
  Pain cannot be relieved with simple pain medicine.
  You develop symptoms of malabsorption (see Malabsorption in Illness section).
- New, unexplained symptoms develop. Drugs used in treatment may produce side effects.

LYMPHOMA, NON-HODGKIN'S
(Lymphosarcoma; Reticulum Cell Sarcoma)

GENERAL INFORMATION

DEFINITION—Malignant tumor of the lymph glands. This is more common than Hodgkin's disease (another form of lymphoma).

BODY PARTS INVOLVED
- Lymphocytes (white blood cells).
- Lymph glands (glands that fight infection and produce immune substances).
- Spleen (a large lymph gland).

SEX OR AGE MOST AFFECTED—All ages, but most common in men in their 40s.

SIGNS & SYMPTOMS
- Swollen, nontender, rubbery, distinct lymph glands anywhere in the body—but most commonly in the armpit, neck or groin.
- Weight loss.
- General ill feeling.
- Anemia.
- Bleeding from the gastrointestinal tract.
- Jaundice (yellow skin and eyes).

CAUSES—Unknown, but research suggests a virus infection may be a factor or suppression of the immune system, particularly after organ transplantation. One type of non-Hodgkin's lymphoma called Burkitt's lymphoma is thought to be caused by the Epstein-Barr virus.

RISK INCREASES WITH—Adults over 40.

HOW TO PREVENT—No specific preventive measures.

WHAT TO EXPECT

DIAGNOSTIC MEASURES
- Your own observation of symptoms.
- Medical history and physical exam by a doctor.
- Laboratory studies of blood and bone marrow.
- Lymphangiogram (see Glossary).
- Biopsy (see Glossary) of lymph node.
- X-rays of various body parts that may be involved.
- CT scan (see Glossary).

APPROPRIATE HEALTH CARE
- Doctor's treatment.
- Radiation therapy and/or anticancer drugs are given for treatment, depending on extent of the disease.
- Bone-marrow transplantation (see in Surgery section) may be considered if other methods fail.

POSSIBLE COMPLICATIONS—Spread of lymphoma to other parts of the body.

PROBABLE OUTCOME—Usually treatable with radiation therapy and anticancer drugs and may result in long-term control or cure. Life expectancy can be normal. The potential for cure varies according to the cell type discovered from biopsy of the lymph node and the extent and spread of disease when diagnosed.

HOW TO TREAT

GENERAL MEASURES
- The more you can learn and understand about a disease, the more you will be able to make informed decisions about where to go for your care, the treatments available, the risks involved, side effects of therapy and expected outcome.
- Try to remain optimistic about your treatment and chances for cure. A good mental attitude is a powerful ally.
- See Resources for Additional Information.

MEDICATION—Your doctor may prescribe anticancer drugs. Medication may cause side effects or adverse reactions in some people. New symptoms may be caused by the medicine, original disorder or a new illness. Side effects caused by medicine usually disappear when your body adjusts to the drug or when the drug is discontinued.

ACTIVITY—Remain as active as your strength allows.

DIET—No special diet.

CALL YOUR DOCTOR IF

- You have symptoms of lymphoma.
- The following occurs during treatment:
  Fever.
  Signs of infection (redness, swelling, pain or tenderness) anywhere in the body.
  Swelling of the feet and ankles.
  Discomfort when urinating or decreased urination in 1 day.
- You think your medicine is causing symptoms.

MALABSORPTION
(Malabsorptive Syndrome)

GENERAL INFORMATION

DEFINITION—Poor absorption of nutrients, vitamins and minerals from the intestinal tract into the bloodstream.

BODY PARTS INVOLVED—Intestinal tract; liver; pancreas.

SEX OR AGE MOST AFFECTED—**x**Both sexes; all ages.

SIGNS & SYMPTOMS
- Diarrhea.
- Weakness.
- Weight loss.
- Gas and vague abdominal discomfort.
- Bad-smelling, copious stools, frequently with mucus.
- Mild anemia (sometimes).

CAUSES
- Deficiency of intestinal enzymes.
- Inadequate digestion caused by disease of the pancreas (such as cystic fibrosis), gallbladder or liver.
- Change in bacteria that normally live in the intestinal tract.
- Disease of the intestinal walls, including worms or parasites, tropical sprue and celiac disease.
- Surgery that reduces the intestinal tract, decreasing the area for absorption.
- HIV and AIDS.

RISK INCREASES WITH
- Family history of malabsorption or cystic fibrosis.
- Excess alcohol consumption.
- Use of drugs, such as mineral oil and other laxatives.
- Travel to foreign countries.
- Intestinal surgery.
- Lactose intolerance.

HOW TO PREVENT
- Avoid prolonged dependence on mineral oil and other laxatives.
- Avoid excess alcohol consumption.

WHAT TO EXPECT

DIAGNOSTIC MEASURES
- Your own observation of symptoms.
- Medical history and physical exam by a doctor.
- Laboratory studies of stool, chromosomes and blood.
- X-rays of the intestinal tract.

APPROPRIATE HEALTH CARE
- Self-care after diagnosis.
- Doctor's treatment.
- Treatment depends on the underlying cause. In most patients, modification to the diet or dietary supplements will restore health.

POSSIBLE COMPLICATIONS
- Prolonged illness.
- Failure to thrive in infants.
- Additional illness caused by nutritional, vitamin or mineral deficiency.
- Anemia.

PROBABLE OUTCOME—The degree to which symptoms can be controlled depends on the cause, but many things are common to all malabsorptive disorders. The onset is usually slow and difficult to diagnose. Disorders may be present for months or years before being recognized. Treatment is long, complicated and may need to be changed often.

HOW TO TREAT

GENERAL MEASURES—Patience and a positive attitude are important in cure.

MEDICATION—Your doctor may prescribe:
- Enzymes to replace missing intestinal enzymes.
- Antispasmodics to reduce discomfort.
- Injections of vitamin B-12 and iron because neither is absorbed well with any malabsorptive disorder.

ACTIVITY—No restrictions. Resume normal activities as soon as symptoms improve.

DIET
- Don't drink alcohol.
- You will need a special diet, depending on the cause of your illness. Your doctor or nutritionist will provide specific information.

CALL YOUR DOCTOR IF

- You or a family member has symptoms of malabsorption.
- Any of the following occur during treatment:
  Black, tarry bowel movements.
  Fever of 101F (38.3C) or higher.
  Severe abdominal pain.
  Muscle cramps.

MALARIA

GENERAL INFORMATION

DEFINITION—An infection caused by a single-cell parasite that is transmitted by the bite of an anopheles mosquito.

BODY PARTS INVOLVED—Blood cells; blood vessels; liver; central nervous system.

SEX OR AGE MOST AFFECTED—Both sexes; all ages.

SIGNS & SYMPTOMS—The first episode of the following symptoms usually occurs about 8 to 30 days after the mosquito bite:
- Headache.
- Fatigue.
- Nausea.
- Hard, shaking chills with fever for 12 to 24 hours.
- Rapid breathing.
- Heavy sweating, accompanied by a drop in temperature.

Episodes may recur every 2 or 3 days until the disease is treated. Without treatment, the disease can continue for years.

CAUSES—There are 4 types of malarial parasites; they are transferred from person to person by a mosquito bite. The mosquito becomes infected with malaria after biting a person with the disease. The organisms multiply in the mosquito, then enter the bloodstream of the next person the mosquito bites.

   Once in a person's bloodstream, the parasites travel to the liver, where they thrive and multiply rapidly. After several days, thousands re-enter the bloodstream and destroy red-blood cells. Some parasites remain in the liver, continue to multiply and are released again at intervals into the bloodstream.

RISK INCREASES WITH
- Crowded or unsanitary living conditions.
- Hot, humid climates.
- Geographic locations, such as Latin America, Asia and Africa. Malaria is uncommon in the U.S., but it often affects travelers or military personnel stationed in foreign countries.

HOW TO PREVENT
- Take antimalaria drugs before visiting an area where malaria is prevalent. Continue to take the drugs after you return. The public health department or your doctor can give you instructions.
- If you are in a mosquito-infested area, destroy mosquito breeding areas, install window screens and mosquito nets over beds, and use insect repellants.
- Call Traveler's Hot Line (404)332-4559 (established by the Centers for Disease Control) for current information about risk of exposure and preventive regimens in the area to which you are traveling.

WHAT TO EXPECT

DIAGNOSTIC MEASURES
- Your own observation of symptoms.
- Medical history and physical exam by a doctor. Tell your doctor of recent travel.
- Laboratory studies, such as studies of blood smears to identify the parasite.

APPROPRIATE HEALTH CARE
- Self-care after diagnosis.
- Doctor's treatment.
- Hospitalization (severe cases).

POSSIBLE COMPLICATIONS
- Anemia caused by blood-cell destruction.
- Clumping of blood cells, which may cause brain or kidney damage.

PROBABLE OUTCOME—Usually curable in 2 weeks with treatment. Malaria can be fatal without treatment in persons who don't receive adequate nourishment or have low resistance to disease.

HOW TO TREAT

GENERAL MEASURES
- Protect yourself from secondary bacterial infection while you are ill with malaria. Wash your hands and bathe often.
- Make your environment mosquito-free so your infection cannot be transmitted to others.
- All cases of malaria are reported to the local health department.

MEDICATION—Your doctor may prescribe antimalaria drugs to kill the parasite.

ACTIVITY—Rest in bed until fever and chills subside. Resume your normal activities gradually as symptoms improve.

DIET—No special diet. Take vitamin and mineral supplements until you recover.

CALL YOUR DOCTOR IF

- You have symptoms of malaria.
- You are weak for a prolonged time after an attack. This may indicate anemia.
- Symptoms of malaria recur after treatment.
- New, unexplained symptoms develop. Drugs used in treatment may produce side effects.

ILLNESS & DISORDERS

MARFAN SYNDROME

GENERAL INFORMATION

DEFINITION—A rare, inherited disorder involving the body's connective tissue. It primarily affects the musculoskeletal system, the cardiovascular system and the eye. The disorder is present from birth and diagnosis can occasionally be made in newborns. However, signs or symptoms sometimes do not become apparent until adolescence or young adulthood and the severity varies greatly.

BODY PARTS INVOLVED—Musculoskeletal; endocrine system and metabolic system.

SEX OR AGE MOST AFFECTED—Newborns of both sexes.

SIGNS & SYMPTOMS
Musculoskeletal:
• Tall stature; thin, gangly body (limb length out of proportion to trunk).
• Long, thin fingers (arachnodactyly); pectus deformity; high arched palate.
• "Double jointed"; joint weakness or looseness.
• Chest deformity.
Cardiovascular:
• Aortic regurgitation; aortic dissection; mitral valve prolapse; mitral regurgitation.
Eyes:
• Dislocation of lens, usually upward; myopia.
• Retinal detachment (uncommon).
• Glaucoma and/or cataracts.
Other:
• Easy bruising (uncommon).
• Excessive bleeding (uncommon).

CAUSES—Inherited disorder in about 85% of cases. Defective gene is believed to reside on chromosome 15. Other cases are spontaneous with no known cause.

RISK INCREASES WITH
• Advanced paternal age may be a risk in those cases that are not clearly inherited.
• Family history of Marfan syndrome.

PREVENTIVE MEASURES
• No prenatal diagnosis is yet available.
• Each child has a 50% chance of inheriting the disorder from an affected parent. Signs and symptoms are variable, however, so children may be more or less severely affected. Get genetic counseling if you have Marfan syndrome or there is a family history of the disorder.

WHAT TO EXPECT

DIAGNOSTIC MEASURES
• Medical history and exam by a doctor.
• There are no specific diagnostic laboratory tests to identify Marfan syndrome. Echocardiogram may be performed to detect heart valve deformities, and an eye examination may be performed. X-rays of spine are needed during growth years to detect scoliosis.

APPROPRIATE HEALTH CARE
• Self-care.
• Doctor's treatment.
• Medical treatment will involve a team approach that involves eye care, cardiac care and orthopedic help. Frequent exams (at least twice a year) while growing, with attention to cardiovascular system and scoliosis.

POSSIBLE COMPLICATIONS
• Bacterial endocarditis.
• Aortic dissection; aortic or mitral valve insufficiency; cardiomyopathy; cardiovascular complications.
• Retinal detachment.

PROBABLE OUTCOME—The prognosis depends to a great extent on the cardiovascular complications (such as rupture of the aorta). Improved surgical techniques on the aorta appear to help in prolonging survival as does the use of medications such as beta-blockers for the heart complications.

HOW TO TREAT

GENERAL MEASURES
• Annual screening echocardiograms are recommended beginning in adolescence.
• Routine eye examinations are recommended.
• Most patients will ultimately require reconstructive cardiovascular surgery.
• Pregnant women with the Marfan syndrome need to be managed as high-risk patients.
• See Resources for Additional Information.

MEDICATION
• No specific medical therapy is available, but drugs are used to try to prevent complications.
• Beta-adrenergic blocking drugs are sometimes used for heart complications.
• Male or female hormones are often administered prior to puberty to help control height.
• Antibiotic therapy may be recommended for some patients.

ACTIVITY
• Fully active unless limited by symptoms.
• Several highly-trained athletes with the Marfan syndrome have suffered sudden death during competition leading to some concern that people with Marfan syndrome should be discouraged from demanding sports.

DIET—No special diet.

CALL YOUR DOCTOR IF

You believe your child has signs or symptoms of Marfan syndrome.

MASTITIS
(Breast Abscess)

GENERAL INFORMATION

DEFINITION—Inflammation and infection in the breast of a woman who has recently given birth. It occurs in about 1% of new mothers and is more likely in women who are breast-feeding. An abscess is a collection of pus that may follow if the mastitis is not treated.

BODY PARTS INVOLVED—Breasts.

SEX OR AGE MOST AFFECTED—Females of childbearing age.

SIGNS & SYMPTOMS—Symptoms may occur anytime while nursing, but usually begin 3 to 4 weeks after delivery. Common symptoms include:
• Fever.
• Tender, swollen, hard, hot breast(s).
• A localized area with increasing redness, pain, tenderness and fluctuance (feels like pushing on an inflated inner tube) indicates an abscess.

CAUSES—Infection from bacteria that enter the mother's breast from the nursing baby's nose or throat. The most-common germs are Staphylococcus aureus and beta-hemolytic streptococcus. Infection with the mumps virus is another cause.

RISK INCREASES WITH
• Abrasion of the nipple.
• Blocked milk ducts from wearing too-tight bras, sleeping on the stomach or waiting too long between feedings.
• Use of an electric or manual breast pump.

HOW TO PREVENT
• Wash nipples before nursing. Wash hands before touching breasts.
• Wear a comfortable bra that is not too tight.
• If a nipple cracks or fissures, apply lanolin cream or other topical medication recommended by your doctor.
• Don't sleep on your stomach.

WHAT TO EXPECT

DIAGNOSTIC MEASURES
• Your own observation of symptoms.
• Medical history and physical exam by a doctor.
• Laboratory blood studies and a culture of breast milk.

APPROPRIATE HEALTH CARE
• Self-care after diagnosis.
• Doctor's treatment.
• Surgery to drain an abscess (rare).

POSSIBLE COMPLICATIONS—It may be necessary to discontinue breast-feeding if the infection is severe enough to require treatment with antibiotics.

PROBABLE OUTCOME—Usually curable in 10 days with treatment.

HOW TO TREAT

GENERAL MEASURES
• Apply an ice pack (ice in a plastic bag, covered with a thin towel) to the engorged breast 3 to 6 times a day. Use for 15 to 20 minutes at a time. Don't use ice packs within 1 hour of nursing—use warm compresses instead.
• Massage nipples with cocoa butter or a cream recommended by the doctor.
• Wear an uplift bra during treatment.
• Continue to breast-feed, even though breasts are infected. Offer the affected breast first to promote complete emptying.
• If an abscess develops, stop breast-feeding on the affected side. Use a breast pump to empty the infected breast regularly, and continue breast-feeding on the unaffected side.

MEDICATION—Your doctor may prescribe:
• Antibiotics to fight infection. Finish the prescription, even if symptoms subside quickly.
• Pain relievers. For minor discomfort, you may use nonprescription drugs such as acetaminophen.

ACTIVITY—Rest in bed until fever and pain diminish.

DIET—No special diet. Drink extra fluids if you have fever.

CALL YOUR DOCTOR IF

• You have symptoms of mastitis.
• Symptoms recur or worsen despite treatment.

MEASLES (Red Measles; Rubeola)

GENERAL INFORMATION

DEFINITION—A viral illness that infects the respiratory tract and skin. This is one of the most contagious diseases known. Measles was once very common, but it is now less common due to immunization. However, recent outbreaks have occurred due to low rates of immunization.

BODY PARTS INVOLVED—Skin; eyes; upper-respiratory tract.

SEX OR AGE MOST AFFECTED—All ages, but most common in children.

SIGNS & SYMPTOMS—Measles symptoms usually occur in the following sequence:
- Fever, often high; fatigue; appetite loss.
- Sneezing and runny nose.
- Harsh, hacking cough.
- Red eyes and sensitivity to light.
- Koplik's spots (tiny white spots) in the mouth and throat; reddish rash on the forehead and around ears that spreads to the body.

CAUSES—Measles is caused by a rubeola virus infection that chiefly affects the skin and respiratory tract. The incubation period after exposure is 7 to 14 days.

RISK INCREASES WITH
- Crowded or unsanitary living conditions.
- Population groups that are not immunized.
- Measles epidemics. The disease becomes more virulent as it spreads.

HOW TO PREVENT
- Immunize children against measles. Prevention is important because measles can have rare, but serious, complications.
- If a person has not been immunized against measles and is exposed to it, a gamma globulin (antibodies) injection may prevent or reduce the severity of the disease.

WHAT TO EXPECT

DIAGNOSTIC MEASURES
- Medical history and exam by a doctor.
- Diagnosis is usually determined by the appearance of the spots; however, laboratory studies may be required to rule out other disorders.

APPROPRIATE HEALTH CARE
- Home care after diagnosis.
- Doctor's treatment.

POSSIBLE COMPLICATIONS
- Ear and chest infections.
- Pneumonia.
- Encephalitis or meningitis.
- Strep throat.
- Death (Rare).

PROBABLE OUTCOME
- Symptoms usually subside after about 3 days.
- A child who has been immunized against measles will probably never develop it. A person who has been passively immunized with gamma globulin is protected against measles for about 3 months.

HOW TO TREAT

GENERAL MEASURES
- Treatment involves rest, relief of symptoms and isolation during the communicable period.
- Use a cool-mist, ultrasonic humidifier to soothe the cough and to thin lung secretions so they can be coughed up more easily. Clean humidifier daily.
- Take morning and evening temperatures; keep a record. If the fever is 101F (38.3C) or higher, reduce it.

MEDICATION
- Your doctor will not prescribe antibiotics for measles, which is a virus. However, if complications arise, such as pneumonia or a middle-ear infection, antibiotics may be necessary.
- Don't give aspirin to a person younger than 18. Use acetaminophen instead to relieve discomfort and reduce fever. Some research shows a link between the use of aspirin in children during a virus illness and the development of Reye's syndrome.

ACTIVITY—Rest until the fever and rash disappear. Encourage a child to rest, but don't force it. Light activities are acceptable once eyes are not painful. Children should not return to school until 7 to 10 days after the fever and rash disappear.

DIET—No special diet. Drink extra fluids, including water, tea, lemonade, cola and fruit juice. Maintaining an adequate fluid intake is very important in keeping lung secretions thin and preventing lung complications.

CALL YOUR DOCTOR IF

- You or your child have symptoms of measles.
- The following occurs during treatment:
  High fever, accompanied by a sore throat.
  Severe headache, even several weeks after infection.
  Earache.
  Convulsion.
  Excessive lethargy or drowsiness.
  Breathing rate above 35 breaths-per- minute or breathing difficulty.

MELANOMA

GENERAL INFORMATION

DEFINITION—A skin cancer that spreads to other areas of the body, primarily the lymph nodes, liver, lungs and central nervous system. Most melanomas begin in a mole or other pre-existing skin lesion.

BODY PARTS INVOLVED—Usually in skin of the head, neck, legs or back. It appears rarely in the eye, mouth, vagina or anus.

SEX OR AGE MOST AFFECTED—Adults.

SIGNS & SYMPTOMS—A flat or slightly raised skin lesion that can be black, brown, blue, red, white or a mixture of all colors. Its borders are often irregular and may bleed.

CAUSES—Uncontrolled growth of cells that give skin its brownish color (melanocytes). When the cells grow down into deep skin layers, they invade blood vessels and lymph vessels and are spread to other body areas.

RISK INCREASES WITH
- Moles on the skin.
- Occupations or activities involving excessive sun exposure, such as farming, construction work, athletics or sunbathing.
- Pregnancy.
- Genetic factors. This is most common in light-complexioned, blonde people. It is rare in black people.
- Radiation treatment or excessive exposure to ultraviolet light, as with sun lamps.
- Family history of melanoma.
- Living in "sunbelt" areas of the U.S.

HOW TO PREVENT
- Protect yourself from excessive sun exposure. Wear broad-rimmed hats and protective clothing. Use SPF 15 or greater sun-block preparations on exposed skin. This is especially important in the adolescent years.
- Examine your skin, including soles of the feet, regularly for changes in pigmented areas. Ask a family member to examine your back. See your doctor about any skin area (especially brown or black) that becomes multicolored, develops irregular edges or surfaces, bleeds or changes in any way. See Skin Examination in Appendix.
- Community provided, skin cancer screening clinics available in some areas.

WHAT TO EXPECT

DIAGNOSTIC MEASURES
- Your own observation of suspicious growths.
- Medical history and physical exam by a doctor.
- Biopsy (see Glossary) of suspicious lesions. The melanoma's depth must be established to determine appropriate treatment.

APPROPRIATE HEALTH CARE
- Doctor's treatment.
- Surgery to remove suspicious skin lesions or to remove nearby lymph glands, if the tumor has spread. Skin graft may be necessary to avoid an unsightly scar. (See Melanoma Removal in Surgery section.)
- Radiation treatment, if the tumor has spread.

POSSIBLE COMPLICATIONS—Fatal spread to lungs, liver, brain or other internal organs.

PROBABLE OUTCOME—Varies greatly. Early melanomas that have not grown downward are curable with surgical removal. Once the tumor has spread to distant organs, this condition is currently considered incurable and fatal in a short time. However, symptoms can be relieved or controlled.

Scientific research into causes and treatment continues, so there is hope for increasingly effective treatment and cure.

HOW TO TREAT

GENERAL MEASURES
- Once diagnosis is made, get frequent body examinations to check for other lesions.
- The more you can learn and understand about a disease, the more you will be able to make informed decisions about where to go for your care, the treatments available, the risks involved, side effects of therapy and expected outcome.
- See Resources for Additional Information.

MEDICATION—Your doctor may prescribe anticancer (chemotherapy) drugs.

ACTIVITY—No restrictions except those involving sun exposure.

DIET—No special diet.

CALL YOUR DOCTOR IF

- You have symptoms of melanoma.
- During treatment, changes occur in another skin area.
- New, unexplained symptoms develop. Drugs used in treatment may produce side effects.

MÉNIÈRE'S DISEASE

GENERAL INFORMATION

DEFINITION—Increased fluid in the inner ear's semicircular canals, which normally help maintain balance. Excess fluid produces pressure in the inner ear, disturbing balance and sometimes reducing hearing.

BODY PARTS INVOLVED—Semicircular canals of the inner ear, usually on one side only (80-85%).

SEX OR AGE MOST AFFECTED
- Both sexes, but slightly more common in women.
- Adults between ages 30 and 60.

SIGNS & SYMPTOMS—The following occur with every acute attack:
- Severe dizziness.
- Vertigo (feeling that you are spinning or everything around you is spinning).
- Noises in the affected ear, such as ringing or buzzing.
- Hearing loss that increases with each attack.
Possible accompanying symptoms:
- Vomiting.
- Sweating.
- Jerky eye movements.
- Loss of balance.

CAUSES—The exact cause is unknown. Suggested causes involve an inner ear response to a variety of injuries. There is an increase in the amount of fluid in the membranous labyrinth (the canals in the inner ear that control balance).

RISK INCREASES WITH
- Stress.
- Allergy.
- Increased salt intake.
- Noise.

HOW TO PREVENT—Avoid risk factors where possible.

WHAT TO EXPECT

DIAGNOSTIC MEASURES
- Your own observation of symptoms.
- Medical history and physical exam by a doctor.
- Diagnostic tests may include laboratory blood studies to rule out other disorders, various hearing tests, MRI (see Glossary) to rule out acoustic tumor.

APPROPRIATE HEALTH CARE
- Self-care after diagnosis.
- Doctor's treatment.
- Treatment usually consists of rest and medication to control the symptoms.
- Surgical procedure on the affected labyrinth may be utilized in some patients with chronic Ménière's.

POSSIBLE COMPLICATIONS
- Permanent hearing loss.
- Chronic noises in the ear.

PROBABLE OUTCOME—Attacks of Ménière's disease usually recur over a period of years. Mild attacks may last a half hour to several days. Severe attacks may last several weeks. Some symptoms can be controlled. The condition is frustrating but not life-threatening.

HOW TO TREAT

GENERAL MEASURES
- Avoid glaring light and don't read during attacks.
- Severe attacks may be accompanied by anxiety attacks or migraines.

MEDICATION—Your doctor may prescribe:
- To treat an acute attack, intravenous atropine or diazepam, or scopolamine via a patch.
- Antinausea drugs.
- Tranquilizers to reduce dizziness.
- Antihistamines, which lessen symptoms in some persons.
- Diuretics to decrease fluid in the inner ear.

ACTIVITY
- Rest quietly in bed until dizziness and nausea disappear.
- Don't walk without assistance.
- Avoid sudden changes in position.
- Don't drive, climb ladders or work around dangerous machinery.

DIET
- Decrease salt intake.
- Limit total intake during an attack because of nausea.

CALL YOUR DOCTOR IF

- You have symptoms of Ménière's disease.
- The following occurs during treatment:
  Decreased hearing in either ear.
  Persistent vomiting.
  Convulsions.
  Fainting.
  Fever of 101F (38.3C) or higher.
- New, unexplained symptoms develop. Drugs used in treatment may produce side effects.

MENINGITIS, ASEPTIC
(Viral Meningitis)

 GENERAL INFORMATION

DEFINITION—Inflammation of the meninges (thin membranes that cover the brain and spinal cord). This is contagious.

BODY PARTS INVOLVED—Brain; spinal cord.

SEX OR AGE MOST AFFECTED—Both sexes; all ages.

SIGNS & SYMPTOMS
- Fever.
- Headache.
- Irritability.
- Eyes that are sensitive to light.
- Stiff neck.
- Vomiting.
- Confusion, lethargy and drowsiness.

CAUSES
- Viruses of several types, including the polio virus.
- Fungi, including yeasts.
- A reaction—probably an autoimmune response—following various viral illnesses, such as measles.

RISK INCREASES WITH
- Recent measles, rubella (German measles) or various types of flu.
- Immunosuppressive treatment, such as for cancer or following an organ transplant.
- Poor nutrition.
- Recent illness that has lowered resistance.
- Meningitis epidemics. The disease becomes more severe as it spreads from person to person.

HOW TO PREVENT—Keep immunizations up to date against all viruses for which vaccines are available.

 WHAT TO EXPECT

DIAGNOSTIC MEASURES
- Your own observation of symptoms.
- Medical history and physical exam by a doctor.
- Laboratory studies, such as blood-cell counts and examination of the cerebrospinal fluid.
- CT scan or MRI (see Glossary for both) of the brain.

APPROPRIATE HEALTH CARE
- Doctor's treatment.
- Hospitalization for most cases.

POSSIBLE COMPLICATIONS
- Permanent brain damage (rare).
- Muscle impairment or paralysis (uncommon).

PROBABLE OUTCOME—Most patients recover fully from viral meningitis without specific therapy—unlike bacterial meningitis, in which antibiotics may be life-saving.

 HOW TO TREAT

GENERAL MEASURES—Treatment involves hospital care for any support measures that might be necessary.

MEDICATION
- If aseptic meningitis is caused by a virus, there is no medication for it. The body defenses will usually cure it.
- Your doctor may prescribe antifungal drugs, such as amphoterecin B, if the meningitis is caused by a fungus; antinausea drugs and stronger pain medications may be needed.
- Avoid aspirin for pain; it may cause bleeding.

ACTIVITY—Rest in bed in a darkened room. Resume your normal activities as soon as symptoms improve.

DIET—No special diet. Drink 6 to 8 glasses of fluid daily, even if you don't feel like it.

 CALL YOUR DOCTOR IF

- You have symptoms of aseptic meningitis.
- New, unexplained symptoms develop. Drugs used in treatment may produce side effects.

MENINGITIS, BACTERIAL
(Spinal Meningitis)

GENERAL INFORMATION

DEFINITION—Bacterial infection or inflammation of the meninges (thin membranes that cover the brain and spinal cord).

BODY PARTS INVOLVED—Central nervous system.

SEX OR AGE MOST AFFECTED—All ages, but more severe in persons under age 2 or over age 60.

SIGNS & SYMPTOMS
- Fever, chills and sweating (may be absent in critically ill persons).
- Headache.
- Irritability.
- Eyes sensitive to light; pupils may be of different size.
- Stiff neck.
- Vomiting.
- Red or purple skin rash.
- Confusion, lethargy, drowsiness or unconsciousness.
- Sore throat or other signs of respiratory illness may precede other symptoms.

CAUSES—Infection caused by bacteria, from the following sources:
- Infection in another body part, such as the lung, ear, nose, throat or sinus, that spreads to the meninges.
- Head injury, such as a fractured skull, that allows infection to enter.

RISK INCREASES WITH
- Newborns and infants.
- Adults over 60.
- Illness that has lowered resistance.
- Poor nutrition.
- Use of drugs that decrease the body's immune responses, such as anticancer drugs.
- Alcoholism.
- Sinus infection or bacterial skin infections around eyes or nose.

HOW TO PREVENT
- Get medical care for treatment of any infection in your body to prevent its spread.
- Avoid contact with anyone who has meningitis (depending on bacterial type). Those who have had close contact with a person with meningitis may need preventive antibiotic treatment even if they have no symptoms.

WHAT TO EXPECT

DIAGNOSTIC MEASURES
- Your own observation of symptoms.
- Medical history and physical exam by a doctor.

- Laboratory studies, such as blood-sugar tests and cultures of throat, blood, nose or other infection sites.
- Lumbar puncture, CT scan (see Glossary for both), x-rays of chest and head.

APPROPRIATE HEALTH CARE
- Doctor's care.
- Hospitalization, often in an Intensive Care Unit.
- Constant nursing to ensure prompt recognition of any possible complications.
- Treatment for any co-existing medical conditions.

POSSIBLE COMPLICATIONS—Death or permanent brain damage—including paralysis, hearing loss, speech difficulty and intellectual impairment—if not treated quickly.

PROBABLE OUTCOME—Full recovery is likely in 2 to 3 weeks with treatment, if no complications arise.

HOW TO TREAT

GENERAL MEASURES—The family should stay in close contact with the patient's doctor and help by making their visits with the patient as supportive as possible.

MEDICATION—Your doctor may prescribe:
- Intravenous antibiotics. Dosage and type will depend on what bacteria is causing meningitis, patient's age and other health factors.
- Corticosteroids.

ACTIVITY—While in the hospital, you will need bed rest in a darkened room. After a 2- to 3-week recovery, you should be as active as your strength allows.

DIET—You may be given intravenous nutrients in the hospital. At home, eat a normal, well-balanced diet. Vitamin and mineral supplements should not be necessary unless you have a deficiency or cannot eat normally.

CALL YOUR DOCTOR IF

- You have symptoms of bacterial meningitis.
- Temperature rises to 101F (38.3C) or higher during treatment.
- New, unexplained symptoms develop. Drugs used in treatment may produce side effects.
- You have had contact with someone who has meningitis.

MENOPAUSE

GENERAL INFORMATION

DEFINITION—The permanent cessation of menstruation. This occurs as early as age 40 or as late as age 55 and usually spans 1 to 2 years. It is usually diagnosed in females after 1 year of absent periods. Menopause is only one event in the "climacteric," a biological change in all body tissue and body systems that occurs in both sexes between the mid-40s and mid-60s. Menopause occurring before age 40 is termed premature and may need medical evaluation.

BODY PARTS INVOLVED—Female reproductive system, with secondary effects in other body parts.

SEX OR AGE MOST AFFECTED—Women, especially between ages 45 and 50.

SIGNS & SYMPTOMS
Physical changes (directly associated with decreased blood levels of female hormones):
- Menstrual irregularity.
- Hot flashes or flushes—sensations of heat spreading from the waist or chest toward the neck, face and upper arms.
- Headaches; dizziness.
- Rapid or irregular heartbeat.
- Vaginal itching, burning or discomfort during intercourse, beginning a few years after menopause.
- Bloating in the upper abdomen; bladder irritability; breast tenderness.
Emotional changes (associated with lower hormone levels and conflicting feelings about aging and loss of fertility):
- Mood changes; pronounced tension and anxiety; sleeping difficulty; depression or melancholy and fatigue.

CAUSES
- A normal decline in ovary function, resulting in decreased levels of the female hormones, estrogen and progesterone.
- Surgical removal of both ovaries.

RISK INCREASES WITH—Menopause is a natural part of the aging process for women.

HOW TO PREVENT—Menopause cannot be avoided, but its effects may be controlled.

WHAT TO EXPECT

DIAGNOSTIC MEASURES
- Medical history and exam by a doctor.
- Laboratory blood studies of hormone levels (sometimes).

APPROPRIATE HEALTH CARE
- Doctor's diagnosis to rule out other causes of menstrual changes.
- Self-care after diagnosis.

- Psychotherapy or counseling, if emotional changes interfere with personal life or work.

POSSIBLE COMPLICATIONS
- Increased irritability and susceptibility to infection in the urinary tract.
- Decreased skin elasticity and vaginal moisture.
- Increased risk of hardening of the arteries, heart disease, stroke and osteoporosis after menopause.
- Changes in feelings of self-worth.

PROBABLE OUTCOME—Menopause is a normal process—not an illness. Most women make an easy transition without crisis.

HOW TO TREAT

GENERAL MEASURES
- Continue to use birth-control measures until 12 months after your last menstrual period.
- Reduce stress in your life.
- If you take estrogen-replacement therapy, have a Pap smear annually or as recommended.
- Lifestyle changes may be brought about by menopause. Stay as healthy and happy as you can and live life to the fullest.
- Consider bone density testing to evaluate risk for osteoporosis.

MEDICATION—Your doctor may prescribe:
- Estrogen replacement therapy (ERT) or it may be referred to as HRT (hormone replacement therapy). Because hormone treatment has benefits as well as risks, learn all you can about replacement therapy before deciding on treatment. ERT helps prevent osteoporosis and coronary heart disease, as well as bringing relief of symptoms of menopause (hot flashes, vaginal dryness).
- Calcium supplements if your diet does not provide at least 1000 mg of calcium a day.
- Vaginal creams to help dryness.

ACTIVITY—No restrictions. Active exercise is beneficial. Weight-bearing activities (such as walking) help strengthen bones.

DIET—No special diet. Increase calcium intake.

CALL YOUR DOCTOR IF

- You have symptoms of menopause. Other causes should be ruled out.
- You experience excessive bleeding, prolonged periods or spotting between your expected periods. These may be signs of other disorders.
- Bleeding appears 6 months or more after your last period.
- New unexplained symptoms develop. Hormones used in treatment may produce side effects.

ILLNESS & DISORDERS

MENORRHAGIA

GENERAL INFORMATION

DEFINITION—A fairly common disorder that is characterized by unusual heavy or prolonged period of menstrual flow. The average amount of blood loss during a normal menstrual period is about two ounces. With menorrhagia, a woman may lose three ounces or more. It rarely signifies a serious underlying disorder.

BODY PARTS INVOLVED—Female reproductive system.

SEX OR AGE MOST AFFECTED—Females from age 12 to 55.

SIGNS & SYMPTOMS
- Anovulation.
- Excessive menstrual flow (varies greatly from woman to woman).
- Menstrual period lasts for more than 7 days.
- Large clots of blood may pass.
- Paleness and fatigue (anemia).

CAUSES
- Imbalance of female hormones (estrogen and progesterone).
- Fibroids (benign uterine tumors).
- Pelvic infection.
- Endometrial disorder.
- Intrauterine device (IUD).
- Hypothyroidism.

RISK INCREASES WITH
- Obesity.
- Estrogen administration (without progestin).
- Young women who have not established a regular ovulation cycle.
- Women approaching menopause.

HOW TO PREVENT—To detect early signs of reproductive system disorders, have an annual pelvic examination with a cervical smear test (Pap smear).

WHAT TO EXPECT

DIAGNOSTIC MEASURES
- Your own observation of symptoms.
- Medical history and physical exam by a doctor.
- Special medical diagnostic tests (e.g., pregnancy test, endometrial biopsy, blood test) to help determine cause of bleeding may be performed.

APPROPRIATE HEALTH CARE
- Treatment usually depends on age of woman, whether or not she wants children and on any underlying disorder.
- Dilatation and curettage (D & C) may be performed.
- Hysterectomy may be considered in persistent cases where fertility is not desired.

POSSIBLE COMPLICATIONS
- Anemia due to excessive blood loss.
- Surgery may be required.

PROBABLE OUTCOME
- Varies with cause of bleeding.
- Patients with hormonal causes usually respond to treatment.

HOW TO TREAT

GENERAL MEASURES
- Wear extra sanitary pads during excessive flow to prevent embarrassment.
- If using an IUD, consider a change to another method of contraception.

MEDICATION—Your doctor may prescribe:
- Hormone therapy to control bleeding.
- Other medications to control the bleeding, if hormones cannot be taken for some reason.
- Iron replacement therapy for anemia.

ACTIVITY—Reducing activities during menstruation and resting with feet up may be helpful.

DIET—No special diet.

CALL YOUR DOCTOR IF

- You have signs or symptoms of menorrhagia.
- Symptoms worsen after treatment begins.
- New or unexplained symptoms develop. Drugs used in treatment may cause side effects.

MENTAL RETARDATION

GENERAL INFORMATION

DEFINITION—A below-average intellectual functioning (an IQ of less than 70) as assessed by a standard IQ test. An IQ of 80 to 130 is considered normal; 100 is average. The impaired intellectual function results in a limited ability to cope with the normal responsibilities of life. Retardation is classified as mild (IQ 50 to 70), moderate (IQ 35 to 49), severe (IQ 20 to 34), or profound (IQ less than 20). Mild retardation is the most common form (over 80% of cases).

SEX OR AGE MOST AFFECTED—Both sexes; all ages.

SIGNS & SYMPTOMS
• Many mildly retarded children are not identified until they enter school. Mental tasks such as math are done more slowly, reading ability is impaired and emotions may be more childlike. May have hyperactivity and/or repetitive involuntary movements.
• May have development delays including speech and language problems, delayed motor skills, sensory defects (slow in responding to people, sounds, toys, etc.), neurological impairments.
• May have seizures, fecal and urinary incontinence, hearing problems.
• Profoundly and severely retarded children are often diagnosed at birth.

CAUSES
• Genetic, inborn errors of metabolism or chromosome disorders. Down syndrome is the most frequent genetic disorder causing retardation.
• Intrauterine–Congenital infections, placental-fetal malfunction, complications of pregnancy.
• Perinatal (just before birth)–Prematurity, postmaturity, birth injury, metabolic disorders.
• Postnatal (after birth)–Endocrine or metabolic disorders, infection, trauma, toxic and other causes of brain damage, abuse.

RISK INCREASES WITH
• Poor prenatal care.
• Family history of mental retardation.
• Lower socioeconomic status.

HOW TO PREVENT
• In some cases, cause is undetermined, and there are no preventive measures.
• Genetic counseling and prenatal genetic diagnosis will help in some cases.
• Proper prenatal care helps, as does avoidance of drugs and alcohol during pregnancy.

WHAT TO EXPECT

DIAGNOSTIC MEASURES
• Your own observation of symptoms.
• Physical exam and mental tests by a doctor.

APPROPRIATE HEALTH CARE—Genetic evaluation and counseling.

POSSIBLE COMPLICATIONS
• Emotional or behavioral problems in the child.
• Coping stresses placed on the family.
• Sexual or other exploitation of the person.

PROBABLE OUTCOME
• Mildly retarded people can learn to live independent, productive lives.
• Moderately retarded people are trainable, but often require protective care (e.g., group home).
• Severely and profoundly retarded people usually require continuous care.

HOW TO TREAT

GENERAL MEASURES
• Special training, education and behavior modification will enhance a retarded child's skills. The retardation cannot be reversed, but much can be done to maximize the child's potential.
• Family support is vital; therapy is helpful to learn to accept and cope with the demands and time-consuming task of caring for the child.
• Support groups for families are helpful.

MEDICATION—Your doctor may prescribe medications for associated medical problems, such as anticonvulsants for seizures. In general, care for retarded people is educational, not medical.

ACTIVITY—As fully active as child's physical condition permits.

DIET—No special diet.

CALL YOUR DOCTOR IF

• You are concerned about your child's development.
• Following diagnosis of mental retardation, any new or unusual signs or symptoms occur in the child or you feel unable to cope.

MIGRAINE

GENERAL INFORMATION

DEFINITION—Migraine refers to a group of symptoms that may occur together. The most noted one is an incapacitating headache, usually on one side of the head, which can last from 2 to 72 hours. Episodes of migraines can occur weekly in some people; others may have less than one a year.

BODY PARTS INVOLVED—Blood vessels, central nervous system, gastrointestinal.

SEX OR AGE MOST AFFECTED
- Both sexes, but more common in females.
- Adolescents and adults.

SIGNS & SYMPTOMS—The nature of attacks varies between persons and from time to time in the same person. Symptoms appear as follows:
- An aura that precedes the headache. This may affect vision, hearing or smell.
- The most common symptom is the inability to see clearly, followed by seeing bright spots and zig-zag patterns. Visual disturbances may last several minutes or hours, then disappear.
- Dull, boring pain in the temple that spreads to the side of the head. Pain becomes intense.
- Nausea and vomiting. In other types of migraine attack, the above symptoms (vision disturbances, headache or vomiting) may be absent; other symptoms may be present.

CAUSES—Exact cause is uncertain. A disturbance in blood circulation in the head accompanies migraine and may be a cause. Attacks may be triggered by:
- Tension. Emotional problems are probably the most common reason for migraine attacks, but headaches don't necessarily coincide with emotional upset. They often occur on weekends when stress is decreased.
- Menstruation; use of oral contraceptives.
- Fatigue; missing meals.
- Consumption of alcohol or certain foods.

RISK INCREASES WITH
Stress; family history of migraines; smoking; excess alcohol consumption; use of many prescription and nonprescription drugs.

HOW TO PREVENT
- Reduce stress in your life where possible (see How to Cope with Stress in Appendix).
- Take a prescription drug to help prevent attacks. Ask your doctor.
- Avoid those factors that trigger attacks.
- Learn to look for warning signs of a headache and do something different (take a walk, etc.).

WHAT TO EXPECT

DIAGNOSTIC MEASURES
- Medical history and exam by a doctor.

- Laboratory blood studies or CT scan (see Glossary) of the head may be done to rule out other disorders.

APPROPRIATE HEALTH CARE
Self-care after diagnosis; doctor's treatment.

POSSIBLE COMPLICATIONS—None expected.

PROBABLE OUTCOME—Symptoms can be controlled with treatment.

HOW TO TREAT

GENERAL MEASURES
- At the first sign of a migraine attack:
  Apply a cold cloth or ice pack to your head or splash your face with cold water.
  Lie down in a quiet, dark room for several hours. Wedge pillows to support head.
  Relax and sleep if possible. Minimize noise, light and odors (especially cooking odors and tobacco smoke). Don't read.
- See Resources for Additional Information.

MEDICATION—A wide variety of drugs can be prescribed for migraine symptoms and prevention. Follow all prescription instructions carefully. Your doctor may prescribe:
- Ergotamines (contain caffeine) in oral form, suppository or inhaler.
- Aspirin, acetaminophen or ibuprofen.
- Drugs that combine acetaminophen and a narcotic (codeine).
- Antihistamines to expand blood vessels.
- Antiemetics to decrease nausea and vomiting.
- Vasoconstrictors to narrow blood vessels.
- Triptans (Imitrex) in self-administered subcutaneous (under the skin) injection or oral tablets.
- Beta-adrenergic or calcium channel blockers or tricyclic antidepressants to prevent attacks, if headaches are so frequent that you can't function normally. These medications may have undesirable side effects and may not help everyone.

ACTIVITY—Rest during attacks; exercise regularly; keep a regular sleep pattern.

DIET
- Don't skip meals. At least snack.
- Because some attacks are caused by foods, avoid or limit: cheese, chocolate, spicy foods, mixed spices, monosodium glutamate (MSG), nitrites or nitrates (used in preserved meats such as bacon, hot dogs or deli meats). Keep a record of what you ate before each attack. Avoid foods that may trigger migraine attacks.
- Avoid alcohol.

CALL YOUR DOCTOR IF

You have a migraine attack that persists longer than 24 hours, despite treatment.

MISCARRIAGE (Spontaneous Abortion)

GENERAL INFORMATION

DEFINITION—Premature termination of a pregnancy before the fetus can survive outside the uterus. It occurs in about 30% of first pregnancies and frequently occurs so early that the woman is unaware that she is pregnant. Most miscarriages occur during the first 14 weeks of pregnancy. Many miscarriages are only "threatened," and the pregnancy continues to term, although symptoms may be the same.

BODY PARTS INVOLVED—Reproductive system.

SEX OR AGE MOST AFFECTED—Women of childbearing age.

SIGNS & SYMPTOMS
- Uterine cramps.
- Vaginal bleeding—from slight to heavy.

CAUSES
During the first 3 months (first trimester):
- An abnormal or defective fetus.
- Uterine abnormalities that prevent the fertilized egg from growing normally.
During the second trimester:
- Uterine abnormalities that cause detachment of the fetus and placenta.
- Severe psychological stress (maybe).
Anytime:
- Use of drugs that harm the fetus.
- Infections, especially virus infections, such as rubella or influenza.

RISK INCREASES WITH
- Stress; smoking; poor nutrition.
- Illness that has lowered resistance.
- Recent serious infection.
- Medical history of endocrine diseases, such as diabetes mellitus or hypothyroidism.

HOW TO PREVENT—During pregnancy:
- Obtain regular medical checkups.
- Eat a normal, well-balanced diet.
- Don't drink alcohol, smoke cigarettes or use recreational drugs. Don't use any medications, including nonprescription drugs, without consulting doctor.

WHAT TO EXPECT

DIAGNOSTIC MEASURES
- Medical history and exam by a doctor.
- Ultrasound (see Glossary).

APPROPRIATE HEALTH CARE
- Self-care.
- Doctor's treatment.
- Surgery: D & C (dilatation and curettage) or D & E (dilatation and evacuation) to remove any remaining tissue or a dead fetus (sometimes).
- Hospitalization (sometimes).
- Psychotherapy or grief counseling may help.

POSSIBLE COMPLICATIONS
- Uterine infection, signaled by fever, chills and aching; hemorrhaging from other body parts.
- "Incomplete" abortion, in which some placenta or fetal tissue remains in the uterus, or missed abortion, in which the fetus dies but remains in the uterus.

PROBABLE OUTCOME
- An inevitable miscarriage cannot be stopped.
- With treatment, a miscarriage is not a life-threatening condition. It usually does not affect a woman's ability to carry a healthy baby to term in the future.
- Feelings of loss and grief are common. If these persist, seek emotional help.

HOW TO TREAT

GENERAL MEASURES
- For a threatened miscarriage, follow your doctor's orders. Bed rest is often enough to stabilize the pregnancy.
- After a miscarriage:
  Expect a small amount of vaginal bleeding or spotting for 8 to 10 days.
  Don't use tampons for 2 to 4 weeks.
  Wait through several normal menstrual cycles (usually 2 to 4) before attempting to become pregnant. Your doctor will advise you.

MEDICATION
- For a threatened miscarriage, medicine usually is not necessary.
- Your doctor may prescribe:
  Oxytocin to control bleeding in some patients.
  Pain medication if needed.
  After a miscarriage, antibiotics for infection.
  Blood transfusions for severe blood loss.
  RhoD (immune globulin) for Rh negative female.

ACTIVITY
- For a threatened miscarriage: Rest in bed until symptoms disappear. Avoid sexual intercourse until the outcome is known.
- After a miscarriage, rest often and reduce activity during the next 48 hours.

DIET
- For a threatened miscarriage, drink fluids only, if bleeding and cramping are severe.
- After a miscarriage, no special diet.

CALL YOUR DOCTOR IF

- Any bleeding occurs during pregnancy.
- Bleeding and cramps worsen during a threatened miscarriage or you pass tissue.
- Fever and chills occur during a threatened miscarriage or following miscarriage.
- Unexplained bruising occurs after a miscarriage.
- Infection develops while you are pregnant.

MITRAL VALVE PROLAPSE

GENERAL INFORMATION

DEFINITION—A fairly common and often benign disorder in which a slight deformity of the mitral valve (situated in the left side of the heart) can produce a degree of leakage (mitral insufficiency). Mitral valve prolapse causes a characteristic heart murmur that may be heard through a stethoscope.

BODY PARTS INVOLVED—Heart.

SEX OR AGE MOST AFFECTED—Both sexes; all ages. It occurs more frequently in young to middle age women.

SIGNS & SYMPTOMS
- Often no symptoms are present and the condition may be discovered on a routine examination.
- Chest pain (sharp, dull or pressing).
- Fatigue, shortness of breath.
- Dizziness.
- Anxiety.
- Lightheadedness when getting up from a chair or bed.
- Palpitations.

CAUSES
- Unknown in many instances.
- Some evidence that the condition is inherited.
- May be associated with congenital heart disease.

RISK INCREASES WITH
- Patients with cardiomyopathy, rheumatic fever or coronary artery disease (see all in Illness section).
- Scoliosis or other skeletal abnormalities.

HOW TO PREVENT—No preventive measures.

WHAT TO EXPECT

DIAGNOSTIC MEASURES
- Your own observation of symptoms.
- Medical history and physical exam by a doctor.

APPROPRIATE HEALTH CARE
- For most patients, no treatment is necessary. Further evaluation may be done every 2-3 years.
- Rarely, heart valve surgery may be considered in select patients.

POSSIBLE COMPLICATIONS
- The risk of complications is very low.
- Mitral regurgitation (blood leaks backward through the mitral valve).
The following are rare:
- Congestive heart disease.
- Stroke.
- Infective endocarditis (inflammation of the internal lining of the heart, particularly heart valves).

PROBABLE OUTCOME—It is usually a benign disorder that does not prevent a normal active life.

HOW TO TREAT

GENERAL MEASURES
- Be reassured that for most people, the condition is benign and requires no treatment except follow-up evaluation.
- Antibiotics may be recommended for any dental cleaning or potentially nonsterile surgeries (urological and intestinal). Ask your doctor.

MEDICATION—Usually no medications are needed. If symptoms (e.g., chest pain) are present, heart drugs or other therapies may be prescribed.

ACTIVITY—No restrictions.

DIET
- No special diet. Keep fluid intake at normal recommended levels.
- For some of the symptoms, such as palpitations, discontinuing caffeine and alcohol may be helpful.

CALL YOUR DOCTOR IF

You have signs or symptoms of mitral valve prolapse.

MOLLUSCUM CONTAGIOSUM

 GENERAL INFORMATION

DEFINITION—A contagious, common, benign virus infection of the skin.

BODY PARTS INVOLVED—Skin anywhere on the body. The virus usually occurs on the face in children. In adults, it usually occurs on the inner thighs, abdomen and genitals.

SEX OR AGE MOST AFFECTED—Both sexes; all ages.

SIGNS & SYMPTOMS—Papules (small, raised bumps on the skin) with the following characteristics:
• Bumps are firm, smooth, domed with a central pit and skin-colored or white. The overlying skin is transparent and thin.
• Bumps are usually 2mm to 3mm in diameter. A few may be as large as 10mm.
• Bumps cause eye irritation if they are on the eyelids.
• Bumps don't hurt or itch.

CAUSES—DNA virus of the pox group. For adults, this virus may be transmitted sexually. For children, transmission can occur from swimming pools. The incubation is 2 weeks to 2 months.

RISK INCREASES WITH
• Immunosuppression from drugs or illness.
• Close contact with an infected person.

HOW TO PREVENT
• For adults, avoid contact with infected people.
• To prevent spread to other parts of the body or to other people, don't scratch bumps.

 WHAT TO EXPECT

DIAGNOSTIC MEASURES
• Your own observation of symptoms.
• Medical history and physical exam by a doctor.

APPROPRIATE HEALTH CARE
• Doctor's treatment to remove the papules with liquid nitrogen, curettage (see Glossary) or topical medication.
• Self-care after removal.

POSSIBLE COMPLICATIONS—Scarring or disfigurement (rare).

PROBABLE OUTCOME—If untreated, a few papules may increase to 20 to 50 lesions in several weeks. They will disappear spontaneously in 10 to 24 months. However, they should be treated to prevent their spread to other persons.

 HOW TO TREAT

GENERAL MEASURES
• After treatment with liquid nitrogen, leave the blisters alone. The tops will come off spontaneously in 7 to 14 days.
• Keep blisters dry. Cover with small adhesive bandages any that may be irritated by clothing.

MEDICATION—Medicine usually is not necessary for this disorder. In some cases, your doctor may apply cantharidin (Cantharone) or other topical medication to kill the virus.

ACTIVITY—No restrictions, except to avoid sexual relations until bumps disappear.

DIET—No special diet.

 CALL YOUR DOCTOR IF

• You have symptoms of molluscum contagiosum.
• The following occurs after treatment:
  Fever.
  Signs of infection (swelling, redness, pain, tenderness or warmth) at the treatment site.

ILLNESS & DISORDERS

MONONUCLEOSIS, INFECTIOUS
(Mono)

 GENERAL INFORMATION

DEFINITION—An infectious viral disease that affects the respiratory system, liver and lymphatic system.

BODY PARTS INVOLVED—Lymph nodes; liver; spleen; throat; bronchial tubes.

SEX OR AGE MOST AFFECTED—Adolescents and young adults (12 to 40 years).

SIGNS & SYMPTOMS
- Fever.
- Sore throat (sometimes severe).
- Appetite loss.
- Fatigue.
- Swollen lymph glands, usually in the neck, underarms or groin.
- Enlarged spleen.
- Enlarged liver.
- Jaundice with yellow skin and eyes (sometimes).
- Headache.
- General aching.

CAUSES—A contagious virus (Epstein-Barr virus) transmitted from person to person by close contact, such as kissing, shared food or coughing.

RISK INCREASES WITH
- Stress.
- Illness that has lowered resistance.
- Fatigue or overwork. The high incidence among college students and military recruits may result from inadequate rest and crowded living conditions.
- High school or college attendance.

HOW TO PREVENT
- Avoid contact with persons having infectious mononucleosis.
- If you have mononucleosis, avoid contact with persons with immune deficiencies to prevent them from getting mononucleosis.

 WHAT TO EXPECT

DIAGNOSTIC MEASURES
- Your own observation of symptoms.
- Medical history and physical exam by a doctor.
- Laboratory blood tests.

APPROPRIATE HEALTH CARE
- Self-care after diagnosis.
- Doctor's treatment.

POSSIBLE COMPLICATIONS
- Ruptured spleen, resulting in emergency surgery (rare).
- Anemia.
- In rare cases, the heart, lungs or central nervous system could become involved, and the disease may prove to be serious.

PROBABLE OUTCOME—Spontaneous recovery in 10 days to 6 months. Fatigue frequently persists for 3 to 6 weeks after other symptoms disappear. A few patients experience a chronic form in which symptoms persist for months or years.

 HOW TO TREAT

GENERAL MEASURES
- No specific cure is available. Extra rest and healthy diet are important. No need for quarantine.
- To relieve the sore throat, gargle frequently with double-strength tea or warm salt water (1 teaspoon of salt to 8 oz. of water).
- Don't strain hard for bowel movements. This may injure an enlarged spleen.
- If you are a student, check on ways to continue school work while you are recovering.

MEDICATION
- For minor discomfort, you may use nonprescription drugs such as acetaminophen. Don't take aspirin because of its suspected association with Reye's syndrome.
- If symptoms are severe, your doctor may prescribe a short course of cortisone drugs.

ACTIVITY
- Rest in bed while you have fever. Complete bed rest is normally not necessary or beneficial. Resume activity gradually.
- Don't participate in contact sports until at least 1 month after complete recovery or when your doctor gives approval.
- Avoid heavy lifting.

DIET—No special diet. You may not feel like eating while you are ill. Maintain an adequate fluid intake. Drink at least 8 glasses of water or juice a day—more during periods of high fever.

 CALL YOUR DOCTOR IF

- You have symptoms of infectious mononucleosis.
- The following occurs during treatment:
  Fever over 102F (38.9C).
  Constipation, which may cause straining.
  Severe pain in the upper left abdomen that lasts for 5 minutes or more.
  Swallowing or breathing difficulty from severe throat inflammation.

MORNING SICKNESS DURING PREGNANCY

GENERAL INFORMATION

DEFINITION—Nausea during pregnancy. This usually occurs in the morning but may occur at any time. Most pregnant women experience at least mild morning sickness.

BODY PARTS INVOLVED—Muscles of the intestinal tract; vomiting center in the hypothalamus gland.

SEX OR AGE MOST AFFECTED—Pregnant women.

SIGNS & SYMPTOMS—Mild to severe nausea—with or without vomiting—usually during the first 12 to 14 weeks of pregnancy.

CAUSES—Major hormone changes that take place to permit normal growth of the fetus. Progesterone and other hormones cause involuntary muscles to relax, probably slowing movement of food through the stomach and intestines. They may also affect the vomiting center in the brain.

In addition, blood sugar is lower during early pregnancy in many women, contributing to gastrointestinal upsets.

RISK INCREASES WITH—Multiple pregnancies (twins, triplets, etc.).

HOW TO PREVENT—Do not let your stomach get empty, eat something every two hours if necessary.

WHAT TO EXPECT

DIAGNOSTIC MEASURES
• Your own observation of symptoms.
• Medical history and physical exam by a doctor.

APPROPRIATE HEALTH CARE
• Self-care after diagnosis.
• Doctor's treatment, if morning sickness becomes disabling.

POSSIBLE COMPLICATIONS—Hyperemesis gravidarum, a condition of pregnancy characterized by severe nausea, vomiting, weight loss and electrolyte disturbance (rare).

PROBABLE OUTCOME—Usually stops after the first 3 to 4 months of pregnancy.

HOW TO TREAT

GENERAL MEASURES
• Keep rooms well-ventilated to prevent accumulation of cooking odors or cigarette smoke.
• Don't smoke cigarettes, and ask your family and friends not to smoke while you are experiencing morning sickness.
• Keep a positive attitude. If you have conflicts that you cannot resolve, ask for help from family, friends or professional counselors.
• Keep a daily record of your weight.

MEDICATION—Medicine is usually not necessary for this disorder. Don't take any medications during pregnancy without consulting your doctor. Your doctor may prescribe a trial of vitamin B-6, which appears safe at the present.

ACTIVITY—No restrictions.

DIET—The following may help minimize nausea:
• Place a small, quick-energy snack, such as soda crackers, at your bedside. Eat it before getting up in the morning.
• Eat a small snack at bedtime and when you get up to go to the bathroom during the night.
• Eat a snack as often as every hour or two during the day. Avoid large meals. Snacks should consist of high-protein foods, such as: peanut butter on apple slices or celery; nuts; a quarter-sandwich; cheese and crackers; milk; cottage cheese; yogurt sprinkled with granola; and turkey or chicken slices. Avoid foods that are high in fat and salt and low in nutrition.

CALL YOUR DOCTOR IF

• You have morning sickness that does not improve, despite the above measures.
• You vomit blood or material that resembles coffee grounds.
• You lose more than 1 or 2 pounds.

MOTION SICKNESS
(Car, Sea or Air Sickness)

GENERAL INFORMATION

DEFINITION—An unpleasant, temporary disturbance that occurs while traveling, characterized by dizziness and stomach upset.

BODY PARTS INVOLVED—Semicircular canals in the inner ear. These fluid-filled canals maintain balance.

SEX OR AGE MOST AFFECTED—Both sexes; all ages.

SIGNS & SYMPTOMS
- Loss of appetite.
- Nausea and vomiting.
- Spinning sensation.
- Weakness and unsteadiness.
- Confusion.
- Yawning.

CAUSES—Motion, especially airplane, boat or car; amusement park ride or swinging. Irregular motion causes fluid changes in the semicircular canals of the inner ear, which transmit signals to the brain's vomiting center.

HOW TO PREVENT
- Don't eat large meals or drink alcohol before and during travel.
- Sit in areas of the airplane (usually over the wings) or boat with the least motion.
- Recline in your seat, if possible.
- Breathe slowly and deeply.
- Avoid areas where others are smoking, if possible.
- On an airplane or bus, turn on the overhead air vent to improve air circulation.
- Don't read.
- Take medication to prevent motion sickness before you travel.
- Some airlines have developed behavior-modification techniques for those who are afraid to fly or have motion sickness. Contact the airline or your travel agent for information.
- Psychological factors contribute to motion sickness. Try to resolve concerns about travel before leaving home. Maintain a positive attitude.
- Consider preventive therapy. One technique involves desensitization (special training for using your eyes that may help avoid the symptoms of motion sickness).

WHAT TO EXPECT

DIAGNOSTIC MEASURES
- Your own observation of symptoms.
- Medical history and physical exam by a doctor, if motion sickness is recurrent and interferes with your life.

APPROPRIATE HEALTH CARE
- Self-care.
- Doctor's treatment, if you have a chronic illness that may be worsened by vomiting.
- Psychotherapy or counseling, if your occupation or lifestyle requires travel and you usually develop motion sickness.

POSSIBLE COMPLICATIONS
- Dehydration from vomiting.
- Falls and injuries from unsteadiness.

PROBABLE OUTCOME—Spontaneous recovery when the trip is over or soon thereafter.

HOW TO TREAT

GENERAL MEASURES
- Once you have the symptoms, try to rest in a dark room with a cool cloth over the eyes and forehead.
- Allowing yourself to vomit can help the nausea. Don't make yourself vomit.

MEDICATION
- For minor discomfort, you may use nonprescription drugs, such as dimenhydrate (Dramamine), or meclizine (Bonine) before and during travel.
- Your doctor may prescribe scopolamine patches to control symptoms. Remove promptly after travel is completed; long-term use is not recommended.

ACTIVITY—To minimize symptoms during travel, rest in a reclining position and fix your gaze on a distant object.

DIET—Eat lightly or not at all before and during brief trips. For longer trips, sip frequently on beverages—don't take large drinks—to maintain your fluid intake. Avoid alcohol, carbonated drinks and extra-cold beverages.

CALL YOUR DOCTOR IF

You plan to travel and have had disabling motion sickness in the past.

MOUTH OR TONGUE TUMOR, BENIGN

 GENERAL INFORMATION

DEFINITION—Abnormal new growth in the mouth or tongue that is unlikely to spread to other body parts. Benign mouth and tongue tumors usually occur singly and grow very slowly over 2 to 6 years.

BODY PARTS INVOLVED—Lips; gums; palate; tongue; membrane covering the lips and cheeks; floor of the mouth.

SEX OR AGE MOST AFFECTED—Adults over 60.

SIGNS & SYMPTOMS—A lump in any part of the mouth or tongue with the following characteristics:
- It may ulcerate and bleed.
- It may interfere with the way dentures fit.
- It may interfere with speech or swallowing.

CAUSES—Unknown, although it is most common in people who smoke cigarettes, cigars or pipes, or use chewing tobacco or snuff.

RISK INCREASES WITH
- Use of tobacco.
- Poorly fitting dentures.

HOW TO PREVENT
- Don't smoke or use tobacco.
- See your dentist for annual dental exams and for problems with denture fit.

 WHAT TO EXPECT

DIAGNOSTIC MEASURES
- Your own observation of symptoms.
- Medical history and physical exam by a doctor.
- Biopsy (see Glossary) of the tumor.

APPROPRIATE HEALTH CARE
- Doctor's or dentist's treatment.
- Self-care after diagnosis.
- Surgery to remove the tumor.

POSSIBLE COMPLICATIONS
- Cancerous change in the tumor (rare).
- Bleeding from the tumor.
- Infection in the tumor.

PROBABLE OUTCOME—Curable with surgical removal. Normal facial appearance can usually be restored by plastic surgery (if needed).

 HOW TO TREAT

GENERAL MEASURES—After surgery, cleanse the mouth 3 to 4 times a day with a soothing salt-water solution (1 teaspoon salt in 8 oz. warm water).

MEDICATION
- For minor discomfort, you may use nonprescription drugs such as acetaminophen.
- Your doctor may prescribe antibiotics, if infection exists.

ACTIVITY—No restrictions.

DIET—A liquid diet may be necessary for several days after surgery (see Liquid Diet in Appendix); no special diet after recovery.

 CALL YOUR DOCTOR IF

- You have symptoms of a mouth or tongue tumor.
- The following occurs after surgery:
  Fever.
  Bleeding at the surgical site.
  Unbearable pain.
- New, unexplained symptoms develop. Drugs used in treatment may produce side effects.

ILLNESS & DISORDERS

MULTIPLE MYELOMA
(Primary Bone-Marrow Cancer)

 GENERAL INFORMATION

DEFINITION—A malignancy beginning in the plasma cells of the bone marrow. Plasma cells normally produce antibodies to help destroy germs and protect against infection. With myeloma, this function becomes impaired, and the body cannot deal effectively with infection.

BODY PARTS INVOLVED—Bone marrow of all bones, but most common in the thigh, back, pelvis or upper arms.

SEX OR AGE MOST AFFECTED—Both sexes, but most common in men between ages 50 and 70.

SIGNS & SYMPTOMS
• Pain in the affected bone. The pain is severe, boring and deep. If the bone collapses, pain spreads to other parts of the body.
• Weight loss.
• Symptoms of anemia, such as weakness, paleness, tiredness and breathlessness.

CAUSES—Unknown. The bone pain is caused by the cancerous abnormal plasma cells. The anemia is caused by damaged red blood cells and decreased platelets.

RISK INCREASES WITH—Immuno-suppression due to disease or drugs.

HOW TO PREVENT—No specific preventive measures.

 WHAT TO EXPECT

DIAGNOSTIC MEASURES
• Your own observation of symptoms.
• Medical history and physical exam by a doctor.
• Laboratory blood studies.
• Biopsy (see Glossary) of bone marrow.
• X-rays of painful bones.
• Plasmapheresis (see Glossary).

APPROPRIATE HEALTH CARE
• Self-care after diagnosis.
• Doctor's treatment.
• Radiation therapy to relieve bone pain.
• Hospitalization in late stages.

POSSIBLE COMPLICATIONS
• Recurrent infections.
• Kidney failure.
• Spontaneous bleeding.

PROBABLE OUTCOME—This condition is currently considered incurable. However, pain can be relieved or controlled. Some persons live up to 5 years after symptoms appear, and medical literature cites a few instances of unexplained recovery.
   Scientific research into causes and treatment continues, so there is hope for increasingly effective treatment and cure.

 HOW TO TREAT

GENERAL MEASURES
• The more you can learn and understand about this disorder, the more you will be able to make informed decisions about where to go for your care, the treatments available, the risks involved, side effects of therapy and expected outcome.
• See Resources for Additional Information.

MEDICATION—Your doctor may prescribe:
• Anticancer and cortisone drugs (chemotherapy).
• Pain relievers.
• Antibiotics to fight infections.
• Blood transfusions if anemia becomes severe.

ACTIVITY—Stay as active as pain or bone complications allow.

DIET—No special diet.

 CALL YOUR DOCTOR IF

• You have symptoms of multiple myeloma.
• The following occurs during treatment:
   Fever.
   Any sign of infection (pain, swelling, redness, tenderness or warmth) anywhere in the body.
   Swelling of the feet and ankles.
   Urination discomfort or decreased urine output in 1 day.
   Unexplained bleeding from any part of the body.
• New, unexplained symptoms develop. Drugs used in treatment may produce side effects.

MULTIPLE SCLEROSIS (MS)

GENERAL INFORMATION

DEFINITION—A chronic disorder affecting many nervous-system functions. One-third of patients have mild, nonprogressive disease. Another third worsen slowly. The rest worsen rapidly.

BODY PARTS INVOLVED—Central nervous system (brain and spinal cord).

SEX OR AGE MOST AFFECTED—Younger adults (ages 20 to 40) of both sexes, but more common in women.

SIGNS & SYMPTOMS
Early stages:
- Vague eye problems, such as intermittent blurred or double vision.
- Weakness; difficulty with walking or balance.
- Vague loss of sensation; numbness; tingling.
Late stages:
- Marked weakness; tremor; speaking difficulty.
- Loss of bladder or bowel control.
- Extreme mood swings.
- Sexual impotence in men.
Signs and symptoms vary widely between persons. Sometimes they are mistakenly attributed to emotions or "nerves."

CAUSES—Unknown. Research suggests multiple sclerosis may be caused by an autoimmune disorder or slow-acting virus.

RISK INCREASES WITH
- Children and adolescents raised in cool climates. Moving to a warmer climate later does not help.
- Family history of the disease.

HOW TO PREVENT—Cannot be prevented at present, but relapses can be shortened by therapy. Avoid infections, which trigger relapses.

WHAT TO EXPECT

DIAGNOSTIC MEASURES
- Medical history and physical exam by a doctor. Consultation with a neurologist is often valuable.
- No specific test is available to diagnose MS. Testing may include CT scan, MRI (see Glossary for both), visual evoked response or VER (electrical response to stimulation of a sensory system), lab studies of spinal fluid.

APPROPRIATE HEALTH CARE
- Self-care after diagnosis.
- Doctor's treatment.
- Self-catheterizations for inadequate bladder emptying (indwelling catheter may be necessary in a few patients).
- Hospitalization or chronic-care facility, depending on the severity of the disease.

POSSIBLE COMPLICATIONS
- Urinary-tract infections caused by bowel and bladder disorders.
- Pressure sores from prolonged bed rest.
- Constipation caused by inactivity.

PROBABLE OUTCOME—Spontaneous recovery sometimes occurs. In most cases, however, multiple sclerosis is incurable. Symptoms can be relieved or controlled, and the condition often remains stable for months or years. Survival of 20 to 30 years is common.
  Scientific research into causes and treatment continues, so there is hope for increasingly effective treatment and cure.

HOW TO TREAT

GENERAL MEASURES
- Emotional support, encouragement, and reassurances are helpful in coping.
- Lead as normal a life as possible; avoid fatigue.
- Avoid warm surroundings, even a hot shower. Heat can temporarily worsen symptoms.
- Have frequent massages, which help prevent contractures (shortening of muscles).
- Avoid stress, which may aggravate symptoms.
- When there is a remission in your symptoms, it is sometimes difficult to determine if it was due to a particular treatment or spontaneous.
- Some unethical medical practitioners offer unproven treatments of no value. Discuss any unconventional treatment with your medical team before investing your money.
- See Resources for Additional Information.

MEDICATION—Your doctor may prescribe:
- Cortisone drugs during periods of relapse or when symptoms worsen.
- Cyclophosphamide, which helps blunt the immune system's response.
- Muscle relaxants to control muscle spasms.
- Interferon and other treatments are under investigation.

ACTIVITY
- A regular program of physical exercise and mental activity is essential. Obtain physical therapy and muscle retraining if needed.
- Take regular rest periods.
- Remain sexually active, if possible. Sexual counseling may be helpful.

DIET—Eat a normal, well-balanced diet that is high in fiber to prevent constipation.

CALL YOUR DOCTOR IF

The following occurs during treatment:
  Breathing or swallowing difficulty.
  Sudden increased weakness.
  Chills and fever or other signs of infection.

MUMPS

GENERAL INFORMATION

DEFINITION—A mild, contagious viral disease that causes painful swelling of the salivary glands.

BODY PARTS INVOLVED—Parotid glands (salivary glands that lie between the ear and jaw). Other organs, including the testicles, ovaries, pancreas, breasts, brain and meninges (membranes that cover the brain) sometimes become involved.

SEX OR AGE MOST AFFECTED—All ages, but most common in children (2 to 12 years). Approximately 10% of adults are susceptible to mumps.

SIGNS & SYMPTOMS
Mumps without complications:
- Inflammation, swelling and pain of the parotid glands. The glands feel firm, and pain increases with chewing or swallowing.
- Fever.
- Headache.
- Sore throat.

Additional symptoms with complications:
- Painful, swollen testicles.
- Abdominal pain, if the ovaries or pancreas are involved.
- Severe headache, if the brain or meninges are involved.

CAUSES—Person-to-person transmission of the mumps virus. The virus can be transmitted anytime from 48 hours before symptoms begin to 6 days after symptoms appear. Virus incubation is 14 to 24 days after contact; the average is 18 days.

RISK INCREASES WITH
- Crowded living conditions.
- Epidemics in a nonvaccinated population.
- Lack of immunization.

HOW TO PREVENT
- Obtain mumps immunizations for children at the appropriate age.
- If you have not had mumps or been vaccinated and a close family member has mumps, your doctor may suggest an antimumps globulin. The injection may prevent the disease—it is not guaranteed.

WHAT TO EXPECT

DIAGNOSTIC MEASURES
- Your own observation of symptoms.
- Medical history and physical exam by a doctor.

APPROPRIATE HEALTH CARE
- Home care after diagnosis.
- Doctor's treatment to confirm the diagnosis and treat complications, if any occur.

POSSIBLE COMPLICATIONS—Mumps rarely has long-term complications. Infections of the brain or meninges (meningo-encephalitis), pancreas, ovaries, breasts or testicles may occur.
- Sterility in males, if both testicles become infected (rare).
- Temporary hearing loss in some adults.

PROBABLE OUTCOME—Spontaneous recovery in about 10 days if no complications occur. After having the disease, a person has lifetime immunity to mumps.

HOW TO TREAT

GENERAL MEASURES
- It is not necessary to isolate the infected person from the family. By the time symptoms appear, the disease has usually already spread.
- Apply heat or ice—whichever feels better—intermittently to the swollen, painful glands (parotid or testicles). Use a hot-water bottle, hot towel or ice pack.
- Stay out of school until no longer contagious (about 9 days after onset of pain).

MEDICATION—Once the disease begins, it must run its natural course. There is no safe, readily available medicine that can kill the virus or keep it from multiplying.
- For minor pain, you may use nonprescription drugs such as acetaminophen. Don't use aspirin.
- Your doctor may prescribe:
  Stronger pain relievers.
  Cortisone drugs, if testicles are involved.

ACTIVITY—Bed rest is not essential and does not reduce the possibility of complications. Allow as much activity as strength and feeling of well-being allow. Patients are no longer contagious when swelling disappears.

DIET—No special diet, but increase daily fluid intake to at least 6 to 8 glasses of liquid, including ginger ale, cola, tea or water. Fruit juices or tart beverages may increase pain.

CALL YOUR DOCTOR IF

- Fever (oral) rises above 101F (38.3C).
- The following occurs during the illness:
  Vomiting or abdominal pain.
  Severe headache that is not relieved by acetaminophen.
  Drowsiness or inability to stay awake.
  Swelling or pain in the testicle.
  Twitching of the face muscles.
  Convulsion.
  Discomfort or redness in the eyes.

MUSCULAR DYSTROPHY

GENERAL INFORMATION

DEFINITION—A gradual deterioration of the body's muscles, especially of the extremities, pelvis and hips, leading to increasing difficulty in walking and moving. Different types of muscular dystrophy exist, depending on the exact genes involved.

BODY PARTS INVOLVED—Different types affect different areas of the body, such as shoulders, hips or face.

SEX OR AGE MOST AFFECTED—It affects males more often than females, usually between ages 5 and 12.

SIGNS & SYMPTOMS
Early symptoms:
- Weakness.
- Duck-like gait.
- Falling and difficulty in getting up.
- Muscles that appear larger and stronger but are weaker than normal.

Late symptoms:
- Muscle deterioration severe enough to require confinement to a wheelchair by age 9 to 12.
- Severe distortion of the body.
- Recurrent respiratory infections.

CAUSES—Inherited. Muscular dystrophy is a genetic abnormality. It is carried by a female who does not have the disease; she passes it to male children. When a woman carrier marries a normal male, half the male children will inherit the condition.

RISK INCREASES WITH—Family history of muscular dystrophy.

HOW TO PREVENT
If you have a family history of muscular dystrophy:
- Obtain genetic counseling prior to starting a family.
- If you are pregnant, consider amniocentesis to determine whether the fetus is male and the disorder is present.
- Carriers can be detected with medical testing, because their blood contains high levels of a particular enzyme.

WHAT TO EXPECT

DIAGNOSTIC MEASURES
- Your own observation of symptoms.
- Medical history and physical exam by a doctor.
- Diagnostic tests may include laboratory studies of muscle enzymes in the blood and muscle biopsy (removal of a small amount of tissue or fluid for laboratory examination that aids in diagnosis).

APPROPRIATE HEALTH CARE
- Home-care.
- Team approach to care so that all needs are met (primary care doctor, neurologist, orthopedic surgeon, physical and occupational therapists, social worker).
- Psychotherapy or counseling to learn ways to cope with disability and to adjust socially.
- Surgical release of contractures or fixation of joints (sometimes).

POSSIBLE COMPLICATIONS
- Frequent fractures or injuries from falls.
- Spinal curvature caused by weakened muscles of the spine.
- Pneumonia caused by weakened chest muscles and a diminished cough response.
- Muscle shortening (contractures).
- Pressure sores.

PROBABLE OUTCOME
This condition is currently considered incurable. Persons with this condition rarely reach adulthood.
Scientific research into causes and treatment continues, so there is hope for better treatment and increased life expectancy.

HOW TO TREAT

GENERAL MEASURES
- The child should learn deep-breathing techniques.
- The child should stay active in school as long as possible.
- Respiratory support at night.
- See Resources for Additional Information.

MEDICATION—Your doctor may prescribe:
- Stool softeners to prevent constipation.
- Medications appropriate for any complications.

ACTIVITY
- The child should be as physically and mentally active as possible. Many devices can help overcome handicaps caused by weakness. Braces may help.
- If the child cannot voluntarily move muscle groups, family members or a visiting nurse should massage and passively exercise them to prevent contractures. Long periods of inactivity or bed rest should be avoided.

DIET—No special diet. Overweight should be avoided, because it adds stress to weakened muscles.

CALL YOUR DOCTOR IF

- You detect symptoms of muscular dystrophy in your child.
- Infection, especially of the lung, occurs after diagnosis. Symptoms include fever, cough and chest pain.

MYASTHENIA GRAVIS

GENERAL INFORMATION

DEFINITION—Disorder of muscles, especially of the face and head, with increasing fatigue and weakness as muscles are used.

BODY PARTS INVOLVED—The muscles around the eyes, mouth and throat, and the extremities.

SEX OR AGE MOST AFFECTED—Both sexes; all ages, but more common in adolescents and young adults and in females.

SIGNS & SYMPTOMS
- Drooping eyelids.
- Double vision (diplopia).
- Loss of normal facial expression.
- Swallowing difficulty.
- Weakness of the arms and legs.
- Difficulty speaking clearly.
- Breathing difficulty.

Most flare-ups appear after a brief period of normal muscle function and worsen as the muscle is used.

CAUSES
- Autoimmune disorder (probably).
- Tumor of the thymus (newborns only).

RISK INCREASES WITH
- Medical history of other autoimmune diseases.
- Some cancers, especially thymus and lung cancer.
- Newborns and infants of mothers with myasthenia gravis. They show symptoms in 2 to 3 weeks.

HOW TO PREVENT—Cannot be prevented at present.

WHAT TO EXPECT

DIAGNOSTIC MEASURES
- Your own observation of symptoms.
- Medical history and physical exam by a doctor.
- Diagnostic tests include laboratory studies of antibodies in the blood, electrical muscle tests, x-rays of the chest and a therapeutic trial of anticholinesterase drugs.

APPROPRIATE HEALTH CARE
- Doctor's treatment.
- Treatment is directed towards controlling symptoms.
- Surgical removal of the thymus gland (thymectomy) (sometimes).
- Acute flare-ups may require emergency care for respiratory distress.

POSSIBLE COMPLICATIONS
- Choking from swallowing difficulty.
- Respiratory paralysis.

PROBABLE OUTCOME—This condition is currently considered incurable. However, symptoms can be relieved or controlled. Worsening may be followed by improvement. Life expectancy is reduced but patients usually live many years with the disease.

Scientific research into causes and treatment continues, so there is hope for increasingly effective treatment and cure.

HOW TO TREAT

GENERAL MEASURES
- To feel more confident about how to treat yourself, ask your doctor about the following:
  About your medications and the importance of compliance.
  How to adjust to progressive fatigue and weakness.
  How to prevent and manage complications.
  How to recognize signs of myasthenic crisis.
- Wear a Medic-Alert (see Glossary) bracelet or neck tag that indicates your medical problem.
- See Resources for Additional Information.

MEDICATION
- Anticholinesterase drugs to restore normal muscle function. Excessive doses may cause weakness.
- Cortisone drugs at times when symptoms worsen.

ACTIVITY
- Plan activities to make the most of energy peaks. Frequent rest periods are important. Day-to-day fluctuations in symptoms are common.
- Avoid strenuous activities and needless exposure to the sun or to cold weather.

DIET—No special diet. Soft diet may be necessary if chewing and swallowing are difficult.

CALL YOUR DOCTOR IF

- You have symptoms of myasthenia gravis.
- You develop swallowing or breathing difficulty. You should have emergency medications (anticholinesterase drugs) available at all times to use if symptoms develop.

MYOCARDITIS

GENERAL INFORMATION

DEFINITION—Inflammation of the heart muscle (myocardium) that usually occurs as a complication of underlying illness, such as hypersensitive immune reactions, injury, radiation therapy, infection or toxic reactions to drugs.

BODY PARTS INVOLVED—Heart muscle.

SEX OR AGE MOST AFFECTED—Both sexes; all ages.

SIGNS & SYMPTOMS
- Fatigue.
- Shortness of breath.
- Irregular heartbeat.
- Fever.
- Other symptoms caused by the underlying disorder.

If myocarditis causes congestive heart failure, the following symptoms may also occur:
- Swollen feet and ankles.
- Distended neck veins.
- Rapid heartbeat, even when at rest.
- Breathing difficulty while resting or lying down.

CAUSES
- Viral infections, such as measles, influenza or adenovirus.
- Bacterial infections, such as tetanus, gonorrhea, typhoid fever, tuberculosis or diphtheria.
- Surgery on the heart.
- Rheumatic fever.
- Parasite infections.
- Radiation therapy for cancers in the chest, such as lung or breast cancer.
- Certain medications.

RISK INCREASES WITH
- Exposure to any of the Causes.
- Excess alcohol consumption.

HOW TO PREVENT
- Don't drink more than 1 or 2 alcoholic drinks, if any, a day.
- Keep immunizations current against diphtheria, tetanus, measles, rubella and polio.

WHAT TO EXPECT

DIAGNOSTIC MEASURES
- Your own observation of symptoms.
- Medical history and physical exam by a doctor.
- Laboratory blood studies.
- ECG (see Glossary), cardiac catheterization and angiography (see Glossary).

APPROPRIATE HEALTH CARE
- Self-care after diagnosis.
- Doctor's treatment.

- Hospitalization for the underlying disorder (frequently).
- Heart transplantation may be the only effective treatment for some types.

POSSIBLE COMPLICATIONS—Even with excellent treatment of the underlying disorder, a few patients develop:
- Congestive heart failure.
- Permanent damage to the heart muscle or valves.
- A blood clot inside the heart muscle that can break away and lodge elsewhere in the body. This may be life-threatening.

PROBABLE OUTCOME—Often curable with detection and treatment of the underlying cause.

HOW TO TREAT

GENERAL MEASURES
- Treatment includes medications for infections, rest and careful management of any complications. Compliance with your treatment plan is important for your recovery.
- See Resources for Additional Information.

MEDICATION—Your doctor may prescribe:
- Cortisone drugs to reduce inflammation.
- Antibiotics to fight infection, if myocarditis is caused by a bacterial infection.
- Appropriate medications, if myocarditis develops into congestive heart failure. These include:
  Diuretics to reduce fluid retention.
  Digitalis to stimulate a stronger heartbeat.
  Anticoagulants to prevent clot formation.
  Medications to reduce the heart's workload.
  Supplemental oxygen if necessary.

ACTIVITY
- Rest in bed until symptoms disappear. Recovery time varies, depending on the underlying cause. Use a bedside commode for bowel movements while at complete bed rest. This causes less stress than a bedpan.
- After recovery, resume your normal activities gradually.

DIET—Eat a low-salt diet.

CALL YOUR DOCTOR IF

- You have symptoms of myocarditis.
- The following occurs during treatment:
  Recurrence of fever or chills.
  Increased shortness of breath.
- New, unexplained symptoms develop. Drugs used in treatment may produce side effects.

NARCOLEPSY

GENERAL INFORMATION

DEFINITION—Rare sleep disorder characterized by uncontrollable episodes of falling asleep at any place or time. After a 10 or 15 minute sleep attack, the person feels rested only briefly, then returns to an uncomfortable feeling of sleepiness. Attacks may occur while driving, talking or working.

BODY PARTS INVOLVED—Central nervous system.

SEX OR AGE MOST AFFECTED
• Both sexes.
• Begins in adolescence or young adulthood and continues throughout life.

SIGNS & SYMPTOMS—Any of the following (10% of people with narcolepsy have all signs):
• Sleep attacks that may occur up to 10 times a day. These can occur during conversations or other activities. An attack leaves the person feeling refreshed, but another may occur again quickly.
• Vivid dreams, sounds or hallucinations at the beginning of a sleep attack or upon awakening.
• Temporary paralysis (sudden loss of muscle strength) when falling asleep or just before complete awakening.
• Momentary paralysis not related to sleep when feeling sudden emotion, such as anger, fear or joy.
• Irresistible drowsiness during the day.

CAUSES—Unknown. Possible involvement of the immune system. Occasionally, it follows brain infection or head injury.

RISK INCREASES WITH
• Family history.
• Either of the following may trigger an attack: Monotonous activity, prolonged laughter.

HOW TO PREVENT—No known preventive measures.

WHAT TO EXPECT

DIAGNOSTIC MEASURES
• Your own observation of symptoms.
• Medical history and physical exam by a doctor.
• EEG (see Glossary).
• Studies in a sleep laboratory (sometimes).

APPROPRIATE HEALTH CARE
• Self-care after diagnosis.
• Doctor's treatment.

POSSIBLE COMPLICATIONS—Accidental injury during a sudden sleep attack.

PROBABLE OUTCOME—This disorder lasts throughout life, but it has no effect on life expectancy. Symptoms can worsen with aging. However, in women, symptoms can improve after menopause. Medication can decrease the frequency of sleep attacks.

HOW TO TREAT

GENERAL MEASURES
• Treatment usually involves regular naps along with medication to help control the drowsiness.
• Wear a Medic-Alert bracelet or pendant (see Glossary).
• See Resources for Additional Information.

MEDICATION—Your doctor may prescribe:
• Stimulants that increase levels of daytime alertness.
• Antidepressants for other symptoms (momentary paralysis).

ACTIVITY
• Don't engage in any activity that carries the risk of injury from a sudden sleep attack. These include activities such as driving long distances, climbing ladders or working around dangerous machinery.
• Exercise can sometimes decrease the number of sleep attacks. Seek to achieve optimal physical fitness.

DIET—No special diet.

CALL YOUR DOCTOR IF

• You have symptoms of narcolepsy.
• New, unexplained symptoms develop. Drugs used in treatment may produce side effects.

NASAL POLYPS

GENERAL INFORMATION

DEFINITION—Nonmalignant growths in the nasal cavities, usually in both sides of the nose. They sometimes grow large and numerous enough to cause nasal distension and enlargement of the bony framework.

BODY PARTS INVOLVED—Nasal mucous membranes.

SEX OR AGE MOST AFFECTED—All ages, but most common in adults.

SIGNS & SYMPTOMS
- Obstruction of air through the nose (chronic "stuffy-nose" feeling).
- Impaired sense of smell.
- Feelings of fullness in the face.
- Nasal discharge (sometimes).
- Facial pain (sometimes).
- Headaches (sometimes).

CAUSES—Chronic infection or allergy in the nose (allergic rhinitis) that causes the nasal mucous membranes to swell and produce excess fluid in the nasal cells.

RISK INCREASES WITH—Sinusitis or chronic nasal infection.

HOW TO PREVENT—Obtain medical treatment for the underlying allergy. Consult your doctor about allergy testing and desensitizing procedures.

WHAT TO EXPECT

DIAGNOSTIC MEASURES
- Your own observation of symptoms.
- Medical history and physical exam by a doctor.
- X-rays of the sinuses and examination with a nasal speculum.

APPROPRIATE HEALTH CARE
- Self-care (only if surgery cannot be performed).
- Doctor's treatment.
- Surgery (a minor procedure) is often required to remove polyps (under local anesthesia).

POSSIBLE COMPLICATIONS
- Repeated infections.
- Nosebleeds.

PROBABLE OUTCOME—Symptoms can be controlled with treatment (usually surgery). Recurrence is common, even with surgical treatment.

HOW TO TREAT

GENERAL MEASURES
- If nosebleeds occur, see treatment described under Nosebleed (in Illness section).
- For information about surgery and postoperative care, see Nasal Polyp Removal in surgery section.

MEDICATION
- For minor pain, you may use acetaminophen. Avoid aspirin, which may increase the tendency to bleed and may cause an allergic reaction.
- Your doctor may prescribe cortisone drugs or suggest cromolyn in nasal spray or oral form for a short while before surgery to shrink the polyps.
- Caution: Don't use over-the-counter decongestant sprays.

ACTIVITY—Resume your normal activities gradually after surgery.

DIET—No special diet.

CALL YOUR DOCTOR IF

- You have symptoms of nasal polyps.
- The following occurs during treatment:
  Nosebleeds that cannot be stopped.
  Fever.
  Pain that persists despite the use of acetaminophen.

ILLNESS & DISORDERS

NASAL SEPTUM, DEVIATED

GENERAL INFORMATION

DEFINITION—Crookedness or other abnormality of the septum, the structure dividing the nose in 2 equal parts.

BODY PARTS INVOLVED—The septum is made of cartilage (farther toward the tip) and bone (closer to the forehead).

SEX OR AGE MOST AFFECTED—Both sexes of adults.

SIGNS & SYMPTOMS
- An apparently crooked nose.
- Obstruction of air through the nostrils.
- Nasal discharge.
- Often, there are no symptoms.

CAUSES
- Rapid growth, especially at puberty.
- Injury.
- Nose surgery.

RISK INCREASES WITH—Those listed in Causes.

HOW TO PREVENT—Protect yourself from nose injury. Wear protective headgear for contact sports or cycling. Buckle your auto seat belt.

WHAT TO EXPECT

DIAGNOSTIC MEASURES
- Your own observation of symptoms.
- Medical history and physical exam by a doctor, including inspection of the nose with a bright light and nasal speculum.

APPROPRIATE HEALTH CARE
- Self-care after diagnosis.
- Doctor's treatment, if symptoms warrant it.
- Surgery to correct the deviation (sometimes). The procedures are:
  Submucosal removal, which relieves obstruction.
  Rhinoplasty, which corrects anatomical deformity.
  Septoplasty, which relieves nasal obstruction and improves appearance.

POSSIBLE COMPLICATIONS
- Recurrent nosebleeds.
- Recurrent nasal or sinus infections.

PROBABLE OUTCOME—Usually curable with surgery. If symptoms are not troublesome, surgery is probably not necessary.

HOW TO TREAT

GENERAL MEASURES—For an explanation of one type of corrective surgery and postoperative care, see Rhinoplasty & Submucosal Removal (in Surgery section).

MEDICATION
- For minor discomfort, you may use nonprescription drugs, such as decongestants, to decrease nasal secretions.
- Your doctor may prescribe antibiotics to fight infection, if necessary.
- Caution: Avoid over-the-counter nasal sprays.

ACTIVITY—No restrictions unless surgery is necessary. If so, resume your normal activities gradually.

DIET—No special diet.

CALL YOUR DOCTOR IF

You have symptoms of a deviated nasal septum, especially recurrent nosebleeds or nasal and sinus infections, and you want to consider corrective surgery.

NEPHROTIC SYNDROME
(Nephrosis)

GENERAL INFORMATION

DEFINITION—A condition that results from damage to the glomeruli (the filtering units of the kidneys). It causes impaired blood to flow from the kidneys back into the body's tissues, leading to swelling throughout the body. In addition, there is an increase of salt and fluid retention, which further aggravates the situation. Nephrotic syndrome is not actually a disease, but a combination of symptoms and signs.

BODY PARTS INVOLVED—Kidneys. Late or complicated stages involve all body cells.

SEX OR AGE MOST AFFECTED—Children and adults. It affects more boys than girls.

SIGNS & SYMPTOMS
- Fluid retention (edema) that appears first as puffy eyes and ankles, then as general puffiness of the skin, and eventually as a swollen abdomen.
- Reduced urine production, sometimes to 20% of normal; frothy urine.
- Appetite loss; weakness; general ill feeling.

CAUSES—May be primary (not always possible to determine the cause) or may occur as a complication of other problems that affect kidney function, such as: diabetes; lupus erythematosus; multiple myeloma; AIDS; glomerulonephritis; autoimmune disorders; serum sickness and other severe allergic disorders; blood clot in the kidney; infections; congenital heart disease; or some medications.

RISK INCREASES WITH
- Family history of nephrotic syndrome (primary form only).
- Pregnancy.
- Exposure to chemical toxins.
- Congestive heart failure.
- Lymphoma.
- Drug addiction.
- Immunosuppression due to illness or drugs.

HOW TO PREVENT—Obtaining prompt treatment for any causes listed, especially skin and throat infections, may lessen risks.

WHAT TO EXPECT

DIAGNOSTIC MEASURES
- Medical history and physical exam by a doctor. Laboratory studies, such as urinalysis and blood studies of protein and cholesterol.
- Kidney biopsy (see Glossary).

APPROPRIATE HEALTH CARE
- Home care after diagnosis.
- Doctor's treatment.

POSSIBLE COMPLICATIONS
- Kidney disease that resembles chronic glomerulonephritis; kidney failure.
- Increased susceptibility to infections.

PROBABLE OUTCOME—Medication and diet can control swelling and reverse kidney abnormalities. Although symptoms usually disappear in 2 weeks with treatment, medication is continued for 6 to 8 weeks. Nephrotic syndrome can be arrested with treatment, but relapses are common and the treatment must be repeated. If kidney failure develops, dialysis or a kidney transplant can prolong life.

HOW TO TREAT

GENERAL MEASURES
- Parents may need counseling and help in learning to manage a chronically ill child.
- During the acute phase: Keep a record of the temperature each morning and evening. Collect all urine passed during each 24 hours and record every amount. Record all fluids consumed also. Portions of the urine may be analyzed in the doctor's office.
- Keep immunizations current, especially influenza and pneumovax.
- See Resources for Additional Information.

MEDICATION—Your doctor may prescribe:
- Cortisone or immunosuppressive drugs to reduce kidney inflammation.
- Diuretics, including potassium-saving diuretics, to reduce fluid retention.
- Antibiotics to control infection.
- Angiotensin I converting enzyme inhibitors often reduce protein loss.
- Supplemental vitamins and iron.

ACTIVITY—Stay in bed (except for trips to the bathroom) until the edema (fluid retention) improves. After the swelling decreases, be as mildly active as your strength allows.

DIET
- Cook and serve food without salt. Avoid salty prepared foods. Reduce fat in the diet.
- You may need to restrict fluid intake. Ask your doctor.
- If you are overweight, try to lose weight.

CALL YOUR DOCTOR IF

The following occurs during treatment:
  Severe headache; convulsion; extreme weakness.
  Signs of infection, such as fever, sores on the skin, cough or burning on urination.
  Failure to pass 1 quart of urine in a 24-hour period. Increased fluid retention.
  Vomiting, diarrhea or nausea.

NOSE FRACTURE

 GENERAL INFORMATION

DEFINITION—Fracture or damage to the bones and cartilage of the nose. This often happens when other facial bones are also fractured.

BODY PARTS INVOLVED—Nose.

SEX OR AGE MOST AFFECTED—Older children (over age 8) and adults. Young children's noses have only cartilage.

SIGNS & SYMPTOMS
* Pain in the nose.
* Nosebleed.
* Swollen, discolored nose.
* Inability to breathe through the nose.
* Crooked or misshapen nose (sometimes).
* Black eyes.

CAUSES—Injury to the nose.

RISK INCREASES WITH—Previous nose injury.

HOW TO PREVENT—Protect your nose from injury, whenever possible. Wear protective headgear for contact sports or when riding motorcycles or bicycles. Wear auto seat belts.

 WHAT TO EXPECT

DIAGNOSTIC MEASURES
* Your own observation of symptoms.
* Medical history and physical exam by a doctor.
* X-ray of the nose.

APPROPRIATE HEALTH CARE
* Self-care after diagnosis of minor injuries.
* Doctor's treatment.
* Emergency-room treatment for heavy bleeding.
* Surgery, if the nose is crooked or breathing is impaired.

POSSIBLE COMPLICATIONS
* Infection of the nose and sinuses.
* Shock from loss of blood (rare).
* Permanent breathing difficulty.
* Permanent change in appearance.
* Deviated nasal septum.

PROBABLE OUTCOME—Minor fractures with no deformity usually heal in 4-6 weeks. Major fractures can be repaired with surgery. If surgery is necessary, it should be done within 2 weeks or not until 6 months after injury.

 HOW TO TREAT

GENERAL MEASURES
* Apply ice packs to the nose immediately after injury to minimize swelling.
* If the nosebleed is heavy or cannot be stopped, obtain emergency medical treatment.

MEDICATION
* For minor discomfort, you may use nonprescription drugs such as acetaminophen (aspirin and ibuprofen interfere with blood clotting).
* Your doctor may prescribe:
  Stronger pain relievers, if needed.
  Antibiotics, if infection develops.

ACTIVITY—Rest until bleeding stops.

DIET—No special diet.

 CALL YOUR DOCTOR IF

* You have symptoms of a fractured nose, especially bleeding that is heavy or cannot be stopped.
* You have had a fractured nose and think surgery is needed.

NOSEBLEED
(Epistaxis)

GENERAL INFORMATION

DEFINITION—Bleeding from the nose.

BODY PARTS INVOLVED—Blood vessels (arteries and veins) in the nose. Nosebleeds occur close to the nose opening or deeper in the nose.

SEX OR AGE MOST AFFECTED—All ages, but twice as common in children as adults.

SIGNS & SYMPTOMS
- Blood oozing from the nostril. If the nosebleed is close to the nostril, the blood is bright red. If the nosebleed is deeper in the nose, the blood may be bright or dark.
- Lightheadedness from heavy blood loss.
- Rapid heartbeat, shortness of breath and pallor (with significant blood loss only).
- Black stool from swallowed blood.

CAUSES
- Injury to the nose or nasal polyps—even simple injury caused by picking the nose.
- Nasal or sinus infection.
- A foreign body in the nose.
- Scarlet fever, malaria or typhoid fever.
- Dry mucous membranes in the nose from any cause, such as low humidity.
- Atherosclerosis; high blood pressure.
- Bleeding tendencies associated with alcoholism, aplastic anemia, leukemia, thrombocytopenia or liver disease.

RISK INCREASES WITH
- Any disorder listed as a cause.
- Hodgkin's disease; scurvy; rheumatic fever.
- Blood disorders, including leukemia and hemophilia.
- Use of certain drugs, such as anticoagulants, aspirin, or prolonged use of nose drops.
- Exposure to irritating chemicals.
- High altitude or dry climate.
- Dry air in airplanes or air conditioned buildings.

HOW TO PREVENT
- Avoid injury if possible.
- Obtain treatment for the underlying cause.
- Humidify the air if you live in a dry climate or at high altitude.
- Avoid picking at nose or vigorous nose blowing.
- Avoid aspirin if you have frequent nosebleeds.

WHAT TO EXPECT

DIAGNOSTIC MEASURES
- Your own observation of symptoms.
- Medical history and exam by a doctor.
- Laboratory blood studies.

APPROPRIATE HEALTH CAR
- Self-care (see General Measures).
- Doctor's treatment.
- Surgery (for severe bleeding only) to tie off the artery feeding the bleeding area.

POSSIBLE COMPLICATIONS—Bleeding severe enough to require transfusion (rare).

PROBABLE OUTCOME—Symptoms can be controlled with treatment. Severe bleeding requires hospitalization and usually is caused by an underlying disorder, such as liver disease, blood disease or hypertension. In these cases, the underlying disorder should be treated also.

HOW TO TREAT

GENERAL MEASURES
Self-care:
- Sit up with your head bent forward.
- Clamp your nose closed with your fingers for 5 uninterrupted minutes. During this time, breathe through your mouth. If blood is coming from one nostril, press firmly on that nostril.
- If bleeding stops and recurs, repeat, but pinch your nose firmly on both sides for 8 to 10 minutes. Holding your nose tightly closed allows the blood to clot and seal the damaged blood vessels.
- You may apply cold compresses at the same time.
- Don't blow your nose for 12 hours after bleeding stops to avoid dislodging blood clot.
- Don't swallow blood. It may upset your stomach or make you "gag," causing you to inhale blood.
- Don't talk (also to avoid gagging).
Medical or emergency-room treatment:
- If self-care is unsuccessful. Gauze packing may be inserted to absorb blood, stop dripping and exert pressure on the ruptured blood vessels.
- Continued or recurrent bleeding may require cauterization (see Glossary).

MEDICATION—Your doctor may prescribe drugs to treat any underlying serious disorder.

ACTIVITY—Resume your normal activities as soon as symptoms improve.

DIET—No special diet.

CALL YOUR DOCTOR IF

- You have a nosebleed that won't stop with self-care described above.
- After the nosebleed, you become nauseous or vomit.
- After the nose has been packed, your temperature rises to 101F (38.3C) or higher.

OBESITY

GENERAL INFORMATION

DEFINITION—A condition of excess body weight. May be defined as: Males over 20% body fat or females over 25% body fat are considered obese. The concept that obesity is a will-power or self-discipline problem is outmoded. However, there is no clear understanding of the biochemical defects that cause it.

BODY PARTS INVOLVED—Total body.

SEX OR AGE MOST AFFECTED—Both sexes; all ages.

SIGNS & SYMPTOMS
• Excessive body fat composition.
• Emotional problems.
• Poor exercise tolerance. Excess weight increases the heart's work.

CAUSES
• Genetic factors.
• Environmental factors: Diet and eating habits, activity levels, stress (emotional and physical), drugs, cultural.
• Metabolic and endocrine disorders.
• Abnormal regulation of body weight to body fat.
• Central nervous system lesions.

RISK INCREASES WITH—Those listed in Causes.

HOW TO PREVENT—Life-long adherence to a program consisting of proper diet and nutrition, exercising, and behavior and lifestyle modification as needed.

OTHER—Surgery to reduce weight, such as bypassing part of the intestine or stomach, cutting away fat, fat suctioning or wiring the jaw shut, are rare, desperate measures.

WHAT TO EXPECT

DIAGNOSTIC MEASURES
• Medical history and exam by a doctor.
• Medical assessment to determine the degree of health risk. The most accurate method of determining body composition remains underwater weighing and skinfold measurements. Also used are BMI (body mass index) and waist to hip ratio (WHR).

APPROPRIATE HEALTH CARE
• Self-care.
• Doctor's treatment (sometimes).
• Psychotherapy or counseling.

POSSIBLE COMPLICATIONS
• Obesity may contribute to the development of diabetes, high blood pressure, heart disease and gallbladder disease. It complicates treatment and decreases survival chances of patients with stroke, kidney disease and other disorders.
• Psychosocial complications (poor self-image, difficulty in getting jobs, lack of social contacts with opposite sex).

PROBABLE OUTCOME—Obesity can be controlled if motivation stays high for life. Long-term management of weight loss is extremely difficult.

HOW TO TREAT

GENERAL MEASURES
• Many commercial and community programs are available that provide help in losing weight. Choose a program whose diet plans meet the recommended guidelines for nutrients, provides exercise and behavior counseling and includes long-term maintenance support.
• Keep diaries for food intake, exercise activities and behavior changes. Review them with your weight loss advisor weekly.
• Several techniques exist for behavioral modification. Determine the type that fits your needs (e.g., assertiveness, rewards, cognitive, substitution, imagery and others).

MEDICATION—Medications are available to help initiate a weight loss program; however, they are only mildly effective and have potentially dangerous side effects and are not useful for long-term weight loss.

ACTIVITY
• Increase your current level of activity. Daily exercise (bicycle riding, walking, swimming and others) helps you lose weight, feel better and control appetite.
• 30 minutes of activity, 5 times a week should be the goal. Keep an activity diary to monitor your progress.

DIET
• Many different diet plans are available to choose from. Diets that are not nutritionally balanced can cause more problems than the obesity. Crash diets and fad diets don't produce long-term results. Schemes which promise easy weight loss are usually unsuccessful.
• During your diet and exercise program, there may be periods when you don't lose weight. This is normal; don't stop the program. Weight loss will begin again in a week or two.
• A realistic weight loss is 1 to 2-1/2 pounds a week. This may seem slow, but 1 pound of fat lost per week totals 52 pounds in 1 year! Keep a food diary to record everything you eat.

CALL YOUR DOCTOR IF

Obesity increases, despite your self-help measures.

OBSESSIVE COMPULSIVE DISORDER

 GENERAL INFORMATION

DEFINITION—A disorder characterized by recurrent, intrusive thoughts (obsessions) and repetitive, ritualistic behaviors (compulsions). The disorder usually begins in adolescence and waxes and wanes throughout life, never going completely away and sometimes becoming more severe. New cases after age 50 are rare.

BODY PARTS INVOLVED—Nervous system.

SEX OR AGE MOST AFFECTED—Both sexes; adolescents and young adults; rarely starts after age 50.

SIGNS & SYMPTOMS
- Obsessions and/or compulsions that consume more than an hour a day and cause significant distress or impairment.
- Obsessions (thoughts) are recurrent and attempts to ignore or resist them are unsuccessful.

Obsessions include:
Thoughts of violence; fear of harming a family member or a friend. Fears of infection (from germs, dirt, etc.). Doubts (is the front door shut, locked; is the iron on). Excessive orderliness or symmetry. Constant brooding (over a word, phrase or unanswerable problem).
- Compulsions (actions) are repetitive, purposeful behaviors in response to the thoughts (obsessions) in an attempt to neutralize the thought.

Compulsions include:
Checking in response to doubt (locks, doors, windows). Excessive hand washing. Counting over and over to a certain number. Hoarding. Repeaters — such as dressing rituals.

CAUSES
- Exact cause is unknown. It may be connected to an imbalance in a brain chemical called serotonin. Serotonin is involved in sending impulses from one nerve cell to the next and in regulating repetitive behavior.
- Certain forms of brain damage (e.g., encephalitis) can result in obsessions.

RISK INCREASES WITH
- People who suffer from phobias and panic attacks or major depression.
- Schizophrenia; organic brain syndrome.
- Family history of the disorder.

HOW TO PREVENT—No specific prevention methods known.

 WHAT TO EXPECT

DIAGNOSTIC MEASURES
- Medical history and exam by a doctor.

- There are no medical tests to diagnose the disorder. Often the patient's description of the behavior offers the best clues to diagnosis.

APPROPRIATE HEALTH CARE
- Treatment is aimed at reducing anxiety, resolving inner conflicts, relieving depression, learning ways of dealing with stress, building self-esteem and understanding the behavior.
- Behavioral therapy (usually a process known as "exposure and response prevention") is used in treatment and is often combined with medications to achieve satisfactory results.
- Group therapy (sometimes). Family therapy is important to help educate relatives.

POSSIBLE COMPLICATIONS
- Incapacity to develop and maintain normal work and personal relationships.
- Depression; psychosis.
- Anxiety and panic-like episodes.
- Housebound lifestyles; indecisiveness.

PROBABLE OUTCOME—Effective and specific therapy is now available, and though it may not lead to a total cure, it can reduce disabling symptoms considerably.

 HOW TO TREAT

GENERAL MEASURES
- This is a complex disorder that usually requires professional help.
- See Resources for Additional Information.

MEDICATION
- Antidepressant, such as clomipramine or fluoxetine, may be prescribed. Complete benefits may not be seen for 10-12 weeks. About 10% of patients are unable to tolerate the side effects of the drugs, but an adverse response to one does not mean there will be problems with the other.
- Antianxiety or tranquilizer drugs may be prescribed.

ACTIVITY—No restrictions.

DIET—With use of some medications, a tyramine free diet may be necessary to prevent precipitation of hypertensive crisis. The doctor will advise you if this is necessary.

 CALL YOUR DOCTOR IF

- You have symptoms of obsessive compulsive disorder.
- Symptoms continue or worsen after an adequate treatment time has elapsed.
- New, unexplained symptoms appear. Drugs used in treatment may produce side effects.

ORAL CANCER

GENERAL INFORMATION

DEFINITION—Growth of malignant cells in the mouth or tongue. These are rare but dangerous. Any sore, ulcer or lump in the mouth that doesn't heal in 2 weeks should be examined by a doctor.

BODY PARTS INVOLVED—Lips; gums; palate; tongue; membranes inside the lip or cheek; floor of the mouth; tonsillar area.

SEX OR AGE MOST AFFECTED—Adults over 40; increasing in young people who chew smokeless tobacco.

SIGNS & SYMPTOMS—A pale lump—usually painless—with a hard rim that appears in any part of the mouth or tongue. It has the following characteristics:
- It enlarges, ulcerates and bleeds easily.
- It may prevent dentures from fitting properly.
- It may make the tongue stiff and difficult to control, causing speaking and swallowing difficulty.

CAUSES—Unknown.

RISK INCREASES WITH
- Use of tobacco in any form (including smokeless).
- Family history of oral cancer.
- Past history of oral cancer.
- Excess alcohol consumption.
- Sun exposure (cancer on the lower lip).

HOW TO PREVENT—Don't use tobacco; and drink alcohol in moderate amounts, if any.

WHAT TO EXPECT

DIAGNOSTIC MEASURES
- Your own observation of symptoms.
- Medical history and physical exam by a doctor.
- Laboratory blood studies.
- Biopsy (see Glossary) of the lump.
- X-rays of the head. Also CT scan or MRI (see Glossary for both) to help rule out spread of the malignancy. The larger the lesion at the time of diagnosis, the greater the chance that it has metastasized (spread) to other areas.

APPROPRIATE HEALTH CARE
- Self-care after diagnosis.
- Doctor's treatment.
- Treatment will vary depending on location of the cancer (lips, tongue, palate, etc.).
- Surgery to remove the cancerous area.
- Radiation therapy and/or anticancer drugs.
- Speech therapy, if surgery impairs speech.

POSSIBLE COMPLICATIONS
- Slow healing after surgery.
- Spread to lymph nodes in the neck, requiring radical head and neck surgery.
- Permanent disfigurement.
- Permanent speech impairment.
- Persistent difficulty in swallowing.

PROBABLE OUTCOME—May be curable with early detection and treatment. Normal facial appearance can often be restored by plastic surgery.

HOW TO TREAT

GENERAL MEASURES
- Discontinue use of tobacco in any form.
- Don't use any mouth rinses that contain alcohol.
- After surgery, cleanse the mouth 3 to 4 times a day with a soothing salt-water solution (1 teaspoon salt to 8 oz. warm water).
- See Resources for Additional Information.

MEDICATION—Your doctor may prescribe:
- Anticancer drugs.
- Pain relievers after surgery.
- Antibiotics, if infection coexists.

ACTIVITY—Resume your normal activities gradually after surgery.

DIET
- Don't drink alcohol.
- No special diet after recovery. A liquid diet (see Liquid Diet in Appendix) may be necessary for several days after surgery.

CALL YOUR DOCTOR IF

- You have signs of a mouth or tongue tumor.
- The following occurs after surgery:
  Increasing pain.
  Fever.
  New lumps.
  Excessive bleeding.

OSGOOD-SCHLATTER DISEASE
(Osteochondrosis)

GENERAL INFORMATION

DEFINITION—A temporary condition of the leg at the knee, characterized by swelling, tenderness and pain.

BODY PARTS INVOLVED—Tibial tubercle, a prominence just below the knee cap attached to a large thigh muscle connecting the bone of the upper leg (femur) to the large bone in the lower leg (tibia). This disorder often affects both knees.

SEX OR AGE MOST AFFECTED—Adolescents of both sexes, but more common in boys than girls. It is uncommon after age 16.

SIGNS & SYMPTOMS
- A slightly swollen, warm and tender bump below the knee.
- Pain with activity, especially straightening the leg against force, as in stair-climbing, jumping or weight-lifting.

CAUSES—Probably results from stress or injury of the tibial tubercle (which is still developing during adolescence). Repeated stress or injury interferes with development, causing inflammation.

RISK INCREASES WITH
- Overzealous conditioning routines, such as running, jumping or jogging.
- Overweight.
- Male between 11 and 18.
- Rapid skeletal growth.

HOW TO PREVENT
- Help an overweight child lose weight.
- Encourage your child to exercise moderately, avoiding extremes.

WHAT TO EXPECT

DIAGNOSTIC MEASURES
- Your own observation of symptoms.
- Medical history and physical exam by a doctor.
- X-ray and bone scan of the knee (sometimes).

APPROPRIATE HEALTH CARE
- Home care after diagnosis.
- Doctor's treatment.
- Initial treatment involves ice, medications (if needed) and decreased exercise.
- The affected leg may be immobilized for 6-8 weeks (reinforced elastic knee support, and rarely, plaster cast or splint).
- Surgery (rarely needed) if conservative measures fail.

POSSIBLE COMPLICATIONS
- Bone infection.
- Recurrence of the condition in adulthood.
- Persisting prominence below the kneecap.

PROBABLE OUTCOME—Usually resolves within 2 years after reaching full skeletal growth.

HOW TO TREAT

GENERAL MEASURES
- Use heat to relieve pain. Warm compresses, heating pads, warm whirlpool baths, heat lamps, diathermy or ultrasound are effective.
- Ice applications may help.
- Use a cushioned knee pad.
- Provide the patient with emotional support and assurances that symptoms will diminish with time.

MEDICATION
- For minor discomfort, you may use nonprescription drugs such as aspirin.
- Your doctor may prescribe cortisone injections, if other treatment fails. Cortisone injections may weaken tendons, so it is better to give the condition more time to heal than to use them.

ACTIVITY
- Resting the affected leg is the most important treatment.
- May require crutches, leg cast or splint, or an elastic knee brace that prevents the knee from bending fully. The child should not participate in sports during treatment. This is temporary, and normal activity can be resumed when inflammation subsides, but treatment often requires 2 to 12 months.
- Avoid jumping activities and activities that cause pain to the leg.

DIET—No special diet, unless the child is overweight. Ask your doctor about a weight reduction diet.

CALL YOUR DOCTOR IF

- Your child has symptoms of Osgood-Schlatter disease.
- The following occurs during treatment:
  Symptoms don't improve in 4 weeks, despite treatment.
  Pain increases.
  Fever.

ILLNESS & DISORDERS

OSTEOARTHRITIS
(Degenerative Joint Disease; Hypertrophic Arthritis)

 GENERAL INFORMATION

DEFINITION—Degeneration of cartilage at a joint and growth of bone "spurs" that inflame surrounding tissue.

BODY PARTS INVOLVED—All joints, but most common in fingers, feet, knees, hips and spine.

SEX OR AGE MOST AFFECTED—Adults over 45.

SIGNS & SYMPTOMS
- Joint stiffness and pain, including backache. Weather changes, especially cold, damp weather, may increase aching.
- Limited movement and loss of dexterity in affected joints.
- No redness, heat or fever in joints (usually).
- Swelling of affected joints (sometimes), especially finger joints.
- Cracking or grating sounds with joint movement (sometimes).

CAUSES—Exact cause is unknown. Appears to be a combination or interaction of mechanical, biologic, biochemical, inflammatory and immunologic factors.

RISK INCREASES WITH
- Obesity.
- Persons with occupations that put stress on joints.
- Stress on joints caused by activity and aging. Most people over age 50 have some osteoarthritis.
- Injury to the joint lining.

HOW TO PREVENT
- Maintain a normal weight for your height and body structure.
- Be physically active, but avoid activities that lead to joint injury, especially after age 40. Try regular stretching or yoga exercises.

 WHAT TO EXPECT

DIAGNOSTIC MEASURES
- Medical history and exam by a doctor.
- Laboratory blood studies to rule out inflammatory forms of arthritis.
- X-rays of painful joints.

APPROPRIATE HEALTH CARE
- Self-care after diagnosis.
- Doctor's treatment.
- An overall treatment plan will involve understanding the disorder, rehabilitation, activities of daily living and medications.
- Acupuncture (sometimes).

- Surgery for osteoarthritis includes arthroplasty (joint replacement) and arthrodesis (immobilization of a joint).

POSSIBLE COMPLICATIONS
- Crippling (sometimes).
- Muscles around affected joints may become smaller and weaker because of decreased use.
- Tends to be progressive.

PROBABLE OUTCOME—Symptoms can usually be relieved, but joint changes are permanent. Pain may begin as a minor irritant, but it can become severe enough to interfere with daily activities and sleep.

 HOW TO TREAT

GENERAL MEASURES
- To relieve pain, apply heat to painful and stiff joints for 20 minutes 2 or 3 times a day. Use hot towels, hot tubs, infrared heat lamps, electric heating pads or deep-heating ointments or lotions. Swim often in a heated pool or spa.
- If osteoarthritis of the neck causes pain in the arms, wear a soft, immobilizing collar (Thomas collar).
- Massage the muscles around painful joints. Massaging the joint itself is not helpful.
- If osteoarthritis affects the spine, sleep on your back on a very firm mattress or place 3/4-inch plywood between your box spring and mattress. Waterbeds help some people.
- Avoid chilling. Wear thermal underwear or avoid outdoor activity in cold weather.
- Keep a positive outlook on life. Remain active to prevent wasting of muscles.

MEDICATION—Your doctor may prescribe:
- Aspirin or other nonsteroidal anti-inflammatory drugs or acetaminophen for pain.
- Cortisone injections in painful, stiff joints. These may provide temporary relief.
- Glucosamine seems to help many people.

ACTIVITY
- Rest is important only during acute phases when joints are very painful. Resume normal activity as soon as symptoms improve.
- Physical therapy for muscle and joint rehabilitation (severe cases only).
- May need to protect joints from overuse (crutches, cane, walker, elastic knee support).

DIET—If you are overweight, lose weight (see Weight Loss Diet in Appendix).

 CALL YOUR DOCTOR IF

- You have joint pain or stiffness.
- New, unexplained symptoms develop.

OSTEOMYELITIS

GENERAL INFORMATION

DEFINITION—Infection of the bone and bone marrow.

BODY PARTS INVOLVED—Any bone in the body. In a child, the femur (upper-leg bone), tibia (lower-leg bone) or humerus or radius (bones in the arm) is usually affected. In an adult, the pelvis or spine is usually affected.

SEX OR AGE MOST AFFECTED
● Both sexes, but more common in males.
● All ages, but most common in rapidly growing children (5 to 14 years).

SIGNS & SYMPTOMS
● Fever. Sometimes this is the only symptom.
● Pain, swelling, redness, warmth and tenderness in the area over the infected bone, especially when moving a nearby joint. Nearby joints—especially the knee—may also be red, warm and swollen.
● If a child is too young to talk, signs of pain are: reluctance to move an arm or leg or refusal to walk; limping; or screaming when the limb is touched or moved.
● Pus drainage through a skin abscess, without fever or severe pain (chronic osteomyelitis only).
● General ill feeling.

CAUSES—Usually staphylococcal infection, but many other bacteria may be responsible. The bacteria may spread to the bone through the bloodstream from the following sources:
● Compound fracture or other injury.
● Boil, carbuncle or any break in the skin.
● Middle-ear infection.
● Pneumonia.

RISK INCREASES WITH
● Illness that has lowered resistance.
● Rapid growth during childhood.
● Diabetes mellitus.
● Implanted orthopedic device (artificial knee).
● Intravenous drug use.

HOW TO PREVENT—Obtain prompt medical treatment of any bacterial infection to prevent its spread to bone or other body parts.

WHAT TO EXPECT

DIAGNOSTIC MEASURES
● Your own observation of symptoms.
● Medical history and physical exam by a doctor.
● Laboratory blood studies and blood cultures to identify the bacteria.
● Radionuclide bone scans, CT or MRI scans (see Glossary for all). X-rays often don't show changes until 2 to 3 weeks after the infection begins.

APPROPRIATE HEALTH CARE
● Doctor's treatment.
● Hospitalization may be necessary for surgery to remove pockets of infected bone and/or to administer high doses of antibiotics sometimes intravenously.
● A previously implanted orthopedic device (artificial knee) may need to be removed (sometimes a replacement can be implanted at the same time).

POSSIBLE COMPLICATIONS
● Abscess that breaks through the skin and won't heal until the underlying bone heals.
● Permanent stiffness in a nearby joint (rare).
● Fracture.
● Loosening of implanted orthopedic device.
● May require amputation if circulation blocked or severe gangrene infection occurs (rare).

PROBABLE OUTCOME—Usually curable with prompt and aggressive treatment.

HOW TO TREAT

GENERAL MEASURES
● Keep the involved limb level or slightly elevated and immobilized with pillows. Don't let it dangle.
● Keep unaffected parts of the body as active as possible to prevent pressure sores during required, prolonged bed rest.

MEDICATION—Your doctor may prescribe:
● Large doses of antibiotics. With powerful new antibiotics, intravenous administration, once a necessity, may no longer be needed. Antibiotics may be necessary—either orally or by injection—for 8 to 10 weeks.
● Pain relievers.
● Laxatives, if constipation develops during prolonged bed rest.

ACTIVITY—Rest in bed until 2 to 3 weeks after symptoms disappear. Resume your normal activities gradually.

DIET—No special diet. Eat heartily. Take vitamin and mineral supplements if needed.

CALL YOUR DOCTOR IF

● You or your child have symptoms of osteomyelitis.
● The following occurs during treatment:
An abscess forms over the infected bone or drainage from an existing abscess increases.
Fever.
Pain becomes intolerable.
● New, unexplained symptoms develop. Drugs used in treatment may produce side effects.

OSTEOPOROSIS

GENERAL INFORMATION

DEFINITION—Loss of normal bone density, mass and strength, leading to increased thinning and vulnerability to fracture.

BODY PARTS INVOLVED—Bones.

SEX OR AGE MOST AFFECTED—Women after menopause.

SIGNS & SYMPTOMS
Early symptoms:
- Backache.
- No symptoms (often).

Late symptoms:
- Sudden back pain with a cracking sound indicating fracture.
- Deformed spinal column with humps.
- Loss of height.
- Fractures occurring with minor injury, especially of the hip or arm.

CAUSES—Loss of bony structure and strength. Factors include:
- Prolonged lack of adequate calcium and protein in the diet.
- Low estrogen levels after menopause.
- Decreased activity with increased age.
- Smoking (possibly).
- Use of cortisone drugs.
- Prolonged disease, including alcoholism.
- Vitamin deficiency (especially of vitamin C).
- Hyperthyroidism.
- Cancer.

RISK INCREASES WITH
- Aging.
- Surgery to remove the ovaries.
- Radiation treatment for ovarian cancer.
- Chronic or recurrent urinary-tract or other pelvic infections.
- Poor nutrition, especially inadequate calcium and protein.
- Body type. Thin women with a small frame are more susceptible.
- Family history of osteoporosis.
- Smoking.
- Heavy drinking of alcohol.
- Long-term use of cortisone drugs.
- High-intensity exercise with subsequent cessation of periods.
- Use of thyroid medications.

HOW TO PREVENT
- Ensure an adequate calcium intake—up to 1500mg a day—with milk and milk products or calcium supplements.
- Regular weight-bearing exercise, such as brisk walking, which is better for preventing osteoporosis than swimming.
- Seek medical advice about taking estrogen, calcium and fluoride after menopause begins or the ovaries have been removed.
- Avoid risk factors where possible.

WHAT TO EXPECT

DIAGNOSTIC MEASURES
- Medical history and exam by a doctor.
- Bone density studies.

APPROPRIATE HEALTH CARE
- Self-care.
- Doctor's treatment.

POSSIBLE COMPLICATIONS
- Bone fracture, especially of the hip or spine, after a fall. Sometimes a bone will break or collapse without injury or a fall.
- Severe, disabling pain.

PROBABLE OUTCOME—Diet, calcium and fluoride supplements, vitamin D, exercise and estrogen can halt—and may reverse—bone deterioration. Fractures will heal with standard treatment.

HOW TO TREAT

GENERAL MEASURES
- Avoid all circumstances that may lead to injury. Stay off icy streets and wet or waxed floors. Hold banisters when using stairs.
- If estrogen is prescribed, get regular medical pelvic exams and Pap smears. Examine your breasts for lumps once a month. Report any vaginal bleeding or discharge.
- Use heat or ice in any form to ease pain.
- Sleep on a firm mattress.
- Use a back brace, if prescribed.
- Use correct posture when lifting.
- See Resources for Additional Information.

MEDICATION
- For minor pain, you may use nonprescription drugs such as acetaminophen.
- Your doctor may prescribe calcium, vitamin-D supplements, estrogen or fluoride.

ACTIVITY—Stay active, but avoid the risk of falls. Exercise—especially weight-bearing exercise, such as walking—helps maintain bone strength.

DIET
- Eat a normal, well-balanced diet high in protein, calcium and vitamin D.
- Reducing diet if you are overweight (see Weight Loss Diet in Appendix).

CALL YOUR DOCTOR IF

- You have symptoms of osteoporosis.
- Pain develops, especially after injury.
- New, unexplained symptoms develop, such as vaginal bleeding. Drugs used in treatment may produce side effects.

OTOSCLEROSIS

 GENERAL INFORMATION

DEFINITION—Slow formation of abnormal spongy bone growth in the middle ear. The growth prevents one of the small bones in the middle ear from vibrating sound waves, leading to hearing loss.

BODY PARTS INVOLVED—Middle-ear bones and nerves in the ear that allow us to hear. Otosclerosis usually affects both ears.

SEX OR AGE MOST AFFECTED
- Both sexes, but twice as likely in females.
- All ages, but most common from ages 15 to 30.

SIGNS & SYMPTOMS
- Slow, progressive hearing loss.
- Ringing in the ears.
- Hearing that is better in noisy environments than quiet ones.

CAUSES—Appears to be inherited. 60% of those affected have positive family history.

RISK INCREASES WITH
- Family history of hearing loss.
- Caucasian heritage. Otosclerosis affects to some degree about 10% of all white people.
- Pregnancy, which may trigger the onset.

HOW TO PREVENT—Cannot be prevented at present. Obtain genetic counseling before starting a family if you or your spouse have otosclerosis.

 WHAT TO EXPECT

DIAGNOSTIC MEASURES
- Your own observation of symptoms.
- Medical history and physical exam by a doctor.
- Laboratory studies such as audiogram and Rinne test (see Glossary for both).

APPROPRIATE HEALTH CARE
- Doctor's treatment.
- Treatment usually involves surgery to remove the stapes (a bone in the middle ear) and replace it with a prosthesis. The hearing is corrected (or partially corrected) in most cases.

POSSIBLE COMPLICATIONS—Total deafness in 10 to 15 years without treatment. The younger the patient, the more rapid the hearing loss.

PROBABLE OUTCOME—In most cases, hearing is at least partially restored with surgery.

 HOW TO TREAT

GENERAL MEASURES
- A hearing aid may be used as an alternative to surgery.
- See Resources for Additional Information.

MEDICATION
- Your doctor may prescribe antibiotics after surgery.
- Treatment with tablets of sodium fluoride. calcium and vitamin D may prevent further hearing loss by hardening the spongy bone.

ACTIVITY—After surgery, resume your normal activities gradually.

DIET—No special diet.

 CALL YOUR DOCTOR IF

- You have symptoms of otosclerosis.
- Signs of infection, such as fever, pain or excessive dizziness, develop after treatment.

ILLNESS & DISORDERS

OVARIAN CANCER

 GENERAL INFORMATION

DEFINITION—A malignant growth in the ovary that is likely to spread to other body parts and threaten life.

BODY PARTS INVOLVED—One or both ovaries. It may spread to the lungs and bone.

SEX OR AGE MOST AFFECTED—Females of all ages, but most common after age 50.

SIGNS & SYMPTOMS—Frequently no symptoms occur until the tumor becomes large.
The earliest symptoms include:
- Vague discomfort in the lower abdomen.
- Gastrointestinal upsets.
- Irregular menstrual periods.

Later symptoms:
- Deep voice.
- Excessive hair growth.
- Unexplained weight loss.
- An enlarged, hard and sometimes tender mass in the lower abdomen.
- Pain with intercourse.
- Anemia.

CAUSES—Unknown.

RISK INCREASES WITH
- Family history of ovarian cancer.
- Late pregnancies (over age 30).
- Never having had children.
- Women who have previously been diagnosed with cancers of the breast, uterus, colon or rectum.

HOW TO PREVENT
- Have yearly pelvic examinations and Pap smears (see Glossary), which offer the best chance of early detection and cure.
- Oral contraceptives may help with prevention.
- Preventive surgery (removal of the ovaries) has been suggested for some women who have mother or sisters with ovarian cancer.

 WHAT TO EXPECT

DIAGNOSTIC MEASURES
- Your own observation of symptoms.
- Medical history and physical exam by a doctor.
- Laboratory blood studies.
- Ultrasound (see Glossary) of the abdomen.
- X-rays of the abdomen.
- Surgical diagnostic procedures, such as culdoscopy (see Glossary) and laparoscopy (see in Surgery section).

APPROPRIATE HEALTH CARE
- Doctor's treatment.
- Surgery to remove the cancerous ovary and other affected areas, including fallopian tubes, uterus and the other ovary (sometimes). In young patients who want to retain reproductive capacity, only the ovary and the tube may be removed.
- Radiation treatment and/or chemotherapy.
- Psychotherapy or counseling to learn to accept and cope with cancer.

POSSIBLE COMPLICATIONS
- Pleural effusion.
- Reaction to radiation and/or anticancer drugs.
- Ascites (fluid in the spaces between tissues and organs in the abdominal cavity).
- Death from spread of cancer to other body parts.

PROBABLE OUTCOME—25% to 50% of women with ovarian cancer survive at least 5 years after treatment. With early diagnosis and aggressive treatment, the long-term survival rate is improving.

 HOW TO TREAT

GENERAL MEASURES
- The more you can learn and understand about ovarian cancer, the more you will be able to make informed decisions about where to go for your care, the treatments available, the risks involved, side effects of therapy and expected outcome.
- See Resources for Additional Information.

MEDICATION—Your doctor may prescribe:
- Anticancer drugs.
- Pain relievers.

ACTIVITY—Be as active as your health permits.

DIET—Eat a normal, well-balanced diet that is high in protein to promote repair of body tissues.

 CALL YOUR DOCTOR IF

- You have symptoms of an ovarian tumor.
- The following occurs after surgery:
Increased pain, swelling, redness or drainage from the surgical wound.
Pain or swelling in the leg.
Signs of infection, such as fever, chills, headache or muscle aches.

OVARIAN TUMOR, BENIGN

GENERAL INFORMATION

DEFINITION—A benign, cystic (saclike) tumor on the ovary that contains fluid or semisolid material. These are usually small, but in some cases they may grow large enough to make a woman appear pregnant. Ovarian tumors are usually benign, but a few undergo malignant change.

BODY PARTS INVOLVED—One or both ovaries.

SEX OR AGE MOST AFFECTED—Females between puberty and menopause.

SIGNS & SYMPTOMS—May not cause symptoms. If symptoms occur, they may include:
• Mild pelvic pain.
• Pain in the lower back.
• Discomfort with sexual intercourse.
• Abnormal menstruation, including changes in menstrual flow, length of periods and intervals between periods.
• Excessive hair growth, deep voice and weight gain (sometimes).
If a large ovarian tumor twists or ruptures, the following will occur in the lower abdomen:
• Severe pain.
• Rigid muscles.
• Swelling.

CAUSES
• Unknown, but it is probably related to abnormalities of female hormone production and secretion.
• Endometriosis.

RISK INCREASES WITH—Unknown.

HOW TO PREVENT—No specific preventive measures.

WHAT TO EXPECT

DIAGNOSTIC MEASURES
• Your own observation of symptoms.
• Medical history and physical exam by a doctor.
• Laboratory blood studies.
• Laparoscopy, a surgical diagnostic procedure. A small tube is inserted in the abdomen under local anesthesia. The tube allows the doctor to see the organs and biopsy or drain the tumor, if necessary.

APPROPRIATE HEALTH CARE
• Doctor's treatment.
• Treatment may not be necessary, except to have regular pelvic examinations so the tumor's growth can be monitored.
• Surgery to remove the tumor or diseased ovary (sometimes).

POSSIBLE COMPLICATIONS—Emergency abdominal surgery caused by twisting, rupture or bleeding of a tumor.

PROBABLE OUTCOME—Most ovarian tumors require no treatment and disappear spontaneously within 2 months.

HOW TO TREAT

GENERAL MEASURES
• Some tumors require surgery to diagnose accurately, rule out malignancy or to treat. If one ovary must be removed, normal conception and childbirth is possible as long as a normal ovary remains on the other side.
• If surgery is required, see Laparotomy (in Surgery section) for an explanation of surgery and postoperative care.

MEDICATION
• Your doctor may prescribe female hormones or clomiphene. These help shrink or destroy some tumors.
• Oral contraceptives are often used as the first step in treatment.

ACTIVITY—No restrictions if surgery is not necessary.

DIET—No special diet.

CALL YOUR DOCTOR IF

• You have symptoms of an ovarian tumor, especially severe pain, rigidity and abdominal distention.
• New, unexplained symptoms develop. Drugs used in treatment may produce side effects.

PAGET'S DISEASE OF BONE
(Osteitis Deformans)

 GENERAL INFORMATION

DEFINITION—A gradual, progressive bone disease, characterized by bones breaking down and regenerating excessively. The new bone is fragile and weak. It is not cancerous.

BODY PARTS INVOLVED—Bones of the skull, spine, legs, collar bone and pelvis.

SEX OR AGE MOST AFFECTED—Both sexes, but most common in men over age 40.

SIGNS & SYMPTOMS
Early stages:
● Mild bone pain or none.
Later stages:
● Affected bones are chronically painful—especially at night—enlarged, misshapen, tender, and the skin over them is warm
● Movement is impaired.
● Spinal curvature compresses sensory nerves.
● Fractures occur from minor trauma and heal slowly with deformity.

CAUSES—Unknown, although a virus may be involved.

RISK INCREASES WITH—Family history of Paget's disease.

HOW TO PREVENT—No specific preventive measures.

 WHAT TO EXPECT

DIAGNOSTIC MEASURES
● Your own observation of symptoms.
● Medical history and exam by a doctor.
● X-rays of affected bones.
● Laboratory blood and urine studies to determine levels of serum alkaline phosphatase and urinary calcium.
● Possibly CT scan or MRI (see Glossary for both). Hearing and vision testing if skull is involved.

APPROPRIATE HEALTH CARE
● Self-care after diagnosis.
● Doctor's treatment.
● Most people do not require treatment other than occasional pain medication.
● Rarely, splinting may be needed for severely affected areas to prevent fractures.
● Bone surgery (sometimes) to correct deformities or treat secondary arthritis.

POSSIBLE COMPLICATIONS
● Visual impairment or hearing loss caused by the skull pressing on the brain.
● High blood pressure; kidney stones; gout; bone cancer.

● Congestive heart failure. The heart is strained by the greatly increased blood flow through diseased bones.
● Misdiagnosis of Paget's disease as an overactive parathyroid gland or spread of cancer from the prostate gland, breast or bone marrow.

PROBABLE OUTCOME—This condition is currently considered incurable. However, symptoms can be relieved or controlled. The disease has a pattern of remissions and flare-ups that become progressively worse. Sometimes adjacent joints become involved. Life expectancy is reduced, but most persons live with the disease for at least 10 to 15 years.
  Scientific research into causes and treatment continues, so there is hope for increasingly effective treatment and cure.

 HOW TO TREAT

GENERAL MEASURES
● Use heat to relieve pain, including hot compresses, hot soaks or heat lamps.
● If you don't have a firm bed, place 3/4-inch plywood under your mattress.
● Accident-proof your home as much as possible. Avoid throw rugs and slippery floors. Install hand rails next to the tub.
● Hearing aid may be useful if hearing loss occurs.

MEDICATION
● Your doctor may prescribe male and female hormones, fluoride, pain relievers, bone building and cytotoxic drugs. All relieve pain, but none cure the disease.
● Try aspirin or nonsteroidal anti-inflammatory drugs for pain.

ACTIVITY
● Rest in bed during active phases. Move or turn often to prevent pressure sores. Resume your normal activities during remissions.
● Avoid excessive physical stress on bones.

DIET—No special diet.

 CALL YOUR DOCTOR IF

● You have symptoms of Paget's disease.
● The following occurs during treatment:
  Fever of 101F (38.3C) or higher.
  Unbearable pain.
  Weight loss.
  Worsening symptoms.
● New, unexplained symptoms develop. Drugs used in treatment may produce side effects.

PANCREAS CANCER

GENERAL INFORMATION

DEFINITION—Uncontrolled growth of malignant cells in the pancreas. This is the 4th leading cause of cancer deaths in the U.S.

BODY PARTS INVOLVED—Pancreas, an organ in the back of the upper abdomen. The pancreas produces intestinal enzymes to help digest food and insulin to control blood sugar.

SEX OR AGE MOST AFFECTED—Men more often than women, between ages 35 and 70.

SIGNS & SYMPTOMS
- Rapid, unexplained weight loss.
- Pain in the back or upper abdomen that is often relieved by bending forward.
- Blood clots in veins anywhere, especially the arms and legs. This is often an early sign.
- Jaundice (yellow skin and eyes) from blockage of the nearby bile duct. Jaundice is usually accompanied by intense itching.
- Depression.

CAUSES—Unknown.

RISK INCREASES WITH
- Chronic pancreatitis.
- Diabetes mellitus.
- Genetic factors. This is more common in blacks than Caucasians.
- Smoking.
- Excess alcohol consumption.
- Geographic location. The incidence is higher in Israel, the U.S., Sweden and Canada than in other parts of the world.
- Poor nutrition, especially a diet high in fat, protein and processed foods containing many food additives.
- Exposure to some industrial chemicals.

HOW TO PREVENT—Cannot be prevented. Avoid risk factors where possible.

WHAT TO EXPECT

DIAGNOSTIC MEASURES
- Your own observation of symptoms.
- Medical history and physical exam by a doctor.
- Laboratory blood-chemistry studies of the pancreas, liver and gallbladder, and blood-sugar tests.
- Needle biopsy (see Glossary) of the liver.
- Exploratory abdominal surgery (laparotomy).
- X-rays of the abdomen, liver, gallbladder and blood vessels (angiography).
- Ultrasound (see Glossary) of the pancreas.
- CT scan (see Glossary) of the pancreas.

APPROPRIATE HEALTH CARE
- Doctor's treatment.

- Treatment will vary depending on overall health, spread of the cancer and location and size of tumor.
- Psychotherapy or counseling to help adjust to incurable illness.
- Chemotherapy and/or radiation therapy.
- Surgery to:
  Remove the tumor, if it is small.
  Relieve any bile-duct blockage.
  Relieve or prevent bowel obstruction.

POSSIBLE COMPLICATIONS
- Hemorrhage into the intestinal tract.
- Pancreas infections.
- Spread of cancer to liver, other abdominal organs and lungs (usually has already occurred by the time of diagnosis).
- Diabetes mellitus.

PROBABLE OUTCOME—This condition is currently considered incurable. Survival chances for more than 1 or 2 years are unlikely. However, symptoms can be relieved or controlled.

Scientific research into causes and treatment continues, so there is hope for increasingly effective treatment and cure.

HOW TO TREAT

GENERAL MEASURES
- The more you can learn and understand about this disorder, the more you will be able to make informed decisions about where to go for your care, the treatments available, the risks involved, side effects of therapy and expected outcome.
- See Resources for Additional Information.

MEDICATION—Your doctor may prescribe:
- Antibiotics for coexisting infections.
- Pain relievers.
- Anticancer drugs.
- Pancreatic enzymes to replace those the pancreas cannot manufacture.
- Sedatives for sleep.
- Antacids.

ACTIVITY—Remain as active as your strength allows.

DIET—No special diet.

CALL YOUR DOCTOR IF

- You have symptoms of pancreas cancer.
- The following occurs during treatment:
  Fever and headache.
  Muscle aches and fatigue.
  Nausea and vomiting.
  Severe abdominal pain and swelling.
  Black, tarry stools.
- New unexplained symptoms develop. Drugs used in treatment may produce side effects.

PANCREATITIS

GENERAL INFORMATION

DEFINITION—Inflammation of the pancreas. Chronic pancreatitis usually follows recurrent attacks of acute pancreatitis, because the pancreas does not recover completely between attacks. It gradually becomes unable to supply digestive juices and hormones necessary for good health.

BODY PARTS INVOLVED—Pancreas.

SEX OR AGE MOST AFFECTED—Adults.

SIGNS & SYMPTOMS
Severe acute pancreatitis:
- Extreme abdominal pain; vomiting; abdominal swelling and gas.
- Fever; muscle aches.
- Drop in blood pressure.

Chronic pancreatitis:
- Persistent, mild or severe pain, often after meals, in the upper abdomen, sometimes radiating to the back or generalized. Pain is aching, burning, gnawing or stabbing. Pain episodes may last days or weeks, but rarely less than 1 day.
- Mild jaundice (yellow skin and eyes, sometimes); rapid weight loss.

CAUSES
- Alcoholism.
- Disease of the gallbladder or bile ducts.
- Obstruction of the pancreatic duct by stones, scarring or slow-growing cancer (rare).
- Abdominal injury.
- Virus infection.
- Hyperlipidemia.
- Tumor.
- Medications.
- Trauma or surgery.

RISK INCREASES WITH
- Poor nutrition; obesity; excess alcohol consumption.
- Use of drugs, such as sulfa drugs, azathioprine, chlorothiazide or cortisone drugs.

HOW TO PREVENT—Don't drink more than 1 or 2 alcoholic drinks—if any—a day.

WHAT TO EXPECT

DIAGNOSTIC MEASURES
- Your own observation of symptoms.
- Medical history and physical exam by a doctor. This may be difficult to diagnose.
- Laboratory studies, such as blood and urine tests and radioisotope scans (see Glossary).
- X-rays of the pancreas.
- CT scan or ultrasound of the pancreas; endoscopy (see Glossary for all).

APPROPRIATE HEALTH CARE
- Doctor's treatment.

- Acute pancreatitis usually requires hospitalization for intravenous fluids, control of pain and vomiting, correction of metabolic abnormalities (replace calcium and magnesium). Surgery may be needed for gallstones, perforated peptic ulcer or to drain a source of infection.
- Chronic pancreatitis may be managed as an outpatient condition with medications, diet controls and abstinence from alcohol.

POSSIBLE COMPLICATIONS
- Diabetes mellitus.
- Chronic calcium deficiency.
- Secondary bacterial infection in the pancreas.
- Massive hemorrhage and destruction of the pancreas.
- Cyst or abscess of the pancreas.

PROBABLE OUTCOME—Acute pancreatitis is often curable with intensive care. Treatment includes resting the gastrointestinal tract completely and providing intravenous fluids and nourishment. About 5% of cases don't respond to treatment and are fatal. Chronic pancreatitis may recur for many years.

HOW TO TREAT

GENERAL MEASURES
- Follow your doctor's instructions. Compliance with your medical treatment plan is essential for the best outcome.
- Stop drinking alcohol. Contact Alcoholics Anonymous or other support groups if you need help.
- Use heat from a heating pad, heat lamp or hot compresses to relieve pain.
- See Resources for Additional Information.

MEDICATION—Your doctor may prescribe:
- Pain relievers.
- Digestive enzymes that the damaged pancreas cannot manufacture.
- Antibiotics, if bacterial infection develops.
- Stomach acid (H2) blockers.
- Insulin if diabetes present.

ACTIVITY—No restrictions.

DIET
- Intravenous fluids during an acute attack, then slowly progressing to oral feedings.
- Abstain totally from drinking alcohol.

CALL YOUR DOCTOR IF

- You have symptoms of acute pancreatitis.
- The following occurs during or after treatment: Jaundice (yellow skin and eyes).
  Fever of 101F (38.3C) or higher.
  Continued weight loss.
  Signs of calcium deficiency, such as muscle cramps or seizures.

PANIC DISORDER

GENERAL INFORMATION

DEFINITION—A severe, spontaneous form of anxiety that is recurrent and unpredictable. Most attacks last 2-10 minutes, but some may extend over an hour or two. This type of anxiety occurs with attack-like symptoms (often during sleep), while chronic anxiety (generalized anxiety) is a persistent state of anxiety.

BODY PARTS INVOLVED—Central nervous system; heart; lungs; skin; hands; feet.

SEX OR AGE MOST AFFECTED—Twice as many females as males; young adults, ages 25-44.

SIGNS & SYMPTOMS
Physical symptoms:
- Palpitations, rapid heart beat; chest pains.
- Shortness of breath; choking feeling; hyperventilation; weakness or faintness; fainting (occasionally); sweating and trembling.
- Numbness and tingling around the mouth, hands and feet.
- Muscle spasm or contractions in the hands and feet.
- Feeling of "butterflies in the stomach".
Emotional symptoms:
- Intense fear of losing one's sense of reason (fear of going crazy); fear of dying; sense of terror, doom or dread.
- Feelings of unreality, loss of contact with people and objects.

CAUSES
- Most often an unresolved emotional conflict or unrecognized conflict. The physical symptoms are a result of the autonomic nervous system being set in motion by the arousal of frightening fantasies, impulses and emotions.
- A variety of disorders can simulate panic attacks (heart rhythm problems, angina, respiratory illness, asthma, obstructive pulmonary disease, endocrine disorders, seizure disorders, stimulating drugs and withdrawal from certain drugs).

RISK INCREASES WITH
- Stress; feelings of guilt; fatigue or overwork; illness; alcohol and drug abuse.
- History of other psychiatric problems, family history of panic disorder.

HOW TO PREVENT—There are no specific measures to prevent a first panic attack; therapy may help prevent additional episodes.

WHAT TO EXPECT

DIAGNOSTIC MEASURES
- Medical history and exam by a doctor.
- Laboratory tests as needed to rule out other disorders.

APPROPRIATE HEALTH CARE
- Self-care.
- Doctor's treatment, if the cause is organic or symptoms are prolonged.
- Psychotherapy or counseling to uncover the emotional conflicts causing the anxiety and finding ways to deal with them.

POSSIBLE COMPLICATIONS
- Chronic anxiety or depression.
- Phobias, including agoraphobia, a fear of being alone or being in public places.
- Drug dependency.

PROBABLE OUTCOME—For many, this disorder may run a limited course with a few attacks and long periods of remission. For others, treatment with psychotherapy and/or medication is effective.

HOW TO TREAT

GENERAL MEASURES
- Talk to a friend or family member about your feelings. This sometimes defuses your anxiety.
- Keep a journal or diary about your anxious thoughts or emotions. Consider the causes and possible solutions.
- Join a self-help group. Call your local mental health society for referrals.
- Learn relaxation techniques. For some, meditation is effective.
- Reduce stress (see How to Cope with Stress in Appendix).
- For hyperventilation symptoms, cover the mouth and nose with a small paper bag and breathe into it for a few minutes.

MEDICATION—Your doctor may prescribe a tricyclic antidepressant, MAO inhibitor, anti-anxiety agent or beta-blocking agent. The medicine may be slowly reduced or discontinued after 6 months to a year to determine if the panic attacks return. If not, the medicine can be discontinued.

ACTIVITY
- Get physical exercise regularly.
- Get adequate rest at night.

DIET—Consider giving up caffeine (coffee, tea, soft drinks). You may experience withdrawal symptoms of headache or tiredness, but they stop in a few days.

CALL YOUR DOCTOR IF

- You have symptoms of panic disorder that don't diminish with self-treatment.
- Treatment program fails after 8 weeks.
- New, unexplained symptoms develop.

PARALYSIS

GENERAL INFORMATION

DEFINITION—The loss of ability to move a part of the body caused by the inability to contract one or more muscles. The condition varies in degree and severity from paralysis of one small muscle to paralysis of almost the total body. The paralysis may be temporary or permanent. Types include: paraplegia (partial or complete paralysis of both legs), quadriplegia (partial or complete paralysis of both arms and legs), and hemiplegia (partial or complete paralysis of one side of the body).

BODY PARTS INVOLVED—Brain; spinal cord; nervous system; muscles.

SEX OR AGE MOST AFFECTED—Both sexes; all ages.

SIGNS & SYMPTOMS—The following vary, depending on the site and extent of damage:
- Loss of movement and sensation in affected arms or legs.
- Loss of urinary and bowel control; impaired sexual function; loss of normal blood pressure; loss of body-temperature control; constipation.
- Difficulty speaking, understanding or recognizing words.
- Blurred, double or decreased vision.

CAUSES—Normally, the brain originates the impulses for muscle movement. These impulses travel via the spinal cord and peripheral nerves to the muscles. Paralysis occurs when there is an injury or disruption in this nerve pathway. Causes include:
- Stroke (most common). Stroke may be caused by bleeding in brain, or blood clot or obstruction of blood vessel to brain.
- Brain: tumor, abscess, hemorrhage, infection (encephalitis).
- Spinal cord: injury (from an accident); pressure on the spinal cord (disk prolapse, cervical osteoarthritis), decompression sickness.
- Disease: multiple sclerosis, poliomyelitis, myelitis, Friedreich's ataxia, meningitis, motor neuron disease.
- Nerve disorders (neuropathies): secondary to disorders such as diabetes mellitus, vitamin deficiency, liver disease, alcoholism, cancer and toxic effects of drugs or metals.
- Muscle disorders such as muscular dystrophy and sometimes, myasthenia gravis.

RISK INCREASES WITH
- Any activity with a high risk of injury.
- Excess alcohol consumption or drug use.

HOW TO PREVENT
- Observe safety precautions; don't take risks.
- Don't dive into shallow water.
- Wear protective headgear during contact sports and while riding a bicycle or motorcycle.

- Obtain medical treatment to control any chronic medical condition.

WHAT TO EXPECT

DIAGNOSTIC MEASURES
- Medical history and exam by a doctor.
- Laboratory studies of blood, urine and cerebrospinal fluid, x-rays of the injured area.

APPROPRIATE HEALTH CARE
- Treatment of any underlying cause.
- Hospitalization; intensive care if paralysis affects the breathing muscles.
- Surgery to limit further spinal-cord damage or to remove bones or a tumor.
- Time in an extended-care facility or special rehabilitation facility (sometimes).
- Physical and occupational rehabilitation.
- Psychotherapy or counseling for depression or for sexual problems.

POSSIBLE COMPLICATIONS—Kidney infections, especially if a urinary catheter is needed; lung infections; constipation; fecal impaction; pressure sores; deep-vein blood clot; depression; limb deformities.

PROBABLE OUTCOME—Depends on the extent of injury. Damaged spinal cord and nerves are limited in their ability to recover.

HOW TO TREAT

GENERAL MEASURES—The more you can learn and understand about your disorder, the more you will be able to make informed decisions about where to go for your care, the treatments available, the risks involved, side effects of therapy and expected outcome.

MEDICATION—Your doctor may prescribe:
- Antibiotics to fight infection.
- Medications to control hypertension, diabetes or other underlying disorders.
- Anticoagulants to prevent blood clot.
- Stool softeners and laxatives.

ACTIVITY—Resume activities gradually to the extent possible. With rehabilitation, many lost functions can be compensated for or restored. Use passive exercise for paralyzed or partially paralyzed muscles to prevent contractures.

DIET
- Eat a high-fiber diet to prevent constipation.
- If you have a urinary catheter, drink up to 16 glasses of water a day to prevent bladder stones and urinary-tract infections.

CALL YOUR DOCTOR IF

Signs of infection occur during treatment.

PARKINSON'S DISEASE

GENERAL INFORMATION

DEFINITION—A disease of the central nervous system that occurs in older adults and is characterized by gradual, progressive muscle rigidity, tremors and clumsiness.

BODY PARTS INVOLVED—Area of the brain that regulates movement; muscles.

SEX OR AGE MOST AFFECTED—Adults over 60.

SIGNS & SYMPTOMS
- Tremors, especially when not moving.
- General muscle stiffness and slowness.
- Awkward or shuffling walk; stooped posture; loss of facial expression; swallowing difficulty.
- Voice changes. The voice becomes weak and high pitched.
- Intellectual ability is unchanged until advanced stages, when it deteriorates slowly.

CAUSES
- Usually unknown. It results from a deficiency of dopamine, a chemical that relays messages across the nerve pathways. It affects the area of the brain responsible for control of voluntary muscle movements and posture.
- Some cases may be caused by: medications, such as phenothiazine tranquilizers; brain injury; tumors; post-influenza encephalitis; slow-virus infection; or carbon-monoxide poisoning (possibly).

RISK INCREASES WITH—Unknown.

HOW TO PREVENT—No specific preventive measures.

WHAT TO EXPECT

DIAGNOSTIC MEASURES
- Medical history and exam by a doctor.
- There are no confirming diagnostic tests for Parkinson's. Diagnosis is usually based on physical examination. Medical tests may be recommended to rule out other disorders.

APPROPRIATE HEALTH CARE
- Doctor's treatment.
- Physical therapy, encouragement, reassurance and treatment of associated conditions (such as depression).
- Counseling to help relieve depression.
- Occupational and speech therapy may be recommended.

POSSIBLE COMPLICATIONS
- Dementia; pneumonia; severe constipation.
- Urine retention caused by medication.
- Falls and fractures; debilitation.

PROBABLE OUTCOME—This condition is currently considered incurable. However, symptoms can be relieved or controlled. Life expectancy is not significantly reduced.

Research utilizing fetal tissue transplantation shows promise for future treatment. This therapy appears to resupply the brain with dopamine-producing cells.

HOW TO TREAT

GENERAL MEASURES
- Gradual restrictions of the disease may frustrate you and cause social withdrawal. Seek professional help and ask your family for support in finding ways to remain active and useful.
- There are numerous techniques you can learn to help you cope with the physical limitations. These can be tailored to your specific needs as symptoms change.
- Compliance with your treatment program (diet, exercise, medications) is important to help you maintain an optimum level of function.
- Accident-proof your home to prevent falls and injuries.
- Wear a Medic-Alert (see Glossary) bracelet or neck tag that indicates your medical problem.
- See Resources for Additional Information.

MEDICATION—Your doctor may prescribe: Anticholinergics; antihistamines; antitremor drugs, such as amantadine; or antiparkinson medications, including bromocriptine, levodopa and carbidopa. New medications are available that can help maintain maximal effectiveness of levodopa and carbidopa. All these decrease tremors and reduce muscle rigidity, but they often have significant side effects.

ACTIVITY—Remain as active as possible and rest often. Physical abilities vary greatly between persons with this disease. The only restrictions are those imposed by muscle rigidity. Physical therapy and exercise help to increase or maintain your mobility.

DIET
- No special diet, but soft foods may be necessary if swallowing becomes difficult. Add bulk or fiber to the diet and increase fluid intake to prevent constipation.
- If eating takes a long time, try eating smaller, more frequent meals.
- Special utensils and drinking cups are helpful if tremors cause too much unsteadiness.

CALL YOUR DOCTOR IF

New, unexplained symptoms develop, especially urination difficulty, confusion or blurred vision.

PARONYCHIA

 GENERAL INFORMATION

DEFINITION—Inflammation of tissue folds that surround the fingernail. The inflammation can be bacterial or fungal and is not contagious.

BODY PARTS INVOLVED—Fingernails.

SEX OR AGE MOST AFFECTED—Both sexes; all ages.

SIGNS & SYMPTOMS
Bacterial paronychia:
- Pain or tenderness, redness, warmth and swelling of tissue adjacent to the fingernail.
- Central whitish area produced by pus.

Fungal paronychia:
- Redness and swelling around the fingernail.
- No pain, warmth, itching or pus.

CAUSES
- Bacterial paronychia is preceded by injury, such as a torn hangnail. The infecting germ is usually Staphylococcus.
- Fungal paronychia is caused by a fungus or yeast infection.

RISK INCREASES WITH
- Injury around the fingernail.
- Occupational exposure to constant wetness (dishwashers, bartenders, housewives).
- Diabetes mellitus.

HOW TO PREVENT
- Protect hands from wetness.
- Leave hangnails alone.
- Avoid fingertip injury.

 WHAT TO EXPECT

DIAGNOSTIC MEASURES
- Your own observation of symptoms.
- Medical history and physical exam by a doctor (sometimes).
- Laboratory studies, such as culture of the discharge, to identify the germ (rare).

APPROPRIATE HEALTH CARE
- Self-care after diagnosis.
- Doctor's treatment.
- If abscesses present, may require incision and drainage.

POSSIBLE COMPLICATIONS—If untreated, may permanently damage the fingernail and nail bed, and the infection may enter bone or bloodstream.

PROBABLE OUTCOME
- Bacterial paronychia is curable with treatment in 2 weeks.
- Fungal paronychia is chronic and may require 6 months to heal.
- Recurrence is common with both forms.

 HOW TO TREAT

GENERAL MEASURES
- Wear heavy-duty vinyl gloves to prevent contact with irritating substances, such as water, soap, detergent, metal scrubbing pads, scouring pads, scouring powder and other chemicals.
- Dry the insides of gloves after use. Discard gloves if they develop a hole. A glove with a hole harms the hand more than not wearing a glove.
- Wear gloves when you peel or squeeze lemons, oranges, grapefruit, tomatoes or potatoes.
- Wear leather or heavy-duty fabric gloves for housework or gardening.
- Use a dishwashing machine or ask someone else to wash dishes.
- Avoid contact with irritating chemicals, such as paint, paint thinner, turpentine, and polish for cars, floors, shoes, furniture or metal.
- Use lukewarm water and very little mild soap to shower or bathe. All soaps are irritating. Expensive soaps offer no more protection against irritation than less-expensive ones.
- For bacterial paronychia, apply warm soaks.

MEDICATION
- For minor pain, you may use nonprescription drugs, such as aspirin or acetaminophen.
- Your doctor may prescribe antibiotics or antifungal medicine (depending on the type of infection).

ACTIVITY—No restrictions.

DIET—No special diet.

 CALL YOUR DOCTOR IF

- You have symptoms of paronychia.
- Fever develops.
- Pain is not relieved by treatment.

PELVIC INFLAMMATORY DISEASE (PID)

 GENERAL INFORMATION

DEFINITION—Infection of the female internal reproductive organs. This is contagious if it is caused by a sexually transmitted organism.

BODY PARTS INVOLVED—Fallopian tubes; cervix; uterus; ovaries; urinary bladder.

SEX OR AGE MOST AFFECTED—Sexually active females after puberty. The peak incidence occurs in late teens and early 20s.

SIGNS & SYMPTOMS
Early symptoms (up to 1 week):
- Pain in the lower pelvis on one or both sides, especially during menstrual periods. Menstrual flow may be heavy.
- Pain with intercourse.
- Bad-smelling vaginal discharge.
- General ill feeling; low fever.
- Frequent, painful urination.

Later symptoms (1 to 3 weeks later):
- Severe pain and tenderness in the lower abdomen; high fever.
- Increased bad-smelling, vaginal discharge.

CAUSES
- Bacterial infection (chlamydia, gonorrhea or mycoplasma) or a virus. This may be transmitted by an infected sexual partner.
- Childbirth; abortion; pelvic surgery.

RISK INCREASES WITH
- Many sexual partners.
- Use of an intrauterine contraceptive device (IUD).
- Previous history of PID or cervicitis.

HOW TO PREVENT
- Use latex condoms, spermicidal creams or sponges to help prevent sexually transmitted infections.
- Oral contraceptives appear to decrease risk.
- Seek routine medical check-ups for sexually transmitted diseases if you have multiple sexual partners. Have your sexual partner evaluated and treated if necessary.

 WHAT TO EXPECT

DIAGNOSTIC MEASURES
- Medical history and exam by a doctor.
- Laboratory blood studies and culture of the vaginal discharge.
- Surgical diagnostic procedures, such as laparoscopy or culdocentesis (see Glossary).

APPROPRIATE HEALTH CARE
- Doctor's treatment.
- You may receive treatment as as outpatient if infection is mild. You must adhere to treatment and medication schedule. Close medical follow up care is necessary.

- Hospitalization may be required for severe illness, further diagnostic studies, suspected abscess or appendicitis, failure to comply or failure to respond to outpatient therapy, or pregnancy.
- Surgery to drain a pelvic abscess (sometimes).
- Hysterectomy may be recommended for older patients who desire no more children.
- Psychotherapy or counseling, if infertility occurs.

POSSIBLE COMPLICATIONS
- Pelvic abscess and rupture. This can be life-threatening.
- Adhesions (bands of scar tissue) inside the pelvis.
- Infertility; ectopic pregnancy.
- Recurrence.

PROBABLE OUTCOME—Usually curable with early treatment and avoidance of further infection. The illness lasts from 1 to 6 weeks, depending on its severity. Poorer prognosis if treated late and unsafe lifestyle continues.

 HOW TO TREAT

GENERAL MEASURES
- Use heat such as warm baths to relieve pain. This may reduce the bad odor of the vaginal discharge, as well as relax muscles and relieve discomfort. Sit in a tub of hot water for 10 to 15 minutes as often as needed.
- Use sanitary pads to absorb the discharge or menstrual flow.
- Don't douche during treatment.

MEDICATION—Your doctor may prescribe:
- Intravenous antibiotics to fight infection if hospitalization is required. Oral antibiotics may be necessary for about 1 month following hospitalization.
- Oral antibiotics for early or mild PID.
- Pain relievers.

ACTIVITY—Avoid sexual intercourse until you are well. Rest in bed until the fever subsides. Sit and lie in different positions until you find one that is comfortable for you. Allow several weeks for recovery.

DIET—No special diet.

 CALL YOUR DOCTOR IF

- Symptoms recur after treatment.
- New, unexplained symptoms develop.

PENIS CANCER

GENERAL INFORMATION

DEFINITION—An uncommon malignant tumor of the penis.

BODY PARTS INVOLVED—Penis, including the glans (tip), corona (rounded border of the glans) or prepuce (foreskin covering the glans).

SEX OR AGE MOST AFFECTED—Men over age 50.

SIGNS & SYMPTOMS
Early stages:
• A small circular lesion (resembles a pimple) or persistent, painless sore on the penis. The lesion is easily visible in a circumcised male but it may go unnoticed in an uncircumcised male.
Later stages:
• Pain, bleeding or discharge from the tumor.
• Discomfort with urination.
• Enlarged lymph nodes in the groin.

CAUSES—Unknown, but penile cancer is rare in men circumcised at birth or shortly thereafter. This may explain why it is rare among Jews, Muslims and other cultures where early circumcision is customary.

RISK INCREASES WITH
• Previous leukoplakia of the penis, balanitis or epithelial horn on the penis.
• Personal uncleanliness, especially of the genitals, in uncircumcised males.

HOW TO PREVENT
• Consider having male children circumcised soon after birth.
• Examine the penis and testicles monthly to detect possible cancers early, when treatment is most successful. Seek medical treatment for any sign of infection or sore on the penis.

WHAT TO EXPECT

DIAGNOSTIC MEASURES
• Your own observation of symptoms.
• Medical history and physical exam by a doctor.
• Laboratory studies, such as culture of the tumor discharge, urinalysis and blood tests.
• Biopsy (see Glossary)
• CT scan (see Glossary) and a lymph node biopsy may be necessary to see if the cancer has spread.

APPROPRIATE HEALTH CARE
• Self-care after diagnosis.
• Doctor's treatment.
• Treatment will depend on stage of the cancer.
• Hospitalization and surgery to remove the tumor. Local tumors of the foreskin may require circumcision only. Invasive tumors require total removal of the penis and regional lymph nodes.
• Radiation therapy may be recommended if the cancer has not spread.
• Psychotherapy or counseling after surgery to learn to cope with an altered self-image.

POSSIBLE COMPLICATIONS—This spreads quickly to nearby lymph nodes but slowly to distant sites or organs. Many men delay treatment due to denial or fear of disfigurement and loss of sexual function. This increases the likelihood the cancer will spread and cause death.

PROBABLE OUTCOME—The 5-year survival rate is about 50%, even with treatment. Recurrence remains a possibility after treatment.

HOW TO TREAT

GENERAL MEASURES
• A bladder catheter will be necessary for a prolonged period—sometimes permanently—after surgery and irradiation treatment.
• The more you can learn and understand about this disorder, the more you will be able to make informed decisions about where to go for your care, the treatments available, the risks involved, side effects of therapy and expected outcome.
• See Resources for Additional Information.

MEDICATION—Your doctor may prescribe:
• Pain relievers, if necessary.
• Anticancer drugs for widespread cancer. However, the effectiveness of presently available drugs is only temporary.

ACTIVITY—Resume your normal activities as soon as possible after treatment. Sexual relations are possible if enough penile tissue remains following surgery.

DIET—No special diet.

CALL YOUR DOCTOR IF

• You have any lump or sore on the penis.
• Excessive bleeding occurs at the surgical site.
• New, unexplained symptoms develop. Drugs used in treatment may produce side effects.

PERICARDITIS, ACUTE

GENERAL INFORMATION

DEFINITION—Inflammation of the pericardium (thin membrane around the heart). This is not contagious or cancerous, unless caused by the spread of cancer from somewhere else.

BODY PARTS INVOLVED—Pericardium.

SEX OR AGE MOST AFFECTED—Both sexes; all ages.

SIGNS & SYMPTOMS
- Dull or sharp pain in the front of the chest, radiating to the neck and shoulder. The pain worsens with movement and eases when sitting up or leaning forward.
- Rapid breathing.
- Cough.
- Fever and chills.
- Weakness.
- Anxiety.
- The most important signs are apparent only with medical examination.

CAUSES—Sometimes unknown. The most common known causes are:
- Viral, bacterial, tuberculous, amebic, toxoplasmosis or fungal infection.
- Rheumatic fever and other diseases of connective tissue, such as lupus erythematosus.
- Chronic kidney failure.
- Complication of a heart attack.
- Complication following heart surgery.
- Complication of a chest injury, including use of a cardiac catheter.
- Spread of cancer to the pericardium.
- Drug induced.
- Radiation therapy.

RISK INCREASES WITH
- Recent illness, such as a heart attack, viral illness or rheumatic fever.
- Medical history of tuberculosis.

HOW TO PREVENT—No specific preventive measures except medical treatment of the disorders that cause pericarditis.

WHAT TO EXPECT

DIAGNOSTIC MEASURES
- Your own observation of symptoms.
- Medical history and physical exam by a doctor.
- Diagnostic tests may include chest x-ray, chest CT scan or MRI, ECG, echocardiogram, heart catheterization (see Glossary for all).
- Pericardiocentesis (fluid removal from the pericardial sac) may be diagnostic or therapeutic (for complications).

APPROPRIATE HEALTH CARE
- Doctor's treatment.
- Surgery (sometimes) to remove fluid through a needle if fluid collects in the pericardium.
- Self-care.

POSSIBLE COMPLICATIONS
- Chronic pericarditis.
- Recurrence.
- Pericardial effusion (fluid in the pericardial sac).
- Cardiac tamponade (effusion that impairs heart function).

PROBABLE OUTCOME—Usually curable in 6 months unless pericarditis is caused by cancer. After cure, there should be no functional disability.

HOW TO TREAT

GENERAL MEASURES
- Home care is usually sufficient, unless there are complications. Treatment is aimed at relieving symptoms and managing the underlying disease.
- Apply a heating pad or warm compresses to the chest to relieve pain.
- See Resources for Additional Information.

MEDICATION—Your doctor may prescribe:
- Anti-inflammatory therapy with aspirin.
- Steroid drugs for severe forms of pericarditis.
- Stronger pain medications (if aspirin doesn't control the pain).
- Antibiotics, if bacterial infection present.
- Amphotericin B, if fungal infection present.
- Antitubercular drugs, if tuberculous pericarditis.

ACTIVITY
- Rest in bed until fever and pain subside.
- Resume your normal activities gradually.
- Resume sexual relations when fever and pain disappear.

DIET—No special diet. Ask your doctor about a weight loss diet if you are overweight.

CALL YOUR DOCTOR IF

- You have symptoms of pericarditis.
- The following occurs during treatment:
  Fever.
  Shortness of breath and rapid heartbeat.
  Cough with blood.
  Unexplained weight loss.
  Pain not controlled by acetaminophen.
- New, unexplained symptoms develop. Steroids used in treatment may produce side effects, especially restlessness.

PERIODONTITIS
(Gum Inflammation)

 GENERAL INFORMATION

DEFINITION—Inflammation and infection of the gums, causing loss of supporting bone. Periodontitis is responsible for more tooth loss than tooth decay. It is not contagious.

BODY PARTS INVOLVED—Gums; jaw bones.

SEX OR AGE MOST AFFECTED—Adults over age 20.

SIGNS & SYMPTOMS
● Unpleasant taste in the mouth.
● Bad breath.
● Loosening of teeth in the sockets.
● Aching teeth and gums when eating hot, cold or sweet food.
● If an abscess develops, tenderness, swelling, pain and fever will also occur.

CAUSES—Plaque (a sticky deposit of food, bacteria and mucus) destroys bone that surrounds and supports teeth. Poor dental hygiene causes the accumulation of plaque.

RISK INCREASES WITH—Illness that has lowered resistance.

HOW TO PREVENT
● Practice good oral hygiene (see General Measures).
● Avoid sweet snacks, which contribute to plaque formation.
● Visit your dentist regularly to have teeth cleaned. Ask your dentist about the level of fluoride in local drinking water. Fluoride supplements may provide added protection.

 WHAT TO EXPECT

DIAGNOSTIC MEASURES
● Your own observation of symptoms.
● Medical history and physical exam by a dentist.
● X-rays of the mouth.

APPROPRIATE HEALTH CARE
● Self-care after diagnosis.
● Dentist's care.
● Surgery to remove unhealthy gum tissue and reshape underlying bone to eliminate pockets.

POSSIBLE COMPLICATIONS—Without treatment, teeth loosen so much in their bony sockets that they must be extracted.

PROBABLE OUTCOME—Usually curable with a combination of dental treatment and strict adherence to a good oral-hygiene program (see General Measures).

 HOW TO TREAT

GENERAL MEASURES
● To brush teeth: Scrub the clear, sticky plaque off teeth daily with a soft toothbrush. A soft brush is less likely to damage teeth and gums than a hard brush. Place the brush at the gum line and gently rotate it, pointing the bristles toward the gum. Brush one section of teeth at a time.
● To floss teeth: Wind waxed or unwaxed dental floss around one finger on each hand. Force the dental floss between teeth. Gently clean the tooth surfaces with a back-and-forth, sawing motion at the gum line. Floss between all lower teeth, using your fingers as guides. Next, loosen the floss and place it on the tops of your thumbs. Floss between all upper teeth, using your thumbs as guides.

MEDICATION—For minor pain, you may use nonprescription drugs such as acetaminophen.

ACTIVITY—No restrictions.

DIET—No special diet, except to avoid sweets.

 CALL YOUR DENTIST IF

You have symptoms of periodontitis.

PERIPHERAL NEUROPATHY
(Peripheral Neuritis)

 GENERAL INFORMATION

DEFINITION—A group of symptoms caused by abnormalities in sensory or motor nerves.

BODY PARTS INVOLVED—Many nerves that end in muscles, blood vessels and skin. This usually affects fingers, toes, hands, feet, lower arms and legs, and may affect bladder or bowel control.

SEX OR AGE MOST AFFECTED—Adults of both sexes.

SIGNS & SYMPTOMS—Symptoms usually appear gradually over many months:
- Tingling and numbness that begins in the hands and feet and spreads gradually.
- Gradual muscle weakness throughout the body—often in same place on both sides.
- Shooting pains that are often worse at night. Pains are aggravated by touch or temperature changes.
- Painless ulcers on the toes or fingers.
- Pale, dry skin that becomes sensitive to touch.
- Weight loss.
- Severe back pain or loss of bladder or bowel control, if caused by intervertebral disk disease.

CAUSES
- Reactions to drugs or chemicals, including: emetine; hexobarbital; sulfonamides; phenytoin; nitrofurantoin; heavy metals; carbon monoxide; solvents; or industrial poisons. Interactions of drugs required by people with cardiovascular disease sometimes cause symptoms.
- Complication of an underlying disorder, such as: diabetes mellitus; alcoholism; vitamin deficiency; vitamin B-12 deficiency anemia; or thyroid disorder.
- Poor nutrition.
- Malabsorption disorders.
- Autoimmune reaction.
- Trauma or pressure on a nerve.
- Excessive vomiting, including early pregnancy vomiting.
- Decreased thyroid function.
- Acute porphyria.
- Complication of dialysis treatment.
- Cancer.
- Ruptured intervertebral disc.
- Some hereditary disorders.

RISK INCREASES WITH
- Adults over 60.
- Use of drugs listed in Causes, especially multiple medications.
- Exposure to chemicals listed in Causes.
- Poor nutrition, such as in alcoholism.
- Poor control of diabetes.
- Family history of neuropathies.

HOW TO PREVENT—Avoid as many causes and risks as possible.

 WHAT TO EXPECT

DIAGNOSTIC MEASURES
- Medical history and exam by a doctor.
- Laboratory studies of blood, urine, vitamin B-12 levels, thyroid function and spinal fluid.
- Electromyography (see Glossary) and nerve conduction studies.

APPROPRIATE HEALTH CARE
- Doctor's care.
- Hospitalization (sometimes).
- Surgery to relieve pressure, if nerves are compressed.

POSSIBLE COMPLICATIONS—Chronic pain and disability.

PROBABLE OUTCOME—Mild cases can be cured if the underlying cause is diagnosed and treated. Serious cases may be incurable but treatment can help symptoms improve.

 HOW TO TREAT

GENERAL MEASURES
- Most important aspect of treatment is to identify the underlying cause and correct it if possible.
- Biofeedback training to learn relaxation techniques that relieve pain may be helpful.
- Inspect hands and feet daily for wounds.
- Keep feet clean and toenails trimmed properly; wear shoes that fit well.

MEDICATION
- For minor pain, you may use nonprescription drugs such as aspirin or acetaminophen.
- The medication gabapentin is sometimes helpful in treating this condition.
- Your doctor may prescribe medications to treat underlying disorders.

ACTIVITY
- If peripheral neuropathy is interfering with normal activities, physical therapy may help.
- If you have difficulty maintaining balance, walk with a cane or other support.
- Install rails next to the bathtub.

DIET—No special diet. Vitamin and mineral supplements probably will be necessary. Pyridoxine (vitamin B-6) may help.

 CALL YOUR DOCTOR IF

- You have symptoms of peripheral neuropathy.
- Symptoms (especially muscle weakness) persist or worsen, despite treatment.
- You develop a severe bruise or open sore.

PERITONITIS

GENERAL INFORMATION

DEFINITION—A serious infection or inflammation of part or all of the peritoneum, the covering of the intestinal tract.

BODY PARTS INVOLVED—Abdomen, including intestines and peritoneum (a thin membrane that covers all the organs and walls of the abdomen).

SEX OR AGE MOST AFFECTED—Both sexes; all ages.

SIGNS & SYMPTOMS
• Pain in one area or throughout the abdomen. Pain usually starts suddenly and becomes increasingly severe. Pain may be cramp-like at first, and then steady. The patient often prefers to lie quietly on the back because movement or pressure on the abdomen increases pain.
• Shoulder pain (sometimes).
• Chills and fever (often high).
• Dizziness and weakness.
• Rapid heartbeat.
• Low blood pressure.

CAUSES—Intense inflammation of the peritoneum lining that occurs when foreign material enters the abdominal cavity. Foreign material includes bacteria or gastrointestinal contents, such as digestive juices, blood, partly digested food or feces. These materials enter the abdomen following:
• Rupture or perforation of any organ in the abdomen, such as an inflamed appendix, peptic ulcer or infected diverticulum or gallbladder.
• Injury to the abdominal wall, such as from a knife or bullet wound.
• Pelvic inflammatory disease.
• Rupture of an ectopic pregnancy.

RISK INCREASES WITH
• Delay in treatment of causes listed above.
• Recent abdominal surgery.
• Corticosteroid therapy.
• Advanced liver disease.

HOW TO PREVENT—Obtain prompt medical treatment for underlying disorders.

WHAT TO EXPECT

DIAGNOSTIC MEASURES
• Your own observation of symptoms.
• Medical history and physical exam by a doctor.
• Laboratory white-blood-cell count to detect inflammation, red-blood-cell count to detect bleeding and measurement of fluid and electrolyte levels.
• Surgical diagnostic procedures, such as passing a small needle into the abdomen to obtain fluid, blood or other material.

• CT scan (see Glossary) and x-rays of the abdomen.

APPROPRIATE HEALTH CARE
• Doctor's treatment.
• Hospitalization is usually necessary to treat this condition and any underlying problem. You may require therapy for dehydration, respiratory support and blood transfusions.
• Surgery may be necessary to repair the organ damage or injury that allowed foreign material into the abdomen.

POSSIBLE COMPLICATIONS
• Shock.
• Blood poisoning (septicemia).
• Intestinal obstruction caused by later adhesions (bands of scar tissue).
• Kidney or liver failure.

PROBABLE OUTCOME—Usually curable with early diagnosis and treatment. Treatment delay and complications can be fatal. Outcome dependent on age, duration of illness, cause and any pre-existing condition.

HOW TO TREAT

GENERAL MEASURES—Early diagnosis and treatment of the underlying disorder, such as appendicitis, ulcer or ectopic pregnancy, are essential. If abdominal pain develops, don't waste valuable time with home treatments—especially laxative use. Laxatives may cause inflamed abdominal organs to rupture.

MEDICATION—Your doctor may prescribe:
• Antibiotics to fight infection.
• Pain relievers (sometimes) after diagnosis or surgery.

ACTIVITY—Rest in bed after treatment until symptoms disappear. If surgery is necessary, resume your activities gradually after surgery.

DIET—Don't eat or drink anything (so the intestinal tract can rest) until the acute infection subsides. You will be given intravenous nourishment and fluids. Oral feedings will resume when your system can tolerate them.

CALL YOUR DOCTOR IF

• You have symptoms of peritonitis. This is an emergency!
• The following occurs during treatment: Constipation.
Signs of new infection, including fever, chills, muscle aches, dizziness, headache and increasing abdominal pain.
• New, unexplained symptoms develop. Drugs used in treatment may produce side effects.

PERSONALITY DISORDERS

 ## GENERAL INFORMATION

DEFINITION—A group of conditions that are not illnesses, but ways of behaving. Characteristics include relatively fixed, inflexible and maladaptive patterns of behavior that cause trouble with relationships, work and the law. Individuals with these conditions feel their behavior patterns are normal and "right."

SEX OR AGE MOST AFFECTED—Both sexes; all ages.

SIGNS & SYMPTOMS
- **Paranoid**—Shows unwarranted suspiciousness and distrust of others; is defensive, oversensitive.
- **Schizoid and schizotypal**—Cold emotionally; has difficulty forming relationships; is withdrawn, shy superstitious, socially isolated.
- **Compulsive**—Perfectionist, rigid in habits, indecisive; needs control.
- **Histrionic**—Dependent, immature, excitable, vain; constantly craves stimulation and attention; communicates by appearances or behavior.
- **Narcissistic**—Has an exaggerated sense of one's own importance; is preoccupied with power; lacks interest in others; demands attention; feels entitled to special consideration.
- **Avoidant**—Fears and overreacts to rejection; has low self-esteem; is socially withdrawn, dependent.
- **Dependent**—Passive, overaccepting, unable to make decisions; lacks confidence.
- **Passive-aggressive**—Stubborn, sulking; fears authority; proscrastinates; is chronically late, argumentative, helpless, clinging.
- **Antisocial**—Selfish, callous, promiscuous, impulsive, reckless; unable to learn from experience; fails at school and work.
- **Borderline**—Impulsive; has unstable and intense interpersonal relationships; displays inappropriate anger, fear and guilt; lacks self-control; has identity problems; may self-mutilate (cut or burn oneself to relieve tension); is suicidal (sometimes).

CAUSES—Unknown. Theories include biological, social and psychological factors.

RISK INCREASES WITH
- History of abuse as a child.
- Family history of mood disorders.

HOW TO PREVENT—No specific preventive measures. Early diagnosis and counseling may lessen the severity of the disorder.

 ## WHAT TO EXPECT

DIAGNOSTIC MEASURES
- Observation of symptoms by other people.
- Medical and behavior history, physical exam and psychological evaluation by a therapist.

APPROPRIATE HEALTH CARE—Doctor's treatment. Psychological counseling.

POSSIBLE COMPLICATIONS
- Difficulty maintaining personal relationships and jobs; anxiety and depression.
- Drug abuse.
- Noncompliance with treatment.
- Suicide.

PROBABLE OUTCOME—Therapy can be effective for some patients and bring about a gradual change in personality and behavior. For others prognosis is guarded, and for some the outcome is poor.

 ## HOW TO TREAT

GENERAL MEASURES
- Treatment requires a trusting relationship between the therapist and patient. This can be difficult as motivation for treatment often comes from someone other than the person with the disorder.
- Psychological treatment may include family and group therapy, group living situations and self-help groups. Behavior-changing techniques involve the learning of social skills, reinforcement of appropriate behavior, setting limits on inappropriate behavior, learning to express feelings, self-analysis of behavior and accepting accountability for actions.

MEDICATION
- No medication will cure or treat a personality disorder. Drugs may be prescribed for treatment of additional illnesses:
  Antidepressants for depression; anxiety medications;
  Antipsychotic drugs for psychoses.

ACTIVITY—No restrictions.

DIET—No special diet.

 ## CALL YOUR DOCTOR IF

- You or a family member has symptoms of a personality disorder.
- Symptoms continue to worsen after treatment has started.
- New, unexplained symptoms develop. Drugs used in treatment may produce side effects.

PHARYNGITIS

GENERAL INFORMATION

DEFINITION—A very common throat inflammation and infection, usually from a virus.

BODY PARTS INVOLVED—Throat area, including tonsils.

SEX OR AGE MOST AFFECTED
- Both sexes.
- All ages except infancy.

SIGNS & SYMPTOMS
- Sore throat.
- Swallowing difficulty.
- Tickle or "lump" in the throat.
- Fever.
- Swollen glands in the neck (sometimes).
- Throat may be red or covered with a grayish membrane (sometimes).
- Generalized aching.

CAUSES—Infection from viruses or bacteria. Following are the most common germs.
- Viruses—Epstein-Barr and many types of respiratory viruses.
- Bacteria—streptococci, gonococci, Haemophilus, pneumococci or staphylococci.

RISK INCREASES WITH
- Illness that has lowered resistance.
- Fatigue or overwork.
- Diabetes mellitus.
- Immune deficiencies.
- Smoking.
- Excess alcohol consumption.
- Oral sex.
- Epidemics, during which all persons are at increased risk.
- Close quarters, such as in military recruits, schools, day care centers.

HOW TO PREVENT
- Avoid close contact with anyone with a sore throat.
- Keep immunizations, including diphtheria, up to date.

WHAT TO EXPECT

DIAGNOSTIC MEASURES
- Your own observation of symptoms.
- Medical history and physical exam by a doctor.
- Laboratory throat culture and blood count.

APPROPRIATE HEALTH CARE
- Self-care after diagnosis.
- Doctor's treatment.
- Hospitalization for pharyngitis caused by diphtheria or hemophilus bacteria (rare).

POSSIBLE COMPLICATIONS
- Epiglottitis, leading to complete breathing obstruction.
- Pneumonia.
- Rheumatic fever, scarlet fever or glomerulonephritis, if pharyngitis is caused by strep bacteria and does not receive adequate antibiotic treatment.
- Ear infection.
- Sinusitis or rhinitis.

PROBABLE OUTCOME—Spontaneous recovery for most cases of viral pharyngitis. Other cases are curable with antibiotics.

HOW TO TREAT

GENERAL MEASURES
- Home care is usually sufficient.
- Use gargles to relieve throat pain. Prepare double-strength tea, hot or cold, or a salt-water solution (1 teaspoon salt in 8 oz. warm water). Use to gargle as often as you wish.
- Use a cool-mist, ultrasonic humidifier to increase air moisture. This will relieve the dry, tight feeling in the throat. Clean humidifier daily.
- If the glands are large and tender, apply moist, warm soaks at least 4 times a day for 30 to 60 minutes. The compresses will be more effective if they are kept warm. Be careful not to burn the skin.
- Replace your toothbrush. It may harbor germs.
- Until infection is gone, use separate washcloths; don't share food.

MEDICATION
- For minor discomfort, you may use nonprescription drugs such as acetaminophen. Don't give aspirin to a child for any viral illness. Studies link its use with the development of Reye's syndrome.
- Your doctor may prescribe antibiotics. Be sure to finish entire course of prescribed antibiotics to avoid complications.

ACTIVITY—Limited activity is necessary until symptoms disappear.

DIET—Extra fluids are necessary. Drink at least 8 glasses of fluid daily, more for high fevers. If swallowing solid food is painful, try a liquid or soft diet for a few days.

CALL YOUR DOCTOR IF

- You have symptoms of pharyngitis.
- The following occurs during treatment:
  Breathing or swallowing difficulty.
  Fever; severe headache.
  Thick mucus drainage from the nose.
  Cough that produces green, yellow, brown or bloody sputum.
  Skin rash.
  Dark urine.
  Chest pain.

PHEOCHROMOCYTOMA

GENERAL INFORMATION

DEFINITION—A tumor of the core (medulla) of the adrenal glands. The tumor is usually benign and does not spread to other organs.

BODY PARTS INVOLVED—Adrenal medulla.

SEX OR AGE MOST AFFECTED—Adults of both sexes between ages 30 and 50.

SIGNS & SYMPTOMS
- Rapid heartbeat following exercise, emotional upset or exposure to cold.
- Tremors and nervousness.
- Feelings of impending doom.
- Feelings of hunger.
- Episodes of flushing.
- Sweating; paleness.
- Weakness and fatigue; nausea; vomiting.
- Very high blood-pressure spikes, accompanied by headaches.
- Unexplained weight loss.
Episodes of at least some of these symptoms may occur several times a day or only occasionally (up to 2 months apart).

CAUSES—The hormones adrenalin and noradrenalin, produced by the core of each adrenal gland, work with the central nervous system to control heart rate, blood pressure and other vital body functions. When a tumor (the pheochromocytoma) exists—even though it is benign—excess hormones are produced. The excess hormones cause symptoms. Cause of the tumor is unknown.

RISK INCREASES WITH
- Pregnancy.
- Family history of pheochromocytoma.

HOW TO PREVENT—No specific preventive measures.

WHAT TO EXPECT

DIAGNOSTIC MEASURES
- Your own observation of symptoms.
- Medical history and physical exam by a doctor.
- Laboratory studies of urine and blood to measure catecholamine levels. Catecholamines are breakdown products of hormone production.
- MRI and nuclear imaging techniques (see Glossary).

APPROPRIATE HEALTH CARE
- Doctor's treatment.
- Surgery to remove the tumor. The tumor is usually removed through an abdominal incision after several days of study and pretreatment with medications that block release of hormones during surgery.

POSSIBLE COMPLICATIONS
- Stroke caused by very high blood pressure during an episode.
- Kidney, brain, heart damage and death caused by unrecognized and untreated pheochromocytoma.

PROBABLE OUTCOME—Usually curable with surgery.

HOW TO TREAT

GENERAL MEASURES—For a description of abdominal surgery and postoperative care, see Laparotomy in Surgery section.

MEDICATION—Your doctor may prescribe:
- Alpha- and beta-adrenergic blockers before surgery to suppress the effect of hormones.
- Drugs to treat high blood pressure.

ACTIVITY—No restrictions after recovery from surgery.

DIET—Prior to surgery, a high salt diet may be recommended to increase blood volume.

CALL YOUR DOCTOR IF

- You have symptoms of pheochromocytoma.
- New, unexplained symptoms develop. Drugs used in treatment may produce side effects.

PHOBIAS

GENERAL INFORMATION

DEFINITION—A type of anxiety that involves persistent, irrational or an exaggerated fear of a particular object, situation, activity, setting or even a bodily function (all of which are not basically dangerous or an appropriate source for anxiety). Most people with phobias recognize that the fear is inappropriate to the situation. Phobias are classified as:
- Social (fear of embarrassment in social situations such as public speaking or using public bathroom).
- Agoraphobia (fear of being alone or fear of public places).
- Simple (fear of a particular stimulus such as animals, insects, heights, flying, closed places, etc.).

BODY PARTS INVOLVED—Nervous system.

SEX OR AGE MOST AFFECTED—Females more than males; usually late adolescent or young adulthood.

SIGNS & SYMPTOMS—Anxiety symptoms occur when exposed to, or thinking of, the phobic stimulus:
- Palpitations.
- Sweating.
- Tremors.
- Flushing.
- Nausea.
- Experiencing negative thoughts and scary images.

CAUSES—Exact cause is unknown. Possibly a learned response (conditioning) such as being raised by someone with a similar fear or having an early frightening experience that has become associated with the object or situation. Other theories focus on the phobia as having a symbolic meaning.

RISK INCREASES WITH
- Family history of anxiety.
- Separation anxiety in childhood.
- Presence of another psychiatric disorder.
- Perfectionist type individual.

HOW TO PREVENT—No specific preventive measure to prevent the phobia. Techniques are available to prevent or control the reaction.

WHAT TO EXPECT

DIAGNOSTIC MEASURES
- Your own observation of symptoms.
- Medical and social history and physical exam by a doctor (sometimes).

APPROPRIATE HEALTH CARE
- Self-care.
- Psychotherapy or counseling for severe phobias and for phobias that are life-style restricting. Several different types of therapy are used such as desensitization or flooding (see Glossary for both).
- Fear of flying clinics are available in many communities.

POSSIBLE COMPLICATIONS
- Life-style constrictions brought on by avoidance of the phobic stimulus. Agoraphobia in particular restricts an individual's activities and is severely disabling.
- Dependence on drugs or alcohol to overcome anxiety.

PROBABLE OUTCOME
- Simple phobias—some spontaneously stop as a person ages; others don't cause any impairment if the object can be avoided (such as fear of snakes); for some, the people go through their fearful situations (such as flying); and others can be cured with treatment.
- Social phobias—may be overcome with treatment.
- Agoraphobia—person becomes more and more homebound without treatment (is often associated with panic disorder).

HOW TO TREAT

GENERAL MEASURES
- If you feel your fear taking hold:
  Shift your thoughts from negative—"The dog will bite"—to something realistic and positive—"The dog is on a leash."
  Do something manageable—count backward from 1000, read a book, talk aloud, take deep-measured breaths.
  Practice relaxation techniques.
- Join a support group if available.
- See Resources for Additional Information.

MEDICATION—Your doctor may prescribe tranquillizers for a short period of time.

ACTIVITY—No restrictions.

DIET—No special diet. Avoid caffeine.

CALL YOUR DOCTOR IF

- You feel any phobia is restricting or disrupting your life.
- Symptoms of the phobia return after treatment.

PHOTOSENSITIVITY

GENERAL INFORMATION

DEFINITION—Abnormal sensitivity to sunlight (a reaction may occur after only a few minutes exposure).

BODY PARTS INVOLVED—Skin in areas most exposed to sunlight.

SEX OR AGE MOST AFFECTED—Both sexes; all ages.

SIGNS & SYMPTOMS
- A burning reaction similar to those that follow prolonged sun exposure.
- Red skin rash, sometimes with small blisters.
- Dizziness, nausea, vomiting.

CAUSES—An interaction between photosentizing substances and sunlight causes the cutaneous (skin) reaction. Photosentizing possibilities include:
- The reaction is often produced when certain substances are combined with ultraviolet light. Among those substances are common drugs, taken orally, including antibiotics, sulfonamides, tolbutamide, chlorpropamide, chlorothiazides, tetracycline, griseofulvin, nalidixic acid, psoralens, nonsteroidal anti-inflammatories, anticancer drugs, estrogens, progestins, chlordiazepoxide, cyclamates, phenothiazines, thiazide diuretics. Chemicals in externally applied substances including perfume and after-shave lotions; coal tar products; soaps containing halogenated bacteriostatic agents; even some sunscreen products (containing PABA, PABA esters, cinnamates, benzophenones) can cause a photosensitive reaction.
- Lupus erythematosus (systemic or discoid).
- Porphyria.

RISK INCREASES WITH
- Spring and summer seasons.
- Exposure to the sun between 11:00 a.m. and 2:00 p.m.

HOW TO PREVENT
- Stay out of the sun when possible if you have a history of photosensitivity.
- When exposed to the sun, use sunscreen lotions with a sun-protective factor (SPF) of 15 or more; wear protective, light colored clothing (including gloves) and broad-brimmed hat.

WHAT TO EXPECT

DIAGNOSTIC MEASURES
- Your own observation of symptoms.
- Medical history and physical exam by a doctor.
- Determine any underlying cause such as drugs, cosmetics or a medical disorder. Photopatch testing can be used to identify photoallergic causes.

APPROPRIATE HEALTH CARE
- Self care after diagnosis.
- Doctor's treatment.
- Eliminate the photosensitizing agent (change medications if necessary).

POSSIBLE COMPLICATIONS—Recurrence of the rash and other symptoms when exposed to the sun—even for short periods—especially in spring and summer.

PROBABLE OUTCOME—Curable with elimination of photosensitizing agent. Medications may be required to resolve severe reactions.

HOW TO TREAT

GENERAL MEASURES
- Stay out of the sun during the hours of strongest ultraviolet light (11 a.m. to 2 p.m.).
- If you must go out in the sun, wear protective clothing and the most protective sunscreen preparation available.

MEDICATION—Your doctor may prescribe:
- Corticosteroids for severe reactions (oral or topical).
- Antihistamines for itching symptoms.
- Sunscreens for prevention (ones that block both ultraviolet A and B; without PABA as an ingredient).

ACTIVITY—No restrictions, except to avoid prolonged sun exposure.

DIET—No special diet. Drink extra fluids to prevent dehydration.

CALL YOUR DOCTOR IF

- You have symptoms of photosensitivity.
- New, unexplained symptoms develop. Drugs used in treatment may produce side effects.

PICA

GENERAL INFORMATION

DEFINITION—Craving or eating bizarre substances that have no food value.

BODY PARTS INVOLVED—Brain; gastrointestinal tract.

SEX OR AGE MOST AFFECTED—Children between ages 1 and 6 and pregnant women. Pica does not apply to infants and children up to about 18 months old who "put everything" in the mouth. That is normal.

SIGNS & SYMPTOMS
- Eating nonfood substances, such as starch, clay, ice, plaster, paint, hair or gravel.
- Abdominal pain (sometimes).

CAUSES
- Instinctive need to replace minerals absent in the diet. This is especially true of eating clay for iron content.
- Psychological factors that are not well-understood, related to substandard housing, low income or emotional deprivation.

RISK INCREASES WITH
- Family history of pica.
- Poor nutrition.
- Poverty.
- Mental retardation.
- Anemia or iron deficiency.

HOW TO PREVENT
- Remove substances from the reach of children.
- Repaint homes in which lead-base paints have been used. Don't use older baby cribs painted with lead-base paint.
- Provide a well-balanced diet for yourself and your children.
- Provide a loving, supportive home environment for your children.

WHAT TO EXPECT

DIAGNOSTIC MEASURES
- Your own observation of symptoms.
- Medical history and physical exam by a doctor.
- Laboratory blood studies to detect anemia and measure fluids and electrolytes.
- X-rays of the abdomen.

APPROPRIATE HEALTH CARE
- Self-care after diagnosis.
- Doctor's treatment.
- Psychotherapy or counseling.

POSSIBLE COMPLICATIONS
- Lead poisoning from paint or plaster.
- Intestinal infections or parasites from soil.
- Anemia.
- Malnutrition.
- Intestinal obstruction.

PROBABLE OUTCOME—Pica during pregnancy usually ends with childbirth. Other forms can be controlled with treatment.

HOW TO TREAT

GENERAL MEASURES
- If the craving is due to a deficiency of an element, such as iron, treatment involves iron replacement.
- Other treatment steps:
  Proper supervision of young children.
  Examine your home environment and family interactions. If you feel they are not what they should be, seek ways to create a healthier atmosphere. Consult a counselor, if necessary.
  Behavior modification therapy whereby parents learn to encourage the child's acceptable behaviors through positive reinforcement and unacceptable behavior by providing the child with distractions.

MEDICATION—Your doctor may prescribe iron or other supplements if needed.

ACTIVITY—No restrictions.

DIET—Provide a well-balanced diet. Vitamin and mineral supplements may be necessary. If you need help planning meals, consult the home-extension service, a dietitian or a visiting nurse.

CALL YOUR DOCTOR IF

- Your child has symptoms of pica.
- You are pregnant and have symptoms of pica.
- Pica does not improve in 2 weeks, despite treatment.

PILONIDAL CYST

 GENERAL INFORMATION

DEFINITION—A small, hair-containing skin sac at the base of the spine. The cyst looks like a small opening—sometimes no more than a dimple—with a few hairs protruding. It is prone to infection. Pilonidal cysts are uncommon in black people.

BODY PARTS INVOLVED—Skin.

SEX OR AGE MOST AFFECTED—Both sexes, but more common in men. Cyst infections usually begin in young adulthood (ages 18 to 40).

SIGNS & SYMPTOMS—No symptoms when not infected. When infected, it causes:
- Pain, redness, tenderness and swelling in the area.
- Fever and chills.
- Discharge of pus.

CAUSES—The cyst is a minor abnormality that occurs during fetal development. Infection is usually caused by staphylococcal bacteria.

RISK INCREASES WITH
- Heavy perspiration. Obesity increases perspiration.
- Tight clothing.

HOW TO PREVENT
- Bathe or shower daily to keep the area clean. Hot tub baths seem more effective in preventing infection of the cyst.
- Wear light, loose-fitting clothing.
- Avoid overweight.

 WHAT TO EXPECT

DIAGNOSTIC MEASURES
- Your own observation of symptoms.
- Medical history and physical exam by a doctor.
- Laboratory culture of the discharge.

APPROPRIATE HEALTH CARE
- Self-care after diagnosis.
- Doctor's treatment.
- Treatment for infected cysts usually consists of incision and drainage of the abscess, or occasionally, surgical excision of the whole infected area.

POSSIBLE COMPLICATIONS—Spread of infection (rare).

PROBABLE OUTCOME—Infection curable with antibiotic treatment and surgery.

 HOW TO TREAT

GENERAL MEASURES
- If the cyst is infected, take warm baths to relieve pain. Sit in a tub of warm water for 10 to 15 minutes as often as it feels good.
- If surgery is necessary, see Pilonidal Cyst Removal (in Surgery section) for an explanation of the surgery and postoperative care.

MEDICATION—Your doctor may prescribe antibiotics to fight infection.

ACTIVITY—No restrictions, unless the cyst becomes infected. Then, limit activities until the infection is cured.

DIET—Lose weight if you are overweight.

 CALL YOUR DOCTOR IF

- You have symptoms of a pilonidal cyst. It should be diagnosed.
- After diagnosis, a cyst shows signs of infection.

ILLNESS & DISORDERS

PINWORMS
(Enterobiasis)

GENERAL INFORMATION

DEFINITION—Infestation with intestinal parasites, a common occurrence in children. Pinworm infestations are more a nuisance than a major health problem.

BODY PARTS INVOLVED—Cecum (pouchlike beginning of the large intestine on the right side to which the appendix is attached); large intestine; anus; skin around the anus.

SEX OR AGE MOST AFFECTED—All ages, but most common in children.

SIGNS & SYMPTOMS
- Skin irritation and painful itching around the anus, especially during sleep.
- Restless sleep.
- Vaginal discharge, itching and discomfort, if pinworms migrate into the vaginal opening.
- Poor appetite and stomach pain (rare).
- Paleness (sometimes).

CAUSES—Infestation of the cecum by a very small worm (oxyuria) that measures only 10mm in its adult form.

Pinworms travel from the cecum to the rectum to lay eggs around the anus and buttocks. The tiny eggs are picked up on the fingers by scratching.

Eggs are transferred to others on toilet seats or by hand-to-hand or hand-to-mouth contact. They also drift in the air, where they are inhaled or swallowed.

Eggs hatch in the small intestine. The larvae travel to the cecum, where they mature, mate and repeat the cycle.

RISK INCREASES WITH
- Groups of children, as in schools or large families.
- Poor personal hygiene.
- Warm climate.

HOW TO PREVENT
- Wash hands carefully after using the toilet and before meals.
- Keep the nails short and clean.
- Wash the anus and genitals at least once a day. Rinse well, preferably under a shower.
- Have children wear snug cotton underpants day and night, and change them daily.
- Don't scratch the anus or put fingers near the nose or mouth.
- Use very hot water to wash dishes.

WHAT TO EXPECT

DIAGNOSTIC MEASURES
- Your own observation of symptoms.

- Medical history and physical exam by a doctor.
- Microscopic study of the worms or eggs.

APPROPRIATE HEALTH CARE
- Home care after diagnosis.
- Doctor's treatment with medication.

POSSIBLE COMPLICATIONS—No serious complications expected.

PROBABLE OUTCOME—Usually curable in one treatment—two treatments at the most. Treatment should include all family members at once. Recurrence is common.

If worms reappear soon after treatment, they usually represent a new infection—not treatment failure.

HOW TO TREAT

GENERAL MEASURES
- The following should be done on the day the family is treated with medicine:
  Clean the house with extra care. Wash the sheets and clothing with extra bleach or ammonia, or boil them.
  Scrub washable toys. Sterilize metal toys and similar objects in a hot oven.
  Cut and clean fingernails.
  Change towels.
  Scrub toilet bowls.
  Take extra-long showers.
- About 2 weeks after treatment, your doctor will probably check to be sure all parasites have been destroyed.

MEDICATION
- Your doctor may prescribe antiworm medicine. Follow directions carefully. Take the medicine on an empty stomach. The medicine may cause nausea, vomiting and diarrhea. It is not absorbed by the stomach or intestines, so the bowel movement following treatment will probably be the color of the medicine.
- Nonprescription creams or lotions to relieve itching may be helpful.

ACTIVITY—No restrictions.

DIET—No special diet.

CALL YOUR DOCTOR IF

- Anyone in your family has symptoms of pinworms.
- Pinworms reappear after treatment.
- You think medicine is causing side effects that don't disappear quickly.

PITUITARY GLAND, UNDERACTIVE
(Hypopituitarism)

GENERAL INFORMATION

DEFINITION—Underactivity of the pituitary gland, resulting in inadequate amounts of hormones produced by the pituitary.

The anterior lobe of the pituitary produces the following hormones:
- Growth hormone.
- Prolactin, which stimulates breasts to produce milk.
- Thyroid-stimulating hormone.
- Adrenal-stimulating hormone.
- Ovarian- or testicular-stimulating hormones.

The posterior lobe of the pituitary gland produces two hormones:
- Antidiuretic hormone, which affects the kidneys in regulating concentration and quantity of urine.
- Oxytocin, which stimulates contractions of the uterus during childbirth and releases milk during breast-feeding.

BODY PARTS INVOLVED—Pituitary gland and body parts mentioned above.

SEX OR AGE MOST AFFECTED—Both sexes; all ages.

SIGNS & SYMPTOMS
- Menstrual irregularities.
- Impotence; infertility.
- Low blood sugar and weakness; low blood pressure.
- Intolerance to cold and stress.
- Retarded growth in children (evident after age 6 months).
- Lack of secondary sexual features that develop in puberty, such as voice changes, breast development and growth of pubic hair.
- Mental changes, including psychosis.
- Extreme lethargy.
- Persistent headaches.
- Increased quantity and frequency of urination.

CAUSES
- Unknown (sometimes).
- Serious head injury with pressure (usually from bleeding) on the pituitary gland.
- Reduced blood supply to the pituitary gland in a mother following severe hemorrhage and shock during childbirth.
- Tumor of the pituitary gland.
- Infection in the brain.
- Aneurysm of blood vessels in the base of the brain.

RISK INCREASES WITH
- Family history of pituitary disorders.
- Pregnancy.

HOW TO PREVENT—Obtain medical treatment for any underlying injury, infection or tumor, if possible.

WHAT TO EXPECT

DIAGNOSTIC MEASURES
- Your own observation of symptoms.
- Medical history and physical exam by a doctor.
- Laboratory blood studies of hormone levels and function.
- CT scan (see Glossary) of the head, x-ray of the skull.

APPROPRIATE HEALTH CARE
- Treatment is aimed at treating the cause of the pituitary failure and providing adequate hormone replacement.
- Surgery to remove underlying tumors or blood clots, if necessary.

POSSIBLE COMPLICATIONS—Hormonal failure with serious consequences without treatment.

PROBABLE OUTCOME—Usually treatable with surgery or replacement therapy of pituitary, thyroid, adrenal and sex hormones.

HOW TO TREAT

GENERAL MEASURES
- This disorder requires close medical supervision and continuing treatment.
- Wear a Medic-Alert (see Glossary) bracelet or neck pendant indicating your hormone deficiencies and their proper treatment.

MEDICATION—Your doctor may prescribe:
- Hormones to replace those the pituitary is not producing.
- Pain relievers after surgery.
- Antibiotics or antiviral medications, if infection is causing the disorder.

ACTIVITY—Stay as active as your condition allows. A regular exercise program is encouraged. Consult your doctor.

DIET—No special diet.

CALL YOUR DOCTOR IF

- You have symptoms of an underactive pituitary gland.
- After surgery, you develop signs of infection, such as fever, lethargy and muscle aches.
- New, unexplained symptoms develop. Drugs used in treatment may produce side effects.

PITUITARY TUMOR

GENERAL INFORMATION

DEFINITION—Abnormal growth in the pituitary gland, which leads to overactivity of other endocrine glands. Pituitary tumors may be benign or malignant—but even malignant pituitary tumors rarely spread to other body parts.

BODY PARTS INVOLVED—Pituitary gland, located at the base of the brain.

SEX OR AGE MOST AFFECTED—Both sexes and all ages, but most common between ages 30 and 50.

SIGNS & SYMPTOMS
- Blurred vision, double vision, dizziness or a drooping eyelid caused by tumor pressure on nerves to the eye.
- Headache in the forehead.
- Nausea and vomiting.
- Seizures.
- Runny nose.
- Excessive thirst.
- Menstrual changes.
- Unexplained weight gain.
- Retarded or excessive growth in children.
- Low blood sugar.
- Low blood pressure.
- Loss of peripheral vision.
- Symptoms of abnormalities in other endocrine glands. See Hyperthyroidism, Hyperparathyroidism, Cushing's Syndrome and Ovarian Tumor (all in Illness section).

CAUSES—Unknown, but it may be caused by a dominant genetic trait. The pituitary gland is divided into two parts, the anterior (front) lobe and posterior (rear) lobe. Two main types of tumor occur, pituitary adenomas (usually nonmalignant) and craniopharyngioma.

RISK INCREASES WITH—Unknown.

HOW TO PREVENT—No specific preventive measures.

WHAT TO EXPECT

DIAGNOSTIC MEASURES
- Your own observation of symptoms.
- Medical history and physical exam by a doctor.
- Laboratory studies of cerebrospinal fluid and blood.
- X-rays of the skull.
- CT scan, angiogram (see Glossary for both).
- Vision studies.

APPROPRIATE HEALTH CARE
- Doctor's treatment.
- Treatment may involve surgery to remove the tumor, radiation treatment, hormone therapy or a combination of all three. Surgery is a delicate procedure because of the location of the pituitary (close to the brain); you may require open brain surgery.

POSSIBLE COMPLICATIONS
- Vision loss.
- Loss of sense of smell.
- Extreme hormone imbalance.

PROBABLE OUTCOME—Curable with surgery if the tumor has not spread from the pituitary gland.

HOW TO TREAT

GENERAL MEASURES
- If surgery is required, the family should maintain an optimistic outlook, stay in close contact with the patient's doctor and help by making their visits with the patient as supportive as possible.
- Wear a Medic-Alert (see Glossary) type bracelet or neck tag that indicates your medical problem and the medications you take.

MEDICATION—Your doctor may prescribe:
- Pain relievers.
- Hormone replacement medication for life. This may require frequent dosage adjustments.
- Anticancer drugs.

ACTIVITY—Resume your normal activities gradually after surgery.

DIET—Restricted while you are in the hospital; after surgery, you may return to a regular diet.

CALL YOUR DOCTOR IF

- You have symptoms of a pituitary tumor.
- The following occurs after surgery:
  Bleeding at the surgical site.
  Signs of general infection, such as fever, chills, muscle aches and headache.
  Clear discharge from the nose.

PITYRIASIS ALBA

GENERAL INFORMATION

DEFINITION—A benign disorder of the skin in which skin temporarily loses pigmentation in patches.

BODY PARTS INVOLVED—Skin of the cheeks and arms.

SEX OR AGE MOST AFFECTED—Occurs most in children, but may occur up to age 25.

SIGNS & SYMPTOMS—Skin lesions with the following characteristics:
- Lesions are small white patches with vague borders. They sometimes have pinpoint-sized white papules (small, raised bumps).
- Patches are most apparent in summer because the lesions cannot tan, and tanning heightens the contrast between the areas.
- One person may have 1 to 12 patches at a time.
- Patches feel smooth.
- Patches may itch occasionally, but they are not painful.

CAUSES—Unknown. The tendency may be inherited.

RISK INCREASES WITH—Family history of allergies of any kind.

HOW TO PREVENT—No specific preventive measures.

WHAT TO EXPECT

DIAGNOSTIC MEASURES
- Your own observation of symptoms.
- Medical history and physical exam by a doctor.

APPROPRIATE HEALTH CARE
- Self-care after diagnosis.
- Doctor's treatment.

POSSIBLE COMPLICATIONS—None expected.

PROBABLE OUTCOME—Patches may come and go for years. Between ages 20 and 30, they disappear completely.

HOW TO TREAT

GENERAL MEASURES
- No truly effective therapy available.
- Use sunscreen or protective clothing to prevent sunburn in affected areas.

MEDICATION
- Lubricating cream application may improve roughness or dryness, but does not improve the color.
- Use of coal-tar preparations may be helpful.
- Your doctor may prescribe prescription or nonprescription topical steroid medicine to control itching and prevent papules (raised, discolored skin growths).

ACTIVITY—No restrictions.

DIET—No special diet.

CALL YOUR DOCTOR IF

- You have symptoms of pityriasis alba.
- New, unexplained symptoms develop. Drugs used in treatment may produce side effects.

ILLNESS & DISORDERS

PITYRIASIS ROSEA

GENERAL INFORMATION

DEFINITION—A noncontagious, inflammatory skin disorder with a faint rash that lasts 3 to 4 weeks or longer.

BODY PARTS INVOLVED—Skin, especially of the chest and abdomen.

SEX OR AGE MOST AFFECTED—All ages, but most common in adolescents and young adults.

SIGNS & SYMPTOMS
- A faint rash often found in skin creases of oval or round, pale-pink or light-brown areas. One larger patch (the "herald patch") may appear first. They may evolve into a Christmas tree pattern on the chest or back.
- Mild fatigue.
- Itching, usually mild.
- Occasional slight fever and headache.

CAUSES—Unknown, but may be caused by a virus or autoimmune disorder.

RISK INCREASES WITH—Fall and spring seasons.

HOW TO PREVENT—Cannot be prevented at present.

WHAT TO EXPECT

DIAGNOSTIC MEASURES
- Your own observation of symptoms.
- Medical history and physical exam by a doctor to rule out other disorders.

APPROPRIATE HEALTH CARE
- Self-care after diagnosis.
- Doctor's treatment, if severe itching occurs.

POSSIBLE COMPLICATIONS—Secondary bacterial infection of the rash area.

PROBABLE OUTCOME
- Pityriasis rosea usually runs its natural course in 5 weeks to 4 months. No medication or treatment is available to shorten its course but itching and discomfort can be relieved.
- The skin eruptions won't leave scars unless complicated by a secondary infection. New rash areas continue to break out for several weeks. Once over, one episode seems to confer lifelong immunity.
- Although pityriasis is probably caused by an infectious agent, it is not contagious. Even close family contacts are unlikely to develop the disease.

HOW TO TREAT

GENERAL MEASURES
- Treatment is focused on relieving the itching.
- Bathe as usual with a mild soap. Use warm water, as hot water may intensify the itching. Oatmeal baths may help. You don't need to sterilize the tub or shower after bathing.
- Expose the skin to moderate amounts of sunlight. This may decrease the rash.

MEDICATION
- For minor discomfort, you may use nonprescription drugs, such as:
  Calamine lotion to decrease itching.
  Acetaminophen to reduce fever.
  Steroid cream to control severe itching (a rare symptom).
  Acetaminophen to reduce fever.
- Your doctor may prescribe other topical steroids and/or antihistamines.

ACTIVITY—Usually no restrictions.

DIET—No special diet.

CALL YOUR DOCTOR IF

- You have symptoms of pityriasis rosea.
- The following occurs during treatment:
  Fever over 101F (38.3C).
  Signs of infection (warmth, redness, tenderness, pain and swelling) in the rash area.

PLACENTA PREVIA

GENERAL INFORMATION

DEFINITION—A placenta attachment that is too low in the uterus and covers the cervix. This can be life-threatening to the unborn child. It occurs to some degree in 1 of 200 pregnancies.

BODY PARTS INVOLVED—Uterus; placenta (the organ that transfers nourishment and oxygen from mother to fetus); cervix (opening to the uterus).

SEX OR AGE MOST AFFECTED—Pregnant women.

SIGNS & SYMPTOMS
- Sudden, painless bleeding during the second or third trimester of pregnancy—especially the last 13 weeks. Bleeding may begin moderately and become severe.
- Abnormal fetal position in the uterus.

CAUSES—Normally, placenta attaches high on the uterus wall, away from the cervix. In placenta previa, the placenta covers the cervix partially or completely. Any change in the cervix, such as the softening and dilating that occurs close to delivery, can cause the placenta to bleed as it separates from the uterus.

RISK INCREASES WITH
- Fibroid tumors of the uterus.
- Diabetes mellitus.
- Previous uterine surgery.
- Smoking.
- Multiple previous pregnancies and deliveries.
- Mothers over age 35.
- Prior placenta previa.

HOW TO PREVENT
- Don't smoke during your pregnancy.
- Get good prenatal care during a pregnancy. It can't prevent previa, but can help prevent complications.

WHAT TO EXPECT

DIAGNOSTIC MEASURES
- Your own observation of symptoms, especially of vaginal bleeding during pregnancy.
- Medical history and physical exam by a doctor.
- Laboratory blood tests to determine the amount of blood loss.
- Amniocentesis, and ultrasonography (see Glossary for both) to determine the exact location of the placenta.

APPROPRIATE HEALTH CARE
- Doctor's treatment.
- Hospitalization.
- Surgery to deliver the fetus by cesarean section (sometimes). Vaginal delivery is possible if the placenta separation is small or the cervix is covered only partially.

POSSIBLE COMPLICATIONS
- Premature delivery or fetal death, if extensive placenta previa develops before the expected delivery date.
- Hazardous blood loss, requiring blood transfusions for the mother.

PROBABLE OUTCOME—With prompt care, mothers and most infants survive without complications. In some cases, delivery is necessary before the fetus is mature enough to survive.

HOW TO TREAT

GENERAL MEASURES
- Have regular checkups during pregnancy. If signs of placenta previa appear, be prepared to go to the hospital early for observation and possible delivery. Arrange for fast transportation to the hospital in case of emergency, especially massive bleeding.
- A marginal placenta previa requires bed rest in the hospital until bleeding stops. If bleeding stops, you may get up—but you should stay in the hospital until delivery. If you leave the hospital, your life and that of your child will be at risk. Massive bleeding can occur before you can get back to the hospital.
- If you are near the expected delivery date and studies reveal more than a marginal or low-lying placenta, immediate Cesarean section is necessary—even though the child is below optimal size and development.

MEDICATION—Only minimal analgesic medications—if any—will be used in delivery to increase the child's survival chances. Blood transfusions may be necessary.
Don't use aspirin during pregnancy—it increases the risk of bleeding.

ACTIVITY—Rest in bed until bleeding stops or you deliver your child.

DIET—While you are bleeding and as long as surgery is being considered, drink liquids only. Eating solid food before surgery can cause anesthesia problems.

CALL YOUR DOCTOR IF

You have symptoms of placenta previa. Report any bleeding immediately. This is an emergency!

PLEURAL EFFUSION
(Empyema; Hemothorax)

 GENERAL INFORMATION

DEFINITION—An abnormal accumulation of fluid in the pleural space. Pleura are the thin membranes that line the lungs and chest cavity. Normally the fluid in this area provides lubrication and allows smooth, uniform contractions of the lungs during breathing. Types of pleural effusion include: empyema, characterized by an accumulation of pus due to infection, and hemothorax, the presence of blood in the pleural space.

BODY PARTS INVOLVED—Lung; pleura.

SEX OR AGE MOST AFFECTED—Both sexes; all ages.

SIGNS & SYMPTOMS
- No symptoms sometimes (with small effusions).
- Chest pain. Pain varies from vague discomfort to stabbing pain. It is often worse with coughing or breathing. Pain may extend to the lower chest wall or abdomen.
- Dry cough.
- Rapid, shallow breathing.
- Chills.
- Fever.
- Extreme fatigue.
- Bad breath.
- Weight loss.
- Night sweats.

CAUSES—A complication of:
- Lung or chest infections, such as pneumonia, tuberculosis or lung abscess.
- Collapsed lung or chest injury.
- Malignancy in other parts of the body.
- Collagen vascular disease, such as systemic lupus erythematosus.
- Infection in another part of the body that has spread to the chest.
- Congestive heart failure.
- Kidney disorders.
- Liver disorders.

RISK INCREASES WITH
- Recent illness (see Causes).
- Smoking.
- Wet, cold climates.

HOW TO PREVENT—Obtain medical treatment for any serious disorder or infection that may lead to pleural effusion.

 WHAT TO EXPECT

DIAGNOSTIC MEASURES
- Your own observation of symptoms.
- Medical history and physical exam by a doctor.
- Laboratory culture of pleural fluid obtained by thoracentesis (needle inserted into the chest to withdraw fluid).
- X-ray and ultrasound (see Glossary) of the chest.

APPROPRIATE HEALTH CARE
- Self-care after diagnosis.
- Doctor's treatment.
- Treatment usually consists of surgery to open the infected cavity and drain any pus or blood, and sometimes insertion of tubes to allow further drainage.

POSSIBLE COMPLICATIONS
- Meningitis.
- Pericarditis.
- Endocarditis.
- Brain abscess.

PROBABLE OUTCOME—Successful treatment depends on discovery and treatment of the underlying disorder.

 HOW TO TREAT

GENERAL MEASURES
- Use an ultrasonic cool-mist humidifier to loosen bronchial secretions so they may be coughed up more easily. Clean humidifier daily.
- Practice these breathing exercises:
  Purse your lips and breathe forcefully against resistance (as if blowing out a candle) 10 times. Repeat every hour.
  Take 10 deep breaths every hour.
  - Don't smoke.

MEDICATION
- Your doctor may prescribe antibiotics to fight infection. The type of antibiotic will depend on the type of germ responsible and sensitivity studies (see Glossary).
- For minor pain, you may use nonprescription drugs such as acetaminophen.

ACTIVITY—Reduce activity until the pain and fever are gone. Gradually return to normal activity. Allow 2 months for recovery.

DIET—No special diet. Take vitamin supplements. Increase fluid intake.

 CALL YOUR DOCTOR IF

- You have symptoms of empyema.
- The following occurs during treatment:
  Fever.
  Pain increases.
  Breathlessness worsens.
  Cough becomes dry and nonproductive.
  Fingernails or toenails turn blue or dark.
  Blood appears in the sputum.

PLEURISY

GENERAL INFORMATION

DEFINITION—Inflammation and irritation of the pleura, a thin, two-layered membrane that lines the lung and chest cavity. Pleurisy is not a disease, but may be a manifestation of many different diseases.

BODY PARTS INVOLVED—Pleura.

SEX OR AGE MOST AFFECTED—Both sexes; all ages.

SIGNS & SYMPTOMS
- Sudden chest pain that worsens with breathing and coughing. The pain varies from vague discomfort that occurs only with deep breathing or coughing to intense, stabbing pain. Pain is usually over the area of pleura inflammation, but it may also occur in the lower chest or abdomen.
- Fever (sometimes).
- Discomfort on moving the affected side.
- Rapid, shallow breathing.
- If fluid develops at the site of inflammation between the two membrane layers, the liquid is called pleural effusion. When this happens, the pleurisy pain usually subsides, but breathlessness worsens.

CAUSES—Complication of:
- Lung or chest infections, such as pneumonia or tuberculosis.
- Viral infection.
- Bronchiectasis.
- Collapse of part of the lung.
- Blood clot in the lung.
- Injury to the chest or rib fracture.
- Cancer in other parts of the body.
- Collagen vascular disease, such as systemic lupus erythematosus or rheumatoid arthritis.
- Congestive heart failure.
- Kidney and liver disorders.

RISK INCREASES WITH
- Obesity.
- Smoking.
- Use of immunosuppressive drugs.

HOW TO PREVENT—Obtain medical treatment for the underlying disorder.

WHAT TO EXPECT

DIAGNOSTIC MEASURES
- Your own observation of symptoms.
- Medical history and physical exam by a doctor.
- Laboratory blood studies to detect infection or autoimmune disease.
- X-rays of the chest.
- Biopsy (sometimes).
- Examination of pleural fluid (if any).

APPROPRIATE HEALTH CARE
- Self-care after diagnosis.
- Doctor's treatment.

POSSIBLE COMPLICATIONS
- Pneumonia.
- Lung compression or collapse and impaired breathing from leakage of pleural effusion.
- Scarring and adhesions at the site of inflammation, restricting lung expansion.

PROBABLE OUTCOME—Successful treatment of pleurisy depends on successful treatment of the disorder causing it. Often, symptoms without complications clear completely and spontaneously in 2 weeks.

HOW TO TREAT

GENERAL MEASURES
- For chest pain, wrap the entire chest firmly with 2 or 3 nonadhesive, 6-inch-wide elastic bandages.
- For coughing, use a cool-mist, ultrasonic humidifier to help loosen bronchial secretions so they can be coughed up easily. Clean humidifier daily. Holding a pillow firmly against the chest wall helps facilitate coughing.

MEDICATION
- Your doctor may prescribe antibiotics, bronchodilators, or pain relievers after diagnosis of the underlying disorder.
- You may take simple pain relievers, such as acetaminophen or aspirin, to relieve pain if no complicating disorders exist.

ACTIVITY—Reduce activity until pain and fever disappear. Then resume normal activities gradually.

DIET—No special diet.

CALL YOUR DOCTOR IF
- You have symptoms of pleurisy.
- The following occurs during treatment:
  Fever.
  Increased pain.
  Increased breathlessness.
  Cough that is dry and nonproductive.
  Blue or dark fingernails, toenails or lips.
  Blood in the sputum.

PNEUMOCONIOSIS

GENERAL INFORMATION

DEFINITION—Inflammation of the lung caused by breathing industrial dusts. Inhalation of such particles continuously for many years may cause little patches of irritation to form in one or both lungs. The scar tissue formed by the irritation may make the lungs less flexible and porous. Pneumoconiosis is not contagious.

BODY PARTS INVOLVED—Lungs.

SEX OR AGE MOST AFFECTED—Men over age 40.

SIGNS & SYMPTOMS
Early symptoms:
Shortness of breath; cough that produces little or no sputum; general ill feeling.
Late symptoms:
- Fitful sleep; appetite and weight loss; chest pain; hoarseness; coughing blood.
- Symptoms of congestive heart failure.
- Bluish nails.
- Shadows on the lungs (on chest x-rays).

CAUSES—Exposure to small particles of industrial dusts cause the following forms of pneumoconiosis:
- Coal dust causes black-lung disease (coal miner's pneumoconiosis, anthracosis).
- Beryllium and its compounds once used in manufacturing fluorescent lamp bulbs, ceramics and chemicals cause berylliosis.
- Talc, iron, cotton, synthetic fiber and aluminum dusts cause a rare form.
- Asbestos and silica cause asbestosis and silicosis.

RISK INCREASES WITH
- Poor nutrition; smoking.
- Excess alcohol consumption.
- Amount of dust inhaled over the years.

HOW TO PREVENT
- Practice safety during exposure to industrial dusts, wear a protective mask or external-air-supplied hood. Get an x-ray once a year.
- Participate in a physical exercise program to maintain good cardiopulmonary fitness.
- Avoid lung irritants like secondhand cigarette smoke or dust. Don't smoke.

WHAT TO EXPECT

DIAGNOSTIC MEASURES
- Medical history and exam by a doctor.
- X-ray of chest and pulmonary function studies.

APPROPRIATE HEALTH CARE
- Self-care after diagnosis.
- Doctor's treatment.
- Treatment is directed to relieving symptoms and treating complications.

POSSIBLE COMPLICATIONS
- Congestive heart failure.
- Lung collapse; pleurisy.
- Tuberculosis in the late stages.
- Cancer.

PROBABLE OUTCOME—This condition is currently considered incurable. However, symptoms can be relieved or controlled. It reduces life expectancy, but many patients live into their 60s and 70s. Research into causes and treatment continues, so there is hope for increasingly effective treatment and cure.

HOW TO TREAT

GENERAL MEASURES
- The following measures may relieve symptoms and protect against recurrent lung infections:
  Obtain medical treatment for any respiratory infection, including the common cold.
  Consider moving to a warm, dry climate if your disease is advanced.
  Practice bronchial drainage. Your doctor will provide instructions.
  Use a cool-mist or ultrasonic humidifier to loosen bronchial secretions so they may be coughed up easily. Clean humidifier daily.
  Stop smoking.
- Wear a Medic-Alert (see Glossary) bracelet or neck tag that indicates your medical problem and any medications you take.

MEDICATION
- Your doctor may prescribe:
  Antibiotics for infections.
  Bronchodilators (inhaled or oral) with inhalation therapy (supervised at first by an inhalation therapist) to open bronchial tubes.
- For minor discomfort, you may use nonprescription drugs, such as acetaminophen or aspirin.

ACTIVITY
- Rest in bed with infections.
- After treatment, conserve energy when necessary, attempt physical conditioning to the extent possible.

DIET—No special diet.

CALL YOUR DOCTOR IF

- The following occurs during treatment:
  Temperature spike of 101F (38.3C) or more.
  Increased chest pain or breathlessness.
  Blood in sputum.
  Continuing weight loss.
- New, unexplained symptoms develop.

PNEUMONIA, BACTERIAL

GENERAL INFORMATION

DEFINITION—Infection and inflammation of the lungs with bacteria. This is not usually contagious.

BODY PARTS INVOLVED—Lungs; bronchial tubes.

SEX OR AGE MOST AFFECTED—All ages, but most severe in young children and adults over age 60.

SIGNS & SYMPTOMS
- High fever (over 102F or 38.9C) and chills.
- Shortness of breath.
- Cough with sputum that may contain blood or blood streaks (rusty color).
- Rapid breathing.
- Chest pain that worsens with inhalations.
- Abdominal pain.
- Fatigue.
- Bluish lips and nails (rare).

CAUSES—Infection with bacteria, such as streptococci, staphylococci, hemophilus, Enterobacteriaceae, pseudomonas (also Legionella, which causes Legionnaire's disease, and Mycoplasma pneumonia; see both in Illness section).

RISK INCREASES WITH
- Newborns and infants.
- Adults over 60.
- Use of anticancer drugs.
- Smoking.
- Illness that has lowered resistance, such as: heart disease; recent surgery; cancer; tuberculosis; congestive heart failure; diabetes; alcoholism; chronic lung disease, or asthma.
- Poor general health from any cause.
- Crowded or unsanitary living conditions.
- Alcoholism.
- Hospitalization.

HOW TO PREVENT
- Obtain prompt medical treatment for respiratory infections.
- Arrange for pneumococcal and influenza immunizations of persons at risk.
- Avoid risk factors where possible.

WHAT TO EXPECT

DIAGNOSTIC MEASURES
- Your own observation of symptoms.
- Medical history and physical exam by a doctor.
- Laboratory studies, such as a sputum culture, blood culture and blood count.
- X-rays of lungs and lung scan.

APPROPRIATE HEALTH CARE
- Self-care after diagnosis.
- Doctor's treatment.

- Hospitalization for moderate to severe cases. May need breathing support, intravenous fluids, suctioning of fluids from the lung and intravenous medications.
- For mild cases, may be treated at home.

POSSIBLE COMPLICATIONS
- Pleurisy.
- Pleural effusion (fluid between the membranes that cover the lung).
- Spread of infection to the brain or meninges (meningitis).
- Pulmonary abscess.

PROBABLE OUTCOME—Usually curable in 1 to 2 weeks with treatment, but may take longer for the very young or elderly.

HOW TO TREAT

GENERAL MEASURES
- Use a cool-mist, ultrasonic humidifier to increase air moisture. Putting medicine in the humidifier probably will not help. Clean humidifier daily.
- Don't suppress the cough with medicine if the cough produces sputum or mucus. It is useful in ridding the body of lung secretions.
- Suppress the cough with medicine if it is dry, nonproductive and painful.
- Use a heating pad or hot compresses to relieve chest pain.
- See Resources for Additional Information.

MEDICATION
- Your doctor may prescribe antibiotics to fight infection.
- You may use nonprescription drugs, such as acetaminophen, to relieve minor discomfort.

ACTIVITY—Rest in bed until fever declines and pain and shortness of breath disappear. After treatment, resume normal activity as soon as possible.

DIET—No special diet. Increase fluid intake; drink at least 1 glass of water or other beverage every hour. Extra fluid helps thin lung secretions so they are easier to cough up.

CALL YOUR DOCTOR IF

- You have symptoms of pneumonia.
- The following occurs during treatment:
  Fever.
  Pain not relieved by heat or prescribed medication.
  Increased shortness of breath.
  Dark or bluish fingernails, skin or toenails.
  Blood in the sputum.
  Nausea, vomiting or diarrhea.
- New, unexplained symptoms develop. Drugs used in treatment may produce side effects.

PNEUMONIA, MYCOPLASMA
(Primary Atypical Pneumonia; "Walking Pneumonia"; Eaton-Agent Pneumonia)

 GENERAL INFORMATION

DEFINITION—Contagious lung inflammation caused by mycoplasma bacteria. This germ can cause infection in other body parts.

BODY PARTS INVOLVED—Upper-respiratory system.

SEX OR AGE MOST AFFECTED—All ages, but most common in children (1 to 12 years).

SIGNS & SYMPTOMS
- Cough (with or without sputum).
- Fever.
- Labored breathing.
- Chest pain.
- Abdominal pain.
- Bluish skin (severe cases).

CAUSES—Preceding mycoplasma infection in the nose, throat or bronchial tubes.

RISK INCREASES WITH
- Stress.
- Illness that has lowered resistance.
- Exposure to cold, harsh weather.
- Unsanitary living conditions.
- Close living conditions (military barracks, college dorms).
- Immunosuppression due to illness or drugs.

HOW TO PREVENT—Avoid exposure to persons who are ill with respiratory infections.

 WHAT TO EXPECT

DIAGNOSTIC MEASURES
- Your own observation of symptoms.
- Medical history and physical exam by a doctor.
- Laboratory culture of sputum and blood studies.
- Chest x-rays.

APPROPRIATE HEALTH CARE
- Home care after diagnosis.
- Doctor's treatment.
- Hospitalization of seriously ill children.
- For most patients, treatment can usually be done at home.

POSSIBLE COMPLICATIONS—Prolonged illness.

PROBABLE OUTCOME—This form of pneumonia is characteristically slow to heal. It is usually curable in 4 to 6 weeks with treatment. Lungs should not have residual scars.

 HOW TO TREAT

GENERAL MEASURES
- Use a cool-mist, ultrasonic humidifier to increase air moisture. Putting medicine in the humidifier probably will not help. Clean humidifier daily.
- Don't suppress the cough with medicine if it produces sputum or mucus. Coughing is useful in ridding the body of lung secretions.
- Suppress the cough with medicine if it is dry, nonproductive and painful. Consult your doctor about a cough suppressant.
- Use a heating pad on low heat or hot compresses to relieve chest pain.
- Catch sneezes and coughs with disposable tissue.
- See Resources for Additional Information.

MEDICATION—Your doctor may prescribe:
- Antibiotics, such as erythromycin or tetracycline, to fight infection. They will shorten duration of fever and other symptoms, but you can carry the organism for weeks in spite of treatment.
- Cough medicine to make the cough more tolerable.
- Nose drops, sprays or oral decongestants to reduce congestion in the upper-respiratory system.

ACTIVITY—Bed rest is necessary until fever subsides. Normal activities should be resumed gradually.

DIET—No special diet. Increase fluids to at least 1 glass of water or other beverage every hour. Extra fluid helps thin lung secretions so they can be coughed up more easily .

 CALL YOUR DOCTOR IF

- You or your child have symptoms of mycoplasma pneumonia.
- The following occurs during treatment:
  Fever.
  Pain that is not relieved by heat or prescribed medication.
  Increased shortness of breath.
  Dark or bluish fingernails, skin or toenails.
  Blood in the sputum.
  Nausea, vomiting or diarrhea.
- New, unexplained symptoms develop. Drugs used in treatment may produce side effects.

PNEUMONIA, PNEUMOCYSTIS CARINII

GENERAL INFORMATION

DEFINITION—Inflammation of the lung caused by a protozoan single-celled microscopic organism. This is an opportunistic germ, one that the body usually wards off, but which infects the body when there is breakdown and failure of the immune system as with AIDS, Hodgkin's disease and other causes of immune system failure.

BODY PARTS INVOLVED—Lower-respiratory system (bronchial tubes and lungs).

SEX OR AGE MOST AFFECTED—All ages, both sexes, but most common in adult men.

SIGNS & SYMPTOMS
- Slow onset of dry, nonproductive cough.
- Fever.
- Air hunger.
- Shortness of breath.
- Rapid heart rate.
- Anxiety.
- Purple lips and fingernails.

CAUSES—The protozoan Pneumocystis carinii is transmitted from person to person.

RISK INCREASES WITH
- AIDS.
- Hodgkin's disease.
- Cancer chemotherapy.
- Taking cortisone or corticosteroid medicines.
- Blood transfusions.
- X-ray treatments.

HOW TO PREVENT—Will be dependent on your risk factors and whether you have had previous infection with Pneumocystis carinii pneumonia.

WHAT TO EXPECT

DIAGNOSTIC MEASURES
- Your own observation of symptoms.
- Medical history and physical exam by a doctor.
- Arterial blood gases.
- X-rays.
- Stained specimen of sputum obtained by bronchoscopy or lung biopsy to identify the organism.

APPROPRIATE HEALTH CARE
- Doctor's treatment.
- Treatment may be done at home for mild cases; for moderate to severe infection, you will be hospitalized. You may require mechanical breathing support.

POSSIBLE COMPLICATIONS
- Prolonged illness, sometimes fatal.
- Side effects of medication, especially skin rash and low white blood-cell count.

PROBABLE OUTCOME—Outcome is variable depending on general health and degree of infection.

HOW TO TREAT

GENERAL MEASURES—No special self-care measures.

MEDICATION—Your doctor may prescribe:
- Antibiotics, such as trimethoprim/sulfamethoxazole or pentamidine (oral or aerosol).
- Corticosteroids.
- Cough medicine to make the cough more tolerable.
- Nose drops, sprays or oral decongestants to reduce congestion in the upper-respiratory system.
- New drugs that are currently being investigated.
- Preventive medications for HIV or AIDS patients.

ACTIVITY—Bed rest is necessary until fever subsides. Normal activities should be resumed gradually.

DIET—No special diet. Increase fluids to at least 1 glass of water or other beverage every hour. Extra fluid helps thin lung secretions so they can be coughed up more easily .

CALL YOUR DOCTOR IF

- You have symptoms of pneumocystis pneumonia.
- The following occurs during treatment:
  Fever.
  Pain that is not relieved by heat or prescribed medication.
  Increased shortness of breath.
  Dark or bluish fingernails, skin or toenails.
  Blood in the sputum.
  Nausea, vomiting or diarrhea.
- New, unexplained symptoms develop. Drugs used in treatment may produce side effects.

PNEUMONIA, VIRAL

 GENERAL INFORMATION

DEFINITION—An acute lung infection caused by a virus. The infection causes tissues of the lungs to become inflamed and filled with fluid.

BODY PARTS INVOLVED
- Lower respiratory tract (bronchial tubes, bronchioles and lungs).
- Upper respiratory tract (nose, throat, tonsils, sinuses, trachea and larynx).

SEX OR AGE MOST AFFECTED—Both sexes; all ages.

SIGNS & SYMPTOMS
- Fever and chills.
- Muscle aches and fatigue.
- Cough, with or without sputum or "croup."
- Rapid, labored (sometimes) breathing.
- Chest pain.
- Sore throat.
- Loss of appetite.
- Enlarged lymph glands in the neck.

CAUSES—Virus infections, including influenza, chickenpox and respiratory syncytial virus (RSV) (especially in adults), respiratory viruses, measles and cytomegalovirus (especially in infants).

RISK INCREASES WITH
- Newborns and infants.
- Adults over 60.
- Asthma.
- Cystic fibrosis.
- Inhalation of a foreign body into the lung.
- Smoking.
- Crowded or unsanitary living conditions.

HOW TO PREVENT
- Annual flu vaccines recommended for high-risk people (heart or lung disease, other chronic diseases, medical personnel and over age 65).
- Measles vaccination for children.

 WHAT TO EXPECT

DIAGNOSTIC MEASURES
- Your own observation of symptoms.
- Medical history and physical exam by a doctor.
- Laboratory blood studies.
- X-rays of the chest.

APPROPRIATE HEALTH CARE
- Self-care after diagnosis.
- Doctor's treatment.
- Hospitalization (rare).

POSSIBLE COMPLICATIONS—Secondary bacterial infections of the lungs.

PROBABLE OUTCOME—Usually curable in a few days to a week. Post-viral fatigue is common.

 HOW TO TREAT

GENERAL MEASURES
- Use a cool-mist, ultrasonic humidifier to increase air moisture. Putting medicine in the vaporizer probably will not help. Clean humidifier daily.
- Use a heating pad or warm compresses on the chest to relieve chest pain.
- Coughing and deep breathing is encouraged to help clear secretions. Dispose of secretions carefully.

MEDICATION
- Your doctor may prescribe:
  Antiviral medication such as amantadine or rimantadine.
  Acyclovir for herpes or varicella (chickenpox) infection
  Aerosolized ribavirinor for RSV infection.
  Antibiotics to fight secondary bacterial infections.
- For minor pain and fever, you may use nonprescription drugs, such as acetaminophen or decongestant nose drops, nasal sprays or tablets.

ACTIVITY—Bed rest is necessary until fever, pain and shortness of breath have been gone at least 48 hours. Then normal activity may be resumed slowly. Many people are fatigued and weak for up to 6 weeks after recovery, so don't expect a quick return to normal strength.

DIET—No special diet, but do everything possible to maintain a normal intake of nutritious foods and drinks. Drink at least 1 full glass of fluid each hour. This helps thin lung secretions so they are easier to cough up.

 CALL YOUR DOCTOR IF

- You have symptoms of pneumonia.
- The following occurs during treatment:
  Temperature spikes over 102F (38.9C).
  Intolerable pain, despite medication and heat treatment.
  Increasing shortness of breath.
  Increasing blueness of nails and skin.
  Blood in the sputum.
  Nausea, vomiting or diarrhea.

PNEUMOTHORAX

GENERAL INFORMATION

DEFINITION—Collapse of part or all of a lung caused by pressure from free air in the chest between the two layers of the pleura (thin membranes that cover the lung). The pain is sometimes confused with a heart attack.

BODY PARTS INVOLVED—Lung; pleura.

SEX OR AGE MOST AFFECTED—All ages, but most common in active young men (20 to 40 years).

SIGNS & SYMPTOMS—The following symptoms vary according to the degree of lung collapse and extent of underlying lung disease. Symptoms may be less acute if the pneumothorax develops slowly:
- Sharp chest pain. Pain may extend to a shoulder or across the chest or abdomen.
- Shortness of breath.
- Dry, hacking cough (occasionally).

CAUSES
Spontaneous pneumothorax:
- Rupture of a small air sac in the lung resulting from asthma, lung abscess or empyema, or physical exertion, such as diving, high-altitude flying or stretching. Causes related to activity occur most often in healthy persons.

Pneumothorax due to trauma:
- Penetrating wounds to the chest, which permit outside air to rush into the pleural space and cause the lung to collapse.
- Complication of removing fluid from the lung (thoracentesis).

RISK INCREASES WITH
- Chest injury.
- Chronic lung disease.
- Smoking.
- Exercise, stretching.
- Diving.
- High altitude flying.
- Cancer.

HOW TO PREVENT
- Obtain medical treatment for lung disorders, such as asthma or emphysema.
- Don't smoke.

WHAT TO EXPECT

DIAGNOSTIC MEASURES
- Your own observation of symptoms.
- Medical history and physical exam by a doctor.
- X-rays of the chest to confirm the diagnosis and determine the size of the pneumothorax.

APPROPRIATE HEALTH CARE
- Self-care after diagnosis.
- Doctor's treatment.
- Treatment depends on the size of the pneumothorax and the condition of the lungs. The disorder may heal itself, but hospitalization and treatment may be necessary to remove the air.

POSSIBLE COMPLICATIONS
- Pulmonary edema.
- Lung infection.
- Repeated pneumothorax requiring surgery.

PROBABLE OUTCOME—A small pneumothorax is inconsequential and heals itself. However, if the collapse is extensive and it occurs in middle-aged or older adults whose lungs are damaged by asthma, chronic bronchitis or emphysema, it can lead to respiratory failure and critical illness.

HOW TO TREAT

GENERAL MEASURES
- Don't smoke; try not to cough; avoid loud talking, laughing or singing.
- You may be more comfortable if you rest in a sitting position.
- If at home, monitor your blood pressure, pulse rate and respirations.

MEDICATION—Medication usually is not necessary. However, you may use nonprescription drugs, such as acetaminophen, for minor pain. For severe pain, your doctor may prescribe stronger pain relievers.

ACTIVITY—Stay as active as your strength allows. Rest often. Resume your normal activities as soon as possible. Allow about 2 weeks for recovery.

DIET—No special diet.

CALL YOUR DOCTOR IF

- You have symptoms of pneumothorax.
- The following occurs during treatment:
  Temperature rises to 101F (38.3C).
  Chest pain or shortness of breath increases.
  Painful, debilitating coughing or sputum production begins.

POISON IVY, OAK, SUMAC

GENERAL INFORMATION

DEFINITION—A type of contact dermatitis. The skin reaction (sometimes severe) results from contact with an oily substance (resin) produced by these three plants. This particular allergic reaction is the most common in the U.S. and about 50% of the population has developed an allergy to these plants.

BODY PARTS INVOLVED—Skin.

SEX OR AGE MOST AFFECTED—Both sexes; all ages.

SIGNS & SYMPTOMS—Skin rash with the following characteristics:
- Bright red papules and plaques (see Glossary for both) that develop 24 to 48 hours (sometimes may take several days) after contact.
- Weeping, crusting and swelling.
- Intense itching and burning.
- The rash forms a linear pattern.
- Blistering (the fluid in blisters is not contagious).
- Enough of the oily resin remains on hands or clothing so that the rash is carried to other body parts, such as the face or genitalia.

CAUSES—Allergic reaction from contact with any part of poison ivy, poison oak or poison sumac plants. They grow as vines or bushes and have three leaflets (poison ivy and poison oak) or a row of paired leaflets (poison sumac). They produce a potent resin (or oil) that is responsible for the problem. A reaction may also occur from touching contaminated clothing, equipment (hunting, golf or athletic) or animals such as pets; and from smoke these plants give off when burned (may affect the face, eyelids, throat and lungs).

RISK INCREASES WITH
- Spring and summer (though plants are dangerous year round).
- Lack of protective clothing.

HOW TO PREVENT
- Learn to identify and avoid contact with these plants.
- When walking in areas where these plants grow, wear shoes, socks, long pants, long sleeved shirts and sometimes, gloves. Wash this clothing as soon thereafter as possible.
- If you are exposed, washing the skin immediately with soap and water and sponging with rubbing alcohol may prevent the rash.

WHAT TO EXPECT

DIAGNOSTIC MEASURES
- Your own observation of symptoms.
- Medical history and physical exam by a doctor (sometimes).

APPROPRIATE HEALTH CARE
- Self-care.
- Doctor's treatment for severe cases.

POSSIBLE COMPLICATIONS—Development of a secondary bacteria infection.

PROBABLE OUTCOME—Itching, redness and swelling are often improved by the second day, and complete healing occurs within 7-14 days.

HOW TO TREAT

GENERAL MEASURES
- Sweating and heat make the itching worse, so stay cool if possible.
- Apply cool compresses to the affected area (see Soaks in Appendix).
- A soothing bath helps. Use Aveeno (a commercial product) or baking soda (about a half cup) per bath.
- Wash all clothing and shoes and any equipment that came in contact with the plant oils with soap and water.
- Give pets a warm, soapy bath to remove any oil from the fur.

MEDICATION
- You may use calamine lotion to relieve the itching; oral antihistamines may be helpful also.
- Your doctor may prescribe topical or oral corticosteroids for severe symptoms.

ACTIVITY—No restrictions. Avoid activities that can cause sweating. This can worsen itching.

DIET—No special diet.

CALL YOUR DOCTOR IF

- If the rash seems severe.
- If swelling or pain develops around the eyes, nose or genitals.
- Rash worsens or doesn't improve with self-care methods.

POLYARTERITIS NODOSA
(Polyarteritis; Necrotizing Angiitis)

GENERAL INFORMATION

DEFINITION—A disorder of connective tissue that is one of several related diseases of collagen tissue. Collagen is a protein molecule that forms the major part of all connective tissue. Polyarteritis causes inflammation of small and medium arteries, decreasing the blood supply to tissues supplied by the affected blood vessels. It is not contagious. The course may be acute, with fever, weight loss and rapid deterioration. If the course is chronic, body tissues will waste away over several years.

BODY PARTS INVOLVED—All body parts.

SEX OR AGE MOST AFFECTED
- Both sexes, but more common in men.
- All ages, but most common in adults under age 50.

SIGNS & SYMPTOMS—Varies, depending on which organ is affected by the decreased blood supply. The most common include:
- Chest pain (heart involvement).
- Shortness of breath (lung involvement).
- Abdominal pain (intestinal and liver involvement).
- Blood in the urine (kidney involvement).
- Numbness and tingling of the hands and feet (nerve involvement).

CAUSES—This is considered a disease of autoimmunity or hypersensitivity, although the cause is uncertain. In many persons, no predisposing factors can be found. Following are the most common preceding factors:
- Bacterial infections.
- Viral infections.
- Use of certain drugs, including sulfa drugs, penicillin, antithyroid drugs, gold and thiazide diuretics.
- Vaccines.
- HIV (AIDS).

RISK INCREASES WITH
- Family history of collagen or hypersensitivity disease.
- Smoking.

HOW TO PREVENT—No specific preventive measures.

WHAT TO EXPECT

DIAGNOSTIC MEASURES
- Your own observation of symptoms.
- Medical history and physical exam by a doctor.
- Laboratory studies of kidneys and blood, including sedimentation rate (see Glossary).
- Angiography (see Glossary).

APPROPRIATE HEALTH CARE
- Self-care after diagnosis.
- Doctor's treatment.
- Hospitalization for intensive treatment (severe cases).
- Surgery to remove part of the intestines, if they are involved.

POSSIBLE COMPLICATIONS—Kidney failure and death, despite treatment.

PROBABLE OUTCOME—This condition is currently considered incurable. However, symptoms may be relieved or controlled. With treatment, over 50% of patients survive 5 years or more. Without treatment, few patients live beyond 5 years.

Scientific research into causes and treatment continues, so there is hope for increasingly effective treatment and cure.

HOW TO TREAT

GENERAL MEASURES
- Learn about side-effects for any medicines prescribed for you.
- You have a high risk for infections, so avoid crowds when possible and stay away from individuals with a known infection.
- See arthritis in Resources for Additional Information.

MEDICATION—Your doctor may prescribe:
- Cortisone drugs in high doses until acute symptoms diminish. Then symptoms may be controlled by alternate day cortisone.
- Drugs to treat disorders of organs involved with this serious disease, such as heart medications for heart involvement or antihypertensives for high blood pressure.
- Immunosuppressive drugs—either alone or with steroids—if other drugs fail. These drugs pose additional risks, including severe generalized septic bacterial infections.

ACTIVITY—Resume your normal activities gradually as symptoms improve.

DIET—Low-salt diet if you have high blood pressure (see Low-Salt Diet in Appendix).

CALL YOUR DOCTOR IF

- You have symptoms of polyarteritis.
- New, unexplained symptoms develop. Drugs used in treatment may produce side effects.

POLYCYSTIC OVARIAN SYNDROME
(Stein-Leventhal Syndrome)

GENERAL INFORMATION

DEFINITION—Ovary enlargement from many small cysts. The surface of the ovaries becomes too thick to allow ovulation (the monthly release of the egg from the ovary). Women with this problem cannot become pregnant without treatment.

BODY PARTS INVOLVED—Ovaries.

SEX OR AGE MOST AFFECTED—Females.

SIGNS & SYMPTOMS
- Irregular menstrual bleeding, usually a lighter flow.
- Increased time between periods, often up to several months.
- Increased hair growth on the face, arms, legs and from pubic area to navel.
- Enlarged clitoris.
- Increased sex drive.
- Higher energy level.
- Obesity.
- Acne.

CAUSES—An imbalance between the pituitary gonadotropin luteinizing hormone (LH) and follicle-stimulating hormone (FSH), resulting in a lack of ovulation and an increased testosterone production.

RISK INCREASES WITH
- Endometrial hypoplasia or carcinoma.
- Obesity.
- High-blood pressure.
- Diabetes mellitus.
- Breast cancer.

HOW TO PREVENT—Cannot be prevented at present. Get appropriate cancer screening tests to reduce risk factors.

WHAT TO EXPECT

DIAGNOSTIC MEASURES
- Your own observation of symptoms.
- Medical history and physical exam by a doctor.
- Laboratory studies of blood hormone levels and pelvic ultrasound; endometrial biopsy (see Glossary for both) to rule out hyperplasia or cancer.

APPROPRIATE HEALTH CARE
- No ideal medical treatment exists; drugs prescribed for the disorder will be determined by severity of symptoms and whether there is a desire for pregnancy.
- Surgery to remove a small section from each ovary may be recommended in patients not helped by drugs.

POSSIBLE COMPLICATIONS
- Permanent hormone imbalance.
- Infertility.
- Increased likelihood of uterine cancer and breast cancer.

PROBABLE OUTCOME—Hormone therapy and surgery usually decrease masculine characteristics and often restore fertility. Some signs and symptoms may never disappear completely.

HOW TO TREAT

GENERAL MEASURES—You may need professional help if you want to remove excess hair from your face, arms and legs (techniques can include bleaching, electrolysis, plucking, waxing and depilation).

MEDICATION—Your doctor may prescribe:
- Progestin or oral contraceptives for patients not desiring pregnancy.
- Clomiphene citrate or other hormones for patients who desire pregnancy.
- Drugs for excess hair (hirsutism). A few drugs have been tried, but the success rate is not high, and side-effects are numerous.

ACTIVITY—No restrictions on activity, including sexual intercourse.

DIET—No special diet. Weight loss recommended if you are overweight.

CALL YOUR DOCTOR IF

- You have symptoms of polycystic ovarian syndrome.
- Your periods become profuse or more frequent than usual.
- You develop a lump or swelling in the breast.
- Symptoms recur after treatment or surgery.
- You want a referral to remove excess body hair.
- New, unexplained symptoms develop. Drugs used in treatment may produce side effects.

POLYCYTHEMIA

GENERAL INFORMATION

DEFINITION—An increase in red blood cells in the body. The disease has 3 forms:
- Polycythemia vera, which involves overproduction of red blood cells, white blood cells and platelets.
- Secondary polycythemia (pseudo-polycythemia), which is a complication of diseases or factors other than blood-cell disorders.
- Stress polycythemia (pseudo-polycythemia), which involves decreased blood plasma.

BODY PARTS INVOLVED—Blood-forming organs: bone marrow; spleen; lymph glands; lymph channels.

SEX OR AGE MOST AFFECTED—Adults of both sexes, but more common in men; usually over age 50.

SIGNS & SYMPTOMS—Some patients have no symptoms. Others have any of the following:
- Fatigue; headache; drowsiness; dizziness.
- Itching or flushed skin.
- Enlarged spleen.
- Unexplained bleeding.

CAUSES
- Polycythemia vera: unknown.
- Secondary polycythemia: congenital heart disease; chronic lung disease; cigarette or cigar smoking; living at high altitude.
- Stress polycythemia: use of diuretic drugs; smoking; dehydration.

RISK INCREASES WITH
- Smoking.
- Heart or lung disease.
- Stress.
- Family history of polycythemia.

HOW TO PREVENT
- Polycythemia vera cannot be prevented at present.
- To help prevent secondary polycythemia or stress polycythemia:
  Don't smoke.
  Avoid dehydration.
  Obtain medical treatment for heart or lung disease.

WHAT TO EXPECT

DIAGNOSTIC MEASURES
- Your own observation of symptoms.
- Medical history and physical exam by a doctor.
- Laboratory studies of bone marrow and blood (red-blood-cell count, measurement of hematocrit).
- X-ray of the kidneys.
- Radioactive chromium studies.

APPROPRIATE HEALTH CARE
- Doctor's treatment.
- Treatment steps will be individualized depending on your age, disease duration, type of polycythemia, complications and disease activity.
- Possible treatment steps to keep the hematocrit range near normal and prevent clotting or hemorrhage are: Phlebotomy (withdrawal of excess blood); radioisotope therapy; and drug therapy. The treatment chosen will depend upon symptoms and response to treatment. More than one form of treatment may be needed.

POSSIBLE COMPLICATIONS
- Clots in veins or arteries.
- Gout.
- Stroke.
- Heart attack.
- Peptic ulcer.
- Kidney stones.
- Leukemia.

PROBABLE OUTCOME
- Polycythemia vera is incurable, but symptoms can be controlled. With treatment, average survival ranges from 7-15 years, with some patients living 20 or more years.
- Other forms of polycythemia can be cured if the causes can be eliminated.

HOW TO TREAT

GENERAL MEASURES
- Stop smoking. Consult your doctor about recommendations for a cessation program.
- Adherence to your treatment plan brings about improved survival and well-being.

MEDICATION—Your doctor may prescribe:
- Aspirin to decrease clotting and reduce the chance of stroke or heart attack may be recommended.
- Radioactive phosphorus or cytotoxic drugs.
- Allopurinol for elevated uric acid.
- Anti-itching medications.
- H2-receptor or antacids for hyperacidity.

ACTIVITY—After treatment, resume normal activity as soon as possible.

DIET—No special diet. Drink 6 to 8 oz. of fluid every 2 hours to maintain adequate body fluid.

CALL YOUR DOCTOR IF

- You have symptoms of polycythemia.
- You have symptoms of complications (refer to specific disorder in this book).
- New, unexplained symptoms develop. Drugs used in treatment may produce side effects.

POLYMYALGIA RHEUMATICA OR TEMPORAL ARTERITIS
(Giant-Cell Arteritis; Cranial Arteritis)

GENERAL INFORMATION

DEFINITION—Inflammatory disease of the large arteries, especially those in the head and neck. Symptoms of polymyalgia rheumatica (stiffness and pain in muscles) and temporal arteritis (inflammation of the walls of the arteries that pass over the temples in the scalp) are the same, so the two diseases may be identical.

BODY PARTS INVOLVED—Muscles; temporal arteries; eyes; connective tissue.

SEX OR AGE MOST AFFECTED—Adults over 50. The disease occurs 4 times more often in women than men.

SIGNS & SYMPTOMS—The following symptoms may resemble those of an infection such as influenza.
• Low fever.
• Muscle stiffness, aches and pains—especially in the morning. The muscles involved are usually those of the trunk, upper arms and legs.
• Severe, throbbing headache (usually in one temple).
• Redness, swelling, tenderness and pulsating nodules along the temporal artery on one side of the head.
• Appetite loss.

CAUSES—An autoimmune disorder in which the body's immune system attacks and destroys its own tissues (especially connective tissue). The underlying cause is unknown.

RISK INCREASES WITH—Adults over 60, especially women.

HOW TO PREVENT—No specific preventive measures.

WHAT TO EXPECT

DIAGNOSTIC MEASURES
• Your own observation of symptoms.
• Medical history and exam by a doctor.
• Laboratory studies, such as sedimentation rate (see Glossary), white-blood-cell count and blood tests for anemia.
• Biopsy (see Glossary) of a small amount of tissue or fluid of the temporal artery and muscle.

APPROPRIATE HEALTH CARE
• Self-care after diagnosis.
• Doctor's treatment for this disorder or problems associated with it. These may include heart disease, high blood pressure or decreased blood supply to the bowel.
• Surgery, if the bowel develops intestinal gangrene.

POSSIBLE COMPLICATIONS
• Without treatment: Loss of vision (if blood vessels to the eyes are involved, it's an emergency); coronary artery disease; stroke; poor blood circulation to the arms and legs.
• With treatment: Cortisone drugs may be necessary for many months. Complications of long-term cortisone use are significant, including osteoporosis and peptic-ulcer disease.

PROBABLE OUTCOME—Usually curable, but relapse is possible.

HOW TO TREAT

GENERAL MEASURES
• Apply heat to the painful side of the head. You may use warm compresses or a heat lamp.
• Gently massage the back of the neck and sore muscles.
• See Arthritis in Resources for Additional Information.

MEDICATION—Your doctor may prescribe:
• Cortisone drugs in high doses until the acute phase ends. These dramatically relieve symptoms by altering the inflammation causing them. For continuing treatment with cortisone, the lowest possible single dose taken every other day may keep symptoms under control.
• Immunosuppressive drugs, either alone or with corticosteroids, if other treatment is not successful.
• Heart medications (if the heart is involved).
• Antihypertensive drugs (if high blood pressure is part of the problem).

ACTIVITY—No restrictions.

DIET—No special diet.

CALL YOUR DOCTOR IF

• You have symptoms of polymyalgia rheumatica and temporal arteritis.
• The following occurs during treatment:
  Temperature of 101F (38.3C).
  Blood in the urine.
  Shortness of breath.
  Chest pain.
  Bloody bowel movements.
  Severe abdominal pain.
  Any illness with fever.
• New, unexplained symptoms develop. Drugs used in treatment may produce side effects.

POLYMYOSITIS & DERMATOMYOSITIS

GENERAL INFORMATION

DEFINITION—Inflammation of connective tissue, with degenerative changes in the muscles (polymyositis) and skin (dermatomyositis). This causes weakness and muscle wasting, especially in the arms and legs. This disease has many similarities to rheumatoid arthritis and lupus erythematosus.

BODY PARTS INVOLVED—Muscles, including large muscles of the skeleton and tiny muscles that control small arteries; skin; connective tissue.

SEX OR AGE MOST AFFECTED
- Twice as common in women as men.
- All ages, but most likely to begin between ages 30 and 50.

SIGNS & SYMPTOMS—Sudden or slow onset of the following:
- Weakness in the pelvic-girdle and shoulder-girdle muscles.
- Skin rash that may itch on the face, shoulders, arms and over joints.
- Cold hands and feet.
- Frequent falls and difficulty in getting up.
- Speaking or swallowing difficulty.
- Infection with fever, muscle weakness, weight loss and joint pain (sometimes) preceding other symptoms.

CAUSES—Probably a disease of hypersensitivity or autoimmunity, although the cause is uncertain. This disease has been associated with the use of certain drugs and preceding bacterial infections, viral infections and vaccines.

RISK INCREASES WITH
- Allergies.
- Use of sulfa drugs, penicillin, antithyroid drugs, gold and thiazide diuretics.
- Family history of hypersensitivity diseases.
- Cancer of the lung, colon or breast.

HOW TO PREVENT—No specific preventive measures.

WHAT TO EXPECT

DIAGNOSTIC MEASURES
- Medical history and exam by a doctor.
- Laboratory studies to measure antinuclear antibodies (ANA) and muscle enzymes.
- Surgical diagnostic procedures, such as biopsy of muscle and electromyography (see Glossary for both).

APPROPRIATE HEALTH CARE
- Doctor's treatment.
- Hospitalization during early, active phases.
- Surgery, if intestinal obstruction occurs.
- Physical therapy and rehabilitation.

POSSIBLE COMPLICATIONS
- Muscle and body wasting; congestive heart failure; high blood pressure.
- Intestinal obstruction.
- Kidney damage.
- Pneumonia; respiratory problems.
- Cancer.

PROBABLE OUTCOME—The disease may begin suddenly or gradually. Muscle weakness may be severe and progressive. Some symptoms can be controlled with treatment. Patients with cardiac or pulmonary involvement tend to have more severe symptoms that are somewhat resistant to treatment. Remissions or spontaneous recovery can occur—especially in children. Research into causes and treatment continues, so there is hope for increasingly effective treatment and cure.

HOW TO TREAT

GENERAL MEASURES
- Care can usually be managed at home. In time, a wheelchair may be required or confinement to bed due to the muscle weakness.
- Passive exercise should be provided to prevent contractures (muscle shortening).
- Cool-water compresses may relieve itching.
- See Muscular Dystrophy in Resources for Additional Information.

MEDICATION—Your doctor may prescribe:
- Cortisone drugs in high doses until acute symptoms diminish, then in lower doses.
- Cytotoxic or immunosuppressive drugs, if other treatment is not effective.
- Medications to help control itching.
- Pain medications if needed.

ACTIVITY
- Restrict activities during acute phase. Bed rest is recommended. Pace activities to counteract muscle weakness.
- If confined to bed, the patient should be moved frequently to prevent pressure sores.

DIET—No special diet. Salt restriction diet might prevent fluid retention. Ask your doctor.

CALL YOUR DOCTOR IF

The following occurs during treatment:
Blood in the urine.
Shortness of breath.
Chest pain.
Bloody bowel movements.
Severe abdominal pain.
Fever.

PORPHYRIA

GENERAL INFORMATION

DEFINITION—Any of a group of rare inherited disorders characterized by excessive formation and excretion of porphyrins (chemicals in all living things). This disease is often mistakenly attributed to emotions.

BODY PARTS INVOLVED—Central nervous system; skin; liver; digestive system.

SEX OR AGE MOST AFFECTED
• Both sexes, but more common and severe in females.
• All ages, but less likely in older adults.

SIGNS & SYMPTOMS
• Chest or abdominal pain.
• Mental changes, including depression and mania.
• Skin changes, including itching and blistering.
• Leg pain.
• Muscle cramps and weakness.
• Numbness and tingling in the feet and hands.
• Excessive hair growth.

CAUSES—An inherited disturbance in the metabolism of porphyrins.

RISK INCREASES WITH
• Family history of porphyria.
• Use of drugs, such as birth-control pills, alcohol, barbiturates. These don't cause the disease, but they may trigger attacks.
• Exposure to sunlight. This may trigger attacks.

HOW TO PREVENT
• Cannot be prevented at present. To reduce the frequency and severity of attacks:
  Avoid all drugs, including nonprescription medicines, until you talk with your doctor.
  Don't take birth-control pills.
  Avoid bright sunlight.
• Any person with a family history of porphyria should seek genetic counseling before starting a family.

WHAT TO EXPECT

DIAGNOSTIC MEASURES
• Your own observation of symptoms.
• Medical history and physical exam by a doctor.
• Laboratory studies to measure porphyrins in the urine, blood and stool.

APPROPRIATE HEALTH CARE
• Doctor's treatment.
• Psychotherapy or counseling.
• Hospitalization during attacks for supportive care.

POSSIBLE COMPLICATIONS
• Many complications may be associated with this disorder. Most are reversible, but some may be permanent. The complications can cause physical symptoms and disorders as well as psychological problems.
• If you are a woman and your disease is severe, pregnancy may not be advisable. Talk to your doctor.

PROBABLE OUTCOME—This condition is currently considered incurable, but many patients live a normal life-span with the disorder, especially those who have no symptoms or minor symptoms. For others, symptoms can be relieved or controlled.

Scientific research into causes and treatment continues, so there is hope for increasingly effective treatment and cure.

HOW TO TREAT

GENERAL MEASURES
• Avoid bright sunlight. If you must be in bright sun, use a hat and protective clothing.
• See Resources for Additional Information.

MEDICATION
• Don't take any medicine until you ask your doctor.
• Your doctor may prescribe:
  Intravenous glucose or hemin (an enzyme-inhibitor derived from processed red blood cells) to help prevent or treat acute attacks.
  Tranquilizers to decrease anxiety.
  Medications to inhibit ovulation may help reduce premenstrual attacks.
  Beta-carotene to reduce photosensitivity.

ACTIVITY—No restrictions except for sunlight restrictions.

DIET
• High carbohydrate diet.
• Avoid alcohol. It precipitates attacks.

CALL YOUR DOCTOR IF

• You have symptoms of porphyria.
• Dark urine or other symptoms of an attack recur.

POSTPARTUM DEPRESSION
(Postnatal Depression)

GENERAL INFORMATION

DEFINITION—Depression beginning up to 6 weeks following childbirth.

BODY PARTS INVOLVED—Brain.

SEX OR AGE MOST AFFECTED—Females of childbearing age.

SIGNS & SYMPTOMS
- Feelings of sadness, hopelessness or gloom.
- Appetite and weight loss.
- Sleep disturbances or frightening dreams.
- Loss of energy; fatigue.
- Slow speech and thought.
- Frequent headaches and other physical discomfort.
- Confusion about one's ability to improve life.

CAUSES—It's common for mothers to experience some degree of depression during the first weeks after birth. Pregnancy and birth are accompanied by sudden hormonal changes that affect emotions.

Additionally, the 24-hour responsibility for a newborn infant represents a major psychological and lifestyle adjustment for most mothers—even after the first child.

These physical and emotional stresses are usually accompanied by inadequate rest until the baby's routine stabilizes, so fatigue and depression are not unusual.

RISK INCREASES WITH
- Stress.
- Lack of sleep.
- Poor nutrition.
- Lack of support from one's partner, family or friends.
- Pre-existing neurosis or psychosis.

HOW TO PREVENT—Cannot be prevented, but can be minimized with rest, an adequate diet and a strong emotional support system.

WHAT TO EXPECT

DIAGNOSTIC MEASURES
- Your own observation of symptoms.
- Medical history and physical exam by a doctor.

APPROPRIATE HEALTH CARE
- Self-care after diagnosis.
- Doctor's treatment.
- Psychotherapy or counseling, if depression persists.
- Hospitalization (severe cases only).

POSSIBLE COMPLICATIONS
- Lack of bonding between mother and infant, which is harmful to both.
- Serious depression that may be accompanied by aggressive feelings toward the baby, a loss of pride in appearance and home, loss of appetite or compulsive eating, withdrawal from others or suicidal tendencies.

PROBABLE OUTCOME—With support from friends and family, mild postpartum depression usually disappears quickly. If depression becomes severe, a mother may not be able to care for herself and the baby, and rarely, hospitalization may be necessary. Medication, counseling and support from others usually cure even severe depression in 3 to 6 months.

HOW TO TREAT

GENERAL MEASURES
- Don't feel guilty if you have mixed feelings about motherhood. Adjustment and bonding take time.
- Schedule frequent outings, such as walks and short visits with friends or family. These help prevent feelings of isolation.
- Have your baby sleep in a separate room. You will sleep more restfully.
- Ask for daytime help from family or friends who will shop for you or care for the baby while you rest.
- If you feel depressed, share your feelings with your partner or a friend who is a good listener. Talking with other mothers can help you keep problems in perspective.
- If depression becomes severe and hospitalization is necessary, choose a facility close enough to home so you can continue a close relationship with your baby.

MEDICATION—Your doctor may prescribe antidepressant drugs. These are often effective when used for 3 to 4 weeks. Any medication use must be carefully considered if you are breast-feeding.

ACTIVITY—No restrictions. Resume your normal activities as soon as possible.

DIET—No special diet.

CALL YOUR DOCTOR IF

- You have postpartum depression and additional life changes occur, such as divorce, career change or moving.
- Postpartum depression does not improve in 4 to 6 weeks.
- You seriously consider suicide. This is an emergency!

POST-TRAUMATIC STRESS DISORDER (PTSD)

GENERAL INFORMATION

DEFINITION—A type of anxiety seen in people who experience an event that would be extremely distressing to most human beings. Such events (natural disasters, murder, rape, war, imprisonment, torture, car accidents) produce psychological stress in anyone. Some people do not recover normally. PTSD is characterized by a persistent re-experiencing of the trauma and other associated symptoms. The symptoms may begin right after the event or may develop several months later.

BODY PARTS INVOLVED—Nervous.

SEX OR AGE MOST AFFECTED—Both sexes; all ages (children often are affected).

SIGNS & SYMPTOMS
- Recurrent, intrusive and distressing recollections of the event.
- Recurrent dreams relating to the event.
- A sense of reliving the event (flashbacks).
- Chronic anxiety.
- Insomnia.
- Difficulty in concentrating.
- Memory impairment.
- A sense of personal isolation.
- Diminished interest in activities.
- Phobic reactions to situations, or avoidance of activities, that recall memories of the event.
- Emotional effects (irritable, restless, tremulous, explosive outbursts of behavior, a deadening of feelings, painful guilt feelings).

CAUSES—Exposure to an overwhelming event. A variety of factors seem to combine to produce PTSD:
- The event's suddenness and unexpectedness.
- Bloody and brutal event.
- More prolonged and chronic stress during the event.
- Psychological and constitutional strengths and weaknesses of the victim.
- Bodily injury (especially head injury).
- Type and availability of social support.

RISK INCREASES WITH—People with a history of childhood neglect or dysfunctional families, children of alcoholic parents or childhood abuse, low educational attainment.

HOW TO PREVENT—Crisis intervention immediately after a traumatic event may prevent the development of PTSD.

WHAT TO EXPECT

DIAGNOSTIC MEASURES
- Your own observation of symptoms.
- Medical history and physical exam by a doctor.
- Laboratory and medical tests as needed to rule out any brain disorder.
- Psychiatric exam and psychological testing.

APPROPRIATE HEALTH CARE
- Psychotherapy and counseling. Several different methods of therapy are available including behavior therapy, desensitization (see Glossary for both), hypnosis and others. Individual or group therapy as needed.
- Psychiatric hospitalization for suicidal patient or one who is severely dysfunctional with activities of daily living.

POSSIBLE COMPLICATIONS
- Chronic PTSD, which can lead to loss of job, marital conflicts and disability.
- Injury to self during a re-enactment of the trauma.
- Drug or alcohol dependency.
- Suicide.

PROBABLE OUTCOME—For some patients, the symptoms disappear spontaneously after 6 months; additional patients can be helped with treatment, while in others, the disorder may run a chronic course for months or years.

HOW TO TREAT

GENERAL MEASURES
- Make a commitment to yourself to work on the problem.
- Learn relaxation techniques. They are particularly helpful, especially in helping with sleep problems.
- Support groups are highly effective and available through Veterans Administrative Centers and community crisis centers.

MEDICATION—Your doctor may prescribe antianxiety or antidepressant drugs for short periods of time.

ACTIVITY—No restrictions. A routine physical exercise program is helpful in relieving some stress.

DIET—No special diet.

CALL YOUR DOCTOR IF

- You have symptoms of post-traumatic stress disorder.
- Symptoms don't improve or worsen after treatment begins.
- New, unexplained symptoms develop. Drugs used in treatment may produce side effects.

POTASSIUM IMBALANCE

GENERAL INFORMATION

DEFINITION—Above (hyperkalemia) or below (hypokalemia) normal levels of potassium in the blood, body fluids and body cells. Potassium, along with sodium and calcium, maintains normal heart rhythm, regulates the body's water balance and is responsible for muscle contractions and nerve impulses.

BODY PARTS INVOLVED—Blood, which affects all body cells and body fluids.

SEX OR AGE MOST AFFECTED—Both sexes; all ages.

SIGNS & SYMPTOMS
Hyperkalemia:
- Weakness and paralysis.
- Dangerously rapid, irregular heartbeat or slow heartbeat (sometimes).
- Nausea and diarrhea.

Hypokalemia:
- Weakness and paralysis.
- Low blood pressure.
- Life-threatening rapid, irregular heartbeat. This is more severe than with hyperkalemia.

CAUSES
Hyperkalemia:
- Chronic kidney disease with kidney failure. Failing kidneys eliminate potassium too slowly, causing an excess in the body.
- Use of oral potassium supplements.
- Burns or crushing injuries. These may release potassium from body tissues into body fluids.
- Addison's disease.
- Using ACE Inhibitors for hypertension or to protect kidney function.

Hypokalemia:
- The use of diuretic drugs for hypertension or heart failure.
- Prolonged loss of body fluids from vomiting or diarrhea.
- Chronic kidney disease with kidney failure. At certain stages, this may cause the body to lose potassium.

RISK INCREASES WITH
- Diabetes mellitus.
- Adrenal disease.
- Use of drugs, such as diuretics, ACE inhibitors, potassium supplements and digitalis. Low potassium levels especially in persons who take digitalis often lead to serious heartbeat disturbances.

HOW TO PREVENT
- If you have a disorder or take drugs that affect potassium levels , learn as much as you can about your condition, your drugs and how to prevent a potassium imbalance.
- If you take digitalis and diuretics, have frequent blood studies to monitor potassium levels.

- Obtain medical care for prolonged vomiting or diarrhea.

WHAT TO EXPECT

DIAGNOSTIC MEASURES
- Your own observation of symptoms, especially muscle weakness and heart-rhythm changes.
- Medical history and physical exam by a doctor.
- Laboratory blood and urine studies of potassium and other electrolytes.
- ECG (see Glossary).

APPROPRIATE HEALTH CARE
- Self-care after diagnosis.
- Doctor's treatment.
- May be treatable at home with diet or potassium supplements, could require hospitalization for intravenous therapy (severe cases of either too much or too little potassium).

POSSIBLE COMPLICATIONS—Cardiac arrest and death.

PROBABLE OUTCOME—Usually can be corrected with treatment of the underlying disorder.

HOW TO TREAT

GENERAL MEASURES
- If you take diuretics and digitalis, your friends and family members should learn cardiopulmonary resuscitation (CPR). Learn to count your own pulse at the wrist or neck.
- Don't take potassium supplements without your doctor' approval.

MEDICATION—Your doctor may prescribe:
- Oral potassium supplements to raise low levels.
- Diuretics to increase urination and decrease high potassium levels.
- Intravenous fluids to correct a serious imbalance.
- Medications appropriate for the underlying disease.

ACTIVITY—Resume your normal activities as soon as symptoms improve.

DIET—Depends on the condition. Mild hypokalemia can be corrected by increasing consumption of potassium-containing foods, such as orange juice, bananas, melon, carrots, tomato juice, papaya.

CALL YOUR DOCTOR IF

You have symptoms of a potassium imbalance or are having problems with a disorder that affects potassium levels.

PREMATURE EJACULATION

 GENERAL INFORMATION

DEFINITION—Male orgasm and ejaculation following brief sexual stimulation, prior to satisfactory arousal and orgasm in the sexual partner. This is a common disorder affecting all age groups and usually caused by psychological problems.

BODY PARTS INVOLVED—Brain and central nervous system; reproductive system.

SEX OR AGE MOST AFFECTED—Male adolescents and adults.

SIGNS & SYMPTOMS
- Repeated episodes of premature ejaculation.
- Feelings of self-doubt, inadequacy and guilt.

CAUSES
- Poor relationship or communication with the sexual partner.
- Fear of impregnating the partner.
- Fear of contracting a sexually transmitted disease.
- Anxiety about sexual performance.
- Cultural or religious conflicts.
- Belief that sex is sinful or dirty.
- Rarely may be due to underlying neurological disorder (e.g., prostatitis).

RISK INCREASES WITH—Listed with Causes.

HOW TO PREVENT—See suggestions in General Measures.

 WHAT TO EXPECT

DIAGNOSTIC MEASURES
- Your own observation of signs.
- Medical history and physical exam by a doctor.
- Any laboratory test results are usually normal, since most males with this problem are healthy individuals.

APPROPRIATE HEALTH CARE
- Self-care after diagnosis.
- Doctor's treatment, if self-help measures fail.
- Counseling from a qualified sex therapist if other methods are not successful.

POSSIBLE COMPLICATIONS
- Low self-esteem.
- Damage to marital or interpersonal relationships.

PROBABLE OUTCOME—Usually curable in most people within 6 months after recognition and treatment.

 HOW TO TREAT

GENERAL MEASURES—The following methods are recommended by sex researchers and therapists Masters and Johnson. These measures usually lead to ejaculatory control for 5 to 10 minutes or longer:
- Sensate-focus exercises, in which each partner caresses the other's body without intercourse to learn relaxed, pleasurable aspects of touching.
- Mutual physical examination of each other's bodies to acquaint both partners thoroughly with anatomy. This helps reduce shameful feelings about sex.
- Stop-and-start technique, in which the man is stimulated through controlled intercourse or masturbation until he feels an impending ejaculation. Stimulation is stopped, then resumed in 20 to 30 seconds.
- Squeeze technique, in which the woman squeezes her partner's penis with her thumb and forefinger when he feels an impending ejaculation. When ejaculatory feelings pass, intercourse is resumed. This is repeated as often as necessary until the man can control ejaculation to the satisfaction of both partners.

MEDICATION—Medicine usually is not necessary for this disorder.

ACTIVITY—No restrictions.

DIET—No special diet.

 CALL YOUR DOCTOR IF

You have had repeated episodes of premature ejaculation and want professional guidance to solve the problem.

PREMATURE LABOR

GENERAL INFORMATION

DEFINITION—Labor that begins before the 37th week of pregnancy.

BODY PARTS INVOLVED—Female reproductive system.

SEX OR AGE MOST AFFECTED—Pregnant females.

SIGNS & SYMPTOMS
- Uterine contractions at regular intervals that begin before the fetus is mature, usually before the due date of delivery.
- Passage of bloody mucus (sometimes).
- Flow of fluid (amniotic fluid) from the uterus (sometimes). This may occur with a gush or may be only a continuous watery discharge.

CAUSES
- Premature rupture of the membranes (the "water breaks").
- Illness of the mother, including preeclampsia, high blood pressure or diabetes.
- Abnormal shape or size of the uterus.
- Weak cervix.
- Hormone imbalance.
- Vaginal infection that spreads to the uterus.
- Large fetus or more than one fetus.
- Abnormalities of the placenta, such as placenta previa.
- Excessive amniotic fluid.

RISK INCREASES WITH
- Poor nutrition, especially when associated with weight loss.
- Previous premature labor.
- Smoking.
- Injury to the uterus.
- Excess alcohol consumption.
- Urinary-tract infection.
- Use of mind-altering drugs, such as narcotics, psychedelics, hallucinogens, marijuana, sedatives, hypnotics or cocaine.
- Adolescent mothers.

HOW TO PREVENT
- Obtain good prenatal care throughout pregnancy.
- Don't smoke, use mind-altering drugs or drink alcohol during pregnancy.
- Eat a normal, well-balanced diet during pregnancy. Take prenatal vitamin and mineral supplements, if your doctor prescribes them.
- Don't use medications of any kind, including nonprescription drugs, without consulting your doctor.
- If you have a weak cervix, which is sometimes evident before pregnancy, ask your doctor about a minor operation to strengthen the cervix.
- Rest more and decrease activity in the 3rd trimester, especially if you have blood spotting or irregular contractions.

WHAT TO EXPECT

DIAGNOSTIC MEASURES
- Your own observation of watery vaginal drainage or regular uterine contractions.
- Medical history and exam by a doctor.
- Laboratory blood studies.
- Amniocentesis (in Surgery section) to determine fetal maturity.
- Ultrasound (see Glossary) to determine fetal maturity and position.

APPROPRIATE HEALTH CARE
- Doctor's treatment.
- Hospitalization may be necessary and treatment provided for any underlying risk factors (infections, dehydration).

POSSIBLE COMPLICATIONS
- Premature infant.
- Uterine infection after delivery.
- Fetal death.

PROBABLE OUTCOME—Labor can often be stopped with treatment to allow more time for the fetus to mature. However, if the membranes have ruptured or the placenta has separated from the uterus, labor must proceed, sometimes by Cesarean section. The outcome depends on fetal maturity.

HOW TO TREAT

GENERAL MEASURES—Don't douche or use tampons to absorb fluid or blood. This increases the risk of infection.

MEDICATION—Your doctor may prescribe:
- Medication to stop labor or hasten maturity of fetal lungs.
- Antibiotics to fight infection, if it develops.
- No sedatives and pain relievers. These are withheld to give the fetus the greatest chance for survival.

ACTIVITY—Complete bed rest is necessary when premature labor begins. Discontinue all physical activities. Avoid any sexual activity.

DIET—Once labor begins, drink only clear liquids until after delivery.

CALL YOUR DOCTOR IF

- You have symptoms of premature labor. Call immediately. This is an emergency!
- During pregnancy, you think you have a urinary-tract infection.
- After delivery, you have abdominal pain, chills and fever, headache, muscle aches or a bad-smelling vaginal discharge.
- New, unexplained symptoms develop.

PREMENSTRUAL SYNDROME (PMS)

 GENERAL INFORMATION

DEFINITION—Symptoms that begin 7 to 14 days prior to a menstrual period and usually stop when menstruation begins.

BODY PARTS INVOLVED—Gastrointestinal system; central nervous system; skin; reproductive system; breasts.

SEX OR AGE MOST AFFECTED—About half of all women experience PMS at some time—some very frequently. The peak incidence occurs between ages 25 and 40.

SIGNS & SYMPTOMS
- Nervousness and irritability.
- Dizziness or fainting.
- Emotional instability.
- Increased or decreased sex drive.
- Headaches.
- Tender, swollen breasts.
- Bloating, constipation, diarrhea or other digestive disturbances.
- Fluid retention that causes puffiness in the ankles, hands and face.
- Higher incidence of minor infections such as colds.
- Acne outbreaks.
- Decreased urination.

CAUSES—Unknown, but appear to be fluctuations in the circulating level of hormones (especially estrogen and progesterone). These fluctuations cause retention of sodium in the bloodstream, resulting in edema in body tissues including the brain. Increased levels of prostaglandin (a chemical) in the bloodstream may be a factor.

RISK INCREASES WITH
- Stress may precipitate.
- Caffeine and high fluid intake seem to worsen symptoms.
- PMS increases with age.
- PMS can occur with other disorders such as depression.

HOW TO PREVENT—No specific preventive measures. Try to avoid stressful situations at expected time of PMS. Also share your feelings and needs with a close friend or spouse.

 WHAT TO EXPECT

DIAGNOSTIC MEASURES
- Your own observation of symptoms.
- Medical history and physical exam by a doctor.

APPROPRIATE HEALTH CARE
- Self-care.
- Doctor's treatment.

POSSIBLE COMPLICATIONS—Emotional stress caused by symptoms severe enough to disrupt a woman's life.

PROBABLE OUTCOME—Present treatments may or may not be effective. Medication can relieve some symptoms. However, many new treatments are in the experimental stage, offering hope for the future.

 HOW TO TREAT

GENERAL MEASURES
- Treatment steps may involve diet, exercise and lifestyle changes. There are no medications clearly indicated for PMS.
- Reduce stress whenever possible (see How to Cope with Stress in Appendix).
- Learn relaxation techniques. Cut back on your schedule during these days if feasible.
- Stop smoking.
- Join a support group. Talking about your PMS problems with others can help.
- See Resources for Additional Information.

MEDICATION—Ask your doctor. These are used with varying degrees of success:
- Tranquilizers or sedatives to relieve tension.
- Nonsteroidal anti-inflammatory drugs to decrease prostaglandin levels.
- Diuretics to reduce fluid retention.
- Pain medications such as acetaminophen or ibuprofen.
- Vitamin B-6, vitamin E, magnesium.
- Bromocriptine for breast tenderness (rare).
- Antianxiety drugs.
- Danazol for total symptom complex.
- Oral contraceptives may help.
- Other medications are undergoing study and may be more effective.

ACTIVITY
- Begin a regular, aerobic exercise program (walking, biking, etc.).
- Get enough sleep at night.

DIET
- Decrease salt intake during the premenstrual phase.
- Eat a low-fat, high- complex carbohydrate diet.
- Eat frequent small meals.
- Limit intake of caffeine (coffee, soft drinks, tea and chocolate). Abstain from alcohol.

 CALL YOUR DOCTOR IF

- You have symptoms of PMS that interfere with normal activities or relationships, and self-care is not sufficient.
- Symptoms don't improve, despite treatment.
- New, unexplained symptoms develop. Drugs used in treatment may produce side effects.

PRIAPISM

 GENERAL INFORMATION

DEFINITION—A painful and persistent erection of the penis without sexual arousal or desire. It is a rare but serious condition that requires immediate attention so that a permanent injury does not occur to the penis and impair the patient's ability to have a normal erection.

BODY PARTS INVOLVED—Penis.

SEX OR AGE MOST AFFECTED—Males; young adult.

SIGNS & SYMPTOMS—A prolonged, painful, tender erection unaccompanied by sexual arousal.

CAUSES—Blood becomes trapped in the penis causing its engorgement.

RISK INCREASES WITH
- Damage to the nerves that control the supply of blood to the penis.
- Blood disease (leukemia, sickle cell anemia).
- Prolonged sexual activity.
- Pelvic hematoma or cancer.
- Inflammation, injury or infection of the male genitalia.
- Certain medications (e.g., chlorpromazine, methaqualone, prazosin, tolbutamide, trazodone, and some corticosteroids, anticoagulants and antihypertensives).
- Spinal tumor.

HOW TO PREVENT
- Avoid drugs (when possible) that may cause the problem.
- Avoid excessive sexual stimulation.

 WHAT TO EXPECT

DIAGNOSTIC MEASURES
- Your own observation of symptoms.
- Medical history and physical exam by a doctor.

APPROPRIATE HEALTH CARE
- Emergency treatment is necessary because of the risk of permanent damage to the penis.
- Treatment possibilities include surgery; injection of anesthesia into the spinal cord; or withdrawal of blood from the penis through a wide bore needle.
- Any underlying cause will also need treatment.

POSSIBLE COMPLICATIONS—Permanent impotence.

PROBABLE OUTCOME—With prompt, effective medical treatment, a patient may eventually have normal erections again, and sex life should not be adversely affected.

 HOW TO TREAT

GENERAL MEASURES—No measures other than emergency medical care.

MEDICATION—Your doctor may prescribe:
- Pain medicine.
- Drugs to reduce blood pressure or thin the blood.

ACTIVITY—Bed rest until relieved.

DIET—No special diet.

 CALL YOUR DOCTOR IF

You have an erection that persists for no apparent reason. Do not waste time trying to get it down with cold compresses. Go to an emergency room if unable to reach doctor's office immediately.

PRICKLY HEAT
(Miliaria Rubra)

 GENERAL INFORMATION

DEFINITION—A skin disorder characterized by a noninflammatory, itchy rash caused by obstructed sweat-gland ducts.

BODY PARTS INVOLVED—Skin.

SEX OR AGE MOST AFFECTED—All ages, but most common in infants.

SIGNS & SYMPTOMS—Clusters of vesicles (small, fluid-filled skin blisters that may come and go within a matter of hours) or red rash without vesicles in areas of heavy perspiration.

CAUSES—Obstruction of sweat-gland ducts for unknown reasons.

RISK INCREASES WITH
- Obesity
- Stress.
- Hot, humid weather.
- Genetic factors, such as fair, sensitive skin.
- Plastic undersheets.

HOW TO PREVENT—Avoid risk factors.

 WHAT TO EXPECT

DIAGNOSTIC MEASURES
- Your own observation of symptoms.
- Medical history and physical exam by a doctor (severe cases only).

APPROPRIATE HEALTH CARE
- Home care.
- Doctor's treatment, if home care fails.

POSSIBLE COMPLICATIONS—Secondary skin infection.

PROBABLE OUTCOME—Usually curable with treatment. Recurrence is common.

 HOW TO TREAT

GENERAL MEASURES
- Take frequent cool showers or tub baths.
- Apply lubricating ointment or cream to skin 6 or 7 times a day.
- Use cool-water soaks to relieve itching and hasten healing. Pat skin dry, and dust with cornstarch after and between soaks.
- Wear cotton socks and leather-soled footwear rather than shoes made of man-made materials.
- Expose the affected skin to air as much as possible.
- Don't use binding materials, such as adhesive tape, or wear tight clothing.
- Change diapers on infants as soon as they are wet.
- Avoid sunburn once you have had prickly heat. The body's inflammatory reaction to sunburn may trigger a new outbreak of prickly heat.
- Provide cool, dry environment.

MEDICATION
- Your doctor may suggest nonprescription steroid cream to apply 2 or 3 times a day.
- Oral antibiotics may be prescribed if there is a secondary bacterial infection.

ACTIVITY—Decrease activity during hot, humid weather or until skin heals.

DIET—No special diet.

 CALL YOUR DOCTOR IF

Prickly heat doesn't improve in 10 days, despite home care.

PROCTITIS

GENERAL INFORMATION

DEFINITION—Inflammation of the rectum and tissues around the anus.

BODY PARTS INVOLVED—Anus; rectum.

SEX OR AGE MOST AFFECTED—Adolescents and adults of both sexes, but more common in males around age 30.

SIGNS & SYMPTOMS
- Rectal pain.
- Constant urge to have a bowel movement, often when little or no stool is present.
- Blood or mucus discharge from the rectum.
- Cramping pain in the left lower abdomen.
- Fever.

CAUSES
- Gonorrhea.
- Syphilis (usually secondary).
- Herpes simplex.
- Candidiasis.
- Chlamydia.
- Papilloma virus.
- Amebiasis.
- Nonspecific sexually transmitted infection.
- Radiation therapy.

RISK INCREASES WITH
- Male-to-male sexual activity.
- Use of laxatives.
- Rectal injury, rectal medications.
- Radiation therapy.
- Endocrine disorders.
- Ulcerative colitis (early stages).
- Chronic constipation.
- Cancer of the rectum.
- Food allergy.

HOW TO PREVENT
- Avoid anal intercourse.
- Practice safe sex methods. Unsafe sexual activity may make you more at risk for HIV infection.
- To prevent constipation, establish a regular pattern for bowel movements. Eat a diet high in fiber and drink lots of fluids.
- Don't use laxatives regularly.
- Don't eat foods to which you are sensitive.
- Sexually transmitted diseases, such as gonorrhea and syphilis, must be reported to the local health department to prevent their spread. Information is kept confidential.

WHAT TO EXPECT

DIAGNOSTIC MEASURES
- Your own observation of symptoms.
- Medical history and physical exam by a doctor.
- Laboratory studies, such as: blood counts; tests for gonorrhea, syphilis and other sexually transmitted diseases; and stool cultures.
- Surgical diagnostic procedures such as proctoscopy or sigmoidoscopy to rule out other disorders (see Glossary for both).

APPROPRIATE HEALTH CARE
- Self-care after diagnosis.
- Doctor's treatment.
- Surgery to remove any underlying tumor.

POSSIBLE COMPLICATIONS—Anal scarring and stricture (permanent narrowing of the anus).

PROBABLE OUTCOME—The outcome of proctitis depends on the treatment of the underlying cause. Infections can usually be cured with antibiotics. Symptoms of other disorders can be relieved or controlled with treatment.

HOW TO TREAT

GENERAL MEASURES
- Keep the anal area clean with frequent bathing.
- Take sitz baths often to relieve pain. Sit in a tub of hot water for 10 to 15 minutes as often as necessary.

MEDICATION
- You may use nonprescription topical anesthetics to relieve discomfort.
- Your doctor may prescribe:
  Antibiotics for sexually transmitted infections.
  Acyclovir for herpes simplex infection.
  Steroid suppositories to reduce inflammation from other causes.

ACTIVITY—No restrictions.

DIET
- Eat a high-fiber diet.
- Drink at least 8 glasses of water a day.
- Don't eat foods to which you are sensitive.

CALL YOUR DOCTOR IF

- You have symptoms of proctitis, or symptoms recur after treatment.
- New, unexplained symptoms develop. Drugs used in treatment may produce side effects.

ILLNESS & DISORDERS

PROSTATE CANCER

GENERAL INFORMATION

DEFINITION—Growth of malignant cells in the prostate gland, the gland at the base of the urinary bladder in men that helps form semen. Many prostate cancers grow very slowly and never cause symptoms or spread.

BODY PARTS INVOLVED—Prostate.

SEX OR AGE MOST AFFECTED—Men over age 50.

SIGNS & SYMPTOMS
Early stages:
• No symptoms (usually). Most prostate cancers are discovered during a routine rectal examination.
Later stages:
• Urinary obstruction.
• Pain in the low back or pelvis from spread of cancer.

CAUSES—Unknown. Prostate cancer does not seem to be related to an enlarged prostate, a common condition in older men.

RISK INCREASES WITH
• Genetic predisposition.
• Hormonal influences.
• Exposure to cancer causing chemicals.
• Sexually transmitted disease.

HOW TO PREVENT—No specific method. A yearly rectal examination after age 40 is the best way to detect early prostate cancer.

WHAT TO EXPECT

DIAGNOSTIC MEASURES
• Your own observation of symptoms, especially urinary obstruction.
• Medical history and physical exam by a doctor, including rectal examination.
• Diagnostic tests may include digital rectal examination (DRE), core-needle biopsy, prostatic-specific-antigen (PSA) and transrectal ultrasound. For staging to determine any spread of the cancer, a bone scan, measurement of serum prostatic acid phosphatase, biopsy of prostate tissue and of lymph node tissue.

APPROPRIATE HEALTH CARE
• Doctor's treatment.
• Surgery is usually recommended, unless pre-existing medical conditions, such as chronic heart, lung, kidney or liver disease, or advanced age prohibit it.
• Surgery to remove the prostate gland and testes (sometimes), if the cancer has not spread. (See 2 topics on Prostate Gland Removal in Surgery section.)
• Radiation or hormone treatment, if the cancer has spread or for patients unable to undergo surgery.
• Psychotherapy or counseling, if sexual difficulties occur after treatment.

POSSIBLE COMPLICATIONS
• Fatal spread to bone, bladder and other organs.
• Urinary incontinence.
• Sexual impotence after surgery (sometimes).

PROBABLE OUTCOME—Often curable with surgery if treated before cancer spreads. Even after spread, therapy can relieve symptoms and prolong life.

HOW TO TREAT

GENERAL MEASURES
• The more you can learn and understand about prostate cancer, the more you will be able to make informed decisions about where to go for your care, the treatments available, the risks involved, side effects of therapy and expected outcome.
• See Resources for Additional Information.

MEDICATION—Your doctor may prescribe:
• Hormones (usually estrogens or leutinizing-hormone-releasing hormone) to slow malignant growth in bones. Other chemotherapy treatment is not effective with prostate cancer.
• Analgesics to control pain.

ACTIVITY—Resume your normal activities gradually after surgery. Resume sexual relations when able.

DIET—No special diet.

CALL YOUR DOCTOR IF

• You have symptoms of prostate cancer.
• During treatment, any sign of urinary-tract infection occurs, such as: frequent, difficult or painful urination; fever and chills; aching around the genitals or rectum; or backache.
• New, unexplained symptoms develop. Drugs used in treatment may produce side effects.

PROSTATE, ENLARGED (Prostate Hypertrophy; Benign Prostatic Hypertrophy; BPH)

GENERAL INFORMATION

DEFINITION—Enlargement of the prostate (a gland surrounding the neck of the bladder and urethra in the male). The enlargement does not cause problems unless it obstructs the flow of urine from the bladder.

BODY PARTS INVOLVED—Prostate gland; bladder; urethra.

SEX OR AGE MOST AFFECTED—Men over age 50.

SIGNS & SYMPTOMS
- Increased urinary urgency and frequency, especially at night.
- Weak urinary stream.
- Straining and dribbling on urination.
- Feeling that the bladder cannot be emptied completely.
- Urine of abnormal color.
- Impotence (rarely).
- Burning on urination.

CAUSES—Exact cause unknown, may be due to hormonal changes that accompany aging.

RISK INCREASES WITH—Aging.

HOW TO PREVENT—No specific prevention known. Appears to be a part of the aging process. An herb, saw palmetto seems to slow the growth of the prostate in many men.

WHAT TO EXPECT

DIAGNOSTIC MEASURES
- Your own observation of symptoms.
- Medical history and physical exam by a doctor. The degree of difficulty BPH is causing you should be determined with a question and answer interview about your specific symptoms. This can help in making treatment decisions, and then after treatment, provide a good indication of degree of improvement.
- Diagnostic tests may include digital rectal examination, a urinary flow rate with post-void residual and a cystourethroscopy (visual examination, with a lighted instrument, of the inside of the urinary bladder and urethra).
- Intravenous pyelogram, biopsy or ultrasound may be used (see Glossary for all).

APPROPRIATE HEALTH CARE
- Doctor's treatment. Urinary retention, hydronephrosis (kidney disorder), azotemia (excess urea in the blood) and worsening obstructive symptoms are the usual indications for treatment.

- Surgery, transurethral resection of the prostate (TURP), may be recommended. Complications are rare, but are of great concern to patients. Balloon dilatation of the prostate is sometimes temporarily effective in patients with mild obstruction. New surgery methods using lasers are under development. (See 2 topics on Prostate Gland Removal in Surgery section.)
- Treatment with medications is an option.

POSSIBLE COMPLICATIONS—About 11-13% of males with BPH will be found to have clinically undetectable prostate cancer.

PROBABLE OUTCOME—Symptoms in the majority of patients remain stable, while 10-20% will need treatment.

HOW TO TREAT

GENERAL MEASURES
- Urinate as soon as you feel the urge. Don't let the bladder become too full before emptying it.
- For an explanation of surgery and postoperative care, see Prostate Gland Removal in Surgery section.

MEDICATION
- Your doctor may prescribe:
  Finasteride (brand name Proscar) for treatment of mild to moderate disease.
  Alpha-adrenergic blockers, hormonal agents and anti-androgens to improve urinary flow and other symptoms.
  Antibiotics if you develop a urinary-tract infection.
- Saw palmetto.
- Read labels on all nonprescription medicines. Avoid those that state "not recommended if you have prostatic hypertrophy" (examples are antidiarrheals and antihistamines).

ACTIVITY—No restrictions on activities; however, avoid when possible, long bus, train or plane rides unless restrooms are available so you can urinate at any time.

DIET—No special diet. Avoid spicy foods and pepper, which irritate the urethra.

CALL YOUR DOCTOR IF

- You cannot urinate.
- You develop fever.
- You have an enlarged prostate and the symptoms are worsening.

PROSTATITIS

GENERAL INFORMATION

DEFINITION—Inflammation or infection of the prostate (the gland surrounding the neck of the bladder and urethra). Prostatitis is not contagious. It may rarely accompany cancer of the prostate.

BODY PARTS INVOLVED—Prostate gland.

SEX OR AGE MOST AFFECTED—Male adolescents and adults.

SIGNS & SYMPTOMS
- Urgency to urinate.
- Burning with urination.
- Frequent urination; waking to urinate at night.
- Difficulty starting urination and emptying the bladder completely.
- Fever; chills.
- Pain between the scrotum and anus.
- Joint and muscle aches.
- Blood in the urine (sometimes) or semen.
- Low back pain.
- Pain with a doctor's rectal examination.

CAUSES
- Bacterial infection, usually from gram-negative germs such as those found in feces. These may reach the prostate through the bloodstream, the lymphatic system or directly from the urethra.
- The cause of nonbacterial infections is unknown.

RISK INCREASES WITH
- Recent urinary-tract infection.
- Smoking.
- Excess alcohol consumption.

HOW TO PREVENT—Men who have never had prostatitis are less likely to develop it if they are sexually active. Men who have prostatitis at least once may decrease the likelihood of recurrence by increasing sexual activity.

WHAT TO EXPECT

DIAGNOSTIC MEASURES
- Your own observation of symptoms.
- Medical history and physical exam by a doctor.
- Laboratory studies, such as urinalysis and culture of secretions obtained at the time of the doctor's prostate exam.

APPROPRIATE HEALTH CARE
- Self-care after diagnosis.
- Doctor's treatment. Treatment usually involves medications, rest and adequate fluid intake.
- Hospitalization for 3 to 4 days in serious cases if blood poisoning is suspected.
- Surgery to drain an abscess of the prostate (rare).

POSSIBLE COMPLICATIONS—If untreated, may lead to:
- Blood poisoning.
- Chronic bacterial or nonbacterial prostate infections. These have similar symptoms, but they are more likely to recur and respond less readily to treatment.

PROBABLE OUTCOME—Usually curable with treatment, but recurrence is common.

HOW TO TREAT

GENERAL MEASURES
- Sit in a tub with 6 or 8 inches of warm water (106F or 41.1C) for 15 minutes at least 3 times a day. Use a whirlpool bath, if possible.
- Reduce stress in your life (see How to Cope with Stress in Appendix).

MEDICATION—Your doctor may prescribe:
- Antibiotics to fight infection (usually for at least 30 days).
- Pain relievers.
- Stool softeners to avoid constipation.
- Drugs to reduce fever if needed.

ACTIVITY—Rest in bed until fever and pain subside. Then resume your normal activities gradually. The ability to be sexually active during acute prostatitis depends on the degree of disability.

DIET—No special diet, but don't drink alcohol, coffee or eat spicy foods, chocolate or tomato products. These irritate the urethra. Drink 8 to 10 glasses of water a day to ensure an adequate urine flow.

CALL YOUR DOCTOR IF

- You have symptoms of prostatitis.
- Symptoms worsen or you have fever during treatment.
- Symptoms don't improve after 3 days of treatment.
- Symptoms recur after treatment.

PRURITIS ANI
(Anal Itching)

 GENERAL INFORMATION

DEFINITION—Intense chronic itching of the anus and skin around the anus.

BODY PARTS INVOLVED—Anus.

SEX OR AGE MOST AFFECTED—Both sexes; all ages.

SIGNS & SYMPTOMS
- Itching, often intense and worse at night.
- Redness of skin around the anus.
- Abrasion of the skin due to scratching.

CAUSES
- Yeast infection.
- Pinworms, scabies, lice.
- Contact dermatitis caused by soaps, contraceptive foams or jellies, perfumed toilet paper, deodorant sprays, douches or underwear made of synthetic fabric.
- Various skin disorders, including psoriasis or seborrheic dermatitis.
- Vaginal discharge or skin atrophy in women caused by low estrogen levels.
- Chronic diarrhea.
- Excessive coffee intake.
- Unknown (often).

RISK INCREASES WITH
- Stress.
- Diabetes mellitus.
- Excessive sweating.
- Overweight.

HOW TO PREVENT
- Keep the body clean with regular showers or baths.
- Cleanse carefully after bowel movements with moistened tissue.
- Avoid contact with substances to which you are sensitive (see Causes).
- Avoid tight underclothing made from synthetic material.

 WHAT TO EXPECT

DIAGNOSTIC MEASURES
- Your own observation of symptoms.
- Medical history and physical exam by a doctor.
- Laboratory studies, such as cultures for fungi, or microscopic examinations for pinworm eggs or scabies in skin burrows.

APPROPRIATE HEALTH CARE
- Self-care after diagnosis.
- Doctor's treatment, if self-care is not successful.

POSSIBLE COMPLICATIONS
- Skin damage, allowing secondary bacterial infection to develop.
- Skin thickening and chronic inflammation.

PROBABLE OUTCOME—Symptoms can be controlled with treatment, even if the cause cannot be determined. Problem may recur.

 HOW TO TREAT

GENERAL MEASURES
- Keep showers or baths brief to minimize dryness and soap irritation. Use plain, unscented soap if any.
- Keep the rectal area clean, dry and cool. Wear loose clothing and underclothing. Clean carefully after bowel movements, using moist tufts of cotton or plain soap and water.
- Don't use irritants listed as causes.
- Wear underwear with a cotton crotch or underwear made of cotton, rather than nylon or other synthetics.
- Use plain, noncolored, nonscented toilet tissue.
- Use talcum powder in the area of itching.
- Women may be more comfortable using tampons for menstrual periods, rather than sanitary napkins.
- Wear soft mittens at night, if scratching while asleep.
- If you are unable to completely empty rectum with bowel movement, use a small plain water enema (infant bulb syringe) after each bowel movement. This may prevent irritation.

MEDICATION
- You may use nonprescription cortisone ointment or cream. Apply 3 times a day and rub in gently until it disappears. Avoid laxatives.
- Your doctor may prescribe more potent topical cortisone drugs.

ACTIVITY—Avoid activities that cause excessive perspiration.

DIET—Try eliminating spicy or highly seasoned foods, such as citrus, vitamin C, tomato products, coffee, beer, cola, to see if there is improvement. These can irritate mucous membranes of the anus.

 CALL YOUR DOCTOR IF

- You have symptoms of pruritis ani that persist, despite self-care.
- You develop a fever.
- The irritated area seems infected.

ILLNESS & DISORDERS

PRURITIS VULVAE

GENERAL INFORMATION

DEFINITION—An acute or chronic disorder of the skin around the vulva (the vaginal lips). This disorder is characterized by severe itching. It is not contagious. In most instances, it is a symptom of an underlying disorder, and in others, the cause is unknown.

BODY PARTS INVOLVED—Vulva and skin surrounding the vulva and anus.

SEX OR AGE MOST AFFECTED—Female adolescents and adults, especially after menopause.

SIGNS & SYMPTOMS
- Intense itching, sensitivity and irritation in the genital area. The skin may be dry.
- Burning feeling in the genital area.
- Thin, white vaginal discharge (sometimes).
- Discomfort during sexual intercourse.

CAUSES
- Skin disease, such as psoriasis or lichen planus.
- Systemic disease, such as diabetes.
- Atrophy and dryness caused by estrogen deficiency.
- Skin reaction to irritants, such as: toilet tissue; sanitary pads; soap; douches; deodorants; powders; perfume; and fabric.
- Systemic allergies, including food allergies.
- Disorder of the vagina or rectum, such as vaginitis or hemorrhoids.
- Unknown causes in some cases.

RISK INCREASES WITH
- Stress.
- Days prior to menstruation.
- Hot, humid weather.
- Diabetes mellitus.
- Lack of urinary or bowel control.

HOW TO PREVENT
- Wear cotton underpants rather than nylon.
- Avoid contact with irritants listed above.
- Obtain medical treatment for underlying causes.

WHAT TO EXPECT

DIAGNOSTIC MEASURES
- Your own observation of symptoms.
- Medical history and physical exam by a doctor.
- Diagnostic tests may include laboratory study of vaginal secretions, and if needed, a biopsy (see Glossary) of the vulva.

APPROPRIATE HEALTH CARE
- Self-care.
- Doctor's treatment for any underlying cause and more severe symptoms.

POSSIBLE COMPLICATIONS
- Secondary bacterial infection of the inflamed skin.
- Chronic course.

PROBABLE OUTCOME—Home treatment usually provides relief in 4 to 7 days. If medical treatment becomes necessary, allow 2 weeks for recovery.

HOW TO TREAT

GENERAL MEASURES
- Wear cotton underclothes.
- Keep the area as dry and cool as possible. Wear loose clothing.
- Don't scratch the itchy area. Scratching will aggravate soreness and irritation.
- Wash the genital area with water and unscented soap only once a day.
- Use a lubricant, such as K-Y Lubricating Jelly or baby oil, during intercourse.
- After urinating or having a bowel movement, clean the genital area gently with absorbent cotton or antiseptic wipes. Wipe from front to back (vagina to anus).
- During menstruation, use tampons rather than sanitary napkins until the disorder heals.
- Sit in bathtub of warm water several times a day to help relieve itching.

MEDICATION
- You may use low-potency, nonprescription steroid creams or ointments.
- Your doctor may prescribe:
  More potent steroid creams or lotions to reduce inflammation. These require 24 to 36 hours to provide relief.
  Ointments that contain hormones.
  Medications for any bacterial or fungal infections.

ACTIVITY—Avoid overexertion, heat and excessive sweating.

DIET
- Avoid foods to which you may be allergic. If you are unsure, try eliminating suspected foods from your diet to see if symptoms get better. Then slowly introduce the foods back into your diet.
- Avoid coffee or other caffeine beverages, tomatoes and peanuts.

CALL YOUR DOCTOR IF

- You have symptoms of pruritis vulvae.
- Symptoms don't improve in 2 weeks, despite treatment.
- Scratching leads to skin infection.
- New, unexplained symptoms develop. Drugs used in treatment may produce side effects.

PSEUDOGOUT

GENERAL INFORMATION

DEFINITION—An acute, inflammatory form of arthritis that usually involves the large joints of the body. Pseudogout, like gout, involves deposits of crystals in and around the joints. It is usually characterized by acute attacks, but often the disease may progress without the attacks.

BODY PARTS INVOLVED—Large joints (most often, the knee, wrist, ankle).

SEX OR AGE MOST AFFECTED—Elderly; more common in men than women.

SIGNS & SYMPTOMS
- Acute attacks of swelling and pain in one or more of the joints.
- Joints involved most often are the knee (50% of the time), ankle, wrist and shoulder.
- Attacks may last for two or more days.
- Freedom from pain or less severe pain between attacks.
- Limitation of motion of a joint.
- Fever.

CAUSES—Deposition of crystals formed of calcium pyrophosphate dihydrate (CPPD) in the synovial (joint fluid). Why the crystals form is unknown.

RISK INCREASES WITH
- Trauma.
- Aging.
- Patients hospitalized for other medical or surgical illnesses.
- Metabolic diseases (e.g., hypothyroidism, hyperthyroidism, gout, amyloidosis).

HOW TO PREVENT
- None known to prevent original disorder.
- Attacks may be triggered by stress, trauma, surgery, severe dieting, thiazide therapy and alcohol abuse. Avoid any of these when possible.

WHAT TO EXPECT

DIAGNOSTIC MEASURES
- Your own observation of symptoms.
- Medical history and physical exam by a doctor.
- Diagnosis is made by microscopic examination of a sample of joint fluid. This will distinguish it from gout, which is caused by different urate crystals.

APPROPRIATE HEALTH CARE
- Doctor's treatment.
- If appropriate, treatment for any underlying metabolic disorder.
- Drainage of the inflamed joint if needed.

POSSIBLE COMPLICATIONS
- Recurrences of the attacks.
- Permanent joint damage.

PROBABLE OUTCOME—Prognosis for relief in acute attacks is excellent.

HOW TO TREAT

GENERAL MEASURES—Moist, warm compresses applied to affected joint may be helpful.

MEDICATION—Your doctor may prescribe:
- Nonsteroidal anti-inflammatory drugs to promptly control acute attacks.
- Intravenous colchicine for persistent pain (rarely needed). Oral colchicine may help prevent acute attacks. Ask your doctor.
- Corticosteroid injection into the joint to help relieve symptoms.

ACTIVITY
- Avoid putting weight on affected joint during acute attack.
- Once pain subsides, begin range of motion exercises or isometric exercises to maintain strength.

DIET—Avoid excess consumption of alcohol and foods that contain purines (sardines, anchovies, liver, sweet breads).

CALL YOUR DOCTOR IF

- You have signs or symptoms of pseudogout.
- Symptoms worsen after treatment begins.
- New or unexplained symptoms develop. Drugs used in treatment may cause side effects.
- Temperature goes over 101F (38.3C).

ILLNESS & DISORDERS

PSEUDOMEMBRANOUS ENTEROCOLITIS

GENERAL INFORMATION

DEFINITION—A rare, severe illness in the small and large intestines. It usually follows 5 to 7 days after extensive gastrointestinal surgery and antibiotic treatment in a person who was debilitated before surgery. It is characterized by inflammation and tissue death of the lining membrane and deeper layers of the intestine.

BODY PARTS INVOLVED—Large and small intestines.

SEX OR AGE MOST AFFECTED—Adults, especially those over age 60.

SIGNS & SYMPTOMS
• Watery diarrhea (sometimes bloody) with abdominal cramps.
• Fever; nausea and vomiting.
• Drop in blood pressure, sometimes to shock levels, with weak pulse and rapid heartbeat.
• Disorientation.
• Symptoms may begin during the antibiotic treatment or may appear 1-10 days after the treatment has stopped.

CAUSES—Infection from bacteria, usually Clostridium difficile, which manufactures a toxin that causes the symptoms; or from the staphylococcus germ. These germs normally inhabit the intestinal tract. They cause enterocolitis when other normal bacterial of the intestinal tract have been killed by heavy use of broad-spectrum antibiotics. This upsets the bacterial balance of the intestinal tract. The illness usually occurs as a complication of surgery.

RISK INCREASES WITH
• Adults over 60.
• Recent surgery with a drop in blood pressure during surgery.
• Kidney failure.
• Obesity; poor nutrition.
• Use of antibiotics, especially lincomycin, clindamycin, ampicillin, chloramphenicol, cephalosporins, penicillin or sulfa drugs.

HOW TO PREVENT—No specific preventive measures.

WHAT TO EXPECT

DIAGNOSTIC MEASURES
• Your own observation of symptoms.
• Medical history and exam by a doctor.
• Laboratory culture of the stool, biopsy (see Glossary) of the membrane lining of the large intestine through a colonoscope (see Glossary).
Note: A barium enema should not be administered. It may cause intestinal perforation.

APPROPRIATE HEALTH CARE
• Doctor's treatment.
• The most important aspect of treatment is to discontinue use of the antibiotic causing the illness.
• Hospitalization for intravenous nutrition and intensive care in moderate to severe cases.

POSSIBLE COMPLICATIONS—The following occur only if the problem is not recognized and treated:
• Shock and severe dehydration.
• Peritonitis caused by perforation of the intestine.

PROBABLE OUTCOME—Symptoms will usually disappear in 1 to 2 weeks after the offending antibiotic is discontinued. A substitute antibiotic is usually not prescribed; the body's defense mechanisms must take over for the withdrawn antibiotic. The worst cases are fatal.

HOW TO TREAT

GENERAL MEASURES—While in the hospital, you will be monitored closely for any changes in your vital signs, electrolyte imbalances, your fluid intake and output (including fluid lost in stools), signs of possible shock and your level of consciousness.

MEDICATION
• Your doctor may prescribe:
Cholestyramine, vancomycin or metronidazole to prevent secondary, nonbacterial infections that occur when the balance of intestinal organisms is upset.
High doses of cortisone for a short time to decrease inflammation.
• Don't take antidiarrheal drugs unless prescribed by your doctor. They may contribute to intestinal perforation.

ACTIVITY—Rest in bed until all symptoms of the illness disappear. Flex legs often while in bed to decrease the likelihood of deep-vein blood clots. Resume normal activities gradually.

DIET—Intravenous nourishment will be necessary at first, progressing to a liquid diet, a soft diet and finally to a normal diet.

CALL YOUR DOCTOR IF

• You have symptoms of pseudomembranous enterocolitis following intestinal surgery.
• Symptoms return after treatment.
• New, unexplained symptoms develop. Drugs used in treatment may produce side effects.

PSITTACOSIS
(Parrot Fever; Ornithosis)

 GENERAL INFORMATION

DEFINITION—An infectious form of pneumonia transmitted by birds.

BODY PARTS INVOLVED—Lungs.

SEX OR AGE MOST AFFECTED—Both sexes; all ages.

SIGNS & SYMPTOMS
- Fever and chills.
- General ill feeling.
- Appetite loss.
- Cough without sputum that progresses to cough with occasional discolored sputum.
- Shortness of breath.

CAUSES—Infection by the organism, Chlamydia. Microscopic chlamydia organisms are not bacteria, viruses or fungi. However, they can be destroyed with antibiotics.

Psittacosis is found in psittacine birds (parrots, parakeets, lovebirds), poultry, pigeons, canaries and some sea birds. Germs enter the human body by inhalation of air that contains the germ or by a bite from an infected bird. Incubation is 1 to 3 weeks after exposure.

RISK INCREASES WITH—Exposure to birds, especially in zoos, pet shops or on farms.

HOW TO PREVENT
- Avoid dust from bird feathers and cage contents.
- Don't handle any sick bird. Imported psittacine birds must be treated for 45 days with feed that contains chlortetracycline. This eliminates the organisms from the birds' blood and feces.

 WHAT TO EXPECT

DIAGNOSTIC MEASURES
- Your own observation of symptoms.
- Medical history and physical exam by a doctor.
- Diagnosis is suggested by symptoms and history of exposure to birds. Firm diagnosis is determined by recovery of the organism from mice, eggs or tissue culture inoculated with the patient's blood or sputum.

APPROPRIATE HEALTH CARE
- Self-care after diagnosis.
- Doctor's treatment.
- Treatment involves medication (sometimes intravenous) and supportive care for symptoms.

POSSIBLE COMPLICATIONS—Severe or fatal pneumonia.

PROBABLE OUTCOME—Usually curable in 7 to 14 days with early diagnosis and treatment. Fever may remain for 2 or 3 weeks before falling slowly, unless antibiotics are used.

 HOW TO TREAT

GENERAL MEASURES
- Use a cool-mist, ultrasonic humidifier to increase air moisture and loosen lung secretions. Use pure water; don't put medication in the humidifier. Clean humidifier daily.
- Use a heating pad or warm, moist compresses on the chest to relieve pain.
- Don't smoke.

MEDICATION
- Your doctor may prescribe tetracycline (an antibiotic) for at least 10 days to control fever and other symptoms.
- Don't suppress the cough if it produces sputum. It is performing a useful function in ridding the lungs of mucus. If the cough is nonproductive and painful, you may suppress it with prescribed medication.
- For minor pain, take nonprescription drugs such as aspirin or acetaminophen.

ACTIVITY—Bed rest is necessary until the fever, pain and shortness of breath have been gone at least 48 hours. Then normal activities may be resumed gradually. Fatigue and weakness may persist for a long time, so don't expect a quick return to normal strength.

DIET—No special diet. Increase fluid intake to at least 1 glass of fluid every hour. This helps to thin lung secretions so they can be coughed up more easily.

 CALL YOUR DOCTOR IF

- You have symptoms of psittacosis.
- The following occurs during treatment:
  Fever.
  Pain is not relieved by heat or prescribed medication.
  Shortness of breath increases.
  Fingernails become dark or bluish.
  Blood appears in the sputum.
  Nausea, vomiting or diarrhea occur.

PSORIASIS

GENERAL INFORMATION

DEFINITION—A chronic, scaly skin disorder characterized by frequent remissions and recurrences.

BODY PARTS INVOLVED—Skin, especially of the scalp, elbows, knees, chest, back, arms, legs, toenails, fingernails and fold between the buttocks.

SEX OR AGE MOST AFFECTED—Begins in late childhood or young adulthood and continues throughout life.

SIGNS & SYMPTOMS
- Skin areas that are slightly raised, have red borders and are covered with large white or silver-white scales. The areas crack and become painful.
- Itching (sometimes).
- Joint pain.

CAUSES—Unknown, but probably caused by autoimmune disorder.

RISK INCREASES WITH
- Family history of psoriasis.
- Rheumatoid arthritis.
- Local injury.
- Infections (viral and bacterial) elsewhere in the body.
- Stress.
- Cold climates.
- Genetic factors. Persons with psoriasis have HLA antigens, and the incidence is highest among Caucasians.
- AIDS.

HOW TO PREVENT—Cannot be prevented at present.

WHAT TO EXPECT

DIAGNOSTIC MEASURES
- Your own observation of symptoms.
- Medical history and physical exam by a doctor.
- Skin biopsy (see Glossary) if needed to confirm diagnosis.

APPROPRIATE HEALTH CARE
- Self-care after diagnosis.
- Doctor's treatment.
- No permanent cure exists. Steps in treatment depend on the type of psoriasis, extent of the disease, your response to it, and affect on your lifestyle.
- Psychotherapy or counseling (sometimes) to help in adapting to the disorder.

POSSIBLE COMPLICATIONS
- Secondary bacterial infection in the affected area.
- Pustular psoriasis.
- Psoriatic arthritis.

PROBABLE OUTCOME—Symptoms can be controlled but not cured. The disease may have long periods of inactivity. In women, severity decreases during pregnancy.

HOW TO TREAT

GENERAL MEASURES
- Maintain good skin hygiene with daily baths or showers.
- Avoid skin injury, including harsh scrubbing, which can trigger new outbreaks.
- Avoid skin dryness to decrease the frequency of recurrences. To reduce scaling, use nonprescription waterless cleansers and hair preparations containing coal tar or cortisone.
- Expose skin to moderate amounts of sunlight as often as possible.
- Oatmeal baths may loosen scales. Use 1 cup of oatmeal to a tub of warm water.
- Get counseling for any psychological problems caused by psoriasis.
- See Resources for Additional Information.

MEDICATION—Your doctor may prescribe the following to decrease inflammation and scaling:
- Ointments containing coal tar.
- Topical cortisone drugs to use under plastic dressings.
- Immunosuppressive drugs (severest cases).
- PUVA (combination of a medication and exposure to ultraviolet light-wavelength A).
- Combination of tar baths with UVB (ultraviolet therapy-wavelength B).
- Antihistamines to relieve itching.
- For pustular psoriasis—etretinate, isotretinoin or oral methotrexate.

ACTIVITY—No restrictions.

DIET—No special diet.

CALL YOUR DOCTOR IF

- You have symptoms of psoriasis, or symptoms recur after treatment.
- During an outbreak, pustules erupt on the skin, accompanied by fever, muscle aches and fatigue.
- New, unexplained symptoms develop. Drugs used in treatment may produce side effects.

PSORIATIC ARTHRITIS

 ## GENERAL INFORMATION

DEFINITION—Joint inflammation that accompanies psoriasis lesions in nearby nails and skin.

BODY PARTS INVOLVED
- Joints in any part of the body, but most likely in finger joints and low-back and neck joints in the spine.
- Skin or nails that have psoriasis lesions and are close to the affected joint. Sometimes additional skin sites include the scalp, navel, underarm and groin.

SEX OR AGE MOST AFFECTED—Usually begins between ages 30 and 35 and continues intermittently throughout life.

SIGNS & SYMPTOMS
- Pain, swelling, restricted movement, tenderness and warmth in the affected joint.
- Scaling skin.
- Pitted, ridged, yellow nails.
- Tiredness and fever (sometimes).

CAUSES
- Predisposition to psoriatic arthritis may be hereditary.
- Immunological response to a streptococcal infection.
- Unknown (usually).
- Physical or emotional trauma (rare).

RISK INCREASES WITH
- Strep infections (rare).
- Family history of rheumatoid arthritis or psoriasis.

HOW TO PREVENT—No specific preventive measures. Always obtain prompt antibiotic treatment for strep infections.

 ## WHAT TO EXPECT

DIAGNOSTIC MEASURES
- Your own observation of symptoms.
- Medical history and physical exam by a doctor.
- Laboratory blood studies to detect a rheumatic factor and measure antinuclear antibodies (ANA).
- X-ray.

APPROPRIATE HEALTH CARE
- Self-care after diagnosis.
- Doctor's treatment. Treatment is directed at control of skin lesions and joint inflammation.

POSSIBLE COMPLICATIONS—Progression to chronic arthritis and severe crippling may occur (rare).

PROBABLE OUTCOME—This condition is currently considered incurable. It is characterized by acute flare-ups and remissions. However, symptoms can be relieved or controlled, and medical literature cites a few instances of unexplained recovery.

Scientific research into causes and treatment continues, so there is hope for increasingly effective treatment and cure.

 ## HOW TO TREAT

GENERAL MEASURES
- Immobilize inflamed joints with splints.
- Use heat to relieve joint pain. Hot soaks, whirlpool treatments, heat lamps, ultrasound or diathermy are all effective.
- Schedule periods for regular, moderate exposure to sunlight. If heat does not help, try cold compresses.
- PUVA therapy, high intensity ultraviolet light along with psoralen medication, is effective for the skin lesions.
- See Resources for Additional Information.

MEDICATION
- For minor discomfort, you may use nonprescription drugs such as aspirin.
- To reduce joint inflammation, your doctor may prescribe:
  Nonsteroidal anti-inflammatory drugs.
  Cortisone injections into inflamed joints (occasionally).
  Immunosuppressive drugs (sometimes) such as methotrexate.

ACTIVITY—Rest inflamed joints during flare-ups, then resume your normal activities gradually. Try to increase outdoor activity in sunshine.

DIET—No special diet.

 ## CALL YOUR DOCTOR IF

- You have symptoms of psoriatic arthritis.
- New, unexplained symptoms develop. Drugs used in treatment may produce side effects.

PTOSIS

GENERAL INFORMATION

DEFINITION—Drooping of the upper eyelid, partially or completely covering the eye.

BODY PARTS INVOLVED—Upper eyelid; eye.

SEX OR AGE MOST AFFECTED—Both sexes; all ages.

SIGNS & SYMPTOMS—Drooping of one or both eyelids, accompanied by poor blinking reflexes. The extent of droop may vary at different times of the day.

CAUSES—May be present at birth or may accompany other problems, including:
- Paralysis of nerve fibers to the eyelids.
- Myasthenia gravis.
- Muscular dystrophy.
- Diabetes.
- Brain tumor.
- Birth injury.
- Head or eyelid injury.
- Tumor in the upper lobe of a lung.

RISK INCREASES WITH
- Adults over 60.
- Family history of ptosis.

HOW TO PREVENT—No specific preventive measures.

WHAT TO EXPECT

DIAGNOSTIC MEASURES
- Medical history and physical exam by a doctor.
- Your own observation of symptoms.
- X-rays of various body regions to look for the underlying cause.

APPROPRIATE HEALTH CARE
- Self-care after diagnosis.
- Doctor's treatment. Some ophthalmologists recommend keeping the lid raised with a support that is part of eyeglasses.
- Surgery to strengthen the muscles of the eyelid (sometimes).

POSSIBLE COMPLICATIONS
- Permanent disfigurement.
- Irritation and infection in the eye caused by poor blinking reflexes and continuous contact between the eyelid and eye surface.
- Visual disturbance.

PROBABLE OUTCOME—Sometimes curable if the underlying cause can be corrected by surgery or medication.

HOW TO TREAT

GENERAL MEASURES
- Keep the eye moist with nonprescription, artificial tears.
- Wear safety goggles to protect the eye from injury when exposed to dust or flying debris.

MEDICATION—Medicine usually is not necessary for ptosis, but it may be necessary for the underlying disorder.

ACTIVITY—No restrictions.

DIET—No special diet.

CALL YOUR DOCTOR IF

- You have symptoms of ptosis.
- Ptosis worsens or vision is affected.

PUERPERAL INFECTION
(Puerperal Fever; Postpartum Infection)

GENERAL INFORMATION

DEFINITION—Infection of the birth canal after the first 24 hours following delivery of a baby.

BODY PARTS INVOLVED—Any or all: vagina; vulva; perineum (area between the vagina and rectum); cervix, uterus; peritoneum (membrane that covers abdominal organs).

SEX OR AGE MOST AFFECTED—Females of childbearing age.

SIGNS & SYMPTOMS
- Unexplained fever and chills for 2 or more days after the first postpartum day (first day after delivery).
- Headache; muscle aches.
- Appetite loss.
- Rapid heartbeat.
- Soft, large, tender uterus.
- Vaginal discharge with an unpleasant odor.
- Abdominal pain.

CAUSES—Infection by bacteria normally found in a healthy vagina. These bacteria can infect the uterus, vagina, adjacent tissues and kidney, especially in conjunction with risk factors.

RISK INCREASES WITH
- Insertion of a fetal scalp electrode during labor.
- Anemia, either pre-existing or from loss of blood during delivery.
- Toxemia during pregnancy.
- Long delay between rupture of the placental membranes and delivery (greater than 24 hours).
- Prolonged labor.
- Traumatic delivery.
- Repeated vaginal examinations with unsterile equipment during labor.
- Retained fragments of placenta in the uterus.
- Excessive bleeding after delivery.

HOW TO PREVENT
- Avoid anyone with an active infection for the last 2 weeks of pregnancy.
- Notify your doctor as soon as placental membranes rupture (your "water breaks"). Don't have sexual intercourse after membranes rupture.
- Wash the perineal area often during the first week after delivery.
- Ask your prenatal care doctor for a culture for group D strep at 28-34 weeks of pregnancy for screening purposes.

WHAT TO EXPECT

DIAGNOSTIC MEASURES
- Medical history and physical exam by a doctor.
- Laboratory blood studies, blood culture and culture of the vaginal discharge.

APPROPRIATE HEALTH CARE
- Doctor's treatment.
- Hospitalization for intensive treatment.
- Surgery to remove fragments of placenta (sometimes).

POSSIBLE COMPLICATIONS
- Deep-vein blood clot in the pelvis.
- Blood poisoning.
- Shock.
- Infection in your newborn infant.

PROBABLE OUTCOME—Usually curable in 7 to 10 days with intensive treatment. Without treatment, complications can be severe and sometimes fatal.

HOW TO TREAT

GENERAL MEASURES
- To relieve pain, place a heating pad or hot-water bottle on the abdomen or back.
- Take frequent hot baths to relax muscles and relieve pain.
- Use sanitary pads rather than tampons for the vaginal discharge.
- If you plan to breast-feed, use a breast pump to express milk until the infection heals.

MEDICATION—Your doctor may prescribe:
- Antibiotics in high doses—intravenously, if necessary.
- Codeine and acetaminophen to reduce fever and pain.
- Anticoagulants to prevent blood-clot formation.

ACTIVITY
- Rest in bed, except to use the bathroom, until fever and other signs of infection subside. You will probably be more comfortable if you lie on your left side.
- Abstain from sexual relations until signs of infection have been gone at least 7 days.

DIET—Drink lots of fluids to prevent dehydration from high fever. Vitamin and mineral supplements should not be necessary unless you are anemic.

CALL YOUR DOCTOR IF

- You have symptoms of a puerperal infection even several hours after delivery.
- You faint.
- You develop a skin rash.
- New, unexplained symptoms develop. Drugs used in treatment may produce side effects.
- Symptoms of infection recur after treatment.

ILLNESS & DISORDERS

PULMONARY EDEMA

GENERAL INFORMATION

DEFINITION—A set of dramatic, life-threatening symptoms caused by congestive heart failure.

BODY PARTS INVOLVED—Lungs and heart.

SEX OR AGE MOST AFFECTED—Adults over 40.

SIGNS & SYMPTOMS—The following symptoms often begin suddenly in the middle of the night and worsen rapidly:
• Extreme shortness of breath, sometimes with wheezing.
• Rapid breathing.
• Restlessness and anxiety.
• Paleness.
• Sweating.
• Bluish nails and lips.
• Low blood pressure.
• Cough. This may be unproductive at first, but later it can produce a frothy, blood-stained sputum.

CAUSES—Failure of the heart's left ventricle to pump well enough to supply all body cells with oxygen. The underlying cause of heart failure includes many forms of heart disease, especially heart rhythm disturbances or hypertension with atherosclerosis or narrowing of the aortic valve.

RISK INCREASES WITH
• Adults over 60.
• Stress.
• Recent heart attack.
• High blood pressure or any form of heart disease.
• Obesity.
• Smoking.
• Fatigue or overwork.

HOW TO PREVENT—If you have any form of heart disease, obtain prompt treatment for less dramatic signs of congestive heart failure. The treatment may include a low-salt diet, smoking cessation, maintenance of an ideal weight, adequate rest and prescription drugs.

WHAT TO EXPECT

DIAGNOSTIC MEASURES
• Your own observation of symptoms.
• Medical history and physical exam by a doctor.
• Laboratory blood studies and ECG (see Glossary), chest x-ray, pulmonary function studies and pulmonary arterial catheterization (a study to evaluate function of the heart).

APPROPRIATE HEALTH CARE
• Doctor's treatment.
• Treatment is designed to reduce the excess fluid, improve lung and heart function and correct any underlying disorder.

POSSIBLE COMPLICATIONS
• Death (if treatment is delayed or unsuccessful).
• Misdiagnosis as asthma, resulting in inappropriate treatment.

PROBABLE OUTCOME—In most cases, symptoms can be controlled with treatment. The treatment for pulmonary edema usually brings dramatic and effective relief. However, the underlying heart disease causing pulmonary edema will require lifelong treatment.

HOW TO TREAT

GENERAL MEASURES—Self-care is not appropriate for pulmonary edema. This is a medical emergency requiring intensive medical care. Delay can lead to death.

MEDICATION—Your doctor may prescribe:
• Narcotics to relieve anxiety, decrease blood flow to the lung and reduce oxygen demand of the body.
• Diuretics to decrease excess fluid circulating in the bloodstream and lessen fluid accumulated in the lungs.
• Digitalis to stimulate a stronger heartbeat.
• Antibiotics (if pulmonary edema has been triggered by infection).
• Medications such as beta-blockers, ACE inhibitors, nitrates and calcium-channel blockers to reduce workload on the heart.
• Supplemental oxygen.

ACTIVITY—Rest in bed until your condition stabilizes. After treatment, resume your normal activities gradually. Resume sexual relations when symptoms disappear and strength returns.

DIET—Your doctor may recommend a low-salt, low-fat diet (see both in Appendix).

CALL YOUR DOCTOR IF

You have symptoms of pulmonary edema. This is an emergency!

PULMONARY EMBOLISM

 ## GENERAL INFORMATION

DEFINITION—A blood clot or fat cells (rarely) in one of the arteries carrying blood to the lungs. The blood clot begins in a deep vein of the leg or pelvis. A fat embolus usually begins at a fracture site. The embolus moves through the bloodstream, passing through the heart and lodging in the branch of an artery that nourishes the lungs. This blockage decreases breathing ability and sometimes destroys lung tissue.

BODY PARTS INVOLVED—Veins, especially veins in the legs; pulmonary artery and smaller artery branches that nourish the lungs; broken bone.

SEX OR AGE MOST AFFECTED—All ages, but most common in adults.

SIGNS & SYMPTOMS
- Sudden shortness of breath.
- Faintness or fainting.
- Pain in the chest.
- Cough (sometimes with bloody sputum).
- Rapid heartbeat.
- Low fever.

These symptoms are often preceded by swelling and pain in the leg.

CAUSES—Deep-vein thrombosis, which can occur anytime that blood pools in a vein.

RISK INCREASES WITH
- Adults over 60.
- Any injury or illness that requires prolonged bed rest.
- Sitting in one position for prolonged periods, as on airplane flights.
- Recent surgery.
- Congestive heart failure.
- Heart rhythm disturbances.
- Polycythemia; hemolytic anemia.
- Bone fractures.
- Obesity; smoking.
- Pregnancy.
- Use of oral contraceptives, especially in women who smoke.

HOW TO PREVENT
- Avoid prolonged bed rest during illnesses. Wear elastic stockings during recuperation—in or out of bed.
- Start moving lower limbs and walking as soon as possible after surgery.
- Don't smoke, especially if you are a woman 35 or older who takes birth-control pills.
- Avoid needless surgery. Get a second opinion.
- When traveling, stand and walk every 1 to 2 hours.
- Aspirin has generally not been shown to be effective in preventing venous clots.

 ## WHAT TO EXPECT

DIAGNOSTIC MEASURES
- Your own observation of symptoms.
- Medical history and exam by a doctor.
- Laboratory blood studies to measure coagulation factors and prothrombin time.
- X-rays of the chest.
- Radioactive lung scan and arterial blood gases.

APPROPRIATE HEALTH CARE
- Doctor's treatment.
- Treatment is aimed at maintaining adequate cardiovascular and pulmonary functions (during resolution of the clot) and preventing recurrence.
- Surgery may be necessary to tie off the big vein leading to the heart and lungs (vena cava) or insertion of a filter to trap recurrent clots (rare).

POSSIBLE COMPLICATIONS
- Rapid death from a large clot that obstructs more than 50% of the blood to the lungs.
- Massive bleeding in the lungs caused by smaller clots.

PROBABLE OUTCOME—Usually curable in 10 to 14 days with intensive care.

 ## HOW TO TREAT

GENERAL MEASURES
- Wear elastic stockings or leg wraps with elastic bandages.
- Don't sit with your legs or ankles crossed.
- Elevate your feet higher than your hips when sitting for long periods.
- Elevate the foot of your bed.

MEDICATION—Your doctor may prescribe:
- Anticoagulant drugs to dissolve and prevent clots. The anticoagulant level must be monitored to keep it in a safe range.
- Oxygen, if needed.
- Antibiotics if septic emboli.

ACTIVITY—Rest in bed until all symptoms and signs of clot inflammation disappear. While in bed, move your legs often to stimulate circulation.

DIET—No special diet.

 ## CALL YOUR DOCTOR IF

The following occurs during treatment:
Chest pain.
Coughing up blood.
Shortness of breath.
Increased swelling and pain in the leg, despite treatment.

ILLNESS & DISORDERS

PURPURA, ALLERGIC
(Anaphylactoid Purpura; Henoch-Schönlein Purpura)

 GENERAL INFORMATION

DEFINITION—A common allergic disorder involving sudden bleeding into the skin or intestines.

BODY PARTS INVOLVED
* Joints (usually knees, ankles, hips, wrists and elbows).
* Skin of the legs, thighs and abdomen.
* Gastrointestinal tract.
* Kidneys.

SEX OR AGE MOST AFFECTED—Both sexes; all ages, most common in children and boys twice as often as girls.

SIGNS & SYMPTOMS
* Sore throat about 2 weeks prior to other symptoms.
* Itching skin rash that seems to be just beneath the skin surface. The rash usually consists of large hives with small bruises or blood spots in the centers. The rash is most often on the buttocks and upper thighs in children and on the feet and ankles of adults, but it may be scattered over the body.
* Joint pain and inflammation at the knees, ankles, hips, wrists or elbows.
* Cramping abdominal pain and vomiting.
* Diarrhea; low fever.
* Protein and blood in the urine.

CAUSES—Purpura is probably an autoimmune reaction in the inflamed small blood vessels throughout the body. The allergic trigger is not known, but attacks often follow an upper-respiratory infection or the use of some drugs, especially sulfa drugs.

RISK INCREASES WITH
* Recent illness, especially a bacterial sore throat.
* Use of sulfa drugs.

HOW TO PREVENT
* Don't allow your child to be exposed to respiratory infections, if possible.
* Obtain prompt medical treatment of any bacterial throat infection.
* Avoid the use of any drug that has triggered allergic purpura in your child. Consult the doctor before giving any medication to a child.

 WHAT TO EXPECT

DIAGNOSTIC MEASURES
* Your own observation of symptoms.
* Medical history and exam by a doctor.
* Laboratory blood studies and blood-clotting studies.

APPROPRIATE HEALTH CARE
* Home care after diagnosis.
* Doctor's treatment.
* Care can usually be given at home, but complications may require hospitalization.
* Treatment involves the elimination of any possible offending drug and supportive therapy to relieve symptoms.

POSSIBLE COMPLICATIONS
* Kidney failure, resulting from kidney inflammation and damage.
* Permanent joint deformity.

PROBABLE OUTCOME—Allergic purpura usually lasts 1 to 3 weeks. Some children only have a few spots and fever. Others require hospitalization for severe abdominal pain and kidney inflammation.
   Most children with allergic purpura recover completely. In a few, however, allergic purpura recurs or persists for years.

 HOW TO TREAT

GENERAL MEASURES—Use warm soaks (see Soaks in Appendix) to relieve joint pain.

MEDICATION—Your doctor may prescribe:
* Cortisone drugs or immunosuppressive drugs, such as cyclophosphamide, to suppress inflammation. Effectiveness of treatment varies.
* Antihistamines to relieve itching.

ACTIVITY—If the child has fever or pain, encourage bed rest. The child may sit up for meals and walk to the bathroom. When fever and pain are gone, the child may gradually resume normal activities as strength and well-being allow.

DIET—The child should eat a normal, well-balanced diet. Vitamin and mineral supplements should not be necessary unless the child shows evidence of deficiency.

 CALL YOUR DOCTOR IF

* Your child has symptoms of allergic purpura.
* The following symptoms occur during treatment:
   Unrelenting abdominal pain.
   Blood in the stool.
   Black, tarry bowel movements.
   New bleeding under the skin.
   Blood in the urine.

PYLORIC STENOSIS, CONGENITAL
(Hypertrophic Pyloric Stenosis)

 GENERAL INFORMATION

DEFINITION—A condition of infancy in which encircling muscles at the end of the stomach enlarge and cause obstruction.

BODY PARTS INVOLVED—Pylorus (a muscular tube that carries food from the stomach to the small intestine).

SEX OR AGE MOST AFFECTED
• Both sexes, but more common in firstborn males.
• Usually begins between 2 and 5 weeks of age, but can occur as late as 4 months.

SIGNS & SYMPTOMS
• Recurrent vomiting after feedings that becomes increasingly forceful.
• Hard, olive-sized mass in the upper abdomen (sometimes).
• No pain or fever. Infant seems happy but hungry after vomiting.
• Constipation.
• Gradual weight loss and dehydration.

CAUSES—The muscular band that encircles the pylorus thickens and eventually closes off the outlet from the stomach.

RISK INCREASES WITH—Family history of pyloric stenosis.

HOW TO PREVENT—Cannot be prevented at present.

 WHAT TO EXPECT

DIAGNOSTIC MEASURES
• Your own observation of symptoms.
• Medical history and physical exam by a doctor.
• Barium-swallow x-ray or ultrasound (see Glossary) may be used for confirmation.

APPROPRIATE HEALTH CARE
• Doctor's treatment.
• Surgery to cut the thickened muscle (pyloromyotomy)
• Hospitalization for about 3 days after surgery.

POSSIBLE COMPLICATIONS—Weight loss, dehydration, shock and death without treatment.

PROBABLE OUTCOME—Curable with surgery. The child usually recovers quickly.

 HOW TO TREAT

GENERAL MEASURES—After surgery:
• A firm ridge will appear at the incision site. This is a healthy sign and requires no treatment.
• Wash the incision site gently several times a day.
• If the baby seems uncomfortable, apply warm compresses to the incision site.

MEDICATION—Intravenous fluids and electrolytes until the baby is ready for surgery. Medication is usually not necessary after surgery.

ACTIVITY—No restrictions.

DIET—The baby may tolerate small feedings of half-strength formula while awaiting surgery—check with your doctor. If not, formula will be given by stomach tube.

 CALL YOUR DOCTOR IF

• Your baby vomits repeatedly.
• The following occurs after surgery:
  Swelling, redness, bleeding or drainage at the surgical site.
  Temperature rises to 101F (38.3C).

RABIES (Hydrophobia)

GENERAL INFORMATION

DEFINITION—A serious virus infection of the central nervous system, transmitted by the bite of infected animals. Rabies occurs rarely in the United States, but there is still public fear and substantial prevention efforts continue.

BODY PARTS INVOLVED—Brain and central nervous system; body parts bitten by the rabid animal.

SEX OR AGE MOST AFFECTED—Both sexes; all ages.

SIGNS & SYMPTOMS—In two-thirds of patients, symptoms may appear 1 to 3 months after the bite. Sometimes it can be as short as 5 days or as long as 5 years.
Early symptoms are:
- Restlessness and irritability.
- Fatigue.
- Slight fever.
- Cough.
- Sore throat.
- Increased saliva and tears.

2 to 10 days later:
- Violent spasms of throat muscles that make swallowing impossible.
- Hyperactivity and violent behavior.
- Confusion.
- High fever.
- Irregular heartbeat.
- Irregular breathing.

CAUSES
- A virus in the saliva of infected animals passes to humans through broken skin or a mucous membrane. The virus travels slowly from the bite area to the brain.
- Animals that are commonly infected include dogs (especially wild dogs), bats, skunks, foxes, coyotes and raccoons. Cats can become infected, sometimes from contact with a rabid bat (such as playing with one that is ill and on the ground). Other animals can also be infected, so consult your local health department after any animal bite.

RISK INCREASES WITH—Professions or activities that may involve exposure to wild animals (cave exploration, hunting, farm or ranch workers, forest rangers, some laboratory workers, veterinarians).

HOW TO PREVENT
- Vaccinate your dog or cat against rabies.
- Report stray animals in the neighborhood, and teach children to avoid them.
- Have a rabies immunization, if your work involves animals.
- Keep tetanus immunizations up-to-date.
- Avoid wild animals. In the U.S., bats, skunks and raccoons are the most likely to be infected, but any carnivore can carry the disease.

WHAT TO EXPECT

DIAGNOSTIC MEASURES
- Medical history and exam by a doctor.
- Diagnostic tests may include laboratory blood tests and fluid and electrolyte measurements.
- Pathological exam of the animal's tissue and your own observation of the animal's behavior. Determine if the animal was provoked. Attacking animals are more likely to be infected.

APPROPRIATE HEALTH CARE
- Treatment will be determined by type of exposure (bite or nonbite), the possibility of rabies in the type of animal, circumstances of the biting incident, and vaccination status of animal.
- Surgery to clean and repair the bite wound (sometimes).
- Hospitalization, if symptoms develop.

POSSIBLE COMPLICATIONS—Once symptoms begin, survival is unlikely.

PROBABLE OUTCOME—Rabies can be prevented with early treatment following bites.

HOW TO TREAT

GENERAL MEASURES
- Wash the bite area for 10 minutes with soap and water to remove all saliva.
- Cover the wound with a clean bandage.
- Call your doctor or local emergency room for advice.
- Call your local animal-control center to catch the animal, if possible.
- If the animal is killed, remove the head and refrigerate or freeze it until it can be examined by pathologists.
- Don't panic. The incubation period allows time for diagnosis and treatment.

MEDICATION—Your doctor may prescribe one of the following:
- Injections of rabies-immune globulin.
- Injections of human-diploid-cell-strain vaccine, if the animal is proven rabid.
- Tetanus booster. Painful injections in the abdomen are no longer necessary.

ACTIVITY—No restrictions unless symptoms begin. If they do, bed rest in a hospital is necessary.

DIET—No special diet during treatment before symptoms begin. Intravenous fluids and nutrients are necessary during hospitalization.

CALL YOUR DOCTOR IF

Anyone is bitten by an animal.

RADIATION SICKNESS

GENERAL INFORMATION

DEFINITION—Side effects that accompany radiation treatment for cancer or aftereffects of accidental exposure to radiation.

BODY PARTS INVOLVED—Depends on the location of treatment or exposure. See Signs & Symptoms below.

SEX OR AGE MOST AFFECTED—Both sexes; all ages.

SIGNS & SYMPTOMS—The following vary widely, and are often temporary, depending on the radiation dosage and area radiated:
- Nausea, vomiting and diarrhea.
- Headache.
- Fatigue and shortness of breath.
- Rapid heartbeat.
- Yeast infection in the mouth.
- Dry mouth and loss of taste.
- Swallowing difficulty.
- Worsening of tooth or gum disease.
- Hair loss; dry cough.
- Heart inflammation with chest pain.
- Burning, inflammation or scarring of skin.
- Permanent skin darkening.
- Bleeding spots anywhere under the skin.
- Anemia; sexual impotence.

CAUSES—Radiation damage to the immune system and to healthy tissues.

RISK INCREASES WITH—For radiation treatment:
- Poor nutrition.
- Illness that has lowered resistance.

HOW TO PREVENT
- Have a thorough dental checkup to detect tooth or gum disease before head or neck radiation.
- Eat well before radiation treatment to be in optimal nutritional condition.
- If you work around radiation, learn and observe safety regulations.

WHAT TO EXPECT

DIAGNOSTIC MEASURES
- Laboratory blood studies of hemoglobin, platelet counts and white-blood-cell counts.
- X-rays of treated areas and dosimetry (detects and measures exposure to radiation).

APPROPRIATE HEALTH CARE
- Doctor's treatment.
- Psychotherapy or counseling to reduce the stress of radiation treatment.
- Hospitalization for radiation treatment or complications.
- Bone marrow transplant for severe exposure.

POSSIBLE COMPLICATIONS
- Susceptibility to infections due to decreased resistance.
- Sterility or birth defects may occur.
- Increased susceptibility to cancer—especially bone-marrow cancer or leukemia.
- With radiation treatment, other complications depend on the area involved. Your doctor will explain possible complications. Modern radiation equipment makes serious complications unlikely.

PROBABLE OUTCOME
- With radiation treatment, most side effects or complications disappear gradually afterward.
- With radiation accidents not severe enough to cause immediate death, side effects may not appear for years.

HOW TO TREAT

GENERAL MEASURES
- During radiation treatment, keep medical personnel informed of how you are feeling. Treatments can sometimes be adjusted or interrupted until you feel better.
- If you lose your hair, consider wearing a wig until hair growth resumes.
- Use effective birth-control measures to prevent pregnancy until it is determined that it is safe to have children.

MEDICATION—Your doctor may prescribe:
- Antinausea drugs.
- Pain relievers.
- Blood transfusions for anemia.
- Antibiotics to fight infections.
- Antidiarrheal medications.
- Sedatives if sleeping is a problem.

ACTIVITY—Be as active as your strength allows. Rest often.

DIET—Eat a balanced diet. You may temporarily need a liquid diet (see Liquid Diet in Appendix) or want to prepare food in a blender if you have trouble swallowing. Intravenous feeding or use of a small stomach tube is also possible until you resume normal eating. A dietitian can help.

CALL YOUR DOCTOR IF

- You are accidentally exposed to radiation.
- You feel very ill during radiation treatment, especially if you have unexpected symptoms.
- You develop signs of infection, such as fever and chills, muscle aches, headache and dizziness, during or after exposure or treatment.
- New, unexplained symptoms develop. Drugs in treatment may produce side effects.

ILLNESS & DISORDERS

RAPE CRISIS SYNDROME

GENERAL INFORMATION

DEFINITION—The physical and emotional aftereffects of rape. The term rape refers to forcible sexual intercourse with an unwilling partner. Rape involves varying degrees of physical and psychological trauma. In the majority cases the rapist is a man and the victim is a woman.

BODY PARTS INVOLVED—Genitals; rectum; mouth; brain.

SEX OR AGE MOST AFFECTED—All ages and both sexes, but more common in females.

SIGNS & SYMPTOMS
Immediately following rape:
- Physical injuries such as cuts, bruises or other injuries, including vaginal and rectal tears.
- Fear, anger, crying or unusual behavior such as laughter.
- No outward emotional signs (sometimes).

Aftereffects (may be weeks to months):
- Feelings of self-blame and guilt.
- Depression and withdrawal, even from family and friends.
- Mood swings; feelings of grief, shame, revenge.
- Loss of appetite.
- Fear of intercourse, fear of men.
- Nightmares, sleep disorders.
- Fear of being alone.

CAUSES—Rape is extremely traumatizing. All rape victims suffer physical and psychological aftereffects.

RISK INCREASES WITH—Any victim of rape or attempted rape.

HOW TO PREVENT
- The scope of rape prevention is complex and involves individuals, society and government.
- There is no prevention for rape crisis syndrome.

WHAT TO EXPECT

DIAGNOSTIC MEASURES—A general physical examination and pelvic examination will be conducted (these exams follow specific medical guidelines). A report is normally made to local law enforcement personnel.

APPROPRIATE HEALTH CARE
- Emergency medical assessment and care will be provided for your physical injuries.
- Medical personnel will discuss with you the risks of pregnancy, sexually transmitted diseases, HIV/AIDS, hepatitis B and other infections; what preventive measures there are available; and what follow-up tests may be required.

POSSIBLE COMPLICATIONS
- Pregnancy.
- Sexually transmitted disease.
- Emotional trauma that may last years.

PROBABLE OUTCOME—Most victims take a long time to feel like they are normal again, some never do, and some say that they are a completely changed person.

HOW TO TREAT

GENERAL MEASURES
- Ask for assistance from a Rape Crisis Center (or similar agency). They can provide immediate support and help you through the urgent medical, emotional and legal necessities.
- Arrange for counseling or psychological help. This is important for your emotional recovery. Don't just try to put the matter out of your mind and don't try to "go it alone." Suppressing your feelings can increase distress.
- Keeping a journal or diary about your feelings, thoughts and reactions may be helpful. Talk over your feelings with trusted friends and family.
- Prepare yourself as much as possible for legal proceedings that force you to relive the trauma and may cause additional emotional upsets.

MEDICATION—Your doctor may prescribe:
- Antibiotics, if venereal infection is suspected or diagnosed.
- Hormones to prevent pregnancy ("day-after pill").
- Sedatives or tranquilizers for a short time to reduce anxiety.
- Tetanus prophylaxis.

ACTIVITY—Resume your normal life as quickly as possible.

DIET—No special diet.

CALL YOUR DOCTOR IF

- You or someone you know has been raped.
- Emotional and/or physical problems worsen, or are not improved with treatment.

RAYNAUD'S PHENOMENON

GENERAL INFORMATION

DEFINITION—Primary Raynaud's is a disorder of the circulatory system that affects blood circulation to fingers and occasionally toes. Secondary Raynaud's is a circulatory-system disorder that occurs as a complication of other diseases, medications or activities.

BODY PARTS INVOLVED—Small arteries to the hands and feet.

SEX OR AGE MOST AFFECTED—Both sexes; primary Raynaud's is more common in females under 40; secondary is more common in adults over 40.

SIGNS & SYMPTOMS
Early symptoms:
• Fingers that turn pale when exposed to cold or stress. Paleness is followed by a bluish tinge, then redness. Pain, numbness and tingling accompany the color changes. Warmth relieves these symptoms.
Late symptoms:
• Chronic infections around fingernails and toenails.
• Ulcers on the fingertips caused by inadequate blood circulation in the fingers. Symptoms develop gradually over a period of years but may begin suddenly.

CAUSES—Spasms of arteries that supply blood to the fingers and toes caused by extreme sensitivity to cold. The sensitivity may be due to poor function of the autoimmune system. With primary Raynaud's, there is no known cause. Secondary type can be linked to an underlying disorder, a medication or an activity.

RISK INCREASES WITH
Primary:
Stress; cold, wet weather.
Secondary:
• Scleroderma, rheumatoid arthritis, lupus erythematosus or other connective-tissue disorders.
• Buerger's disease or cor pulmonale.
• Low levels of thyroid hormone.
• Certain medications, including ergot preparations, antihypertensives, alpha- and beta-adrenergic blockers, and some cancer drugs.
• Smoking (impairs circulation to extremities).
• Occupations that involve work with heavy equipment that vibrates forcefully.
• Occupations that involve physical stress to the fingers (typists, piano players).

HOW TO PREVENT
• Don't smoke. Tobacco triggers the problem. This disease is rare among nonsmokers.
• Avoid exposure to all cigarette smoke.

WHAT TO EXPECT

DIAGNOSTIC MEASURES
• Medical history and exam by a doctor.
• Laboratory blood studies, cold challenge test (putting hands in 10-15C water).
• X-rays of the hands and feet.

APPROPRIATE HEALTH CARE
• Self-care after diagnosis.
• Doctor's treatment.
• Surgery to sever sympathetic nerves to the involved extremities. Surgery usually relieves symptoms for 1 to 2 years before they recur.

POSSIBLE COMPLICATIONS
• Permanent weakness and numbness in the toes and fingers.
• Gangrene and amputation (worst cases only).
• Raynaud's phenomenon may progress to disease.

PROBABLE OUTCOME
• Most persons cope well with primary Raynaud's and live a normal life span. In about half of the patients, the disease may improve or disappear after several years.
• Secondary Raynaud's may be curable if the underlying cause can be cured.

HOW TO TREAT

GENERAL MEASURES
• Stop smoking.
• Avoid exposure to cold in any form. Wear mittens or gloves in cold environments.
• Wear comfortable shoes and wool socks.
• Avoid stressful situations.
• To stop an attack, briskly swing the arms in 360-degree circles (as if to release an underhand pitch) for a minute or two. This can help bring blood into constricted vessels.
• Move to a warm climate, if possible.
• Biofeedback training may be helpful.
• Avoid vasoconstrictive drugs.

MEDICATION—Your doctor may prescribe:
• Vasodilator drugs to dilate the small arteries and improve circulation.
• Sedatives to reduce stress.

ACTIVITY—No restrictions, except to keep warm. Avoid chilling while participating in sports.

DIET—No special diet.

CALL YOUR DOCTOR IF

• You have symptoms of Raynaud's disease or phenomenon.
• Discomfort worsens, despite treatment.
• Ulcers that do not heal appear on fingers or toes.

ILLNESS & DISORDERS

RECTAL PROLAPSE
(Procidentia)

GENERAL INFORMATION

DEFINITION—Protrusion of rectal tissues outside the anus. Partial prolapse is protrusion of the mucosa alone, complete prolapse (procidentia) is protrusion of the entire thickness of the rectum.

BODY PARTS INVOLVED—Anus and rectum.

SEX OR AGE MOST AFFECTED—Adults, usually over age 60, and children ages 1 to 3. Rectal prolapse in infants can be a sign of cystic fibrosis.

SIGNS & SYMPTOMS
- A vague sense of fullness in the lower abdomen or rectal area.
- A mucus discharge—sometimes tinged with blood—from the rectum.
- A firm mass of tissue that can be felt at the anus after a bowel movement.
- Pain when having bowel movements.

CAUSES
- Weak pelvic or rectal muscles.
- Weak anal sphincter.
- Unknown, particularly in children.

RISK INCREASES WITH
- Cystic fibrosis (children).
- Aging.
- Previous surgery on the rectum or vagina.
- Prolonged constipation and straining to have bowel movements.
- Multiple sclerosis.
- Stroke or paralysis.
- Neurological disease.
- Pertussis.
- Nutritional disorders.

HOW TO PREVENT
- Practice perineal strengthening exercises—lie down with back on mattress; pull in abdomen and squeeze while taking a deep breath; or repeatedly squeeze and relax your buttocks while sitting in a chair.
- Do not strain when having bowel movements. Avoid constipation and diarrhea.

WHAT TO EXPECT

DIAGNOSTIC MEASURES
- Your own observation of symptoms.
- Medical history and physical exam by a doctor.
- Examination of the rectal area by anoscope or sigmoidoscope (see Glossary for both).

APPROPRIATE HEALTH CARE
- Treatment varies according to underlying cause. Any causes of straining need to be corrected.
- In children, prolapse is usually temporary.
- Occasionally minor prolapse can often be reversed by gently pushing the protruding tissue back into the rectum.
- Strapping the buttocks together firmly between bowel movements often cures the condition.
- For other patients, the excess tissue can be surgically cut out (excised) or tied off with special rubber bands causing the tissue to wither in a few days.
- Surgery to strengthen tissues that support the rectum (sometimes).
- For people who are unable to have surgery, a wire or synthetic plastic loop can be inserted to circle the sphincter to constrict the anus and prevent prolapse.

POSSIBLE COMPLICATIONS
- Ulceration and bleeding in tissue that protrudes permanently.
- Bowel incontinence.
- Recurrence of rectal prolapse.

PROBABLE OUTCOME—Good prognosis with treatment. In children, usually complete recovery.

HOW TO TREAT

GENERAL MEASURES—Use sanitary napkins or absorbent pads to absorb the mucus discharge.

MEDICATION—Your doctor may prescribe stool softeners to prevent constipation.

ACTIVITY
- Avoid standing or walking for long periods; this increases abdominal pressure.
- Practice perineal and pelvic-strengthening exercises to help prevent a recurrence.

DIET—Drink at least 8 glasses of water a day and eat a diet high in fiber to prevent constipation.

CALL YOUR DOCTOR IF

- Rectal tissue remains outside the anus.
- Rectal pain or bleeding occur.
- Fever or chills develop, indicating infection.

REITER'S SYNDROME

GENERAL INFORMATION

DEFINITION—An inflammatory disease characterized by a complex of symptoms resembling those of arthritis, urethritis, conjunctivitis and psoriasis.

BODY PARTS INVOLVED—Joints; eyes, including white eye covering; urethra and head of the penis; skin.

SEX OR AGE MOST AFFECTED—Male adolescents and young adults (12 to 40 years). This is rare in women and children.

SIGNS & SYMPTOMS
- Inflammation of the urethra and discharge within 7 to 14 days after sexual intercourse.
- Frequent urinary urgency.
- Small ulcers inside the mouth, tongue and on the penis tip.
- Low fever.
- Red eyes.
- Painful joints, especially toes, legs, hips and back.
- Aching in the pelvis.
- Skin lesions similar to psoriasis on the soles, palms and around fingernails and toenails.

CAUSES—Unknown. The predisposition is inherited, and two forms are recognized: Sexually transmitted (Chlamydia infection most often implicated) and dysenteric (follows a gastrointestinal bacterial infection).

RISK INCREASES WITH
- Recent gastrointestinal illness with diarrhea.
- Previous sexually-transmitted infections.
- Family history of Reiter's syndrome.
- Genetic factors.

HOW TO PREVENT—Use condoms for sexual intercourse.

WHAT TO EXPECT

DIAGNOSTIC MEASURES
- Your own observation of symptoms.
- Medical history and physical exam by a doctor.
- Laboratory blood studies and culture of the urethral discharge and x-rays.

APPROPRIATE HEALTH CARE
- Doctor's treatment for diagnosis and supervision of treatment.
- There is no treatment to cure Reiter's. Symptoms are usually managed with medication.
- Treatment for sexually transmitted disease with antibiotics for patients and their sexual partners. Patients with guilt or anxiety feelings about sexually transmitted disease should seek counseling or psychological help.
- Usually, no treatment is needed for eye symptoms, unless severe or chronic.

POSSIBLE COMPLICATIONS—Stiffening and effusion (fluid) of joints.

PROBABLE OUTCOME—Arthritis symptoms may continue up to 4 months, others disappear sooner. Most patients recover in 2 to 16 weeks with no residual signs of the disease, but some persons have recurrent flare-ups and remissions.

HOW TO TREAT

GENERAL MEASURES
- To relieve foot pain, wear cushion pads and arch supports in your shoes.
- Use a firm mattress on your bed.
- If joint impairment is chronic, ask your doctor about occupational therapy.

MEDICATION—Your doctor may prescribe:
- Nonsteroidal anti-inflammatory drugs.
- Antibiotics, such as tetracyclines, for urethritis.
- Steroid eye drops if eye symptoms are severe.

ACTIVITY
- Stay as active as your condition allows, but avoid sexual excitement and activity during the illness.
- Exercise the affected joints according to instructions from your doctor or physical therapist. Don't immobilize affected joints.

DIET—No special diet.

CALL YOUR DOCTOR IF

- You have symptoms of Reiter's syndrome.
- Symptoms recur after recovery.
- New, unexplained symptoms develop. Drugs used in treatment may produce side effects.

RENAL FAILURE, ACUTE
(Kidney Failure, Acute)

 GENERAL INFORMATION

DEFINITION—Sudden failure of the kidneys to function. Kidneys normally help rid the body of waste products, and when they fail, the waste products build up and cause symptoms that vary in severity. This usually has a short, relatively severe course, but often is curable.

BODY PARTS INVOLVED—Kidneys.

SEX OR AGE MOST AFFECTED—Both sexes; all ages.

SIGNS & SYMPTOMS
Early stages:
- Little or no urine output.
Later stages:
- Nausea, vomiting, diarrhea and appetite loss.
- Mental changes, including irritability, drowsiness, stupor or coma.
- Convulsions; severe itching.
- High or low blood pressure.
- Unexplained bruising, bleeding spots under the skin or spontaneous bleeding.
The symptoms of the underlying cause (see list below) will also be present.

CAUSES—Conditions in the kidney, or in other areas of the body, that cause the kidneys to stop functioning. This leads to a buildup of waste products in the blood and tissues. Underlying conditions include:
- Shock with very low blood pressure.
- Blood poisoning (septicemia).
- Congestive heart failure.
- Fluid and electrolyte imbalance.
- Blood-transfusion reaction.
- Severe accident with extensive muscle injury.
- Acute glomerulonephritis.
- Multiple myeloma.
- Obstruction of blood vessels that supply the kidney.
- Kidney stones that obstruct both ureters or the urethra.
- Prostate enlargement.
- Use of certain medications, including anticancer drugs, kanamycin, amphotericin B, anticonvulsants, nonsteroidal anti-inflammatory drugs (NSAID's), or excessive vitamin D.
- Overdose of many poisons or drugs, especially mind-altering drugs.

RISK INCREASES WITH
- Persons with one kidney.
- Recent surgery.
- Accidents with severe injuries.
- Medical history of conditions affecting the kidney, such as diabetes or gout.

HOW TO PREVENT—No specific preventive measures. Avoid causes and risk factors when possible.

 WHAT TO EXPECT

DIAGNOSTIC MEASURES
- Medical history and exam by a doctor.
- Laboratory blood counts and blood and urine tests that measure kidney function and fluid and electrolyte balance.
- ECG (see Glossary).
- Needle biopsy (see Glossary) of kidneys.
- X-rays of the abdomen, kidneys, ureters and bladder to detect kidney stones.

APPROPRIATE HEALTH CARE
- Doctor's treatment.
- Surgery, if surgery can correct cause.
- Hospitalization for fluid and electrolyte therapy and kidney dialysis (sometimes).
- Dialysis (see Glossary) may be required until the kidneys recover function.

POSSIBLE COMPLICATIONS
- Congestive heart failure.
- Increased risk of infections.
- Chronic kidney failure.

PROBABLE OUTCOME—If the underlying condition can be controlled and the kidney failure can be treated promptly, complete recovery is likely. If not, the disorder can lead to chronic kidney failure or death.

 HOW TO TREAT

GENERAL MEASURES
- Follow your doctor's instructions. Compliance with your medical treatment plan is essential.
- See Resources for Additional Information.

MEDICATION—Your doctor may prescribe:
- Medications appropriate to control the underlying condition.
- Antibiotics if infection develops.

ACTIVITY—Rest in bed until the condition is cured. Then resume your normal activities as soon as symptoms improve.

DIET—Food and water intake is rigorously controlled to prevent fluid and electrolyte imbalance, and to minimize buildup of body wastes. A diet high in carbohydrates and low in protein (main source of waste products) to reduce workload for kidneys may be part of the treatment.

 CALL YOUR DOCTOR IF

The following occurs during treatment:
Chills, fever, headache or muscle aches.
Shortness or breath.
Unexpected bleeding from any body opening.

RENAL FAILURE, CHRONIC (Uremia)

GENERAL INFORMATION

DEFINITION—Inability of the kidneys to eliminate the body's waste products. Kidneys normally help rid the body of waste products, and when they fail, the waste products build up and cause symptoms that vary in severity. Chronic kidney failure usually develops gradually.

BODY PARTS INVOLVED—Kidneys, which eventually affect all body systems.

SEX OR AGE MOST AFFECTED—Both sexes; all ages.

SIGNS & SYMPTOMS—None or few symptoms until 60% to 75% of kidney filtration fails. Then, 1 or more of the following:
- Listlessness, mental confusion and drowsiness; high blood pressure.
- Shortness of breath or bad breath.
- Inflamed, bleeding gums and mouth ulcers.
- Abdominal pain; itching skin.
- Numbness, tingling and burning in the legs and feet; muscle cramps.
- Decreased sex drive.
- Cessation of menstruation; unusual bleeding.
- Anemia, with paleness and fatigue.
- Muscle and bone pain. Bones break easily.

CAUSES
- Collagen diseases, such as systemic lupus erythematosus.
- Chronic glomerulonephritis.
- Chronic urinary-tract infections.
- Congenital kidney abnormalities, such as polycystic kidney disease.
- Kidney damage due to diabetes mellitus.
- Urinary-tract obstruction.
- Overdose of many drugs and chemicals, especially phenacetin or streptomycin.
- Blood-vessel diseases, such as hardening of the arteries in or leading to the kidney.

RISK INCREASES WITH—Any of the conditions listed in Causes.

HOW TO PREVENT—Obtain medical treatment for underlying diseases that lead to uremia before uremia results.

WHAT TO EXPECT

DIAGNOSTIC MEASURES
- Laboratory blood and urine studies of kidney function.
- X-rays of abdomen, kidneys, ureters and bladder to detect kidney stones, ECG (see Glossary).
- Kidney biopsy (see Glossary).

APPROPRIATE HEALTH CARE
- Doctor's treatment.
- Treatment will be determined by cause.

- Surgery, if the cause can be corrected by surgery.
- Emergency hospitalization for fluid and electrolyte therapy and kidney dialysis (sometimes).
- Dialysis (artificial methods of removing waste products from the blood) may be required until the kidneys recover their function.

POSSIBLE COMPLICATIONS
- Pericarditis.
- Myocarditis.
- Pneumonia.
- Pancreatitis.
- Hormone deficiencies.
- Fluid and electrolyte imbalance.
- Gastrointestinal ulcers.

PROBABLE OUTCOME—Kidney transplants can sometimes cure younger patients. Otherwise, kidney failure is a condition that worsens gradually, although a near-normal lifespan is possible if the condition stabilizes. Kidney dialysis treatment can improve and prolong life for several years.

HOW TO TREAT

GENERAL MEASURES
- Weigh daily and keep a record.
- Measure the fluids you drink and the urine you pass each day. Keep a record, and take it with you to doctor visits. You should pass about 2500cc or more of urine a day. If you pass less, decrease fluid intake so intake does not exceed output by more than 800cc a day. For example, if you pass 2000cc in 24 hours, don't drink more than 2800cc in the next 24 hours.
- See Resources for Additional Information.

MEDICATION—Your doctor may prescribe:
- Diuretics to reduce fluid accumulation.
- Iron and folic-acid supplements for anemia.
- Stool softeners to prevent constipation.
- Digitalis for congestive heart failure.

ACTIVITY—You must reduce activity. Don't become overheated or fatigued. Sleep more at night, and take rests during the day. If you are confined to bed, flex your legs often to reduce the chance of blood clots in leg veins.

DIET—Eat a low-salt, low-potassium, low-protein diet with added fiber. Eat frequent small, high-calorie meals.

CALL YOUR DOCTOR IF

The following occurs during treatment:
Fever, vomiting or diarrhea.
Urine output of less than 2000cc.
Severe headache or convulsion.

ILLNESS & DISORDERS

RESPIRATORY SYNCYTIAL VIRUS (RSV)

GENERAL INFORMATION

DEFINITION—A contagious, viral infection that occurs in epidemics, usually in the fall, winter and early spring. In healthy adults and older children, the symptoms are usually mild, but in infants and young children, they can be serious.

BODY PARTS INVOLVED—Upper and lower respiratory tracts.

SEX OR AGE MOST AFFECTED—Both sexes; all ages; most common in infants and children (it is the major cause of respiratory tract infections in this age group).

SIGNS & SYMPTOMS
Early symptoms:
- Runny nose.
- Low grade fever.
- Decrease in appetite.
- Cough, sometimes with wheezing.
- Lethargy.

Later symptoms (may occur early in infant with underlying cardiac or respiratory disease):
- Infant or child refuses to eat.
- Ear ache.
- Cough and wheezing increases.
- Difficulty breathing.
- Listlessness; excessive sleeping.
- Spells of apnea (in premature infants or those under 6 weeks).

CAUSES—The virus is transmitted from person-to-person by respiratory secretions (exhaled, coughed or sneezed). Reinfection is common, but the symptoms are milder.

RISK INCREASES WITH
- Infants and young children.
- School or day care. Adults who are caring for small children are often infected.
- Medical personnel.

HOW TO PREVENT
- Studies show that few children under 4 have escaped contracting some form of RSV, even if it is mild. As with any situation involving a viral epidemic: careful attention to hand washing, proper disposal of any paper tissues used for nasal or throat secretions, and covering your mouth when coughing or sneezing.
- A vaccine was temporarily available but has been withdrawn due to adverse reactions.

WHAT TO EXPECT

DIAGNOSTIC MEASURES
- Your own observation of symptoms.
- Medical history and physical exam by a doctor. The symptoms are similar to many other disorders (common cold and flu), but knowing

there is an RSV epidemic in the community helps makes the diagnosis more likely.
- Laboratory studies of blood and respiratory secretions from the nose or throat.

APPROPRIATE HEALTH CARE
- Doctor's treatment.
- Hospitalization for severe symptoms with close observation for respiratory problems. May require respiratory support.

POSSIBLE COMPLICATIONS
- Pneumonia.
- Bronchiolitis.

PROBABLE OUTCOME—Mild cases usually resolve in 7-12 days (5 days for adults with reinfections) without any special treatment. More severe cases are curable with hospitalization and treatment for complications.

HOW TO TREAT

GENERAL MEASURES
- Hospitalization of an infant or young child is traumatic for parents and children. Stay in close communication with the doctor. Provide reassurance to the child, cuddle an infant, provide diversion activities suitable to the child's condition.
- For home care: provide supportive measures, including rest, extra fluids to drink, humidify the air with a cool-mist, ultrasonic humidifier. Clean humidifier daily.

MEDICATION—Your doctor may prescribe:
- Ribavarin (an antiviral drug) for severe symptoms.
- Oxygen for hospitalized patient.
- Theophylline or adrenergic drugs for wheezing.

ACTIVITY—In mild cases treated at home, have the infant or child get extra rest.

DIET—No special diet. Drink plenty of fluids.

CALL YOUR DOCTOR IF

- You or your child has symptoms of respiratory syncytial virus.
- Any of the following occur during treatment:
  Temperature rises.
  Cough or wheezing worsens.
  Increased difficulty in breathing.
  Unusual tiredness or weakness.
  Infant refuses any foods or liquids.
  Excessive sleeping or periods of sleep apnea (breathing stops for a period of time).

RETINAL DETACHMENT

 GENERAL INFORMATION

DEFINITION—A separation or tear of the retina (the light-sensitive tissue at the back of the eye) from the remainder of the eye. Retinal detachment is a medical emergency.

BODY PARTS INVOLVED—Eye.

SEX OR AGE MOST AFFECTED—All ages and both sexes, but more common in men.

SIGNS & SYMPTOMS—The following usually affect one eye, but sometimes both are affected:
• Light flashes in the field of vision.
• Floating spots in the field of vision.
• Blurred vision.
• Wavy visual images (sometimes).
• Gradual loss of vision. This may not be noticed because it is so gradual.
• No pain.

CAUSES
• Eye injury (break or tear in the retina).
• Inherited tendency (possibly).
• Degenerative changes of aging.

RISK INCREASES WITH
• Age.
• Diabetes mellitus.
• Vascular disease.
• Previous retinal detachment.
• Family history of retinal detachment.
• Extreme nearsightedness (myopia).
• Complications of eye surgery.
• Tumors or inflammation.

HOW TO PREVENT
• Patients at risk should have regular eye examinations.
• If you have diabetes mellitus or vascular disease, obtain medical treatment to control the disorder.

 WHAT TO EXPECT

DIAGNOSTIC MEASURES
• Your own observation of symptoms.
• Diagnosis is determined by an ophthalmoscopy exam of the eye.

APPROPRIATE HEALTH CARE
• Doctor's (ophthalmologist's) treatment.
• Treatment will depend on location and severity of the detachment.
• An eye shield may be needed if there was trauma to the eye.
• Surgery to reattach the retina using special lasers or cryotherapy (using below freezing temperatures), or by changing the shape of the eye (sometimes).

POSSIBLE COMPLICATIONS
• Without treatment: Partial or complete blindness in the affected eye.
• With delayed treatment: Detachment that extends to the macula (the area of most detailed vision). This causes permanent loss of detailed (central) vision.

PROBABLE OUTCOME—Often treatable with early surgical treatment.

 HOW TO TREAT

GENERAL MEASURES—The following instructions apply after surgery:
• Both eyes will be patched for a time. Your family and friends can help overcome this stress by providing companionship and assistance.
• Use dark glasses after the patches are removed.
• Don't rub your eyes.
• Don't bend over.
• Avoid straining, such as from constipation, heavy lifting or harsh coughing. This may increase pressure in the eyes.

MEDICATION—Your doctor may prescribe:
• Mydriatic eye drops to dilate the pupil. Dilation reduces eye activity during healing. If you cannot instill the drops, ask someone to be available to help at the appropriate times.
• Sedatives or tranquilizers to reduce anxiety during convalescence.

ACTIVITY—After surgery, lie on your back in bed with your head elevated. Move your legs frequently to prevent blood clots from forming in deep veins. Resume your normal activities when your ophthalmologist considers it safe.

DIET—No special diet.

 CALL YOUR DOCTOR IF

• You have flashes or floating spots in your field of vision. Do not delay in getting medical help.
• Any sign of infection (bleeding, redness, pain, swelling or fever) occurs after surgery.
• Your vision worsens after full recovery from surgery.

REYE'S SYNDROME

GENERAL INFORMATION

DEFINITION—A rare disease in children and adolescents that involves inflammation of the brain and other major organs, mainly the liver, which is damaged due to fatty deposits.

BODY PARTS INVOLVED—Brain; liver; kidneys; heart.

SEX OR AGE MOST AFFECTED—Children from infancy through adolescence.

SIGNS & SYMPTOMS
- Vomiting.
- Lethargy.
- Drowsiness.
- Confusion.
- Delirium.
- Personality changes (irritability, combativeness).
- Seizures.
- Weakness and paralysis in an arm or leg.
- Double vision.
- Speech impairment.
- Coma.

CAUSES—Unknown. Reye's syndrome usually follows a virus infection. Some studies link it to the use of aspirin during a viral illness, especially chickenpox and influenza.

RISK INCREASES WITH
- Recent illness, such as chickenpox, influenza or other respiratory illness.
- Use of aspirin.

HOW TO PREVENT—Don't give a child under the age of 18 aspirin for any illness with fever until the doctor has diagnosed it. If the illness is diagnosed as viral, never use aspirin.

WHAT TO EXPECT

DIAGNOSTIC MEASURES
- Your own observation of symptoms.
- Medical history and physical exam by a doctor.
- Laboratory studies, such as blood studies of liver function and an analysis of cerebrospinal fluid and EEG (see Glossary).

APPROPRIATE HEALTH CARE
- Doctor's treatment.
- Hospitalization, with specific treatment determined by severity of the illness. May involve feeding tube, urinary catheter, mechanical breathing support, kidney dialysis, blood transfusion, cardiovascular monitoring, and therapies to reduce pressure on the brain.
- Home care during convalescence.

POSSIBLE COMPLICATIONS
- Permanent brain damage, coma or death caused by pressure on the brain.
- Pneumonia.
- Respiratory failure.
- Heart rhythm problems or heart attack.

PROBABLE OUTCOME—With treatment, the majority of patients will have a mild illness. Most recover completely, but some have varying degrees of brain damage.

HOW TO TREAT

GENERAL MEASURES
- The family should maintain an optimistic outlook, stay in close contact with the patient's doctor and help by making their visits with the patient as supportive as possible.
- See Resources for Additional Information.

MEDICATION—Your doctor may prescribe:
- Intravenous fluids.
- Anticoagulant drugs to prevent blood-clot formation during prolonged bed rest.
- Drugs, such as dexamethasone, to reduce cerebral swelling.
- Antibiotics to fight secondary bacterial infections, if they develop.
- Newer drugs such as L-Carnitine that are being studied.

ACTIVITY—Bed rest is necessary until the acute stage is over. Normal activities may then be resumed gradually.

DIET—Nothing by mouth initially. After recovery, no special diet required.

CALL YOUR DOCTOR IF

- Your child has symptoms of Reye's syndrome. Call at the first sign of confusion, lethargy or other mental changes!
- After hospitalization, any symptoms of Reye's syndrome recur or the child develops fever.
- New, unexplained symptoms develop. Drugs used in treatment may produce side effects.

RH INCOMPATIBILITY
(Erythroblastosis Fetalis)

 GENERAL INFORMATION

DEFINITION—Incompatibility between an infant's blood type and that of the mother, resulting in destruction of the infant's red blood cells (hemolytic anemia) after birth by antibodies from the mother's blood.

BODY PARTS INVOLVED—Blood of pregnant mother and fetus.

SEX OR AGE MOST AFFECTED—Newborn infants only.

SIGNS & SYMPTOMS
Signs during pregnancy:
• Decreased fetal growth.
• Decreased fetal movement.
Signs in a newborn:
• Paleness.
• Jaundice (yellow skin and eyes) that begins within 24 hours after delivery.
• Unexplained bruising or blood spots under skin.
• Tissue swelling (edema).
• Breathing difficulty or seizures.
• Lack of normal movement; poor reflexes.

CAUSES—The fetus of an Rh-negative (blood type) mother and an Rh-positive father may be Rh-positive. During delivery, a small amount of the infant's blood is absorbed by the mother through the placenta, stimulating her body to produce antibodies against Rh-positive blood. The antibodies are produced after delivery, so the first infant is not affected. With succeeding pregnancies, the antibodies in the mother's blood destroy fetal blood cells. In pregnancy, anti-Rh antibodies cross the placenta and destroy fetal blood cells. The resulting anemia can cause fetal death. If the fetus survives, antibodies can cross to baby during birth, producing jaundice and other symptoms.

RISK INCREASES WITH
• Each pregnancy after the first involving different blood types.
• Previous blood transfusions. These might have contained unidentified, incompatible blood types.

HOW TO PREVENT
• Obtain prenatal care throughout pregnancy. Early care is essential to determine the risk of Rh incompatibility.
• Special anti-Rh gamma globulin is given to the mother at 28 weeks gestation and within 72 hours after delivery, miscarriage, ectopic pregnancy or abortion. This prevents formation of antibodies that might affect future infants.
• Amniocentesis beginning at 28 weeks if indicated by elevated antibody titers in the mother.

 WHAT TO EXPECT

DIAGNOSTIC MEASURES
• Medical history and physical exam by a doctor. Tell your doctor if you have had a miscarriage or abortion.
• Blood tests to: type mother's, father's and infant's blood; measure the mother's Rh-positive antibodies; and detect hemolytic anemia in the infant's blood.
• Amniocentesis (see Glossary).

APPROPRIATE HEALTH CARE
• Doctor's treatment.
• Intrauterine transfusions (sometimes).
• Transfusion to exchange completely the infant's blood after birth.
• Hospitalization.

POSSIBLE COMPLICATIONS
• Permanent neurological damage.
• Blood-transfusion reaction.

PROBABLE OUTCOME—With prompt recognition of the disorder, damage to the infant can be prevented with exchange transfusions.

 HOW TO TREAT

GENERAL MEASURES—If you have an Rh-negative blood type:
• Tell any doctor or medical professional who treats you. Make sure this information is in your medical records.
• Wear a Medic-Alert bracelet or pendant (see Glossary).

MEDICATION—If you are pregnant and have Rh-negative blood type, you will be prescribed an anti-Rh gamma globulin injection at 28 weeks and again within 72 hours after delivery or termination of a pregnancy for any reason. You may also have antibody titer drawn during pregnancy to see if you are producing anti-Rh antibodies.

ACTIVITY—No restrictions after treatment.

DIET—The infant may be breast-fed or bottle-fed normally.

 CALL YOUR DOCTOR IF

Your baby has any of the following after returning home:
• Fever or jaundice (yellow skin or eyes).
• Poor appetite or poor weight gain.
• Excessive crying that does not stop when the baby is held.

RHEUMATIC FEVER

GENERAL INFORMATION

DEFINITION—An inflammatory complication of Group A streptococcal infections that affects many parts of the body, especially the joints and heart. Strep infections are contagious, but rheumatic fever is not.

BODY PARTS INVOLVED—Joints; heart and heart valves; skin and brain (sometimes).

SEX OR AGE MOST AFFECTED—Both children and adults.

SIGNS & SYMPTOMS
- Joint inflammation, characterized by pain, redness, swelling and warmth that can move from one joint to another. Wrists, elbows, knees or ankles are most often affected. Joint inflammation usually subsides in 10 to 14 days, but without treatment, other joints may become inflamed.
- Fever; fatigue; paleness.
- Appetite loss; general ill feeling.
- Abdominal pain; chest pain.
- Mild skin rash on chest, back, abdomen.
- Small, painless bumps just under the skin in bony areas such as the elbows or knees.

If the heart is involved:
- Shortness of breath.
- Fluid retention that causes swelling of the legs and back.
- Rapid heartbeat, especially when lying down.
- Uncontrollable arm and leg movement (chorea).

CAUSES—Rheumatic fever is caused by a preceding strep infection, usually in the throat, that occurs 1 to 6 weeks prior to the onset of symptoms. It is probably an autoimmune disorder in which antibodies produced to attack the strep bacteria also attack tissues of the joints or heart.

RISK INCREASES WITH
- Poor nutrition.
- Family history of rheumatic fever.
- Crowded or unsanitary living conditions.
- Tendency to upper respiratory infections.
- Untreated strep infections or incomplete treatment.

HOW TO PREVENT
- Request a throat culture for strep for any throat infection, especially in a child.
- Obtain prompt antibiotic treatment of any strep infection, including those of the skin. Strep infections must be treated with antibiotics, usually penicillin, for 10 days orally or by long-lasting injection.

WHAT TO EXPECT

DIAGNOSTIC MEASURES
- Medical history and exam by a doctor.
- Laboratory studies, such as blood studies, a throat culture and ECG (see Glossary).
- X-rays of the chest and heart.

APPROPRIATE HEALTH CARE
- Doctor's treatment.
- Home care after diagnosis (mild cases).
- Hospitalization (severe cases).

POSSIBLE COMPLICATIONS
- Permanently damaged heart valves, leading to congestive heart failure.
- Subsequent attacks of acute rheumatic fever.

PROBABLE OUTCOME—Strep infections are usually curable with treatment. Rheumatic fever is treatable, but not curable. It will subside in 2-12 weeks. In some cases, rheumatic fever may damage the heart valves. A damaged valve can be replaced with surgery. In rare cases, rheumatic fever is fatal even with treatment.

HOW TO TREAT

GENERAL MEASURES
- Take the patient's temperature and count the pulse; keep a record for your doctor.
- Use a cool-mist, ultrasonic humidifier if the patient has a sore throat or cough.
- Good dental hygiene is important.
- See Resources for Additional Information.

MEDICATION—Your doctor may prescribe:
- Steroids (anti-inflammatory drugs) or aspirin to reduce inflammation.
- Diuretics to reduce fluid retention.
- Antibiotics to fight any remaining strep bacteria.

ACTIVITY—The patient should restrict activity only if heart failure is present.

DIET
- A liquid or soft diet (see both in Appendix) in the early stages, progressing to a normal diet high in protein, calories and vitamins.
- A low-salt diet may be recommended.

CALL YOUR DOCTOR IF

- The following symptoms occur during treatment:
  Swelling of the legs or back.
  Shortness of breath.
  Vomiting, diarrhea or cough.
  Severe abdominal pain or fever.
- New, unexplained symptoms develop. Drugs in treatment may produce side effects.

RINGWORM

GENERAL INFORMATION

DEFINITION—Fungus (tinea) infection of the skin. This is transmitted by person-to-person contact or by contact with infected surfaces, such as towels, shoes or shower stalls.

BODY PARTS INVOLVED—Ringworm can involve the scalp (tinea capitis); skin (tinea corporis); groin skin (tinea cruris); nails (tinea unguium); feet (tinea pedis); skin with beard (tinea barbae)

SEX OR AGE MOST AFFECTED— Adolescents and adults. It is more common in males than females.

SIGNS & SYMPTOMS—Lesions that itch (sometimes) and have the following characteristics:
- On the scalp, lesions cause patchy hair loss and scaling scalp.
- On body skin, lesions are red, circular, flat, scaling and have well-defined borders.
- On the bearded area of the face, lesions cause an itchy, scaling rash under the beard.
- On the feet: see Athlete's Foot in the Illness section.
- Of the nails: see Paronychia in the Illness section.

CAUSES—Fungus infection with one or more of 5 different fungi.

RISK INCREASES WITH
- Crowded living conditions.
- Contact with infected animals.
- Day care centers or schools.
- Immunosuppression due to illness or drugs.
- Chronic moisture and chafing of the skin.

HOW TO PREVENT—The fungi are so prevalent that total prevention is impossible. To minimize risk:
- Get treatment for pets that have skin problems.
- Carefully dry feet after bathing in tub or shower or swimming.
- Good personal hygiene.
- Don't share headgear (hats, combs, brushes).
- Avoid tight shoes or underwear that may rub or chafe the skin.

WHAT TO EXPECT

DIAGNOSTIC MEASURES
- Your own observation of symptoms.
- Medical history and physical exam by a doctor.
- Microscopic exam of skin scrapings in potassium hydroxide solution.
- Laboratory culture of skin scrapings.
- Examination with ultraviolet light (Wood's lamp) for ringworm on the scalp.

APPROPRIATE HEALTH CARE
- Self-care after diagnosis.
- Treatment is usually with topical medications; other specific care depends on location of infection.

POSSIBLE COMPLICATIONS—Secondary bacterial infection of ringworm lesions.

PROBABLE OUTCOME—Usually curable with treatment, but may take weeks to months depending on location. Recurrence is common and ringworm becomes chronic in 20% of cases.

HOW TO TREAT

GENERAL MEASURES
- For infection on the body: Carefully launder all clothing, towels or bed linens that have touched the lesions.
- Keep the skin dry. If the area is red, swollen and weeping, use compresses made of 1 teaspoon salt to 1 pint water. Apply 4 times a day for 2 to 3 days before starting the local antifungal medication.
- For infection of the scalp, shampoo the hair every day. Have the hair cut short, but don't shave the scalp (wear clothing that can be sterilized). Repeat this procedure every 2 weeks, or whenever the hair grows back.
- For infected beard, let beard grow. If necessary for you to shave, use electric shaver and not a blade.

MEDICATION—Your doctor may prescribe:
- Topical antifungal drugs in the form of creams, lotions or ointments. Treatment may continue after symptoms disappear to eradicate the fungi and prevent recurrence.
- In widespread infections or nail infections, an oral antifungal (usually griseofulvin) may be prescribed.

ACTIVITY—No restrictions.

DIET—No special diet.

CALL YOUR DOCTOR IF

- You have symptoms of ringworm.
- Ringworm lesions become redder, painful and ooze pus.
- Symptoms don't improve in 3 or 4 weeks, despite treatment.
- New, unexplained symptoms develop. Drugs used in treatment may produce side effects.

ROCKY MOUNTAIN SPOTTED FEVER
(Tick Typhus)

 ## GENERAL INFORMATION

DEFINITION—An acute illness with fever caused by an organism transmitted by infected ticks. This is not contagious from person to person. The disease was named for the geographic site of its original discovery.

BODY PARTS INVOLVED—Skin; central nervous system; gastrointestinal tract; muscles.

SEX OR AGE MOST AFFECTED—Both sexes; all ages, more likely to occur in children and young adults.

SIGNS & SYMPTOMS—The following occur 2 to 5 days after a tick bite:
- Fever, often high, with chills.
- Red skin rash that begins on hands and feet and spreads to ankles, wrists, legs, trunk and abdomen.
- Headache.
- Muscle aches and weakness; stiff back.
- Nausea and vomiting.
- Mental confusion; coma.

CAUSES—Rickettsia organisms that live inside ticks. People are infected through tick bites, usually in the spring or summer. Rickettsia also infect rodents, squirrels and chipmunks.

The disease occurs in about 40 states of the U.S., especially on the Eastern seaboard from Georgia to Maryland, and in heavy brushy areas, such as Long Island. The tick is found in urban areas as well as rural. The disease can be transmitted by transfusion of contaminated blood.

RISK INCREASES WITH
- Outdoor activities in tick-infested areas.
- Contact with dogs.

HOW TO PREVENT
- Wear protective clothing in tick-infested areas and use insect repellant.
- During outdoor activity, carefully inspect the body frequently to remove ticks. Don't crush them during removal as the whole tick must be removed. Hold a lighted cigarette near the tick, or apply gasoline, kerosene or oil to the tick's body. Pull it off with tweezers.
- No vaccine is currently available, but research continues.

 ## WHAT TO EXPECT

DIAGNOSTIC MEASURES
- Your own observation of symptoms.
- Medical history and physical exam by a doctor.
- Laboratory studies, such as blood counts, serological tests (see Glossary) and skin biopsy (see Glossary). The history of a tick bite or travel to a tick-infested area helps confirm diagnosis.

APPROPRIATE HEALTH CARE
- Doctor's treatment. This may be a medical emergency.
- Patients with mild disease may be treated at home; but more likely, the infection will require hospitalization (may need mechanical breathing support, blood transfusions and close watch for complications such as kidney failure).

POSSIBLE COMPLICATIONS
- Brain infection.
- Seizures.
- Kidney failure.
- Hepatitis.
- Rocky Mountain spotted fever is often fatal if untreated (due to pneumonia or heart failure).

PROBABLE OUTCOME—Curable if antibiotic treatment is begun in the early stages.

 ## HOW TO TREAT

GENERAL MEASURES—If the patient is hospitalized, the family should maintain an optimistic outlook, stay in close contact with the patient's doctor and help by making their visits with the patient brief and as supportive as possible.

MEDICATION—Your doctor may prescribe antibiotics, such as tetracycline, doxycycline or chloramphenicol.

ACTIVITY—Rest in bed until fever and other symptoms disappear.

DIET—No special diet. Critically ill patients may require intravenous feedings. In others, small frequent meals may be necessary.

 ## CALL YOUR DOCTOR IF

- You have symptoms of Rocky Mountain spotted fever.
- New, unexplained symptoms develop. Drugs used in treatment may produce side effects.

ROSEOLA INFANTUM
(Exanthem Subitum)

 GENERAL INFORMATION

DEFINITION—A common, contagious childhood disease characterized by high fever and skin rash.

BODY PARTS INVOLVED—Skin; central nervous system.

SEX OR AGE MOST AFFECTED—Infants and young children (1 to 3 years).

SIGNS & SYMPTOMS
- Fever, often high, for several days to 1 week.
- Irritability.
- Drowsiness.
- Flat, reddish skin rash after 4 or 5 days of high fever. When the rash appears, fever and other symptoms disappear.

CAUSES—It is caused by a herpes virus (type 6). Incubation is 5 to 15 days.

RISK INCREASES WITH
- Day care center.
- Exposure to others in public places.

HOW TO PREVENT—Avoid exposure if possible.

 WHAT TO EXPECT

DIAGNOSTIC MEASURES
- Your own observation of symptoms.
- Medical history and physical exam by a doctor.
- Laboratory studies, such as urinalysis and blood counts, to rule out other reasons for high fever (such as middle-ear infection, meningitis, pneumonia or urinary-tract infection).

APPROPRIATE HEALTH CARE
- Home care after diagnosis.
- Doctor's treatment.

POSSIBLE COMPLICATIONS
- Convulsions caused by high fever (they will not cause brain damage and will cease after fever subsides). Roseola's high fevers are a common cause of febrile convulsions during the first two years of life. They can be frightening, especially for the parents, but they are not harmful. It is the body's response to the rapid changes in temperature.
- Infection of the brain (rare).

PROBABLE OUTCOME—Spontaneous recovery in 1 week. The rash may last 2 days, but sometimes it comes and goes in only a few hours.

 HOW TO TREAT

GENERAL MEASURES
- There is no specific treatment for roseola. Rest at home is sufficient until symptoms disappear.
- Lukewarm water baths or a sponge bath may be used to reduce fever if it reaches 102F (38.9C) or higher.

MEDICATION
- For minor discomfort and to reduce fever, you may use nonprescription drugs such as acetaminophen. Antibiotics don't help. Don't give a child younger than 18 aspirin for fever. It has been linked to Reye's syndrome.
- Anticonvulsant medication (if child has seizure) may be prescribed.

ACTIVITY—The child should rest in bed until fever disappears.

DIET—Encourage fluid intake. The child should eat a normal, well-balanced diet. Continue baby-vitamin supplements if the child is accustomed to taking them.

 CALL YOUR DOCTOR IF

- High fever.
- Twitching or other signs of a convulsion begin.
- The child refuses liquids.
- The child cries loudly and persistently and does not stop when picked up.
- The child is listless and has a stiff neck.

ILLNESS & DISORDERS

ROUNDWORMS
(Ascariasis)

GENERAL INFORMATION

DEFINITION—Intestinal parasites shaped like earthworms that can be seen easily without a microscope. Roundworms thrive in the gastrointestinal tract (and sometimes the lungs). They are contagious. The infection is most common in rural southwestern United States.

BODY PARTS INVOLVED—Gastrointestinal tract; lungs (sometimes).

SEX OR AGE MOST AFFECTED—All ages, but most common in children.

SIGNS & SYMPTOMS
- Irritability.
- Restlessness at night.
- Erratic or poor appetite.
- Frequent fatigue.
- Weight loss or lack of weight gain.
- Colicky abdominal discomfort.
- Diarrhea (sometimes).
- Cough and wheezing (rare).
- Worms may sometimes be seen in bowel movements or in the child's bed. Rarely, one may be vomited.
- Fever.

CAUSES—A parasite called Ascaris whose eggs enter the human body through contaminated water, food or soil-contaminated hands.

RISK INCREASES WITH—Crowded or unsanitary living conditions.

HOW TO PREVENT
- Wash hands frequently—always before eating.
- Keep fingers away from the mouth.
- Have pets treated for worms. Avoid strange animals.

WHAT TO EXPECT

DIAGNOSTIC MEASURES
- Your own observation of symptoms.
- Medical history and physical exam by a doctor.
- Laboratory studies of the stool or a study of an adult worm, if passed, to identify the worm; x-ray of the lungs (sometimes).

APPROPRIATE HEALTH CARE
- Home care after diagnosis.
- Treatment can be given at home and involves antiworm drugs and other hygienic care.

POSSIBLE COMPLICATIONS—If untreated:
- Worms migrate to other body parts.
- Intestinal obstruction (rare).
- Malnutrition in children.

PROBABLE OUTCOME—Usually curable in 1 week with treatment

HOW TO TREAT

GENERAL MEASURES
- Wash hands carefully after using the toilet or before meals. Keep fingers away from the mouth. Keep nails short and clean.
- Wash the anus and genitals with warm soap and water at least twice a day. Rinse well, preferably under a shower. Don't take tub baths.
- If possible, boil all soiled linen, nightclothes, underwear, towels and washcloths that have been used by anyone with roundworms. Fabrics that cannot be boiled can be soaked in an ammonia solution (1 cup of household ammonia to 5 gallons of cold water).
- After treatment, scrub all toilet seats, bathroom floors and fixtures. Vacuum rugs, table tops, curtains, sofa and chairs carefully. Sterilize metal toys or similar objects in a hot oven.

MEDICATION—Your doctor may prescribe drugs to kill roundworms, such as pyrantel pamoate, piperazine or mebendazole (this medication may cause fetal abnormalities; don't use it if you are pregnant). These drugs can be effective after a single dose.

ACTIVITY—Patient may resume normal activities as soon as symptoms improve.

DIET—No special diet.

CALL YOUR DOCTOR IF

- You or your child have symptoms of roundworms.
- Roundworms reappear after treatment.
- New, unexplained symptoms develop. Drugs used in treatment may produce side effects.

RUBELLA (German Measles)

GENERAL INFORMATION

DEFINITION—A mild, contagious virus illness. Immunization has significantly decreased the number of cases in the U.S. Rubella is likely to cause serious birth defects to the unborn baby of a pregnant woman who develops the disease in the first 3 or 4 months of pregnancy.

BODY PARTS INVOLVED—Skin; lymph glands behind the ears and in the neck.

SEX OR AGE MOST AFFECTED—All ages, but most common in children.

SIGNS & SYMPTOMS—Symptoms are usually quite mild.
- Fever.
- Muscle aches and stiffness, especially in the neck.
- Fatigue.
- Headache.
- Reddish rash on the head and body after the 2nd or 3rd day. The rash lasts 1 or 2 days.
- Swollen lymph glands, especially behind the ears and at the back and sides of the neck.
- Joint pain (adults).

CAUSES—RNA virus spread by person-to-person contact. Patients are contagious from 1 week before the rash appears until 1 week after it fades.

RISK INCREASES WITH
- Springtime weather when epidemics are common.
- Inadequate immunization.
- Crowded living conditions.
- School or day care.
- Immunosuppression due to illness or drugs.

HOW TO PREVENT
- Children should be immunized against rubella at approximately 12-15 months of age and a booster given at ages 5-6 or ages 11-15.
- Nonpregnant women of childbearing age should be immunized if they have not had rubella or been immunized. Pregnancy should be prevented for 3 months following immunization. (If you don't know whether or not you have had rubella, your doctor or local health department can determine it from a blood test.)
- A person, especially a pregnant woman who is exposed to rubella, who has not had it or been immunized, should receive a gamma globulin (antibodies) injection. If taken soon after exposure, the gamma globulin may prevent or reduce the severity of the disease.
- A person should not be immunized if he or she has an altered autoimmune system, as with cancer; currently takes cortisone or anticancer drugs; is receiving radiation therapy; or has an illness with fever.

WHAT TO EXPECT

DIAGNOSTIC MEASURES
- Medical history and exam by a doctor.
- Diagnostic laboratory tests normally not needed for rubella; however, culture of the throat, blood, urine or cerebrospinal fluid can confirm the presence of the virus.

APPROPRIATE HEALTH CARE
- Self-care.
- Doctor's treatment.

POSSIBLE COMPLICATIONS
- In a pregnant woman, miscarriage or birth defects in the newborn child.
- Encephalitis, thrombocytopenia, agranulocytosis (all very rare).

PROBABLE OUTCOME—Spontaneous recovery in 1 week in children, longer in adults.

HOW TO TREAT

GENERAL MEASURES
- Usually no specific treatment is required; extra rest (if needed) and extra fluid intake are recommended.
- Be sure to contact any pregnant woman who has been exposed to the patient. Exposure includes contact with the infected person 1 week prior to, during or 1 week after the infection. This woman should consult her prenatal doctor immediately.

MEDICATION—For minor discomfort, you may use nonprescription drugs such as acetaminophen. Don't give aspirin to a person younger than 18. Research shows a link between the use of aspirin in children during a virus illness and the development of Reye's syndrome (a type of encephalitis).

ACTIVITY—Get extra rest until the fever disappears. Then limit activities until the day after the rash disappears. Don't expose yourself to others until 1 week after the rash disappears.

DIET—No special diet.

CALL YOUR DOCTOR IF

- You have symptoms of rubella.
- The following occurs during treatment:
  High fever.
  Red eyes.
  Cough or shortness of breath.
  Severe headache, drowsiness, lethargy or convulsion.
- Unusual bleeding occurs 1 to 4 weeks after the illness (bleeding gums, nose, uterus or scattered blood specks on the skin).

ILLNESS & DISORDERS

SALIVARY GLAND DISORDERS

GENERAL INFORMATION

DEFINITION—Infections are caused by an infectious organism other than the virus that causes mumps. A tumor is an abnormal growth in the salivary gland. Most salivary gland tumors are benign and require several years to develop. Even malignant tumors rarely spread to distant body parts. Salivary duct stone is a tiny hard particle that forms in a salivary gland duct (usually a salivary gland under the tongue). Chemicals in the saliva cause crusting in the duct.

BODY PARTS INVOLVED—Salivary glands and ducts.

SEX OR AGE MOST AFFECTED—Adults of both sexes.

SIGNS & SYMPTOMS
Infection:
- Pain and swelling of parotid (behind ear) or sublingual (under tongue) salivary glands.
- Pain and swelling of lymph glands in the neck (below jaw); fever.
- Bitter pus in the mouth from infected gland.

Tumor:
- A soft, painful swelling or firm mass above the angle of either jaw or in the floor of the mouth.

Stones:
- Pain and swelling in the salivary gland (between ear and jaw), especially with meals.
- Redness and tenderness in the floor of the mouth and under the jaw.
- Swollen, tender lymph glands in the neck or under the jaw; fever (if infection is present).

CAUSES
- Infections—Bacterial infection caused by staphylococci or another bacteria.
- Tumors—Unknown.
- Stones—Chemical change of unknown cause in salivary-gland secretions.

RISK INCREASES WITH
- Adults over 60; smoking; dehydration.
- Poor oral hygiene; poor nutrition; dentures.
- Recent or chronic illness.
- Use of drugs that cause a dry mouth.

HOW TO PREVENT—Some disorders can't be prevented, but the risk can be minimized by:
- Not smoking and keeping the mouth healthy.
- Visit your dentist regularly for checkups.

WHAT TO EXPECT

DIAGNOSTIC MEASURES
- Medical history and exam by a doctor.
- Laboratory studies.
- For tumors—X-rays of the salivary glands and chest, MRI, CT scan, ultrasound (see Glossary), technetium 99 (radioisotope scan method).

APPROPRIATE HEALTH CARE
- Doctor's treatment.
- Infections are treated with antibiotics.
- Tumors are treated with surgery to remove the tumor and lymph glands in the neck, if malignant cells have spread.
- Surgery to remove the stone—generally under local anesthesia.

POSSIBLE COMPLICATIONS
- Infections—Complete, permanent blockage of the salivary gland duct (will require surgery).
- Tumors—Infection at the surgical site; disfigurement after surgery; spread to other organs.
- Stones—Recurrence of the stone. If it recurs, a surgeon can permanently open the duct so saliva drains from the gland into the mouth.

PROBABLE OUTCOME
- Infections—Usually curable in 2 weeks with treatment. If the gland becomes blocked with a stone or scar tissue, surgery is necessary before the infection can clear.
- Tumors—Benign tumors are usually curable with surgery alone; malignant salivary tumors are usually curable with surgery, radiation treatment and anticancer drugs.
- Stones—Many stones pass spontaneously. Others are usually curable with surgery.

HOW TO TREAT

GENERAL MEASURES
- Apply warm or cool soaks (see Soaks in Appendix), whichever feels better.
- After surgery, keep the mouth clean with salt-water mouthwashes. At least 3 or 4 times a day, rinse the mouth with a solution of 1 teaspoon salt in 8 oz. of warm water.

MEDICATION
- Your doctor may prescribe:
  Antibiotics to fight bacterial infection.
  Pain relievers.
  Anticancer drugs, if surgery and radiation treatment don't destroy a malignant tumor.
- For minor pain, you may use nonprescription drugs such as acetaminophen.

ACTIVITY—No restrictions.

DIET
- With infections, usually no special diet. Drink at least 6 to 8 glasses of fluid a day.
- After surgery, a liquid diet (see Liquid Diet in Appendix) will be necessary until mouth heals.

CALL YOUR DOCTOR IF

- The infection does not improve in 4 days or symptoms worsen or fever persists.
- After surgery, signs of infection develop in your mouth, including increased warmth, redness, pain or tenderness and swelling.
- New, unexplained symptoms develop.

SALMONELLA INFECTIONS

GENERAL INFORMATION

DEFINITION—A general infection caused by organisms in the salmonella family. A relatively mild Salmonella infection may be mistaken for simple gastroenteritis.

BODY PARTS INVOLVED—Gastrointestinal tract; lymphatic system.

SEX OR AGE MOST AFFECTED—Both sexes; all ages.

SIGNS & SYMPTOMS
- Diarrhea, often accompanied by abdominal cramps. In mild cases, diarrhea may be only 2 or 3 loose bowel movements a day. In severe cases, it may be watery diarrhea as often as every 10 or 15 minutes.
- Vomiting (occasionally); fever.
- Blood in the stool (sometimes).

CAUSES
- Infection with Salmonella bacteria after eating food such as meat, poultry, raw milk or eggs, or drinking water that contains the bacteria. Salmonella bacteria survive freezing, but thorough cooking kills them. Pet turtles and other animals can also carry Salmonella bacteria.
- Salmonella epidemics often occur when many people eat the same contaminated food at a picnic, social gathering or restaurant. The infection can be transmitted from person to person.

RISK INCREASES WITH
- Recent gastrointestinal illness.
- Crowded or unsanitary living conditions.
- Infancy; old age.
- Immunosuppression due to illness or drugs.
- Anemia or malignancy.

HOW TO PREVENT
- Proper cooking, handling, storage and refrigeration of poultry, meat, eggs, etc. Additional information available from the National Center for Nutrition, (800)366-1655.
- Avoid animals that could be infected.
- Drink only pasteurized milk.
- Wash your hands after bowel movements and before handling food.
- Isolate anyone in the family who has the infection.
- Get medical advice about preventive antibiotics before traveling in countries with unsanitary water and food supplies.

WHAT TO EXPECT

DIAGNOSTIC MEASURES
- Your own observation of symptoms.
- Medical history and exam by a doctor.
- Laboratory stool studies and blood culture.

APPROPRIATE HEALTH CARE
- Self-care.
- Doctor's treatment, if symptoms continue longer than 48 hours or for complications.
- Hospitalization (rare).

POSSIBLE COMPLICATIONS
- Dehydration from excessive diarrhea and vomiting. Severe dehydration can be fatal, especially in infants and persons over 60.
- Infection of other organs, such as the kidneys, gallbladder, spleen and lungs, from salmonella bacteria in the bloodstream (rare).

PROBABLE OUTCOME—Most salmonella infections are mild and curable with treatment in 24 to 48 hours. Patients with severe infections require hospitalization and isolation. The infection may last 2 to 3 weeks.

HOW TO TREAT

GENERAL MEASURES
- Isolate the ill person, if possible.
- Use a heating pad or hot-water bottle to relieve abdominal cramps.
- If diarrhea is severe, use a bedside commode.

MEDICATION—Medicine is usually not necessary for mild cases. Antidiarrhea medications may retard recovery. For severe cases, your doctor may prescribe antidiarrhea medication, antibiotics to fight infection and intravenous fluids for severe dehydration.

ACTIVITY—Restrict activity, except for trips to the bathroom, until at least 3 days after diarrhea, fever and other symptoms disappear. Then resume normal activities gradually.

DIET—Drink diluted electrolyte solutions, such as Gatorade or Pedialyte, until diarrhea stops. Then eat a high-calorie, well-balanced diet. Vitamin and mineral supplements may be helpful after prolonged illness.

CALL YOUR DOCTOR IF

- An infant has symptoms of a Salmonella infection and shows signs of dehydration, such as dry, wrinkled skin, decreased urination or dark urine.
- You have symptoms of a Salmonella infection that persist longer than 48 hours.
- The following occurs during the illness: Fever of 102F (38.9C) or higher; jaundice (yellow skin or eyes); cough with blood; worsening diarrhea.

SCABIES

GENERAL INFORMATION

DEFINITION—A disease of the skin caused by a mite (the "itch" mite) with a characteristic pattern of distribution. Scabies is contagious from person to person (by shared clothing or bed linen) and from one site to another in the same person. It may be misdiagnosed as poison ivy, eczema, allergies or other skin conditions.

BODY PARTS INVOLVED—Skin of the finger webs and folds under the arms, breasts, elbows, genitals and buttocks.

SEX OR AGE MOST AFFECTED—Both sexes; all ages.

SIGNS & SYMPTOMS
• Small, itchy blisters (usually in a thin line) in several parts of the body. The blisters break easily when scratched.
• Broken blisters leave scratch marks and thickened skin, crisscrossed by grooves and scaling.

CAUSES—A mite, Sarcoptes scabiei, that burrows into deep skin layers, where the female mite deposits eggs. Eggs mature into adult mites in 3 weeks. Mites are 0.1mm in diameter and can only be seen under a microscope. Scratching collects mites and eggs under the fingernails, so they spread to other parts of the body.

RISK INCREASES WITH
• Crowded or unsanitary living conditions.
• Contact with an infested person (usually by physical contact, but mites can pass by just standing close to infected person).

HOW TO PREVENT
• Avoid contact with persons or linen and clothing that you suspect may be infected with scabies.
• Maintain personal cleanliness:
  Bathe daily, or at least 2 to 3 times a week.
  Wash hands before eating.
  Launder clothes often.

WHAT TO EXPECT

DIAGNOSTIC MEASURES
• Your own observation of symptoms.
• Medical history and physical exam by a doctor. The diagnosis is confirmed by discovering the mite, lifting it from its burrow and identifying it under a microscope.

APPROPRIATE HEALTH CARE
• Self-care after diagnosis.
• Doctor's treatment. Medicine used for treatment is very effective.

POSSIBLE COMPLICATIONS
• Secondary bacterial infection of mite-infested areas of inflammation.
• A rare form of scabies (Norwegian) may occur in immunocompromised patients.

PROBABLE OUTCOME—Itching usually disappears quickly, and evidence of the disease is gone in 1 to 2 weeks with treatment. In some cases, re-treatment is necessary in 20 days.

HOW TO TREAT

GENERAL MEASURES
• Wash clothing and bedding after your treatment.
• Extensive cleaning and fumigating of furniture and other items is unnecessary, since scabies only survive a short time off the body.

MEDICATION—Your doctor may prescribe:
• An insecticide lotion such as permethrin, lindane, crotamiton, or 5% sulfur ointment. (Infants and pregnant women may need a pediculicide that is less toxic, such as a 6% solution of sulfur).
  Bathe thoroughly before applying the prescribed medicine.
  Apply from the neck down, and cover the entire body.
  Wait 15 minutes before dressing.
  Leave medicine on the skin for 12-24 hours before bathing.
  Your family or other close contacts should be treated at the same time.
  You may need to repeat in 1 week.
• Topical steroids or other drugs to relieve the itching.
• Antibiotic ointments or oral antibiotics if a secondary bacteria infection develops.

ACTIVITY—No restrictions.

DIET—No special diet.

CALL YOUR DOCTOR IF

• You have symptoms of scabies.
• After treatment, the lesions show signs of infection (redness, pus, swelling or pain).
• New, unexplained symptoms develop. Drugs used in treatment may produce side effects.

SCARLET FEVER

GENERAL INFORMATION

DEFINITION—A childhood disorder characterized by a bright red rash. Scarlet fever is preceded by a streptococcal throat infection. Both are very contagious for 2 to 3 weeks. Scarlet fever is far less common and less dangerous than it once was.

BODY PARTS INVOLVED—Throat; tonsils; skin.

SEX OR AGE MOST AFFECTED—Children and adolescents, especially between ages 2 and 10.

SIGNS & SYMPTOMS—Symptoms may vary from person to person. Following is the usual course of the disease:
• Day 1—Fever as high as 104F (40C); a red sore throat; swollen tonsils (tonsils may have a whitish coating); enlarged lymph glands in the neck; cough; vomiting.
• Day 2—Bright red rash on the face, except around the mouth.
• Day 3—Reddened tongue and rash in body creases, spreading to the neck, chest, back, then the entire body. The rash resembles a sunburn with bumps.
• Day 6—Faded rash and skin that begins peeling, continuing for 10 to 14 days.

CAUSES
• Streptococcal infection caused by a specific type of germ that manufactures a scarlet-fever toxin (poison). The bacteria are spread in droplets coughed or breathed into the air.
• Very few strep infections progress to scarlet fever, because everyone is not susceptible to the rash-producing toxin. In one family, one child may contract scarlet fever, another may have a strep throat only, and a third may carry the germ and transmit it to others without being sick.

RISK INCREASES WITH
• Family history of recurrent strep infections.
• Recent impetigo.
• Crowded or unsanitary living conditions.
• Exposure to others in public places.
• Age (2-10).

HOW TO PREVENT—Cannot be prevented completely, because some healthy persons are carriers of the strep germ without being ill. However, partial preventive measures include:
• Antibiotic treatment for at least 10 days for any strep infection.
• Avoidance of persons with sore throats.

WHAT TO EXPECT

DIAGNOSTIC MEASURES
• Your own observation of symptoms.
• Medical history and physical exam by a doctor.
• Laboratory throat culture.

APPROPRIATE HEALTH CARE
• Home care after diagnosis.
• Doctor's treatment.

POSSIBLE COMPLICATIONS—Without treatment:
• Rheumatic fever.
• Impaired hearing.
• Glomerulonephritis.
• Meningitis.
• Pneumonia.
• Encephalitis.

PROBABLE OUTCOME—Usually curable in 10 days or more with treatment. Scarlet fever is not as prevalent as it once was, and it is rarely fatal. With antibiotic treatment, the severity and likelihood of complications decrease.

HOW TO TREAT

GENERAL MEASURES
• Care may be given at home.
• Use a cool-mist, ultrasonic humidifier to relieve the dry, tight feeling in the throat. Clean humidifier daily.
• Use moist, warm soaks to relieve tender, enlarged glands in the neck.
• Isolate the ill person from other people, including family members.

MEDICATION
• Your doctor may prescribe penicillin to shorten the course of scarlet fever and prevent complications. If the patient is allergic to penicillin, other antibiotics, such as erythromycin, are also effective. Finish the entire course of the medicine, even if the symptoms disappear.
• Use acetaminophen for pain relief and fever.

ACTIVITY—Bed rest is necessary until all signs of illness have disappeared.

DIET—No special diet. Drink plenty of fluids.

CALL YOUR DOCTOR IF

• You or your child have symptoms of strep throat or scarlet fever.
• The following occurs during treatment:
  Temperature becomes normal for 2 days, then fever develops again.
  New symptoms begin, such as: nausea; vomiting; earache; cough; headache; thick, colored, nasal drainage; chest pain; or labored breathing.

ILLNESS & DISORDERS

SCLERITIS

GENERAL INFORMATION

DEFINITION—Deep, localized inflammation of the sclera, the outermost white layer of tissue covering the eyeball. Scleritis is not contagious.

BODY PARTS INVOLVED—Sclera, which includes the conjunctiva and cornea. Scleritis may affect one or both eyes.

SEX OR AGE MOST AFFECTED—All ages, but most common in adults from ages 30 to 60.

SIGNS & SYMPTOMS
- Eye pain (usually dull).
- Purple-red, inflamed areas in one or more areas of the white of the eye.
- Partial vision loss (sometimes).

CAUSES—Unknown, but scleritis frequently occurs with rheumatoid arthritis, Crohn's disease and other connective-tissue disorders. It is probably an autoimmune disorder.

RISK INCREASES WITH
- Rheumatoid arthritis.
- Crohn's disease (regional ileitis).
- Chronic gastrointestinal disorder.

HOW TO PREVENT—No specific preventive measures.

WHAT TO EXPECT

DIAGNOSTIC MEASURES
- Your own observation of symptoms.
- Medical history and physical exam by a doctor.

APPROPRIATE HEALTH CARE
- Self-care after diagnosis.
- Doctor's treatment.
- Surgery to close a perforation, if perforation occurs as a complication.

POSSIBLE COMPLICATIONS
- Rupture of the scleral tissue, perforating the eyeball and causing loss of the eye. The eye can sometimes be saved with surgery after perforation.
- Cataracts or glaucoma as a result of the treatment required.

PROBABLE OUTCOME—Outcome is variable. It is sometimes recurrent, chronic and progressive. If partial vision loss occurs, it is usually permanent.

HOW TO TREAT

GENERAL MEASURES—Use warm-water soaks (see Soaks in Appendix) to relieve pain.

MEDICATION
- Your doctor may prescribe immunosuppressive drugs, oral cortisone drugs or cortisone eye drops to reduce inflammation.
- For minor pain, you may use nonprescription drugs, such as acetaminophen.

ACTIVITY—Reduce normal activity until inflammation subsides.

DIET—No special diet.

CALL YOUR DOCTOR IF

- You have symptoms of scleritis.
- The following occurs during treatment:
  Symptoms don't improve in 48 hours.
  Temperature rises to 100F (37.8C) or higher.
  Pain becomes worse.
  Vision is affected.

SCLERODERMA
(Progressive System Sclerosis)

 GENERAL INFORMATION

DEFINITION—A rare, connective tissue disease in which the skin and other body parts gradually degenerate, thicken and become stiff (*sclero* means thickening and *derma* means skin).

BODY PARTS INVOLVED—Skin; joints; digestive system, especially the esophagus; intestinal tract; heart; kidneys; lungs; blood vessels; fingers; toes.

SEX OR AGE MOST AFFECTED—Adults of both sexes, but more common in women between ages 30 and 50.

SIGNS & SYMPTOMS
- Fingers—hardening and thickening of the skin, stiffness, poor circulation, numbness and fingertip ulceration.
- Digestive system—swallowing difficulty, poor food absorption, bloating after eating, weight loss, heartburn and a feeling that food sticks in the chest.
- Skin—hardening and thickening, especially in the face, which becomes tight and loses its elasticity.
- Muscle aches; weakness and fatigue.
- Joint pain, stiffness and swelling; anemia.

CAUSES—Unknown, but may be an autoimmune disorder in which the body's immune system attacks its own tissues. The connective tissue (the framework for all body tissues and blood vessels) thickens, becoming stiff and inflexible.

RISK INCREASES WITH—Unknown.

HOW TO PREVENT—Cannot be prevented.

 WHAT TO EXPECT

DIAGNOSTIC MEASURES
- Medical history and exam by a doctor.
- Laboratory blood tests to detect anemia and measure antibodies.
- Urinalysis to detect red cells in the urine.
- ECG (see Glossary), lung function tests; barium enema; and skin biopsy (see Glossary).
- X-rays of the hands, esophagus and chest.

APPROPRIATE HEALTH CARE
- Self-care during treatment.
- Treatment program will vary.
- Psychotherapy or counseling to adjust to living with an incurable disease.
- Home care usually. Rarely, hospitalization for heart, lung or kidney complications or for surgical procedure (e.g., on the esophagus).

POSSIBLE COMPLICATIONS
- Bleeding tendencies.
- Heart-rhythm disturbances.
- Congestive heart failure.
- Kidney failure.
- High blood pressure.
- Lung destruction.
- Poor wound healing and gangrene.

PROBABLE OUTCOME—The course of the disorder is variable and unpredictable. It is often slowly progressive and affects the heart, lungs and kidneys. In some, the disease may remain limited and nonprogressive for long periods of time.

 HOW TO TREAT

GENERAL MEASURES
- Because of poor circulation, wear warm clothing, especially socks and gloves. Avoid exposure to extreme cold.
- Protect yourself from burns and cuts.
- Sleep on 2 or 3 pillows, or raise the head of your bed 5 to 8 inches to prevent stomach acid from rolling back into the esophagus.
- Learn biofeedback techniques to increase circulation to the extremities.
- Don't smoke.
- Use heat to relieve joint stiffness.
- See Resources for Additional Information.

MEDICATION
- You may take nonprescription antacids to relieve heartburn or indigestion, and aspirin or ibuprofen for muscle aches and joint pain.
- Use lotions, lubricants and bath oil on skin.
- Your doctor may prescribe cortisone drugs to relieve inflammatory symptoms and antibiotics to fight infections. There is no one drug that is helpful for this disorder.

ACTIVITY
- Be as active as your strength permits; avoid fatigue.
- Regular exercise (or movement) can help keep the skin flexible, maintain good blood circulation and prevent fixed joints. Physical therapy may help preserve muscle strength. Ask your doctor.

DIET—Eat frequent, small meals to minimize bloating, heartburn and gastrointestinal discomfort. A soft diet is sometimes recommended. Use additional fluids to help with swallowing. Consult a dietitian.

 CALL YOUR DOCTOR IF

The following occurs during treatment:
Unexplained bruising or bleeding under skin.
Slow healing of a wound.

SCOLIOSIS
(Curvature of the Spine)

GENERAL INFORMATION

DEFINITION—A painless bending and twisting of the upper spinal column, which is sometimes progressive and distorts the chest and back.

BODY PARTS INVOLVED—The thoracic (middle spine) or the lumbar (lower spine).

SEX OR AGE MOST AFFECTED
• Adolescents.
• Both sexes, but more common in girls.

SIGNS & SYMPTOMS
Early stages:
• No obvious symptoms or signs, but scoliosis can be detected by a doctor or school nurse with a simple screening test.
Later stages:
• Visible curving of the upper body. The spine becomes S-shaped or rotated.
• Shoulders become uneven and rounded.
• Sunken chest.
• Swayback.
• One side of the pelvis thrusts forward.
• Back pain.

CAUSES—Usually unknown. Scoliosis is sometimes a result of:
• Diseases of the central nervous system, such as polio or muscular dystrophy.
• Congenital defects of the spine.
• Uneven leg length.

RISK INCREASES WITH—Family history of scoliosis.

HOW TO PREVENT—Cannot be prevented at present.

WHAT TO EXPECT

DIAGNOSTIC MEASURES
• Your own observation of symptoms.
• Medical history and physical exam by a doctor.
• X-ray of the back.

APPROPRIATE HEALTH CARE
• Doctor's treatment and regular examinations.
• Many cases of scoliosis are minor and require little treatment except physical therapy aimed at strengthening back muscles and improving posture.
• For children needing further treatment, it usually involves wearing a orthopedic back brace (sometimes for several years). Newer type braces are less visible and permit the person to wear regular clothes.

• For adults needing treatment, exercises to strengthen back muscles are recommended (exercises will not correct the curvature). A brace is not effective in adults since the spine has stopped growing.
• If legs are of unequal length, a shoe lift for the shorter leg may be prescribed.
• Surgery to correct the deformity (severe cases only).

POSSIBLE COMPLICATIONS
• Severe distortion of the spine and ribs.
• Social embarrassment.
• Breathing difficulty.
• Lung infection.
• Congestive heart failure.

PROBABLE OUTCOME—When diagnosed early, scoliosis can usually be corrected completely. Often a back brace may be required and worn daily for several years.

HOW TO TREAT

GENERAL MEASURES—A teenager may be embarrassed to wear a brace. Be sure your teenager understands that the brace is temporary. Explain the eventual consequences of not wearing the brace. Insist on keeping doctor appointments for follow-up evaluation.

MEDICATION—Medicine doesn't correct this disorder. For minor discomfort from muscle imbalance or complications, you may use nonprescription drugs, such as aspirin or acetaminophen.

ACTIVITY—Consult your doctor. Special exercises may be part of therapy. If a brace is necessary, sports participation will be restricted. Some activities such as swimming and horseback riding may be recommended since they tone and strengthen the back.

DIET—No special diet.

CALL YOUR DOCTOR IF

You suspect your child is developing scoliosis.

SEASONAL AFFECTIVE DISORDER

GENERAL INFORMATION

DEFINITION—A seasonal disruption of mood that occurs during the winter months and ceases with the advent of spring. Symptoms usually begin in September when days begin to shorten, and last through the winter into March when the days begin to lengthen again. Light plays a big part in its origin and in its treatment. In rarer instances, the seasonal disorder symptoms occur in the summer months and may be caused by an intolerance to heat.

BODY PARTS INVOLVED—Nervous.

SEX OR AGE MOST AFFECTED—Adults and children and is more common in women.

SIGNS & SYMPTOMS
Experienced at the start of winter:
• Depression; tiredness; sluggishness.
• Increased appetite (especially for carbohydrates); weight gain.
• Irritability; needing more sleep; feeling less cheerful; socializing less.
• Difficulty in coping with life as a result of these changes.

CAUSES—The pineal gland (one of the body's clocks) in the brain releases a hormone called melatonin that can adversely affect our moods. Very little melatonin is secreted in light (daytime) and its peak production is usually at night, between 2 and 3 a.m. Winter months (with their longer nights) cause extra production of melatonin, so the level in the body is increased. The average nighttime illumination in homes or offices is not adequate to counteract this affect.

RISK INCREASES WITH
• Geographical location (people in northern latitudes more susceptible).
• Other depressive illness.

HOW TO PREVENT—No measures known.

WHAT TO EXPECT

DIAGNOSTIC MEASURES
• Medical history and exam by a doctor.
• Diagnosis can be difficult. The same symptoms can arise from other types of depression. Laboratory blood studies may be done to rule out other medical disorders. Diagnosis usually requires a three-year mood disturbance pattern, with the onset occurring in the autumn and a remission in the spring.

APPROPRIATE HEALTH CARE
• Self-care.
• Doctor's treatment.
• Therapies continue to evolve for treatment of people with moderate to severe symptoms, but they usually involve extending the day artificially in various ways with light therapy (phototherapy). Duration and intensities of the therapy may vary for individuals and they need to be worked out with you and your medical team. Even though these light sources are commercially available, it is recommended that they not be used without medical advice. Examples include:
   Sitting in a very bright light (equivalent to 10 100 watt bulbs or more) for an hour in the morning and evening.
   Installing a computerized system of lighting in a patient's bedroom that creates an artificial dawn. The light goes from very dim to bright like a sunrise.
   Wearing a visor cap with small battery-powered lights that provide illumination falling directly on the eyes.
• For some patients the light therapy doesn't work and they may require other forms of treatment such as drugs or psychotherapy.

PROBABLE OUTCOME—With correct diagnosis and treatment, symptoms can be minimized.

POSSIBLE COMPLICATIONS—Continuation of the symptoms and lifestyle disruptions.

HOW TO TREAT

GENERAL MEASURES
• Mild symptoms may be resolved with simple measures: keep drapes and blinds open in your house; sit near windows and gaze outside frequently; turn on bright lights on cloudy days; keep a diary or journal of your mood changes so that any changes or patterns can be evaluated; don't isolate yourself (visit friends, see shows, etc.).
• See Resources for Additional Information.

MEDICATION—Antidepressants may be prescribed for patients who do not respond to other forms of therapy.

ACTIVITY
• Stay as active as your energy permits. Physical activity is therapeutic for mood disorders.
• Get outside as much as possible, especially in the early morning light.
• Try to take a vacation in the winter months instead of the summer.

DIET—No special diet.

CALL YOUR DOCTOR IF

Symptoms continue or worsen despite treatment.

SEBACEOUS CYST
(Epidermoid Cyst; Wens)

 GENERAL INFORMATION

DEFINITION—A dome-shaped cyst filled with semisolid material (keratin, the same material that forms skin, hair and nails). The name sebaceous cyst is in error, because a real sebaceous cyst would be filled with material called sebum and manufactured in hair follicles.

BODY PARTS INVOLVED—Skin of the trunk, face, neck and scalp.

SEX OR AGE MOST AFFECTED—All ages, but most common in adolescents and adults.

SIGNS & SYMPTOMS—A cyst with the following characteristics:
• The cyst has sloped shoulders or a dome-shaped, nodular appearance and a smooth surface.
• The cyst is whitish or skin-colored.
• Cysts range from 1cm to 4cm in diameter.
• If the cyst becomes injured or infected, it may become bright red and painful.

CAUSES—Sebaceous cysts are caused by plugged ducts in malformed hair follicles. They may enlarge from hormonal stimulation or injury.

RISK INCREASES WITH
• Skin injury.
• Hormonal stimulation at puberty.

HOW TO PREVENT—Cannot be prevented at present.

 WHAT TO EXPECT

DIAGNOSTIC MEASURES
• Your own observation of symptoms.
• Medical history and physical exam by a doctor.

APPROPRIATE HEALTH CARE
• Self-care.
• Doctor's treatment.
• Cysts can be removed through a simple incision in the skin lying over the cyst, the sac is removed and the incision is stitched with sutures. If the entire cyst wall is removed, recurrence is unlikely.

POSSIBLE COMPLICATIONS
• Infection of a cyst.
• Injury to a cyst, causing rupture or inflammation.

PROBABLE OUTCOME—Cysts that cause no symptoms require no medical treatment. Those that are unsightly or are repeatedly injured can be removed.

 HOW TO TREAT

GENERAL MEASURES—Before surgery, apply warm compresses to the cyst to reduce inflammation and size.

MEDICATION—Medicine usually is not necessary for this disorder. If a cyst becomes infected, your doctor may prescribe antibiotics.

ACTIVITY—No restrictions.

DIET—No special diet.

 CALL YOUR DOCTOR IF

• After removal, signs of infection (pain, redness, warmth and increased tenderness) occur at the surgical site.
• Fever of 101F (38.3C) or higher develops.
• The treated area does not appear to be healing well within 1 week.
• You are taking antibiotics, and new, unexplained symptoms develop. Antibiotics may produce side effects.

SEIZURE DISORDER (Epilepsy)

 GENERAL INFORMATION

DEFINITION—A disorder of brain function characterized by sudden seizures, brief attacks of inappropriate behavior, change in one's state of consciousness or bizarre movements. There are several different categories: mild types that can go almost unnoticed and severe types that can cause serious harm if they are not treated. Not all seizures are convulsions. A convulsion involves the nerves that control movement. Convulsions cause jerking, spastic muscle movement, altered consciousness and sometimes, loss of consciousness.

BODY PARTS INVOLVED—Nervous system.

SEX OR AGE MOST AFFECTED—Both sexes; all ages. Seizures usually begin between ages 2 and 14.

SIGNS & SYMPTOMS
- Simple partial seizures:
  Tingling sensation in arm, finger or foot.
  Perception of a bad odor. Sees flashing lights.
  Remains conscious.
- Complex partial seizures:
  Remains conscious, but sits motionless.
  Strange, repetitive or inappropriate
  movements or behaviors.
- Generalized convulsive seizures:
  Sense or aura preceding the seizure. May cry
  out and fall to the ground unconscious. Loss
  of urinary and bowel control. Muscle spasms;
  may bite tongue. Thrashing movements;
  jerking of limbs. Deep sleep after the
  convulsion; awakens with headache and lack
  of memory about the episode.
- Generalized nonconvulsive (absent) seizures;
  (most common in children):
  Remains conscious. Stares into space;
  appearance of daydreaming. Rhythmic
  blinking. Unawareness of the seizure.

CAUSES—More than 50 brain disorders, but the organic cause can be determined in only 25% of cases. Common causes include:
- Brain damage at or before birth; lack of oxygen during pregnancy, labor or delivery.
- Severe head injury; stroke; brain infection; brain tumor or an expanding lesion that compresses the brain (occasionally).
- Lead poisoning.
- Meningitis; encephalitis; measles.

RISK INCREASES WITH
- Family history of seizure disorders.
- Breech-birth (slightly).

HOW TO PREVENT—No specific preventive measures. Avoid head injuries.

 WHAT TO EXPECT

DIAGNOSTIC MEASURES
- Medical history and exam by a doctor.
- Laboratory blood studies, EEG (see Glossary), x-rays of the head, CT or MRI scan.

APPROPRIATE HEALTH CARE
- Doctor's treatment; counseling.
- Rarely, when all else fails, brain surgery.

POSSIBLE COMPLICATIONS
- Continuing seizures (despite treatment).
- Seizures can be life-threatening if they occur in hazardous situations (driving or swimming).

PROBABLE OUTCOME—Epilepsy is incurable, except in relatively rare cases where epilepsy is caused by treatable brain damage, tumors or infection. However, anticonvulsant drugs can prevent most seizures and allow a near-normal life. Newer drugs are helping many patients who have not responded to standard treatments.

 HOW TO TREAT

GENERAL MEASURES
- Wear a Medic-Alert (see Glossary) bracelet or pendant that shows you have epilepsy.
- Avoid any circumstance that has triggered a seizure previously.
- In event of seizure, loosen clothing, lay person flat and protect from injury. Although frightening, seizures are rarely harmful in themselves.

MEDICATION—Your doctor will prescribe anticonvulsant drugs. Your response to treatment will be monitored. Medication changes or adjustments are often necessary.
  Learn as much as you can about your medication. The drugs used cause significant side effects, in addition to suppressing seizures. Drugs may be withdrawn gradually after freedom from seizures for a period of time. Many people (especially children) can then stay free of seizures without medication.

ACTIVITY—No restrictions. Most states allow persons with epilepsy to drive a vehicle after being seizure-free for 1 year.

DIET
- Usually no special diet. Avoid alcohol or illicit drugs which can trigger seizures.
- For some patients, whose seizures aren't controlled by drugs, may be prescribed a ketogenic (very high-fat) diet. It is difficult to swallow and not always effective.

 CALL YOUR DOCTOR IF

New, unexplained symptoms develop during treatment for epilepsy.

SEXUAL DYSFUNCTION, FEMALE

 GENERAL INFORMATION

DEFINITION—Female sexual dysfunction may involve an inability to experience sexual pleasure (arousal dysfunction); or an inability to achieve orgasm (orgasmic dysfunction).

BODY PARTS INVOLVED—Brain and central nervous system; autonomic nervous system.

SEX OR AGE MOST AFFECTED—Sexually active women.

SIGNS & SYMPTOMS
- Lack of sexual desire; inability to enjoy sex.
- Lack of vaginal lubrication.
- Failure to achieve orgasm, even when sexually aroused.

CAUSES
- Inadequate or ineffective foreplay.
- Psychological problems, including depression, poor self-esteem, sexual abuse or incest. Feelings of shame or guilt about sex. Fear of pregnancy. Stress and fatigue.
- Two-career marriages (work, children and household tasks leave little energy for sex).
- Acute illness or chronic illness.
- Inexperience or inadequate information about sexuality on the part of either partner.
- Repressed anger toward the sexual partner that may result from feelings of being used as a sexual object, physical or emotional abuse, jealousy or fears of disloyalty, or lack of true intimacy.
- Drug abuse including alcohol.
- Gynecologic factors (infection or other disorders).
- Aging (sexual desire may decline).
- Children (hormonal changes in pregnancy cause many women to lose interest in sex).
- Surgery on the reproductive organs.

RISK INCREASES WITH
- Use of some medications, such as MAO inhibitors, antidepressants, beta-adrenergic blockers, narcotics, barbiturates and for some women, use of birth-control pills.
- Couple discrepancies in expectations and attitudes towards sex.
- Proximity of other people in the home (children, mother-in-law).

HOW TO PREVENT
- Talk with your partner about your needs.
- Seek counseling to resolve feelings.

 WHAT TO EXPECT

DIAGNOSTIC MEASURES
- Medical history and exam by a doctor.
- Diagnostic tests may include laboratory blood tests and other studies to rule out physical causes of arousal or orgasmic dysfunction.
- If no physical problems are found, a detailed sexual history is the most important tool for determining an appropriate treatment program.

APPROPRIATE HEALTH CARE
Possible treatment methods:
- For childhood sexual abuse problems—psychotherapy or counseling.
- For arousal dysfunction—relaxation techniques, sensate focus exercises, counseling (usually with a sex therapist).
- For orgasmic problems—self stimulation, new behavior patterns and sexual homework with partner (usually in conjunction with sex therapy.
- For medication caused problems—change in dosage, discontinuing or different medication.
- Other problems—family therapy, sensate conditioning, referral to sex therapist.

POSSIBLE COMPLICATIONS
- Permanent inability to enjoy sex.
- Damage to interpersonal relationships.

PROBABLE OUTCOME—Best predictors of positive outcome are the desire to change and an overall healthy relationship. Arousal dysfunction is more difficult to treat and outcome may vary.

 HOW TO TREAT

GENERAL MEASURES
- Self-help suggestions for you and your partner:

Admit the problem and try to establish open communication with your partner. Pretending to have orgasms leaves the problem unsolved.

Reduce stress in your life (see How to Cope with Stress in Appendix).

Spend time together as a couple that is nonsexual; go on regular dates. Spend time touching or cuddling that doesn't lead to sex.

Don't let age stop you from enjoying sex. You are never too old for sexual activities.

MEDICATION—Medication is not necessary unless the sexual problem is due to some underlying medical condition.

ACTIVITY—No restrictions. Exercise regularly to reduce stress and improve your self-image. A healthy body and mind promote enjoyable sex.

DIET
Eat a well-balanced diet. Vitamin and mineral supplements may be helpful. Weight loss program may be recommended if either partner is overweight. Avoid alcohol.

 CALL YOUR DOCTOR IF

You have sexual problems and you want help in resolving them.

SHOCK

GENERAL INFORMATION

DEFINITION—Blood pressure that is too low for the body to maintain vital functions. Shock does not include a person's reaction to emotional trauma, which is a totally different disorder.

BODY PARTS INVOLVED—Heart; blood vessels; blood.

SEX OR AGE MOST AFFECTED—Both sexes; all ages.

SIGNS & SYMPTOMS
- Cold hands and feet.
- Fast, weak pulse.
- Disorientation or confusion.
- Anxiety with feelings of impending doom.
- Skin that is pale, moist and sweaty.
- Shortness of breath and rapid breathing.
- Lack of urination.
- Low blood pressure. This may be so low that it cannot be measured by usual means.

CAUSES
- Sudden loss of blood from injury or disorders, such as bleeding peptic ulcer, ruptured aneurysm or ruptured ectopic pregnancy (hypovolemic shock).
- Fluid loss, such as occurs with severe burns, fluid and electrolyte imbalance, or peritonitis.
- Impaired heart pumping function from heart attack, heart rhythm irregularities, pericarditis or pulmonary embolism (cardiogenic shock).
- Blood poisoning, which causes blood vessels to greatly expand, such as occurs with toxic shock syndrome or major infections (septic shock).
- Some endocrine diseases, such as Addison's disease or diabetes mellitus.

RISK INCREASES WITH
- Recent serious injury; recent surgery.
- Childbirth.
- Anemia; infection; cancer.
- Use of drugs that cause anaphylactic (allergic) shock as an adverse reaction, such as penicillin, local anesthetics and many others.
- Overdose of mind-altering drugs.
- Excess alcohol consumption.

HOW TO PREVENT—Avoid causes and risk factors when possible.

WHAT TO EXPECT

DIAGNOSTIC MEASURES
- Medical history and physical exam by a doctor.
- Laboratory blood studies to measure the amount of blood in circulation and to measure fluids and electrolytes.

APPROPRIATE HEALTH CARE
- Doctor's treatment.
- Surgery to stop hemorrhaging.
- Hospitalization for intravenous fluids and medications to raise blood pressure and treat the underlying cause.

POSSIBLE COMPLICATIONS
- Cardiac arrest.
- Respiratory arrest.
- Permanent brain damage.

PROBABLE OUTCOME—Usually curable with early diagnosis and treatment. Without treatment, shock can be fatal.

HOW TO TREAT

GENERAL MEASURES—If you observe signs of shock in someone, do the following until medical help arrives:
- Stop external bleeding by applying pressure.
- Keep the victim lying down with legs elevated. Cover the victim for warmth.
- Make sure the victim's airway is open to allow breathing. If breathing stops, give mouth-to-mouth resuscitation. If breathing and pulse stop, give cardiopulmonary resuscitation.

MEDICATION—Depends on the underlying disorder:
- If shock is from blood or fluid loss, treatment includes blood transfusion or intravenous fluids.
- If blood pressure is at a life-threatening low level, hypertensive drugs to raise blood pressure may be given.
- If infection is present, antibiotics will be used.

ACTIVITY—Rest in bed until completely recovered. Move legs actively while in bed to decrease the likelihood of deep-vein blood clots.

DIET—No special diet.

CALL YOUR DOCTOR IF

- You have symptoms of shock or observe them in someone else. Call immediately. This is a life-threatening emergency!
- New, unexplained symptoms develop. Drugs used in treatment may produce side effects.

SHOULDER, FROZEN
(Adhesive Capsulitis)

 GENERAL INFORMATION

DEFINITION—Pain and stiffness in the shoulder joint that progresses to inability to use the shoulder. In this case, "frozen" does not relate to freezing temperatures.

BODY PARTS INVOLVED—Shoulder tendons, bursa, joint capsule, muscles, blood vessels and nerves.

SEX OR AGE MOST AFFECTED—All ages, but most common in athletic adolescents and young adults.

SIGNS & SYMPTOMS
Early stages:
• Pain in the shoulder, often slight, that progresses to severe pain that interferes with sleep and normal activities. Pain worsens with shoulder movement.
• Stiffness in the shoulder that prevents normal movement. Reduced movement increases stiffness.
Later stages:
• Pain in the arm or neck.
• Inability to move the shoulder.
• Intolerable shoulder pain.

CAUSES—Minor shoulder injury or inflammation, such as bursitis or tendinitis, that worsens from lack of use. Adhesions (constricting bands of tissue) form with disuse in 7 to 10 days. Adhesions increase disuse. After 3 weeks of disuse, adhesions grow so severe that the joint cannot move.

RISK INCREASES WITH
• Neglect of minor injuries, including bursitis or tendinitis.
• Poor physical conditioning and occasional athletic activity.
• Diabetes mellitus.
• Peripheral vascular disease.
• Immobilization.
• Sedentary workers.
• Extreme or traumatic sports.

HOW TO PREVENT
• Obtain medical treatment for bursitis and tendinitis, including exercises to prevent formation of adhesions.
• Do regular stretching exercises.

 WHAT TO EXPECT

DIAGNOSTIC MEASURES
• Your own observation of symptoms.
• Medical history and physical exam by a doctor.
• X-rays of the shoulder (arthrography) or MRI (see Glossary) of the shoulder.

APPROPRIATE HEALTH CARE
• Self-care after diagnosis.
• Doctor's treatment, including manipulation of the shoulder to break up adhesions. This is done in a hospital or outpatient surgical facility under general anesthesia.
• Physical therapy and exercises.
• Surgery may be necessary in severe cases to remove adhesions or repair the capsule.

POSSIBLE COMPLICATIONS
• Permanent shoulder disability and pain without treatment or with delayed treatment.
• Tearing of the shoulder capsule due to weakness and scar tissue.

PROBABLE OUTCOME—Usually curable with treatment and rehabilitation (but may take several months). Some heal spontaneously.

 HOW TO TREAT

GENERAL MEASURES
• Wearing a sling may help ease discomfort.
• Application of heat (warm compresses or heating pad) to the affected area helps relieve pain. For some patients, ice may be more helpful.

MEDICATION
• Your doctor may prescribe:
Nonsteroidal anti-inflammatory drugs. Injections of cortisone and local anesthesia into joints to reduce pain and inflammation.
• For minor pain, you may use nonprescription drugs such as aspirin.

ACTIVITY
• Physical therapy and passive shoulder exercises.
• Resume your normal activities as soon as symptoms improve.

DIET—No special diet. Vitamins and mineral supplements don't help unless you can't eat a normal, well-balanced diet.

 CALL YOUR DOCTOR IF

• You have symptoms of a frozen shoulder.
• You have persistent shoulder pain, indicating possible bursitis or tendinitis.
• New, unexplained symptoms develop. Drugs used in treatment may produce side effects.

SICKLE-CELL DISEASE

GENERAL INFORMATION

DEFINITION—An inherited blood disorder that causes anemia, episodes of severe pain, low resistance to infection and chronic poor health. Sickle-cell trait (also called carriers) is a benign condition and never progresses to sickle-cell anemia.

BODY PARTS INVOLVED—Bone marrow; lymph glands; spleen; liver; thymus.

SEX OR AGE MOST AFFECTED—Usually begins around 6 months of age and lasts a lifetime.

SIGNS & SYMPTOMS
- Anemia with shortness of breath, rapid heartbeat, fatigue and jaundice.
- Episodes of pain in joints, chest, abdomen and back.
- Frequent infections, especially pneumonia.
- Nerve impairment.
- Delayed growth and development.
- Skin ulcers, especially on the legs.

CAUSES—This disease is hereditary and occurs mostly in black people. If both parents are carriers of the defective gene, there is a 1 in 4 chance each child will have the disease. The anemia results from red blood cells that contain an abnormal type of hemoglobin called hemoglobin S. Red blood cells change from round to sickle shapes, which causes blockage in the capillaries making the blood more viscous.

RISK INCREASES WITH
- Family history of sickle-cell anemia.
- The following may aggravate symptoms: Ascending to high altitude, as in driving up a mountain or flying; pregnancy; surgery; injury; infection.

HOW TO PREVENT
- If you have a family history of sickle-cell anemia, ask for testing. If you and your partner both have the gene, obtain genetic counseling before starting a family.
- Tests in early pregnancy to determine if unborn child has inherited the double-dose gene (both parents are carriers).

WHAT TO EXPECT

DIAGNOSTIC MEASURES
- Medical history and exam by a doctor.
- Laboratory blood studies. Simple screening tests are also available. They may be done at birth if there is a family history of sickle-cell anemia.
- X-rays, MRI or CT scan (see Glossary for both) of bones and lungs.

APPROPRIATE HEALTH CARE
- Doctor's treatment. Seek a doctor with special knowledge of this condition.
- Treatment at home involves general health care maintenance and prompt treatment of any infection and sickle-cell crises.
- Hospitalization may be required at times.
- Get regular eye exams to check for eye complications.
- Psychotherapy or counseling may be helpful.

POSSIBLE COMPLICATIONS
- Persons with sickle-cell trait may be at risk of death while engaged in strenuous exercise.
- Infections of lungs and bones; kidney failure; eye disease; stroke.
- Impaired growth; gallstones; enlarged heart.

PROBABLE OUTCOME—Sickle-cell anemia is incurable and life expectancy is reduced. However, life span has gradually increased to over 40 years with increasingly effective treatments. People with the disorder can lead productive lives and are able to hold jobs, raise families and maintain a normal lifestyle.

HOW TO TREAT

GENERAL MEASURES
- Maintain immunization schedule, including a pneumonia vaccine. Promptly treat infections.
- Practice good oral hygiene and get regular dental checkups.
- Parents should avoid being too overly protective. Most everyday activities are tolerated without problems.
- Wear a Medic-Alert bracelet or pendant (see Glossary).
- See Resources for Additional Information.

MEDICATION—No medications are yet available to control this condition. For severe attacks, intravenous fluids, blood transfusions, antibiotics and pain relievers may be used. Prophylactic penicillin may be started in infancy.

ACTIVITY
- Avoid strenuous exercise and exposure to cold temperatures. Rest in bed during acute attacks.
- Activity may be limited due to chronic anemia and poor muscular development.

DIET—Drink at least 8 glasses of water a day—more if you have a fever. This helps keep blood cells from collecting and blocking capillaries.

CALL YOUR DOCTOR IF

- You want to know if you have the sickle-cell gene.
- Symptoms recur after a period of remission or you develop fever or other signs of infection.

SILICOSIS

GENERAL INFORMATION

DEFINITION—Inflammation of the lung due to breathing silica (quartz) dust. Silicosis is the most common form of pneumoconiosis (a group of lung diseases caused by inhaling certain mineral dusts).

BODY PARTS INVOLVED—Lungs.

SEX OR AGE MOST AFFECTED—Men and women over age 40.

SIGNS & SYMPTOMS
Early symptoms:
- Shortness of breath.
- Cough that produces little or no sputum.
- General ill feeling.

Late symptoms:
- Fitful sleep; appetite loss.
- Chest pain; hoarseness.
- Coughing blood.
- Symptoms of heart failure; bluish nails.

CAUSES—Chronic inhalation of small particles of free crystalline silica (silicon dioxide). Usually takes 20 to 30 years of exposure, but possibly less than 10 years if exposure is extremely high.

RISK INCREASES WITH
- Work such as mining, granite-cutting, manufacturing pottery, metal-grinding, tunneling and sand-blasting.
- Poor nutrition; smoking.

HOW TO PREVENT
- During exposure to silica, wear a protective mask or external-air-supplied hood.
- Don't smoke.
- Participate in a regular physical exercise program to maintain cardiopulmonary fitness.

WHAT TO EXPECT

DIAGNOSTIC MEASURES
- Medical history and exam by a doctor.
- X-ray of the chest, pulmonary function tests and bronchoscopy (see Bronchoscopy in Surgery section).

APPROPRIATE HEALTH CARE
- Self-care after diagnosis.
- Doctor's treatment.
- There is no overall effective treatment available for silicosis. Treatment is directed to relieving respiratory symptoms, manage complications and prevent infections.

POSSIBLE COMPLICATIONS
- Tuberculosis (late stages of silicosis).
- Heart failure due to lung disease.
- Lung collapse; pleurisy; lung cancer.

PROBABLE OUTCOME—This condition is currently considered incurable. Life expectancy is reduced. Silicosis causes increasing respiratory disability. However, symptoms can be relieved or controlled. Scientific research into causes and treatment continues, so there is hope for increasingly effective treatment.

HOW TO TREAT

GENERAL MEASURES
- No effective treatment is known for silicosis.
- The following measures may relieve symptoms and protect against recurrent lung infections:
  Obtain medical treatment for any respiratory infection, including the common cold.
  Prevent infections by avoiding crowds and persons with respiratory infections.
  Get influenza and pneumococcal vaccinations.
  Consider moving to a warm, dry climate if you have advanced disease.
  Chest physical therapy (such as controlled coughing) and bronchial drainage help clear secretions. Get medical training about these procedures.
  Use a cool-mist, ultrasonic humidifier to loosen bronchial secretions so they may be coughed up easily. Clean humidifier daily.
- See Resources for Additional Information.

MEDICATION
- Your doctor may prescribe:
  Antibiotics for infections.
  Bronchodilators (inhaled or oral) with inhalation therapy (supervised at first by an inhalation therapist) to open bronchial tubes to the maximum.
- For minor discomfort, you may use nonprescription drugs, such as acetaminophen or aspirin.

ACTIVITY
- Rest in bed with infections.
- After treatment, resume normal activity as soon as symptoms improve. Pace yourself, rest often and plan daily activities to minimize breathing difficulties.

DIET—No special diet. Maintain high fluid intake.

CALL YOUR DOCTOR IF

- You have symptoms of silicosis.
- The following occurs during treatment:
  Fever.
  Increased chest pain or breathlessness.
  Blood in the sputum.
  Continuing weight loss.
  Confusion or lethargy.
- New, unexplained symptoms develop. Drugs used in treatment may produce side effects.

SINUSITIS

GENERAL INFORMATION

DEFINITION—Inflammation of the sinuses adjacent to the nose. The disorder may be acute (usually caused by an allergy or virus) or chronic (often a bacterial infection such as Staphylococcus).

BODY PARTS INVOLVED—The 8 sinuses (mucosa-lined air pockets) located within the facial bone structure and connected to the nose. Usually involved are the ethmoidal sinuses, located between the eyes; and the maxillary sinuses, located in the cheekbone.

SEX OR AGE MOST AFFECTED—Both sexes; all ages.

SIGNS & SYMPTOMS
- Nasal congestion with green-yellow (sometimes blood-tinged) discharge.
- Feeling of pressure inside the head.
- Headache that is worse in the morning or when bending forward. With chronic sinusitis, the headache may occur daily for weeks at a time.
- Cheek pain that may resemble a toothache.
- Post-nasal drip.
- Cough (sometimes) that is usually nonproductive.
- Tiredness; lack of energy; disturbed sleep (sometimes); fever (sometimes); eye pain.

CAUSES—The sinuses add moisture (by producing mucus) to the air we breath. With sinusitis, the normal draining of this mucus is disrupted; fluid accumulates and becomes infected. Common causes include:
- Allergies; acute or chronic rhinitis (hay fever).
- Environmental irritants (tobacco smoke, dry air, other pollutants).
- Nasal polyps; deviated septum.
- Viral infection; fungal infection; surgical packing.

RISK INCREASES WITH
- Illness that has lowered resistance.
- Exposure to infected people.
- Immunosuppression due to illness or drugs.
- Swimming or diving injury.
- Abscessed tooth.

HOW TO PREVENT—Try to prevent the respiratory conditions that usually precede sinusitis (allergies, colds, flu), and if they do occur, treat them promptly. Avoid smoking.

WHAT TO EXPECT

DIAGNOSTIC MEASURES
- Medical history and exam by a doctor.
- Diagnostic tests (depending on severity of infection and chronicity) may include laboratory blood studies, culture of mucus, endoscopy (see Glossary), x-rays or CT scan (see Glossary) of the sinuses.

APPROPRIATE HEALTH CARE
- Self-care.
- Doctor's treatment.
- Chronic sinusitis not responding to other treatment may require surgery to drain blocked sinuses.

POSSIBLE COMPLICATIONS
- Meningitis or brain abscess (rare).
- Infection of bone or bone marrow (rare).
- Infections of the eye.

PROBABLE OUTCOME—Acute sinusitis usually clears up in 3 weeks with treatment. Recurrence is common and may lead to chronic sinusitis, which may require prolonged treatment with antibiotics (4-6 weeks).

HOW TO TREAT

GENERAL MEASURES
- Warm moist air may help relieve sinus congestion. Use a vaporizer or breathe steam from a pan of boiled water (after removing it from the heat).
- Use warm compresses to relieve pain in the sinuses and nose.
- Don't allow other persons to use your nose drops. They will be contaminated.
- Avoid decongestant nose drops or sprays. Use prescribed drops only for the recommended time. They can interfere with normal nasal and sinus function and become addictive, causing a rebound phenomenon (see Glossary). Ask your doctor about using saline nose drops (they are usually safe).

MEDICATION
- Your doctor may prescribe: Nasal sprays, nose drops or oral decongestant medicine to reduce congestion. Antibiotics for any bacterial infection (antibiotics are not effective against viral infections).
- Antihistamines for allergies.
- Antihistamine nasal sprays such as Cromolyn.
- Antifungal medicine for any fungal infection.
- For minor pain, you may use nonprescription drugs such as acetaminophen.

ACTIVITY—Resume normal activities slowly.

DIET—No special diet, but drink extra fluids to help thin secretions.

CALL YOUR DOCTOR IF

The following occurs during treatment: Fever; bleeding from the nose; severe headache. Swelling of the face (forehead, eyes, side of the nose or cheek). Blurred vision or other eye symptoms.

SJÖGREN'S SYNDROME

GENERAL INFORMATION

DEFINITION—The second most common autoimmune, rheumatic disorder (after rheumatoid arthritis). It may be a primary disorder or be associated with other connective tissue disorders (rheumatoid arthritis, scleroderma, systemic lupus erythematous, polymyositis).

BODY PARTS INVOLVED—May involve only the exocrine (mucus secreting) glands or involve other organs, such as the lung or kidneys.

SEX OR AGE MOST AFFECTED—Average age of occurrence is 50 and 90% of patients are female.

SIGNS & SYMPTOMS
- Dryness of the eyes that can cause foreign body sensation, gritty feeling, redness, burning, sensitivity to light, itching, a sensation of a "film" across the vision field and eye discharge.
- Dryness of the mouth that can cause difficulty in swallowing and talking, abnormal taste or smell, thirst, ulcers, dental cavities.
- Dryness of the vagina that can cause painful intercourse.
- Dryness of the upper respiratory tract that can cause nosebleeds, hoarseness, chronic nonproductive cough, ear infection, other respiratory infections.
- Parotid gland enlargement (sometimes referred to as "chipmunk face").
- Joint inflammation.
- Other symptoms include hair loss, generalized itching, fatigue, low-grade fever, muscle pain.

CAUSES—Unknown. Genetic, immunologic, hormonal and environmental factors may contribute to its development. Viral infection may trigger disorder in susceptible individual.

RISK INCREASES WITH
- Family history of autoimmune disorders.
- Rheumatoid arthritis.
- Scleroderma.
- Systemic lupus erythematosus.
- Polymyositis.

HOW TO PREVENT—No specific measures.

WHAT TO EXPECT

DIAGNOSTIC MEASURES
- Medical history and exam by a doctor.
- Tests may include the Schirmer's test to measure quantity of tears produced in 5 minutes, other eye examinations, salivary flow studies, lip biopsy, and studies of the blood and urine.

APPROPRIATE HEALTH CARE
- Doctor's treatment.
- Treatment is directed to relieving the dryness of the eyes, mouth and other body parts.

POSSIBLE COMPLICATIONS
- Pulmonary infection.
- Increased disability.
- Renal failure (rare).
- Lymphoma (rare).

PROBABLE OUTCOME—Sjögren's syndrome is a chronic disorder and the prognosis is often related to an associated disorder. Treatment can relieve symptoms and help prevent complications.

HOW TO TREAT

GENERAL MEASURES
- Meticulous oral hygiene is important. Regular dental visits should be scheduled.
- Wear sunglasses when outside to help protect eyes from dust, wind and strong light. Special moisture chamber spectacles may be helpful.
- Avoid rubbing the eyes.
- Soft contact lenses may be prescribed.
- Use a cool-mist, ultrasonic humidifier in the home. Clean humidifier daily.
- Avoid prolonged hot showers or baths.
- Warm compresses or heating pad may help ease joint pain or swollen gland discomfort.
- Avoid decongestants and antihistamines. They cause dry mouth.
- See Resources for Additional Information.

MEDICATION—Your doctor may prescribe:
- Artificial tears for eye dryness.
- Methylcellulose swab or spray for mouth dryness.
- Normal saline solution drops or aerosolized spray for respiratory dryness.
- K-Y Jelly as a lubricant for vaginal dryness.
- Corticosteroids and immunosuppressants for patients with severe symptoms.
- Nystatin for mouth infections.

ACTIVITY—No restrictions, but may be limited by symptoms.

DIET
- Avoid sugar, which contributes to dental caries.
- To ease mouth dryness, chew sugarless gum or suck on sugarless candies.
- Drink plenty of fluids, especially at mealtime.
- If mouth soreness prevents eating regular foods, drink high-calorie, high-protein liquid supplements to prevent malnutrition.

CALL YOUR DOCTOR IF

Symptoms worsen or don't improve with treatment.

SKIN CANCER, BASAL-CELL

GENERAL INFORMATION

DEFINITION—Skin cancer affecting skin's basal layer. Basal-cell skin cancer invades areas under skin, but rarely does it spread to distant areas.

BODY PARTS INVOLVED—Skin of face, ears, backs of hands, shoulders and arms.

SEX OR AGE MOST AFFECTED
- Both sexes.
- Adults 40 and older.

SIGNS & SYMPTOMS—A small skin lesion that does not heal in 3 weeks with the following characteristics:
- The lesion appears flat and "pearly." Its edges are translucent and rounded or rolled. The edges may have small, curvy, new blood vessels. The ulcer in the center is dimpled. Lesion size varies from 4mm to 6mm, but it may grow larger if untreated.
- The lesion occurs on skin that is exposed to the sun and shows evidence of sun damage.
- The lesion grows slowly. It does not hurt or itch. It may alternately crust and heal.

CAUSES—Skin damage from sun that occurs many years prior to the cancer's appearance.

RISK INCREASES WITH
- Adults over 60.
- Exposure to excess sunlight.
- Fair skin complexion.

HOW TO PREVENT
- Limit exposure to sun. Protect skin from sun exposure with a hat, clothing and sunscreen with protective factor of 15 or more.
- Perform a skin self-exam once a month (see Skin Self-exam in Appendix).

WHAT TO EXPECT

DIAGNOSTIC MEASURES
- Your own observation of symptoms.
- Medical history and physical exam by a doctor.
- Pathological exam of tissue after removal to confirm diagnosis.

APPROPRIATE HEALTH CARE
- Treatment selection varies with appearance, extent and location of the lesion.
- Removal of cancer by one of the following methods. The treatment method is chosen in a doctor-patient conference:
1. Curettage and electrodesiccation—local anesthetic applied, then cutting out or shaving of lesion, followed by high-frequency electrical current to destroy tissue with heat.
2. Surgical excision—local anesthetic is applied, then skin is marked for surgery, and a scalpel is used for the excision.

3. Moh's surgery—a specialized type of excisional surgery used to treat high-risk cancers.
4. Cryosurgery—use of liquid nitrogen to freeze and kill the cells. A local anesthetic is sometimes used.
5. Laser treatment—is being used in some medical centers.
6. Radiation treatment—used if tumor location requires it, such as locations near lips and eyelids.

POSSIBLE COMPLICATIONS—Without treatment, cancers may enlarge, ulcerate and disfigure. Less than 1% spread to other sites, but they should be removed to prevent local damage.

PROBABLE OUTCOME—Curable with proper treatment. Over a third of the patients will develop a new lesion within 5 years.

HOW TO TREAT

GENERAL MEASURES—After surgery:
- Apply rubbing alcohol to the scab twice a day.
- Apply an adhesive bandage to the scab during the day. Leave it uncovered at night.
- Wash the wound as usual. Dry gently and completely after bathing or swimming.

MEDICATION
- For minor pain, you may use nonprescription drugs, such as acetaminophen or aspirin.
- Your doctor may prescribe an antibiotic ointment to prevent wound infection.

ACTIVITY—No restrictions.

DIET—No special diet.

CALL YOUR DOCTOR IF

- You have symptoms of basal-cell skin cancer.
- The wound bleeds after surgery and the bleeding cannot be stopped by applying pressure for 10 minutes.
- The wound shows signs of infection, such as pain, redness, swelling or increased tenderness.

ILLNESS & DISORDERS

SKIN CANCER, SQUAMOUS-CELL

GENERAL INFORMATION

DEFINITION—A malignant growth of the epithelial layer (external surface) of the skin.

BODY PARTS INVOLVED—Skin in areas exposed to the sun, such as the face, ears, hands or arms.

SEX OR AGE MOST AFFECTED—Adults over 40.

SIGNS & SYMPTOMS—A small, disfiguring, scaling, raised bump on the skin with a crusting ulcer in the center. The bump doesn't hurt or itch.

CAUSES
- Excessive exposure to sunlight.
- Skin damaged by radiation.
- Immunosuppression due to illness or drugs.
- Exposure to coal tar, other oil and tar derivatives.

RISK INCREASES WITH
- Adults over 60.
- Light complexion.
- Recent illness with chronic skin ulcers from any cause.
- Outdoor occupation.
- Occupation or treatment requiring exposure to X-rays.
- Actinic keratosis (see in Illness section).

HOW TO PREVENT
- Wear sunscreen (sun-protective factor of 15 or more) or hat and protective clothing to protect skin from sun damage.
- Perform monthly self-exams of your skin, especially if you have had previous skin cancers (see Skin Self-exam in Appendix).

WHAT TO EXPECT

DIAGNOSTIC MEASURES
- Your own observation of symptoms.
- Medical history and physical exam by a doctor.
- Biopsy (see Glossary).

APPROPRIATE HEALTH CARE
- Doctor's treatment.
- Treatment selection varies with appearance, extent and location of the lesion.
- Removal of cancer by one of the following methods. The treatment method is chosen in a doctor-patient conference:
1. Curettage and electrodesiccation—local anesthetic applied, then cutting out or shaving of lesion, followed by high-frequency electrical current to destroy tissue with heat.
2. Surgical excision—local anesthetic, then skin is marked for surgery, and a scalpel is used for the excision.
3. Moh's surgery—a specialized type of excisional surgery used to treat high-risk cancers.
4. Cryosurgery—use of liquid nitrogen to freeze and kill the cells. A local anesthetic is often used.
5. Laser treatment—is being used in some medical centers.
6. Radiation treatment—used if tumor location requires it, such as locations near lips and eyelids.

POSSIBLE COMPLICATIONS
- Must be treated again in 10% of cases.
- Cancer will spread to other tissue if untreated (rare).

PROBABLE OUTCOME—Curable with appropriate treatment.

HOW TO TREAT

GENERAL MEASURES
After surgery:
- Apply diluted hydrogen peroxide or sterile saline solution to the scab twice a day.
- Apply an adhesive bandage to the scab during the day. Leave it uncovered at night.
- Wash the wound as usual. Dry gently and completely after bathing or swimming.

MEDICATION
- For minor discomfort, you may use nonprescription drugs such as acetaminophen.
- Your doctor may prescribe topical antibiotic ointment or cream to prevent infection after surgery.

ACTIVITY—After treatment, resume normal activity as soon as possible.

DIET—No special diet.

CALL YOUR DOCTOR IF

- You have symptoms of squamous-cell skin cancer.
- The following occurs after treatment:
  Redness, swelling, bleeding or tenderness at the treatment site.
  Pain that is not controlled by nonprescription pain relievers.
- The sore has not healed 3 weeks after treatment.

SKIN LESIONS, BENIGN

GENERAL INFORMATION

DEFINITION—Noncancerous growths or areas of pigment or color change on the skin.

BODY PARTS INVOLVED—Skin.

SEX OR AGE MOST AFFECTED—Both sexes; all ages.

SIGNS & SYMPTOMS—Benign skin lesions fall into the following categories:
- Tags—Soft, flesh-colored buds, often on stalks, found on the neck, armpits or groin.
- Moles—Flat or raised lesions with clearly defined borders. Moles may be black, blue, red, yellow or brown.
- Cherry spots—Pinhead-sized, bright-red lesions on the chest or back.
- Strawberry marks—Bright-red raised areas in infants that grow until they are removed.
- Keloids—Thick, pale, irregular growths that begin at the site of a scar and gradually increase in size.
- Dermatofibromas—Rounded nodules, usually brownish and usually on the legs.
- Freckles—Flat, brownish spots of pinhead-size or larger.

CAUSES—Unknown, but most people have a few benign skin lesions.

RISK INCREASES WITH
- Family history of benign skin lesions.
- Pregnancy or use of oral contraceptives (brownish, freckle-like patches only).

HOW TO PREVENT—To decrease freckles, avoid excessive sun exposure. Other forms cannot be prevented.

WHAT TO EXPECT

DIAGNOSTIC MEASURES
- Your own observation of symptoms.
- Medical history and physical exam by a doctor.
- Rarely, skin biopsy (see Glossary).

APPROPRIATE HEALTH CARE
- Self-care after diagnosis.
- Doctor's treatment.
- Surgery to remove lesions that enlarge, bleed, change color, are slow to heal or are unsightly. (See Skin Lesion Removal in Surgery section.)
- Radiation treatment following removal of keloids to prevent their recurrence.

POSSIBLE COMPLICATIONS
- Malignant change in moles.
- Bleeding in strawberry marks.

PROBABLE OUTCOME—Treatment is usually unnecessary because most skin lesions are harmless. Suspicious or unsightly lesions can be removed surgically. If the affected area is large or in a prominent place, plastic surgery may be necessary after removal.

HOW TO TREAT

GENERAL MEASURES
- Examine skin lesions—especially those that are constantly rubbed or irritated by clothing—regularly for signs of growth, color change, pain, infection or bleeding. (See Skin Self-exam in Appendix.)
- If a lesion is removed, cover the area with a clean dressing and protect against injury. Ointments are rarely needed.

MEDICATION—Medicine usually is not necessary for this disorder. Makeup may be helpful in covering unsightly blemishes.

ACTIVITY—No restrictions.

DIET—No special diet.

CALL YOUR DOCTOR IF

You have a skin lesion that enlarges, bleeds, changes color, is painful or doesn't heal.

SLEEP APNEA

GENERAL INFORMATION

DEFINITION—Episodes of cessation of breathing, during sleep, that last 10 seconds or longer.

BODY PARTS INVOLVED—Central nervous system.

SEX OR AGE MOST AFFECTED—All ages, but most common in adults over 60.

SIGNS & SYMPTOMS
- Long periods (up to 1 or 2 minutes) of not breathing while asleep. Sleep apnea must be observed by others—it is most reliably recorded in a sleep laboratory.
- Choking while asleep caused by obstruction in the back of the throat from the uvula and other loose tissue. This causes cycles of sleep, choking, startled awakening, drowsiness and sleep. The cycles often continue throughout the day because poor sleep causes chronic sleepiness.

CAUSES
- Unknown (often).
- Airway obstruction, especially in obese patients.
- Chronic respiratory-system disease.
- Central-nervous-system disorder, such as a brain tumor, viral brain infection or stroke.

RISK INCREASES WITH
- Stress, including anxiety and depression.
- Persons with high blood pressure, cardiovascular or arteriovascular disease.
- Senility; obesity; smoking; excess alcohol consumption; use of mind-altering drugs; hypothyroidism.

HOW TO PREVENT—If you have an underlying disease listed as a cause of sleep apnea, avoid as many risk factors as possible to decrease the chance of triggering the disorder.

WHAT TO EXPECT

DIAGNOSTIC MEASURES
- Observation of symptoms by someone close to you.
- Medical history and exam by a doctor.
- Laboratory studies to measure oxygen in blood, chest-wall movement and air flow through nose.
- EEG (see Glossary).
- Studies in a sleep laboratory.

APPROPRIATE HEALTH CARE
- Doctor's treatment.
- Treatment choice will depend on severity of apnea, any health problems, and level of daytime functioning.
- Steps should be taken to improve any underlying medical problems.

- A special dental appliance may be prescribed.
- Continuous positive airway pressure (CPAP)—patient wears a mask over nose and mouth during sleep while a small air-compressor forces air into the nasal passages keeping the airway open. It is an effective treatment for many patients.
- Treatment can include surgery, such as tonsillectomy, uvulopalatopharyngoplasty (to enlarge the larynx) or tracheostomy (rare).

POSSIBLE COMPLICATIONS
- Excessive daytime sleepiness (EDT), due to lack of sleep, may lead to accidents, inattentiveness and lowered work productivity.
- Increased risk of stroke and heart attack.
- Heartbeat irregularities and congestive heart failure.

PROBABLE OUTCOME—Treatment measures, other than surgery and weight loss in an obese patient, are directed at controlling the sleep apnea rather than curing it. Lifelong compliance to therapy is usually necessary.

HOW TO TREAT

GENERAL MEASURES
- If sleep apnea occurs only when you sleep on your back, sew a ping-pong ball or tennis ball to the back of your pajamas. This forces you to sleep on your side.
- Drugs such as sedatives, hypnotics, barbiturates, narcotics, and alcohol should be avoided. Get medical advice about withdrawing medications that may be causing sleep apnea.

MEDICATION—Medicine usually is not necessary for this disorder; however, protriptyline may be helpful for a small number of patients to help control daytime sleepiness.

ACTIVITY
- No restrictions. Engage in regular physical exercise to become physically fit, but don't exercise vigorously before bedtime.
- Be cautious about driving and hazardous activities if you suffer from daytime sleepiness.

DIET
- Lose weight if you are obese (see Weight Loss Diet in Appendix). Obesity may be the cause of the apnea
- Avoid alcohol.

CALL YOUR DOCTOR IF

- You suspect you have sleep apnea.
- You observe signs of sleep apnea in another family member.

SMALL-INTESTINE TUMOR
(Small-Bowel Neoplasms)

GENERAL INFORMATION

DEFINITION—Abnormal new growth in the small intestine or spread of abnormal cell growth from surrounding body structure. Most are benign; only 10% of small-intestine tumors are cancerous. Small-intestine tumors are uncommon compared to large intestine tumors.

BODY PARTS INVOLVED—Small intestine.

SEX OR AGE MOST AFFECTED—All ages, but most likely in adults.

SIGNS & SYMPTOMS
- No symptoms (50% of the time with benign tumors).
- Tiredness.
- Paleness.
- Blood in stools or black, tarry stools.
- Unexplained weight loss.
- Jaundice (yellow skin and eyes).

CAUSES—Unknown.

RISK INCREASES WITH
- Celiac disease.
- Regional enteritis.
- Gardner syndrome.
- Peutz-Jeghers syndrome.
- Immunosuppression due to illness or drugs.

HOW TO PREVENT—No specific preventive measures.

WHAT TO EXPECT

DIAGNOSTIC MEASURES
- Your own observation of symptoms.
- Medical history and physical exam by a doctor.
- Laboratory blood studies for anemia.
- X-rays of the intestinal tract (upper and lower GI series).
- Abdominal ultrasound and CT scan; endoscopy and enteroscopy (see Glossary for all). Tests are done to determine any cancerous growth and spread.

APPROPRIATE HEALTH CARE
- Doctor's treatment.
- Surgery to remove the tumor if it is benign and causing symptoms and for malignant tumors.
- Radiation treatment (sometimes).
- Self-care after surgery or during treatment.

POSSIBLE COMPLICATIONS—Intestinal obstruction. Symptoms are: distended abdomen; severe colicky pain; nausea, vomiting; fever.

PROBABLE OUTCOME—With surgery the prognosis for benign tumors is good; with malignant tumors, the prognosis depends on the type of malignancy found and if it can be completely removed with surgery.

HOW TO TREAT

GENERAL MEASURES
- The more you can learn and understand about this disorder, the more you will be able to make informed decisions about where to go for your care, the treatments available, the risks involved, side effects of therapy and expected outcome.
- See Resources for Additional Information.

MEDICATION—Your doctor may prescribe:
- Anticancer drugs.
- Cortisone drugs to reduce bowel inflammation that may cause obstruction.

ACTIVITY—No restrictions. Resume normal activities as soon as possible after surgery.

DIET—Your doctor may prescribe a special diet following surgery or during treatment with radiation or anticancer drugs.

CALL YOUR DOCTOR IF

- You have symptoms of a tumor of the small intestine.
- You have symptoms of intestinal obstruction (see Possible Complications).
- New, unexplained symptoms develop during treatment. Drugs used in treatment may produce side effects.

SNAKEBITE

GENERAL INFORMATION

DEFINITION—Bite from a poisonous snake. Bites on the extremities are most common, but bites on the head and trunk are most dangerous. Not all bites involve actual injection of venom.

BODY PARTS INVOLVED—Exposed skin; blood; lymphatic system.

SEX OR AGE MOST AFFECTED—Both sexes; all ages.

SIGNS & SYMPTOMS—Will vary depending on the species. May include:
- Severe pain and swelling around the bite.
- Weakness and dizziness.
- Irregular heart beat.
- Excessive sweating.
- Low blood pressure and shock.
- Nausea and vomiting.
- Numbness and tingling around the mouth and in the hands and feet.
- Breathing difficulty.
- Blurred vision.
- Seizures; coma.
- Fever; headache.
- Multiple fang marks and small cuts, if the bite is from a coral snake. Symptoms may not appear for 3 to 4 hours.
- Deep single or double fang marks, if the bite is from another snake. Symptoms begin quickly.
- Skin discoloration that resembles bruising around the bite.
- Bleeding spots under the skin all over the body.

CAUSES—Bite from a poisonous snake, including pit vipers (rattlesnake, copperhead, water moccasin) and coral snake. Coral snakes are nocturnal and placid (their bites are less common than pit vipers).

RISK INCREASES WITH
- Outdoor activities during warm months in areas where poisonous snakes are abundant.
- Risk-taking behaviors; alcohol consumption.

HOW TO PREVENT—Wear protective shoes, boots and clothing for hiking, camping, fishing and hunting. Prevent complications by carrying a snakebite kit and instructions. Avoid alcohol while participating in these outdoor activities.

WHAT TO EXPECT

DIAGNOSTIC MEASURES
- If possible, identify the snake, but don't waste time looking for it.
- Physical exam, laboratory blood studies, urinalysis and other tests as needed to monitor vital signs.

APPROPRIATE HEALTH CARE
- Administer first aid, then emergency room care for treatment and monitoring. Remove rings or constrictive items close to the bite. Place affected part at same level as the heart. Immobilize the patient horizontally and transport to medical care immediately. Do not give alcohol, do not apply ice, do not apply a tourniquet. Skin incisions are not recommended unless the person has medical training.
- Hospitalization for mechanical breathing support if needed, dialysis treatment if kidneys stop working, cardiac and neurological monitoring.
- Surgical debridement (removal of dead or contaminated tissue) after 3 or 4 days.

POSSIBLE COMPLICATIONS
- Gangrene, requiring amputation of the affected part.
- Aspiration pneumonia.
- Shock.
- Convulsions.

PROBABLE OUTCOME—Usually curable with early and proper medical care. Often with bites from poisonous snakes, little or no venom is injected.

HOW TO TREAT

GENERAL MEASURES—Don't panic! Venom will spread more quickly through the body if the victim runs or becomes excited.

MEDICATION—Your doctor may prescribe:
- Antivenin to neutralize snake poison.
- Tetanus booster injection.
- Antibiotics to prevent infection.
- Pain relievers. (Narcotics cannot be used for coral-snake bites. They may cause shock.)

ACTIVITY—Resume normal activities as soon as symptoms improve.

DIET—No special diet.

CALL YOUR DOCTOR IF

- You or someone you are with receives a snakebite.
- New, unexplained symptoms develop. Drugs used in treatment may produce side effects.

SODIUM IMBALANCE

GENERAL INFORMATION

DEFINITION—Above normal sodium level (hypernatremia) or below normal sodium level (hyponatremia) in the blood. Sodium helps regulate the body's water balance, maintains normal heart rhythm, and is responsible for the conduction of nerve impulses and the contraction of muscles.

BODY PARTS INVOLVED—All body cells.

SEX OR AGE MOST AFFECTED—Both sexes; all ages.

SIGNS & SYMPTOMS
- Confusion.
- Restlessness and anxiety.
- Weakness.
- Muscle cramps (usually in the legs).
- Changes in pulse rate and blood pressure.
- Tissue swelling (edema).
- Stupor or coma (if severe imbalance).
Sodium imbalance may be part of a disease with other symptoms that predominate, such as fever, vomiting, diarrhea or excessive sweating.

CAUSES
Hyponatremia:
- Prolonged loss of body fluids from vomiting or diarrhea.
- Addison's disease.
- Congestive heart failure.
- Prolonged, excessive drinking of water. (This is usually a psychiatric condition.)
- Some cancers of the adrenal glands.
- Infections with high fever.
Hypernatremia:
- Inability to drink water, as with stroke or gastrointestinal diseases.
- Use of cortisone drugs.
- Excessive intake of salty food or liquid, as in near-drowning in salt water.

RISK INCREASES WITH
- Diabetes mellitus.
- Congestive heart failure.
- Use of diuretics.
- Kidney diseases. Healthy kidneys can usually control sodium levels.

HOW TO PREVENT—Because sodium disturbance is the result of underlying disease, obtain early medical treatment to prevent a sodium imbalance.

WHAT TO EXPECT

DIAGNOSTIC MEASURES
- Your own observation of symptoms.
- Medical history and physical exam by a doctor.
- Laboratory blood and urine studies of sodium and other electrolytes.

APPROPRIATE HEALTH CARE
- Self-care after diagnosis and treatment.
- Doctor's treatment.
- If a drug is the cause for sodium imbalance (above or below normal), it may be discontinued or dosage lowered.
- For below normal sodium levels, water restriction is usually the therapy. This will increase the sodium levels in the body. It is important that the treatment not overcorrect the sodium levels as that can be dangerous.
- For above normal levels of sodium, administration of fluids (such as dextrose in water) to return sodium levels to normal is the usual therapy.

POSSIBLE COMPLICATIONS—Shock and death.

PROBABLE OUTCOME—Usually can be corrected with intravenous fluids and treatment of the underlying disorder.

HOW TO TREAT

GENERAL MEASURES—If you have a disorder or take drugs that affect sodium balance, learn as much as possible about your drugs, your condition and how to prevent a sodium imbalance.

MEDICATION—Your doctor may prescribe:
- Intravenous sodium if sodium levels are low.
- Diuretics to decrease high sodium levels.
- Medications to correct underlying disorders.

ACTIVITY—Limit activity until stable, or underlying condition resolved or controlled. Resume your normal activities after recovery.

DIET—No special diet for low sodium levels. Most persons with high sodium levels benefit from a low-salt diet (see Reduced Sodium Diet in Appendix). Low-salt diets contain enough sodium to prevent hyponatremia. However, sodium levels are not influenced by diet alone.

CALL YOUR DOCTOR IF

- You have symptoms of a sodium imbalance.
- You are having problems with a disorder that affects sodium levels.

SORES, PRESSURE
(Bed Sores; Decubitus Ulcers)

 GENERAL INFORMATION

DEFINITION—Skin ulcerations, usually in an area of pressure over a bony prominence. Pressure sores are not contagious or cancerous.

BODY PARTS INVOLVED—Skin over pressure points in the lower back, buttocks, elbows, knees, shoulders, heels, ankles and other areas with bony prominences.

SEX OR AGE MOST AFFECTED—All ages, but most likely in the elderly.

SIGNS & SYMPTOMS—Spots of skin that are red and shiny. Spots progress to blisters, then ulcers, leading to a breakdown of tissue under the ulcer. Ulcers are usually painless.

CAUSES—Constant pressure on the skin, especially over bony areas. Pressure reduces the blood supply, causing death in the tissue layers. Pressure sores usually develop in persons who cannot move because of chronic illness or disability that confines them to bed.

RISK INCREASES WITH
- Adults over 60.
- Poor circulation.
- Decreased or absent sensation.
- Malnutrition.
- Obesity.
- Illness or accident requiring prolonged bed confinement, especially with unsanitary living conditions and wrinkled or wet bed linen.

HOW TO PREVENT—Provide good nursing care for the disabled, including the following:
- Daily skin inspection in good light.
- Frequent changes of position in bed (hourly may be necessary).
- Control of fecal or urinary incontinence.
- Protective, soft padding, such as gel flotation pads or sheepskin, over bony areas.
- A water mattress, egg-crate rubber mattress or alternating-pressure mattress.
- Specialized air bed.
- Dry, clean, smooth bed linen.
- Frequent inspection of skin areas at risk.

 WHAT TO EXPECT

DIAGNOSTIC MEASURES
- Your own observation of symptoms.
- Medical history and physical exam by a doctor.

APPROPRIATE HEALTH CARE
- Home care.
- Doctor's treatment.
- Surgery to remove dead tissue (sometimes).

POSSIBLE COMPLICATIONS
- Local or general infection.
- Infection of bone (osteomyelitis) adjacent to the ulcer.

PROBABLE OUTCOME—Usually curable with treatment. Sores may heal very slowly. Healing time varies with the site and size of the ulcer and the patient's general health.

 HOW TO TREAT

GENERAL MEASURES
- Provide good nursing care for the patient (see How to Prevent).
- Provide warm whirlpool treatments, if a pressure sore is on an arm, hand, foot or leg.
- Apply lotions or ointment if prescribed by your doctor. Apply a thin layer of the cream, ointment or lotion 3 or 4 times daily. A heavy layer wastes medicine and is no more beneficial than a thin layer. Rub in gently for several minutes until it disappears.
- Use saline or peroxide on gauze pad to clean the sore and pat dry. Avoid harsh soaps, tincture of benzoin or hexachlorophene.
- Special dressings for sores may be prescribed.

MEDICATION
- Your doctor may prescribe:
  Antibiotics to fight infection.
  Ointments, dressings and drying agents, such as zinc oxide, granulated sugar, povidone-iodine packs or 3% hydrogen peroxide.
- Avoid harsh soaps, tincture of benzoin or hexachlorophene.

ACTIVITY
- Change the position of an immobilized patient every 1-2 hours. A wheelchair patient should change position every 10-15 minutes.
- Passive or active exercises (if the patient is able).

DIET—Normal, well-balanced diet that includes extra protein. Vitamin and mineral supplements may be necessary.

 CALL YOUR DOCTOR IF

- You have symptoms of pressure sores or observe them in someone else.
- The following occurs during treatment:
  Skin inflammation or breakdown.
  Signs of infection, such as: pain, redness, tenderness, swelling or increased warmth of the affected area.
  Fever.

SPINAL-CORD TUMOR

GENERAL INFORMATION

DEFINITION—An abnormal growth that compresses the spinal cord or its nerve roots. The growth may be benign or malignant—but a nonmalignant tumor may be as disabling as a malignant tumor unless treated appropriately.

BODY PARTS INVOLVED—Spinal cord; nerves below the level of the spinal-cord tumor.

SEX OR AGE MOST AFFECTED—All ages, but most common in adults.

SIGNS & SYMPTOMS
- Progressive weakness, numbness and wasting of muscles whose nerve supply comes from the affected area of the spinal cord.
- Difficult urination or bowel movements; incontinence.
- Chronic back pain.

CAUSES—Tumors originating in the spinal cord (primary tumors) are rare—especially in childhood or old age—and their cause is unknown.
A spinal-cord tumor usually results from cancer that has spread from another part of the body, such as: lung; breast; intestinal tract; prostate; kidney; thyroid; or lymphatic system.

RISK INCREASES WITH—Cancer in any of the body parts listed above.

HOW TO PREVENT
- Because spinal-cord tumors frequently result from the spread of cancer, be alert to early symptoms of cancer in other organs.
- Don't smoke.
- Eat a high-fiber diet to reduce the likelihood of intestinal cancer.
- Be alert to enlargement of the thyroid gland.
- For men over 45, request a prostate exam with your annual physical.
- For women, practice breast self-exam (see Breast Self-exam in Appendix).

WHAT TO EXPECT

DIAGNOSTIC MEASURES
- Your own observation of symptoms.
- Medical history and physical exam by a doctor.
- Laboratory studies of blood and spinal fluid.
- X-rays of the spine, biopsy, MRI or CT scan, radionuclide bone scan and myelogram (see Glossary for all).

APPROPRIATE HEALTH CARE
- Self-care after diagnosis and treatment.
- Doctor's treatment.
- Treatment will depend on the results of all the diagnostic studies and may include surgery to remove tumors and surrounding bone that compress the spinal cord, radiation therapy and chemotherapy.

POSSIBLE COMPLICATIONS—Total paralysis caused by a blockage of blood vessels that nourish spinal-cord cells.

PROBABLE OUTCOME
- The success of treatment depends on the type, size and location of the growth.
- Surgery to remove bone surrounding the cord can relieve pressure on spinal nerves and nerve pathways. This operation generally relieves pain and other symptoms immediately, but may impair motor functions. Physical therapy and rehabilitation may restore lost function.
- If the tumor originated on the exterior of the spinal cord and has not spread, surgery restores a normal life expectancy.

HOW TO TREAT

GENERAL MEASURES
- The more you can learn and understand about this disorder, the more you will be able to make informed decisions about where to go for your care, the treatments available, the risks involved, side effects of therapy and expected outcome.
- See Resources for Additional Information.

MEDICATION—Your doctor may prescribe:
- Pain relievers.
- Cortisone drugs to decrease swelling around the tumor and reduce pressure on the spinal cord.
- Anticancer drugs, if the tumor is malignant.

ACTIVITY—Activity levels will depend on your physical status. Be as active as your energy and mobility permit.

DIET—Eat a normal, well-balanced diet. Vitamin and mineral supplements should not be necessary unless you show evidence of deficiency or cannot eat normally.

CALL YOUR DOCTOR IF

You have any symptoms of a spinal-cord tumor.

SPOROTRICHOSIS

GENERAL INFORMATION

DEFINITION—An infectious fungal disease that causes ulcers and abscesses of the skin, lymph nodes and lymph channels. Farm laborers and gardeners, especially those handling rosebushes, sphagnum moss or barberry bushes, are most often infected. Sporotrichosis is not contagious from person to person.

BODY PARTS INVOLVED—Skin; lymph system; lungs; joints; bones (rare).

SEX OR AGE MOST AFFECTED—Adults of both sexes, but more common in men.

SIGNS & SYMPTOMS
Early stages:
• A small, movable, nontender nodule appears under the skin of the fingers. The nodule enlarges slowly, becomes pink and ulcerates.
In a few days or weeks:
• Dark nodules appear along the lymphatic channel that drains the area.
• Cough with sputum begins, if the organism reaches the lungs (rare).
• Usually no other symptoms—unlike other fungal diseases, which cause fever, chills, a general ill feeling and appetite loss.

CAUSES—Infection by a fungus, Sporothrix schenckii, that lives in soil, sphagnum moss, weeds and decaying organic vegetation.

RISK INCREASES WITH
• Medical history of sarcoidosis or tuberculosis.
• Occupations that involve work with plants and soil, such as farming, nursery work and horticulture.
• Immunosuppression due to illness or drugs.

HOW TO PREVENT—Wear gloves when working with soil.

WHAT TO EXPECT

DIAGNOSTIC MEASURES
• Your own observation of symptoms.
• Medical history and physical exam by a doctor.
• Laboratory culture of pus from the lesions. No skin test is available to diagnose sporotrichosis. Additional tests may be done to rule out other disorders such as tuberculosis, sarcoidosis, bacterial osteomyelitis and neoplasia.

APPROPRIATE HEALTH CARE
• Self-care after diagnosis.
• Doctor's treatment.
• May be treated at home with medication.
• Hospitalization, if complications occur.
Surgery may be recommended for patient with bone and joint disease or pulmonary lesions.

POSSIBLE COMPLICATIONS—Spread of the fungi throughout the body, causing widespread, life-threatening infection.

PROBABLE OUTCOME—With treatment, usually curable within 1 to 2 months after lesions heal—but recovery may require 6 or 7 months.

HOW TO TREAT

GENERAL MEASURES
• Because sporotrichosis is not contagious, the patient does not need to be isolated.
• Cover lesions with loose-fitting bandages to prevent secondary infection with bacteria.

MEDICATION—Your doctor may prescribe:
• Saturated solution of potassium iodide. Dilute this in water, fruit juice or other beverages and take 3 times a day after meals. Drink this with a straw to prevent discoloration of the teeth.
• Antifungal medicine, such as amphotericin B. This medication is potent and may cause severe adverse reactions. It is reserved for serious cases. Hospitalization is necessary so the drug can be administered intravenously.

ACTIVITY—No restrictions unless you develop signs of widespread infection.

DIET—No special diet.

CALL YOUR DOCTOR IF

• You have symptoms of sporotrichosis.
• The following occurs during treatment:
  Unexplained weight loss.
  Fever of 101F (38.3C) orally.
• New, unexplained symptoms develop.
Antifungal drugs used in treatment may produce side effects, including skin rash, tongue and mouth irritation and cough.

SPRAINS & STRAINS (Pulled Muscle)

GENERAL INFORMATION

DEFINITION—A sprain is a stretched or torn ligament. A strain is a stretched or torn muscle or tendinous attachment. Sprains occur most often in ankles, knees, wrist or fingers, although any joint can be sprained. Sprained joints can function, but only with pain.

BODY PARTS INVOLVED—Muscles, tendons and any ligament attached to any joint. Ligaments are the fibrous, elastic connective bands that attach bone to bone (tendons connect muscle to bone).

SEX OR AGE MOST AFFECTED—Both sexes; all ages.

SIGNS & SYMPTOMS
- Pain or tenderness in the area of injury; severity varies with the extent of injury.
- Swelling of the affected joint.
- Redness or bruising in the area of injury, either immediately or several hours after injury.
- Loss of normal mobility in the injured joint.

CAUSES—Strains usually are associated with overuse injuries. Sprains usually occur secondary to trauma (fall, twisting injury or automobile accident). The ankle is injured most often because of its anatomical weakness, its exposed position and the stress it sustains in athletic and recreational activities. It is difficult to differentiate sprains from strains.

RISK INCREASES WITH
- Trauma.
- Excessive exercise; poor conditioning; obesity.
- Poor fitting shoes and high heeled shoes.
- High risk activities (skateboarding), contact sports, ice and roller skating.

HOW TO PREVENT
- Maintain good level of physical fitness.
- Wrap weak joints with support bandages before strenuous activity.
- Stretch muscles before and after exercise.
- Strengthen weak muscles with rehabilitative exercises to prevent a recurrence.
- Accident-proof your home.

WHAT TO EXPECT

DIAGNOSTIC MEASURES
- Medical history and exam by a doctor.
- Depending on the extent of the injury, x-rays of the injured area, CT scan or MRI (see Glossary for both).

APPROPRIATE HEALTH CARE
- Self-care if the injury is not severe.
- Doctor's treatment if the joint cannot move or bear weight normally.
- Surgery may be necessary to repair badly torn ligaments.

- A cast may be necessary for severe sprains or following surgery. Following cast removal, you will wear support bandages for a while. Air cast type devices are very effective.

POSSIBLE COMPLICATIONS
- Permanent weakness or instability if the sprain is severe or a joint is sprained repeatedly.
- Arthritis.

PROBABLE OUTCOME—With appropriate treatment and rest, 6-8 weeks for recovery. May take longer depending on severity of the injury.

HOW TO TREAT

GENERAL MEASURES
- RICE therapy—rest, ice, compression, elevation.
- Apply ice to the injured joint during the first 24 hours. Place ice in a plastic bag and separate it from the skin with a thin towel. Hold it against the joint with your hand or an elastic bandage. Keep the ice pack on the joint up to 2 hours at a time either constantly or intermittently depending on your ability to tolerate the cold. Continue the ice treatment at 2-hour intervals for 24 hours.
- After 24 hours, may continue ice treatment or switch to heat.
- To use heat, soak the joint in hot water or apply heat for 15 minutes every 2 hours or whenever possible. Don't apply heat during the first 24 hours. It may increase bleeding and swelling and prolong healing time.
- Compression with an elastic (Ace) bandage.
- Whenever possible, elevate the joint (especially while sleeping) so fluid can drain and diminish swelling.
- Learn how to use crutches, if needed.

MEDICATION—You may use nonprescription pain relievers such as acetaminophen or ibuprofen. If the sprain is severe, your doctor may prescribe a stronger pain reliever.

ACTIVITY
- Allow the joint to rest 1 or 2 days. Then begin exercising the joint gently, without putting weight on it.
- Physical therapy may be recommended to regain strength and normal use of the joint.

DIET—No special diet.

CALL YOUR DOCTOR IF

- You have a sprained joint that won't bear weight or move normally.
- Pain becomes intolerable.
- Swelling or bruising increases, despite treatment.

STOMACH CANCER
(Gastric Carcinoma)

 GENERAL INFORMATION

DEFINITION—Uncontrolled growth of malignant cells in the stomach. Unfortunately, most people do not have symptoms until the disease is advanced. The incidence of stomach cancer has decreased about 50% over the last 25 years, perhaps due to diet changes. It is a common disorder in Japan.

BODY PARTS INVOLVED—Stomach.

SEX OR AGE MOST AFFECTED—Adults over age 40 and is twice as common in men as women.

SIGNS & SYMPTOMS
Early stages:
• Vague symptoms of indigestion, such as fullness, burping, nausea and poor appetite.
Later stages:
• Unexplained weight loss.
• Vomiting blood.
• Black stools.
• Fullness after eating small amounts.
• Anemia.
• Pain in the upper abdomen.
• Mass in the upper abdomen that can be felt (sometimes).

CAUSES—Unknown. Some evidence suggests that a lack of fresh fruits and vegetables may be a factor.

RISK INCREASES WITH
• Males over age 40.
• Family history of stomach cancer.
• Pernicious anemia.
• Excess alcohol consumption.
• Chronic gastritis.
• Absence of normal stomach acid, previous stomach surgery or partial stomach removal.
• Diet that includes many smoked, pickled and salted foods; low amounts of protein and low amounts of fresh fruits and green, leafy vegetables.

HOW TO PREVENT
• Don't ignore symptoms of indigestion that last more than a few days.
• Eat a nutritious, well-balanced diet.
• Decrease alcohol consumption if you drink more than 1 or 2 drinks a day.
• Examine stool yearly or more often with home tests for blood in the stool.

 WHAT TO EXPECT

DIAGNOSTIC MEASURES
• Your own observation of symptoms.
• Medical history and physical exam by a doctor.

• Laboratory blood studies for anemia, stomach tests for acid and stool tests for bleeding.
• Surgical diagnostic procedures such as biopsy through a gastroscope (see Glossary).
• CT (see Glossary) and x-rays of the stomach, esophagus and small intestine.

APPROPRIATE HEALTH CARE
• Doctor's treatment.
• Surgery to remove part or all of the stomach is the recommended treatment if the cancer has not spread.
• Anticancer drugs (chemotherapy) treatment may achieve a temporary response.

POSSIBLE COMPLICATIONS
• Internal bleeding.
• Misdiagnosis as a stomach ulcer (symptoms are similar).
• Fatal spread to liver, bones and lungs.

PROBABLE OUTCOME—This condition is currently considered incurable. The 5-year survival rate is low even with treatment. Scientific research into causes and treatment continues, so there is hope for increasingly effective treatment and cure.

 HOW TO TREAT

GENERAL MEASURES
• The more you can learn and understand about this disorder, the more you will be able to make informed decisions about where to go for your care, the treatments available, the risks involved, side effects of therapy and expected outcome.
• See Resources for Additional Information.

MEDICATION—Your doctor may prescribe:
• Anticancer drugs (sometimes).
• Pain relievers.

ACTIVITY—As tolerated by your energy level.

DIET—Eat frequent small meals of soft foods. Try to maintain high calorie intake.

 CALL YOUR DOCTOR IF

• You have symptoms of stomach cancer.
• Indigestion occurs after surgery and does not respond to medication in a few days.
• New, unexplained symptoms develop. Drugs used in treatment may produce side effects.

STRABISMUS

GENERAL INFORMATION

DEFINITION—Lack of coordinated muscle movement or focusing ability between the eyes, causing the eyes to point in different directions. One or both eyes may turn inward (crossed eyes) or outward ("walleye"). Eye alignment is not fully mature at birth. A true developmental eye drift typically shows up from birth to 3 or 4 months of age, but may occur in childhood or later.

BODY PARTS INVOLVED—Eyes; brain area that controls vision.

SEX OR AGE MOST AFFECTED—Both sexes; all ages.

SIGNS & SYMPTOMS
- Uncoordinated eye movements. This is sometimes evident only when looking in certain directions.
- Double vision (sometimes).
- Vision in one eye only, with loss of depth perception.

CAUSES—In most cases, strabismus is congenital (present at birth) and the cause is unknown. Eye movement is controlled by brain signals to four muscles around each eye. Loss of coordinated movement results from:
- Muscle imbalance between the eyes.
- Lack of equal focusing ability in the eyes. The brain cannot tolerate differing focused images, so it ignores signals from one field of vision. The weaker eye eventually becomes useless from disuse, and a "lazy" or wandering eye results.
- Brain damage or head injury (rare).

RISK INCREASES WITH
- Family history of strabismus.
- Down syndrome
- Thyroid disease.
- Eye tumor.
- Damage to fetal central nervous system.
- Birth trauma.
- Eye disuse.

HOW TO PREVENT—No specific preventive measures.

WHAT TO EXPECT

DIAGNOSTIC MEASURES
- Your own observation of symptoms. Note particularly if a young child covers one eye—this may indicate the eyes are not focusing together.
- Medical history and physical exam by a doctor, including tests of visual acuity, retina examination, total neurological exam and muscle tests.

APPROPRIATE HEALTH CARE
- Home care after diagnosis.
- Doctor's (ophthalmologist) treatment.
- Treatment has 3 goals—to obtain the best possible vision, gain the best eye alignment, provide the best opportunity for binocular vision.
- Treatment may include corrective glasses or an eye patch over the stronger eye to correct focusing imbalance (these force the weak eye to work), eye-muscle exercises, botulinum toxin (currently used only in adults) or surgery to correct the condition of the eye muscles. Sometimes a second operation is required. (See Strabismus Surgery in Surgery section.)
- Optional therapy involves the use of eyeglasses overlaid with thin plastic prisms. These are used by the patient prior to surgery and help determine the amount of surgical adjustment needed on the eye muscles.

POSSIBLE COMPLICATIONS
- Loss of normal vision in one eye.
- Psychological distress from an unattractive facial appearance.

PROBABLE OUTCOME—With early diagnosis, strabismus can be corrected with glasses, an eye patch, eye exercises or surgery. Without prompt treatment, vision loss in one eye may become permanent.

HOW TO TREAT

GENERAL MEASURES
- Carefully follow your doctor's instructions about the use of eye patches. If you cover the good eye for too long a period, that eye may develop vision problems.
- Bandages are frequently unnecessary following surgery to correct strabismus. An antibiotic ointment is given to put in the child's eyes.

MEDICATION—Medicine usually is not necessary for this disorder unless botulinum toxin injections are recommended. They are injected into an eye-turning muscle, outside the eye, through an electromyographic needle.

ACTIVITY—No restrictions. Protect your child against falls or injury while he or she adjusts to an eye patch.

No special diet.

CALL YOUR DOCTOR IF

Your child has symptoms of strabismus. Early diagnosis is vital to detect and treat underlying causes and prevent severe vision disability.

STREP THROAT
(Streptococcal Sore Throat)

GENERAL INFORMATION

DEFINITION—Infection and inflammation of the pharynx by streptococcal bacteria. Strep throat is contagious. One out of 4 family members usually catches it within 2 to 7 days after exposure. Infection can be present in individuals with no symptoms but who can still spread the germs (carrier state)

BODY PARTS INVOLVED—Throat; tonsils.

SEX OR AGE MOST AFFECTED—Both sexes; all ages, but most common in children.

SIGNS & SYMPTOMS
- Rapid onset of throat pain.
- Throat pain that is worse when swallowing.
- Appetite loss.
- Headache.
- Fever.
- General ill feeling.
- Ear pain when swallowing (sometimes).
- Tender, swollen glands in the neck.
- Bright-red tonsils that may have specks of pus.

CAUSES—Streptococcal bacteria. It is spread by person-to-person contact via drops of saliva or nasal secretions (droplets are exhaled, coughed or sneezed).

RISK INCREASES WITH
- Recent strep infection in the household.
- Smoking.
- Fatigue.
- Crowded living conditions (military recruits).
- Day care center or school.
- Immunosuppression due to illness or drugs.
- Diabetes mellitus.
- Recent illness.

HOW TO PREVENT—Avoid contact with infected people.

WHAT TO EXPECT

DIAGNOSTIC MEASURES
- Your own observation of symptoms.
- Medical history and physical exam by a doctor.
- Laboratory studies, such as a throat culture and blood count. A throat culture is the only way to diagnose a strep throat infection. This is an inexpensive, quick, painless procedure in a doctor's office.

APPROPRIATE HEALTH CARE
- Self-care after diagnosis.
- Doctor's treatment.

POSSIBLE COMPLICATIONS
- Ear infection.
- Sinusitis.
- Rheumatic fever.
- Glomerulonephritis.

PROBABLE OUTCOME—Usually curable in 10 to 12 days with antibiotic treatment (which also helps prevent any complications). Symptoms are usually better in 2-3 days of treatment.

HOW TO TREAT

GENERAL MEASURES
- Use a cool-mist, ultrasonic humidifier to provide moisture. This relieves the dry, tight feeling in the throat. Clean humidifier daily.
- Use warm soaks to relieve pain in swollen glands.
- Isolation techniques are unnecessary.

MEDICATION—Your doctor may prescribe penicillin or another antibiotic to take orally or by injection. It is important to finish the medication, even if the symptoms have disappeared.

ACTIVITY—After treatment, resume normal activity as symptoms improve. Children may return to school 2 days after beginning antibiotics and fever is normal for 24 hours.

DIET—A liquid diet may be necessary while the throat is sore. Drink as many fluids as possible, including milk shakes, soups, tea, carbonated drinks and iced coffee. Any type and amount of solid food is acceptable as long as it can be swallowed without too much pain.

CALL YOUR DOCTOR IF

- You have symptoms of a strep throat.
- The following occurs during treatment:
  Temperature is normal for 1 or 2 days, then fever develops.
  New symptoms appear, such as: nausea; vomiting; earache; cough; swollen glands; skin rash; severe headache; nasal drainage; or shortness of breath.
  Joints become red or painful.
  Dark urine, rash, chest pain or fatigue (may occur as much as 3 to 4 weeks later).

STROKE (Cerebrovascular Accident)

GENERAL INFORMATION

DEFINITION—A sudden decrease in the blood supply to part of the brain, damaging the area so it cannot function normally.

BODY PARTS INVOLVED—Central nervous system; musculoskeletal system.

SEX OR AGE MOST AFFECTED—Adults over 60.

SIGNS & SYMPTOMS—The following symptoms may vary according to the site of brain damage:
- Inability to speak; inability to move part of the body; loss of consciousness.
- Sudden heaviness in an arm or leg or numbness and inability to control muscles.
- Headache; vision disturbances; confusion; dizziness; loss of bowel and bladder control.

CAUSES—Usually hardening of the arteries (atherosclerosis) or high blood pressure. These may result in the following:
- Thrombosis, in which blood flow is blocked by a narrow or closed artery.
- Embolism, in which a small part of an artery wall or a small blood clot from a diseased artery or heart travels to the brain.
- Cerebral hemorrhage, in which a blood vessel to the brain ruptures and bleeds into surrounding brain tissue.
- Rupture of an aneurysm of a small artery to the brain.

RISK INCREASES WITH
- Smoking; obesity; diet that is high in fat or salt; high blood pressure.
- Diabetes mellitus; coronary artery disease; previous transient ischemic attacks (TIA).
- Family history of stroke; excess alcohol consumption; age over 60.

HOW TO PREVENT
- Exercise regularly; eat a diet that is low in fat; don't smoke.
- Control of any chronic disorder (e.g., diabetes).
- Have your blood pressure checked regularly. If it is high, see your doctor.
- Get medical advice about taking 1 aspirin tablet daily. Studies indicate this may affect blood clotting enough to decrease the chance of cerebral thrombosis or embolism.
- If you have blockage of a carotid artery, surgery can reduce the chance of having a future stroke.

WHAT TO EXPECT

DIAGNOSTIC MEASURES
- Medical history and exam by a doctor.
- Laboratory studies of spinal fluid and blood.
- X-rays of the head, ECG and CT scan (see Glossary for both).

APPROPRIATE HEALTH CARE
- Doctor's treatment.
- Immediate transport to an emergency room. Some hospitals have instituted protocols for early treatment with clot busting medicines.
- Hospitalization for acute care (with close monitoring of cardiac and pulmonary function; electrolyte and fluid levels).
- Surgery (sometimes) to remove a clot in an artery to the brain.
- Nursing-home care (sometimes).
- After the acute period, physical therapy, occupational therapy and speech therapy.

POSSIBLE COMPLICATIONS
- Pneumonia; depression.
- Pressure sores from prolonged bed rest.
- Permanent or temporary loss of memory.
- Permanent paralysis or disability.

PROBABLE OUTCOME
- Stroke causes death, permanent damage or disability in 2/3 of all cases. In the rest, recovery without long-term disability is possible.
- A mild stroke may be the forerunner of more severe attacks. For stroke survivors, partial disability may last for months.

HOW TO TREAT

GENERAL MEASURES
- Once the acute period of a stroke is over, the follow-up care will depend on the degree of disability. The patient and the family should be involved in the aspects of rehabilitation that are planned by the doctor and the support team.
- Ongoing care at home or in a facility.

MEDICATION—Your doctor may prescribe:
- Anticoagulant drugs to reduce the chance of clot formation.
- Antihypertensive drugs, for high blood pressure.
- Pain medicine as needed.
- Stool softeners to aid bowel movements.

ACTIVITY
- If you have lost muscle control, therapy will help you to regain basic skills, such as eating, dressing and toilet functions.
- Following a stroke, consider installing ramps at entries to the house and hand bars next to tubs and toilets.

DIET—At first, may require feeding tube, then progress to pureed, soft or regular diet. Eat a diet that is low in salt and low in fat.

CALL YOUR DOCTOR IF

- You have symptoms of a stroke or observe them in someone else. This is an emergency!
- The following occurs during treatment: Fever; pressure sores; worsening symptoms.

STYE
(Hordeolum)

 GENERAL INFORMATION

DEFINITION—A small abscess of hair-follicle glands in the eyelid.

BODY PARTS INVOLVED—Eyelid; eyelashes; conjunctiva (white of the eye).

SEX OR AGE MOST AFFECTED—Both sexes; all ages.

SIGNS & SYMPTOMS
• Redness, swelling, warmth, tenderness or pain on the edge of the top or bottom eyelid. The head of the sty is usually on the outside, but it may be on the underside of the lid.
• Increased tear production.
• Sensitivity to bright light.
• A gritty feeling in the eye.

CAUSES—Bacterial infection (usually staphylococcal). The infection may be limited to the eyelid or may have spread from somewhere else in the body.

RISK INCREASES WITH
• Eye irritation from smoking.
• Exposure to cosmetics, chemical or environmental irritants.
• Blepharitis (infection of eyelid margin).
• Contact lens wearer.

HOW TO PREVENT—General good hygiene including a mild shampoo used on eyelashes when bathing or washing face.

 WHAT TO EXPECT

DIAGNOSTIC MEASURES
• Your own observation of symptoms.
• Medical history and physical exam by a doctor.
• Laboratory culture of the discharge from the sty.

APPROPRIATE HEALTH CARE
• Self-care.
• Doctor's treatment.
• Surgery to drain the abscess (sometimes).

POSSIBLE COMPLICATIONS—Spread of infection to other glands in the eyelid.

PROBABLE OUTCOME—Usually curable once the stye discharges its pus. They frequently recur, even with treatment.

 HOW TO TREAT

GENERAL MEASURES
• Use warm-water soaks to relieve pain and inflammation and hasten healing. Apply soaks for 20 minutes, then rest at least 1 hour. Repeat as often as needed.
• Don't squeeze the stye. It will soon open and release the pus, bringing relief from the pain.

MEDICATION
• Your doctor may prescribe topical antibiotic ointments or creams, such as erythromycin or bacitracin. Apply according to package instructions.
• Sometimes oral antibiotics are necessary and sometimes prolonged treatment is required.

ACTIVITY—No restrictions.

DIET—No special diet.

 CALL YOUR DOCTOR IF

• A ripened sty does not drain spontaneously or after gentle removal of the affected eyelash.
• Pain occurs in the eye.
• Vision changes.

SUBARACHNOID HEMORRHAGE

GENERAL INFORMATION

DEFINITION—Sudden bleeding into the subarachnoid space (the area between 2 of the membranes that cover the brain). The space is normally filled with cerebrospinal fluid.

BODY PARTS INVOLVED—Brain; meninges (membranes that cover the brain); blood vessels to the brain.

SEX OR AGE MOST AFFECTED—All ages, but most common in adults aged 25 to 50.

SIGNS & SYMPTOMS
- Acute, severe headache, often followed by unconsciousness.
- Drowsiness, dizziness, convulsions or coma.
- Eye pain with extreme sensitivity to light.
- Vomiting.
- Rapid heartbeat and breathing.
- Stiff neck with pain on movement.
- Fever.
- Numbness, weakness or inability to move an arm or leg.

CAUSES
- Head injury (the most common cause).
- Hardening of the arteries.
- Infection in any part of the central nervous system.
- Rupture of an aneurysm (weakened part of an artery) that has been present since birth. Rupture is often preceded by high blood pressure or hardening of the arteries.
- Bleeding disorder, such as sickle-cell anemia, leukemia or any bleeding that is a side effect of prescription drugs.

RISK INCREASES WITH
- Atherosclerosis (hardening of the arteries) or high blood pressure.
- Family history of bleeding disorders.
- Cerebral aneurysms (run in families).
- Polycystic disease of the kidneys.

HOW TO PREVENT
- Avoid head injury. Use seat belts in cars, protective head gear in contact sports and helmets while biking.
- Obtain medical treatment for an existing aneurysm or arteriovenous malformation.

WHAT TO EXPECT

DIAGNOSTIC MEASURES
- Your own observation of symptoms.
- Medical history and physical exam by a doctor.
- Laboratory studies of blood and cerebrospinal fluid.
- X-rays of the skull.
- CT scan and myelography (see Glossary for both).

APPROPRIATE HEALTH CARE
- Doctor's treatment.
- Surgery to stop bleeding and remove collected blood.
- Hospitalization required with treatment directed toward preventing complications.
- Surgery to stop bleeding and remove collected blood.

POSSIBLE COMPLICATIONS—Death or permanent disability. Early diagnosis and treatment can influence outcome.

PROBABLE OUTCOME—If surgery is possible, recovery chances are good. Partial paralysis, weakness or numbness, and speech and visual difficulties may remain in some cases. The damaged area of the brain cannot be restored. However, undamaged areas of the brain often can be taught the lost functions. This usually requires rehabilitation, including physical therapy, occupational therapy or speech therapy. Determination and a positive attitude greatly affect the success of the rehabilitation process.

HOW TO TREAT

GENERAL MEASURES
- Once the acute period of a subarachnoid hemorrhage is over, the follow-up care will depend on the degree of disability. The patient and the family should be involved in the aspects of rehabilitation that are planned by the doctor and the medical support team.
- Ongoing care may be provided at home or the patient may need to be cared for in an extended care facility.

MEDICATION—Your doctor may prescribe cortisone drugs to reduce brain swelling and pressure.

ACTIVITY
- Strict bed rest until source of hemorrhage is eliminated.
- Following treatment, if you have lost some motor functions, occupational and physical therapists will help you use the affected limbs to regain basic skills, such as eating, dressing and toilet functions.
- After recovery, resume as many of your former activities as your strength and sense of well-being allow. Allow 6 to 12 months for recovery.

DIET—As tolerated at first. May require feeding tube or intravenous feedings.

CALL YOUR DOCTOR IF

- You have any symptoms of a subarachnoid hemorrhage. This is an emergency!
- Symptoms recur after surgery.

SUBCONJUNCTIVAL HEMORRHAGE

GENERAL INFORMATION

DEFINITION—Sudden appearance of blood in the white area of the eye. Although the bleeding may appear frightening, it is not painful or serious.

BODY PARTS INVOLVED—Conjunctiva, the transparent membrane that covers the white of the eye.

SEX OR AGE MOST AFFECTED—Both sexes; all ages, including newborns.

SIGNS & SYMPTOMS—A small, painless collection of bright red blood over the white of the eye. Swelling may occur in the affected area of the conjunctiva. The blood changes color gradually to brown or green before disappearing. The condition doesn't interfere with vision.

CAUSES—Usually spontaneous bleeding with no known cause. It may follow coughing, sneezing, vomiting or direct injury to the eye. The blood vessels of the conjunctiva are fragile and frequently leak.

RISK INCREASES WITH
• Use of mind-altering drugs.
• Use of anticoagulant drugs.

HOW TO PREVENT—No specific preventive measures.

WHAT TO EXPECT

DIAGNOSTIC MEASURES
• Your own observation of symptoms.
• Medical history and physical exam by a doctor (sometimes).

APPROPRIATE HEALTH CARE
• Self-care after diagnosis.
• Doctor's treatment, if there has been injury or a change in vision.

POSSIBLE COMPLICATIONS—None expected.

PROBABLE OUTCOME—The blood should be absorbed in 2 or 3 weeks. It is very unlikely that any scarring will occur.

HOW TO TREAT

GENERAL MEASURES
• No specific measures are necessary.
• Compresses don't help or hasten the healing.

MEDICATION—Medicine is usually not necessary for this disorder.

ACTIVITY—No restrictions.

DIET—No special diet.

CALL YOUR DOCTOR IF

You have symptoms of subconjunctival hemorrhage, especially if you have eye pain or your vision changes.

SUBDURAL HEMORRHAGE & HEMATOMA

GENERAL INFORMATION

DEFINITION—Bleeding (hemorrhage) that causes blood to collect and clot (hematoma) beneath the outermost of 3 membranes that cover the brain (meninges).

There are 2 types of subdural hematomas. An acute subdural hematoma occurs soon after a severe head injury. A chronic subdural hematoma is a complication that may develop weeks after a head injury. The injury may have been so minor that the patient does not remember it.

BODY PARTS INVOLVED—Brain; meninges; blood vessels to the brain.

SEX OR AGE MOST AFFECTED—Both sexes; all ages.

SIGNS & SYMPTOMS
- Recurrent headaches that worsen each day.
- Fluctuating drowsiness, dizziness, mental changes or confusion.
- Weakness or numbness on one side of the body.
- Vision disturbances.
- Vomiting without nausea.
- Pupils of different size (sometimes).

CAUSES—Head injury.

RISK INCREASES WITH—Injuries occur more often after:
- Use of anticoagulant drugs.
- Excess alcohol consumption.
- Use of mind-altering drugs.

HOW TO PREVENT—Avoid head injury in the following ways:
- Use seat belts in motor vehicles.
- Wear protective head gear during contact sports, or while riding a bicycle or motorcycle.
- Don't drink alcohol or use mind-altering drugs and drive.

WHAT TO EXPECT

DIAGNOSTIC MEASURES
- Your own observation of symptoms.
- Medical history and physical exam by a doctor.
- Laboratory studies of blood and cerebrospinal fluid.
- Hospital diagnostic tests, such as x-ray, arteriography, radionuclide scan and CT scan (see Glossary for all).

APPROPRIATE HEALTH CARE
- Doctor's treatment.
- Hospitalization for emergency treatment.
- Surgical exploration and removal of the clot.

POSSIBLE COMPLICATIONS—Death or permanent brain damage, including partial or complete paralysis, behavioral and personality changes, and speech problems.

PROBABLE OUTCOME—The degree of recovery depends upon general health, age, severity of the injury, rapidity of the treatment, and extensiveness of the bleeding or clot. After the clot is removed, brain tissue that has been compressed usually expands slowly to fill its original space. The outlook is good under the best circumstances.

HOW TO TREAT

GENERAL MEASURES—There is no self-treatment. These suggestions apply to care at home following surgery.

MEDICATION—Your doctor may prescribe drugs to reduce swelling inside the skull.

ACTIVITY—During recovery—stay as active as your strength allows. Work and exercise moderately. Rest when you tire. If your speech or muscle control has been damaged, you may need physical therapy or speech therapy.

DIET—Most likely will require intravenous or tube feeding during acute phase and then shift to regular food as tolerated.

CALL YOUR DOCTOR IF

- You have had a head injury—even if it seems minor—and you develop any symptoms of subdural hemorrhage. This is an emergency!
- The following occurs during or after treatment: Fever.
  Surgical wound becomes red, swollen or tender.
  Headache worsens.

SUNBURN

GENERAL INFORMATION

DEFINITION—Inflammation of the cells of the skin that follows overexposure to the sun, sun lamps or occupational light sources.

BODY PARTS INVOLVED—Exposed skin.

SEX OR AGE MOST AFFECTED—Both sexes; all ages.

SIGNS & SYMPTOMS
* Red, swollen, painful and sometimes blistered skin; fever (occasionally).
* Nausea and vomiting (severe burns).
* Delirium (severe, extensive burns).

CAUSES—Excess exposure to ultraviolet (UV) light. This is not screened out by thin clouds on overcast days, but it is partially screened by smoke and smog. A great deal of ultraviolet light reflects from snow, water, sand and sidewalks.

RISK INCREASES WITH
* Fair skin, blue eyes, and red or blonde hair.
* Exposure to industrial light sources, such as welding arcs.
* Photosensitivity—some drugs, including sulfa, tetracyclines or oral contraceptives, and the chemicals in some substances applied to the skin (perfumes, after shaves, soaps) heighten sensitivity to the sun's ultraviolet rays.

HOW TO PREVENT
* Avoid sun exposure from noon to 3 p.m. Sun exposure is more intense at high altitudes, tropical locations and near snow or water.
* Wear a hat with a 3" brim and long-sleeved shirts and long pants.
* Use a sun-block preparation for outdoor activity. Products with a sun-protective factor (SPF) of 15 or more protect almost totally. Those with lower values offer partial protection and allow minimal tanning. Some of these resist water and perspiration, but reapply them after swimming or after prolonged exposure. Baby oil, mineral oil or cocoa butter offer no protection from the sun.
* For maximum protection, use a physical-barrier agent such as zinc-oxide ointment. Reapply after swimming and at frequent intervals during exposure. Barrier agents are especially helpful on skin areas that are most susceptible to burns, such as the nose, ears, backs of the legs and back of the neck.
* Wear muted colors such as tan. Avoid brilliant colors and whites.
* If you take prescription drugs, ask your doctor or pharmacist if they cause photosensitivity.

WHAT TO EXPECT

DIAGNOSTIC MEASURES—Medical history and physical exam by a doctor (sometimes).

APPROPRIATE HEALTH CARE
* Self-care for minor sunburn.
* Doctor's treatment for severe sunburn.

POSSIBLE COMPLICATIONS
* Skin changes leading to skin cancer, including life-threatening malignant melanoma.
* Keratoses, premalignant skin lesions.
* Premature wrinkling and loss of skin elasticity.
* Temporary delirium in worst cases.

PROBABLE OUTCOME—Spontaneous recovery in 3 days to 3 weeks, depending on the severity of the sunburn.

HOW TO TREAT

GENERAL MEASURES
* To reduce heat and pain, dip gauze or towels in cool water and lay these on the burned areas.
* After skin swelling subsides, apply cold cream or baby lotion.
* For badly blistered skin, apply a light coating of petroleum jelly. This prevents anything from sticking to the blisters.
* Soak in a tub of cool water to which colloidal oatmeal (Aveeno) or baking soda has been added. Pat skin dry, do not rub. Avoid soap.

MEDICATION
* Use nonprescription drugs, such as aspirin, acetaminophen or ibuprofen, to relieve pain and reduce fever. nonprescription burn remedies that contain local anesthetics, such as benzocaine or lidocaine, may be useful, but they produce allergic reactions in some. Aerosols are easier to use than creams or ointments (to avoid contact with your eyes, don't spray directly on your face; spray some on a cotton pad and apply to your face).
* Your doctor may prescribe pain relievers or cortisone drugs to use briefly.

ACTIVITY—Rest in any comfortable position until fever and discomfort diminish. Cover yourself with an upside-down "cradle" or tent of cardboard or other material to keep bed linens off the burned skin. If your legs are burned and your feet swollen, raise your legs above heart level while you are resting.

DIET—No special diet. Increase fluid intake.

CALL YOUR DOCTOR IF

The following occurs after sunburn:
* Extensive blistering (if blisters seem to spread, you may have an infection).
* Oral temperature rises to 101F (38.3C).
* Vomiting, diarrhea or delirium.
* Pain and fever that persist longer than 48 hours.

SYPHILIS

GENERAL INFORMATION

DEFINITION—A contagious, sexually-transmitted disease that causes widespread tissue destruction. Syphilis is known as the "great mimic," because its symptoms resemble those of many other diseases.

BODY PARTS INVOLVED—Genitals; skin; central nervous system.

SEX OR AGE MOST AFFECTED
- Newborns (0 to 2 weeks) born to mothers with syphilis (congenital form).
- Persons of all ages and both sexes who have sexual contact (contagious form).

SIGNS & SYMPTOMS
First stage (contagious; appears 3 to 6 days after contact):
- A painless, red sore (chancre) on the genitals, mouth or rectum. The sore usually affects the penis in males and vagina or cervix in females.
Second stage (contagious; begins 6 or more weeks after the chancre appears):
- Enlarged lymph glands in the neck, armpit or groin.
- Headache.
- Rash on skin and mucous membranes of the penis, vagina or mouth. The rash has small, red, scaly bumps.
- Fever (sometimes).
Third stage (noncontagious; may appear years after the first and second stages):
- Mental deterioration.
- Sexual impotence.
- Loss of balance.
- Loss of feeling or shooting pains in the legs.
- Heart disease.

CAUSES—The infecting germ for both forms is Treponema pallidum.
- The congenital form is spread to the fetus through the bloodstream.
- The contagious form is spread by intimate sexual contact with someone who has syphilis in the first or second stages.

RISK INCREASES WITH
- Many sexual partners.
- Male-to-male sexual activity.

HOW TO PREVENT
- Obtain blood serum test for syphilis early in pregnancy. If infected, consult your doctor immediately for treatment.
- Use latex condoms during intercourse.
- Avoid any sexual contact if you suspect a partner is infectious.

WHAT TO EXPECT

DIAGNOSTIC MEASURES
- Your own observation of symptoms.
- Medical history and physical exam by a doctor.
- Laboratory studies, such as a blood serum test for syphilis, a microscopic exam of discharge from the chancre and a study of spinal fluid. Tests are repeated after treatment.

APPROPRIATE HEALTH CARE—Doctor's treatment.

POSSIBLE COMPLICATIONS—Widespread tissue destruction and death without treatment.

PROBABLE OUTCOME—Usually curable in 3 months with treatment. In spite of treatment, syphilis returns within 1 year in 10% of patients. If this happens, re-treatment is necessary.

HOW TO TREAT

GENERAL MEASURES
- Ensure that all your sexual partners obtain treatment. The public health department will work with you to notify contacts confidentially and help them obtain treatment.
- After treatment, have blood studies done each month for 6 months to check for recurrence. Then repeat blood studies every 3 months for 2 years.
- See Sexually Transmitted Diseases in Resources for Additional Information.

MEDICATION—Your doctor will probably prescribe:
- Penicillin by injection unless you are allergic to it. If penicillin cannot be used, other antibiotics can be equally as effective.
- Topical medications as needed for skin symptoms.

ACTIVITY—Avoid sexual intercourse for at least 2 months after treatment begins. Then use latex condoms during sexual intercourse.

DIET—No special diet.

CALL YOUR DOCTOR IF

- You have symptoms of syphilis.
- The following occurs during or after treatment: Fever.
  Skin rash, sore throat or swelling in any joint, such as the ankle or knee.
- New, unexplained symptoms develop. Drugs used in treatment may produce side effects.
- You once had syphilis and have not had a medical checkup in the past year.
- You have had sexual contact with someone who has syphilis.

TAPEWORM
(Taenia Saginata)

GENERAL INFORMATION

DEFINITION—An infestation of the intestinal tract by the tapeworm, a parasite. They are typically acquired from eating undercooked meat or fish. This is not contagious from person to person.

BODY PARTS INVOLVED—Intestinal tract.

SEX OR AGE MOST AFFECTED—Both sexes; all ages.

SIGNS & SYMPTOMS—Most people with this problem have no symptoms. However, some experience the following:
• Pain in the upper abdomen.
• Diarrhea.
• Unexplained weight loss.
• Symptoms of anemia (weakness, fatigue and shortness of breath).
• Bowel movements containing worm eggs and worm body parts.

CAUSES—Intestinal parasites: Taenia saginata from beef, Taenia solium from pork, and Diphyllobothrium from fish. People become infected by eating improperly cooked or raw food infected with the parasite.

RISK INCREASES WITH—Travel to Africa, the Middle East, Europe, Mexico, Latin America, Japan, Africa, Russia, Asia and South America. This disorder is uncommon in the U.S.

HOW TO PREVENT
• Cook beef, pork, and fish thoroughly. Additional information available from the National Center for Nutrition (800)366-1655 or the Department of Agriculture Meat and Poultry Hotline (800)535-4555.
• Buy only meat that has been inspected.

WHAT TO EXPECT

DIAGNOSTIC MEASURES
• Your own observation of symptoms.
• Medical history and physical exam by a doctor.
• Laboratory stool studies to identify the worm.

APPROPRIATE HEALTH CARE—Doctor's treatment.

POSSIBLE COMPLICATIONS—Anemia.

PROBABLE OUTCOME—Usually curable in 1 day with treatment.

HOW TO TREAT

GENERAL MEASURES
• Wash your hands before eating.
• Have all family members examined by a doctor for possible infection.

MEDICATION—Your doctor will prescribe an anthelmintic drug to kill the parasite. The drug cures with a single dose. Laboratory studies should be repeated in 3-6 weeks to make sure disorder is cured.

ACTIVITY—No restrictions.

DIET—No special diet.

CALL YOUR DOCTOR IF

• You have symptoms of a tapeworm.
• New, unexplained symptoms develop. Drugs used in treatment may produce side effects.

TAY-SACHS DISEASE

GENERAL INFORMATION

DEFINITION—An inherited, rare disorder of the central nervous system in infants and young children. It causes progressive impairment and early death. Less than 100 children are born with the disease each year in the U.S.

BODY PARTS INVOLVED—Brain and central nervous system.

SEX OR AGE MOST AFFECTED—Infants and young children (up to age 5).

SIGNS & SYMPTOMS—The child seems normal at birth. Between 3 and 6 months, the following symptoms begin to appear:
- Loss of alertness and retarded mental development.
- Loss of muscle strength, such as difficulty sitting up or turning over.
- Deafness.
- Blindness.
- Severe constipation caused by an impaired nerve supply to the colon.
- Seizures.

CAUSES—An inherited disease resulting from a recessive gene that causes enzyme deficiency. If both parents have the gene, they have a 25% chance of having a child with Tay-Sachs disease. If only one parent is a carrier, the children will not have the disease. The gene occurs in 1 out of 60 people of Ashkenazim Jewish or French Canadian ancestry.

RISK INCREASES WITH—Genetic factors. Most parents who carry the recessive gene are of Eastern European Jewish origin (Ashkenazi).

HOW TO PREVENT
- Obtain genetic screening for children in families with Tay-Sachs.
- Obtain genetic counseling if you or your spouse have a family history of Tay-Sachs or are of Ashkenazi background.
- If you are expecting a child and have a family history of Tay-Sachs, consider amniocentesis (see Glossary) to detect if the fetus has the disease.

WHAT TO EXPECT

DIAGNOSTIC MEASURES
- Your own observation of symptoms.
- Medical history and physical exam by a doctor.
- Laboratory blood tests to detect the hexosaminidase A enzyme deficiency.

APPROPRIATE HEALTH CARE
- Doctor's treatment.
- Time in an extended-care facility for basic care if parents are unable to provide it at home.
- Psychotherapy or counseling for parents and siblings to learn to cope with the distress produced by this condition.

POSSIBLE COMPLICATIONS
- Pneumonia.
- Pressure sores.

PROBABLE OUTCOME—Death usually occurs before age 5.

HOW TO TREAT

GENERAL MEASURES
- If you care for your child at home, you will need training on how to do suctioning, postural drainage, tube feeding and how to provide good skin care to prevent pressure sores. Ask your doctor for information about getting the help you need.
- Seek out support groups for families of Tay-Sachs victims.
- See Resources for Additional Information.

MEDICATION—Your doctor may prescribe:
- Anticonvulsants to control seizures.
- Stool softeners and laxatives to relieve constipation.
- Other medicines to control complicating disorders as they arise.

ACTIVITY—In the early stages, encourage the child to be as active as possible. Increasing mental, nervous and muscular deficiencies will eventually confine the child to bed much of the time.

DIET—Provide adequate fluids and a normal, high-fiber diet to minimize constipation. Feeding by tube usually becomes necessary as the disease progresses.

CALL YOUR DOCTOR IF

- You are concerned about your infant's mental and physical development.
- You think you or any member of your family carries the abnormal gene. A genetic counselor can advise you on how to prevent having children with this disease.

ILLNESS & DISORDERS

TEAR DUCT INFECTION OR BLOCKAGE
(Dacryocystitis or Dacryostenosis)

GENERAL INFORMATION

DEFINITION—Infection of the tear duct, sac or gland is called dacryocystitis. The germs that cause the infection can be spread to other people.

Scarring, blockage or narrowing of the tear duct—usually from inherited abnormality or prior infection—is called dacryostenosis.

BODY PARTS INVOLVED—Eye; tear (nasolacrimal) gland, sac or duct.

SEX OR AGE MOST AFFECTED
• Inherited blockage of the tear duct usually appears in infants at 3 to 12 weeks.
• Infection of the tear duct or sac occurs in all ages, but it is most common in children.
• Blockage caused by infection can occur at any age following an infection.

SIGNS & SYMPTOMS—The following symptoms may apply to either blockage or infection:
• Persistent tearing of one or both eyes.
• Drainage of mucus and pus instead of water from the tear duct. The drainage may flow spontaneously or with pressure on the area.
• Pain, redness or swelling beneath the eye suggesting infection.
• Redness and swelling of the tear duct.
• Redness of the white of the eye surrounding the tear duct.

CAUSES—Obstruction of the tear duct resulting from the following:
• Inherited abnormality.
• Bacterial infection of the duct.
• Sinus or nasal infection, especially chronic nasal infection.
• Nasal polyps.
• Eye injury.
• Eye infection, including severe pink eye (conjunctivitis).
• Fracture of the nose or facial bones.

RISK INCREASES WITH
• Newborns and infants, especially those with a family history of blocked tear ducts.
• Recent infection, such as those listed above.

HOW TO PREVENT—Obtain prompt medical treatment for eye, nose or sinus infections.

WHAT TO EXPECT

DIAGNOSTIC MEASURES
• Your own observation of symptoms.
• Medical history and physical exam by a doctor.

APPROPRIATE HEALTH CARE
• Often requires no treatment other than massage.
• Home care after diagnosis.
• Doctor's treatment.
• Surgery to dilate and probe the tear-duct canal. In infants, this usually requires a brief general anesthesia in an out-patient surgical facility. In adults, it is often done in the doctor's office with local anesthesia.
After dilation, the tear-duct system is irrigated with saline. (See Tear Duct, Opening of in Surgery Section.)
• Complete obstruction may require a surgical opening from the eye into the nasal passage.

POSSIBLE COMPLICATIONS
• Without treatment, an obstruction may cause chronic infection.
• Without treatment, infection may spread to the cornea and other parts of the eye or permanently scar the tear duct.

PROBABLE OUTCOME
• Infection is usually curable with antibiotics.
• Obstruction is usually curable with dilation of the duct or surgery. Allow 3 weeks for recovery.

HOW TO TREAT

GENERAL MEASURES
• For obstruction (if surgery is not necessary): Massage the tear duct twice a day with fingertips to milk the contents.
• For infection: Relieve pain by applying warm soaks (see Soaks in Appendix).

MEDICATION—Your doctor may prescribe oral or topical antibiotics for infection.

ACTIVITY—Reduce activity during treatment for the infection. Avoid swimming and contact sports.

DIET—No special diet.

CALL YOUR DOCTOR IF

• You have symptoms of a tear-duct infection or blockage.
• You have a temperature of 101F (38.3C) or more.
• Symptoms don't improve, despite treatment.
• Your vision is affected.

TEETHING
(Cutting Teeth; Tooth Eruption)

GENERAL INFORMATION

DEFINITION—Sequential appearance of baby teeth and adult teeth. New teeth erupt continually from age 6 months to 3 years. Between ages 6 and 12, children lose baby teeth, which are replaced with adult teeth. On average, the first set of teeth is complete soon after the second birthday.

BODY PARTS INVOLVED—Mouth; teeth.

SEX OR AGE MOST AFFECTED—Both sexes of children from ages 6 months to 3 years and 6 to 12 years.

SIGNS & SYMPTOMS
- Excess saliva production, drooling and chewing on anything the baby can hold.
- Pain. (This symptom cannot be proven, but probably does occur.)
- Gums may become red or swollen.
- Fretfulness; clinging.
- Irritability; difficulty in sleeping.
- Crying more than usual.
- Teething should not be considered the only reason for fever, vomiting, diarrhea, prolonged loss of appetite, earache, convulsions, cough or diaper rash. These are possible symptoms of an illness. Consult your doctor.

CAUSES—Normal physiological development.

RISK INCREASES WITH—Teething problems are not related to any known risk factor.

HOW TO PREVENT—Teething problems cannot be prevented, but symptoms can be relieved.

WHAT TO EXPECT

DIAGNOSTIC MEASURES—Your own observation of teething symptoms.

APPROPRIATE HEALTH CARE
- Home care for teething discomfort.
- Doctor or dentist's treatment (complications only).

POSSIBLE COMPLICATIONS
- If not cared for properly, baby teeth may decay and need filling.
- Teething may be misdiagnosed as a fever-causing illness.

PROBABLE OUTCOME—Teething discomfort can be partially relieved.

HOW TO TREAT

GENERAL MEASURES
- The sequence of normal tooth eruption in children is:
  First teeth (lower front teeth) at about 6 months, sooner in girls than boys.
  First adult teeth at about age 6.
  Bicuspids (side teeth) between ages 10 and 12.
  Permanent molars at about age 12.
- Home-care:
  Rub the child's gums with your finger; this is very comforting.
  Freeze a coarse washcloth and allow the child to chew it.
  Offer the child a teething biscuit or teething ring (you may chill it).
  Keep the child amused or occupied.
  Clean new teeth and gums with a cotton swab and water or use your finger with a soft washcloth wrapped around it. Wait until the child is 2 or 3 years old before brushing teeth regularly. By this age, children want to imitate parents by brushing teeth.
- Begin regular dental visits at age 2 or 3.
- At age 5, explain to the child that losing baby teeth is normal. This prevents the child from becoming concerned when tooth loss begins.

MEDICATION—Medicine usually is not necessary for teething discomfort. Acetaminophen in proper dosages, or a cream or ointment rubbed on the gums to ease discomfort may be recommended by your doctor.

ACTIVITY—No restrictions.

DIET—No special diet. Chewing on teething biscuits or zwieback toast may help some infants.

CALL YOUR DOCTOR IF

- The child's temperature rises above normal.
- Signs of infection, such as pain, pus, excessive swelling or very red gums, occur at the site of the erupting tooth.

ILLNESS & DISORDERS

TELOGEN EFFLUVIUM

 GENERAL INFORMATION

DEFINITION—Generalized hair loss in which numerous, scattered hair follicles simultaneously change from the growing phase to the resting stage of the hair-growth cycle. Persons with telogen effluvium rarely progress to significant baldness and it is not contagious.

BODY PARTS INVOLVED—Hair; scalp.

SEX OR AGE MOST AFFECTED—Both sexes and all ages but most common in young females (age 8 through adolescence).

SIGNS & SYMPTOMS
- Hair loss of 4 to 5 times the normal rate. Normal hair loss is approximately 400 hairs a day, mostly during washing or brushing.
- No itching or pain.

CAUSES
- Hormonal changes, such as those that occur during adolescence, following childbirth or after discontinuing use of oral contraceptives.
- Severe psychological stress—including that of serious illness, such as high fever, heart attack or stroke.

RISK INCREASES WITH
- Stress.
- Pregnancy.
- Menopause.

HOW TO PREVENT—No specific preventive measures.

 WHAT TO EXPECT

DIAGNOSTIC MEASURES
- Your own observation of symptoms.
- Medical history and physical exam by a doctor (severe, prolonged cases only).

APPROPRIATE HEALTH CARE—Self-care.

POSSIBLE COMPLICATIONS—None expected.

PROBABLE OUTCOME—Spontaneous recovery in 6 to 12 months.

 HOW TO TREAT

GENERAL MEASURES
- Continue to wash and brush your hair as usual.
- Confront and define areas of conflict in your family life, occupational and leisure-time activities. If you cannot resolve conflicts, ask for help from family, friends or competent counselors.
- Aim for a balance of work, recreation, reflection and rest.
- Concentrate on feeling positive. A good attitude toward yourself and others is a powerful asset.

MEDICATION—Medicine usually is not necessary for this disorder.

ACTIVITY—No restrictions. Engage in a regular exercise program at least 3 times a week to reduce stress and maintain good overall fitness.

DIET—No special diet or supplements. Eat a normal, well-balanced diet to provide the nutrients necessary for healthy hair growth.

 CALL YOUR DOCTOR IF

- Hair loss doesn't improve in 4 months.
- Signs of infection (pain, redness, tenderness, swelling) begin at the site of hair loss.

TEMPOROMANDIBULAR JOINT SYNDROME
(Myofascial Pain-Dysfunction Syndrome)

GENERAL INFORMATION

DEFINITION—Pain and inflammation in the temporomandibular joint (TMJ), the joint on either side of the jaw that opens and closes the mouth, and adjoining muscles.

BODY PARTS INVOLVED—
Temporomandibular joint; facial muscles; sensory nerves.

SEX OR AGE MOST AFFECTED—Adults of both sexes, but more common in women.

SIGNS & SYMPTOMS
- Dull, aching pain on one side of the jaw (below the ear) that radiates to the temples, back of the head and along the jaw line.
- Tenderness of the muscles used to chew.
- "Clicking" or "popping" sounds when opening the mouth.
- Inability to open the jaw completely.
- Headache and toothache.
- Aching back, shoulders or neck.
- Pain brought on by yawning.

CAUSES
- Faulty alignment ("bite") between the upper and lower jaws (disk derangement).
- Displacement of the joint as a result of jaw, head or neck injuries.
- TMJ inflammation.
- Myofacial pain dysfunction.
- Hypermobility or hypomobility of the TMJ.

RISK INCREASES WITH
- Grinding or clenching teeth.
- Tension of the masticatory (chewing) muscles.
- Stress.
- Poorly aligned teeth.
- Poorly fitting dentures.
- Osteoarthritis or rheumatoid arthritis.

HOW TO PREVENT—Don't grind your teeth. Learn techniques for relaxing muscles and relieving tension, such as biofeedback, meditation and exercise.

WHAT TO EXPECT

DIAGNOSTIC MEASURES
- Your own observation of symptoms.
- Medical history and physical exam by a doctor or dentist.
- Jaw range-of-motion studies, dental x-rays, arthroscopy and MRI (see Glossary for both).

APPROPRIATE HEALTH CARE
- Self-care after diagnosis.
- Treatment program may involve correction of occlusal disorders, attainment of normal muscle function, pain control, stress management and behavior modification.

- Psychotherapy or counseling, including biofeedback training, to learn new ways to cope with stress.
- Correction of poorly aligned teeth with braces or other orthodontic device.
- A dentist may manufacture, fit and install a night-guard prosthesis to prevent tooth-grinding while asleep. A night-guard prosthesis consists of removable splints that fit over the tops of the teeth to eliminate incorrect biting pressure.
- Rarely, surgery may be recommended for severe cases that do not respond to simpler measures. Be sure you understand all aspects involved with surgery and seek a second opinion.

POSSIBLE COMPLICATIONS
- Loss of joint range-of-motion.
- Secondary degenerative joint disease.
- Depression and chronic pain syndrome.

PROBABLE OUTCOME—With conservative treatment, symptoms can usually be controlled within 3 months.

HOW TO TREAT

GENERAL MEASURES
- Ice and/or heat may be of slight benefit in relieving discomfort, but will not cure. Try one and then the other to see what works best for you.
- Massage the TMJ muscle area.
- Don't chew gum.
- Don't use a pillow for sleeping. Roll up a towel and place it under your neck. Sleep on your back.
- Try to limit jaw movements and learn to relax the jaw. Block a yawn by putting your fist under your chin.

MEDICATION
- Your doctor may prescribe:
  Tranquilizers or muscle relaxants for a short time.
  Nonsteroidal anti-inflammatory drugs.
- For minor pain, you may use nonprescription drugs, such as aspirin or acetaminophen.

ACTIVITY—No restrictions.

DIET—Eat a soft diet until symptoms subside. Avoid hard, chewy foods such as bagels.

CALL YOUR DOCTOR IF

- You have symptoms of temporomandibular joint syndrome.
- Symptoms do not improve or worsen after self-care treatment.
- New, unexplained symptoms develop. Drugs used in treatment may produce side effects.

TENDINITIS

GENERAL INFORMATION

DEFINITION—Painful inflammation of a tendon (tendinitis) and the lining of the tendon sheath (tenosynovitis). They most often occur simultaneously. Normally, tendon fibers merge into muscle fibers. A typical skeletal muscle has a tendon on each end that attaches to bone. The force of a muscle contraction is transmitted through the tendon to produce movement.

BODY PARTS INVOLVED—Common sites are the shoulder (rotator cuff), elbow, heel (Achilles' tendon), knee or hamstring.

SEX OR AGE MOST AFFECTED—
Adolescents and adults.

SIGNS & SYMPTOMS—Symptoms may begin slowly or occur gradually over a 24 hour period after overuse of the affected joint:
- Restricted movement.
- Tenderness and swelling around the inflamed tendon.
- Weakness in the tendon.
- Pain in the affected joint (achy or burning).

CAUSES
- Injury, usually from strenuous athletic activity.
- Musculoskeletal disorders, including congenital defects and rheumatism.
- Poor posture.

RISK INCREASES WITH
- Overuse of certain tendons and joints from participation in active, competitive sports.
- Incorrect movement and strain during activity. For example, repeatedly holding and swinging a golf club or tennis racket incorrectly may cause tendinitis at the elbow (see Tennis Elbow in Illness section).

HOW TO PREVENT
- Precondition your body and build up strength gradually for a sport before beginning it on a regular, competitive basis.
- Warm up before each workout.
- Learn the proper techniques for any sport you intend to play regularly.

WHAT TO EXPECT

DIAGNOSTIC MEASURES
- Medical history and exam by a doctor.
- Diagnostic tests usually unnecessary (x-rays do not show ligaments and tendons).

APPROPRIATE HEALTH CARE
- Self-care for mild cases.
- Doctor's treatment.
- Physical therapy for more severe injuries.

POSSIBLE COMPLICATIONS
- Chronic soreness; possible reinjury.

- Large deposits of calcium in the inflamed tendon, leading to permanent impairment ("frozen joint").

PROBABLE OUTCOME—Usually curable with treatment and rest of the tendon. Healing time varies with degree of injury; may range from a few days to 6 weeks.

HOW TO TREAT

GENERAL MEASURES—Treatment varies with the cause, severity and duration of the condition. Use the RICE therapy (rest, ice, compression, elevation):
- With severe pain, stiffness and tenderness, relax completely with the injured area resting on a pillow until pain becomes more bearable. Elevate the injured area.
- Apply ice packs to the affected area during the acute stage or after receiving injections.
- After using ice, wrap the area in an elastic bandage. Do this for several days. It helps keep swelling down and eases discomfort.
- When pain diminishes, you may temporarily want to use a sling or splint for upper extremity injury or use crutches, canes or braces for lower extremity injury.
- After the acute phase, apply heat. Take hot showers, soak in bath tub, apply hot compresses, use a heat lamp or heating pad.
- Chronic tendinitis may require lifestyle changes to prevent recurring joint irritation.

MEDICATION
- You may use ibuprofen, naproxen or aspirin for pain and inflammation. Acetaminophen helps pain, but not the inflammation.
- Your doctor may prescribe:
  Injections of local anesthetics.
  Injections of cortisone into painful and calcified tendons. This reduces pain and inflammation and allows movement, preventing a frozen joint.
  Stronger pain or anti-inflammatory drugs.

ACTIVITY
- Resume your normal activities as soon as symptoms improve.
- Once pain is gone, begin range-of-motion and stretching exercises on the affected joint.

DIET—No special diet.

CALL YOUR DOCTOR IF

- You have symptoms of tendinitis that don't resolve with self-care.
- If the injured joint area appears distorted or discolored.
- Pain and swelling increases, despite treatment.

TENNIS ELBOW
(Epicondylitis)

GENERAL INFORMATION

DEFINITION—Inflammation of bony areas of the elbow.

BODY PARTS INVOLVED—Elbow muscles, tendons and epicondyle (a bony prominence on either side of the elbow where muscles of the forearm attach to the bone of the upper arm).

SEX OR AGE MOST AFFECTED—Adults (20 to 40 years).

SIGNS & SYMPTOMS
• Pain and tenderness over the epicondyle.
• Weak grip.
• Pain when twisting the hand and arm, as in using a screwdriver or playing tennis.

CAUSES—Partial tear of the tendon and attached covering of the bone caused by:
• Chronic stress on the tissues that attach the forearm muscles to the elbow area.
• Sudden strain on the forearm.

RISK INCREASES WITH
• Occupations that require strenuous or repetitive forearm movement, such as mechanics or carpentry.
• Participation in sports that require strenuous or repetitive forearm movement, such as tennis.
• Poor physical conditioning.

HOW TO PREVENT
• Don't play sports, such as tennis, for long periods until you are in excellent condition. Take frequent rest periods.
• Tennis racquets can aggravate tennis elbow. Choosing a different size or type (larger, more flexible, larger grip) may help.
• Get professional help if you are just learning tennis. Technique and conditioning are important in preventing injuries.
• Do forearm conditioning exercises to build your strength gradually.
• Warm up slowly and completely before participating in sports, especially before competition.

WHAT TO EXPECT

DIAGNOSTIC MEASURES
• Your own observation of symptoms.
• Medical history and physical exam by a doctor.
• Diagnostic tests are usually not necessary (x-rays are usually always negative).

APPROPRIATE HEALTH CARE
• Self-care after diagnosis. Treatment normally consists of medications and supportive care.
• Doctor's treatment.
• Physical therapy.
• If other methods of treatment fail, surgical release of the tendon at the epicondyle may be necessary.

POSSIBLE COMPLICATIONS—Complete ligament tear, requiring surgery to repair.

PROBABLE OUTCOME—Usually curable, but treatment may require 3 to 6 months.

HOW TO TREAT

GENERAL MEASURES
• Use heat or ice to relieve pain. Use warm soaks, a heat lamp or soak in a whirlpool or use cold compresses or ice packs (whichever seems to help the most).
• Apply a forearm band (tennis elbow splint) around the thickest portion of the forearm.
• You may receive diathermy, ultrasound or massage treatments. These help bring quicker symptom relief and healing.
• Massage therapy and manipulation.
• You may need to wear a forearm splint to immobilize the elbow. Do the following exercise 3 or 4 times a day while wearing the splint: Stretch your arm, flex your wrist, then press the back of your hand against a wall. Hold for 1 minute.
• Consider using a tennis-elbow strap when you resume normal activity after treatment.

MEDICATIONS—Your doctor may prescribe:
• Nonsteroidal anti-inflammatory drugs to reduce inflammation.
• Injections of anesthetics or cortisone drugs. Cortisone reduces inflammation and anesthetics temporarily relieve pain. Caution: Repeated injections may weaken the muscle ligament.

ACTIVITY—Don't repeat the activity that caused tennis elbow until symptoms disappear. Then resume your normal activities gradually after proper conditioning.

DIET—No special diet.

CALL YOUR DOCTOR IF

• You have symptoms of tennis elbow.
• Symptoms don't improve in 2 weeks, despite treatment.

TESTES, UNDESCENDED
(Cryptorchidism)

GENERAL INFORMATION

DEFINITION—A disorder present at birth in which one or both testicles have not descended from the pelvis into their normal position in the scrotum. In some boys, they descend spontaneously without treatment by age 1.

BODY PARTS INVOLVED—One or both testes (testicles); scrotum; spermatic cord.

SEX OR AGE MOST AFFECTED—Male infants and children.

SIGNS & SYMPTOMS
* Scrotum appears undeveloped on one or both sides.
* Testicle can't be felt in its normal position in the scrotum.

CAUSES
* Unknown, but probably related to hormone deficiency in the mother or fetus.
* Presence of fibers that interrupt its route and cause it to remain in the groin.

RISK INCREASES WITH—Family history of undescended testes.

HOW TO PREVENT—No specific preventive measures.

WHAT TO EXPECT

DIAGNOSTIC MEASURES
* Your own observation of symptoms.
* Medical history and physical exam by a doctor.
* Ultrasound or CT scan (see Glossary for both) if testis cannot be felt.

APPROPRIATE HEALTH CARE
* Doctor's treatment.
* Treatment will be determined by type of cryptorchidism. If the testis lies in the scrotum at times and then retracts occasionally, the problem normally resolves itself by puberty. Other forms are treated with hormones or by surgery.
* Surgery to move the testes into the scrotum. Surgery is the only treatment for those who don't respond to hormone treatment. Surgery ideally should be performed at a young age (less than 18 months) to help preserve reproductive function. (See Testicle Fixation in Surgery section.)

POSSIBLE COMPLICATIONS
* Increased possibility of testicular cancer.
* Sterility or reduced fertility rate.
* Psychological problems associated with an altered male self-image, if the problem is not corrected.
* Lack of normal sexual development, if testes are not present.
* Hernia development.

PROBABLE OUTCOME—Usually curable if treated with surgery or hormones. The prognosis for future fertility may be 80% if one testicle is involved and 50% if both are involved.

HOW TO TREAT

GENERAL MEASURES
* If a testis appears to be missing after birth, check periodically to see if it has descended on its own accord.
* There is no need to discuss the problem with the child and cause him undue worry.

MEDICATION—Your doctor may prescribe human chorionic gonadotrophins by injection. These are usually given 3 times a week for 4 to 6 weeks. This treatment causes testes to descend normally in about 25% of cases.

ACTIVITY—No restrictions.

DIET—No special diet.

CALL YOUR DOCTOR IF

Your child has undescended testes. Call as soon as you identify this abnormality.

TESTICLE TORSION

GENERAL INFORMATION

DEFINITION—Twisting of the spermatic cord of the testicle, damaging the testicle—sometimes irreversibly. Testicle torsion usually occurs on one side only. Prompt treatment is necessary to salvage the affected testicle.

BODY PARTS INVOLVED—Testicle; spermatic cord; blood supply to each.

SEX OR AGE MOST AFFECTED—Males of all ages, but most common in adolescents (12 to 20 years).

SIGNS & SYMPTOMS
- Sudden pain in one testicle.
- Swelling, redness and tenderness of the scrotum.
- Nausea and vomiting.
- Sweating.
- Rapid heartbeat, if pain is severe.

CAUSES—Usually unknown. It is occasionally present at birth, or may rarely be caused by an injury or sudden, forceful contraction of muscles attached to the testicle and spermatic cord.

RISK INCREASES WITH—Unknown.

HOW TO PREVENT—Wear an athletic supporter or cup when participating in contact sports to prevent genital injury.

WHAT TO EXPECT

DIAGNOSTIC MEASURES
- Your own observation of symptoms.
- Medical history and physical exam by a doctor.
- Ultrasound (sometimes) (see Glossary).

APPROPRIATE HEALTH CARE
- Doctor's treatment.
- Immediate surgery to untangle the twisted spermatic cord and to attach the affected testicle to the inside scrotal wall, which prevents recurrence. The surgeon will probably operate on the unaffected testicle also to prevent torsion.

POSSIBLE COMPLICATIONS—Death of cells in the testicle caused by a diminished or blocked blood supply. This strangulation requires removal of the affected testicle and spermatic cord.

PROBABLE OUTCOME—Sometimes the torsion will correct itself, symptoms will disappear and no treatment will be needed. However, the testicle is usually injured beyond repair unless surgery is done within 3 to 4 hours after symptoms begin.

If one testicle must be removed, the remaining healthy testicle should provide enough hormones for normal male maturation, sex life and reproduction.

HOW TO TREAT

GENERAL MEASURES
- After surgery, use ice packs to relieve pain and swelling. Wrap the ice in plastic. Apply it to the affected side, separating the ice from the skin with a cloth towel. Apply ice 5 to 10 minutes at a time. Repeat as often as necessary.
- Return to your doctor for suture removal in about 7 days.

MEDICATION—After surgery, your doctor may prescribe pain relievers.

ACTIVITY—Resume your normal activities gradually after surgery.

DIET—No special diet.

CALL YOUR DOCTOR IF

- You have symptoms of testicular torsion. This is an emergency!
- Signs of infection begin after surgery. These include fever, chills, muscle aches, headache, dizziness and a general ill feeling.
- Excessive bleeding occurs at the surgical site.

ILLNESS & DISORDERS

TESTICULAR CANCER

GENERAL INFORMATION

DEFINITION—Uncontrolled growth of malignant cells in the testicle. It is rare, but is the most common form of cancer in young men. There are several types of testicular cancer, some more dangerous than others.

BODY PARTS INVOLVED—Testicles (usually one only).

SEX OR AGE MOST AFFECTED—Older adolescent and young adult males (ages 20-40).

SIGNS & SYMPTOMS
- A firm swelling in one testicle discovered by accident or by self-examination.
- No pain (usually).
- Sense of fullness in the scrotum.

CAUSES—Unknown.

RISK INCREASES WITH
- Undescended testicle(s) in infancy even if the testicle was surgically moved into the scrotum.
- Caucasian race.

HOW TO PREVENT—Males should examine testicles routinely at least once a month (see Testicular Self Examination in Appendix). This will not prevent the cancer, but may detect a tumor early enough to provide assurance of cure.

WHAT TO EXPECT

DIAGNOSTIC MEASURES
- Your own observation of symptoms. Testicular self-examination (see Appendix) is the most important diagnostic measure.
- Medical history and physical exam by a doctor.
- Diagnostic tests may include ultrasound, CT scan (see Glossary for both) of scrotum and abdomen, chest x-ray, radioimmune assay (a special laboratory blood study) and pedal lymphangiography (x-ray of the lymph glands). Tests are to verify the diagnosis and to determine if cancer has spread.

APPROPRIATE HEALTH CARE
- Doctor's treatment.
- Surgery to remove the cancerous testicle is the main form of treatment (see Testicle Removal in Surgery section).
- Radiation therapy or chemotherapy following surgery for some types of tumors.

POSSIBLE COMPLICATIONS—Without treatment, some tumors may spread to other parts of the body.

PROBABLE OUTCOME—Most types of testicular tumors are curable with surgery and other treatment. A few types are extremely malignant and have a high death rate unless discovered and treated early.

Removal of one testicle does not interfere with normal sexual function or the ability to have children.

HOW TO TREAT

GENERAL MEASURES
- The more you can learn and understand about this disorder, the better you will be able to make informed decisions about where to go for your care, the treatments available, the risks involved, side effects of therapy and expected outcome.
- See Resources for Additional Information.

MEDICATION
- Your doctor may prescribe anticancer drugs for some types of tumors.
- Pain medicine if needed.

ACTIVITY
- Resume your normal activities as soon as possible. Radiation and chemotherapy may cause temporary fatigue requiring extra rest.
- Resume sexual relations when you are able. Contraception may be necessary for 12 to 18 months because some forms of treatment cause temporary genetic damage to sperm in the remaining testicle.

DIET—No special diet.

CALL YOUR DOCTOR IF

- You have a firm swelling or mass in the scrotum.
- New, unexplained symptoms develop. Drugs used in treatment may produce side effects.

TETANUS
(Lockjaw)

GENERAL INFORMATION

DEFINITION—An infection in a wound or injury that causes severe muscle spasms. Tetanus is not contagious from person to person.

BODY PARTS INVOLVED—Injured tissue; muscles throughout the body, especially the jaw, neck, back and abdomen.

SEX OR AGE MOST AFFECTED—Both sexes; all ages.

SIGNS & SYMPTOMS
- Stiffness of the jaw.
- Muscle pain, irritability and frequent, severe spasms.
- Severe swallowing difficulty.
- Fever.
- Difficulty using chest muscles to breathe.
- Fast pulse.
- Profuse sweating.

CAUSES—Bacteria (Clostridium tetani) that are present almost everywhere—especially in soil, manure or dust. Bacteria may enter through any break in the skin, including burns or puncture wounds. Toxins produced by the bacteria travel to nerves that control muscle contraction, producing muscle spasms and seizures.

RISK INCREASES WITH
- Diabetes mellitus.
- Adults over 60.
- Lack of up-to-date tetanus immunizations.
- Warm, humid weather.
- Crowded or unsanitary living conditions, especially for newborn infants born to nonimmunized mothers.
- Use of street drugs administered with unclean needles and syringes.
- Burns, surgical wounds and skin ulcers.

HOW TO PREVENT—Obtain tetanus immunizations. These consist of 3 immunization shots, starting at 2 months of age with boosters at 18 months, 5 years, and every 10 years afterwards. An additional booster shot may be necessary at the time of injury. Private doctors or local health departments may provide immunizations at little or no cost.

WHAT TO EXPECT

DIAGNOSTIC MEASURES
- Your own observation of symptoms.
- Medical history and physical exam by a doctor.
- Laboratory blood and culture studies.

APPROPRIATE HEALTH CARE
- Doctor's treatment.
- Hospitalization in a quiet, dark room. Treatment may include the use of breathing tubes, a respirator, intravenous fluid support, and medications.
- Surgery to remove infected tissue.

POSSIBLE COMPLICATIONS
- Pneumonia.
- Pressure sores.
- Irregular heartbeat.
- Respiratory paralysis and death.

PROBABLE OUTCOME—The death rate from tetanus is 50%. With early diagnosis and treatment, however, full recovery is likely. Allow 4 weeks for recovery.

HOW TO TREAT

GENERAL MEASURES—Provide the patient with reassurance and psychological support. Despite the seriousness of tetanus, patients are usually conscious.

MEDICATION—Your doctor may prescribe:
- Antitoxins to neutralize the nerve toxin.
- Muscle relaxants to control spasms.
- Sedatives to relieve anxiety.
- Anticonvulsants for seizures.
- Antibiotics for infections.

ACTIVITY—During hospitalization, bed rest is necessary with as little disturbance as possible. During recovery, activities should be resumed gradually.

DIET—During hospitalization, intravenous fluids will be necessary because of swallowing difficulty.

CALL YOUR DOCTOR IF

- You have symptoms of tetanus or observe them in someone else. Call immediately. This is an emergency!
- You or someone in your family needs basic or booster tetanus immunizations.
- You have a puncture wound or injury that breaks the skin, and you have not had an immunization or booster in 5 years.

THALASSEMIA
(Mediterranean Anemia; Hereditary Leptocytosis)

 GENERAL INFORMATION

DEFINITION—An inherited form of anemia in which red blood cells contain less hemoglobin than normal. Types are:
- Alpha-thalassemia—Found in populations from the Chinese subcontinent (Malaysia, Indochina, Africa). It is less common than the beta type.
- Beta-thalassemia—Found in Mediterranean area and Africa. If a person inherits one defective gene, it is called beta thalassemia minor (or trait); with two defective genes (one from each parent), it is called beta thalassemia major (or Cooley's anemia) and is a more serious disorder; a milder form also exists, betathalassemia intermedia.

BODY PARTS INVOLVED—Blood.

SEX OR AGE MOST AFFECTED—Both sexes; all ages.

SIGNS & SYMPTOMS—The minor form may produce no symptoms. When symptoms occur, they may include:
- Fatigue.
- Paleness.
- Breathlessness.
- Irregular heartbeat, especially with exertion.
- Bloody or dark urine.
- Jaundice (yellow skin and eyes).
- Leg ulcers.
- Enlarged spleen.

CAUSES—Inheritance of a defective gene that affects hemoglobin production. Hemoglobin in healthy people has two pairs of protein chains (alpha and beta); with thalassemia, one of the protein chains is reduced and causes an imbalance between the two chains in the hemoglobin produced.

RISK INCREASES WITH
- Poor nutrition, especially a diet likely to produce other anemias.
- Obesity.
- Family history of thalassemia.
- Genetic factors, including absence of the gene necessary to manufacture hemoglobin-A. The disorder first appeared in persons of Mediterranean heritage; it also affects people from the Middle East and Far East.

HOW TO PREVENT
- Cannot be prevented at present, especially if the mother and father have thalassemia or the thalassemia genetic trait. If you have a family history of thalassemia, obtain genetic counseling before having children.
- Prenatal screening is available.

 WHAT TO EXPECT

DIAGNOSTIC MEASURES
- Medical history and exam by a doctor.
- Laboratory blood tests and bone-marrow examinations.

APPROPRIATE HEALTH CARE
- Doctor's treatment.
- Hospitalization for transfusions as needed.
- Surgery to remove the spleen.
- Iron chelation therapy for excess iron in the blood.
- Bone-marrow transplant.

POSSIBLE COMPLICATIONS
- Susceptibility to infections, worsening of anemia, jaundice, leg ulcers, cholelithiasis, pathologic fractures, impaired growth rate, delayed or absent puberty, cardiac disease.
- Repeated transfusions increase the risk of transfusion reaction.

PROBABLE OUTCOME—Varies. This condition is currently considered incurable. However, symptoms can be relieved or controlled. It usually causes death by early adulthood or middle age, depending on the severity of the symptoms. Some forms are consistent with a normal or nearly normal lifespan. Scientific research into causes and treatment continues, so there is hope for increasingly effective treatment.

 HOW TO TREAT

MEDICATION—Your doctor may prescribe:
- Antibiotics for infections.
- Folic acid supplements.
- Deferoxamine by injection for iron chelation therapy. Vitamin C is usually prescribed to patients on this therapy.

ACTIVITY
- Avoid strenuous sports activities.
- Activity levels will depend on the disorder.

DIET—No special diet. Don't take iron supplements; they make symptoms worse. Drinking tea may help reduce the iron in the blood.

 CALL YOUR DOCTOR IF

- You have symptoms of anemia (fatigue, paleness, irregular heartbeat, breathlessness).
- You want genetic counseling.

THORACIC-OUTLET OBSTRUCTION SYNDROME (Cervical-Rib Syndrome)

 ## GENERAL INFORMATION

DEFINITION—Pain and weakness from compression of nerves in the neck that affect the shoulders, arms and hands.

BODY PARTS INVOLVED—Nerves and blood vessels that supply the neck, shoulders, arms and hands.

SEX OR AGE MOST AFFECTED—Adults between ages 35 and 55, usually women.

SIGNS & SYMPTOMS
- Pain, numbness and tingling in the neck, shoulders, arms and hands.
- Weakness in the arms and hands.
- Poor blood circulation, characterized by coldness, swelling and blueness in the hands and fingers (rare).
- Absent pulse in the wrist when raising the arm and turning the head toward the opposite shoulder.

CAUSES—The nerves and blood vessels that supply the shoulder, arms and hands start in the neck and pass as a bundle near the cervical ribs and collarbone. Pressure on this nerve and blood-vessel bundle creates symptoms. Pressure may be caused by:
- An extra rib in the lower neck or overdeveloped neck muscles.
- Muscle weakness and drooping in the shoulder.
- Injury from overextending the arm or shoulder.
- Tumor that has spread to the head and neck area from another part of the body.

RISK INCREASES WITH
- Fracture of clavicle or first rib.
- Body building with muscle bulk in thoracic outlet area.
- Rapid weight loss combined with vigorous physical exertion or exercise.

HOW TO PREVENT
- Avoid shoulder and neck injury whenever possible. Wear seat belts and use padded headrests in cars.
- Don't use mind-altering drugs or drink excessive amounts of alcohol.

 ## WHAT TO EXPECT

DIAGNOSTIC MEASURES
- Your own observation of symptoms.
- Medical history and physical exam by a doctor.
- X-ray, arteriogram (see Glossary), venogram (x-ray of a vein filled with contrast medium) and CT scan (see Glossary).

APPROPRIATE HEALTH CARE
- Doctor's treatment.
- Treatment usually involves physical therapy and exercises unless there is an obvious bony abnormality.
- Surgery to relieve pressure on the nerves and blood vessels.

POSSIBLE COMPLICATIONS
- Postoperative pain or abnormal sensation in arm and hand.
- Recurrence of the disorder.

PROBABLE OUTCOME—Usually curable in most patients with physical therapy or surgery.

 ## HOW TO TREAT

GENERAL MEASURES—Use heat to relieve pain. Use a heating pad, heat lamp, hot showers or warm compresses.

MEDICATION
- You may use nonprescription drugs, such as acetaminophen or aspirin, to relieve pain. Medication cannot correct the underlying condition.
- Your doctor may prescribe antispasmodics and muscle relaxants.

ACTIVITY
- Physical therapy and exercises will be prescribed to promote shoulder muscle function and improve any posture faults. These are usually recommended for 2 to 3 months.
- Avoid straining or heavy activity for 3 months.

DIET—No special diet. If overweight, a weight-reducing diet is recommended.

 ## CALL YOUR DOCTOR IF

- You have symptoms of thoracic-outlet obstruction syndrome.
- Symptoms don't improve in 2 weeks, despite treatment.

THROMBOCYTOPENIA

GENERAL INFORMATION

DEFINITION—A decrease in the circulating number of platelet cells in the blood. Platelets play a vital role in the control of bleeding by plugging any small breaks that occur in the walls of blood vessels. With thrombocytopenia, there is a tendency to bleed, particularly from the smaller blood vessels. This causes abnormal bleeding into the skin and other body parts.

BODY PARTS INVOLVED—Blood, which affects all body parts.

SEX OR AGE MOST AFFECTED—Both sexes; all ages.

SIGNS & SYMPTOMS
- Petechiae (round, nonraised, purple-red spots on the skin).
- Bruising tendency; bleeding in mouth or nose;
- Heavy or prolonged menstrual periods; blood in the urine (if bleeding is prolonged).

CAUSES
- Congenital (present at birth).
- Decreased or defective production of platelets in the marrow.
- Sometimes the cause is unknown (idiopathic).

RISK INCREASES WITH
- Acute infection; HIV infection.
- Taking aspirin or other nonsteroidal anti-inflammatory drugs; taking drugs such as quinidine, sulfa preparations, oral antidiabetic agents, gold salts, rifampin, etc.
- Hypersplenism; hypothermia; blood transfusion.
- Excess alcohol consumption.
- Pre-eclampsia.
- Other diseases such as systemic lupus erythematosus, anemia, leukemia, cirrhosis.
- Exposure to x-ray or radiation.

HOW TO PREVENT
- Avoid medications, when possible, that are a risk factor.
- For patients with thrombocytopenia, avoid trauma and seek treatment if trauma occurs.

WHAT TO EXPECT

DIAGNOSTIC MEASURES
- Medical history and exam by a doctor.
- Laboratory blood studies that show low number of platelets.

APPROPRIATE HEALTH CARE
- No treatment may be necessary in some cases and the thrombocytopenia is allowed to run its course.
- Other treatment programs vary depending on the underlying cause.
- Discontinuance of the offending drug in drug-induced thrombocytopenia.

- Surgery to remove the spleen.
- Platelet transfusions for patients with serious hemorrhage or anticipating major surgery and in some chronic thrombocytopenic patients.

POSSIBLE COMPLICATIONS
- Stroke (cerebral hemorrhage) severe blood loss.
- Pneumococcal infection.
- Adverse effects of drug therapy.

PROBABLE OUTCOME
- For acute cases, particularly in children, most recover within two months.
- Chronic cases may have remissions and relapses, some recover spontaneously.

HOW TO TREAT

GENERAL MEASURES
- To stop bleeding at any accessible site, apply cold compresses or ice packs and pressure until bleeding stops. If nosebleeds are a problem, humidify your air. Use a cool-mist, ultrasonic humidifier. Clean humidifier daily.
- Inform any doctor or dentist who treats you that you have thrombocytopenia.
- Avoid surgery, including dental surgery, unless it is essential. Practice good dental hygiene. Also, avoid injections. If a shot is necessary, apply pressure continuously to the injection site for 5 minutes.
- Monitor your skin condition. Look for any signs of petechiae (round, nonraised, purple-red spots on the skin) or bruising. Have someone else check the skin areas you cannot see.
- Avoid injury whenever possible.
- Wear a Medic-Alert (see Glossary) bracelet or neck tag that indicates your medical problem and any medications you take.

MEDICATION—Your doctor may prescribe: Corticosteroids at time of diagnosis and in relapsing cases; gamma globulin during acute phase of a severe episode; immunosuppressive therapy in persistent cases.

ACTIVITY
- Bed rest during acute phase.
- Limit activity to prevent injury.
- Avoid contact and high risk sports.

DIET—No special diet.

CALL YOUR DOCTOR IF

- The following occurs during treatment:
  Bleeding that can't be stopped.
  Enlargement of the abdomen.
  Black, tarry stools or vomit that looks like coffee grounds.
  A rash (described under Signs & Symptoms)—especially with fever.
- New, unexplained symptoms develop.

THROMBOPHLEBITIS, SUPERFICIAL
(Phlebitis; Phlebothrombosis)

 GENERAL INFORMATION

DEFINITION—Inflammation and small blood clots in a superficial vein, usually in the legs, primarily caused by infection or injury. This type of inflammation seldom causes clots to break loose and flow in the bloodstream, unlike deep-vein thrombosis.

BODY PARTS INVOLVED—Superficial veins, usually in the legs.

SEX OR AGE MOST AFFECTED
• Both sexes, but more common in females.
• All ages, but most common in adults.

SIGNS & SYMPTOMS
• Hardness of superficial vein (cord-like).
• Redness, tenderness and pain in the affected area.
• Fever (sometimes).

CAUSES—Increased fibrin and clotting of red blood cells in a vein due to impaired blood flow. This prevents blood from returning to the heart. The blood below the clot stays there forcing fluid into the tissues, causing swelling (edema). The veins and surrounding area may become inflamed and tender.
• Illness or surgery with long bed confinement.
• Injury or infection that damages a vein.
• Congestive heart failure.

RISK INCREASES WITH
• Smoking; obesity.
• Use of birth-control pills. Combining birth-control pills and smoking greatly increases risk.
• Occupations requiring long periods of standing or sitting.
• Illness with prolonged bed confinement.
• Varicose veins; surgery, trauma, burns, infections; pregnancy; intravenous drug abuse; blood vessel disorders.

HOW TO PREVENT
• Don't smoke if you take birth-control pills.
• If confined to bed for any reason, move the legs as much as possible to prevent pooling of blood in the veins.
• Avoid using any drug intravenously.
• Hospitalized patients should take preventive measures including medications, special stockings or compression boots.

 WHAT TO EXPECT

DIAGNOSTIC MEASURES
• Medical history and exam by a doctor.
• Laboratory blood studies, if the cause is not immediately apparent.

APPROPRIATE HEALTH CARE
• Doctor's treatment.
• Treatment usually involves rest and elevation of the extremity, sometimes medications depending on the cause.

POSSIBLE COMPLICATIONS
• May lead to deep vein thrombosis (clots within the deep veins).
• If there is an infection and it remains untreated, it could lead to blood poisoning.

PROBABLE OUTCOME—Usually curable in 2 weeks.

 HOW TO TREAT

GENERAL MEASURES
• Wearing elastic stockings or using a wrapped elastic bandage may hasten the blood flow through the veins, relieving discomfort and helping prevent further clot formation. Don't wear garters or knee-high hosiery.
• To relieve pain, use wrapped soaks (see Soaks in Appendix).
• Stop smoking and stop taking birth-control pills. If you continue both, the next episode of vein clots may be a dangerous, deep-vein clot.

MEDICATION—Your doctor may prescribe:
• Nonsteroidal anti-inflammatory drugs, including aspirin, to decrease inflammation and pain.
• Antibiotics, if bacterial infection is suspected (rare).
• Anticoagulant drugs (occasionally).
• Topical ointments to relieve any itching.

ACTIVITY—Bed rest with the affected limb elevated may be helpful for 1 or 2 days. Move the feet, ankles and legs often. When the inflammation begins to subside, resume normal activity slowly. Rest often. Don't sit or stand for prolonged periods, and don't cross legs.

DIET—No special diet.

 CALL YOUR DOCTOR IF

• You have symptoms of superficial thrombophlebitis.
• The following occur during treatment:
  Fever of 102F (38.9C) or higher.
  Intolerable pain.
  Coughing blood.
  Shortness of breath.
  Chest pain.
  Swelling of leg or foot.
• New, unexplained symptoms develop. Drugs used in treatment may produce side effects.

THROMBOSIS, DEEP-VEIN

GENERAL INFORMATION

DEFINITION—A blood clot that forms inside a deep vein. It may partially or completely block blood flow, or break off and travel to the lung. This is different from clots in superficial veins, where clots rarely break off.

BODY PARTS INVOLVED—Usually lower legs (calves) or lower abdomen, but occasionally affects other veins in the body.

SEX OR AGE MOST AFFECTED—All ages, but most common in persons over age 60.

SIGNS & SYMPTOMS
- Sometimes no symptoms.
- Swelling and pain in the area drained by the vein, usually the ankle, calf or thigh. Swelling in the leg includes everything below the clot, extending to the toes.
- Tenderness and redness of the affected parts.
- Soreness or pain when walking. The soreness does not disappear with rest.
- Pain when raising the leg and flexing the foot (sometimes).
- Fever (sometimes).
- Increased heartbeat (sometimes).

CAUSES—Pooling of blood in the vein, which triggers blood-clotting mechanisms. The pooling may occur after prolonged bed rest following surgery, or from debilitating illness, such as heart attack, stroke or bone fracture.

RISK INCREASES WITH
- Persons over 60; obesity; smoking.
- Use of estrogen in oral contraceptives or for replacement after menopause. This is especially hazardous if estrogen use is combined with smoking.
- Surgery; trauma; pregnancy; cancer.
- Disorders such as heart failure, stroke and polycythemia.

HOW TO PREVENT
- Avoid prolonged bed rest during illnesses. Start moving the lower limbs as soon as possible after any surgical procedure or during any bed-confining illness.
- On long auto or airplane trips, exercise your legs at least every 1 or 2 hours.
- Stop smoking, especially if you take estrogen.

WHAT TO EXPECT

DIAGNOSTIC MEASURES
- Medical history and exam by a doctor.
- Laboratory studies, such as venography (x-ray study of the veins), ultrasound and plethysmography (see Glossary for both).

APPROPRIATE HEALTH CARE
- Doctor's treatment.
- If the clots are small, confined to the calf and the patient is mobile, no treatment may be necessary. The clots often break up spontaneously.
- Hospitalization required for some patients for anticoagulant injections and observation for complications.
- For certain patients, a surgical procedure to insert a filtering device ("umbrella") into the vena cava (main vein to lungs) to trap clots before they reach the lungs.
- Self-care after hospitalization.

POSSIBLE COMPLICATIONS—Pulmonary embolism, in which the clot breaks away and travels to the lung. The lung's blood supply is blocked, causing affected lung tissue to die.

PROBABLE OUTCOME—Usually curable with anticoagulant treatment, if pulmonary embolism can be avoided.

HOW TO TREAT

GENERAL MEASURES—The following suggestions apply after hospitalization or if the condition can be treated safely at home:
- Wear fitted elastic stockings or wrapped elastic bandages, but don't wear garters or knee-high hosiery.
- Don't cross your legs or ankles while sitting, lying in bed or traveling.
- Elevate the feet higher than the hips when sitting for long periods.
- Elevate the foot of the bed.

MEDICATION—Your doctor may prescribe:
- Intravenous anticoagulant to prevent the extension of the clots.
- Thrombolytic drugs, which dissolve the clots.
- Oral anticoagulants may be necessary for 6 months or longer. To minimize the danger of pulmonary embolism, blood tests to monitor the anticoagulant level are mandatory.

ACTIVITY—Rest in bed until all signs of inflammation have disappeared. While resting, make it a habit to move leg muscles, bend ankles and wiggle toes.

DIET—No special diet.

CALL YOUR DOCTOR IF

- You have symptoms of deep-vein thrombosis.
- The following occurs during treatment:
  Unexpected bleeding anywhere.
  Chest pain.
  Coughing up blood.
  Shortness of breath, despite treatment.
- New, unexplained symptoms develop. Drugs used in treatment may produce side effects.

THROMBOSIS & EMBOLUS, ARTERIAL

 ## GENERAL INFORMATION

DEFINITION—Blood clot formation in an artery (thrombosis) that may travel to distant organs (embolus).

BODY PARTS INVOLVED—Large or medium arteries anywhere in the body, especially arteries in the neck or arteries to the brain, intestine, legs, arms or kidney.

SEX OR AGE MOST AFFECTED—Adults of both sexes.

SIGNS & SYMPTOMS—The following depend on where the embolus lodges:
- Brain: blindness, speaking difficulty, partial paralysis, hearing loss, headache and dizziness.
- Extremities: pain in the arm or calf after exercise (subsides with rest); weakness, numbness, burning and tingling sensations; weak or absent pulse beyond the blocked blood flow. These symptoms subside with rest.
- Intestine: abdominal pain; nausea; vomiting; and shock.

CAUSES—Clots may form with any condition that damages the smooth lining of the heart or that of a blood vessel. As the clot grows, small or large portions break away and are carried by the bloodstream to the brain, abdomen, extremities or other areas.
Conditions that damage the blood-vessel lining include:
- Atherosclerosis (hardening of the arteries).
- Injury to a blood vessel from accident or surgery.
- Heart valve disease.
- Heart attack.
- Atrial fibrillation.

RISK INCREASES WITH
- Adults over 60.
- Smoking.
- High blood pressure.
- Diabetes mellitus.
- Previous transient ischemic attacks.

HOW TO PREVENT
- If you have high blood pressure or diabetes mellitus, adhere to your treatment program to control the disease.
- Take anticoagulant drugs for a short time after injury or surgery to prevent blood clots.
- Exercise regularly to keep blood vessels healthy.

 ## WHAT TO EXPECT

DIAGNOSTIC MEASURES
- Your own observation of symptoms.
- Medical history and physical exam by a doctor.
- Venography or arteriography (see Glossary for both).
- Surgery to repair or replace damaged blood vessels or to remove an embolus by suction or bypass.

APPROPRIATE HEALTH CARE
- Self-care after diagnosis.
- Doctor's treatment.
- Surgery to repair or replace damaged blood vessels or to remove an embolus by suction or bypass.

POSSIBLE COMPLICATIONS—Tissue death or gangrene in cells deprived of oxygen by a clot.

PROBABLE OUTCOME—Depends on the organs affected, size of the affected blood vessel and size of the embolus. Early treatment is essential. Clots can sometimes be removed with surgery, relieving symptoms. Clots to the brain, kidney and intestines may cause death or permanent disability.

 ## HOW TO TREAT

GENERAL MEASURES—Follow suggestions under Diet and Activity to maintain a healthy lifestyle.

MEDICATION—Your doctor may prescribe:
- Anticoagulants to thin the blood and reduce the chance of embolus.
- Vasodilators to widen blood vessels.

ACTIVITY—Complete rest is necessary until circulation is re-established by surgery or other treatment.

DIET—No special diet during recovery. However, atherosclerosis and diabetes require dietary control.

 ## CALL YOUR DOCTOR IF

- You have symptoms of arterial thrombosis or embolus.
- Symptoms return after surgery.
- New, unexplained symptoms develop. Drugs used in treatment may produce side effects.

ILLNESS & DISORDERS

THRUSH

GENERAL INFORMATION

DEFINITION—A common fungus infection of the mouth.

BODY PARTS INVOLVED—Mouth; gums; tongue; soft palate; cheeks; lips.

SEX OR AGE MOST AFFECTED—Newborns and infants, but may also affect older children and adults.

SIGNS & SYMPTOMS—Patches appear in the mouth with the following characteristics:
- Patches are white to creamy yellow and slightly raised. They are similar to milk curds, but they don't wipe off.
- Patches are not painful unless they are rubbed off. Then they leave small, painful ulcers.
- The mouth is dry.

CAUSES—A fungus called Candida albicans. It is usually present in small numbers in the mouth, but certain factors may cause it to multiply out of control:
- Treatment with antibiotics. This may upset the natural balance of organisms in the mouth and allow thrush to develop.
- Birth. Newborns may acquire the infection during passage through the birth canal, especially if the mother has a vaginal yeast infection. Thrush appears within hours or up to 7 days after birth.
- Aging. Older persons develop thrush because of lower natural resistance.

RISK INCREASES WITH
- Poor nutrition.
- Illness that has lowered resistance.
- HIV infection (thrush in adults is part of the criteria for diagnosis).
- Diabetes.
- Irritation from dentures.
- Immunosuppression due to illness or drugs.
- Chronic use of steroid medication (oral or inhaled).

HOW TO PREVENT
- Good oral hygiene.
- Avoid unnecessary antibiotics.

WHAT TO EXPECT

DIAGNOSTIC MEASURES
- Your own observation of symptoms.
- Medical history and physical exam by a doctor.
- Scraping of the plaque and the material examined under a microscope.

APPROPRIATE HEALTH CARE
- Self-care.
- Doctor's treatment if self-care is not successful.
- Treatment is aimed at improving the underlying condition that predisposes the patient to the infection and relieving the symptoms of thrush.

POSSIBLE COMPLICATIONS—Can spread to vagina, skin, larynx, gastrointestinal tract or respiratory system.

PROBABLE OUTCOME—Treatment usually clears this infection in 3 days. It is not dangerous or serious, but it has a tendency to recur.

HOW TO TREAT

GENERAL MEASURES—If an infant has the infection, boil bottle nipples separately for 20 minutes before the final sterilization.

MEDICATION
- A dilution of hydrogen peroxide as a mouth rinse will soothe the discomfort.
- Your doctor may prescribe:
  A throat lozenge of clotrimazole dissolved in the mouth for a course of treatment.
  Nystatin suspension to be applied to the lesions.
  Oral ketoconazole for more severe disorder.
- Anticandidal creams to be applied under dentures or at the corners of the mouth.

ACTIVITY—No restrictions.

DIET—No changes in infants. Older children and adults should maintain an adequate fluid intake with milk, liquid gelatin, ice cream, custard, water, tea or other beverages and foods that are easy to swallow. Use a straw for drinking if the patches are painful.

CALL YOUR DOCTOR IF

- You or your child has symptoms of thrush.
- Signs of dehydration (sunken eyes, poor elasticity of the skin and lethargy) appear in a child.
- An infant fails to gain weight or an unexplained weight loss occurs in an older person.
- Fever develops.
- Lesions on the skin or vagina appear.
- Signs of secondary bacterial infection (pain, redness, tenderness, swelling) occurs in the mouth.

THUMB-SUCKING

GENERAL INFORMATION

DEFINITION—Placing the finger or thumb on the roof of the mouth behind the teeth and sucking with lips and teeth closed. Thumb sucking is common and is a behavior, not a disorder.

BODY PARTS INVOLVED—Mouth; teeth; tongue; pharynx; finger or thumb.

SEX OR AGE MOST AFFECTED—Children of both sexes up to age 12; but most common in young children.

SIGNS & SYMPTOMS—Sucking of the thumb (most likely to occur before going to sleep, watching TV, or when hungry, ill or tired).

CAUSES—Thumb sucking is one of the first coordinated acts that an infant can do that brings comfort, pleasure and satisfies a need for extra sucking. Thumb sucking that persists beyond infancy (particularly into preschool years) might suggest a situational disorder.

RISK INCREASES WITH
- Addition of a new baby brother or sister in the family.
- Infant senses a withdrawal of parents' interest or attention.

HOW TO PREVENT
- Thumb sucking is normal and does not cause serious damage until the permanent teeth begin cutting through gums at age 6 or 7. Most children have outgrown the habit by this age. If not, parents should work with the child to change the habit for the sake of appearance and dental health.
- Provide other comfort mechanisms early in infancy, such as pacifiers if you desire.

WHAT TO EXPECT

DIAGNOSTIC MEASURES
- Your own observation of symptoms.
- Medical history and physical exam by a doctor or dentist (sometimes).

APPROPRIATE HEALTH CARE
- Home care.
- Doctor's or dentist's treatment (sometimes).
- Psychotherapy or counseling (prolonged or excessive thumb-sucking only).

POSSIBLE COMPLICATIONS—Protruding front teeth. Thumb sucking may put enough pressure on front teeth to move them forward eventually.

PROBABLE OUTCOME—In most cases, the habit is given up spontaneously, especially if has not become an issue between parents and child.

HOW TO TREAT

GENERAL MEASURES
- No treatment or action is usually necessary. Methods such as punishment, shaming and reminders are usually of no avail. Other methods also are not particularly successful (mittens, bad-tasting substances on the thumb, elbow splints, etc.) and may cause additional trauma.
- For a child over 6 or 7 who sucks the fingers or thumb:
  Give the child extra attention. Observe if conflicts or anxiety-producing situations provoke sucking. Help the child explore other solutions to stress.
  If the child decides to try to stop sucking, help the child set goals. Give rewards for any progress toward the goal. Reward is not a bribe, but something earned through effort.

MEDICATION—Medicine usually is not necessary for this disorder.

ACTIVITY—No restrictions.

DIET—No special diet.

CALL YOUR DOCTOR IF OR DENTIST IF

- Your child wishes to stop and behavior-modification efforts (rewards for progress) have not solved the problem. The dentist may fit a training device in the child's mouth to prevent the thumb from touching the roof of the mouth.
- The child becomes intolerant of the training device or it loosens.
- The sucking behavior does not diminish in 6 months, despite treatment.

THYROID NODULE

GENERAL INFORMATION

DEFINITION—A benign or malignant nodule involving the thyroid gland in the front of the neck. Benign tumors are much more common and are unlikely to spread to other body parts. These growths may be cystic or solid (thyroid adenoma). Malignant thyroid nodules can spread and threaten life. Early symptoms of both types are the same.

BODY PARTS INVOLVED—Thyroid gland in the front of the neck.

SEX OR AGE MOST AFFECTED
• Both sexes, but benign nodules are more common in women than men.
• All ages, but malignant nodules are more likely in children between ages 4 and 7.

SIGNS & SYMPTOMS
• Swelling or lump in the thyroid gland.
• Pain and tenderness in the thyroid gland.
• Swallowing difficulty.
• Hoarseness.
• Breathing difficulty (rare).
• Symptoms of hypothyroidism or hyperthyroidism (both in Illness section).

CAUSES—Unknown.

RISK INCREASES WITH
• Radiation treatment during childhood—even in small doses—to the head, neck and upper chest.
• Family history of thyroid tumors.
• Iodine deficiency.

HOW TO PREVENT—Avoid radiation treatments to the neck for acne, tonsillitis, enlarged thymus gland or other minor conditions.

WHAT TO EXPECT

DIAGNOSTIC MEASURES
• Your own observation of symptoms.
• Medical history and physical exam by a doctor.
• Laboratory tests, such as thyroid scans, needle biopsy, ultrasound (see Glossary for all), and x-rays. Tests help rule out cancer and avoid unnecessary surgery.

APPROPRIATE HEALTH CARE
• Treatment varies and may involve one or a combination of therapies.
• Suppressive doses of thyroid hormone may be used for some cases, both as an aid in diagnosis and as a treatment. If nodules increase in size, surgery is recommended.

• Surgery to aspirate a cystic tumor or to remove a solid tumor and the affected lobe of the thyroid (near-total thyroidectomy; lobectomy).
• Radioactive iodine treatment.

POSSIBLE COMPLICATIONS
• Spread of a malignant tumor to adjacent parts, requiring radical surgery to remove lymph nodes and muscles of one side of the neck.
• Hypothyroidism or hypoparathyroidism, caused by inadvertent injury to the thyroid or parathyroid glands during surgery.
• Permanent hoarseness and loss of voice following surgery for some thyroid cancers.

PROBABLE OUTCOME—Usually curable with surgery or a combination of surgery and radioactive-iodine treatment.

HOW TO TREAT

GENERAL MEASURES
• For an explanation of surgery and postoperative care, see Thyroidectomy (in Surgery section).
• See Resources for Additional Information under Cancer and Thyroid.

MEDICATION—Your doctor may prescribe:
• Antithyroid medications or replacement thyroid hormone.
• Radioactive iodine to treat cancer (I-131).
• Pain relievers.

ACTIVITY
• Resume your normal activities as soon as symptoms improve after surgery.
• Speech therapy may be recommended if the voice is affected after surgery.

DIET—No special diet.

CALL YOUR DOCTOR IF

• You have symptoms of thyroid nodules or thyroid enlargement.
• The following occurs after surgery:
  Symptoms of hypothyroidism (fatigue, puffy face, rapid weight gain, coarse hair and decreased sex drive).
  Bleeding, pain or swelling at the surgical site.
  Fever.
  Twitching muscles.
  Breathing difficulty.
• New, unexplained symptoms develop. Drugs used in treatment may produce side effects.

THYROIDITIS

GENERAL INFORMATION

DEFINITION—Inflammation of the thyroid gland.

BODY PARTS INVOLVED—Thyroid gland, a hormone-producing organ at the base of the neck, next to the trachea (windpipe).

SEX OR AGE MOST AFFECTED—Middle-aged persons of both sexes between ages 30 and 50, but more common in women.

SIGNS & SYMPTOMS
- Enlarged, painful, tender thyroid gland.
- Fever.
- Pain in the jaw or ears (sometimes).
- Hyperthyroidism (rapid heartbeat, nervousness, tremor and rapid weight loss).

CAUSES
- Disorder of the autoimmune system (especially Hashimoto's and postpartum thyroiditis).
- Various viruses, such as mumps or influenza.
- Bacterial infection of the thyroid gland (rare).

RISK INCREASES WITH
- Recent illness, such as tuberculosis or any infection.
- Pregnancy.
- Family history of thyroiditis.
- Previous thyroid disorders.

HOW TO PREVENT—No specific preventive measures.

WHAT TO EXPECT

DIAGNOSTIC MEASURES
- Your own observation of symptoms.
- Medical history and physical exam by a doctor.
- Laboratory blood counts and thyroid radioiodine uptake and scan, and rarely, ultrasound (see Glossary).

APPROPRIATE HEALTH CARE
- Self-care after diagnosis.
- Doctor's treatment. Consultation with an endocrinologist may be valuable.
- Drug treatment will depend on type of thyroiditis.
- Surgery to relieve pressure on adjacent areas of the neck or to drain an abscess (rare).

POSSIBLE COMPLICATIONS—Permanent loss of thyroid function, requiring lifelong thyroid-hormone replacement.

PROBABLE OUTCOME—Usually curable with treatment. Some persons recover spontaneously. Regular medical follow-up is recommended after the condition is apparently cured.

HOW TO TREAT

GENERAL MEASURES
- Follow instructions from your doctor about medications and follow-up studies to determine the effectiveness of the treatment.
- See Resources for Additional Information.

MEDICATION—Your doctor may prescribe:
- Antithyroid medication or thyroid replacement hormones, depending on the activity of your thyroid hormones.
- Beta-adrenergic blockers to suppress symptoms of an overactive thyroid.
- Antibiotics to fight infection, if necessary.
- Cortisone drugs to decrease inflammation (rare).
- Aspirin in high doses to help inflammation subside.
- Pain medication if needed.

ACTIVITY—Resume your normal activities as soon as symptoms improve.

DIET—No special diet.

CALL YOUR DOCTOR IF

- You have symptoms of thyroiditis.
- The following occurs during treatment: Fever and redness of the thyroid gland. Lethargy.
- New, unexplained symptoms develop. Drugs used in treatment may produce side effects.

ILLNESS & DISORDERS

TINEA VERSICOLOR

 GENERAL INFORMATION

DEFINITION—A yeast infection of the skin that changes the color of skin it affects.

BODY PARTS INVOLVED—Skin of the chest, back, shoulders, upper arms, trunk or groin. This rarely affects the face.

SEX OR AGE MOST AFFECTED— Adolescents and adults.

SIGNS & SYMPTOMS—Lesions with the following characteristics:
* Lesions on exposed skin are white; on covered areas, they are brown or brownish red.
* Lesions are flat with clearly defined borders. They don't scale unless scraped.
* Lesions begin at 3 to 4mm in diameter and spread. They often join together to form large patches.

CAUSES—A developing stage of the yeast, Pityrosporum orbiculare. High heat and high humidity favor the growth of this yeast. The infection is contagious, but how it spreads is unknown.

RISK INCREASES WITH—Environmental exposure to heat and high humidity.

HOW TO PREVENT—No specific preventive measures.

 WHAT TO EXPECT

DIAGNOSTIC MEASURES
* Your own observation of symptoms.
* Medical history and physical exam by a doctor.
* Laboratory culture of scrapings for positive diagnosis.

APPROPRIATE HEALTH CARE
* Doctor's treatment.
* Self-care after diagnosis.
* Numerous topical medicines are effective in clearing tinea versicolor.

POSSIBLE COMPLICATIONS—Unlimited recurrence without treatment.

PROBABLE OUTCOME—Untreated tinea versicolor persists indefinitely but seems to come and go at times. It frequently recurs, even with treatment. Following treatment, the white patches will remain for months after the yeast infection has been cured.

 HOW TO TREAT

GENERAL MEASURES
* Apply medicine with cotton balls to affected parts as prescribed. Rinse off in 30 minutes if you wish.
* Expose affected skin to air as much as possible.
* Repeat treatment prior to tanning season each year.

MEDICATION—Your doctor may recommend selenium sulfide shampoo, clotrimazole, miconazole or ketoconazole cream to apply to affected areas.

ACTIVITY—No restrictions.

DIET—No special diet.

 CALL YOUR DOCTOR IF

* You have symptoms of tinea versicolor.
* Infection doesn't improve despite treatment.

TINNITUS

GENERAL INFORMATION

DEFINITION—A persistent sound heard in one or both ears when there is no environmental noise. Tinnitus can be an extremely common symptom of nearly all ear disorders as well as many other medical problems.

BODY PARTS INVOLVED—Ears.

SEX OR AGE MOST AFFECTED—Both sexes; all ages.

SIGNS & SYMPTOMS—A noise that may be ringing, buzzing, roaring, whistling or hissing sound, and be heard in one or both ears. The sound may be continuous, intermittent or synchronized with the heartbeat.

CAUSES—Normally the acoustic nerve transmits impulses to the brain as a result of vibrations produced by external sound waves. With tinnitus, for reasons not fully understood, the nerve transmits impulses that originate inside the head or within the ear itself.

RISK INCREASES WITH
- Hearing loss.
- Labyrinthitis.
- Meniere's disease.
- Otitis media or externa.
- Otosclerosis (disorder of the middle ear).
- Ototoxicity (having a poisonous effect on the ear).
- Earwax blockage.
- Aneurysm or tumor in the head (rare).
- Foreign body in the ear.
- Certain medications (antibiotics, aspirin, diuretics and others).
- High or low blood pressure.
- Head trauma.
- Anemia.
- Hypothyroidism or hyperthyroidism.
- Allergies.
- Changes in barometric pressure, such as when flying.

PREVENTIVE MEASURES—No specific prevention known. Avoid the risk factors where possible.

WHAT TO EXPECT

DIAGNOSTIC MEASURES
- Your own observation of symptoms.
- Medical history and physical exam by a doctor.

APPROPRIATE HEALTH CARE—A thorough medical examination is conducted to be sure all possible causes have been sought out and corrected with appropriate treatment.

POSSIBLE COMPLICATIONS—There are usually no medical complications. Psychological problems may develop due to feelings of distress for those who find the noise intolerable.

PROBABLE OUTCOME—Treatment of an underlying disorder may help, but often there is no cure and learning to cope is the only therapy. Some people tolerate the condition much better than others.

HOW TO TREAT

GENERAL MEASURES
- If tinnitus continues following medical treatment for underlying disorder, the treatment is basically finding methods that help you cope with the constant noise.
- Try to ignore the sound by directing your attention to other things and activities.
- Play music in the background during the day and while falling asleep.
- Don't smoke. Get help with a cessation program if you need it.
- A hearing aid for any associated deafness may help mask tinnitus.
- Wear a tinnitus suppressor or masker, a device that fits in the ear like a hearing aid and presents a more pleasant sound.
- Electrical stimulation with cochlear implant may reduce tinnitus, but is appropriate for severe deafness only.
- See Resources for Additional Information.

MEDICATION—Medications do not help tinnitus.

ACTIVITY—Avoid getting overfatigued as it may worsen the tinnitus.

DIET—Cutting back on caffeine and chocolate may help some patients.

CALL YOUR DOCTOR IF

- You or a family member has symptoms of tinnitus.
- Feelings of distress about tinnitus worsen.

ILLNESS & DISORDERS

TOENAIL, INGROWN

GENERAL INFORMATION

DEFINITION—A condition in which the sharp edge of a nail grows into the flesh of a toe, usually the great (big) toe.

BODY PARTS INVOLVED—Toes.

SEX OR AGE MOST AFFECTED—All ages, but most common in adolescents and adults.

SIGNS & SYMPTOMS—Pain, tenderness, redness, swelling and heat in the toe where the sharp nail edge pierces the surrounding fold of tissue. Once tissue surrounding the nail becomes inflamed, infection usually develops in the injured area.

CAUSES—An ingrown toenail is likely to accompany one of the following conditions:
• The nail formation is more curved than normal.
• The toenail is clipped back too far, allowing tissue to grow up over it.
• Shoes fit poorly, forcing the toe of the shoe against the nail and surrounding tissue.
• The person participates in activities that require sudden stops ("toe jamming").

RISK INCREASES WITH—Any of the circumstances listed as causes.

HOW TO PREVENT
• Wear roomy, well-fitting shoes.
• Cut toenails carefully. Persons with diabetes mellitus or peripheral vascular disease should be especially careful in trimming toenails. Foot injury is dangerous with these disorders because of impaired blood circulation to the feet.

WHAT TO EXPECT

DIAGNOSTIC MEASURES
• Your own observation of symptoms.
• Medical history and physical exam by a doctor.

APPROPRIATE HEALTH CARE
• Self-care.
• Doctor's treatment.
• Surgery to remove the nail.

POSSIBLE COMPLICATIONS—Chronic infection that cannot be cured without surgery.

PROBABLE OUTCOME—Curable with treatment. Oral antibiotics usually relieve symptoms of infection within 1 week. Sometimes part or all of the toenail is removed surgically.

HOW TO TREAT

GENERAL MEASURES—The following home treatment is appropriate either before or after surgery:
• Use immersion soaks (see Soaks in Appendix).
• Lift the nail corners free of surrounding inflamed tissue by wedging a small piece of cotton under the nail around the edges. Protect the inflamed tissue from further injury.

MEDICATION—Your doctor may prescribe antibiotics to fight infection.

ACTIVITY—Resume your normal activities as soon as symptoms improve. You may need to wear a shoe with the toe cut out until the toe heals.

DIET—No special diet.

CALL YOUR DOCTOR IF

• You have symptoms of an ingrown toenail.
• The following occurs during treatment or after surgery:
Fever.
Increased pain.
Signs of infection (pain, redness, tenderness, swelling or heat) in the toe.

TONGUE INFLAMMATION
(Glossitis)

GENERAL INFORMATION

DEFINITION—Acute or chronic inflammation of the tongue from a variety of causes. This is sometimes contagious, but not cancerous.

BODY PARTS INVOLVED—Tongue and adjacent parts of the mouth.

SEX OR AGE MOST AFFECTED—Both sexes; all ages.

SIGNS & SYMPTOMS—Any of the following:
- Bright red, swollen tongue.
- Ulcers on the tongue.
- Hairy-looking tongue.
- A tongue with red tip and edges.

CAUSES
- Infections, including herpes.
- Burns.
- Injury from jagged teeth, ill-fitting dentures, mouth-breathing or repeated biting during convulsive seizures.
- Excessive consumption of alcohol, tobacco, hot food or spices.
- Poor dental health.
- Allergy to toothpaste, mouthwash (especially mouthwash containing peroxide), candy, dye or material used in dental work.
- Lack of B-vitamins, resulting in pellagra, B-12-deficiency anemia or iron-deficiency anemia.
- Adverse reaction to antibiotic drugs.

RISK INCREASES WITH
- Poor nutrition, especially vitamin deficiencies.
- Smoking.
- Chemical or environmental exposure to irritating or corrosive chemicals.
- Alcoholism.
- Anxiety or depression.
- Diabetes mellitus.

HOW TO PREVENT
- Practice good oral hygiene. Brush teeth and tongue at least twice a day, and floss teeth daily. Get regular dental checkups.
- Don't smoke.
- Prevent tongue injury by wearing protective headgear for contact sports or cycling.

WHAT TO EXPECT

DIAGNOSTIC MEASURES
- Your own observation of symptoms.
- Medical history and exam by a doctor.
- Laboratory blood studies or biopsy (see Glossary) to determine any underlying disorder.

APPROPRIATE HEALTH CARE
- Self-care.
- Doctor's treatment if self-care doesn't relieve symptoms.

POSSIBLE COMPLICATIONS—Tongue inflammation can become chronic if not adequately treated.

PROBABLE OUTCOME—Usually curable in 2 weeks with treatment.

HOW TO TREAT

GENERAL MEASURES
- Treatment will be directed at the underlying cause along with self-help measures.
- Observe if there is an association between eating specific foods and tongue inflammation. Irritating foods may include chocolate, citrus, acid foods (vinegar, pickles), salted nuts or potato chips.
- Rinse mouth 3 or more times a day with a salt solution (1/2 teaspoon salt to 8 oz. water).
- If tongue inflammation is caused by a rough tooth or denture, consult your dentist. Inflammation won't heal until the cause is eliminated.

MEDICATION
- For minor pain, you may use nonprescription drugs, such as anesthetic mouthwashes or acetaminophen.
- For infection and pain, your doctor may prescribe antibiotics or topical anesthetics.

ACTIVITY—No restrictions.

DIET—No special diet, except to avoid foods that aggravate inflammation. Drink as many fluids and eat as well-balanced a diet as possible while healing. To minimize pain, sip liquids through straws. Foods that cause the least pain are milk, liquid gelatin, yogurt, ice cream and custard.

CALL YOUR DOCTOR IF

- Fever develops.
- Symptoms don't improve in 3 days despite treatment.
- Pain is unbearable and isn't relieved by treatment.
- Skin rash appears.
- Weight loss occurs.
- Tongue swells and interferes with swallowing.

TONSILLITIS

GENERAL INFORMATION

DEFINITION—Inflammation of the tonsils (lymph glands located at the back of the throat). Tonsils are small at birth, enlarge during childhood, and become smaller at puberty. Tonsils normally help prevent infection in the sinuses, mouth and throat from spreading to other body parts. Tonsillitis is contagious.

BODY PARTS INVOLVED—Tonsils; pharynx.

SEX OR AGE MOST AFFECTED—All ages, but most common in children between ages 5 and 10.

SIGNS & SYMPTOMS
- Throat pain, either mild or severe.
- Swallowing difficulty.
- Chills and fever as high as 104F (40C) or more.
- Swollen lymph glands on either side of the jaw.
- Headache.
- Ear pain.
- Cough (sometimes).
- Vomiting (sometimes).
- Very young child refuses to eat.

CAUSES—Bacterial (usually streptococcal) or viral infection of the tonsils.

RISK INCREASES WITH
- Crowded or unsanitary living conditions.
- Exposure to others in public places.

HOW TO PREVENT—Avoid exposure to people with upper-respiratory infections.

WHAT TO EXPECT

DIAGNOSTIC MEASURES
- Your own observation of symptoms.
- Medical history and physical exam by a doctor.
- Laboratory throat culture. Family members should be cultured also, so that carriers can be treated at the same time.

APPROPRIATE HEALTH CARE
- Home care.
- Treatment is usually with antibiotics and self-care. Surgery to remove the tonsils for repeated acute tonsillitis or for chronic tonsillitis. (See Tonsil & Adenoid Removal in Surgery section.)

POSSIBLE COMPLICATIONS
- Abscess of the tonsils and nearby throat area, requiring surgery to drain.
- Chronic tonsillitis, with a recurrent sore throat and greatly enlarged tonsils, caused by repeated attacks.

- Rheumatic fever, if the bacterial infection is streptococcal and it is not treated with antibiotics, or if antibiotics are discontinued before 10 days.

PROBABLE OUTCOME—Usually spontaneous recovery. Symptoms generally begin to improve in 2 to 3 days, but treatment may last longer.

If attacks of tonsillitis are so severe and frequent that they affect one's general health or interfere with schooling, hearing or breathing, your doctor may recommend surgery to remove the tonsils.

A tonsillectomy involves small risk, but the risk increases with age.

HOW TO TREAT

GENERAL MEASURES
- Use a cool-mist, ultrasonic humidifier to relieve throat irritation and cough. Clean humidifier daily.
- Prepare a soothing tea or other gargle. Double the usual strength of tea. This may be gargled warm or cold as often as is soothing.

MEDICATION
- If the tonsillitis is caused by a streptococcal infection, your doctor will prescribe penicillin or other antibiotics for at least 10 days.
- To relieve pain, you may use acetaminophen.

ACTIVITY
- Keep the patient away from others until fever, pain and other symptoms disappear.
- Bed rest, except to use the bathroom, is necessary until fever subsides. Normal activity may be resumed when temperature has been normal for 2 or 3 days.

DIET—Increase all fluid intake. While the throat is very sore, use liquid nourishment, such as milk shakes, soups, and high-protein fluids (diet or instant-breakfast milk drinks).

CALL YOUR DOCTOR IF

- You have symptoms of tonsillitis. If tonsils cover the opening of the throat (hold down the tongue with a spoon and look with a flashlight), call your doctor immediately.
- Symptoms worsen or the following occurs during treatment:
  Temperature is normal for 1 or 2 days, then fever returns.
  New symptoms begin, such as: nausea; vomiting; skin rash; thick nasal drainage; chest pain; or shortness of breath.
  There is a convulsion.
  Joints become red or painful.
  Cough produces a discolored (green, yellow, brown or bloody) sputum.

TOOTH ABSCESS
(Periapical Abscess; Periodontal Abscess)

 GENERAL INFORMATION

DEFINITION—An abscess (pus-filled sac) around a tooth root, which is imbedded in bone of the upper or lower jaw.

BODY PARTS INVOLVED—Teeth, gums; jawbone.

SEX OR AGE MOST AFFECTED—Both sexes; all ages.

SIGNS & SYMPTOMS
- Persistent toothache or throbbing, extreme pain upon biting or chewing.
- Swelling and tenderness in the neck glands and on the side of the face.
- Earache.
- Fever.
- General ill feeling.
- Foul taste and bad breath (if the abscess opens spontaneously).

CAUSES—The pulp (nerves and blood vessels that fill the central cavity of a tooth) is invaded by bacteria, usually as a result of dental caries that destroy a tooth's enamel and dentin, or when a tooth is injured. Abscesses also develop from periodontal disease when bacteria invades the pockets between the teeth and gums.

RISK INCREASES WITH
- Tartar beneath the gum.
- Poor nutrition.
- Improper diet.
- Inadequate fluoride in drinking water.

HOW TO PREVENT
- Prevent decay with good brushing and flossing:
Use a soft-bristle toothbrush to remove plaque from the teeth's front and back surfaces, especially at the gum line.
Learn to use dental floss correctly. Ask your dentist or hygienist to demonstrate the technique.
- Use fluoride mouthwash, toothpaste, tablets or liquid supplements if your dentist recommends them.
- Reduce sugar consumption. Tooth decay increases as sugar consumption increases.

 WHAT TO EXPECT

DIAGNOSTIC MEASURES
- Your own observation of symptoms.
- Medical history and physical exam by a dentist.
- X-rays of the mouth.

APPROPRIATE HEALTH CARE—Tooth abscesses can be drained in one of 3 ways:
- If the tooth has poor bone and gum support,

the tooth can be extracted, allowing the abscess to drain through the socket and heal.
- A hole can be drilled through the top of the tooth, and a tiny metal or plastic wick inserted into the narrow nerve canal through the center of the tooth. This allows the abscess to drain.
- An incision can be made in the gum at the site of infection, which dramatically relieves pain and pressure. Your dentist may place a small rubber wick in the incision for a few days. When the infection improves, your dentist can perform root-canal therapy (see Root Canal in Surgery section).

POSSIBLE COMPLICATIONS
- If untreated, the abscess erodes a small channel through the jawbone to the gums surface where it forms a gumboil (swelling). If the gumboil bursts, it lets foul-tasting pus into the mouth.
- Loss of the tooth.
- Spread of infection through the bloodstream to other body parts.

PROBABLE OUTCOME—Curable with treatment.

 HOW TO TREAT

GENERAL MEASURES
- Rinse your mouth with warm water to draw infection from the abscess. Repeat each hour or as often as feels good.
- Don't chew on the affected side of your mouth for at least 2 days.
- If a tube has been used to drain the abscess, keep the small hole free of infection. Carefully remove impacted food.
- If a drain has been placed in gum tissue, return to your dentist in several days to have it removed.

MEDICATION
- For minor pain, you may use nonprescription drugs such as acetaminophen.
- Your doctor or dentist may prescribe:
Antibiotics to control infection.
Pain relievers.

ACTIVITY—Resume your normal activities as soon as possible.

DIET—A liquid diet may be necessary for 1 or 2 days until pain subsides.

 CALL YOUR DENTIST IF

- You have symptoms of a tooth abscess.
- The following occurs during treatment:
Fever spikes to 101F (38.3C) or higher.
Pain becomes unbearable.
- New, unexplained symptoms develop. Drugs used in treatment may produce side effects.

TOOTH DECAY
(Caries; Dental Decay; Cavities)

 GENERAL INFORMATION

DEFINITION—Disintegration of tooth enamel, allowing injury to the dentin (layer below the enamel) and eventual involvement of the pulp (the layer below the dentin), which contains nerves and blood vessels. Tooth decay and the common cold are the most common human disorders.

BODY PARTS INVOLVED—Teeth.

SEX OR AGE MOST AFFECTED—Both sexes; all ages.

SIGNS & SYMPTOMS
• Tooth sensitivity to heat and cold.
• Tooth discomfort after eating sugar.
• Darkening on or between the teeth (cavity) when the decay has progressed enough to be seen. The most common tooth-cavity sites are the gum line, biting surfaces and surfaces between adjacent teeth.
• Unpleasant taste in the mouth and bad breath because of stagnant food and bacteria trapped in the cavity.
• Persistent tooth pain (in the final stages of decay when the pulp becomes inflamed).

CAUSES—Cavities are caused by acid destruction of tooth material. Acid is produced by bacteria in the mouth. The bacteria feed on food debris—usually sugar—and produce the acid that dissolves tooth material.
The combination of sugars from food debris, bacteria and chemicals in the saliva form a substance called plaque. Plaque becomes a localized site of acid production, which forms continuously at the neck of each tooth. This plaque must be thoroughly cleaned away at the gum line daily or it fosters tooth decay.

RISK INCREASES WITH
• Poor nutrition and improper diet.
• Poor dental hygiene.

HOW TO PREVENT
• Brush and floss teeth regularly.
• Consult your dentist about using fluoride mouthwash, liquid, tablets or having fluoride treatments once or twice a year.
• Drinking fluoridated water or taking fluoride supplements during pregnancy has not proven to protect the unborn child's teeth.
• Sealants may help prevent enamel erosion.

 WHAT TO EXPECT

DIAGNOSTIC MEASURES
• Your own observation of symptoms.
• Examination by a dentist. The decayed area feels soft when the dentist probes it with a sharp instrument.
• X-rays of the teeth and mouth.

APPROPRIATE HEALTH CARE
• Self-care.
• Dentist's treatment to remove all decay in the tooth and replace it with a restorative material (filling). The filling prevents further decay.

POSSIBLE COMPLICATIONS
• Abscess around a decayed tooth.
• Death of the tooth, caused by destruction of the tooth pulp that contains the tooth's nerve and blood supply.

PROBABLE OUTCOME—Usually curable with dental treatment.

 HOW TO TREAT

GENERAL MEASURES—No specific instructions except those listed under other headings.

MEDICATION
• For minor pain, you may use nonprescription drugs such as acetaminophen.
• Your dentist may prescribe stronger pain relievers or fluoride supplements.

ACTIVITY—No restrictions.

DIET—For 48 hours after your dentist fills the decayed tooth, don't put pressure on the tooth, as by eating apples, hard candy, raw vegetables or chewing on ice. Avoid very hot or cold foods. The tooth remains sensitive for 48 hours to 10 days after a cavity has been filled.

 CALL YOUR DENTIST IF

• You have symptoms of tooth decay.
• The following occurs after treatment:
Fever.
Increased pain that is not relieved by nonprescription medication.
Discomfort with hot or cold food that persists longer than 2 weeks after the filling procedure.
Brown spots on the tops of any other teeth.

TOOTH GRINDING
(Bruxism)

GENERAL INFORMATION

DEFINITION—The habit of grinding teeth. Tooth-grinding is often done while asleep, but grinding or tapping teeth during the day is also common. Continual tooth-grinding may erode gums and supporting bones in the mouth.

BODY PARTS INVOLVED—Teeth; gums; temperomandibular joints.

SEX OR AGE MOST AFFECTED—Both sexes; all ages.

SIGNS & SYMPTOMS
- Frequent contraction of muscles on the side of the face.
- Annoying, tooth-grinding noises at night. These may be loud enough to awaken others.
- Upon waking, teeth feel loose or sore.
- Slight throbbing of jaw.
- Damaged teeth, supporting gums and bone (apparent in a dental exam).
- Headaches.

CAUSES
- Anxiety.
- Unconscious attempts to correct a faulty "bite" (contact between upper and lower teeth when jaws are closed).

RISK INCREASES WITH
- Stress.
- Anxiety.
- Alcoholism.

HOW TO PREVENT—Avoid stressful situations if possible (see How to Cope with Stress in Appendix)

WHAT TO EXPECT

DIAGNOSTIC MEASURES
- Your own observation of symptoms.
- Medical history and physical exam by a dentist.
- X-rays of the mouth.

APPROPRIATE HEALTH CARE
- Self-care after diagnosis.
- Dentist's care. Your dentist may manufacture, fit and install a night-guard prosthesis to prevent tooth-grinding while asleep. A night-guard prosthesis consists of removable splints that fit over the tops of the teeth to eliminate incorrect biting pressure.
- Biofeedback training (relaxation exercises) or counseling to learn ways to cope more effectively with stress.

POSSIBLE COMPLICATIONS
- Without treatment, teeth, bones and gums may erode from the pressure of grinding.
- May lead to temporomandibular joint syndrome.

PROBABLE OUTCOME—Usually curable in 6 months with treatment.

HOW TO TREAT

GENERAL MEASURES
- Try to keep your jaw relaxed with your teeth slightly apart.
- Be sure you are using good posture. Don't hunch over your work area, don't cradle a phone between your shoulder and your ear, use proper chair height.
- Use warm compresses on your jaw area. This can help relax the clenching muscles.

MEDICATION—Medicine usually is not necessary for this disorder. Your doctor may prescribe a tranquilizer or a sedative for short-term treatment in certain cases.

ACTIVITY—Maintain a regular exercise routine. It is helpful to relieve stress.

DIET
- Avoid alcohol.
- Avoid (or decrease) your intake of caffeine.
- Don't chew gum or nibble on pencils.

CALL YOUR DENTIST IF

- You grind your teeth at night.
- You develop pain around the ears, dizziness or ringing in the ears.
- You develop pain or clicking in the jaw.
- You lose or break your night-guard prosthesis.

TORTICOLLIS
(Wryneck)

GENERAL INFORMATION

DEFINITION—Shortened neck muscles or chronic neck-muscle spasm that causes the head to turn and bend.

BODY PARTS INVOLVED—Brain and central nervous system; muscular system.

SEX OR AGE MOST AFFECTED—Both sexes, but more common in adults age 30-60, or children under age 10. One form is congenital and affects newborns.

SIGNS & SYMPTOMS—The following may be permanent or intermittent:
- Head that turns sideways and bends down.
- Neck-muscle spasm that is sometimes painful.

CAUSES
- Birth defect.
- Injury to neck muscles or vertebrae at birth or later.
- Neck-muscle inflammation.
- Cervical spine injury.
- Organic central nervous system disorder.
- Tumor.
- Stress and psychological conflict may cause intermittent torticollis.

RISK INCREASES WITH
- Tumors in soft tissues or bones of the neck.
- Traumatic delivery of newborn.
- Psychiatric illness.
- Trauma.
- Medications (phenothiazines, butyrophenones).
- Family history of torticollis.
- Hyperthyroidism.
- Brain diseases or infections.

HOW TO PREVENT—No specific prevention. Stress-related forms may be prevented with stress-reduction techniques, including biofeedback.

WHAT TO EXPECT

DIAGNOSTIC MEASURES
- Your own observation of symptoms.
- Medical history and physical exam by a doctor.
- Laboratory blood tests for infection and inflammation.
- X-rays of the spinal column in the neck. CT scan or MRI to help rule out other disorders (see Glossary for both).

APPROPRIATE HEALTH CARE
- Self-care after diagnosis.
- Doctor's treatment.
- Congenital torticollis is initially treated with physical therapy including daily passive therapy for at least a year. If therapy is not successful, then surgery to lengthen neck muscles is performed.
- For other forms of torticollis, various drug therapies are available that may help, along with physical therapy and massages.
- Neck brace or collar or ultrasound therapy may be recommended.
- Surgical procedure to denervate the neck muscles for some patients.

POSSIBLE COMPLICATIONS—Without treatment, the congenital form becomes permanent, causing an unattractive, abnormal appearance of the head and neck.

PROBABLE OUTCOME
- Congenital torticollis can usually be corrected with muscle-stretching exercises or surgery.
- Other forms will improve or heal with treatment. Healing time varies. Some cases require treatment for several years.

HOW TO TREAT

GENERAL MEASURES
- Relieve pain from neck spasms with heat or massage. Take hot showers or use hot compresses, deep-heating ointments or heat lamps.
- Follow your doctor's instructions regarding massage or physical therapy. Compliance with your medical treatment plan is essential for the best outcome.

MEDICATION—Your doctor may prescribe:
- Anticholinergics, benzodiazepines, muscle relaxants, or tricyclic antidepressants (drug possibilities to help reduce the symptoms).
- Multiple injections of botulinum toxin type A into the neck muscles..

ACTIVITY—Normal actvities may be resumed as soon as symptoms improve.

DIET—No special diet.

CALL YOUR DOCTOR IF

- Your infant has symptoms of torticollis.
- You have neck pain or spasms that persist longer than 1 week.

TOXEMIA OF PREGNANCY
(Pre-eclampsia & Eclampsia)

 GENERAL INFORMATION

DEFINITION—A serious disturbance in blood pressure, kidney function and the central nervous system that may occur from the 20th week of pregnancy until 7 days after delivery.

BODY PARTS INVOLVED—Female reproductive system; kidneys; brain and central nervous system; blood and blood vessels.

SEX OR AGE MOST AFFECTED—Pregnant females.

SIGNS & SYMPTOMS
Mild pre-eclampsia:
- Significant blood-pressure rise, even if still in the normal range.
- Puffiness in the face, hands and feet that is worse in the morning.
- Excessive weight gain (more than a pound a week during the last trimester).
- Protein in the urine.

Severe pre-eclampsia:
- Continued blood-pressure rise.
- Continued swelling and puffiness.
- Blurred vision.
- Headache.
- Irritability.
- Abdominal pain.

Eclampsia:
- Worsening of above symptoms.
- Muscle twitching.
- Seizures.
- Coma.

CAUSES—Unknown. Believed to be caused by a substance or toxin produced by the placenta.

RISK INCREASES WITH
- Poor nutrition.
- Diabetes mellitus.
- Previous high blood pressure.
- Chronic kidney disease.
- First pregnancy. Toxemia during one pregnancy does not mean it will recur with subsequent pregnancies.
- Smoking.
- Excess alcohol consumption.
- Use of mind-altering drugs.
- Family history of eclampsia or pre-eclampsia.

HOW TO PREVENT
- Obtain good prenatal care throughout pregnancy.
- Don't smoke, use mind-altering drugs or drink alcohol during pregnancy.
- Eat a normal, well-balanced diet during pregnancy. Take prenatal vitamin and mineral supplements if your doctor prescribes them.
- Don't use medications of any kind, including nonprescription drugs, without consulting your doctor.

 WHAT TO EXPECT

DIAGNOSTIC MEASURES
- Your own observation of symptoms.
- Medical history and physical exam by a doctor.
- Laboratory blood studies, 24 hour urine study and others to rule out complications.

APPROPRIATE HEALTH CARE
- Doctor's treatment.
- Treatment will depend on severity. Home care for mild symptoms, hospital care if condition deteriorates, and early delivery if situation is severe. Eclampsia, because of seizure activity, is more likely to require hospital care and rapid delivery (often cesarean section).

POSSIBLE COMPLICATIONS
- Stroke.
- Increased risk of high blood pressure unrelated to pregnancy after age 30.
- Seizures.
- Pulmonary edema.

PROBABLE OUTCOME—If diagnosed and treated throughout pregnancy, toxemia usually disappears without complications within 7 days after delivery. It is fatal in rare cases. If toxemia causes premature labor, the newborn's survival chances depend on its maturity. Fetal death is common.

 HOW TO TREAT

GENERAL MEASURES
- Weigh yourself daily and keep a record.
- Ask your doctor about testing for urine protein at home.

MEDICATION—Your doctor may prescribe:
- Antihypertensive drugs to lower blood pressure.
- Anticonvulsants to prevent seizures.

ACTIVITY—Rest often—this is important in controlling toxemia. Rest on your left side to help circulation.

DIET—A special diet is usually necessary. Ask your doctor.

 CALL YOUR DOCTOR IF

- You have symptoms of mild toxemia at any stage of pregnancy.
- The following occurs during treatment:
  Severe headache or vision disturbance.
  Weight gain of 3 or more pounds in 24 hours.
  Nausea, vomiting and diarrhea.
  Cramping abdominal pains.
  Excessive irritability.

ILLNESS & DISORDERS

TOXIC SHOCK SYNDROME (TSS)

 GENERAL INFORMATION

DEFINITION—A form of blood poisoning caused by poisons (toxins) released by staphylococcal bacteria. Menstrual toxic shock involves the female reproductive system and respiratory system. Nonmenstrual toxic shock can affect both sexes.

BODY PARTS INVOLVED—Reproductive system (females); respiratory system; soft tissues of the body.

SEX OR AGE MOST AFFECTED—All ages and both sexes, but most common in women of childbearing age (up to 15% of cases occur in males).

SIGNS & SYMPTOMS
- Sudden, high fever in a previously healthy person.
- Vomiting and watery diarrhea.
- Rash that resembles sunburn.
- Low blood pressure.
- Thirst.
- Rapid pulse.
- Feeling of impending doom.
- Mental changes, such as confusion.
- Extreme fatigue and weakness.
- Headache.
- Sore throat.

CAUSES—Some strains of staphylococcal bacteria produce toxins that enter the bloodstream, causing sudden symptoms. Most serious cases have come from staphylococci in the vagina of women using tampons. Toxic shock syndrome can also arise from wounds or infections in the throat, skin, lungs or bone.

RISK INCREASES WITH
- Continuous or prolonged use of highly absorbable tampons during menstrual periods.
- Staphylococcal infections.
- Postpartum women.
- Postoperative patients, particularly after nasal surgery.
- Severe burns, boils or abscesses.

HOW TO PREVENT
- Seek early medical care for any wound that appears infected.
- Females:
  Change tampons frequently, and alternate them at night with sanitary napkins.
  Don't use superabsorbent tampons. Use those made of cotton.
  Don't use tampons if you have a skin infection, especially near the genitals.
  Wash hands thoroughly before inserting tampons. Staphylococci are commonly found on hands.

 WHAT TO EXPECT

DIAGNOSTIC MEASURES
- Your own observation of symptoms.
- Medical history and physical exam by a doctor.
- Laboratory blood studies and mucosal cultures.

APPROPRIATE HEALTH CARE
- Doctor's treatment.
- Immediate hospitalization for intravenous fluids to administer antibiotics and correct fluid and electrolyte loss and dehydration. Also to manage kidney or cardiac problems and provide mechanical breathing support if needed.
- Tampons, diaphragms or other foreign bodies are removed at once.

POSSIBLE COMPLICATIONS
- Severe shock.
- Kidney failure.
- Congestive heart failure.
- Respiratory distress.
- Loss of hair and nails.
- Recurrence of TSS.
- Mortality may be as high as 15% in severe cases.

PROBABLE OUTCOME—Most patients recover with early diagnosis and prompt hospital treatment, but some cases are fatal. Skin of the palms and soles often peels during recovery.

 HOW TO TREAT

GENERAL MEASURES—The family should maintain an optimistic outlook, stay in close contact with the patient's doctor and help by making their visits with the patient as supportive as possible.

MEDICATION—Your doctor may prescribe:
- Antibiotics, usually intravenous, for infection.
- Intravenous fluids and electrolytes.

ACTIVITY—Resume your normal activities as soon as symptoms improve.

DIET—No special diet after recovery. Intravenous nourishment is usually necessary during hospitalization.

 CALL YOUR DOCTOR IF

- You have symptoms of toxic shock syndrome. Call immediately! Shock develops rapidly.
- New, unexplained symptoms develop. Drugs used in treatment may produce side effects.

TOXOPLASMOSIS

 GENERAL INFORMATION

DEFINITION—A protozoan infection found in humans and many species of mammals and birds. There are several types that occur in humans: congenital toxoplasmosis (passed from infected mother to her unborn child); ocular toxoplasmosis (also called retinochoroiditis, which usually results from congenital toxoplasmosis, but symptoms may not occur until ages 20-40); acute toxoplasmosis in a basically healthy individual; acute toxoplasmosis in an immunocompromised individual (person with AIDS, cancer or on immunosuppressant drugs).

BODY PARTS INVOLVED—Nerves, heart, gastrointestinal, skin.

SEX OR AGE MOST AFFECTED—Both sexes: all ages.

SIGNS & SYMPTOMS
- No symptoms usually (80-90% of patients).
- Fever; tiredness; swollen lymph glands.
- Muscle aches; sore throat; rash (sometimes).
- Retinitis (inflammation of the retina).

CAUSES—The protozoan, Toxoplasma gondii, usually transmitted by:
- Eating undercooked meats from infected animals.
- Cats that harbor the germ can excrete it in their stools; humans who handle cat litter (or fail to wash their hands after handling it) may become infected. Children who eat soil contaminated with feces can become infected.
- Blood transfusion.
- An infected pregnant woman can transmit it to her unborn child (often with severe effects).

RISK INCREASES WITH
- Immunosuppression due to illness or drugs.
- Contact with cats.
- Improper food preparation.

HOW TO PREVENT
- Avoid eating raw or undercooked meats, unpasteurized milk, uncooked eggs. Use proper techniques for preparation and storage of meat products. Wash hands carefully after handling raw meats.
- A pregnant woman should have laboratory blood test early in pregnancy to determine if she has antibodies to toxoplasmosis (about 55% of the U.S. population have them, which means they were infected at some time). She should be tested again at 16-18 weeks of pregnancy to determine if she has acquired an infection, and if so, may consider a therapeutic abortion.
- Immunocompromised persons and pregnant women should avoid contact with cat feces.
- Protect children's play area, including sand boxes, from cat and dog feces.
- Change cat litter boxes daily.

 WHAT TO EXPECT

DIAGNOSTIC MEASURES
- Medical history and exam by a doctor.
- Laboratory studies to detect the infection.

APPROPRIATE HEALTH CARE
- Treatment is usually unnecessary for a healthy, nonpregnant individual who has no symptoms. For a child under age 5 medications will be prescribed to prevent eye complications.
- Pregnant female—Your doctor will discuss treatments, risks and outcomes.
- Immunocompromised patient—Treatment is with medication.
- Newborns with infection are treated with medications (with or without symptoms as the germs can multiply after birth).

POSSIBLE COMPLICATIONS
- For pregnant female—When infection occurs early in pregnancy: miscarriage, stillbirth, various chronic disorders (seizures) and birth defects (blindness, deafness) in the newborn (some may not be apparent for years). An infection later in pregnancy usually has no ill effects.
- For immunocompromised patient—Lung and heart damage, brain inflammation, recurrence.
- For nonimmunocompromised patient (basically healthy)—Rarely, may develop lung or brain inflammation. Younger children (under 5) may develop eye inflammation.

PROBABLE OUTCOME—The majority of infected persons have no symptoms and those with mild symptoms recover spontaneously with no aftereffects.

 HOW TO TREAT

GENERAL MEASURES
- Follow instructions in How to Prevent.
- If you are prescribed drugs, your doctor will do frequent blood tests to monitor side effects.

MEDICATION—Your doctor may prescribe:
- Pyrimethamine, sulfadiazine or trisulfapyrimidines for 3-4 weeks.
- Folinic acid to reduce the side effects of pyrimethamine.
- Corticosteroids for inflammation.

ACTIVITY—Level of activity will be determined by severity of symptoms.

DIET—No special diet.

 CALL YOUR DOCTOR IF

- Symptoms worsen or don't improve after diagnosis and treatment.
- New, unexplained symptoms develop.

TRANSIENT ISCHEMIC ATTACK (TIA)

GENERAL INFORMATION

DEFINITION—A temporary decrease in the blood supply to part of the brain. The affected part of the brain is temporarily unable to function normally.

BODY PARTS INVOLVED—Blood vessels to the brain and the part of the brain supplied by the affected blood vessels.

SEX OR AGE MOST AFFECTED—Adults over age 40.

SIGNS & SYMPTOMS—The following symptoms are brief, lasting from several minutes to a few hours.
- Loss of muscle function on one side of the body.
- Headache.
- Dizziness.
- Tingling in the arms and legs.
- Numbness.
- Vision disturbance or temporary blindness in one eye.
- Confusion.
- Faintness without loss of consciousness.
- Slurred speech or inability to speak.

CAUSES—TIA's are caused by a partial blockage in a small artery in the brain or a larger artery (usually the carotid artery in the neck) that supplies blood to brain arteries. The blockage is often caused by a small clot from heart or blood vessel that breaks away and is carried into the brain. This temporarily decreases blood flow to an area of the brain and causes strokelike symptoms.

RISK INCREASES WITH
- Smoking.
- Personal or family medical history of high blood pressure and atherosclerosis.
- Diabetes.
- Heart attack.
- Cardiac disease.
- Polycythemia.

HOW TO PREVENT
- Exercise at least 3 times a week to maintain good cardiovascular fitness.
- Follow recommendations under Diet.
- Don't smoke.
- Have your blood pressure checked regularly. If it is high, consult your doctor for treatment to reduce it.
- Daily aspirin may help, ask your doctor.

WHAT TO EXPECT

DIAGNOSTIC MEASURES
- Your own observation of symptoms.
- Medical history and physical exam by a doctor.
- Laboratory blood studies.
- ECG (see Glossary); x-rays of the heart, lungs and blood flow (angiography) and ultrasound (see Glossary).

APPROPRIATE HEALTH CARE
- Self-care after diagnosis.
- Treatment may include medications, control of risk factors (diabetes, hypertension, cardiac disease, etc.), and lifestyle changes.
- Surgery (endarterectomy) to remove plaques (fatty deposits) from carotid arteries in the neck.

POSSIBLE COMPLICATIONS—Stroke. Without treatment, about 50% of persons who have TIA's have strokes within 5 years.

PROBABLE OUTCOME
- Transient ischemic attacks are often signals of an impending stroke. They should be treated to reduce the risk of future stroke, which may cause serious and permanent brain damage.
- TIA's are likely to recur. A person may have several attacks daily or only 2 or 3 over several years. The symptoms of each attack may be similar or quite different from others. In some patients symptoms appear repeatedly without leaving permanent damage.

HOW TO TREAT

GENERAL MEASURES
- Stop smoking. Get counseling, join support group or find other methods to help you quit.
- Follow your doctor's instructions. Compliance with your medical treatment plan is essential for the best outcome.

MEDICATION—Your doctor may prescribe:
- Anticoagulants, such as warfarin, to decrease the formation of blood clots.
- Daily aspirin. Aspirin can decrease blood-clotting enough to reduce the likelihood of TIA's developing into stroke. The aspirin seems more effective in men than women.

ACTIVITY—If you have frequent TIA's, don't drive, work in high places or operate machinery.

DIET—Eat a normal, well-balanced diet that is low in salt and fat, especially saturated fat. (See both diets in Appendix.)

CALL YOUR DOCTOR IF

- You have your first symptoms of a TIA.
- Symptoms of a TIA recur after diagnosis and persist longer than 2 hours.

TRENCH MOUTH
(Necrotizing Ulcerative Gingivitis; Vincent's Disease)

GENERAL INFORMATION

DEFINITION—Infection of tissue between the teeth. This is not contagious or cancerous.

BODY PARTS INVOLVED—Gums. If untreated, trench mouth can spread to: lymph glands in the neck; tonsils; vocal cords; bronchial tubes; rectum; or vagina.

SEX OR AGE MOST AFFECTED—Both sexes and all ages, but most common in young adults (20 to 40 years).

SIGNS & SYMPTOMS
- Painful gums.
- Gums that bleed when pressed.
- Excess salivation.
- Bad breath.
- Ulcers covered with gray membrane on the gums.
- Swallowing difficulty.
- Speaking difficulty.

CAUSES—Abnormal growth of fusiform bacillus and a spirochete. These are small organisms that usually exist harmlessly in the crevices of the gums.

RISK INCREASES WITH
- Poor nutrition.
- Illness that has lowered resistance.
- Smoking.
- Stress.
- Poor oral hygiene. Tartar, plaque or food debris between teeth.

HOW TO PREVENT
- Maintain good oral hygiene.
To brush teeth: Scrub clear, sticky plaque off teeth daily with a soft toothbrush. Place the brush at the gum line and gently rotate, pointing bristles toward the gum. Brush one section of teeth at a time. Then brush tongue. A soft brush is less likely to damage teeth and gums than a hard brush.
To floss: Use waxed or unwaxed dental floss according to instructions on the package label or your dentist's instructions.
- Eat a well-balanced diet.
- Don't smoke.

WHAT TO EXPECT

DIAGNOSTIC MEASURES
- Your own observation of symptoms.
- Medical history and physical exam by a doctor.
- Diagnosis is determined by examination of the gums and culture of the lesions.

APPROPRIATE HEALTH CARE
- Self-care after diagnosis.
- Doctor's treatment.
- Removal of dead tissue may be recommended as a treatment.

POSSIBLE COMPLICATIONS—Surgery may be necessary to trim rough, infected gums.

PROBABLE OUTCOME—Usually curable in 2 weeks with treatment. Follow-up with frequent dental checkups, up to once a month, after treatment.

HOW TO TREAT

GENERAL MEASURES
- Rinse your mouth every 2 hours, alternating the following rinses:
  Mixture of 1 teaspoon salt in large glass of very warm water.
  Mixture of equal parts 2% hydrogen peroxide and warm water.
- Don't smoke.
- Avoid any gum irritation until gums heal completely.

MEDICATION
- Your doctor may prescribe penicillin or another antibiotic to fight infection.
- You may use nonprescription drugs, such as acetaminophen, for minor pain.

ACTIVITY—Rest at home for the first 2 days of treatment, then resume normal activities.

DIET
- A liquid diet may be necessary for 2 or 3 days because of gum tenderness. When pain subsides, eat many fresh fruits and vegetables. Don't eat spicy or hot (temperature) food.
- Drink juices and 4 to 6 glasses of water each day. Don't drink carbonated beverages or alcohol.

CALL YOUR DOCTOR OR DENTIST IF

- You have symptoms of trench mouth.
- The following occurs during treatment:
  Fever.
  Swelling of neck or face.
  Swallowing difficulty.
  Inability to eat.

TRICHINOSIS

GENERAL INFORMATION

DEFINITION—Infection caused by larvae of parasites that live in the intestines of pigs (rarely, meat of bears and some marine animals).

BODY PARTS INVOLVED—Gastrointestinal tract (where larvae enter); lymphatic system and bloodstream (through which they are transported); large muscles of the body, especially the diaphragm (muscle used in breathing that separates the chest from the abdomen); arms and legs (in which they become embedded).

SEX OR AGE MOST AFFECTED—Both sexes; all ages.

SIGNS & SYMPTOMS
Early stages (usually begin in 7 to 10 days):
• Appetite loss, nausea, vomiting, diarrhea and abdominal cramps.
Later stages:
• Puffy eyelids and face.
• Muscle pain.
• Itching, burning skin.
• Sweating.
• High fever (102F to 104F or 38.9C to 40C).
Late stages:
• Symptoms subside, but some muscle tissues remain permanently infected with microscopic cysts. In rare cases, these cause heart and central nervous system disorders.

CAUSES—Infection with a parasite, Trichinella spiralis, which is transmitted to people when they eat infected animals. Thorough cooking kills the parasite and makes infected meat safe to eat. The parasites pass from animal to animal in contaminated food (usually raw garbage).

RISK INCREASES WITH
• Eating improperly cooked or raw pork.
• Use of immunosuppressive drugs.

HOW TO PREVENT—Don't eat raw or undercooked pork meats (including ready-to-eat pork sausage). Cook all meats thoroughly.

WHAT TO EXPECT

DIAGNOSTIC MEASURES
• Your own observation of symptoms.
• Medical history and physical exam by a doctor.
• Diagnostic tests for early diagnosis are not available. A muscle biopsy during the 4th week of infection may show larvae or cysts. The parasite is rarely found in blood, stool or cerebrospinal fluid.

APPROPRIATE HEALTH CARE
• Self-care after diagnosis.
• Treatment is usually done at home with medication and rest.

POSSIBLE COMPLICATIONS—Overwhelming infection, which can lead to:
• Congestive heart failure.
• Respiratory failure.
• Permanent damage to central nervous system.
• Kidney damage.
• Sinusitis.

PROBABLE OUTCOME—Usually curable in most persons with antiparasitic drugs and, in severe cases, expert supportive care. Some deaths have been reported, usually due to cardiac failure or pneumonia.

HOW TO TREAT

GENERAL MEASURES
• Reduce high fever with sponge bath or a tepid bath.
• Medical personnel report all cases of trichinosis to the local health department.

MEDICATION
• Your doctor may prescribe:
Antihelmintic drugs (usually thiabendazole) to kill the parasites.
Corticosteroids for patients with severe allergic symptoms or with central nervous system involvement.
• You may take nonprescription drugs, such as acetaminophen, to reduce fever and discomfort.

ACTIVITY—Limit activity until symptoms subside. If confined to bed, move legs frequently to reduce the likelihood of deep-vein blood clots. Resume normal activities gradually.

DIET—No special diet.

CALL YOUR DOCTOR IF

• You have symptoms of trichinosis.
• The following occur during treatment:
Fever over 104F (40C).
Irregular heartbeat.
Shortness of breath.
Puffy ankles.
• New, unexplained symptoms develop. Drugs used in treatment may produce side effects, especially nausea, vomiting, skin rash or fever.

TRIGEMINAL NEURALGIA
(Tic Douloureux)

GENERAL INFORMATION

DEFINITION—A nerve condition that causes brief, but often severe, face pain.

BODY PARTS INVOLVED—Nerve branches from the trigeminal or 5th cranial nerve (nerve from the brain that supplies sensation to the face, scalp, teeth, mouth and nose).

SEX OR AGE MOST AFFECTED—Adults over 40, usually men.

SIGNS & SYMPTOMS—Severe face pain, described as "jabbing" or "searing." Pain is often triggered by touching or stroking the face, brushing teeth, shaving, exposure to wind or chewing. Bouts of pain usually last 1 to 15 minutes. Attacks may occur several times a day, or may disappear for weeks or months. Between bouts, there is little or no discomfort.

CAUSES
- Pressure on the nerve from adjacent blood vessels (sometimes).
- Unknown (often).

RISK INCREASES WITH
- Multiple sclerosis.
- Rheumatoid arthritis.
- Sjögren's syndrome (a chronic, inflammatory disorder).

HOW TO PREVENT—No specific preventive measures.

WHAT TO EXPECT

DIAGNOSTIC MEASURES
- Your own observation of symptoms.
- Medical history and physical exam by a doctor.
- X-rays of the head to rule out other conditions, such as brain tumor.

APPROPRIATE HEALTH CARE
- Self-care after diagnosis.
- Doctor's treatment.
- Most patients obtain pain relief with anticonvulsant medication. However, as time goes by, the drugs may become ineffective in some patients and the pain "breaks through."
- Surgical approach to the problem can be effective. Usually involves one of two methods, percutaneous procedures or microvascular decompression. If pain recurs (after a few years) following either procedure, a percutaneous procedure is recommended as further treatment.

DIAGNOSTIC MEASURES
- Your own observation of symptoms.
- Medical history and physical exam by a doctor.
- X-rays of the head to rule out other conditions, such as brain tumor.

POSSIBLE COMPLICATIONS—Interference with normal activities from frequent, severe pain episodes.

PROBABLE OUTCOME—Symptom relief is usually possible with medication; sometimes surgery may be required. A patient may experience pain-free intervals (months to years) and then the pain returns exactly as before.

HOW TO TREAT

GENERAL MEASURES
- Following are suggestions for ways to prevent sudden pain:
  Avoid blasts of hot or cold air.
  Chew on the unaffected side of the mouth.
  Grow a beard.
- Assure good oral health with dental checkups at least twice a year.

MEDICATION—Your doctor may prescribe:
- Carbamazepine, an anticonvulsant; it is effective in treating trigeminal neuralgia.
- Baclofen for people who are sensitive to carbamazepine.
- Gabapentin, a new medicine effective for neuropathies.
- Phenytoin may be prescribed for people who are intolerant to carbamazepine.

ACTIVITY—No restrictions.

DIET—No special diet.

CALL YOUR DOCTOR IF

- You have symptoms of trigeminal neuralgia.
- New, unexplained symptoms develop. Drugs used in treatment may produce side effects.

ILLNESS & DISORDERS

TUBERCULOSIS (TB)

GENERAL INFORMATION

DEFINITION—An acute or chronic, contagious, bacterial infection. TB was once under control, but has resurfaced mainly due to AIDS, poverty, homelessness and abuse of alcohol and other drugs.

BODY PARTS INVOLVED—Lungs primarily, but may spread to other organs. Childhood tuberculosis is usually confined to the middle of the lungs, but it may spread to cause meningitis. Tuberculosis in adults usually affects the top of the lungs.

SEX OR AGE MOST AFFECTED—Both sexes; all ages.

SIGNS & SYMPTOMS
Early stages:
• No symptoms (often).
• Symptoms that resemble those of influenza.
Second stages:
Low fever; weight loss; chronic fatigue; heavy sweating, especially at night.
Later stages:
• Cough with sputum that becomes progressively bloody, yellow, thick or gray.
• Chest pain; shortness of breath; reddish or cloudy urine (sometimes).

CAUSES—Infection by the organism, Mycobacterium tuberculosis. It is transmitted in the air from one person to another. Cattle are also susceptible and can transmit TB through unpasteurized milk.

RISK INCREASES WITH
• Adults over 60.
• Newborns and infants.
• Chronic illness that has lowered resistance.
• Use of cortisone or immunosuppressive drugs. These may reactivate inactive TB.
• Crowded or unsanitary living conditions.
• Alcohol and drug abuse; AIDS; homeless people; foreign born or refugees.
• Health-care workers in prolonged close contact with TB patients.

HOW TO PREVENT
• Vaccination with BCG, a strain of tuberculosis bacteria. This may prevent infection, or shorten and diminish the severity of infection.
• Treatment for several months with isoniazid (INH) if a tuberculin skin test is positive.
• Health authorities recommend vaccination and preventive treatment for the following groups:
Persons who have positive reactions to TB tests, but show no symptoms of disease, especially children under age 5.
Children with negative reactions to TB tests in areas where 20% or more of classmates have positive reactions.
Persons traveling to countries where TB is prevalent.

Persons who must take immunosuppressive or cortisone drugs for a long time.
Postgastrectomy patients whose x-rays show evidence of inactive TB.
Persons with silicosis.

WHAT TO EXPECT

DIAGNOSTIC MEASURES
• Medical history and exam by a doctor.
• Tests may include tuberculin skin test, blood studies, sputum study and chest x-ray. If another disorder is suspected, tests may include a lumbar puncture, bronchoscopy and bone marrow biopsy (see Glossary for all).

APPROPRIATE HEALTH CARE
• Self-care after diagnosis.
• Doctor's treatment.
• Regular follow-up x-rays.

POSSIBLE COMPLICATIONS
• Lung abscess; bronchiectasis; chronic obstructive pulmonary disease.
• Spread of infection to other organs.
• Respiratory failure.

PROBABLE OUTCOME—Usually curable with treatment. Without treatment, it can be fatal. However, recurrent strains have resistance to usual antibiotics.

HOW TO TREAT

GENERAL MEASURES
• It may not be necessary to isolate or hospitalize a person with TB. The disease is usually spread before diagnosis (TB is difficult to catch; lengthy or repeated close contact is usually necessary). Patients are probably not infectious after 10 days to 2 weeks of treatment.
• Occasionally you will need to collect a 24-hour sputum specimen for laboratory analysis to see if TB is still active.
• See Resources for Additional Information.

MEDICATION—Antitubercular drugs, usually for 9-12 months. Several types are given at the same time to avoid bacterial resistance to the drugs. Don't discontinue medications without doctor's approval. A relapse may occur.

ACTIVITY—Limit activities until symptoms disappear and tests show TB germs are gone. You may need to restrict activities for 6 months.

DIET—No special diet.

CALL YOUR DOCTOR IF

• Symptoms persist or worsen.
• New, unexplained symptoms develop. Drugs used in treatment may produce side effects.

TYPHOID FEVER

GENERAL INFORMATION

DEFINITION—A bacterial infection of the gastrointestinal tract. A relatively mild attack may be mistaken for simple gastroenteritis.

BODY PARTS INVOLVED—Gastrointestinal tract; skin; central nervous system.

SEX OR AGE MOST AFFECTED—Both sexes; all ages. Infants and persons over 60 usually have the severest cases.

SIGNS & SYMPTOMS
- Diarrhea. In mild cases, this may be only 2 or 3 loose bowel movements a day. In severe cases, it may be watery diarrhea as often as every 10 or 15 minutes.
- Vomiting.
- Fever.
- Headache.
- Muscle aches.
- Rose-colored skin rash on the abdomen.
- Abdominal cramps (sometimes).
- Blood in the stool (sometimes).

A relatively mild attack may be mistaken for simple gastroenteritis.

CAUSES—Infection with Salmonella typhi, a bacteria found in infected animals and transmitted to persons in contaminated meat or milk. Thorough cooking kills the germ. The infection can also be transmitted by ill persons or nonill carriers who handle food without careful handwashing after bowel movements.

RISK INCREASES WITH
- Illness that has lowered resistance.
- Crowded or unsanitary living conditions.
- Travel to tropical countries.

HOW TO PREVENT
- For travel to countries where typhoid is present, consider vaccination for typhoid (injection or oral form).
- During tropical travel, avoid tap water, salad and raw vegetables, unpeeled fruits and dairy products.
- Avoid poultry or poultry products left unrefrigerated for prolonged period of time.
- Wash your hands after bowel movements and before handling food.

WHAT TO EXPECT

DIAGNOSTIC MEASURES
- Your own observation of symptoms.
- Medical history and physical exam by a doctor.
- Laboratory blood studies.

APPROPRIATE HEALTH CARE
- Doctor's treatment.
- Hospitalization for severe cases; others can be cared for at home.

POSSIBLE COMPLICATIONS
- Dehydration.
- Perforation of the intestines.
- Gastrointestinal hemorrhage or abscess.
- Pneumonia.
- Bone infection.
- Congestive heart failure.
- Hepatitis.

PROBABLE OUTCOME—Usually curable in 2 to 3 weeks with treatment. Without treatment, it can be fatal.

HOW TO TREAT

GENERAL MEASURES—For home-care:
- Isolate ill persons and have them use bedside commodes or a separate bathroom.
- Use a heating pad or hot-water bottle to relieve abdominal cramps.
- Wash hands carefully and often.
- Turn patients frequently in bed.
- Apply lukewarm wet towels to the groin and underarms to reduce fever. Don't use aspirin or acetaminophen; both irritate the gastrointestinal tract. Don't use laxatives.

MEDICATION—Your doctor may prescribe:
- Antibiotics.
- For severe cases, glucocorticoids in addition to antibiotics.

ACTIVITY—Bed rest is necessary until all symptoms have been gone at least 3 days. The legs should be flexed often in bed to prevent formation of deep-vein blood clots.

DIET—A clear-liquid diet (see Liquid Diet in Appendix) is necessary during the diarrhea phase. Later, a high-calorie, well-balanced diet is necessary. Vitamin and mineral supplements may be helpful.

CALL YOUR DOCTOR IF

- You have symptoms of typhoid fever.
- The following occurs during treatment:
  Fever.
  Sore throat.
  Severe cough or coughing up blood.
  Shortness of breath.
  Severe abdominal pain or swelling.
  Rectal bleeding.
  Pain in the calf or leg.
  Headache, earache or swollen joints.

ULCER, PEPTIC (Duodenal Ulcer; Gastric Ulcer)

GENERAL INFORMATION

DEFINITION—An ulcer is a small erosion in the gastrointestinal tract. The most common type, duodenal, occurs in the first 12 inches of small intestine beyond the stomach. Ulcers that form in the stomach are called gastric ulcers. An ulcer is not contagious or cancerous, although some ulcers appear to be caused by an infection. Duodenal ulcers are almost always benign, while stomach ulcers may become malignant.

BODY PARTS INVOLVED—Gastrointestinal tract.

SEX OR AGE MOST AFFECTED—Both sexes (duodenal more common in males); all ages, but most common in adults.

SIGNS & SYMPTOMS
- Pain that has the following characteristics:
  A burning, boring or gnawing feeling that lasts 30 minutes to 3 hours (often interpreted as heartburn, indigestion or hunger).
  Pain is usually in the upper abdomen, but occasionally below the breastbone.
  Pain occurs in some persons immediately after eating; in others, it may not occur until hours later. It frequently awakens one at night.
  Pain comes and goes. Weeks of intermittent pain may alternate with pain-free periods.
  Pain may be relieved by drinking milk, eating, resting or taking antacids.
- Appetite and weight loss (with duodenal, may be weight gain, as person eats more to ease discomfort).
- Recurrent vomiting; blood in the stool; anemia.

CAUSES—The exact cause has not been fully established. An ulcer can develop wherever stomach acid comes in contact with the gastrointestinal lining—especially the lower end of the esophagus, the stomach and the duodenum. A person with an ulcer usually has an overactive stomach that manufactures too much hydrochloric acid. Some ulcers are associated with the bacteria Helicobacter pylori, which when treated prevents any recurrence.

RISK INCREASES WITH
- Family history of ulcers; smoking; excess alcohol consumption (possibly).
- Use of nonsteroidal anti-inflammatory medications (e.g., aspirin) or corticosteroids.
- Zollinger-Ellison syndrome.
- Improper diet, irregular or skipped meals.
- Type O blood (for duodenal ulcers).
- Stress does not cause an ulcer, but may be a contributing factor.
- Chronic disorders such as liver disease, emphysema, rheumatoid arthritis may increase vulnerability to ulcers.

HOW TO PREVENT—Avoid as many risk factors as possible.

WHAT TO EXPECT

DIAGNOSTIC MEASURES
- Medical history and exam by a doctor.
- Laboratory blood and stool studies, endoscopy (see Glossary), x-ray studies with barium meal and sometimes, mucosal biopsy (see Glossary) to rule out cancer.

APPROPRIATE HEALTH CARE
- Self-care after diagnosis; doctor's treatment.
- Hospitalization for bleeding ulcer or severe perforation or obstruction.
- Surgery or other treatments (endoscopic cautery, direct injection of medications and use of lasers) for complications in some patients.

POSSIBLE COMPLICATIONS
- Perforation (erosion of the ulcer through the intestinal wall) with consequent infection or bleeding into the abdomen.
- Hemorrhage into the intestine.

PROBABLE OUTCOME—Most ulcers heal within 2 to 6 weeks with treatment.

HOW TO TREAT

GENERAL MEASURES
- Reduce your use of aspirin or nonsteroidal anti-inflammatory medications.
- Don't smoke.
- Check your stool daily for bleeding. If the stool is black, save a sample for analysis.
- Reduce stress in your life (see How to Cope with Stress in Appendix).
- See Resources for Additional Information.

MEDICATION—Your doctor may prescribe:
- Antacids to neutralize excess stomach acid.
- H-2 blockers to reduce stomach acid.
- Medications to coat the ulcer area.
- Antibiotics for H. pylori bacteria, if present.

ACTIVITY—Resume your normal activities as soon as symptoms improve.

DIET
- Eat a balanced diet of 3 regularly scheduled meals a day. A bland diet is not necessary.
- Avoid caffeine and any food that seems to make symptoms worse. Don't drink alcohol.

CALL YOUR DOCTOR IF

- You have symptoms of an ulcer.
- Vomiting begins that is bloody or looks like coffee grounds.
- Stool is bloody, black or tarry-looking.
- Diarrhea begins that may be caused by antacids.
- Pain is severe, despite treatment.
- You are unusually weak or pale.

URETHRITIS

GENERAL INFORMATION

DEFINITION—Inflammation or infection of the urethra (the tube through which urine travels from the bladder to the outside). Urethritis is frequently accompanied by bladder infection or inflammation (cystitis). The female urethra is much shorter than the male's.

BODY PARTS INVOLVED—Urethra; bladder (sometimes).

SEX OR AGE MOST AFFECTED—All ages and both sexes, but 10 times more common in females.

SIGNS & SYMPTOMS
- Painful or burning urination.
- Discharge that may be cloudy, yellow-green mucus, or may be watery and white.
- Frequent urge to urinate, even when there is not much urine in the bladder.
- Painful sexual intercourse or temporary impotence in males.
- Dribbling of urine (usually in men over 50).
- No symptoms may be present, but both sexes may be carriers of the causative organism.

CAUSES
- The same bacterial infection that causes gonorrhea causes gonococcal urethritis; nonspecific urethritis (also called nongonococcal urethritis) may be caused by a variety of organisms, including bacteria, yeast and chlamydial infection.
- Other causes could be trauma from an injury or surgery, or from an antiseptic.
- Bubble bath and bath oils have been known to cause a urethritis.

RISK INCREASES WITH
- Bacterial infection that spreads and enters the urethra from skin around genitals and anus.
- Bruising during sexual intercourse.
- Contact with an infected sexual partner.
- Use of a urinary catheter.
- Use of drugs to which bacteria causing infection have become resistant.
- Multiple sexual partners.
- Previous kidney stones, prostatitis, epididymitis or genital injury.
- Previous sexually transmitted disease.

HOW TO PREVENT
- For causes related to sexual activity: Drink a glass of water before sexual intercourse, and urinate within 15 minutes afterward. Use a latex condom. Use a water-soluble lubricant e.g., K-Y Lubricating Jelly. Use varying sexual positions to decrease the chance of trauma to the female urethra.
- For causes related only to women: After bowel movements, wipe from front to back and wash with soap and water. Take showers rather than tub baths.
- Drink 8 glasses of water every day.

WHAT TO EXPECT

DIAGNOSTIC MEASURES
- Medical history and exam by a doctor.
- Laboratory blood and urethral discharge studies and urinalysis.

APPROPRIATE HEALTH CARE
- Self-care after diagnosis.
- Doctor's treatment.
- A repeat culture should be done after treatment to verify a cure.

POSSIBLE COMPLICATIONS
- Chronic urethritis and cystitis, if treatment is inadequate.
- Spread of infection to ureters and kidneys.

PROBABLE OUTCOME—With prompt diagnosis and treatment, you will have a relief of symptoms within 24 hours and the problem will resolve without complications.

HOW TO TREAT

GENERAL MEASURES
- To relieve pain, take sitz baths in a tub of hot water for 15 minutes at least twice a day.
- Men: Don't irritate the urethra by pulling the penis skin down to open it and see if the discharge is still present. The penis may be inspected, but don't squeeze it.
- Keep the area around the genitals clean. Use unscented, plain soap.
- Your doctor may recommend testing for sexually transmitted diseases.

MEDICATION—Your doctor may prescribe antibiotics to fight infection. Be sure to finish the dose, even if symptoms subside sooner.

ACTIVITY—No restrictions. Avoid sexual excitement and intercourse until you have been free of symptoms for 2 weeks.

DIET
- Drink 8 glasses of water every day.
- Avoid caffeine and alcohol during treatment.
- Drink cranberry juice to acidify urine. Some drugs are more effective with acid urine.

CALL YOUR DOCTOR IF

- The following occurs during treatment: Oral temperature of 101F (38.3C) or higher. Bleeding from the urethra or blood in urine. No improvement in 1 week, despite treatment.
- New, unexplained symptoms develop. Drugs used in treatment may produce side effects.

ILLNESS & DISORDERS

URINARY CALCULI
(Renal Calculi; Kidney Stones; Bladder Stones)

 GENERAL INFORMATION

DEFINITION—Small, solid particles that form in one or both kidneys and sometimes travel into the ureter (slender muscular tubes that carry urine from the kidneys to the urinary bladder) or to the bladder. Stones vary from the size of a grain of sand to a golf ball and there may be one or several.

BODY PARTS INVOLVED—Kidney, bladder, urethra.

SEX OR AGE MOST AFFECTED—Adults over 30 of both sexes, but more often occurs in men.

SIGNS & SYMPTOMS
- Painful urination; frequent urge to urinate, even if only small amounts of urine pass.
- Episodes of severe, colicky (intermittent) pain every few minutes. The pain usually appears first in the back, just below the ribs. Over several hours or days, the pain follows the stone's course through the ureter toward the groin. Pain stops when the stone passes.
- Frequent nausea.
- Traces of blood in the urine. Urine may appear cloudy or dark.

CAUSES
- Excess calcium in the urine caused by disturbance in the parathyroid gland, which upsets calcium metabolism; or excess calcium or vitamin-D intake.
- Gout (uric-acid stones).
- Blockage of urine from any cause.

RISK INCREASES WITH
- Decreased volume of urine due to dehydration or hot, dry weather.
- Family history of kidney stones; high animal protein diet; sedentary lifestyle.

HOW TO PREVENT
- Drink 3 quarts of fluid, mostly purified water, every day.
- Avoid milk and milk products if you have had a calcium or phosphorus kidney stone.
- Avoid excessive sweating.

 WHAT TO EXPECT

DIAGNOSTIC MEASURES
- Medical history and exam by a doctor.
- Diagnostic tests may include urinalysis and urine culture, x-ray of the abdomen, kidney ultrasound, CT scan, intravenous urography (see Glossary for both).

APPROPRIATE HEALTH CARE
- Self-care after diagnosis.
- Small stone, uncomplicated by obstruction or infection may need no specific treatment.

- Treatment to remove larger stones, if they don't pass spontaneously and are causing complications, infection or severe pain.
- Stones due to excess calcium in the body may require surgical removal of abnormal parathyroid tissue.

POSSIBLE COMPLICATIONS—Urinary-tract infection; damage to the kidney, necessitating surgical removal; recurrence of stones.

PROBABLE OUTCOME—Large stones usually remain in the kidney without symptoms, although they can damage the kidney. Small stones pass easily into the ureter through the urine. Stones that are big enough to pass but not small enough to pass with ease cause excruciating pain. These usually pass in a few days. If the stone stops and blocks urine, it must be removed to prevent further kidney damage.

 HOW TO TREAT

GENERAL MEASURES
- If you are waiting for the stone to pass, watch for it when you urinate. To trap it, urinate each time through a piece of gauze. The stone may pass without discomfort. When it passes, take it to your doctor's office for analysis.
- See Resources for Additional Information.

MEDICATION—Your doctor may prescribe:
- Pain relievers and antispasmodics to relax the ureter muscles and help the stone pass.
- Depending on the type of stone, medication may be prescribed that will stop the growth of existing stones or new stones

ACTIVITY
- If you know you have calculi, avoid situations in which a sudden pain might cause danger, such as climbing ladders.
- During a calculi episode, stay as active as possible. Don't go to bed. Activity may help the stone pass.

DIET
- Drink at least 13 glasses of fluid daily. Most of the fluid should be purified water.
- Low animal fat diet.
- Increase fiber in the diet (especially bran).
- Other dietary restrictions will depend upon type of stone formed. Ask your doctor.

 CALL YOUR DOCTOR IF

- Temperature rises to 101F (38.3C).
- Symptoms of a kidney infection develop (stinging, burning on urination or a frequent urge to urinate).
- New, unexplained symptoms develop.

UTERINE BLEEDING, DYSFUNCTIONAL
(Premenopausal Abnormal Uterine Bleeding)

 GENERAL INFORMATION

DEFINITION—Bleeding that is not related to a woman's normal menstrual pattern and is not associated with tumor, inflammation or pregnancy.

BODY PARTS INVOLVED—Uterus; vagina.

SEX OR AGE MOST AFFECTED—Female adolescents and premenopausal adults.

SIGNS & SYMPTOMS—Bleeding between menstrual cycles. Blood flow may be irregular, prolonged and sometimes profuse.

CAUSES—Usually caused by an overgrowth of the endometrium (lining of the uterus) due to estrogen stimulation.

RISK INCREASES WITH
- Polycystic ovary syndrome.
- Obesity.
- Use of synthetic estrogen without added progestin.
- Women over 35, those with polycystic ovaries, obesity or prolonged abnormal bleeding are at greater risk for having endometrial cancer.

HOW TO PREVENT
- Maintain proper weight.
- Follow medical advice regarding any hormone therapy.

 WHAT TO EXPECT

DIAGNOSTIC MEASURES
- Your own observation of symptoms.
- Medical history and physical exam by a doctor.
- Endometrial aspiration (insertion of a thin tube into the uterus to obtain a sample of the lining) to determine if bleeding is associated with ovulation. This will help determine how to evaluate the cause. Numerous diagnostic tests may have been done previously to rule out other causes of bleeding. Dysfunctional uterine bleeding is the usual diagnosis for patients without discernible causes and is usually not ovulatory.

APPROPRIATE HEALTH CARE
- Self-care after diagnosis.
- Doctor's treatment.
- Treatment is usually with hormonal therapy and lifestyle changes if appropriate.
- If hormonal therapy does not control the bleeding, a dilatation and curettage, often referred to as D & C (dilatation of the cervix and a scraping out of the uterus with a curette), may be performed to check for other problems.

POSSIBLE COMPLICATIONS—Anemia.

PROBABLE OUTCOME—Usually curable in 2 or 3 months, sooner with surgery. Recurrence is common, depending on the underlying cause.

 HOW TO TREAT

GENERAL MEASURES
- Use heat to relieve pain:
  Place a heating pad or hot-water bottle on the abdomen or back.
  Take a hot bath for 10 to 15 minutes as often as needed.
- Stressful situations and emotional turmoil or excessive use of drugs or alcohol can contribute to the problem. Try to resolve any conflicts in your life and get help in discontinuing abusive behaviors.
- Avoid aspirin, especially if you are anemic.

MEDICATION—Your doctor may prescribe:
- Hormones to correct a hormone imbalance.
- Pain relievers if needed.
- Tranquilizers to reduce anxiety (rarely required).
- Avoid aspirin, especially if you are anemic.

ACTIVITY—Stay as active as possible, depending on the underlying condition. Consult your doctor about continuing sexual relations.

DIET—No special diet. Iron supplements may be necessary for anemia.

 CALL YOUR DOCTOR IF

- You have abnormal uterine bleeding.
- The following occurs during treatment:
  Bleeding becomes excessive. (You saturate a pad or tampon more often than once an hour.)
  You develop signs of infection, such as: fever; a general ill feeling; headache; dizziness; or muscle aches.
- New, unexplained symptoms develop. Drugs used in treatment may produce side effects.

ILLNESS & DISORDERS

UTERINE BLEEDING, POSTMENOPAUSAL

 GENERAL INFORMATION

DEFINITION—Unexpected, menstrual-like bleeding that begins 1 or more years after menopause.

BODY PARTS INVOLVED—Vulva (vaginal lips); vagina; cervix (lower third of the uterus); endometrium (inner uterine lining).

SEX OR AGE MOST AFFECTED—Women after menopause.

SIGNS & SYMPTOMS
• Vaginal bleeding, which may be a light-brown discharge or heavy, red bleeding (with or without clots). Mucus may accompany the bleeding. Bleeding episodes vary in length.
• Pelvic pain (sometimes).

CAUSES
• Cancer of the reproductive system.
• Irritation, infection or thinning of the membranes lining the vulva.
• Injury or trauma to the vagina, associated with reduced estrogen levels.
• Polyps or benign tumors of the cervix.
• Polyps on the inner uterine lining, myomas.
• Hormone therapy that stimulates the endometrium (uterine lining), causing sloughing similar to normal menstruation. Estrogens (female hormones) taken irregularly are a common cause of this.
• Disorders of the blood cells, lymphatic system or bone marrow.
• High blood pressure.
• Congestive heart failure.
• Liver disorders.
• Anticoagulant or aspirin-containing drugs.

RISK INCREASES WITH
• Recent vaginal infection.
• Adults over 60, due to fragile blood vessels and thin vaginal lining.

HOW TO PREVENT—No specific preventive measures.

 WHAT TO EXPECT

DIAGNOSTIC MEASURES
• Your own observation of symptoms.
• Medical history and physical exam by a doctor.
• Laboratory blood studies, Pap smear (see Glossary) and endometrial aspiration (insertion of a thin tube into the uterus to obtain a sample of the lining).
• Dilatation and curettage, (D & C) (see Glossary).

APPROPRIATE HEALTH CARE
• Doctor's treatment.
• Specific therapy, usually medications or surgery, is dependent on the cause.

POSSIBLE COMPLICATIONS
• Anemia.
• If cancer is the cause, it may spread to other body parts and cause death.

PROBABLE OUTCOME—Depends on the underlying cause and treatment chosen.

 HOW TO TREAT

NOTE—Follow your doctor's instructions. These instructions are supplemental.

GENERAL MEASURES
• Use heat to relieve pain. Place a heating pad or hot-water bottle on the abdomen or back.
• Take frequent hot baths to relax muscles and relieve discomfort. Sit in a tub of hot water for 10 to 15 minutes as often as necessary.
• Use sanitary pads instead of tampons.

MEDICATION—Your doctor may prescribe:
• Hormones.
• Medication to treat the underlying disorder, such as antihypertensives for high blood pressure.
• Anticancer drugs if a malignancy is diagnosed.

ACTIVITY
• Resume your normal activities as soon as symptoms improve.
• Resume sexual relations as soon as possible after diagnosis and treatment.

DIET—No special diet.

 CALL YOUR DOCTOR IF

• You have postmenopausal vaginal bleeding. Don't delay. This is a warning signal for cancer.
• Bleeding persists for 1 week, despite treatment.
• Your bleeding becomes excessive (saturates a pad more frequently than once each hour).
• You develop signs of infection: fever, a general feeling of ill health, headache, dizziness and muscle aches.
• New, unexplained symptoms develop. Drugs used in treatment may produce side effects.

UTERINE CANCER
(Endometrial Carcinoma)

 GENERAL INFORMATION

DEFINITION—Cancer of the endometrium lining of the uterus.

BODY PARTS INVOLVED—Uterus.

SEX OR AGE MOST AFFECTED—
Postpuberty females; more frequent in postmenopausal women, usually between ages 50 and 60.

SIGNS & SYMPTOMS
Early stages:
• Bleeding or spotting, especially after sexual intercourse. This often occurs after menstrual activity has ceased for 12 months or more. A watery or blood-streaked vaginal discharge may precede bleeding or spotting.
• Enlarged uterus. It is sometimes a large enough mass to be felt externally.
Later stages:
• Spread to other organs, causing abdominal pain, chest pain and weight loss.

CAUSES—Unknown. Appears to be linked to several predisposing factors listed in Risks.

RISK INCREASES WITH
• Diabetes mellitus.
• Obesity.
• High blood pressure.
• Use of estrogen without also using progesterone.
• Family history of breast or ovarian cancer.
• History of uterine polyps, menstrual cycles without ovulation, or other signs of hormone imbalance.
• Delayed menopause.
• Chronic anovulation (absence of ovulation).
• Studies show that use of the drug tamoxifen for breast cancer may increase risk.

HOW TO PREVENT
• See your doctor for pelvic examinations every 6 to 12 months.
• Obtain medical care for any uterine bleeding or spotting after menopause.
• Proper dosages of any female hormones (birth-control or estrogen replacement following menopause). Ask your doctor.

 WHAT TO EXPECT

DIAGNOSTIC MEASURES
• Your own observation of symptoms, especially abnormal bleeding.
• Medical history and physical exam by a doctor.
• Diagnostic tests may be numerous, first to diagnose the cancer, and then to determine any spread to other body organs (staging). May include laboratory blood tests, Pap smear (see Glossary), liver function tests, chest x-ray, CT scan, mammogram, barium enema, MRI, vaginal ultrasound, endometrial biopsy, dilatation and curettage (D & C) (see Glossary for all).

APPROPRIATE HEALTH CARE
• Doctor's treatment.
• Treatment will depend on the extent of the disease and may involve one or a combination of the following: surgery, radiation, hormonal therapy and anticancer drugs (chemotherapy).
• Surgery treatment may involve removing the uterus, and usually, the ovaries and fallopian tubes.
• Psychotherapy or counseling for depression may be recommended.

POSSIBLE COMPLICATIONS—Fatal spread of cancer to the bladder, rectum and distant organs.

PROBABLE OUTCOME—With early diagnosis and treatment, 90% of patients survive at least 5 years.

 HOW TO TREAT

GENERAL MEASURES
• The more you can learn and understand about this disorder, the more you will be able to make informed decisions about where to go for your care, the treatments available, the risks involved, side effects of therapy and expected outcome.
• See Resources for Additional Information.

MEDICATION—Your doctor may prescribe:
• Anticancer drugs, including cortisone drugs.
• Hormone therapy.

ACTIVITY—Resume your normal activities as soon as symptoms improve after treatment. Discuss concerns regarding sexual activity with your partner and doctor. In most cases, full sexual activity after therapy should be resumed as soon as possible.

DIET—No special diet, but eat a well-balanced diet even if you lose your appetite from radiation or drug therapy. Vitamin and mineral supplements are helpful.

 CALL YOUR DOCTOR IF

• You have symptoms of uterine cancer.
• The following occurs after surgery:
   Excessive bleeding (soaking a pad or tampon at least once an hour).
   Signs of infection, such as fever, muscle aches and headache.
• New, unexplained symptoms develop. Drugs used in treatment may produce side effects.

UTERINE PROLAPSE

GENERAL INFORMATION

DEFINITION—A uterus that has fallen or sunk from its normal location, causing it to bulge into the vagina. In its most pronounced form, it projects outside the vagina. Associated with prolapse may be urethrocele and cystocele (urethra and/or bladder bulge along the front wall of the vagina) and rectocele (rectal wall bulges into back wall of vagina).

BODY PARTS INVOLVED—Uterus; ligaments that suspend the uterus; vagina.

SEX OR AGE MOST AFFECTED—Women over age 40.

SIGNS & SYMPTOMS
- Lump in front or back of the vagina, or projecting outside it.
- Vague discomfort in the pelvic region.
- Backache that worsens with lifting.
- Discomfort with urinating.
- Occasional stress incontinence (urine leakage when laughing, sneezing or coughing).
- Difficulty in moving bowels.
- Pain with sexual intercourse.

CAUSES—Prolapse occurs when muscles and ligaments at the base of the abdomen become extremely stretched, usually as a result of childbirth or aging.

RISK INCREASES WITH
- Obesity.
- Repeated childbirth, although one pregnancy and vaginal delivery can weaken the area enough to lead to prolapse eventually.
- Advancing age.
- Conditions that cause increased intra-abdominal pressure such as tumors, chronic coughing, chronic constipation.
- Poor physical fitness.
- Occupations requiring heavy lifting.

HOW TO PREVENT
- Maintain appropriate weight.
- Practice pelvic exercises during pregnancy and after childbirth.
- Eat a normal, well-balanced diet.
- Engage in a regular exercise program to maintain good muscle strength.
- Avoid constipation.

WHAT TO EXPECT

DIAGNOSTIC MEASURES
- Your own observation of symptoms.
- Medical history and physical exam by a doctor.
- Diagnostic tests may include Pap smear, urinalysis, pelvic ultrasound or CT, endometrial biopsy and intravenous pyelogram (see Glossary for all). Most of the tests are to rule out other disorders.

APPROPRIATE HEALTH CARE
- Treatment plan depends on severity of prolapse, age, sexual activity, associated pelvic disorders and desire for future pregnancy.
- Mild symptoms usually treated with exercise program and hormone therapy.
- Pessary (small ring-shaped device that is inserted into the vagina to help maintain the uterus in a normal position) may be prescribed.
- Surgery to remove the uterus (sometimes).

POSSIBLE COMPLICATIONS
- Ulceration of the cervix.
- Increased risk of infection or injury to pelvic organs.
- Urinary tract obstruction.

PROBABLE OUTCOME—Aggressive treatment is not always necessary because prolapse is not a health risk. Exercise can often improve muscle function. If the prolapse is severe, it can be cured with surgery.

HOW TO TREAT

GENERAL MEASURES—Follow your doctor's instructions. Compliance with your medical treatment plan is essential for the best outcome.

MEDICATION—Estrogen therapy can increase blood flow to vaginal tissues and increase supporting tissue strength.

ACTIVITY—No restrictions. If surgery is necessary, resume your normal activities gradually.

DIET
- Lose weight if you are obese (see Weight-Loss Diet in Appendix).
- Eat a diet high in fiber to prevent constipation.

CALL YOUR DOCTOR IF

- You have symptoms of uterine prolapse.
- Symptoms don't improve in 3 months despite treatment or exercise, or symptoms become intolerable and you wish to consider surgery.
- If a pessary is fitted and the following occurs: unusual vaginal bleeding; discomfort; or urination difficulty.

UVEITIS
(Iritis; Cyclitis; Choroiditis; Retinitis)

 GENERAL INFORMATION

DEFINITION—Uveitis is a general term used to describe inflammation of the eye including the iris (iritis), ciliary body (cyclitis), choroid (choroiditis) and retina (retinitis).

BODY PARTS INVOLVED—Eye.

SEX OR AGE MOST AFFECTED—Both sexes; ages.

SIGNS & SYMPTOMS
- Severe eye pain.
- Blurred vision; decreased vision.
- Photophobia (sensitivity to light).
- Eye redness.
- Smaller pupil in the affected eye (sometimes).
- Tears.
- Floating spots in the field of vision.

CAUSES
- Infection (bacteria, virus or fungus) that spreads to the eye from other body parts. Common causes include:
  - Toxoplasmosis.
  - Tuberculosis.
  - Histoplasmosis.
  - Syphilis.
  - Sarcoidosis.
  - Viruses.
- Injury to the eye.
- Autoimmune reaction (possibly).
- Unknown in many cases.

RISK INCREASES WITH
- Rheumatoid arthritis.
- Ulcerative colitis.
- Viral, bacterial, fungal or parasitic infection.
- Other eye disease.

HOW TO PREVENT—Cannot be prevented at present.

 WHAT TO EXPECT

DIAGNOSTIC MEASURES
- Your own observation of symptoms.
- Medical history and special eye exam by a doctor (ophthalmologist).
- Laboratory blood studies and x-rays if an underlying disorder is suspected.

APPROPRIATE HEALTH CARE
- Self-care after diagnosis.
- Doctor's treatment, usually an ophthalmologist.
- Treatment for any underlying condition.

POSSIBLE COMPLICATIONS
- Glaucoma.
- Cataracts.
- Permanent, partial vision loss.

PROBABLE OUTCOME—Vision can usually be preserved with prompt treatment. With infections, uveitis tends to clear up once the infection is treated. Other causes, the outcome is usually dependent on the underlying condition.

 HOW TO TREAT

GENERAL MEASURES—Wear dark glasses—even indoors—until treatment is complete.

MEDICATION—Your ophthalmologist may prescribe:
- Eye drops (mydriatics) that dilate the pupil and prevent scarring. You may need to use eye drops for a long time. Ask your doctor how to instill them in the eye correctly.
- Oral cortisone drugs, cortisone eye drops or injections to reduce inflammation. Discuss the side effects of cortisone drugs with your doctor.

ACTIVITY—No restrictions usually. Don't drive or perform hazardous activities if symptoms are severe or eye medications cause side effects.

DIET—No special diet.

 CALL YOUR DOCTOR IF

- You have symptoms of uveitis—either sudden or gradual. Call immediately.
- Your vision changes in any way.
- New, unexplained symptoms develop. Drugs used in treatment may produce side effects.

VAGINA OR VULVA CANCER

GENERAL INFORMATION

DEFINITION—Uncontrolled growth of malignant cells in the vagina or on the vulva (vaginal lips).

BODY PARTS INVOLVED—Vagina; vulva.

SEX OR AGE MOST AFFECTED—Females of all ages, but the peak incidence is from ages 45 to 65. One type (rhabdomyosarcoma) occurs in children.

SIGNS & SYMPTOMS
- Itching; abnormal vaginal bleeding.
- Discomfort or bleeding with intercourse.
- Small or large, firm, ulcerated, painless lesion of the vulva. Cancers on the vulva have thick, raised edges and bleed easily.
- Uncomfortable urination, if cancer spreads to the bladder.
- Rectal bleeding, if it spreads to the rectum.

CAUSES
- Unknown, except for intrauterine exposure to DES (diethylstilbestrol, a drug prescribed [up to 1971] to control spotting or bleeding in pregnant women).
- A possible connection may be exposure to human papillomavirus (HPV), the cause of venereal warts.

RISK INCREASES WITH
- Family history of cancer of reproductive organs or other cancer.
- Smoking.
- Multiple sex partners.

HOW TO PREVENT
- No specific preventive measures. Have a yearly pelvic exam and Pap smear (see Glossary) to detect the disease during early stages when treatment is most effective.
- Become familiar with the appearance of your genitals. (Use a mirror and examine once a month.)

WHAT TO EXPECT

DIAGNOSTIC MEASURES
- Medical history and exam by a doctor.
- Diagnostic tests may be numerous, first to diagnose the cancer, and then to determine any spread to other body organs (staging). May include laboratory blood tests, Pap smear, chest x-ray, CT scan, mammogram, barium enema, cystoscopy, colposcopy with biopsy, sigmoidoscopy (see Glossary for all).

APPROPRIATE HEALTH CARE
- Doctor's treatment.
- Treatment (surgery, radiation, chemotherapy) depends partly on the location and extent of the disease and the age and physical condition of the patient.

- Surgery (usually) may include vulvectomy, vaginectomy, hysterectomy and lymph node removal. Laser vaporization is often used for treatment of some vulvar cancer.
- Radiation treatment (sometimes). External radiation shrinks the primary tumor. Internal radiation (implants) affects cancer that has spread to adjoining tissues.

POSSIBLE COMPLICATIONS—Fatal spread to other body parts. Common sites of spread are the lymph nodes in the groin, wall of the pelvis, bladder, rectum, bone, lungs or liver.

PROBABLE OUTCOME—This condition is currently considered incurable, but early detection and treatment offer a good chance for normal life expectancy. Symptoms can be relieved or controlled during treatment.

Scientific research into causes and treatment continues, so there is hope for increasingly effective treatment and cure.

HOW TO TREAT

GENERAL MEASURES
- The more you can learn about this disorder, the more you will be able to make informed decisions about where to go for your care, the treatments available, the risks involved, side effects of therapy and expected outcome.
- See Resources for Additional Information.

MEDICATION—Your doctor may prescribe:
- Pain relievers as needed.
- Antibiotics, if urinary-tract infection results from use of a bladder catheter during radiation treatment.
- Stool softeners to prevent constipation.
- Anticancer drugs are usually not prescribed for this disease, with the exception of one type (sarcomas).

ACTIVITY
- After surgery, resume your normal activities gradually, allowing 6 weeks for full recovery. Most patients can be fully active while receiving radiation therapy.
- Resume sexual relations when healing is complete in 8 to 10 weeks.

DIET—No special diet after treatment.

CALL YOUR DOCTOR IF

- You have symptoms of cancer of the vagina or vulva.
- The following occurs at the treatment site after surgery or radiation treatment:
  Signs of infection, such as increasing pain, fever and swelling.
  Excessive bleeding.

VAGINISMUS

GENERAL INFORMATION

DEFINITION—Spasms of the muscles around the opening to the vagina; if severe, may prevent intercourse.

BODY PARTS INVOLVED—Muscles surrounding the vagina and muscles of the lower vagina.

SEX OR AGE MOST AFFECTED—Females of all ages.

SIGNS & SYMPTOMS—Involuntary contraction of the muscles around the vagina and rectum. The vagina closes so tightly that the penis cannot penetrate for sexual intercourse. Also prevents the insertion of any object into the vagina, such as a tampon, diaphragm or speculum (used for medical examination).

CAUSES
- An unconscious desire to prevent penile penetration because of emotional or psychological factors. These may include fear, anxiety, hostility, anger or a distaste for sex.
- An insensitive sexual partner, insufficient or unskillful foreplay or inadequate vaginal lubrication prior to attempted penetration.
- Physical disorders (rare), such as infections, allergic reactions or a rigid, nonperforated hymen.
- Vaginal infection.

RISK INCREASES WITH
- First sexual experiences.
- Previous sexual trauma (incest, rape, sexual abuse).
- Stress.

HOW TO PREVENT—Pelvic examination by a doctor and counseling prior to beginning sexual activity.

WHAT TO EXPECT

DIAGNOSTIC MEASURES
- Your own observation of symptoms.
- Medical history and physical exam by a doctor.
- Diagnostic tests may include pelvic examination to rule out physical disorders (sedation may be necessary for a thorough examination). A sexual history is important and will include early childhood experiences, family attitudes towards sex, previous and current sexual responses, contraceptive practices, reproductive goals, feelings about sexual partner and specifics about the pain you experience.

APPROPRIATE HEALTH CARE
- Self-care after diagnosis.
- Treatment will first take care of any medical problems, followed by therapy to eliminate the muscular spasms and psychological problems.
- For muscular spasms, one type of therapy involves dilating the vaginal opening gently and gradually with rubber or glass dilators. Office treatments will probably be necessary 3 times a week and you should practice at home at least twice a day.
- Psychotherapy or counseling is recommended, in addition to, or if dilating treatment is unsuccessful. This may include sensate focus and improving communication with your partner, plus therapy to resolve any conflicts in your life.

POSSIBLE COMPLICATIONS—Psychological trauma caused by guilt, anxiety, loss of self-esteem and feelings of inadequacy, or interpersonal problems resulting from the disorder.

PROBABLE OUTCOME—Curable if the underlying cause can be cured or a coping method can be developed through medical treatment and psychological counseling.

HOW TO TREAT

GENERAL MEASURES
- Prior to dilation or attempted intercourse, sit in a tub of hot water for 10 to 15 minutes. Baths often relax muscles and relieve discomfort. Repeat baths as often as is helpful.
- Before attempting intercourse, you and your partner should use a lubricant, such as K-Y Lubricating Jelly or baby oil.

MEDICATION—Medicine is usually not necessary for vaginismus, but your doctor may prescribe mild sedatives or tranquilizers for short periods of time.

ACTIVITY—No restrictions.

DIET—No special diet.

CALL YOUR DOCTOR IF

- You have symptoms of vaginismus.
- Symptoms don't improve after 3 weeks, despite treatment
- Symptoms recur after treatment.

VAGINITIS, BACTERIAL
(Gardnerella Vaginitis; Nonspecific Vaginitis)

 GENERAL INFORMATION

DEFINITION—Vaginitis means infection or inflammation of the vagina. Nonspecific vaginitis implies that any of several infecting germs, including Gardnerella, Escherichia coli, Mycoplasma, streptococci or staphylococci, have caused the infection. These infections are contagious.

BODY PARTS INVOLVED—Vagina; urethra; bladder; skin around the genitals.

SEX OR AGE MOST AFFECTED—Female adolescents and adults of all ages; most often occurs during reproductive years.

SIGNS & SYMPTOMS—Severity of the following symptoms varies between women and from time to time in the same woman:
- Vaginal discharge that has an unpleasant odor.
- Genital swelling, burning and itching.
- Vaginal discomfort.
- Change in vaginal color from pale pink to red.
- Discomfort during sexual intercourse.

CAUSES—The organisms normally present in the vagina can multiply and cause infection when the pH and hormone balance of the vagina and surrounding tissue are disturbed.
  E. coli bacteria normally inhabit the rectum and can cause infection if spread to the vagina. The following conditions increase the likelihood of infections:
- General poor health.
- Hot weather, nonventilating clothing, especially underwear, or any other condition that increases genital moisture, warmth and darkness. These foster the growth of germs.
- Poor hygiene (sometimes).

RISK INCREASES WITH
- Diabetes mellitus.
- Menopause.
- Illness that has lowered resistance.
- HIV infection.

HOW TO PREVENT
- Keep the genital area clean. Use plain unscented soap. Be sure sexual partner is clean.
- Take showers rather than tub baths.
- Wear cotton underpants or pantyhose with a cotton crotch.
- Don't sit around in wet clothing, especially a wet bathing suit.
- After urination or bowel movements, cleanse by wiping or washing from front to back (vagina to anus).
- Lose weight if you are obese.
- Avoid vaginal douches, deodorants and bubble baths.

- If you have diabetes, adhere strictly to your treatment program.
- Change tampons or pads frequently.

 WHAT TO EXPECT

DIAGNOSTIC MEASURES
- Your own observation of symptoms.
- Medical history and physical exam (including pelvic exam) by a doctor.
- Laboratory studies, such as a Pap smear (see Glossary) and culture of the vaginal discharge.

APPROPRIATE HEALTH CARE
- Self-care after diagnosis.
- Doctor's treatment.
- Drug therapy will be directed to the specific organism. Your sexual partner may need treatment also. It is best not to do self-treatment for the disorder until the specific cause is determined.

POSSIBLE COMPLICATIONS
- Discomfort and decreased pleasure with sexual activity.
- May indicate an underlying disorder, such as diabetes.

PROBABLE OUTCOME—Usually curable in 2 weeks with treatment. Your sexual partner will need treatment also.

 HOW TO TREAT

GENERAL MEASURES
- Don't douche unless prescribed for you.
- If urinating causes burning, urinate through a tubular device, such as a toilet-paper roll or plastic cup with the end cut out, or pour a cup of warm water over genital area while you urinate.

MEDICATION—Your doctor may prescribe:
- Antibiotics or antifungals to treat the infection.
- Soothing vaginal creams or lotions for nonspecific forms of vaginitis.

ACTIVITY—Avoid overexertion, heat and excessive sweating. Delay sexual relations until after treatment.

DIET—No special diet.

 CALL YOUR DOCTOR IF

- You have symptoms of vaginitis.
- Symptoms persist longer than 1 week or worsen, despite treatment.
- Unusual vaginal bleeding or swelling develops.

VAGINITIS, MONILIAL
(Vaginal Yeast Infection; Vaginal Candidiasis)

 GENERAL INFORMATION

DEFINITION—Infection or inflammation of the vagina caused by a yeast-like fungus (Monilia or Candida albicans). Monilial vaginitis causes at least 50% of infections in the vagina.

BODY PARTS INVOLVED—Vagina and adjacent skin.

SEX OR AGE MOST AFFECTED—Females of all ages, especially after puberty.

SIGNS & SYMPTOMS—Severity of the following symptoms varies between women and from time to time in the same woman:
• White, "curdy" vaginal discharge (resembles lumps of cottage cheese). The odor may be unpleasant, but not foul.
• Swollen, red, tender, itching vaginal lips (labia) and surrounding skin; burning on urination; change in vaginal color from pale pink to red.

CAUSES—Monilia (or Candida) live in small numbers in a healthy vagina, rectum and mouth. When the vagina's hormone and pH balance is disturbed, the organisms multiply and cause infections. Monilial vaginitis tends to appear before menstrual periods and improves as soon as the period begins. Factors that may disturb the vagina's balance include:
• Pregnancy; diabetes mellitus; antibiotic treatment; oral contraceptives.
• High carbohydrate intake, especially sugars and alcohol.
• Hot weather or nonventilating clothing, which increase moisture, warmth and darkness, fostering fungal growth.
• Immunosuppression from drugs or disease.

RISK INCREASES WITH—Factors listed under Causes.

HOW TO PREVENT
• Keep the genital area clean. Use unscented soap. Take showers rather than tub baths.
• Wear cotton underpants or pantyhose with a cotton crotch.
• Don't sit around in wet clothing, especially a wet bathing suit.
• Avoid douches, vaginal deodorants and bubble baths.
• Limit your intake of sweets and alcohol.
• After urination or bowel movements, cleanse by wiping or washing from front to back (vagina to anus).
• If you have diabetes, adhere to your treatment program; lose weight if you are obese.
• Avoid broad-spectrum antibiotics unless necessary. If they are necessary, eat yogurt with live cultures to help prevent a yeast infection.

 WHAT TO EXPECT

DIAGNOSTIC MEASURES
• Medical history and physical exam (including pelvic exam) by a doctor.
• Laboratory studies, such as a Pap smear (see Glossary), and culture and microscopic exam of the vaginal discharge.

APPROPRIATE HEALTH CARE
• Self-care after diagnosis.
• Doctor's treatment.
• Drug therapy will be directed to the specific organism. Your sexual partner may need treatment also. It is best not to do self-treatment for the disorder until the cause is determined.

POSSIBLE COMPLICATIONS—Secondary bacterial infections of the vagina and other pelvic organs.

PROBABLE OUTCOME—Usually curable with 2 weeks of treatment. Recurrence is common.

 HOW TO TREAT

GENERAL MEASURES
• Don't douche unless prescribed for you.
• If urinating causes burning, urinate through a tubular device, such as a toilet-paper roll or plastic cup with the end cut out, or pour a cup of warm water over genital area while you urinate.

MEDICATION—Your doctor may recommend antifungal drugs, either in oral form or in vaginal creams or suppositories (usually). Keep creams or suppositories in the refrigerator. After treatment, you may keep a refill of the medication so you can begin treatment quickly if the infection recurs. Follow the directions carefully. Nonprescription treatments (Gyne-Lotrimin, Mycelex, etc.) are effective.

ACTIVITY—Avoid overexertion, heat and excessive sweating. Delay sexual relations until symptoms cease.

DIET—Increase consumption of yogurt, buttermilk or sour cream. Reduce alcohol and sugars.

 CALL YOUR DOCTOR IF

• You have symptoms of monilial vaginitis.
• Despite treatment, symptoms worsen or persist longer than 1 week.
• Unusual vaginal bleeding or swelling develops.
• After treatment, symptoms recur.

ILLNESS & DISORDERS

VAGINITIS, POSTMENOPAUSAL
(Atrophic Vaginitis)

 GENERAL INFORMATION

DEFINITION—Infection or inflammation of the vagina caused by lowered estrogen levels that upset the vagina's normal hormone and pH balance. Postmenopausal vaginitis is not contagious.

BODY PARTS INVOLVED—Vagina.

SEX OR AGE MOST AFFECTED—Women over age 40.

SIGNS & SYMPTOMS—Severity of the following symptoms varies greatly between women and from time to time in the same woman.
- Bad-smelling vaginal discharge.(sometimes) The discharge is usually thin, whitish and sometimes tinged with blood.
- Genital pain and itching.
- Discomfort during sexual intercourse.
- Change in vaginal color from pale-pink to red.

CAUSES
- Absence of estrogen stimulation causes the vagina to thin and lose elasticity.
- Germs that inhabit the vagina cause infection when the normal physiology of the vagina is disturbed. After menopause, the estrogen level that helped maintain a normal vaginal environment decreases, leaving the vagina more vulnerable to infection. The following conditions increase the likelihood of post-menopausal vaginitis:
- General poor health.
- Hot weather, nonventilating clothing—especially underwear—or any other condition that increases genital moisture, warmth and darkness. These foster growth of germs.

RISK INCREASES WITH
- Diabetes; illness that has lowered resistance.
- More frequent sexual intercourse.

HOW TO PREVENT
- Keep the genital area clean. Use plain unscented soap.
- Take showers rather than tub baths.
- Wear cotton panties or pantyhose with a cotton crotch. Avoid panties made from nonventilating materials, such as nylon.
- Don't sit around in wet clothing—especially a wet bathing suit.
- After urination or bowel movements, cleanse by wiping or washing from front to back (vagina to anus).
- Lose weight if you are obese.
- Avoid frequent douches.
- If you have diabetes, adhere strictly to your treatment program.
- Ask your doctor about replacement estrogen.

 WHAT TO EXPECT

DIAGNOSTIC MEASURES
- Your own observation of symptoms.
- Medical history and physical exam (including pelvic exam) by a doctor.
- Laboratory studies, such as a Pap smear (see Glossary), and microscopic exam and culture of the vaginal discharge and biopsy (see Glossary).

APPROPRIATE HEALTH CARE
- Self-care after diagnosis.
- Doctor's treatment.
- Drug therapy will be directed to the specific organism. Your sexual partner may need treatment also. It is best not to do self-treatment for the disorder until the specific cause is determined.

POSSIBLE COMPLICATIONS—Secondary bacterial infection in any pelvic organ.

PROBABLE OUTCOME—Usually curable in 10 days with treatment.

 HOW TO TREAT

GENERAL MEASURES
- Don't douche unless your doctor recommends it.
- If urinating causes burning, urinate through a tubular device, such as a toilet-paper roll or plastic cup with the end cut out, or pour a cup of warm water over genital area while you urinate.

MEDICATION—Your doctor may prescribe:
- Topical or oral estrogen. If you use a cream or suppository, use a small sanitary pad to protect clothing. Keep creams or suppositories in the refrigerator. After treatment, you may want to keep a refill of the medication so you can begin treatment quickly if the condition recurs. Follow the prescription directions carefully.
- Other creams, ointments or suppositories to suppress the organisms causing the infection.

ACTIVITY—Avoid overexertion, heat and excessive sweating. Delay sexual relations until you are well.

DIET—No special diet.

 CALL YOUR DOCTOR IF

- You have symptoms of vaginitis.
- Symptoms persist longer than 1 week or worsen, despite treatment.
- Unusual vaginal bleeding or swelling develops.
- After treatment, symptoms recur.

VAGINITIS, TRICHOMONAL (Trichomoniasis)

 GENERAL INFORMATION

DEFINITION—Infection or inflammation of the vagina caused by a parasite that lives in the lower genitourinary tract of males and females. This is very contagious between sexual partners. The severity of discomfort varies greatly from woman to woman and from time to time in the same woman. Infected men may have no symptoms.

BODY PARTS INVOLVED—Vagina, urethra and bladder in women; prostate gland and urethra in men.

SEX OR AGE MOST AFFECTED—Adolescents and adults.

SIGNS & SYMPTOMS
- Foul-smelling, frothy vaginal discharge that is most noticeable several days after a menstrual period.
- Vaginal itching and pain.
- Redness of the vaginal lips (labia) and vagina.
- Painful urination, if urine touches inflamed tissue.

CAUSES—Infection from a tiny parasite, Trichomonas vaginalis. The parasite passes from person to person during sexual intercourse. It may live in its host for years without producing symptoms. Then, perhaps from altered resistance, it will suddenly multiply rapidly and cause distressing symptoms. Since it thrives in both the male and female, both sexual partners must receive treatment.

RISK INCREASES WITH—Number of sexual partners.

HOW TO PREVENT—Use latex condoms during sexual intercourse.

 WHAT TO EXPECT

DIAGNOSTIC MEASURES
- Your own observation of symptoms.
- Medical history and physical exam (including pelvic exam) by a doctor.
- Microscopic exam of the vaginal discharge or prostate secretions.

APPROPRIATE HEALTH CARE
- Self-care after diagnosis.
- Doctor's treatment. Both sexual partners require simultaneous treatment.

POSSIBLE COMPLICATIONS—Secondary bacterial infections.

PROBABLE OUTCOME—Usually curable with treatment.

 HOW TO TREAT

GENERAL MEASURES
- Don't douche unless recommended by your doctor.
- Wear cotton panties or pantyhose with a cotton crotch. Avoid panties made from nylon, silk or other nonventilating materials.
- Take showers instead of tub baths.
- If urinating causes burning: Urinate through a tubular device, such as a toilet-paper roll or plastic cup with the end cut out, or pour a cup of warm water over genital area while you urinate.
- Don't sit around in wet clothing, especially in a wet bathing suit.

MEDICATION—Your doctor may prescribe metronidazole for you and your sexual partner or partners. Follow directions carefully. Don't drink alcohol or use vinegar when you take metronidazole. Alcohol or vinegar and metronidazole interact to cause a violent reaction with nausea, vomiting, sweating, weakness and other symptoms.

ACTIVITY—Avoid overexertion, heat and excessive sweating. Delay sexual relations until you are well. Allow about 10 days for recovery.

DIET—No special diet.

 CALL YOUR DOCTOR IF

- You have symptoms of trichomonal vaginitis.
- Symptoms persist longer than 1 week or worsen, despite treatment.
- Unusual vaginal bleeding or swelling develops.
- After treatment, symptoms recur.

VALLEY FEVER
(San Joaquin Valley Fever; Coccidioidomycosis; "Cocci")

 GENERAL INFORMATION

DEFINITION—A pulmonary infection caused by a fungus whose spores are found in soil. Valley fever is not contagious from person to person.

BODY PARTS INVOLVED—Lungs; may spread to skin, bones, membranes of brain.

SEX OR AGE MOST AFFECTED—Both sexes; all ages.

SIGNS & SYMPTOMS—The infection is usually so mild that it produces no symptoms. In a few cases the symptoms may be quite severe. They include:
- Cough; sore throat; chills and fever.
- Chest pain; headache; muscle and joint aches; shortness of breath.
- Skin rash.
- General ill feeling; depression; sweating at night.
- Weight loss; stiff neck (sometimes).

CAUSES—Infection by the fungus, Coccidioides immitis, which thrives in soil, especially soil that lines rodent burrows. Susceptible persons become infected when they breathe the dust from such soil and the fungi lodge in the lungs. Incubation is 1 to 4 weeks after exposure.

RISK INCREASES WITH
- Geographic location. The disease is most common in California's San Joaquin Valley, scattered regions in southern and central Arizona and southwest Texas.
- Occupational or environmental exposure to dust, such as from construction.
- Illness that has lowered resistance, especially uremia, diabetes mellitus, chronic lung disease (asthma), tuberculosis, AIDS, Hodgkin's disease, leukemia or severe burns.
- Use of immunosuppressive drugs, cortisone drugs or antimetabolites.
- Genetic factors. African Americans and Hispanics are more likely to have severe complications from valley fever.

HOW TO PREVENT—Cannot be prevented at present. Face masks offer limited protection against the infinitesimal spores. Efforts to develop a vaccine are unsuccessful so far.

 WHAT TO EXPECT

DIAGNOSTIC MEASURES
- Medical history and exam by a doctor.
- Diagnostic tests may include skin test, laboratory blood studies, sputum cultures and chest x-ray. If diagnosis in doubt, further tests

may include bronchoscopy (see Surgery section) and biopsy (see Glossary) of skin, lung, liver or bone.

APPROPRIATE HEALTH CARE
- Self-care after diagnosis.
- Doctor's treatment.
- Treatment usually involves supportive care at home; hospitalization only for severe cases.

POSSIBLE COMPLICATIONS—Spread of infection throughout the body and severe illness, especially in the brain or membranes that cover the brain.

PROBABLE OUTCOME—Spontaneous recovery in 3 to 6 weeks. Most persons continue to feel ill for 3 to 6 weeks after signs of infection disappear.
   Antifungal drugs are reserved for persons with severe, widespread infection, in which case they are life-saving.

 HOW TO TREAT

GENERAL MEASURES
- Use a cool-mist, ultrasonic humidifier, without medicine added, to increase moisture and help relieve a cough and sore throat. Clean humidifier daily.
- Keep a daily weight chart.

MEDICATION
- Medicine is usually not necessary for mild cases. However, you may use nonprescription nonsteroidal anti-inflammatory medicine for pain, and antitussives for cough if needed.
- For disseminated infection (spread outside the lungs) and for certain patients (infants, patients with pneumonia, coexisting congenital or acquired immunodeficiency, diabetes or pregnancy) antifungal antibiotics should be prescribed.

ACTIVITY—Stay as active as your strength allows. Rest often.

DIET—No special diet.

 CALL YOUR DOCTOR IF

- You have symptoms of valley fever.
- The following occurs during treatment:
   Continued weight loss.
   Fever.
   Diarrhea that cannot be controlled.
   Stiff neck with severe headache.

VARICOSE VEINS

GENERAL INFORMATION

DEFINITION—Veins, usually in the legs, that become permanently dilated and twisted.

BODY PARTS INVOLVED—Veins in the legs, including superficial veins, deep veins and veins that connect superficial and deep veins. Veins in the vaginal lips during pregnancy and those around the anus (hemorrhoids) also may become varicose.

SEX OR AGE MOST AFFECTED—Adults of both sexes.

SIGNS & SYMPTOMS
- Enlarged, snakelike, bluish veins that are visible under the skin upon standing. They appear most often in the back of the calf or on the inside of the leg from ankle to groin.
- Vague discomfort and aching in the legs, especially after standing.
- Fatigue.

CAUSES—The veins of the legs contain one-way valves every few inches to help blood return against gravity to the heart. If the valves leak, blood pressure in the veins prevents blood from draining properly. Valves may fail because of: previous vein disease, such as thrombophlebitis; prolonged standing; or pressure on veins in the pelvis from pregnancy, tumors or fluid in the abdomen.

RISK INCREASES WITH
- Pregnancy.
- Menstrual cycle. Symptoms worsen before and during menstruation.
- Family history of varicose veins.
- Occupations that require prolonged standing.

HOW TO PREVENT—Exercise regularly, especially by walking, swimming or bicycling, to promote good circulation.

WHAT TO EXPECT

DIAGNOSTIC MEASURES
- Your own observation of symptoms.
- Medical history and physical exam by a doctor.
- X-rays of veins (venogram).

APPROPRIATE HEALTH CARE
- Self-care after diagnosis.
- Doctor's treatment.
- Surgical and other methods (if there is pain, recurrent phlebitis, skin changes, or for cosmetic improvement): Ligation and stripping of the saphenous vein; injection of sclerosing solution; stab evulsion phlebectomy (newer procedure with shorter recovery time). For scars, excision of the entire area, followed by skin graft, may be necessary. (See Varicose Vein Removal in Surgery section.)

- Spider veins (idiopathic telangiectases) which may be extensive and unsightly: Intracapillary injections of 1% solution of sodium tetradecyl sulfate (or hypertonic saline 23.4%) using a fine-bore needle. Subsequent treatments may be required until optimal results attained.

POSSIBLE COMPLICATIONS
- Ulcer near the ankle (stasis dermatitis) caused by poor circulation to the skin. This may be slow to heal.
- Deep-vein blood clot.
- Bleeding under the skin or externally.
- Skin problems adjacent to the varicose veins that resemble eczema.

PROBABLE OUTCOME—Symptoms can be controlled with treatment or cured with surgery.

HOW TO TREAT

GENERAL MEASURES—Conservative treatment methods: Frequent rest periods with legs elevated; lightweight, elastic compression hosiery (best put on before getting out of bed); avoid girdles and other restrictive clothing; if itching occurs, use warm, wet dressings.

MEDICATION—Medicine usually is not necessary for this disorder. However, your doctor may inject a chemical into small varicose veins to make them clot and scar (sometimes). Other veins will take over circulation in the area.

ACTIVITY
- Avoid long periods of standing.
- Appropriate exercise routine as part of conservative treatment.
- Walking regimen after sclerotherapy is important to help promote healing.

DIET
- No special diet.
- Weight loss diet recommended, if obesity a problem (see Weight-Loss Diet in Appendix).

CALL YOUR DOCTOR IF

- You have varicose veins.
- After diagnosis, varicose veins begin causing circulation problems in your feet, especially stasis dermatitis.

VITAMIN DEFICIENCIES

GENERAL INFORMATION

DEFINITION—Insufficient intake or absorption of a vitamin. This deficiency is rare in the U.S. and is usually due to failure of the intestine to absorb enough of the vitamin.

BODY PARTS INVOLVED—Total body tissues.

SEX OR AGE MOST AFFECTED—Both sexes; all ages.

SIGNS & SYMPTOMS
- **Vitamin A**—Night blindness, dry eyes, rough skin, loss of appetite, diarrhea, anemia.
- **Vitamin B1**—Loss of sensation in the legs, weakness, congestive heart failure, lack of urinary control, psychosis, abdominal pain.
- **Vitamin B2**—Cracked lips, pallor, sore tongue.
- **Vitamin B3 (Niacin)**—Fatigue and weakness, poor appetite, sore mouth and tongue, indigestion, nausea, vomiting, diarrhea.
- **Vitamin B6**—Dermatitis, sore mouth and tongue, abdominal pain, vomiting, diarrhea.
- **Vitamin B12**—Weakness, sore tongue, nausea, bleeding gums, numbness in hands and feet, jaundice, headache, poor memory, depression.
- **Vitamin C**—Tender legs, bleeding and bruising under the skin, anemia, bleeding gums, loss of teeth, rough skin, increased susceptibility to infection, weakness and fatigue.
- **Vitamin D**—Restlessness, poor sleep habits, profuse sweating, bowed legs in infants, delayed walking in infants, bone pain, muscle weakness.
- **Vitamin E**—Muscle weakness, swelling of the ankles, abdomen and face in infants, anemia in premature infants.
- **Vitamin K**—Unusual bleeding or bruising.

CAUSES
- Inadequate diet.
- Impaired absorption due to disease or use of medications.

RISK INCREASES WITH
- Fad diets.
- Use of several medications.
- Alcohol or drug (including laxative) abuse.
- Malabsorption; disease; pregnancy.
- Poverty; very young or very old.
- Intestinal parasites; gastrointestinal surgery.

HOW TO PREVENT
- Proper diet.
- Supplemental vitamins if needed.

WHAT TO EXPECT

DIAGNOSTIC MEASURES
- Your own observation of symptoms.
- Medical history and physical exam by a doctor.
- Laboratory blood studies; x-rays of bones.

APPROPRIATE HEALTH CARE
- Self-care after diagnosis.
- Doctor's treatment.
- Hospitalization for severe malnutrition and alcoholism.

POSSIBLE COMPLICATIONS
- Vision problems; infections, death, if untreated (Vitamin A deficiency).
- Brain, nerve damage; heart disease (Vitamin B deficiency).
- Bone dislocations, fractures (Vitamin C & D deficiency). Difficult or impossible vaginal childbirth in women with flattened pelvic bones. Cesarean section is usually required (Vitamin D deficiency).
- Chronic anemia (Vitamin E deficiency).
- Severe or fatal hemorrhage (Vitamin K deficiency).

PROBABLE OUTCOME—Usually curable with vitamin supplementation.

HOW TO TREAT

GENERAL MEASURES—No specific instructions except those listed under other headings.

MEDICATION—Your doctor may prescribe vitamin supplements depending on the type of deficiency. Don't take more than the prescribed amount.

ACTIVITY
- Exercise whenever possible. Avoid excessive bed rest.
- Don't drive at night if you have vision problems.
- Handle children carefully to avoid bone or joint injury until deficiency is corrected.

DIET—Eat a well balanced diet that includes foods rich in vitamins. Take prenatal vitamins if you are pregnant. Provide your infant with vitamin supplements or vitamin fortified formula.

CALL YOUR DOCTOR IF

- You or a family member has symptoms of vitamin deficiency.
- Symptoms don't improve in 3 weeks, despite treatment.
- You have unexplained bleeding or bruising.
- Pain or suspected fracture occurs following an injury, even a minor injury.

VITILIGO

GENERAL INFORMATION

DEFINITION—Loss of skin pigmentation in patches. This can affect persons of any race or ethnic group.

BODY PARTS INVOLVED—Skin on the back of the hands, face and armpits.

SEX OR AGE MOST AFFECTED—Late childhood (9 to 12 years) to mid-adulthood.

SIGNS & SYMPTOMS—Macules (small areas of different skin color) or patches with the following characteristics:
- They are flat, white and can't be felt with fingers.
- They spread to form very large, irregularly-shaped areas without pigmentation.
- They are usually on both sides of the body in approximately the same place.
- Their size varies from 2mm or 3mm to several centimeters in diameter.
- They don't hurt or itch.
- Disorder also causes premature graying of hair.

CAUSES—Probably autoimmune disease. The pigment-producing cells (melanocytes) don't function normally, allowing destruction of pigment. Once pigment has been destroyed, melanocytes can't produce more pigment.

RISK INCREASES WITH
- Family history of vitiligo.
- Thyroid or adrenal disease.
- Diabetes mellitus.
- Addison's disease.
- Pernicious anemia.
- Hyperthyroidism and hypothyroidism.
- Myasthenia gravis.
- Unusual physical trauma.

HOW TO PREVENT—Cannot be prevented at present.

WHAT TO EXPECT

DIAGNOSTIC MEASURES
- Your own observation of symptoms.
- Medical history and physical exam by a doctor.
- Microscopic examination of skin scraping.

APPROPRIATE HEALTH CARE
- Self-care.
- Doctor's treatment.
- Skin grafting may be recommended for patients who do not benefit from other therapy.

POSSIBLE COMPLICATIONS—Disorder may never disappear completely, causing permanent disfigurement.

PROBABLE OUTCOME—Treatment is prolonged and often unsatisfactory. Complete and permanent repigmentation is rarely possible. Treatment consists of using an oral medication called psoralens. When discontinued, most of the regained pigmentation is usually lost. It is impossible to predict how much improvement will occur with treatment. Younger individuals (under 30) and those who obtain treatment early usually respond best. Allow 1 year to evaluate results.

HOW TO TREAT

GENERAL MEASURES
- The disorder is benign and usually just a cosmetic problem. Some patients with limited disease may choose to use a make-up product.
- Cover the lesions with waterproof, opaque makeup.
- Apply sunscreen with sunscreen protective factor (SPF) of 15 or greater to protect areas without pigment from sun damage.

MEDICATION—Your doctor may prescribe:
- Psoralens (drugs) along with exposure to ultraviolet A (UVA), which stimulates pigmentation from healthy pigment cells bordering damaged cells. The combination of psoralens and UVA is called PUVA. Results may be disappointing and adverse effects are frequent.
- High-potency topical steroids.
- For extensive vitiligo, application of hydroquinone cream.

ACTIVITY—Avoid excess sun exposure while undergoing any therapy.

DIET—No special diet.

CALL YOUR DOCTOR IF

- You have symptoms of vitiligo.
- New, unexplained symptoms develop. The drug used in treatment may produce side effects.

VOCAL-CORD NODULES
("Singer's Nodes")

 GENERAL INFORMATION

DEFINITION—Nonmalignant overgrowths of tissue on the vocal cords.

BODY PARTS INVOLVED—Larynx (voicebox).

SEX OR AGE MOST AFFECTED—Adults of both sexes.

SIGNS & SYMPTOMS—Persistent hoarseness without pain.

CAUSES—Continued overuse of the voice by singing, shouting, yelling, lecturing or other forms of talking too loudly or too much.

RISK INCREASES WITH
- Smoking.
- Vocal performers or public speakers, such as professional singers, teachers, ministers or auctioneers.

HOW TO PREVENT
- Use voice amplification, such as a microphone or megaphone, when performing or speaking.
- Take voice or speech lessons to learn to make your voice carry with less effort.
- Ask others to remind you when you get overexcited, especially in activities such as sporting events, so you can lower your voice.
- Don't smoke.

 WHAT TO EXPECT

DIAGNOSTIC MEASURES
- Your own observation of symptoms.
- Medical history and physical exam by a doctor, usually an ear, nose and throat specialist.
- Diagnosis may include a biopsy (see Glossary) of the node to rule out cancer.

APPROPRIATE HEALTH CARE
- Self-care after diagnosis.
- Doctor's treatment.
- Surgery to remove nodules (usually).

POSSIBLE COMPLICATIONS
- Without treatment, permanent hoarseness or voice alteration.
- Failure to diagnose larynx cancer, which also begins with hoarseness.

PROBABLE OUTCOME—Curable with a simple surgical procedure.

 HOW TO TREAT

GENERAL MEASURES
- Nodules may disappear if the voice is rested for several months. If you choose this treatment rather than surgery, speak in a whisper or write notes.
- Don't smoke, and avoid smoky environments.

MEDICATION—After surgery:
- Your doctor may prescribe antibiotics to prevent infection.
- You may take mild nonprescription pain relievers, if necessary, such as acetaminophen or aspirin.

ACTIVITY—Don't use your voice after surgery until your doctor determines that healing is complete.

DIET—No special diet.

 CALL YOUR DOCTOR IF

You are hoarse for more than 2 weeks.

VULVOVAGINITIS BEFORE PUBERTY

 GENERAL INFORMATION

DEFINITION—Infection or inflammation of the vagina or vulva before a young girl reaches puberty.

BODY PARTS INVOLVED—Vagina; cervix; vulva (vaginal lips); skin around the genitals.

SEX OR AGE MOST AFFECTED—Female infants and children.

SIGNS & SYMPTOMS
- Redness, pain and itching around the genital area.
- Vaginal discharge, which may or may not smell bad.
- Pain with urination.
- Bleeding from the affected area (sometimes).

CAUSES
- Infections caused by bacteria, parasites (including pinworms), yeast-like fungi or viruses.
- Allergies to synthetic fabrics, soap or other items in contact with the genitals.
- Scratches, abrasions or genital injury from insertion of foreign bodies in the vagina by the child or a playmate.
- Genital injury from sexual abuse.
- Irritation from sources such as bubble bath or bath additives.

RISK INCREASES WITH
- Diabetes mellitus.
- Infrequent bathing or unsanitary living conditions.
- Co-existing pharyngitis or other infection.

HOW TO PREVENT
- Teach the child to wipe from the vagina toward the anus after bowel movements.
- Don't let the child sit around in wet clothing, especially a wet bathing suit.
- Don't use colored or perfumed toilet tissue, scented soap or bubble baths.
- Provide the child with cotton underpants or nylon underpants with a cotton crotch.
- Teach your child to resist and report any attempted sexual contact by another person.

 WHAT TO EXPECT

DIAGNOSTIC MEASURES
- Your own observation of symptoms.
- Medical history and physical exam by a doctor (examination of vagina).
- Diagnostic tests may include laboratory blood studies and culture of the vaginal discharge.

APPROPRIATE HEALTH CARE
- Doctor's treatment, including removal of any foreign object in the vagina.
- Home care after diagnosis.

POSSIBLE COMPLICATIONS—Adhesions (see Glossary).

PROBABLE OUTCOME—Usually curable in 10 days with treatment.

 HOW TO TREAT

GENERAL MEASURES
- Remove the source of any irritation or allergy, such as soap or bubble bath.
- If urinating causes burning, the child may urinate while bathing or urinate through a toilet-paper roll or plastic cup with the end cut out or pour a cup of warm water over genital area while urinating. This prevents urine from stinging inflamed skin.

MEDICATION—Your doctor may prescribe:
- Medication appropriate for the infection, including antibiotics, antifungal or antiparasitic drugs.
- Topical ointments to relieve pain and itching.

ACTIVITY—No restrictions.

DIET—No special diet.

 CALL YOUR DOCTOR IF

- Your child has symptoms of vulvovaginitis.
- You suspect your child has been sexually abused.
- Symptoms don't improve in 7 to 10 days or symptoms worsen, despite treatment.
- Unusual vaginal bleeding or swelling develops.

ILLNESS & DISORDERS

WARTS
(Verruca Vulgaris; Plantar Warts)

GENERAL INFORMATION

DEFINITION—Benign tumors caused by a virus in the outer skin layer. Warts are not cancerous. They are mildly contagious from person to person and from one area to another on the same person.

BODY PARTS INVOLVED—Skin anywhere, but most likely on the fingers, hands and arms.

SEX OR AGE MOST AFFECTED—Most common in children and young adults between ages 1 and 30, but may occur at any age.

SIGNS & SYMPTOMS—A small, raised bump on the skin with the following characteristics:
- Warts begin very small (1mm to 3mm) and grow larger.
- Warts have a rough surface and clearly defined borders.
- They are usually the same color as the skin, but sometimes darker.
- Warts often appear in clusters around a "mother wart."
- If you cut into the wart surface, it contains small black dots or bleeding points.
- Warts are painless and don't itch.
- Plantar warts appear on the soles of the feet.

CAUSES—Invasion of the outer skin layer (epidermis) by the papilloma virus. The virus stimulates some cells to grow more rapidly than normal. Warts are very common. By adulthood, 90% of all people have antibodies to the virus, indicating a history of at least one wart infection.

RISK INCREASES WITH
- Use of public showers.
- Skin trauma.
- Immunosuppression due to drugs or illness.

HOW TO PREVENT
- To keep from spreading warts, don't scratch them. Warts spread readily to small cuts and scratches.
- Protect the skin from injury and wash hands frequently.
- Don't touch warts on other people.
- Don't wear another person's shoes.
- Wear footwear in public locker rooms or showers.

WHAT TO EXPECT

DIAGNOSTIC MEASURES
- Your own observation of symptoms.
- Medical history and physical exam by a doctor.

APPROPRIATE HEALTH CARE
- Home care after diagnosis and treatment.

- Cryotherapy (freezing cells to destroy them). This is an office procedure that doesn't require anesthesia or cause bleeding. Freezing stings or hurts slightly during application, and pain may increase a bit after thawing. Two to 5 weekly treatments are sometimes necessary to destroy the wart.
- Electrosurgery (using heat to destroy cells). This treatment can usually be completed in one office visit, but healing takes longer, and secondary bacterial infections and scarring are more common.

POSSIBLE COMPLICATIONS
- Spread to other body parts.
- Secondary infection of a wart.
- Warts recur after treatment.

PROBABLE OUTCOME—20% of warts disappear spontaneously in 1 month. Without treatment, the remainder disappear in most children in 2 to 3 years.

HOW TO TREAT

GENERAL MEASURES
- If you have cryotherapy, a blister (sometimes with blood) will develop at the treatment site. The roof of the blister will come off without further treatment in 10 to 14 days. You should have little or no scarring. Wash and use make-up or cosmetics as usual. If clothing irritates the blister, cover with a small adhesive bandage. If the blister breaks, the fluid may have active virus and spread to other areas; wash with hot water and soap, dry and cover the area.
- For plantar warts, insert pads or cushion in the shoe to make walking more comfortable.

MEDICATION—Your doctor may prescribe:
- Chemicals, such as mild salicylic acid, to destroy warts. If so, apply twice a day for 4 to 6 weeks.
- Tretinoin (retinoic acid) or benzoyl peroxide to help in treating warts.
- Several new methods are also available for treatment.

ACTIVITY—No restrictions.

DIET—No special diet.

CALL YOUR DOCTOR IF

- You or your child have warts and you want them removed.
- After removal by cryosurgery or electrocautery, signs of infection appear at the treatment site.
- After treatment, fever develops.
- Warts don't disappear completely after treatment.
- Other warts appear after treatment.

WARTS, VENEREAL
(Condylomata Acuminata; Genital Warts; Moist Warts)

 GENERAL INFORMATION

DEFINITION—Warts in the genital area (includes the urethra, genitals and rectum). These are more contagious than other warts. Evidence suggests that the virus that causes venereal warts may also be associated with genital malignancies.

BODY PARTS INVOLVED—Urethra; genitals; rectum.

SEX OR AGE MOST AFFECTED—Both sexes of sexually active adolescents and adults.

SIGNS & SYMPTOMS—Venereal warts have the following characteristics:
- They appear on moist surfaces, especially the penis, entrance to the vagina and entrance to the rectum.
- They are thin, flexible, solid elevations of the skin, growing in stalks or clusters. They are taller than they are wide.
- Each wart measures 1mm to 2mm in diameter, but clusters may be quite large.
- They don't hurt or itch.
- Warts may produce no symptoms, or cause itching, burning, tenderness or pain.

CAUSES—Venereal warts are caused by a subtype of the same virus that causes other warts, human papillomavirus (HPV), but they are more contagious. They spread easily on the skin of the infected person and pass easily to other people. They are usually transmitted sexually, often as a result of poor hygiene. They have an incubation of 1 to 6 months.

RISK INCREASES WITH
- Poor nutrition.
- Other venereal disease.
- Multiple sexual partners.
- Crowded or unsanitary living conditions.
- Poor hygiene.
- Not using condoms.
- In children, warts may be a sign of sexual abuse.

HOW TO PREVENT—To prevent spread of warts to other parts of the body or to other persons:
- Don't scratch warts.
- Avoid sexual activity until warts heal completely.
- Use latex condoms during sexual intercourse.

 WHAT TO EXPECT

DIAGNOSTIC MEASURES
- Your own observation of symptoms.
- Medical history and physical exam by a doctor.
- Sexual partners of infected persons need to be examined also.
- Medical tests including biopsy of tissue, colposcopy, anoscopy and Pap smear (see Glossary for all).

APPROPRIATE HEALTH CARE
- Treatment will be determined by size and location of warts.
- Small warts may be treated with topical applications.
- For larger warts, application of liquid nitrogen to warts (cryotherapy).
- Some larger warts require laser treatment, electrocoagulation or surgical excision.

POSSIBLE COMPLICATIONS
- Female cervical disorders, including cancer.
- In males, urinary obstruction.

PROBABLE OUTCOME—These small warts usually cause no symptoms. If untreated, they probably will disappear eventually. However, because the virus may be associated with genital malignancy, obtain medical treatment. Recurrence is common and retreatment is necessary.

 HOW TO TREAT

GENERAL MEASURES
- These warts are generally treated with chemicals: podophyllin, trichloracetic acid or liquid nitrogen. After applying any of these, wash the treated area according to your doctor's recommendation.
- Follow your doctor's instructions. Compliance with your medical treatment plan is essential for the best outcome.

MEDICATION—Your doctor may prescribe podophyllin, a topical medication. It may be applied by the doctor or you may use it for self-treatment. Follow all instructions carefully. Don't use it if you are pregnant.

ACTIVITY—No restrictions, except to avoid sexual relations until warts are completely gone.

DIET—No special diet.

 CALL YOUR DOCTOR IF

- You have symptoms of venereal warts.
- The following occurs after treatment:
  The treated area becomes infected (red, swollen, painful or tender).
  Fever.
  You feel generally ill.

WHIPLASH
(Acceleration-Deceleration Cervical Injury)

GENERAL INFORMATION

DEFINITION—Injury to the neck caused when it is whipped backward forcefully—usually in an accident.

BODY PARTS INVOLVED—Muscles, tendons, disks and nerves in the neck.

SEX OR AGE MOST AFFECTED—Both sexes; all ages.

SIGNS & SYMPTOMS
- Pain or stiffness in the front and back of the neck—either immediately following or up to 24 hours after injury.
- Dizziness.
- Headache.
- Nausea and vomiting (sometimes).

CAUSES—Injury, usually from contact sports or motor-vehicle accidents.

RISK INCREASES WITH
- Osteoarthritis of the spine.
- Situations that make accidents more likely, such as:
  Driving in rainy, icy or snowy weather.
  "Tail-gaiting" or other poor driving habits.
  Driving after excess alcohol consumption or use of mind-altering drugs.

HOW TO PREVENT—Use the padded headrests in your auto. These have decreased the frequency and severity of auto whiplash injuries. Drive carefully and defensively. Don't drink or use mind-altering drugs and drive.

WHAT TO EXPECT

DIAGNOSTIC MEASURES
- Your own observation of symptoms.
- Medical history and physical exam by a doctor.
- X-rays of the spine and neurological studies to rule out injury to the spine.

APPROPRIATE HEALTH CARE
- Self-care after diagnosis.
- Treatment may involve medications, physical therapy and other supportive therapies.
- Diathermy or ultrasound treatments (see Glossary for both).
- Surgery to remove an injured spinal disk (rare).

POSSIBLE COMPLICATIONS—Temporary numbness and weakness in the arms, if nerve roots are injured. This may persist until recovery.

PROBABLE OUTCOME—Usually curable in 1 week to 3 months with treatment.

HOW TO TREAT

GENERAL MEASURES
- Apply ice packs to the injured area for 10 to 20 minutes each hour during the first 24 hours.
- After 24 hours, use ice packs or heat to relieve pain. Heat may include hot showers twice a day, in which the water beats on your neck and shoulders for 10 to 20 minutes. Between showers, apply hot soaks to the neck, or use a heat lamp several times a day for 10 to 15 minutes.
- Try to improve your posture. Pull in your chin and abdomen when sitting or standing. Sit in a firm chair and force your buttocks to touch the chair's back.
- If symptoms are severe, buy and wear a soft, padded, fabric collar (Thomas collar) until pain subsides.
- Sleep without a pillow. Instead, roll a small towel to 2 inches in diameter, or use a cervical pillow or a Thomas collar. Poor sleeping positions delay healing.
- If you have nerve-root pressure, with numbness and weakness in the hand or arm, a cervical-traction apparatus may be recommended. This can be hung over a doorway.

MEDICATION
- Your doctor may prescribe pain relievers or muscle relaxants (sometimes).
- You may use nonprescription drugs, such as aspirin or acetaminophen, for minor pain.

ACTIVITY—Depends on the severity of symptoms. During the acute or severe stage, rest as much as possible. As symptoms improve, resume normal activity. Avoid lifting heavy objects.

DIET—No special diet. Avoid alcohol.

CALL YOUR DOCTOR IF

- You have a painful neck injury.
- Pain, numbness, tingling or weakness develops in the arm or face.
- New, unexplained symptoms develop. Drugs used in treatment may produce side effects.

WHOOPING COUGH
(Pertussis)

 GENERAL INFORMATION

DEFINITION—A serious, contagious, bacterial infection of the bronchial tubes and lungs. Immunization throughout the world has greatly decreased the incidence of whooping cough.

BODY PARTS INVOLVED—Bronchial tubes; larynx; lungs.

SEX OR AGE MOST AFFECTED—All ages, but most common in children.

SIGNS & SYMPTOMS
Early stages:
- Runny nose.
- Dry cough that progresses to a cough with thick sputum.
- Slight fever.

Later stages:
- Severe, continual coughing bouts that last up to 1 minute. The face turns red or blue from lack of oxygen while coughing. At the end of each coughing effort, the child gasps for breath with a "whooping" sound.
- Vomiting and diarrhea.
- Fever.

CAUSES—Infection with Bordetella pertussis bacteria. The disease is transmitted by direct contact with a contagious person, or by indirect contact, such as breathing air containing infected droplets or handling linen or other contaminated articles. The incubation period is 5 to 7 days.

RISK INCREASES WITH
- Nonimmunized populations.
- Epidemics in late winter or early spring. The bacteria become more virulent as they spread.
- Crowded or unsanitary living conditions.
- Pregnancy.

HOW TO PREVENT
- Obtain immunizations against whooping cough for all children. Immunizations normally begin at 2 months. Immunization after age 5 is not recommended.
- Isolate infected persons.

 WHAT TO EXPECT

DIAGNOSTIC MEASURES
- Your own observation of symptoms.
- Medical history and exam by a doctor.
- Laboratory studies, such as culture of the sputum and x-rays of the chest.

APPROPRIATE HEALTH CARE
- Doctor's treatment.
- Hospitalization with intensive care for severely ill infants. Older children can usually be treated at home.

POSSIBLE COMPLICATIONS
- Children under 1 year of age are subject to severe complications or death.
- Nosebleeds.
- Retinal detachment.
- Seizures and encephalitis.
- Pneumonia.
- Apnea (slowed or stopped breathing).
- Middle-ear infection.
- Ruptured blood vessels in the brain.

PROBABLE OUTCOME—Usually curable in about 6 weeks with treatment (may range from 3 weeks to 3 months). The usual course of illness is: 2 weeks with the noncharacteristic cough; 2 weeks with bouts of the "whooping" cough; and 2 weeks for convalescence. Some persistent coughs may continue for months.

 HOW TO TREAT

GENERAL MEASURES
- Isolate the ill person until fever disappears. Necessary visitors should wear masks.
- During a coughing bout in a baby, raise the foot of the crib. Place the baby face down with the head turned to one side to help drain the lungs. Older children usually prefer to sit up and lean forward during coughing bouts.
- Use a cool-mist, ultrasonic humidifier to soothe the cough and help loosen bronchial and lung secretions. Clean humidifier daily.

MEDICATION
- Don't use cough medicine unless prescribed.
- Your doctor may prescribe:
  Erythromycin started during the incubation period.
  Antibiotics for complications, such as middle-ear infection or pneumonia.

ACTIVITY—Keep the child in bed until the fever disappears. Normal activity should be resumed slowly, according to strength.

DIET
- Encourage extra fluids, such as fruit juice, tea, carbonated drinks and bouillon.
- No special diet. Small, frequent meals may decrease vomiting.

 CALL YOUR DOCTOR IF

- Your child has signs of whooping cough, especially blueness of the face with coughing bouts.
- Fever.
- Vomiting persists more than 1 or 2 days.

WILM'S TUMOR
(Congenital Nephroblastoma)

GENERAL INFORMATION

DEFINITION—A malignant mixed tumor (one that contains several cell types) of the kidney that occurs primarily in children (90% of the time, only one kidney is affected).

BODY PARTS INVOLVED—Kidney.

SEX OR AGE MOST AFFECTED—Both sexes of children under age 7, with a peak incidence between ages 3 and 4. Occasionally doesn't appear until adulthood.

SIGNS & SYMPTOMS
• Enlarged abdomen. A large, firm, smooth tumor can be felt easily within the abdominal wall.
• High blood pressure.
• Blood in the urine (urine may appear cloudy).
• Abdominal pain (sometimes).
• Repeated vomiting.
• Fever.
• Weight loss.

CAUSES—Unknown.

RISK INCREASES WITH—Genetic factors. Wilm's tumor is most likely in children with other congenital abnormalities.

HOW TO PREVENT—Cannot be prevented at present.

WHAT TO EXPECT

DIAGNOSTIC MEASURES
• Your own observation of symptoms.
• Medical history and physical exam by a doctor.
• Laboratory studies, such as 24-hour urine studies.
• Ultrasound, urography, arteriography, vena cavography, retrograde pyelography, CT scan (see Glossary for all) and x-ray.

APPROPRIATE HEALTH CARE
• Doctor's treatment.
• Surgery to remove the affected kidney and adjacent tissue, if the cancer has spread.
• Radiation treatment and anticancer drugs.

POSSIBLE COMPLICATIONS
• Kidney failure.
• Tumor spread to lungs, bones, liver or brain, if untreated.
• Adverse reactions, including hair loss, from radiation treatment and anticancer drugs.

PROBABLE OUTCOME—With appropriate treatment, the outlook is better than for most malignant tumors in children. In most cases, Wilm's tumor is curable with surgery, radiation treatment and anticancer drugs. If the tumor is detected before it spreads, the 5-year-survival rate is 90%.

HOW TO TREAT

GENERAL MEASURES
• The more you can learn and understand about this disorder, the more you will be able to make informed decisions about where to go for care, the treatments available, the risks involved, side effects of therapy and expected outcome.
• See Resources for Additional Information.

MEDICATION—Your doctor may prescribe:
• Anticancer drugs.
• Antinausea drugs.
• Pain relievers.
• Antibiotics, if infection occurs during anticancer drug treatment.
• Stool softeners to prevent constipation following surgery.

ACTIVITY—No restrictions. The child may be as active as strength allows.

DIET—No special diet.

CALL YOUR DOCTOR IF

• Your child has symptoms of Wilm's tumor.
• The following occurs during treatment:
  Vomiting, abdominal pain or constipation.
  Shortness of breath.
  Swelling in feet or ankles.
• New, unexplained symptoms develop. Drugs used in treatment may cause side effects.

ZINC DEFICIENCY

 GENERAL INFORMATION

DEFINITION—Inadequate amounts of zinc in body cells. This affects function of the testes, liver and muscles, and affects the structure of bones, teeth, hair and skin. Zinc is a vital part of many enzymes that facilitate chemical reactions necessary for normal body function—including immune function and skin healing.

BODY PARTS INVOLVED—All body cells.

SEX OR AGE MOST AFFECTED—All ages, but most common in children during periods of rapid growth (10 to 18 years).

SIGNS & SYMPTOMS—.2 or more of the following:
- Poor appetite.
- Poor growth.
- Sensations of unpleasant tastes and odors, and decreased senses of taste and smell.
- Decreased sex drive.
- Darkening of skin all over the body.
- Sparse hair growth.
- Deformed nails.

CAUSES
- Excessive consumption of substances that bind zinc and prevent its absorption from the gastrointestinal tract. These include calcium, vitamin D, high fiber diet and phytate enzyme (found in whole-meal bread).
- Surgical removal of any part of the gastrointestinal tract, especially the stomach.
- Parasite infestation in the gastrointestinal tract.
- Excessive milk consumption in preschool children.

RISK INCREASES WITH
- Alcoholism. Alcohol increases the excretion of zinc.
- Use of cortisone drugs, which increase zinc excretion.
- Pregnancy.
- Diabetes, kidney disease or cirrhosis.
- Burns or major trauma.

HOW TO PREVENT
- Adults should not drink or eat more than the recommended amounts of milk, other dairy products or whole-meal bread. Keep calcium intake at 1500 mg or less daily.
- Don't take large doses of vitamin D supplements.
- Take zinc supplements if you have had gastrointestinal surgery.
- Obtain medical treatment for parasite infections.
- Don't drink more than 1 or 2 alcoholic drinks, if any, a day.

 WHAT TO EXPECT

DIAGNOSTIC MEASURES
- Your own observation of symptoms.
- Medical history and physical exam by a doctor.
- Laboratory blood studies of zinc levels; other tests to determine any underlying disorder.

APPROPRIATE HEALTH CARE
- Home care after diagnosis.
- Doctor's treatment.

POSSIBLE COMPLICATIONS
- Iron-deficiency anemia. Zinc is necessary for iron absorption.
- Poor wound healing.
- Liver and spleen enlargement.
- Excess zinc replacement or overdose may interfere with body's manufacture of necessary enzymes.

PROBABLE OUTCOME—Usually curable in 2 months with zinc supplements and removal or treatment of the underlying causes.

 HOW TO TREAT

GENERAL MEASURES—Follow your doctor's instructions. Compliance with your medical treatment plan is essential for the best outcome.

MEDICATION—Your doctor may prescribe zinc supplements. Take with milk or meals to prevent stomach upset.

ACTIVITY—No restrictions.

DIET—Eat foods high in zinc such as red meat. Avoid excessive intake of whole-meal bread.

 CALL YOUR DOCTOR IF

You or your child have symptoms of zinc deficiency.

ILLNESS & DISORDERS

Surgeries

ABDOMINOPERINEAL RESECTION

 GENERAL INFORMATION

DEFINITION—Removal of cancerous cells in the rectum and anus through an incision in the lower abdomen and the perineum. Enough of the anus and rectum are removed so that the intestines cannot be reconnected. A colostomy (see Colostomy in Surgery section) is performed at the same time so that digestive function is not disrupted.

BODY PARTS INVOLVED—Rectum; anus; sigmoid colon; perineum; abdomen.

REASONS FOR SURGERY—Cancer of the rectum or anus.

SURGICAL RISK INCREASES WITH
- Adults over 60.
- Diabetes mellitus
- Obesity; smoking.
- Poor nutrition.
- Recent illness.
- Alcoholism or other chronic illness.
- Use of some prescription and nonprescription drugs. Inform your doctor of any drugs, medications, or vitamin and herb supplements you are using or have used in the last month.

 WHAT TO EXPECT

WHO OPERATES—Proctologist, general surgeon or colon and rectal surgeon.

WHERE PERFORMED—Hospital.

DIAGNOSTIC TESTS
- Before surgery: Colonoscopy; sigmoidoscopy; barium enema; ultrasound; CT scan (see Glossary for these terms); blood and urine studies.
- After surgery: Laboratory examination of removed tissue; blood studies.

ANESTHESIA—General anesthesia by injection and inhalation with an airway tube placed in the windpipe.

DESCRIPTION OF OPERATION
- An incision is made in the abdomen. The abdominal muscles are divided and the peritoneal cavity is entered. The sigmoid colon is located, isolated and divided. The closer bowel portion is brought to the skin surface for a colostomy.
- The colostomy bag is fitted and placed in position.
- The farther bowel portion is closed and placed deep in the pelvis.
- Incisions are made in the perineum.
- The rectum, anus and end of the bowel (intestine) are isolated and cut free of connective tissue.
- Tubes are left in to allow drainage.
- The skin edges of both incisions are closed with sutures or clips, which usually can be removed in 7 to 10 days after surgery.

POSSIBLE COMPLICATIONS
- Excessive bleeding.
- Impotence.
- Surgical-wound infection.
- Adhesions leading to intestinal obstruction.

AVERAGE HOSPITAL STAY—7 to 10 days.

PROBABLE OUTCOME—Expect complete healing of surgical wounds. You will need to wear an external colostomy pouch to collect bowel movements. Allow about 3 months for recovery from surgery.

 POSTOPERATIVE CARE

GENERAL MEASURES
- A hard ridge should form along each incision. As they heal, the ridges will gradually recede.
- Use an electric heating pad, a heat lamp or a warm compress to relieve incisional pain.
- Ask your surgeon when you may begin to bathe or shower as usual.
- Move and elevate legs often while in bed to decrease the likelihood of deep-vein blood clots.
- An enterostomy specialist (see Glossary) will teach you how to care for your colostomy.

MEDICATION
- Your doctor may prescribe:
  Pain relievers. Don't take prescription pain medication longer than 4 to 7 days. Use only as much as you need.
  Stool softeners to prevent constipation.
  Antibiotics to fight or prevent infection.
- You may use nonprescription drugs, such as acetaminophen, for minor pain. Avoid aspirin.

ACTIVITY
- To help recovery and aid your well-being, resume daily activities, including work, as soon as possible.
- Avoid vigorous exercise for 6 weeks after surgery. Resume driving 2-3 weeks after returning home.

DIET—Clear liquid diet until the gastrointestinal tract functions again. Then eat a well-balanced diet to promote healing. Avoid caffeine and alcohol, and any food or spice that causes painful or unpleasant digestive symptoms. Your doctor may prescribe a special diet.

 CALL YOUR DOCTOR IF

- You experience nausea, vomiting, or constipation; or increased abdominal pain, swelling or bleeding.
- You develop signs of infection, including headache, muscle aches, dizziness, a general ill feeling and fever; or redness, swelling or drainage in the surgical areas.
- New, unexplained symptoms develop. Drugs used in treatment may produce side effects.

ABDOMINOPERINEAL RESECTION

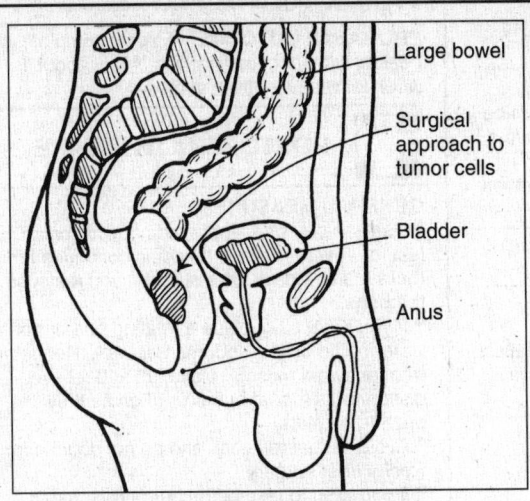

Large bowel

Surgical approach to tumor cells

Bladder

Anus

An illustration of the appearance and anatomical relationships of the large bowel with representation of a large bowel tumor.

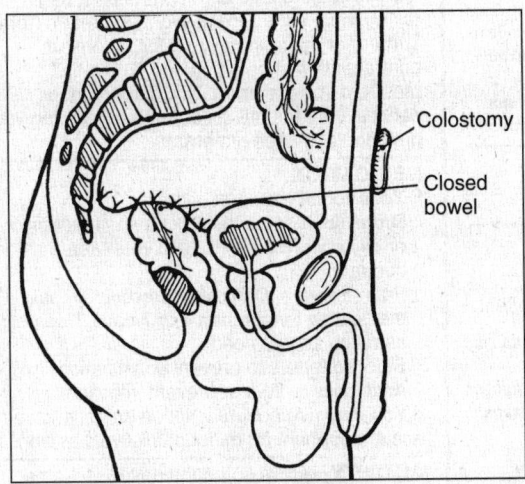

Colostomy

Closed bowel

The colostomy, which protrudes through the abdominal wall and skin.
- The closed distal portion of the bowel.

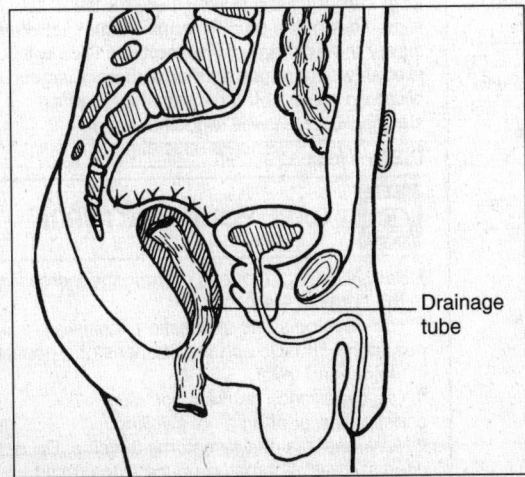

Drainage tube

Tumor removed, along with rectum, bowel and anus.
- Drainage tube left in place to be removed after healing.

SURGERIES

ABORTION
(Suction Curettage)

GENERAL INFORMATION

DEFINITION—Removal of a fetus and accompanying tissue from the uterus. It can be used to terminate a pregnancy, or to remove a fetus that has died in utero, and is usually performed in pregnancies of 12 weeks duration or less.

BODY PARTS INVOLVED—Uterus; placenta; vagina (route for surgery).

REASONS FOR SURGERY
- Missed or incomplete miscarriage.
- Elective termination of pregnancy. The patient should receive competent counseling before making this decision.

SURGICAL RISK INCREASES WITH
- Obesity.
- Smoking.
- Poor nutrition.
- Recent or chronic illness.
- Use of some prescription and nonprescription drugs. Inform your doctor of any drugs, medications, or vitamin and herb supplements you are using or have used in the last month.

WHAT TO EXPECT

WHO OPERATES—General surgeon or obstetrician-gynecologist.

WHERE PERFORMED—Hospital or outpatient surgical facility.

DIAGNOSTIC TESTS
- Before surgery: Pregnancy test; psychological counseling and testing; blood and urine studies.
- After surgery: Laboratory examination of removed tissue.

ANESTHESIA—Local anesthesia by injection; sometimes accompanied by a tranquilizer.

DESCRIPTION OF OPERATION
- The opening of the cervix is dilated by the use of instruments or laminaria (see Glossary).
- A small plastic tube is passed through the vagina and cervix into the uterus. The tube is connected to a suction apparatus.
- Gentle suction through the tube removes the uterine contents. You may feel cramps in the lower abdomen, nausea, sweating and faintness.
- The tube is removed, and the lining of the uterus is scraped with a curette to be sure all the placental tissue is removed.

POSSIBLE COMPLICATIONS
- Excessive bleeding.
- Perforation or infection of the uterus.
- Potential psychological problems.

AVERAGE HOSPITAL STAY—None.

PROBABLE OUTCOME—Expect complete healing without complications. Allow about 1 week for recovery from surgery.

POSTOPERATIVE CARE

GENERAL MEASURES
- Use sanitary pads for bleeding, which may last for several days. If bleeding continues for more than 14 days after surgery, you may use tampons.
- If you have pain, place a heating pad or hot-water bottle on the abdomen or back. Hot baths frequently aid muscle relaxation and relieve discomfort. Repeat baths as often as they provide comfort.
- Avoid sexual relations and do not douche for 2 weeks after surgery.
- If you wish to take birth-control pills, begin taking them either on the night you return from surgery or the next day; a backup form of contraception should be used for the first month. If you prefer an IUD, diaphragm or cervical cap, the fitting can be made during your next doctor's appointment.

MEDICATION
- Your doctor may prescribe:
  Drugs such as methylergonovine (Methergine) or oxytocin (Pitocin) to help your uterus contract.
  Pain relievers. Don't take prescription pain medication longer than 4 to 7 days. Use only as much as you need.
  Stool softeners to prevent constipation.
  Antibiotics to fight or prevent infection.
- You may use nonprescription drugs, such as acetaminophen, for minor pain. Avoid aspirin.

ACTIVITY—Have someone drive you home from surgery. Rest quietly there for the remainder of the day. Resume normal activities slowly the next day, if you feel able. You will probably experience light or moderate vaginal bleeding on and off for 10 to 14 days after surgery. Bed rest will reduce bleeding.

DIET—No special diet.

CALL YOUR DOCTOR IF

- Pain, swelling, redness or drainage increases in the surgical area.
- You develop signs of infection, including headache, muscle aches, dizziness or a general ill feeling and fever.
- You experience nausea, vomiting, constipation or abdominal swelling.
- New, unexplained symptoms develop. Drugs used in treatment may produce side effects.

ABORTION
(Suction Curettage)

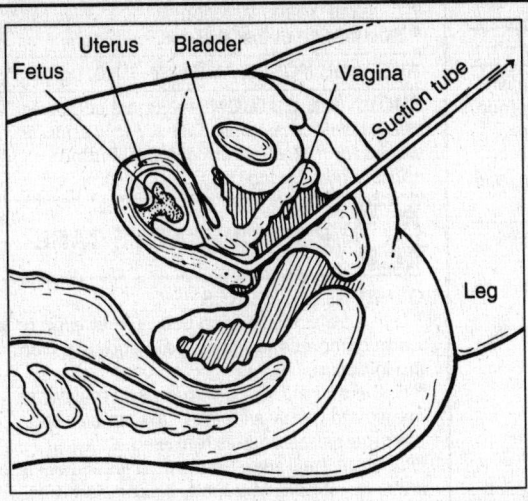

Uterus Bladder
Fetus
Vagina
Suction tube
Leg

A side view of an adult female showing a small fetus within the uterus (womb).
- Suction tube in place. One end of the the tube is attached to the suction machine and the other end is passed through the vagina and cervix into the uterus.

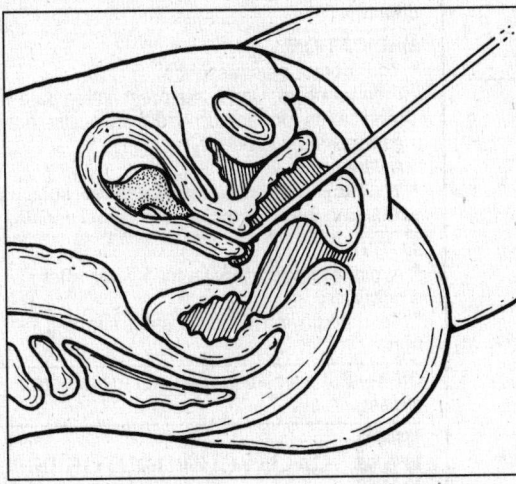

Gentle suction through the tube removes the fetus and placenta.

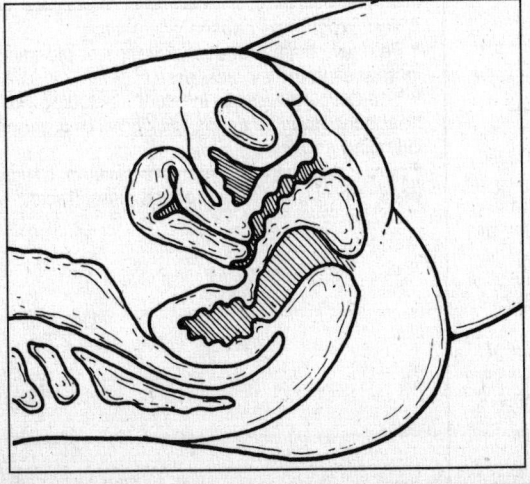

Suction tube removed. Uterus is now empty. Pregnancy terminated.

ABSCESS DRAINAGE

GENERAL INFORMATION

DEFINITION—To open and drain an abscess.

BODY PARTS INVOLVED—Abscesses may occur anywhere in the body. The most common areas include: female breast during lactation; armpit; rectum; vaginal lips; face; area around the tonsils; area under the tongue; scrotum; and arms, legs, hands and feet.

REASONS FOR SURGERY—Treatment of infections. If an abscess breaks open and drains spontaneously, surgery is often still required to assure complete drainage.

SURGICAL RISK INCREASES WITH
- Obesity.
- Smoking.
- Poor nutrition.
- Diabetes mellitus.
- Recent or chronic illness.
- Use of some prescription and nonprescription drugs. Inform your doctor of any drugs, medications, or vitamin and herb supplements you are using or have used in the last month.

WHAT TO EXPECT

WHO OPERATES—Family doctor or general surgeon.

WHERE PERFORMED—Doctor's office, outpatient surgical facility, hospital or emergency room.

DIAGNOSTIC TESTS
- Before surgery: Blood and urine studies (sometimes).
- After surgery: Laboratory examination of removed pus (sometimes).

ANESTHESIA
- Local anesthesia by injection.
- General anesthesia by injection and inhalation.

DESCRIPTION OF OPERATION
- An incision is made over the abscess.
- The incision is spread apart, and a sterile-gloved finger or instrument is inserted inside the abscess to break up small pockets. The pus is drained and the cavity is irrigated.
- Gauze is packed into the space left by the abscess. Sometimes a soft rubber drain may be left in the incision; either method allows the cavity to heal from the bottom outward. The drain is usually removed 24 to 48 hours after surgery.
- The skin is left open to prevent recurrence of the abscess.
- A gauze dressing is applied over the wound.

POSSIBLE COMPLICATIONS
- Excessive bleeding.
- Surgical-wound infection.
- Recurrence of the abscess.

AVERAGE HOSPITAL STAY—0 to 1 day.

PROBABLE OUTCOME—Expect complete healing without complications. Allow about 2 weeks for recovery from surgery. Further surgery may be indicated.

POSTOPERATIVE CARE

GENERAL MEASURES
- Use an electric heating pad, a heat lamp or a warm compress to relieve pain and help clear the infection.
- Bathe and shower as usual. You may wash the wound gently with mild, unscented soap after the gauze drain is removed.
- Change the gauze dressing at least daily after bathing, or more frequently if saturated with drainage.

MEDICATION
- Your doctor may prescribe:
  Pain relievers. Don't take prescription pain medication longer than 4 to 7 days. Use only as much as you need.
  Antibiotics to fight infection.
- You may use nonprescription drugs, such as acetaminophen, for minor pain. Avoid aspirin.

ACTIVITY
- Avoid vigorous exercise for 1 week after surgery.
- Resume driving 1-2 days after returning home.

DIET—Eat a well-balanced diet to promote healing.

CALL YOUR DOCTOR IF

- You experience nausea or vomiting.
- Pain, swelling, redness, drainage or bleeding increases in the surgical area.
- You develop signs of infection, including headache, muscle aches, dizziness or a general ill feeling and fever.
- New, unexplained symptoms develop. Drugs used in treatment may produce side effects.

ABSCESS DRAINAGE

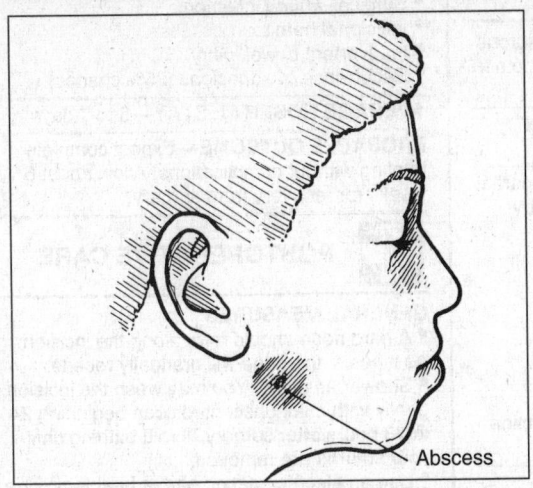

A side view of an adolescent male face showing an abscess.

Abscess

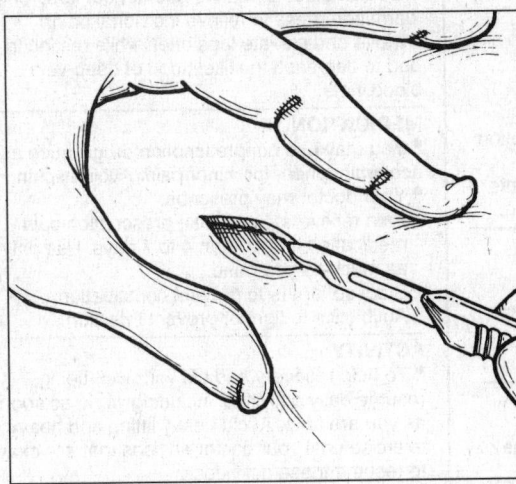

Abscess is incised, the incision spread apart, and finger inserted into abscess cavity to break up small pockets.

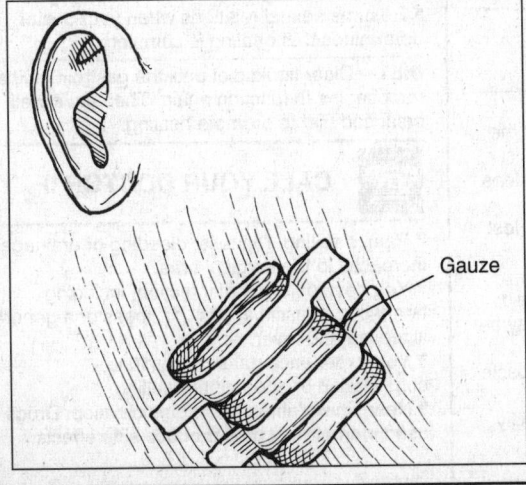

Gauze inserted into space left by the abscess. This provides a drain that allows the abscess cavity to heal from the bottom outward.

Gauze

ADHESIONS, SEPARATION OF (LYSIS OF)

GENERAL INFORMATION

DEFINITION—Separation of adhesions, fibrous bands of tissue that cause parts of the abdomen and pelvis to cling together abnormally.

BODY PARTS INVOLVED—Abdominal or pelvic organs.

REASONS FOR SURGERY—Relief of a partial or complete intestinal obstruction caused by adhesions. Adhesions usually result from:
- Previous abdominal surgery.
- Congenital defects.
- Pelvic inflammatory disease.
- Endometriosis.
- Ruptured ectopic pregnancy.
- Radiation treatment for cancers in the abdomen or pelvis.
- Any ruptured organ that has caused infection and scarring.

SURGICAL RISK INCREASES WITH
- Adults over 60; obesity; smoking.
- Excess alcohol consumption.
- Poor nutrition.
- Diabetes mellitus.
- Recent or chronic illness.
- Use of some prescription and nonprescription drugs. Inform your doctor of any drugs, medications, or vitamin and herb supplements you are using or have used in the last month.

WHAT TO EXPECT

WHO OPERATES—General surgeon.

WHERE PERFORMED—Hospital.

DIAGNOSTIC TESTS
- Before surgery: Blood and urine studies; abdominal x-rays; sometimes, barium enema or small bowel series (see Glossary).
- After surgery: Blood studies.

ANESTHESIA—General anesthesia by injection and inhalation with an airway tube placed in the windpipe.

DESCRIPTION OF OPERATION
- An incision is made in the abdomen over the obstruction.
- The obstruction is isolated and the adhesions are divided carefully.
- The bowel is examined for strangulation (lost blood supply). Any strangulated portion is removed, and the normal ends are joined.
- The abdominal contents are then inspected for undetected disease. Other surgeries may be performed at this time.
- The abdominal contents are replaced. Muscle layers are closed with sutures, and skin is closed with sutures or clips, which can usually be removed in 1 week.

POSSIBLE COMPLICATIONS
- Excessive bleeding; blood clots.
- Surgical-wound infection.
- Incisional hernia.
- Inadvertent bowel injury.
- Recurrence of adhesions (25% chance).

AVERAGE HOSPITAL STAY—5 to 7 days.

PROBABLE OUTCOME—Expect complete healing without complications. Allow about 6 weeks for recovery from surgery.

POSTOPERATIVE CARE

GENERAL MEASURES
- A hard ridge should form along the incision. As it heals, the ridge will gradually recede.
- Shower as usual. You may wash the incision gently with mild, unscented soap beginning 24 to 48 hours after surgery. Avoid bathing until your sutures are removed.
- Use an electric heating pad, a heat lamp or a warm compress to relieve incisional pain.
- Move and elevate legs often while resting in bed to decrease the likelihood of deep-vein blood clots.

MEDICATION
- You may use nonprescription drugs, such as acetaminophen, for minor pain. Avoid aspirin.
- Your doctor may prescribe:
  Pain relievers. Don't take prescription pain medication longer than 4 to 7 days. Use only as much as you need.
  Stool softeners to prevent constipation.
  Antibiotics to fight or prevent infection.

ACTIVITY
- To help recovery and aid your well-being, resume daily activities, including work, as soon as you are able. Avoid heavy lifting and heavy exercise until your doctor advises that it is okay to resume these activities.
- Resume driving 3 weeks after returning home.
- Resume sexual relations when your doctor determines that healing is complete.

DIET—Clear liquid diet until the gastrointestinal tract begins to function again. Then eat a well-balanced diet to promote healing.

CALL YOUR DOCTOR IF

- Pain, swelling, redness, bleeding or drainage increases in the surgical area.
- You develop signs of infection, including headache, muscle aches, dizziness or a general ill feeling and fever.
- You experience nausea, vomiting, constipation or abdominal swelling.
- New, unexplained symptoms develop. Drugs used in treatment may produce side effects.

ADHESIONS, SEPARATION OF (LYSIS OF)

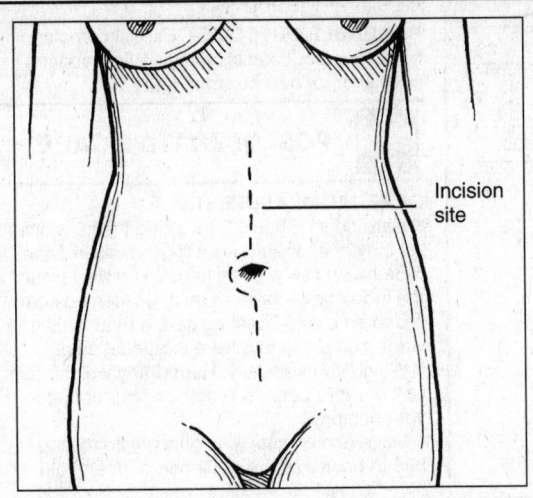

An illustration of the surgical site to enter the abdomen.

Incision site

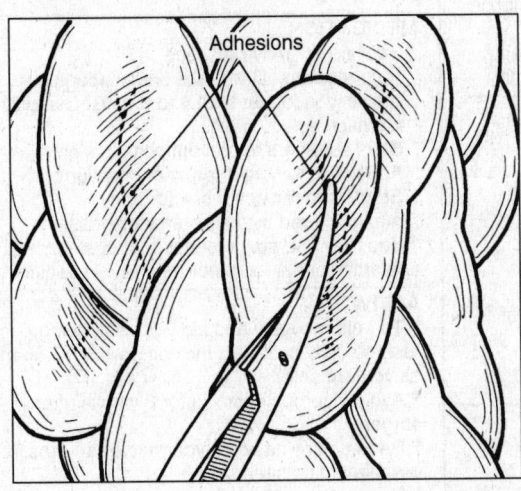

The adhesion causes the small bowel to be obstructed. Here a surgical instrument cuts the adhesions free.

Adhesions

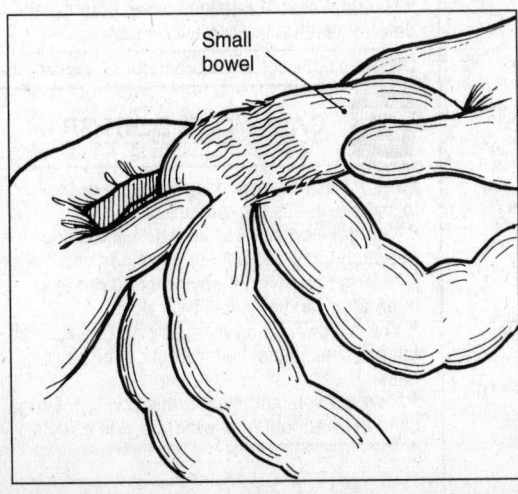

Total bowel is manually inspected for other disease.

Small bowel

SURGERIES

ADRENAL-GLAND REMOVAL
(Adrenalectomy)

 GENERAL INFORMATION

DEFINITION—Removal of one or both of the adrenal glands.

BODY PARTS INVOLVED—Adrenal glands.

REASONS FOR SURGERY
- Cushing's syndrome.
- Pheochromocytoma (a tumor).
- Other adrenal-gland tumors.

SURGICAL RISK INCREASES WITH
- Adults over 60.
- Obesity.
- Smoking.
- Stress.
- Poor nutrition.
- Diabetes mellitus.
- Recent illness.
- Alcoholism or other chronic illness.
- Use of some prescription and nonprescription drugs. Inform your doctor of any drugs, medications, or vitamin and herb supplements you are using or have used in the last month.

 WHAT TO EXPECT

WHO OPERATES—General surgeon.

WHERE PERFORMED—Hospital.

DIAGNOSTIC TESTS
- Before surgery: Blood and urine studies; x-rays of kidneys; CT scan (see Glossary) of adrenal area.
- After surgery: Blood studies; laboratory examination of removed tissue.

ANESTHESIA—General anesthesia by injection and inhalation with an airway tube placed in the windpipe.

DESCRIPTION OF OPERATION
- The adrenal glands can frequently be removed using Laparoscopy (see in Surgery section), rather than open surgery.
- When open surgery is required, the incision may be in the abdomen or the flank (on the back, near the kidneys).
- The adrenal glands are located, isolated, cut free and removed. Tubes are left in to allow drainage.
- The skin incisions are closed with sutures or clips, which usually can be removed about 1 week after surgery.

POSSIBLE COMPLICATIONS
- Excessive bleeding.
- Surgical-wound infection.
- Adrenal-hormone shortage.
- Fluid retention.
- Increased risk of life-threatening infections.

AVERAGE HOSPITAL STAY—7 to 10 days.

PROBABLE OUTCOME—Expect complete healing without complications. Allow about 6 weeks for recovery from surgery.

 POSTOPERATIVE CARE

GENERAL MEASURES
- Hard ridges should form along the incisions. As they heal, the ridges will gradually recede.
- Bathe and shower as usual. You may wash the incisions gently with mild, unscented soap.
- Use an electric heating pad, a heat lamp or a warm compress to relieve incisional pain.
- Weigh yourself daily. Report any weight gain of 2 or more pounds in any 24-hour period to your doctor.
- Move and elevate legs often while resting in bed to decrease the likelihood of deep-vein blood clots.

MEDICATION
- Your doctor may prescribe:
  Pain relievers. Don't take prescription pain medication longer than 4 to 7 days. Use only as much as you need.
  Stool softeners to prevent constipation.
  Antibiotics to fight or prevent infection.
  Steroids to replace those formerly manufactured by the adrenal glands.
- You may use nonprescription drugs, such as acetaminophen, for minor pain. Avoid aspirin.

ACTIVITY
- To help recovery and aid your well-being, resume daily activities, including work, as soon as you are able.
- Avoid vigorous exercise for 6 weeks after surgery.
- Resume driving when your doctor advises that it is okay to do so.
- Resume sexual relations when your doctor determines that healing is complete.

DIET—Your doctor will prescribe a low-salt diet.

 CALL YOUR DOCTOR IF

- Pain, swelling, redness, drainage or bleeding increases in the surgical area.
- You develop signs of infection, including headache, muscle aches, dizziness or a general ill feeling and fever. If any of these develop, even after recovery, call your doctor.
- You experience nausea, vomiting, dizziness, fatigue, weakness, fluid retention, or weight gain.
- New unexplained symptoms develop. Drugs used in treatment may produce side effects.

ADRENAL-GLAND REMOVAL
(Adrenalectomy)

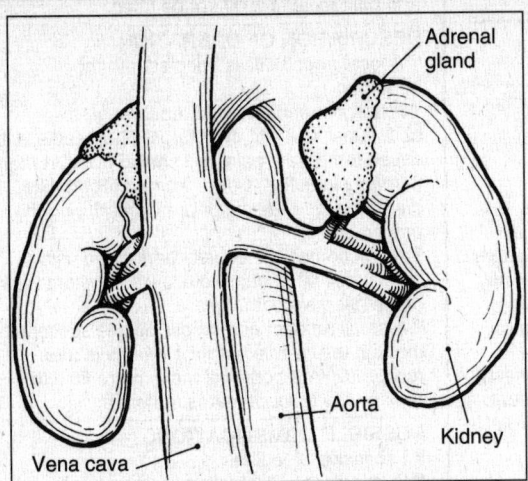

An illustration of the adrenal glands.

Adrenal
gland

Aorta

Kidney

Vena cava

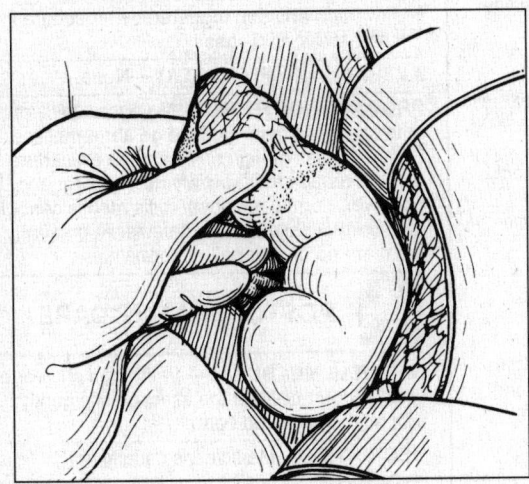

The adrenal gland is freed from the kidney on the left side of the patient.

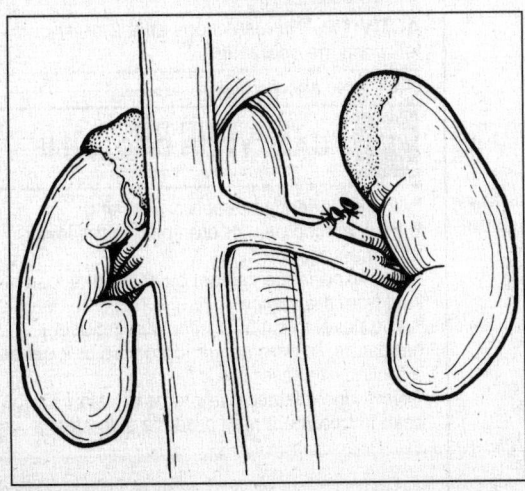

Adrenal glands removed.

AMNIOCENTESIS

GENERAL INFORMATION

DEFINITION—Removal of fluid from the amniotic sac during pregnancy.

BODY PARTS INVOLVED—Uterus; amniotic sac.

REASONS FOR SURGERY—Laboratory examination of amniotic fluid helps diagnose abnormalities of the unborn child. Although genetic testing may be done as early as the 11th week of pregnancy, the best time is usually between the 14th and 20th weeks of pregnancy. There is ample fluid, time to treat certain problems before the baby is born, and enough time exists to terminate the pregnancy if necessary. Amniocentesis may also be done in the third trimester to assess fetal development. Amniocentesis is often done for one or more of the following reasons:
- Mother is over 35 years old.
- Either parent has a chromosome abnormality.
- Mother has previously had a child with a chromosome abnormality, such as Down syndrome.
- Patient had abnormal results from a blood screening test, such as maternal serum alpha-fetoprotein (MSAFP or AFP) test.
- Mother produces antibodies, most commonly to the fetal blood cells, that can cause the unborn child to be very anemic. The amniotic fluid is tested for a chemical (bilirubin) that serves as a marker for fetal anemia.
- To evaluate pregnancy for infection.
- To remove excess amniotic fluid; most commonly in twins when one baby has too much amniotic fluid and the other has too little.
- Mother carries a sex-linked abnormality, and the unborn child's sex must be determined.
- To evaluate fetal lung maturity.
- Unborn child's maturity or other conditions must be determined late in pregnancy.

SURGICAL RISK INCREASES WITH
- Obesity.
- Previous abdominal surgery.
- Previous infection in pelvic organs.

WHAT TO EXPECT

WHO OPERATES—Obstetrician-gynecologist or family doctor.

WHERE PERFORMED—Outpatient surgical facility or hospital.

DIAGNOSTIC TESTS
- Before surgery: Blood and urine studies.
- During surgery: Ultrasonography (see Glossary).
- After surgery: Laboratory examination of the amniotic fluid.

ANESTHESIA—Local anesthesia by injection. To ensure the unborn child's safety, sedatives and pain relievers will not be used.

DESCRIPTION OF OPERATION
- A local anesthetic is injected into the abdomen.
- A hollow needle is inserted through the abdominal wall into the uterus. The needle will cause temporary pain, but should not hurt more than any injection. Some women report mild cramping, or a feeling of pressure, during the procedure.
- Amniocentesis is usually performed using continuous ultrasound to allow a constant view of the needle's path.
- A small amount of amniotic fluid is suctioned through the needle, and the needle is then removed. Your body will make more fluid to replace the amount that is removed.

POSSIBLE COMPLICATIONS
- Excessive bleeding.
- Surgical-wound infection.
- Unwanted abortion triggered by procedure in 1 out of 150 to 200 cases.

AVERAGE HOSPITAL STAY—None.

PROBABLE OUTCOME—More than 95% of amniocentesis tests indicate no abnormalities. Some couples at high risk want the procedure done to reduce their anxiety during pregnancy. However, normal amniocentesis results cannot guarantee a child without defects. At present, there are no tests for all abnormalities.

POSTOPERATIVE CARE

GENERAL MEASURES—Bathe and shower as usual. You may wash the injection site gently with mild, unscented soap.

MEDICATION—Medicine is usually not necessary.

ACTIVITY—No restrictions after 2 or 3 hours following the operation.

DIET—No special diet.

CALL YOUR DOCTOR IF

- You experience nausea or vomiting.
- You develop pain or cramping in the lower abdomen or shoulder.
- You experience vaginal bleeding or a loss of fluid from the vagina.
- You develop signs of infection, including headache, muscle aches, dizziness or a general ill feeling and fever.
- New, unexplained symptoms develop. Drugs used in treatment may produce side effects.

AMNIOCENTESIS

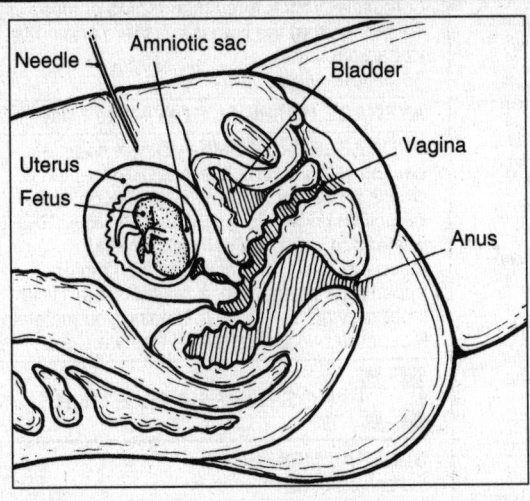

An illustration of the structures near any amniocentesis procedure.
• Hollow needle inserted through the skin and abdominal wall.

Needle
Amniotic sac
Bladder
Vagina
Uterus
Fetus
Anus

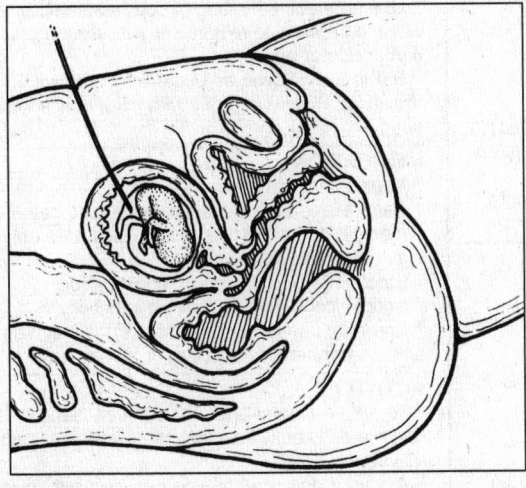

Hollow needle penetrates the cavity of the uterus.

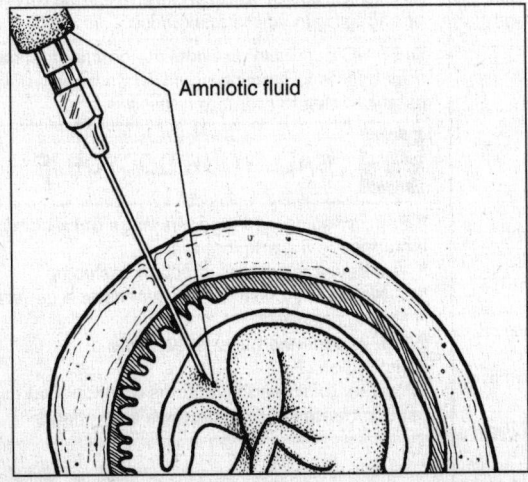

Amniotic fluid suctioned through the needle and collected for study.

Amniotic fluid

AMPUTATION

 GENERAL INFORMATION

DEFINITION—Removal of a limb or appendage.

BODY PARTS INVOLVED—Arms; legs; hands; feet; fingers; or toes.

REASONS FOR SURGERY—Performed when blood circulation to a part of the body is irreversibly interrupted, usually caused by one of the following:
- Injury to blood vessels that cannot be repaired or reconstructed.
- Hardening or obstructions of the arteries.
- Impaired blood circulation as a complication of diabetes mellitus.
- Buerger's disease.; Raynaud's phenomena.
- Severe infection with gangrene.
- Severe frostbite.

SURGICAL RISK INCREASES WITH
- Adults over 60.
- Smoking; obesity; stress; poor nutrition.
- Excess alcohol consumption.
- Newborns and infants.
- Coronary artery disease.
- Diabetes mellitus.
- Disease that increases coagulability of blood.
- Use of some prescription and nonprescription drugs. Inform your doctor of any drugs, medications, or vitamin and herb supplements you are using or have used in the last month.

 WHAT TO EXPECT

WHO OPERATES—General surgeon or orthopedic surgeon.

WHERE PERFORMED—Hospital.

DIAGNOSTIC TESTS
- Before surgery: Blood and urine studies; x-rays of part to be amputated; arterial doppler studies or arteriography (see Glossary for both).
- After surgery: Blood studies.

ANESTHESIA—General anesthesia by injection and inhalation with an airway tube placed in the windpipe.

DESCRIPTION OF OPERATION
- An incision is made around the part to be amputated.
- Tissue, muscles, blood vessels, nerves and bone are severed.
- The bone is filed smooth, and the bone end is covered with connective tissue. Frequently tubes are left in the wound to allow drainage.
- Muscles are closed with large sutures. The skin is closed with fine sutures, which are left in place for 3 to 4 weeks after surgery.
- A snug bandage is often wrapped around the affected area of the body, and may be left in place for several days following surgery.

POSSIBLE COMPLICATIONS
- Excessive bleeding, surgical-wound infection or muscle contractures (shortening of muscles).
- Feelings that the limb is still there and hurts ("phantom limb").
- Pulmonary embolism.

AVERAGE HOSPITAL STAY—2 to 7 days.

PROBABLE OUTCOME—Expect complete healing without complications. Allow about 6 weeks for recovery from surgery. A physical rehabilitation program may be frustrating, but it will lead to improved self-esteem and independence. Depending on the limb or appendage amputated, a prosthesis (artificial limb) may be beneficial in helping you maintain independence and a normal lifestyle.

 POSTOPERATIVE CARE

GENERAL MEASURES
- Don't smoke.
- Use an electric heating pad, a heat lamp or a warm compress to relieve surgical-wound pain, if your doctor approves.
- Bathe and shower as usual. You may wash the surgical wound gently with mild, unscented soap.

MEDICATION
- Your doctor may prescribe:
  Pain relievers. Don't take prescription pain medication longer than 4 to 7 days. Use only as much as you need.
  Stool softeners to prevent constipation.
  Antibiotics to fight or prevent infection.
- You may use nonprescription drugs, such as acetaminophen, for minor pain. Avoid aspirin.

ACTIVITY
- To help recovery and aid your well-being, resume daily activities, including work, as soon as you are able.
- Ask your doctor when you may resume driving or engaging in vigorous exercise.

DIET—Clear liquid diet until the gastrointestinal tract begins to function again. Then eat a well-balanced diet to promote healing.

 CALL YOUR DOCTOR IF

- Pain, swelling, redness, drainage or bleeding increases in the surgical area.
- You develop signs of infection, including headache, muscle aches, dizziness or a general ill feeling and fever.
- You experience nausea, vomiting or constipation.
- New, unexplained symptoms develop. Drugs used in treatment may produce side effects.

AMPUTATION

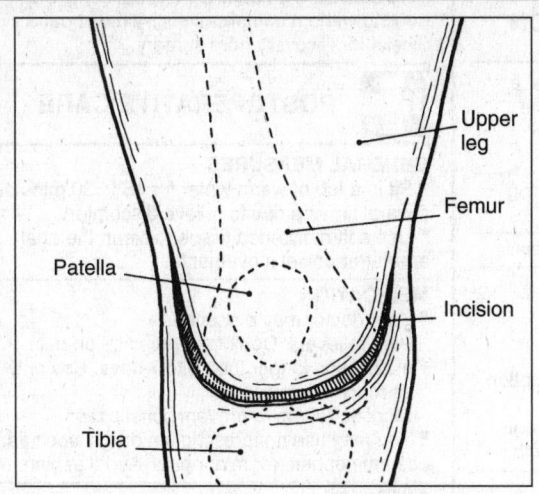

An illustration of a lower leg amputation.

Upper leg

Femur

Patella

Incision

Tibia

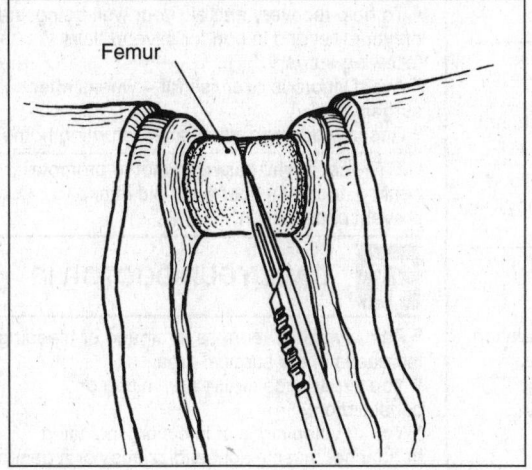

Skin, connective tissue, muscles, blood vessels, nerves, and bone are severed.

Femur

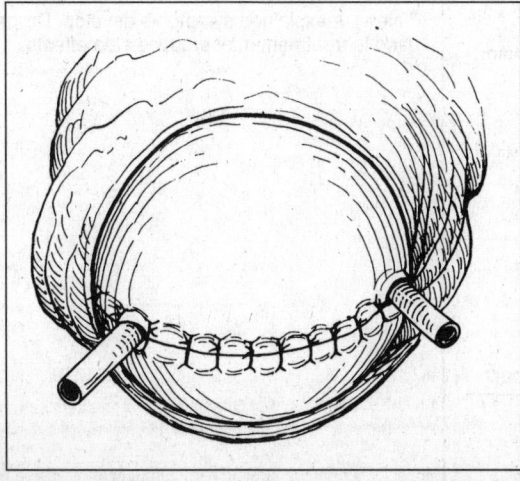

Bone end filed smooth and covered with connective tissue.
- Muscles closed with large sutures, skin closed with fine sutures.
- Drains remain in place.

ANAL FISSURE REMOVAL AND ANAL SPHINCTEROTOMY

GENERAL INFORMATION

DEFINITION—Removal of an anal fissure, a crack or tear in the membrane that lines the anus, and incision of the muscular anal sphincter.

BODY PARTS INVOLVED—Anus and lining membrane; anal muscles (sphincter).

REASONS FOR SURGERY—Relief of pain.

SURGICAL RISK INCREASES WITH
- Obesity; smoking.
- Recent or chronic illness.
- Diabetes mellitus.
- Use of some prescription and nonprescription drugs. Inform your doctor of any drugs, medications, or vitamin and herb supplements you are using or have used in the last month.

WHAT TO EXPECT

WHO OPERATES—General surgeon or proctologist.

WHERE PERFORMED—Hospital or outpatient surgical facility.

DIAGNOSTIC TESTS—Before surgery: Blood and urine studies; anoscopy; sigmoidoscopy (see Glossary for both).

ANESTHESIA
- Local anesthesia by injection.
- Spinal anesthesia by injection.
- General anesthesia by injection and inhalation with an airway tube placed in the windpipe.

DESCRIPTION OF OPERATION
- Sometimes dilatation (see Glossary) of the sphincter muscles is sufficient to treat the problem.
- In other cases, one of the outer sphincter muscles is cut to prevent recurrence.
- Rarely, the fissure is cut from the surrounding tissue and removed.
- Bleeding vessels are tied or closed with electrocauterization.
- A drain or packing is inserted into the surgical area.
- The surgical area is left open to hasten healing. Bandages are applied.

POSSIBLE COMPLICATIONS
- Excessive bleeding or pain.
- Surgical-wound infection.
- Inability to control bowel movements until healing is complete.
- Incontinence, if all or part of sphincter is cut.

AVERAGE HOSPITAL STAY—0 to 1 day.

PROBABLE OUTCOME—Expect complete healing without complications. Allow about 3 weeks for recovery from surgery.

POSTOPERATIVE CARE

GENERAL MEASURES
- Sit in a tub of warm water for 15 to 20 minutes several times a day to relieve discomfort.
- Use soft moistened tissue to clean the anal area after bowel movements.

MEDICATION
- Your doctor may prescribe:
  Pain relievers. Don't take prescription pain medication longer than 4 to 7 days. Use only as much as you need.
  Stool softeners to prevent constipation.
- You may use nonprescription drugs, such as acetaminophen, for minor pain. Avoid aspirin.

ACTIVITY
- To help recovery and aid your well-being, stay off your feet and in bed for several days following surgery.
- Avoid vigorous exercise for 4 weeks after surgery.
- Resume driving 1 week after returning home.

DIET—Eat a well-balanced diet to promote healing. Increase fiber and fluid intake to prevent constipation.

CALL YOUR DOCTOR IF

- Pain, swelling, redness, drainage or bleeding increases in the surgical area.
- You experience nausea, vomiting or constipation.
- You develop signs of infection, including headache, muscle aches, dizziness or a general ill feeling and fever.
- New, unexplained symptoms develop. Drugs used in treatment may produce side effects.

ANAL FISSURE REMOVAL AND ANAL SPHINCTEROTOMY

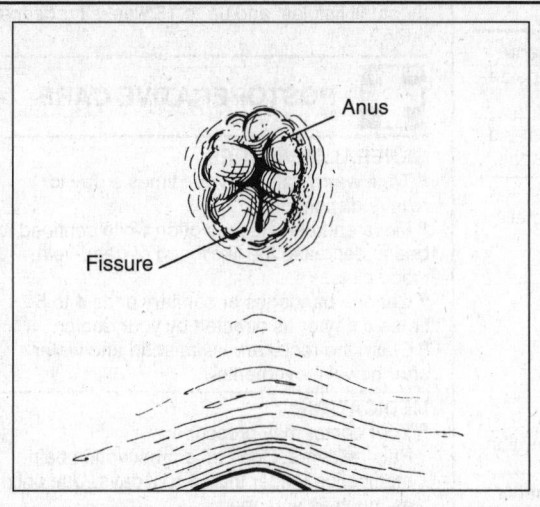

An illustration of an anal fissure. This view places the patient lying on back with legs extended.

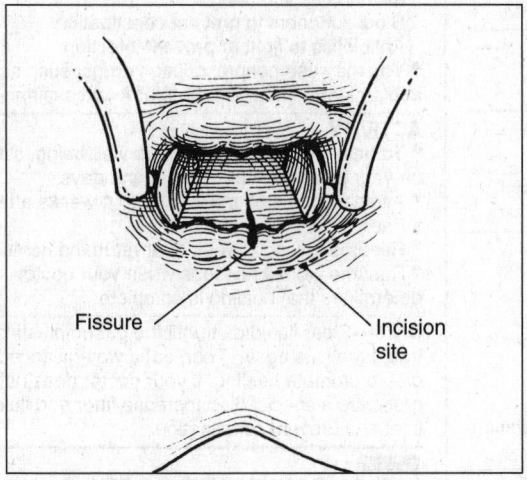

Sphincter muscle is expanded with special instrument. The incision site is indicated above the sphincter muscle.

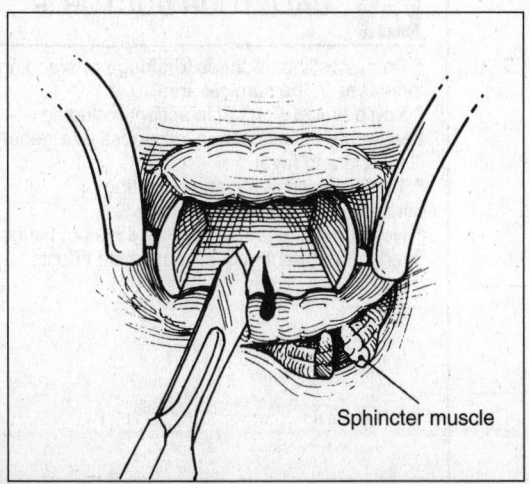

Fissure cut free from surrounding tissue and removed. Sphincter muscle has been cut.

SURGERIES

ANAL FISTULA REPAIR

GENERAL INFORMATION

DEFINITION—Opening or removal of an anal fistula, an abnormal tract extending from inside the rectum to the skin outside of the anus.

BODY PARTS INVOLVED—Rectum; skin and underlying tissue around the rectum and anus.

REASONS FOR SURGERY
- Repeated abscesses in the anal and rectal areas.
- Chronic drainage from a fistula.

SURGICAL RISK INCREASES WITH
- Stress.
- Poor nutrition.
- Recent or chronic illness.
- Obesity.
- Smoking.
- Use of some prescription and nonprescription drugs. Inform your doctor of any drugs, medications, or vitamin and herb supplements you are using or have used in the last month.

WHAT TO EXPECT

WHO OPERATES—General surgeon or proctologist.

WHERE PERFORMED—Outpatient surgical facility or hospital.

DIAGNOSTIC TESTS
- Before surgery: x-rays of lower gastrointestinal tract; colonoscopy (see Glossary).

ANESTHESIA
- Local anesthesia by injection.
- Spinal anesthesia by injection.
- General anesthesia by injection and inhalation with an airway tube placed in the windpipe.

DESCRIPTION OF OPERATION
- Abscesses are drained, if necessary.
- The fistula is located with a delicate probe, and the skin and tissue over the fistula is opened.
- The surgical wound is left open to heal from inside out.
- Occasionally, the internal opening of the fistula may be located very high inside the rectum. In this case, it may be necessary to perform the operation in two stages a few weeks apart.

POSSIBLE COMPLICATIONS
- Excessive bleeding.
- Surgical-wound infection.
- Slow healing or recurrence.

AVERAGE HOSPITAL STAY—0-3 Days.

PROBABLE OUTCOME—Expect complete healing without complications in 4 to 5 weeks for small fistulas, and up to 16 weeks for deeper ones.

POSTOPERATIVE CARE

GENERAL MEASURES
- Take warm baths several times a day to relieve discomfort.
- Move and elevate legs often while confined to bed to decrease the likelihood of deep-vein blood clots.
- Change bandages or sanitary pads 4 to 5 times a day or as directed by your doctor.
- Clean the rectal area with soap and water after bowel movements.

MEDICATION
- Your doctor may prescribe:
  Pain relievers. Don't take prescription pain medication longer than 4 to 7 days. Use only as much as you need.
  Stool softeners to prevent constipation.
  Antibiotics to fight or prevent infection.
- You may use nonprescription drugs, such as acetaminophen, for minor pain. Avoid aspirin.

ACTIVITY
- To help recovery and aid your well-being, stay off your feet and in bed for several days.
- Avoid vigorous exercise for 3 to 4 weeks after surgery.
- Resume driving 1 week after returning home.
- Resume sexual relations when your doctor determines that healing is complete.

DIET—Clear liquid diet until the gastrointestinal tract functions again. Then eat a well-balanced diet to promote healing, if your doctor does not prescribe a special diet. Increase fiber and fluid intake to prevent constipation.

CALL YOUR DOCTOR IF

- Pain, swelling, redness, drainage or bleeding increases in the surgical area.
- You develop signs of infection, including headache, muscle aches, dizziness or a general ill feeling and fever.
- You experience nausea, vomiting or constipation.
- New, unexplained symptoms develop. Drugs used in treatment may produce side effects.

ANAL FISTULA REPAIR

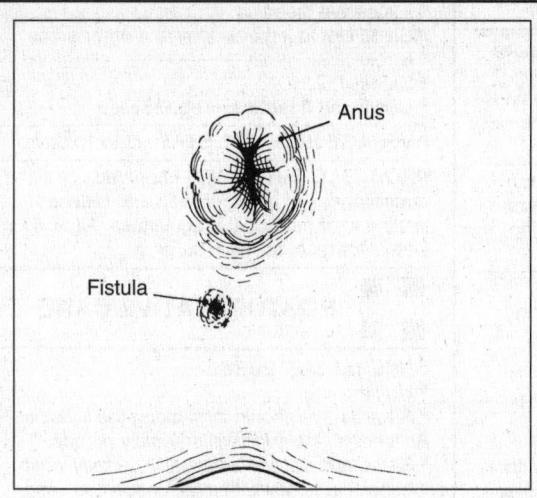

An illustration of an anal fissure. The opening of the tract that appears on the skin may occur in various places in the area surrounding the anus.

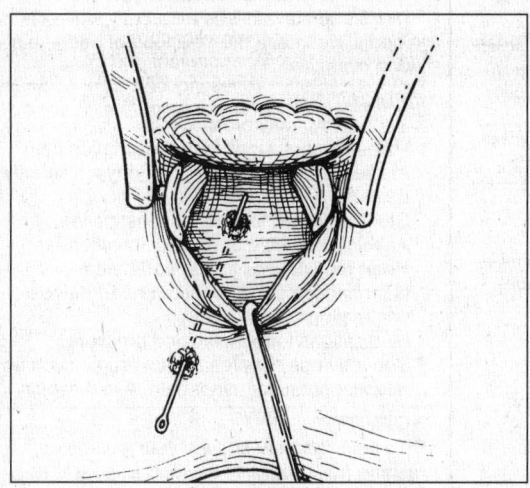

Anus retracted to expose the fistula tract. A probe is inserted to locate the inner opening of the fistula.

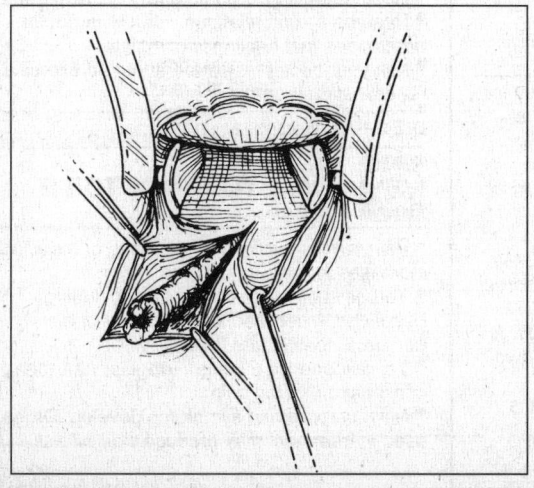

Fistula is opened and the surgical wound is then left open to allow healing from inside out.

ANEURYSM REMOVAL

 GENERAL INFORMATION

DEFINITION—A surgical procedure to remove an aneurysm (a swelling, dilatation or ballooning of a blood vessel due to weakening that is caused by disease, injury or a congenital defect in the artery wall).

BODY PARTS INVOLVED—Aneurysms can form anywhere in the body. The most common sites are the aorta and the arteries supplying the brain.

REASONS FOR SURGERY
- Prevent rupture and uncontrolled bleeding
- Pressure of an aneurysm on surrounding structures.
- Reduce risk of blood clots.

SURGICAL RISK INCREASES WITH
- Obesity; smoking.
- Recent or chronic illness such as heart attack, high blood pressure, thyroid disease, diabetes mellitus or kidney disease.
- Chronic obstructive pulmonary disease (COPD).
- Chronic congestive heart failure (advanced).
- Use of some prescription and nonprescription drugs. Inform your doctor of any drugs, medications, or vitamin and herb supplements you are using or have used in the last month.

 WHAT TO EXPECT

WHO OPERATES—Cardiovascular surgeon, vascular surgeon, or neurosurgeon.

WHERE PERFORMED—Hospital.

DIAGNOSTIC TESTS
- Before surgery: Blood studies; chest x-ray; cardiac catheterization; ECG; sonogram; CT scan; arteriogram (see Glossary for all).
- After surgery: ECG; chest x-ray.

ANESTHESIA—General anesthesia by injection and inhalation with an airway tube placed in the windpipe.

DESCRIPTION OF OPERATION—Surgery for an aneurysm on the heart is described here:
- The patient is connected to the heart-lung equipment to allow the heart to be stopped temporarily so surgery can be performed on the diseased tissue.
- The heart is made to stop by cooling and weak electrical shock.
- The aneurysm is removed along with a border of normal heart tissue.
- The edges of the heart are sewn together. A graft may be sewn into place between the two cut edges.
- The heart is warmed, then the heartbeat is restored by a weak electrical shock.
Note: Coronary artery bypass surgery is frequently performed at the same time.

POSSIBLE COMPLICATIONS
- Surgical wound infection.
- Excessive bleeding.
- Blood clot to leg or kidney and other areas.
- Stroke.
- Kidney failure.
- Continued heartbeat irregularities.

AVERAGE HOSPITAL STAY—7 to 10 days.

PROBABLE OUTCOME—Improved effectiveness of heart function and reduced likelihood of heartbeat irregularities. Allow 6 weeks for recovery from surgery.

 POSTOPERATIVE CARE

GENERAL MEASURES
- No smoking.
- A hard ridge should form along the incision. As it heals, the ridge will gradually recede.
- Bathe and shower as usual. You may wash the incision gently with mild, unscented soap.
- Move and elevate legs frequently while resting in bed to decrease the likelihood of deep-vein blood clots.

MEDICATION
- Your doctor may prescribe:
  Pain relievers. Don't take prescription pain medication longer than 4 to 7 days. Use only as much as you need.
  Stool softeners to prevent constipation.
  Antibiotics to fight or prevent infection.
  Heart medications to prevent rhythm disturbances and strengthen heart muscle contractions.
  Medications to reduce blood pressure.
- You may use nonprescription drugs, such as acetaminophen, for minor pain. Avoid aspirin.

ACTIVITY
- To help recovery and aid your well-being, resume daily activities as soon as possible.
- Resume driving 1 month after returning home.
- Resume sexual relations when your doctor determines that healing is complete.
- Ask your doctor for advice about an exercise rehabilitation program.

DIET—As directed by your doctor.

 CALL YOUR DOCTOR IF

- Pain, swelling, redness, drainage or bleeding increases in the surgical area.
- You develop signs of infection, including headache, muscle aches, dizziness or a general ill feeling and fever.
- You experience a cough, irregular heartbeat, constipation, or leg pain.
- New, unexplained symptoms develop. Drugs used in treatment may produce side effects.

ANEURYSM REMOVAL

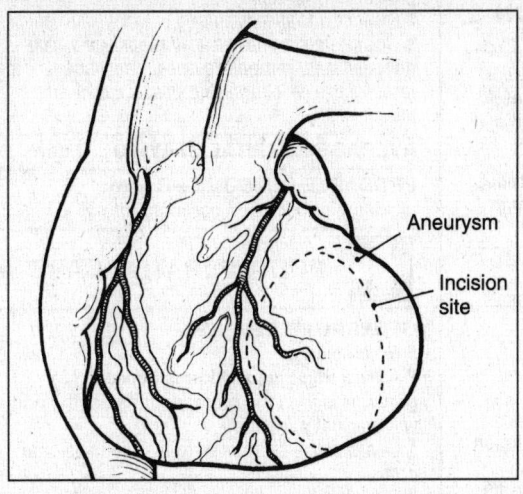

An illustration of the heart as seen after the chest wall has been removed showing the ballooning out of the left ventricle representing the aneurysm as well as the proposed incision site.

Aneurysm

Incision site

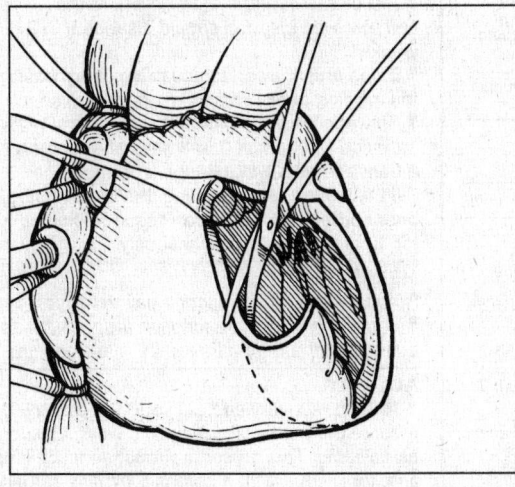

The aneurysm is incised and any blood clot inside is removed. The weakened scarred area is excised and the remaining heart muscle closed in layers.

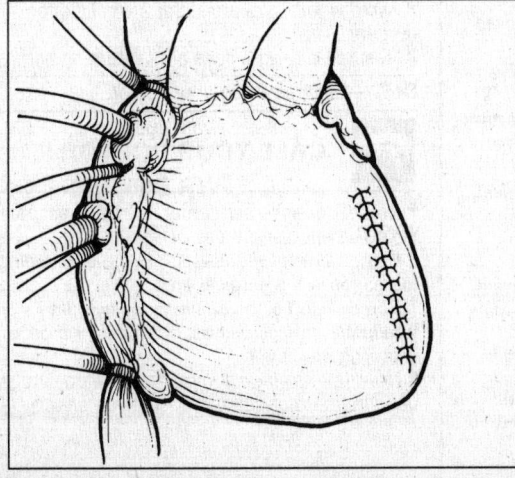

The appearance of the heart after the aneurysm has been excised and the remaining heart muscle closed with the sutures.

ANGIOPLASTY, CORONARY
(Percutaneous Transluminal Coronary Angioplasty)

 GENERAL INFORMATION

DEFINITION—A surgical shaping or alteration of blood vessels. In this procedure, a catheter with an inflatable balloon tip is inserted into a blocked or partially blocked coronary artery.

BODY PARTS INVOLVED—Coronary arteries (the blood vessels that supply nourishment to the heart muscle).

REASONS FOR SURGERY—To remove a block or partial block of a coronary artery.

SURGICAL RISK INCREASES WITH
- Obesity; smoking.
- Excess alcohol consumption.
- Angina (for more than 1 year).
- Calcification of blood vessels.
- Use of some prescription and nonprescription drugs. Inform your doctor of any drugs, medications, or vitamin and herb supplements you are using or have used in the last month.

 WHAT TO EXPECT

WHO OPERATES—Cardiologist or cardiothoracic surgeon.

WHERE PERFORMED—Hospital.

DIAGNOSTIC TESTS
- Before surgery: Heart catheterization with x-ray and fluoroscopic examinations (see Glossary).
- During surgery: X-rays after injection of dye through the catheter into various parts of the heart.

ANESTHESIA—Local, with standby general anesthesia.

DESCRIPTION OF OPERATION
- The cardiac balloon catheter is inserted into an artery in the arm or leg. Fluoroscopy (see Glossary) provides guidance for the catheter to pass through the artery to the heart.
- Blood-pressure readings are taken, and the heart's ability to pump blood is tested.
- The catheter is guided into the coronary-artery system. Fluoroscopy allows identification of any disease in the coronary arteries.
- The catheter is passed through the occlusion, the balloon is inflated, and the occlusion is compressed, allowing blood to flow through once again.
- When all examinations have been completed, the catheter balloon is withdrawn, and the artery is compressed until bleeding stops.

POSSIBLE COMPLICATIONS
- Break or rupture in the dilated artery lining.
- Dislodged plaque that blocks the artery further downstream.

- Coronary spasm.
- Reaction to the dye used in x-ray studies.
- Complete coronary artery blockage which necessitates immediate open-heart surgery to remove the blockage and prevent a heart attack.

AVERAGE HOSPITAL STAY—0 to 1 day.

PROBABLE OUTCOME—Removal of blockage in occluded coronary artery.

 POSTOPERATIVE CARE

GENERAL MEASURES
- No smoking.
- A hard ridge usually forms beneath the puncture site in the groin. As it heals, the ridge will gradually recede.
- Use a warm compress to relieve incisional pain.
- Discoloration under the skin where the catheter was inserted should disappear in 2 weeks.
- Bathe and shower as usual. You may wash the incision gently with mild, unscented soap.
- Between showers, keep the wound dry with a bandage for the first 2 or 3 days after surgery. If a bandage gets wet, change it promptly.
- If the wound bleeds during the first 24 hours after surgery, press a clean tissue or cloth to it for 10 to 15 minutes continuously.

MEDICATION
- Your doctor may prescribe pain relievers.
- You may use nonprescription drugs, such as acetaminophen, for minor pain. Avoid aspirin.

ACTIVITY
- To help recovery and aid your well-being, resume daily activities, including work, as soon as possible. This procedure requires much less time for recovery than coronary bypass surgery.
- Avoid vigorous exercise for 2 weeks after surgery.
- Resume driving 2 days after returning home.

DIET—As directed by your doctor.

 CALL YOUR DOCTOR IF

- You experience sudden or severe chest pain.
- You develop shortness of breath.
- Pain, swelling, redness, drainage or bleeding increases in the surgical area.
- You develop signs of infection, including headache, muscle aches, dizziness or a general ill feeling and fever.
- New, unexplained symptoms develop. Drugs used in treatment may produce side effects.

ANGIOPLASTY, CORONARY
(Percutaneous Transluminal Coronary Angioplasty)

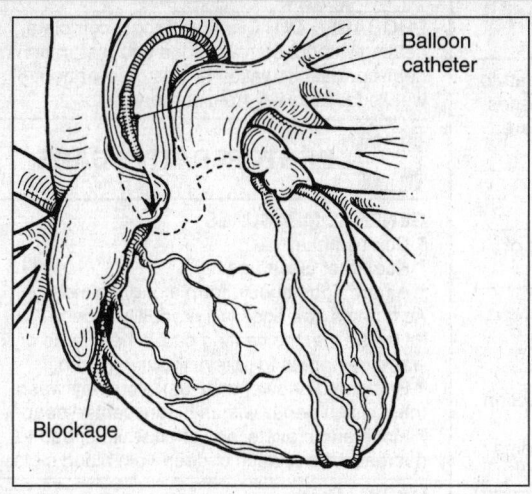

Balloon
catheter

Blockage

An illustration of the cardiac balloon catheter about to enter the right coronary artery.

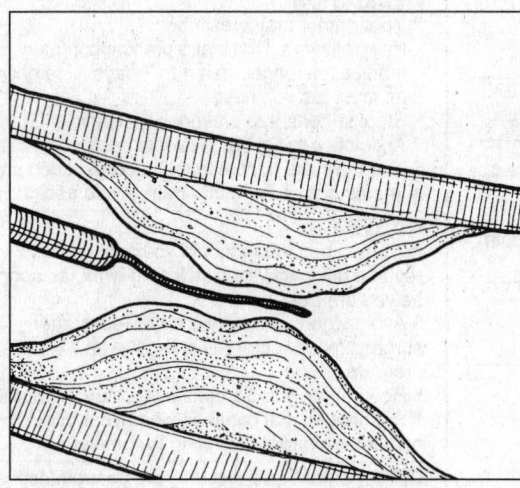

Fluoroscopy allows identification of any disease in the coronary arteries and the catheter is passed through the occlusion.

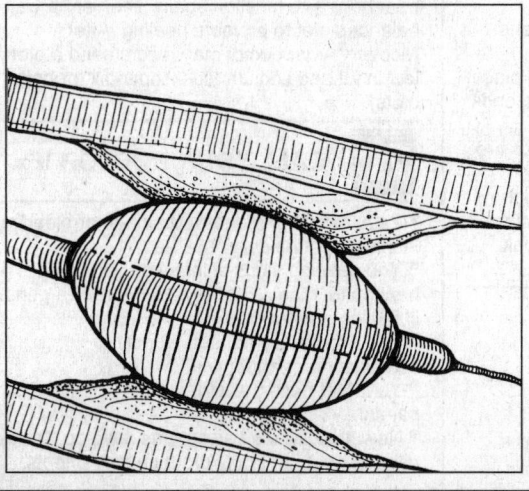

Then the balloon is inflated, the plaque is broken, and the occlusion is dilated allowing blood to flow freely once again. After all examinations have been completed, the catheter balloon is withdrawn.

SURGERIES

AORTO-ILIAC BYPASS GRAFT
(Aortoiliofemoral Reconstruction)

 GENERAL INFORMATION

DEFINITION—Placement of an artificial graft to bypass a blood clot or narrowing in the arteries that supply blood to the abdomen, genital area and legs.

BODY PARTS INVOLVED—Aorta; iliac arteries.

REASONS FOR SURGERY—Restoration of normal blood circulation in the legs.

SURGICAL RISK INCREASES WITH
- Alcoholism; obesity; smoking.
- Diabetes mellitus; coronary artery disease; or atherosclerosis.
- Use of some prescription and nonprescription drugs. Inform your doctor of any drugs, medications, or vitamin and herb supplements you are using or have used in the last month.

 WHAT TO EXPECT

WHO OPERATES—General surgeon or vascular surgeon.

WHERE PERFORMED—Hospital.

DIAGNOSTIC TESTS
- Before surgery: Blood and urine studies; ultrasound; arteriograms (see Glossary for both).
- After surgery: Blood studies.

ANESTHESIA—General anesthesia by injection and inhalation with an airway tube placed in the windpipe.

DESCRIPTION OF OPERATION
- An incision is made in the abdomen.
- The abdominal muscles are separated to expose the abdominal organs, which are inspected for undetected disease. (Other surgeries may be performed at this time.)
- The aorta and iliac arteries are located and clamped to isolate the obstruction.
- An artificial graft is selected and fitted in place. One end fits in the aorta and the other two ends in the iliac arteries.
- The graft is sewn in place and the clamps are released. Blood can now circulate freely.
- The muscles of the abdomen are closed in layers. The skin is closed with sutures or clips, which usually can be removed about 1 week after surgery.

POSSIBLE COMPLICATIONS
- Excessive bleeding.
- Surgical-wound infection; graft infection.
- Incisional hernia.
- Inadvertent injury to the ureter.
- Impotence.
- Occlusion of arteries beyond the grafted vessels.

AVERAGE HOSPITAL STAY—5 to 7 days.

PROBABLE OUTCOME—Expect complete healing without complications and restoration of near-normal circulation to legs. Allow about 6 weeks for recovery from surgery.

 POSTOPERATIVE CARE

GENERAL MEASURES
- Don't smoke.
- Keep feet clean and dry.
- A hard ridge should form along the incision. As it heals, the ridge will gradually recede.
- Use an electric heating pad, a heat lamp or a warm compress to relieve incisional pain.
- Bathe and shower as usual. You may wash the incision gently with mild, unscented soap.
- Move and elevate legs often while in bed to decrease the chance of deep-vein blood clots.

MEDICATION
- Your doctor may prescribe:
  Pain relievers. Don't take prescription pain medication longer than 4 to 7 days. Use only as much as you need.
  Stool softeners to prevent constipation.
  Antibiotics to fight or prevent infection.
- You may use nonprescription drugs, such as acetaminophen, for minor pain. Avoid aspirin.

ACTIVITY
- To help recovery and aid your well-being, resume daily activities, including work, as soon as you are able.
- Avoid vigorous exercise for 6 weeks after surgery. Your doctor will prescribe an exercise program.
- Resume driving 5 weeks after returning home.
- Resume sexual relations when your doctor has determined that healing is complete.

DIET—Clear liquid diet until the gastrointestinal tract begins to function again. Then eat a well-balanced diet to promote healing. After recovery, your doctor may recommend a diet low in fat and sodium (see Appendix for both diets).

 CALL YOUR DOCTOR IF

- Pain, swelling, redness, drainage or bleeding increases in the surgical area.
- You develop signs of infection, including headache, muscle aches, dizziness or a general ill feeling and fever.
- You experience nausea, vomiting, constipation or abdominal swelling.
- Your feet become cold, discolored, numb or painful.
- New, unexplained symptoms develop. Drugs used in treatment may produce side effects.

AORTO-ILIAC BYPASS GRAFT
(Aortoiliofemoral Reconstruction)

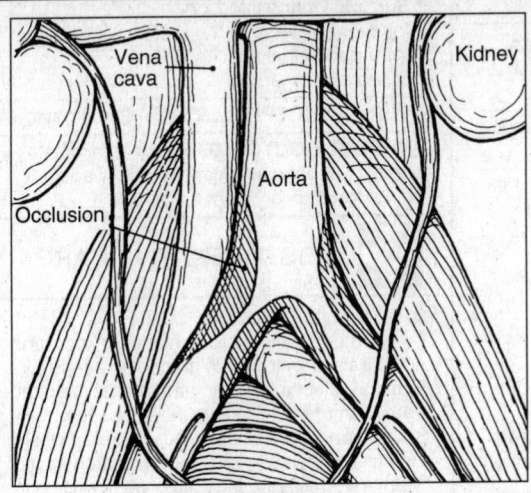

An illustration of the aorta, iliac arteries, and the occlusions to be bypassed.

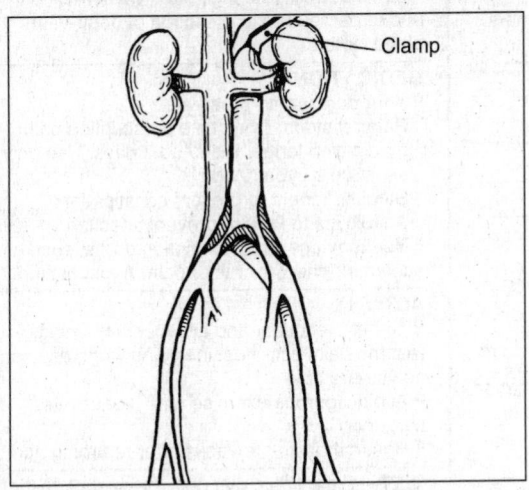

The aorta and iliac arteries are clamped to isolate the obstruction.

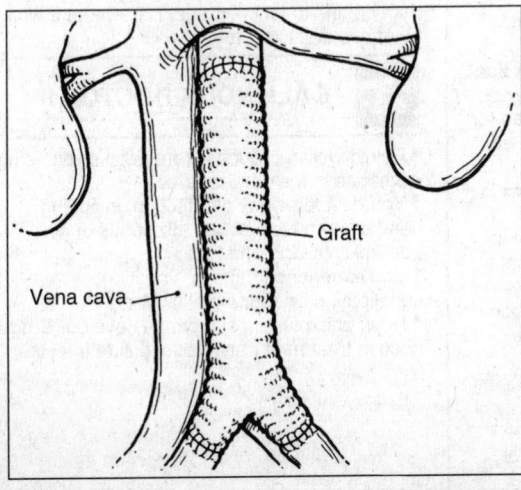

Polyester graft fitted in place. The upper end fits the aorta and the two lower ends fit the iliac arteries.
- After the graft is in place, the clamps are released. Blood can now again circulate freely.

APPENDECTOMY

GENERAL INFORMATION

DEFINITION—Removal of the appendix, an outgrowth of tissue from the cecum, the first part of the large intestine.

BODY PARTS INVOLVED—Appendix; cecum; peritoneum.

REASONS FOR SURGERY—Treatment of an infected appendix. Signs and symptoms of infection can include:
- Abdominal pain; nausea; vomiting.
- Loss of appetite.
- Tenderness in the right lower abdomen.
- Low-grade fever.
- Elevated white blood-cell count.

SURGICAL RISK INCREASES WITH
- Alcoholism; obesity; smoking.
- Chronic heart, lung, liver or kidney disease.
- Use of some prescription and nonprescription drugs. Inform your doctor of any drugs, medications, or vitamin and herb supplements you are using or have used in the last month.

WHAT TO EXPECT

WHO OPERATES—General surgeon.

WHERE PERFORMED—Hospital.

DIAGNOSTIC TESTS
- Before surgery: Blood and urine studies, x-rays of abdomen, ultrasound and CT scan (see Glossary).
- After surgery: Blood studies.

ANESTHESIA
- General anesthesia by injection and inhalation with an airway tube placed in the windpipe or spinal anesthesia.
- Spinal anesthesia by injection.

DESCRIPTION OF OPERATION
- An incision is made in the lower abdomen.
- The abdominal muscles and organs are separated and the appendix is isolated, cut free and removed. The intestine is closed.
- The area around the appendix is inspected for undetected diseases. Other surgeries may be performed at this time.
- Any fluid or pus from the infected appendix is suctioned away.
- Sometimes, a drain is placed in the area left by the removed appendix. The drain is usually removed 2 to 3 days following surgery.
- The abdominal cavity is closed, and the skin is closed with sutures, which usually can be removed 1 week after surgery.
- Alternatively, surgery may be performed using a laparoscope (see Glossary). In this case, several small incisions would be made in the abdomen to facilitate viewing and removal of the appendix.

POSSIBLE COMPLICATIONS
- Excessive bleeding.
- Surgical-wound infection.
- Inadvertent injury to the ureter.
- Intra-abdominal abscess.
- Bowel obstruction.

AVERAGE HOSPITAL STAY—2 to 4 days.

PROBABLE OUTCOME—Expect complete healing without complications. Allow about 3 weeks for recovery from surgery.

POSTOPERATIVE CARE

GENERAL MEASURES
- A hard ridge should form along the incision. As it heals, the ridge will gradually recede.
- Use an electric heating pad, a heat lamp or a warm compress to relieve incisional pain.
- Bathe and shower as usual. You may wash the incision gently with mild, unscented soap.
- Move and elevate legs often while resting in bed to decrease the likelihood of deep-vein blood clots.

MEDICATION
- Your doctor may prescribe:
  Pain relievers. Don't take prescription pain medication longer than 4 to 7 days. Use only as much as you need.
  Stool softeners to prevent constipation.
  Antibiotics to fight or prevent infection.
- You may use nonprescription drugs, such as acetaminophen, for minor pain. Avoid aspirin.

ACTIVITY
- To help recovery and aid your well-being, resume daily activities, including work, as soon as you are able.
- Avoid vigorous exercise for 6 weeks after surgery.
- Resume driving 2 weeks after returning home.

DIET—Clear liquid diet until the gastrointestinal tract begins to function again. Then eat a well-balanced diet to promote healing.

CALL YOUR DOCTOR IF

- Pain, swelling, redness, drainage or bleeding increases in the surgical area.
- You develop signs of infection, including headache, muscle aches, dizziness or a general ill feeling and fever.
- You experience nausea, vomiting, constipation or abdominal swelling.
- New, unexplained symptoms develop. Drugs used in treatment may produce side effects.

APPENDECTOMY

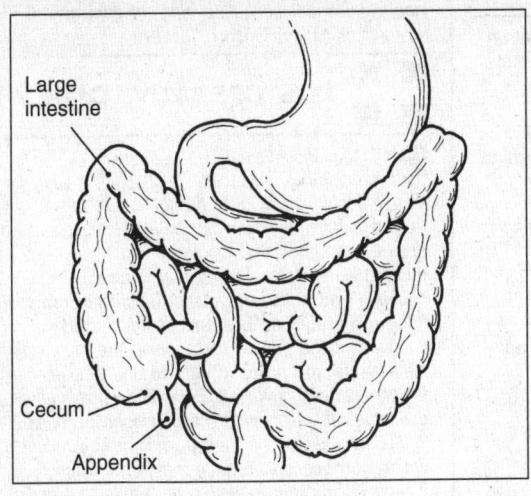

An illustration of the vermiform appendix attached to the cecum (the first part of the large intestine).

Large intestine

Cecum

Appendix

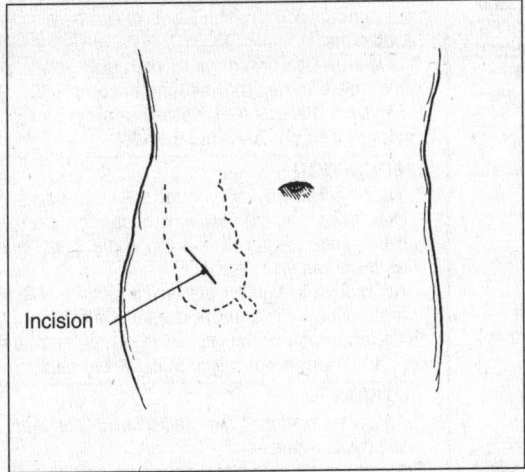

The incision is usually made at a point approximately 2/3 the distance between the navel and the point of the hip.

Incision

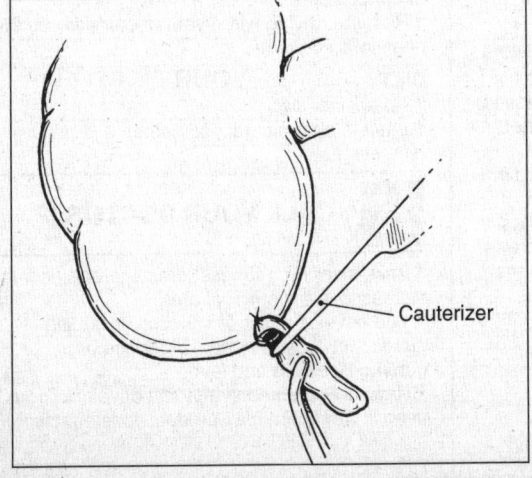

Appendix isolated, cut free and removed. The stump is then cauterized and sterilized to prevent infection.

Cauterizer

ARTHROPLASTY, HIP

GENERAL INFORMATION

DEFINITION—Surgical shaping or reformation of the hip joint. Three types may be used: cup or mold arthroplasty, total hip replacement, and total hip surface replacement. Total hip replacement is described here. In this method, a metal ball replaces the worn head of the thigh bone and a cup (often plastic) replaces the worn socket.

BODY PARTS INVOLVED—Hip joint; muscles, ligaments, bones and bursa forming the hip joint.

REASONS FOR SURGERY—Diseased or injured hip with pain and stiffness causing an altered gait and impaired quality of life.

SURGICAL RISK INCREASES WITH
- Obesity; smoking.
- Excess alcohol consumption.
- Recent or chronic illness; diabetes mellitus.
- Use of some prescription and nonprescription drugs. Inform your doctor of any drugs, medications, or vitamin and herb supplements you are using or have used in the last month.

WHAT TO EXPECT

WHO OPERATES—Orthopedic surgeon.

WHERE PERFORMED—Hospital.

DIAGNOSTIC TESTS
- Before surgery: General history; physical examination; x-rays of joint; CT scan or MRI (see Glossary for both); joint aspiration (to check for active infection); blood and urine studies.
- During surgery: X-rays.
- After surgery: X-rays.

ANESTHESIA
- General anesthesia by injection and inhalation with an airway tube placed in the windpipe.
- Spinal anesthesia by injection.

DESCRIPTION OF OPERATION
- An incision is made over the affected hip.
- The head and neck of the femur are removed.
- The femoral canal is reamed to accept the metal femoral component (head, neck and stem). The femoral component is cemented in place using a special form of bone cement.
- The acetabulum is reamed to accept a plastic cup. The cup is held in place with metal screws.
- The ball and socket are replaced into normal position.

POSSIBLE COMPLICATIONS
- Excessive bleeding; blood clots.
- Surgical-wound infection.
- Dislocation of hip.
- Pneumonia.
- Need for re-operation at a future time.

AVERAGE HOSPITAL STAY—3 to 5 days.

PROBABLE OUTCOME—Expect complete healing without complications. Allow about 6 weeks for recovery from surgery.

POSTOPERATIVE CARE

GENERAL MEASURES
- No smoking.
- Buy and use self-help devices, such as a raised toilet seat, bath bench and long-handled grippers, to limit hip bending.
- Use handrails and wear low shoes.
- Learn and abide by your safe range of motion.
- Cough and deep breathe as instructed.
- A hard ridge should form along the incision. As it heals, the ridge will gradually recede.
- Bathe and shower as usual. You may wash the incision gently with mild, unscented soap.
- Use an electric heating pad, a heat lamp or a warm compress to relieve incisional pain.
- Move and elevate legs often while resting in bed to decrease the likelihood of deep-vein blood clots.
- Use crutches or a cane to walk until your doctor determines that healing is complete.
- Physical therapy may hasten healing and restore strength. Ask your doctor.

MEDICATION
- Your doctor may prescribe:
  Pain relievers. Don't take prescription pain medication longer than 4 to 7 days. Use only as much as you need.
  Antibiotics to fight or prevent infection. Use antibiotics before future dental work.
- You may use nonprescription drugs, such as acetaminophen, for minor pain. Avoid aspirin.

ACTIVITY
- As prescribed and directed by your surgeon and physical therapist.
- Avoid very active sports such as tennis, skiing or contact sports.
- Resume driving when your doctor advises that healing is complete.

DIET
- No special diet.
- Vitamin and mineral supplements (sometimes).

CALL YOUR DOCTOR IF

- Pain, swelling, redness, drainage or bleeding increases in the surgical area.
- You develop signs of infection, including headache, muscle aches, dizziness or a general ill feeling and fever.
- New, unexplained symptoms develop. Drugs used in treatment may produce side effects.

ARTHROPLASTY, HIP

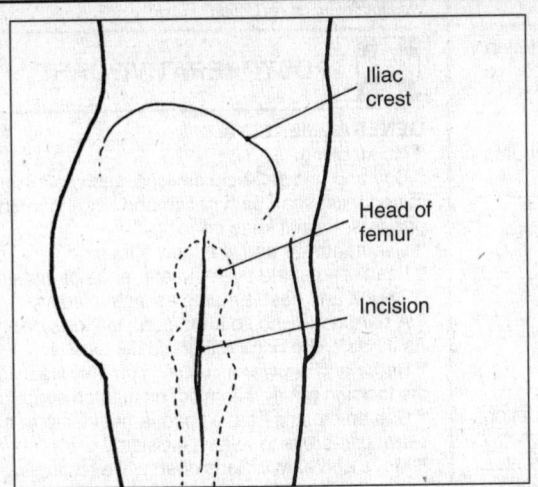

Iliac crest

Head of femur

Incision

An illustration of an incision made over the affected hip showing the head of the femur that is diseased or injured.

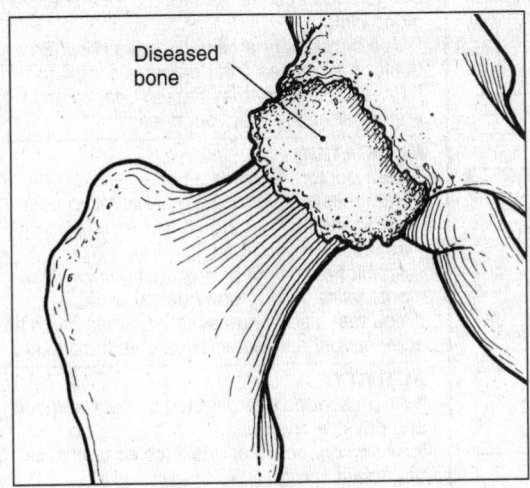

Diseased bone

A closer view of a diseased hip joint. After the diseased bone has been removed, the artificial ball and socket are placed into normal position.

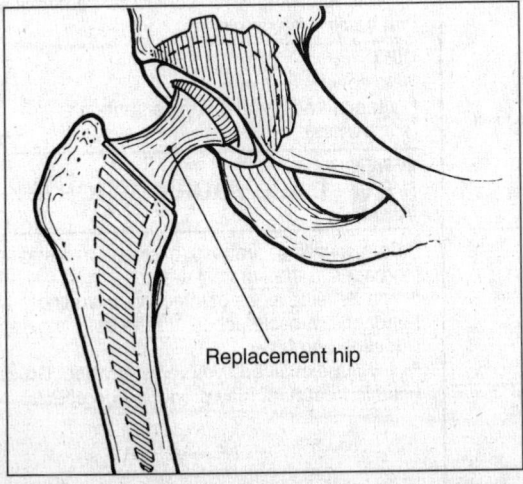

Replacement hip

The appearance of the hip after the metal prosthesis has been inserted.

ARTHROPLASTY, KNEE

GENERAL INFORMATION

DEFINITION—Surgical shaping or reformation of an injured or diseased knee to re-establish a movable joint.

BODY PARTS INVOLVED—Knee joint; muscles, ligaments, bones, cartilage and bursa forming the knee joint.

REASONS FOR SURGERY—Diseased or injured knee causing chronic pain or disability impairing the quality of life.

SURGICAL RISK INCREASES WITH
- Obesity; smoking.
- Excess alcohol consumption.
- Recent or chronic illness.
- Diabetes mellitus.
- Use of some prescription and nonprescription drugs. Inform your doctor of any drugs, medications, or vitamin and herb supplements you are using or have used in the last month.

WHAT TO EXPECT

WHO OPERATES—Orthopedic surgeon.

WHERE PERFORMED—Hospital.

DIAGNOSTIC TESTS
- Before surgery: General history; physical examination; x-rays of joint; MRI or CT scan (see Glossary for both); joint aspiration (to check for active infection); blood and urine studies.
- During surgery: X-rays.
- After surgery: X-rays.

ANESTHESIA—General anesthesia by injection and inhalation with an airway tube placed in the windpipe.

DESCRIPTION OF OPERATION
- An incision is made into the affected knee.
- The arthritic or diseased surfaces of the femoral condyles and tibial plateau are removed.
- The above areas are replaced by durable prosthetic components that are fixed firmly in place with a special form of bone cement.
- The new knee joint may be hinged (for unstable knees) or unhinged.
- The joint is put into a cast.

POSSIBLE COMPLICATIONS
- Excessive bleeding; blood clots.
- Surgical-wound infection.
- Pneumonia.
- Loosening of joint components at a future time.

AVERAGE HOSPITAL STAY—3 to 5 days.

PROBABLE OUTCOME—Expect complete healing without complications. Allow about 6 weeks for recovery from surgery.

POSTOPERATIVE CARE

GENERAL MEASURES
- No smoking.
- Buy and use self-help devices, such as a raised toilet seat, bath bench and long-handled grippers, to limit knee bending.
- Use handrails and wear low shoes.
- Learn and abide by your safe range of motion.
- Cough and deep breathe as instructed.
- A hard ridge should form along the incision. As it heals, the ridge will gradually recede.
- Bathe and shower as usual. You may wash the incision gently with mild, unscented soap.
- Use an electric heating pad, a heat lamp or a warm compress to relieve incisional pain.
- Move and elevate legs often while resting in bed to decrease the likelihood of deep-vein blood clots.
- Use crutches or a cane to walk until your doctor determines that healing is complete.
- Physical therapy may hasten healing and restore strength. Ask your doctor.

MEDICATION
- Your doctor may prescribe:
  Pain relievers. Don't take prescription pain medication longer than 4 to 7 days. Use only as much as you need.
  Antibiotics to fight or prevent infection. Use antibiotics before future dental work.
- You may use nonprescription drugs, such as acetaminophen, for minor pain. Avoid aspirin.

ACTIVITY
- As prescribed and directed by your surgeon and physical therapist.
- Avoid very active sports such as tennis, skiing or contact sports.
- Resume driving when your doctor determines that healing is complete.

DIET
- No special diet.
- Vitamin and mineral supplements (sometimes).

CALL YOUR DOCTOR IF

- Pain, swelling, redness, drainage or bleeding increases in the surgical area.
- You develop signs of infection, including headache, muscle aches, dizziness or a general ill feeling and fever.
- New, unexplained symptoms develop. Drugs used in treatment may produce side effects.

ARTHROPLASTY, KNEE

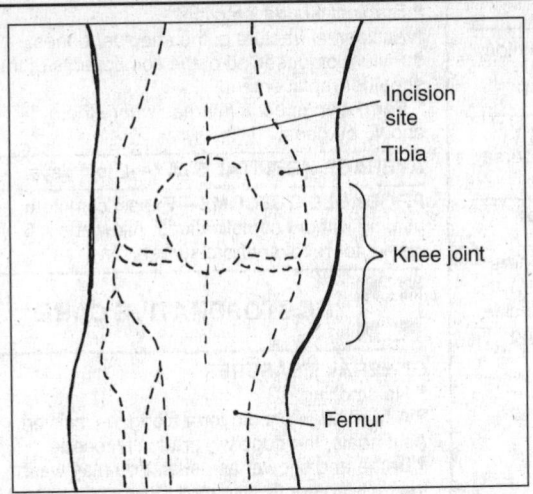

An illustration of the knee joint and a normal site for incision when a replacement procedure is planned.

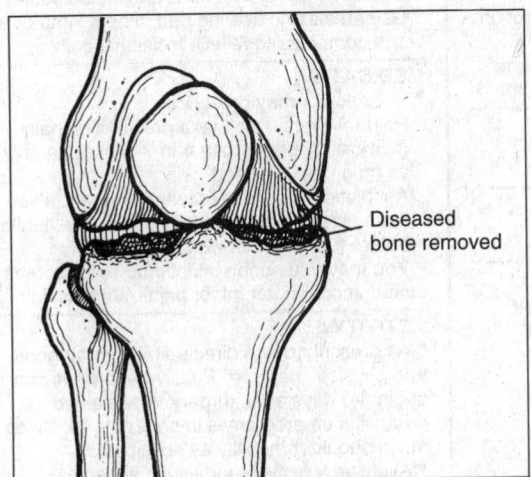

The diseased bone to be removed.

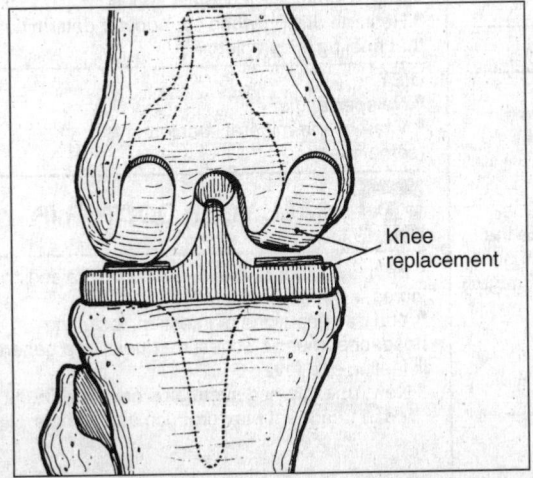

After the diseased surfaces of the femur and tibia have been removed, they are replaced by a durable prosthetic component fixed firmly in place with a special form of bone cement (sometimes).

SURGERIES

ARTHROPLASTY, SHOULDER

GENERAL INFORMATION

DEFINITION—Surgical shaping or reformation of an injured or diseased shoulder to re-establish a movable joint.

BODY PARTS INVOLVED—Shoulder joint; muscles, ligaments, bones, cartilage and bursa forming the shoulder joint.

REASONS FOR SURGERY—Diseased or injured shoulder causing chronic pain or disability impairing the quality of life. Disorders treated include rheumatoid arthritis, osteoarthritis, rotator cuff arthropathy, avascular necrosis, congenital defects, old trauma and failed shoulder prosthesis.

SURGICAL RISK INCREASES WITH
- Obesity; smoking.
- Excess alcohol consumption.
- Recent or chronic illness.
- Diabetes mellitus.
- Use of some prescription and nonprescription drugs. Inform your doctor of any drugs, medications, or vitamin and herb supplements you are using or have used in the last month.

WHAT TO EXPECT

WHO OPERATES—Orthopedic surgeon.

WHERE PERFORMED—Hospital.

DIAGNOSTIC TESTS
- Before surgery: X-rays of joint; CT scan or MRI (see Glossary for both); joint aspiration (to check for active infection); blood and urine studies.
- During surgery: X-rays.
- After surgery: X-rays.

ANESTHESIA—General anesthesia by injection and inhalation with an airway tube placed in the windpipe.

DESCRIPTION OF OPERATION
- An incision is made into the affected shoulder.
- The surgeon will do any repair work necessary; there may be a need to remove tissue fragments, reattach tendons to bones and muscles, stitch or staple torn tissue.
- A total shoulder replacement may be necessary for severe shoulder disability. One type is designed to maintain and reproduce the normal anatomy of the shoulder joint. Another type may be used if there is rotator cuff damage that cannot be repaired.
- The incision is closed with stitches and bandaged. The shoulder is immobilized in a sling, splint or cast that is left on for 2 to 3 weeks.

POSSIBLE COMPLICATIONS
- Excessive bleeding; blood clots.
- Surgical-wound infection.
- Accidental fracture of the shoulder bones.
- Failure or loosening of the components of the shoulder replacement.
- Formation of bone in areas where there should be none.

AVERAGE HOSPITAL STAY—2 to 4 days.

PROBABLE OUTCOME—Expect complete healing without complications. Allow about 6 weeks for recovery from surgery.

POSTOPERATIVE CARE

GENERAL MEASURES
- No smoking.
- A hard ridge should form along the incision. As it heals, the ridge will gradually recede.
- Bathe and shower as usual. You may wash the incision gently with mild, unscented soap.
- Use an electric heating pad, a heat lamp or a warm compress to relieve incisional pain.

MEDICATION
- Your doctor may prescribe:
  Pain relievers. Don't take prescription pain medication longer than 4 to 7 days. Use only as much as you need.
  Antibiotics to fight or prevent infection. If you have an artificial shoulder joint, use antibiotics before future dental work.
- You may use nonprescription drugs, such as acetaminophen, for minor pain. Avoid aspirin.

ACTIVITY
- As prescribed and directed by your surgeon and physical therapist. Passive exercises can begin 3-6 days after surgery. A sustained rehabilitation program is important to regain as much shoulder mobility as possible.
- Avoid very active sports such as tennis, skiing, swimming or contact sports.
- Resume driving when your doctor determines that healing is complete.

DIET
- No special diet.
- Vitamin and mineral supplements (sometimes).

CALL YOUR DOCTOR IF

- Pain, swelling, redness, drainage or bleeding increases in the surgical area.
- You develop signs of infection, including headache, muscle aches, dizziness or a general ill feeling and fever.
- New, unexplained symptoms develop. Drugs used in treatment may produce side effects.

ARTHROPLASTY, SHOULDER

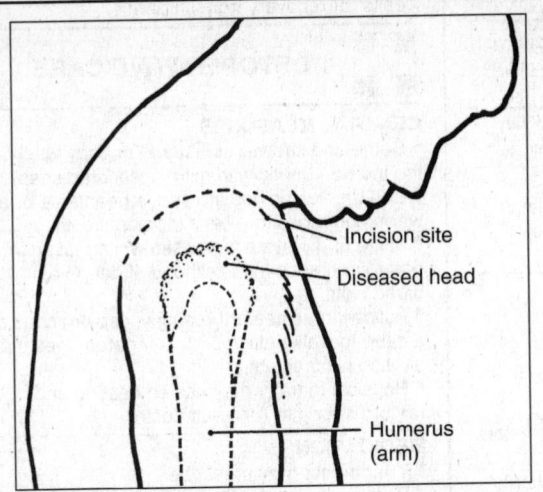

Shoulder is prepared for incision.

Incision site

Diseased head

Humerus
(arm)

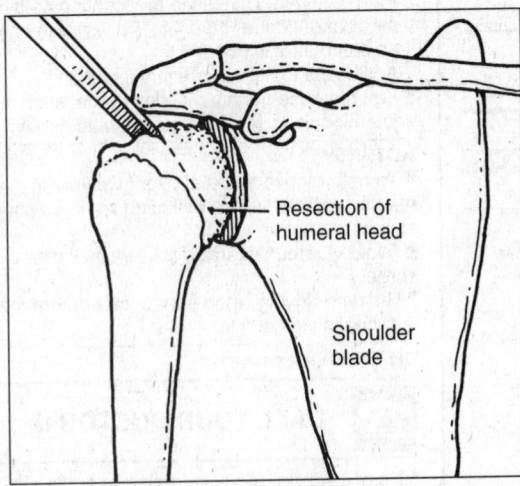

After the humeral head has been surgically exposed, the diseased surface is removed.

Resection of
humeral head

Shoulder
blade

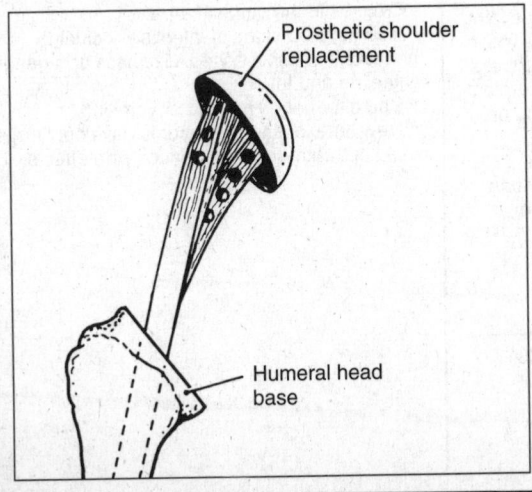

A prosthetic device is inserted into the humeral base. Cement is used to adhere device to the bone. Shoulder is closed and immobilized for a period of time (not illustrated).

Prosthetic shoulder
replacement

Humeral head
base

ARTHROSCOPY

GENERAL INFORMATION

DEFINITION—Visual examination of a joint with an arthroscope, a fiber-optic instrument with a lighted tip.

BODY PARTS INVOLVED—Joint, usually in the knee, but often performed in the shoulder.

REASONS FOR SURGERY
• Diagnosis of disease or injury inside a joint.
• Removal of bone or cartilage or repair of tendons or ligaments.

SURGICAL RISK INCREASES WITH
• Adults over 60.
• Obesity; smoking.
• Poor nutrition.
• Recent or chronic illness.
• Diabetes mellitus.
• Use of some prescription and nonprescription drugs. Inform your doctor of any drugs, medications, or vitamin and herb supplements you are using or have used in the last month.

WHAT TO EXPECT

WHO OPERATES—Orthopedist.

WHERE PERFORMED—Hospital or outpatient surgical facility.

DIAGNOSTIC TESTS
• Before surgery: Blood and urine studies; x-rays of joint.
• After surgery: Blood studies; laboratory examination of removed fluid or tissue.

ANESTHESIA
• Local anesthesia by injection.
• Spinal anesthesia by injection.
• General anesthesia by injection and inhalation with an airway tube placed in the windpipe.

DESCRIPTION OF OPERATION
• A small incision is made at the side of the joint to be examined (several openings may be made for a complete examination). The arthroscope is inserted into the joint. Diagnostic and/or surgical procedures are then performed, depending on the problem.
• The arthroscope is removed. The skin is closed with sutures or clips, which usually can be removed about 7 to 10 days after surgery.

POSSIBLE COMPLICATIONS
• Bleeding into joint.
• Surgical-wound infection.
• Slow healing.

AVERAGE HOSPITAL STAY—0 to 1 day.

PROBABLE OUTCOME—Expect complete healing without complications. Allow about 6 weeks for recovery from surgery.

POSTOPERATIVE CARE

GENERAL MEASURES
• Bathe and shower as usual. You may wash the incision gently with mild, unscented soap.
• Use an electric heating pad, a heat lamp or a warm compress to relieve incisional pain.
• Move and elevate legs often while resting in bed to decrease the likelihood of deep-vein blood clots.
• Following a knee arthroscopy, use crutches or a cane to walk until your doctor determines that healing is complete.
• Physical therapy may hasten healing and restore strength. Ask your doctor.

MEDICATION
• Your doctor may prescribe:
  Pain relievers. Don't take prescription pain medication longer than 4 to 7 days. Use only as much as you need.
  Antibiotics to fight or prevent infection.
• You may use nonprescription drugs, such as acetaminophen, for minor pain. Avoid aspirin.

ACTIVITY
• To help recovery and aid your well-being, resume daily activities, including work, as soon as you are able.
• Avoid vigorous exercise for 6 weeks after surgery.
• Resume driving when your doctor determines that healing is complete.

DIET—No special diet.

CALL YOUR DOCTOR IF

• Pain, swelling, redness, drainage or bleeding increases in the surgical area.
• You develop signs of infection, including headache, muscle aches, dizziness or a general ill feeling and fever.
• You experience nausea or vomiting.
• New, unexplained symptoms develop. Drugs used in treatment may produce side effects.

ARTHROSCOPY

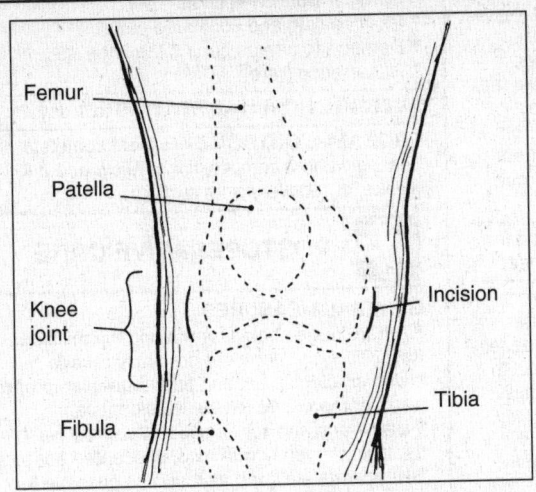

An illustration of the knee joint area frequently examined by arthroscopy.

Femur

Patella

Incision

Knee joint

Tibia

Fibula

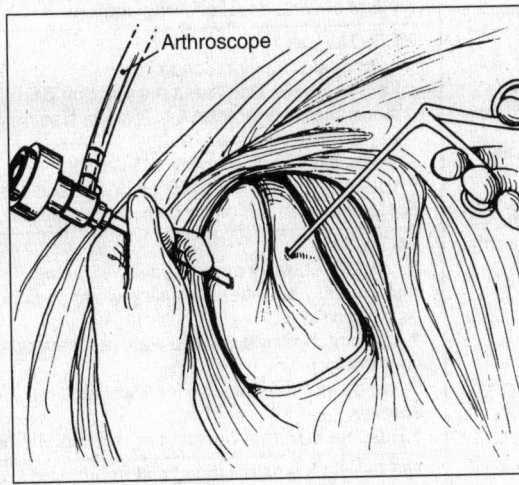

Arthroscope

After an incision is made at the side of the joint to be examined, the arthroscope is inserted into the joint.
- The operator inspects the joint and performs whatever surgical procedures are indicated.

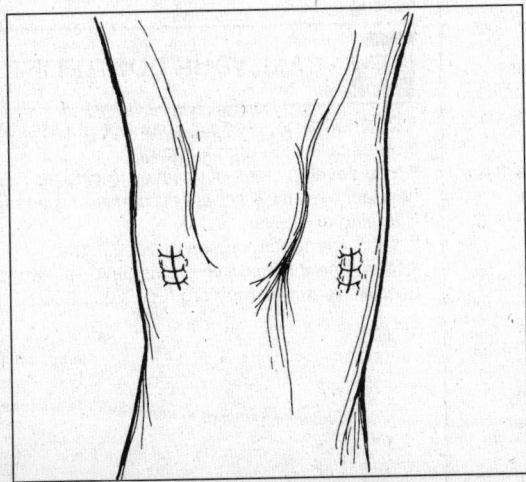

After the arthroscope is removed, the small incisions in the skin are closed.

BAKER'S CYST REMOVAL

GENERAL INFORMATION

DEFINITION—Removal of Baker's cyst, a benign cystic tumor on the back of the knee joint. The cyst consists of accumulated fluid that protrudes between two groups of muscles behind the knee. Baker's cyst may result from injury or from diseases, such as arthritis, gout or inflammation of the membrane lining the knee joint.

BODY PARTS INVOLVED—Space behind the knee joint on either or both sides of the knee.

REASONS FOR SURGERY—If the cyst has resulted from disease, it may disappear after successful treatment of the underlying disease. Often, local steroid injections are successful in treating a Baker's cyst. Otherwise, the cyst is removed when it becomes painful or unsightly. In children, the cyst is usually left to heal by itself, and is not removed unless it presses on nerves or blood vessels.

SURGICAL RISK INCREASES WITH
- Obesity; smoking.
- Poor nutrition.
- Recent or chronic illness.
- Diabetes mellitus.
- Use of some prescription and nonprescription drugs. Inform your doctor of any drugs, medications, or vitamin and herb supplements you are using or have used in the last month.

WHAT TO EXPECT

WHO OPERATES—General surgeon or orthopedist.

WHERE PERFORMED—Outpatient surgical facility or hospital.

DIAGNOSTIC TESTS
- Before surgery: Blood and urine studies; x-rays of both knees; ultrasound; venography; arthrograms (see Glossary for all).
- After surgery: Blood studies.

ANESTHESIA
- Local anesthesia by injection.
- Spinal anesthesia by injection.
- General anesthesia by injection and inhalation with an airway tube placed in the windpipe.

DESCRIPTION OF OPERATION
- An incision is made over the cyst.
- The cyst is located, cut free from surrounding tissue and removed.
- A synthetic patch is sometimes sutured in place to cover the defect left from removal of the cyst.
- The skin is closed with fine sutures, which usually can be removed about 2 weeks after surgery.

POSSIBLE COMPLICATIONS
- Excessive bleeding.
- Surgical-wound infection.
- Slow healing and continued pain.
- Damage to nerves behind the knee.
- Recurrence (rare).

AVERAGE HOSPITAL STAY—0 to 1 day.

PROBABLE OUTCOME—Expect complete healing without complications. Allow about 4 weeks for recovery from surgery.

POSTOPERATIVE CARE

GENERAL MEASURES
- A hard ridge should form along the incision. As it heals, the ridge will gradually recede.
- Use an electric heating pad, a heat lamp or a warm compress to relieve incisional pain.
- Bathe and shower as usual. You may wash the incision gently with mild, unscented soap.
- Keep legs elevated as much as possible for the first several days following surgery.

MEDICATION
- Your doctor may prescribe:
  Pain relievers. Don't take prescription pain medication longer than 4 to 7 days. Use only as much as you need.
  Antibiotics to fight or prevent infection.
- You may use nonprescription drugs, such as acetaminophen, for minor pain. Avoid aspirin.

ACTIVITY
- To help recovery and aid your well-being, resume daily activities, including work, as soon as you are able.
- Use crutches or a cane to walk (as directed by your doctor).
- Avoid vigorous exercise for 6 weeks after surgery.
- Resume driving 2 weeks after returning home.

DIET—Eat a well-balanced diet to promote healing.

CALL YOUR DOCTOR IF

- Pain, swelling, redness, drainage or bleeding increases in the surgical area.
- You develop signs of infection, including headache, muscle aches, dizziness or a general ill feeling and fever.
- You experience nausea or vomiting.
- New, unexplained symptoms develop. Drugs used in treatment may produce side effects.

BAKER'S CYST REMOVAL

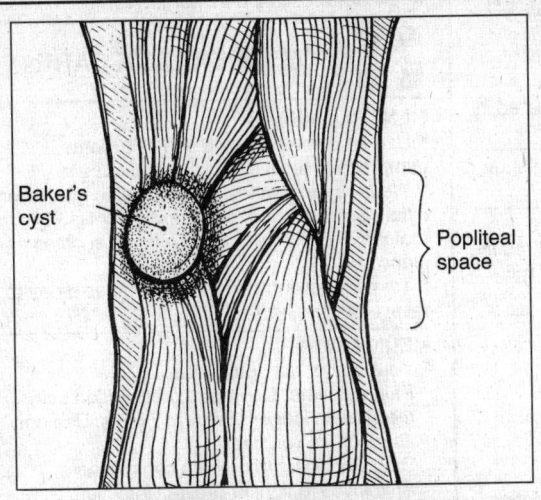

An illustration of a Baker's cyst located in the popliteal space behind the knee joint.

Baker's cyst

Popliteal space

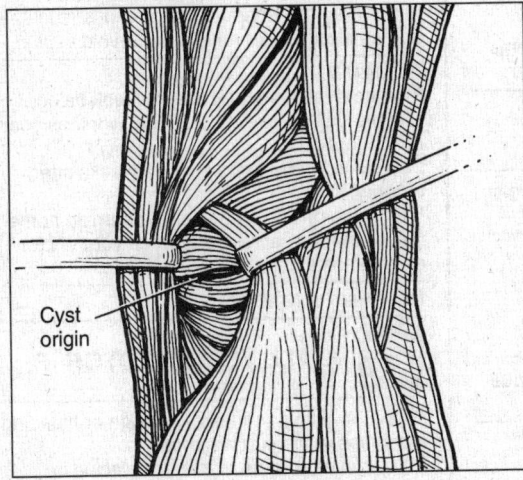

Muscles pulled apart to expose the area where the cyst begins.

Cyst origin

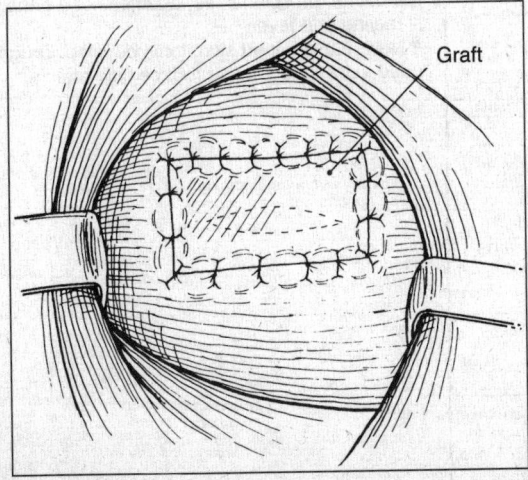

Synthetic patch sutured in place to cover the defect left after surgical removal of the cyst.

Graft

BARTHOLIN'S GLAND, ABSCESS DRAINAGE

GENERAL INFORMATION

DEFINITION—Removal of a blockage of the Bartholin's glands caused by a cyst or an abscess (on accumulation of mucus or infection). These two small glands are located in the base of the vaginal lips.

BODY PARTS INVOLVED—Bartholin's glands; lips of vagina.

REASONS FOR SURGERY—Appropriate treatment of an abscess or cyst which will result in near immediate relief of symptoms and will reduce the risk of subsequent infection.

SURGICAL RISK INCREASES WITH
- Obesity.
- Smoking.
- Poor nutrition.
- Recent illness.
- Alcoholism or chronic illness.
- Diabetes mellitus.
- Use of some prescription and nonprescription drugs. Inform your doctor of any drugs, medications, or vitamin and herb supplements you are using or have used in the last month.

WHAT TO EXPECT

WHO OPERATES—Obstetrician-gynecologist, family doctor or general surgeon.

WHERE PERFORMED—Doctor's office, outpatient surgical facility or hospital.

DIAGNOSTIC TESTS
- Before surgery: Blood and urine studies; laboratory examination of vaginal discharge.
- After surgery: Laboratory examination of pus or secretions from opened glands.

ANESTHESIA
- Local anesthesia by injection.
- Regional anesthesia by injection.

DESCRIPTION OF OPERATION
- A small incision is made in the labia over the area of the abscess. A catheter is placed through the incision, and is allowed to drain into the vagina. The catheter is left in place for approximately 2 weeks.
- The alternate method is marsupialization. In this procedure, the edges of the glands are opened and the linings are folded back and sewn shut. This forms a small pouch that drains easily. Sutures that will be absorbed by the body are used to close the pouch.

POSSIBLE COMPLICATIONS
- Excessive bleeding
- Surgical-wound infection.

AVERAGE HOSPITAL STAY—0 to 1 day.

PROBABLE OUTCOME—Expect complete healing without complications. Allow about 2 weeks for recovery from surgery.

POSTOPERATIVE CARE

GENERAL MEASURES
- Use an electric heating pad or a warm compress to relieve surgical-wound pain.
- Wear cotton panties. Avoid panties made from nylon, polyester, silk or other nonventilating materials. Don't wear tight clothing, such as jeans.
- Take luke-warm baths several times a day to relieve discomfort.

MEDICATION
- Your doctor may prescribe:
  Pain relievers. Don't take prescription pain medication longer than 4 to 7 days. Use only as much as you need.
  Stool softeners to prevent constipation.
  Antibiotics to fight or prevent infection.
- You may use nonprescription drugs, such as acetaminophen, for minor pain. Avoid aspirin.

ACTIVITY
- To help recovery and aid your well-being, resume daily activities, including work, as soon as you are able.
- Avoid vigorous exercise for 4 weeks after surgery.
- Resume driving 4 days after returning home.
- Resume sexual relations when your doctor determines that healing is complete.

DIET—No special diet.

CALL YOUR DOCTOR IF

- Pain, swelling, redness, drainage or bleeding increases in the surgical area.
- You develop signs of infection, including headache, muscle aches, dizziness or a general ill feeling and fever.
- New, unexplained symptoms develop. Drugs used in treatment may produce side effects.

BARTHOLIN'S GLAND, ABSCESS DRAINAGE

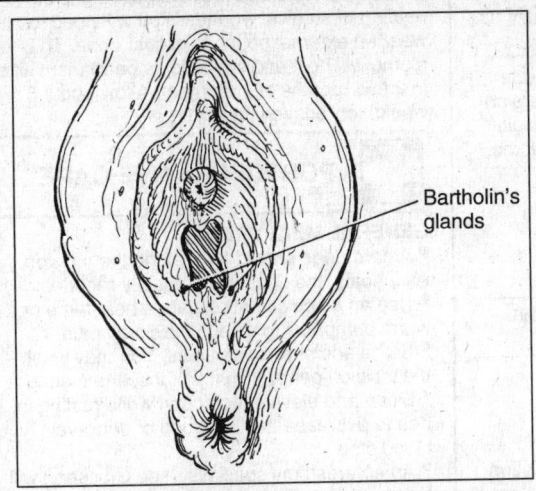

An illustration showing the normal appearance of the Bartholin's glands, which are two small glands located at the base of the vaginal lips.

Bartholin's glands

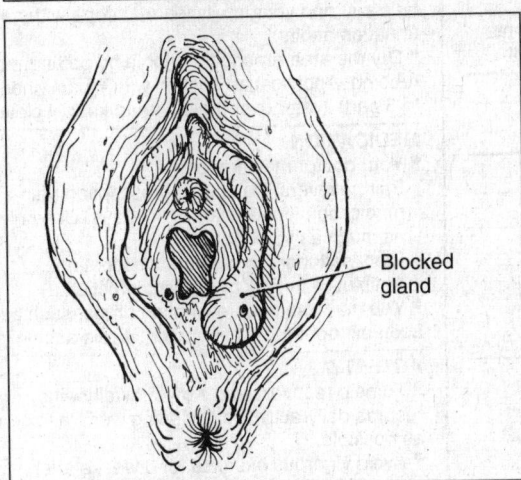

The appearance of a Bartholin's gland which is blocked because of a cyst or abscess.

Blocked gland

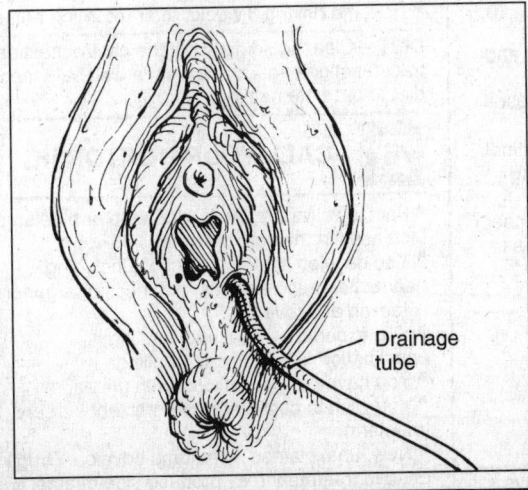

A small incision has been placed in the labia over the area of the abscess. A catheter has been placed in the incision and is allowed to drain into the vagina.

Drainage tube

BLADDER (URINARY) REMOVAL (Cystectomy)

 ## GENERAL INFORMATION

DEFINITION—Removal of the urinary bladder and adjacent tissues and organs, and diversion of the urinary stream. This involves an artificial opening, which is called an "ostomy" or "stoma."

BODY PARTS INVOLVED
* Males: Bladder; prostate; urethra; seminal vesicles; small intestine.
* Females: Urinary bladder; urethra; ureters; cervix; vagina; small intestine.

REASONS FOR SURGERY—Cancer of the bladder.

SURGICAL RISK INCREASES WITH
* Poor nutrition.
* Repeated surgeries on the bladder.
* Diabetes mellitus.
* Use of some prescription and nonprescription drugs. Inform your doctor of any drugs, medications, or vitamin and herb supplements you are using or have used in the last month.

 ## WHAT TO EXPECT

WHO OPERATES—Urologist.

WHERE PERFORMED—Hospital.

DIAGNOSTIC TESTS
* Before surgery: Blood and urine studies; x-rays of kidneys and chest; ultrasound; CT scan; cystoscopy (see Glossary for all).
* During surgery: Cystoscopy (see Glossary).

ANESTHESIA—General anesthesia by injection and inhalation with an airway tube placed in the windpipe.

DESCRIPTION OF OPERATION
* An incision is made in the abdomen. The muscles are separated and the abdominal cavity is entered.
* The blood supply and the ureters are cut and tied.
* The bladder and adjacent tissues and organs are cut free and removed.
* The ureters are diverted through an intestinal pouch (called an ileal conduit) to an opening made in the skin (the stoma).
* The muscles are replaced and sewn together with sutures. The skin is closed with sutures or clips, which usually can be removed about 1 week after surgery.

POSSIBLE COMPLICATIONS
* Excessive bleeding; blood clots.
* Incisional hernia or infection.
* Impotence in males.
* Recurring urinary tract infections.
* Obstruction of the ureter; leakage of urine.

AVERAGE HOSPITAL STAY— 7 to 10 days.

PROBABLE OUTCOME—Expect complete healing of surgical wounds. You will need to wear an external pouch to collect urine. The stoma will heal and shrink to its permanent size in 2 to 4 months after surgery. Allow about 6 weeks for recovery from surgery.

 ## POSTOPERATIVE CARE

GENERAL MEASURES
* A hard ridge should form along the incision. As it heals, the ridge will gradually recede.
* Use an electric heating pad, a heat lamp or a warm compress to relieve incisional pain.
* Bathe and shower as usual. You may wash the incision gently with mild, unscented soap.
* Move and elevate legs often while resting in bed to decrease the likelihood of deep-vein blood clots.
* An enterostomy specialist (see Glossary) will help you and your family learn to cope with new urination habits.
* Dry the area around the stoma by patting, not rubbing. Apply gauze soaked with 1 part vinegar to 3 parts water over the stoma to keep it clean.

MEDICATION
* Your doctor may prescribe:
  Pain relievers. Don't take prescription pain medication longer than 4 to 7 days. Use only as much as you need.
  Stool softeners to prevent constipation.
  Antibiotics to fight or prevent infection.
* You may use nonprescription drugs, such as acetaminophen, for minor pain. Avoid aspirin.

ACTIVITY
* To help recovery and aid your well-being, resume daily activities, including work, as soon as possible.
* Avoid vigorous exercise for 6 weeks after surgery. Avoid heavy lifting indefinitely.
* Resume driving 3 weeks after returning home.

DIET—Clear liquid diet until the gastrointestinal tract functions again. Then eat a well-balanced diet to promote healing.

 ## CALL YOUR DOCTOR IF

* Pain, swelling, redness, drainage or bleeding increases in the surgical area.
* You develop signs of infection, including headache, muscle aches, dizziness or a general ill feeling and fever.
* You experience nausea, vomiting, constipation or abdominal swelling.
* You have pain or difficulty with urination.
* You wish to consider penile implant surgery (if impotent).
* New, unexplained symptoms develop. Drugs used in treatment may produce side effects.

BLADDER (URINARY) REMOVAL
(Cystectomy)

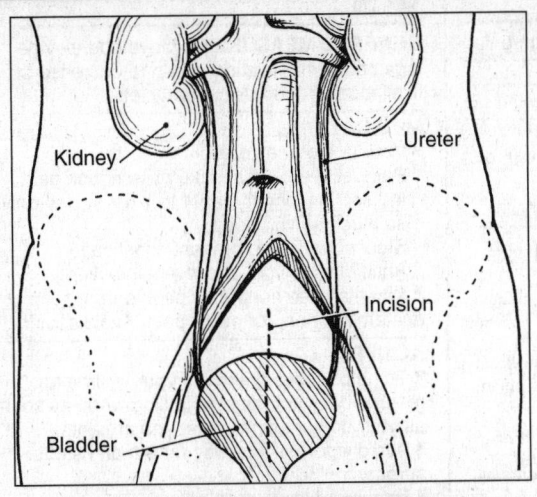

An illustration of the bladder and other parts of the urinary tract.

Kidney

Ureter

Incision

Bladder

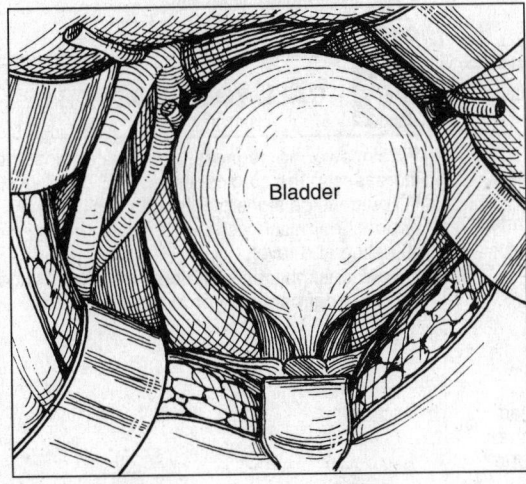

The bladder and adjacent tissues and organs are cut free and removed.
- The ureters are divided through an intestinal pouch to an opening made in the skin.

Bladder

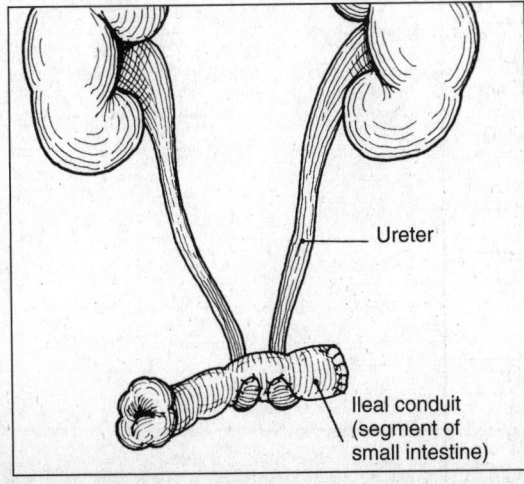

After the bladder has been removed, the kidneys and ureters are connected to an ileal conduit.

Ureter

Ileal conduit (segment of small intestine)

BONE GRAFT

GENERAL INFORMATION

DEFINITION—Filling space between fragments of a broken bone.

BODY PARTS INVOLVED—Bone.

REASONS FOR SURGERY
- Joining of two or more parts of a bone that have broken and not grown back together.
- Fusion of the spine after injury or surgery.

SURGICAL RISK INCREASES WITH
- Adults over 60.
- Obesity.
- Smoking.
- Poor nutrition.
- Recent or chronic illness; diabetes mellitus.
- Use of some prescription and nonprescription drugs. Inform your doctor of any drugs, medications, or vitamin and herb supplements you are using or have used in the last month.

WHAT TO EXPECT

WHO OPERATES—Orthopedist.

WHERE PERFORMED—Hospital.

DIAGNOSTIC TESTS
- Before surgery: X-rays of area to be grafted; blood and urine studies.
- After surgery: Blood studies; x-rays of grafted area.

ANESTHESIA—General anesthesia by injection and inhalation with an airway tube placed in the windpipe.

DESCRIPTION OF OPERATION
- If bone for the graft is to be an autograft (taken from the patient), it is usually removed from the top of the hip bone, the spine, or the ribs. Otherwise, bone is obtained from a bone bank (see Glossary).
- An incision is made over the affected bone. The bone is located and isolated.
- The bone to be grafted is shaped to fit the affected area. Bits and pieces of bone graft are held in place with bone wax or plastic material.
- The skin is closed with sutures or clips, which usually can be removed about 1 week after surgery.
- A splint or plaster cast keeps the affected part rigid and promotes healing (sometimes).

POSSIBLE COMPLICATIONS
- Excessive bleeding.
- Surgical-wound infection.
- Rejection of transplanted bone.

AVERAGE HOSPITAL STAY—7 to 10 days.

PROBABLE OUTCOME—Expect complete healing without complications. Allow about 3 months for recovery from surgery.

POSTOPERATIVE CARE

GENERAL MEASURES—Move and elevate legs often while resting in bed to decrease the likelihood of deep-vein blood clots.

MEDICATION
- Your doctor may prescribe:
  Pain relievers. Don't take prescription pain medication longer than 4 to 7 days. Use only as much as you need.
  Stool softeners to prevent constipation.
  Antibiotics to fight or prevent infection.
- You may use nonprescription drugs, such as acetaminophen, for minor pain. Avoid aspirin.

ACTIVITY
- To help recovery and aid your well-being, resume daily activities, including work, as soon as your doctor advises that you are able.
- Avoid vigorous exercise for 3 months after surgery.
- Resume driving when able.

DIET—No special diet.

CALL YOUR DOCTOR IF

- Pain, swelling, redness, drainage or bleeding increases in the surgical area.
- You develop signs of infection, including headache, muscle aches, dizziness or a general ill feeling and fever.
- New, unexplained symptoms develop. Drugs used in treatment may produce side effects.

BONE GRAFT

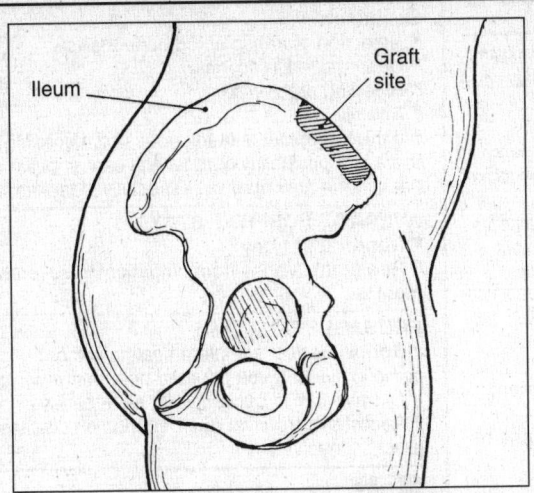

Ileum

Graft site

An illustration of a frequent bone graft site. In this case, located on the crest of the ileum (hip bone).
(These illustrations are used as examples. The principles and techniques are similar for bone grafts in other locations.)

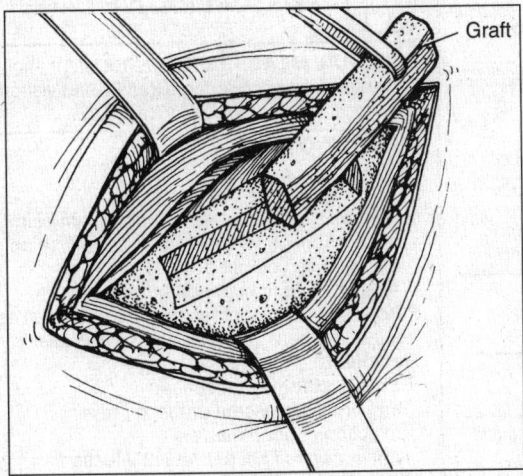

Graft

After muscles and covering tissues are removed, the segment of bone is removed from its normal site.

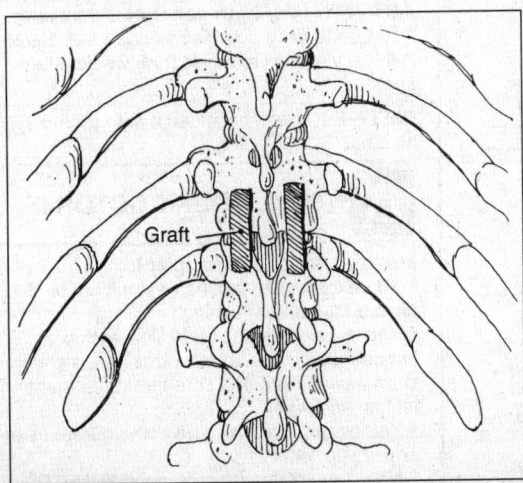

Graft

The bone graft is transplanted to another part of the body (in this example, the spine) where it will provide stabilization.

BONE MARROW TRANSPLANT

GENERAL INFORMATION

DEFINITION—Removal of bone marrow or stem cells (see Glossary) from a donor for introduction into the bloodstream of a recipient. The donor may be a different person than the recipient (allogenic transplant), or may be the same person as the recipient (autologous transplant). The topic of bone marrow and stem cell transplantation is a very complicated one; the information contained herein provides only an overview of the subject. Consult your doctor for additional information.

BODY PARTS INVOLVED
- Donor: Ilium (part of the hip joint); vein.
- Recipient: Vein.

REASONS FOR SURGERY—Replenishment of bone marrow or stem cells which have become weakened or been destroyed by one of the following:
- Acute leukemia or aplastic anemia.
- Multiple myeloma.
- High-dose chemotherapy treatment of some types of cancer.

SURGICAL RISK INCREASES FOR BOTH DONOR AND RECIPIENT WITH
- Obesity; smoking; poor nutrition.
- Recent or chronic illness; diabetes mellitus.
- Use of some prescription and nonprescription drugs. Inform your doctor of any drugs, medications, or vitamin and herb supplements you are using or have used in the last month.

WHAT TO EXPECT

WHO OPERATES—Specially trained oncologist or hematologist.

WHERE PERFORMED—Hospital or outpatient surgical facility.

DIAGNOSTIC TESTS
- Before surgery: Blood and bone marrow studies of both donor and recipient.
- After surgery: Blood studies in recipient to determine success of transplant.

ANESTHESIA—Spinal or general anesthetic.

DESCRIPTION OF OPERATION
- Before surgery, the donor is examined for communicable diseases, and the recipient is treated with immunosuppressive drugs. Sometimes, the recipient also receives chemotherapy or radiation to treat the disease.
- Marrow is harvested from the back of the pelvic bone of the donor with a needle-syringe technique. If stem cells are being harvested, they are usually removed through venous access lines which are placed in surgery under general anesthesia or heavy sedation.
- The bone marrow or stem cells are filtered and then injected into the recipient's vein.

POSSIBLE COMPLICATIONS
Donor: None expected.
Recipient:
- Rejection of transplanted bone marrow.
- Uncontrolled infections.
- Bleeding problems.
- Anemia.
- If the transplant is autologous (from oneself), there is a possibility of receiving cancer cells back in the new marrow, especially in leukemia.

AVERAGE HOSPITAL STAY
- **Donor:** 0 to 1 day.
- **Recipient:** Varies from outpatient to several months.

PROBABLE OUTCOME
- **Donor:** Expect complete healing without complications. If you donated bone marrow, you may have a mild backache for several days.
- **Recipient:** Survival rate depends on disease process involved.

POSTOPERATIVE CARE

GENERAL MEASURES—The recipient should be isolated from attendants, family and visitors to protect the recipient from infection.

MEDICATION—
Donor:
- Your doctor may prescribe:
  Pain relievers. Don't take prescription pain medication longer than 4 to 7 days. Use only as much as you need.
  Antibiotics to fight or prevent infection.
- You may use nonprescription drugs, such as acetaminophen, for minor pain. Avoid aspirin.

Recipient:
- Your doctor may prescribe:
  Immunosuppressant drugs to prevent rejection of bone marrow.
  Antibiotics to fight or prevent infection.

ACTIVITY—For both donor and recipient:
- Return to daily activities as soon as possible.
- Avoid vigorous exercise for 6 weeks after surgery.

DIET—Eat a well-balanced diet to promote healing.

CALL YOUR DOCTOR IF

For both donor and recipient:
- You experience nausea or vomiting; or develop a rash or flushing.
- You develop signs of infection, including headache, muscle aches, dizziness, a cough, shortness of breath, a sore throat or a general ill feeling and fever.
- You experience bleeding from your gums or any of your orifices.
- New, unexplained symptoms develop. Drugs used in treatment may produce side effects.

BONE MARROW TRANSPLANT

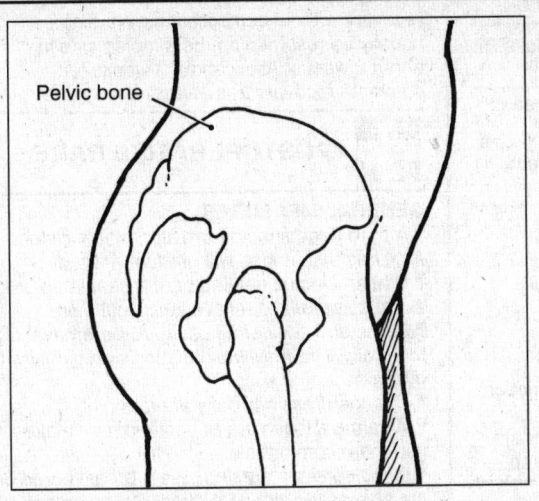

Pelvic bone

Illustration of hip where bone marrow is most often harvested from the donor. The back of the pelvic bone (iliac crest) is the prominent area closest to surface of the skin.

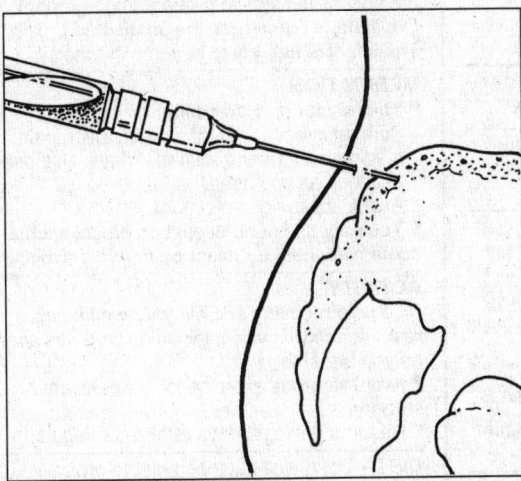

Bone marrow is removed from donor's iliac crest with a needle syringe.

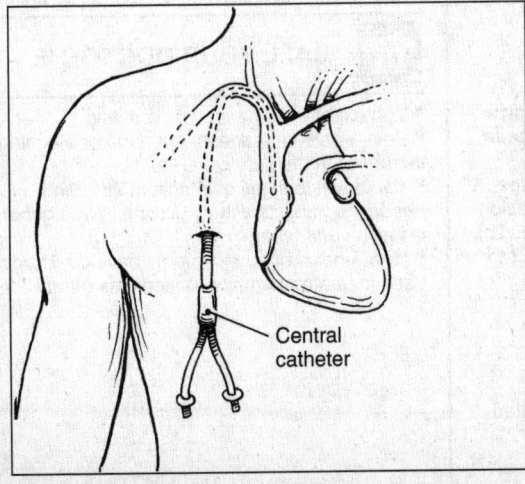

Central catheter

After undergoing a filtering process, the marrow is transfused into the recipient through a central catheter which provides venous access.

BREAST ABSCESS DRAINAGE

GENERAL INFORMATION

DEFINITION—To open and drain an abscess in the female breast.

BODY PARTS INVOLVED—Lactating breast; nipple; lactiferous ducts.

REASONS FOR SURGERY—Relief of pain and prevention of the spread of infection.

SURGICAL RISK INCREASES WITH
- Obesity.
- Smoking.
- Stress.
- Poor nutrition.
- Recent or chronic illness.
- Diabetes mellitus.
- Use of some prescription and nonprescription drugs. Inform your doctor of any drugs, medications, or vitamin and herb supplements you are using or have used in the last month.

WHAT TO EXPECT

WHO OPERATES—General surgeon or obstetrician-gynecologist.

WHERE PERFORMED—Hospital, emergency room, doctor's office or outpatient surgical facility.

DIAGNOSTIC TESTS
- Before surgery: Blood and urine studies; ultrasound; mammogram; aspiration (see Glossary for all).
- After surgery: Laboratory examination of removed pus.

ANESTHESIA
- Local anesthesia by injection.
- General anesthesia by injection and inhalation with an airway tube placed in the windpipe.

DESCRIPTION OF OPERATION
- An incision is made in the breast extending outward from the nipple. The incision is deepened and pus is removed.
- An instrument is forced into the abscess. Pockets of pus are broken up by the surgeon's finger. The opening is enlarged and the area is irrigated with a salt solution.
- Gauze packing is inserted to allow drainage. A small, plastic tube may be placed in the incision to collect additional pus and allow drainage. The drain or gauze packing is usually removed 3 to 5 days following surgery.

POSSIBLE COMPLICATIONS
- Excessive bleeding.
- Surgical-wound infection.
- Slow healing.
- Breast engorgement, if breast is not emptied regularly of milk.
- Recurrence.

AVERAGE HOSPITAL STAY—0 to 2 days.

PROBABLE OUTCOME—Expect complete recovery without complications. Nursing can usually be resumed on the affected side in about 2 weeks. Allow about 3 weeks for complete recovery from surgery.

POSTOPERATIVE CARE

GENERAL MEASURES
- A hard ridge should form along the incision. As it heals, the ridge will gradually recede.
- Use an electric heating pad, a heat lamp or a warm compress to relieve incisional pain.
- Bathe and shower as usual. After removal of the drain, You may wash the incision gently with mild, unscented soap.
- Change dressings daily after bathing.
- Wearing a loose bra at bedtime may make you more comfortable.
- If you continue nursing, use a breast pump on the abscessed side to prevent engorgement. Continue to nurse from the unaffected breast. The infant is unlikely to become infected.

MEDICATION
- Your doctor may prescribe:
  Pain relievers. Don't take prescription pain medication longer than 4 to 7 days. Use only as much as you need.
  Antibiotics to fight infection.
- You may use nonprescription drugs, such as acetaminophen, for minor pain. Avoid aspirin.

ACTIVITY
- To help recovery and aid your well-being, resume daily activities, including work, as soon as you are able.
- Avoid vigorous exercise for 3 weeks after surgery.
- Resume driving 2 days after returning home.

DIET—Eat a well-balanced diet to promote healing. Drink at least 8 glasses of water daily.

CALL YOUR DOCTOR IF

- You experience nausea or vomiting.
- Pain, swelling, redness, drainage or bleeding increases in the surgical area.
- You develop signs of infection, including headache, muscle aches, dizziness or a general ill feeling and fever.
- New, unexplained symptoms develop. Drugs used in treatment may produce side effects.

BREAST ABSCESS DRAINAGE

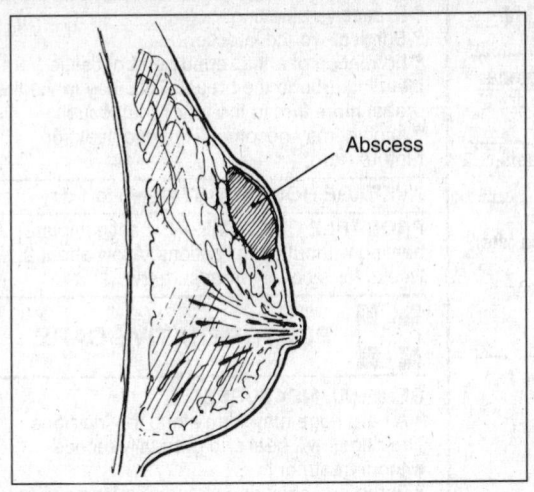

A side illustration of a breast abscess that has become red, warm and fluctuant.

Abscess

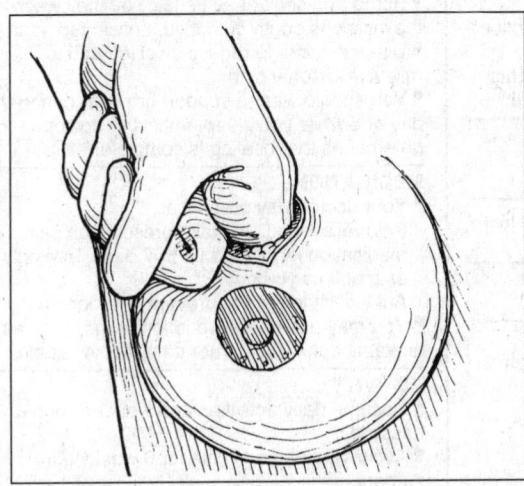

The incision is made into the abscess cavity, a pocket is created, the incision is deepened and pus is removed.

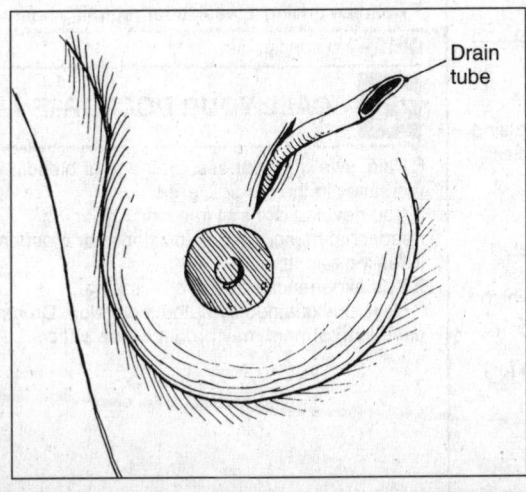

Drain tube

An instrument having been forced into the abscess, pockets of pus are now broken up by the surgeon's finger. The opening is enlarged and the area is irrigated with a salt solution. Gauze packing is inserted for drainage. A small, plastic drain may be placed in the incision to collect additional pus and allow drainage. The drain or gauze packing remains in place for several days and is then removed.

BREAST AUGMENTATION
(Augmentation Mammoplasty)

 GENERAL INFORMATION

DEFINITION—Implantation of artificial material inside the female breasts to enlarge them or give them a different shape.

BODY PARTS INVOLVED—Female breasts; underlying muscles.

REASONS FOR SURGERY
- Restoration of normal breast appearance after a mastectomy.
- Enlargement of the breasts in patients who have less breast tissue than they desire.
- Correction of asymmetry of the breasts.

SURGICAL RISK INCREASES WITH
- Smoking.
- Obesity.
- Excess alcohol consumption.
- Recent or chronic illness.
- Diabetes mellitus.
- Use of some prescription and nonprescription drugs. Inform your doctor of any drugs, medications, or vitamin and herb supplements you are using or have used in the last month.

 WHAT TO EXPECT

WHO OPERATES—Plastic and reconstructive surgeon.

WHERE PERFORMED—Hospital; doctor's office; or outpatient surgical facility.

DIAGNOSTIC TESTS
- Before surgery: Blood studies; mammogram (see Glossary).
- After surgery: Blood studies.

ANESTHESIA
- General anesthesia by injection and inhalation.
- Local anesthesia by injection.

DESCRIPTION OF OPERATION
- Incisions may be made under the breast, through the nipple or in the armpit.
- The breast tissue is brought forward by raising muscles from below the breast or the muscles next to the chest wall.
- A pocket is created, and the implant (a mammary prosthesis filled with saline) is inserted. The procedures are usually repeated on the other breast.
- The skin is closed with sutures or clips, which usually can be removed about 1 week after surgery. A light bandage is applied.
- Occasionally, a drain may be left in place for several days to promote healing.
- A bra or elastic bandage is fitted to give support and to reduce possible bleeding.

POSSIBLE COMPLICATIONS
- Excessive bleeding.
- Surgical-wound infection.
- Formation of a thickened band of tissue from bleeding around the breast. This may make the breast more firm to the touch than usual.
- Implant may become dislodged, leak, or rupture (rare).

AVERAGE HOSPITAL STAY—0 to 1 day.

PROBABLE OUTCOME—Expect complete healing without complications. Allow about 2 weeks for recovery from surgery.

 POSTOPERATIVE CARE

GENERAL MEASURES
- A hard ridge may form along the incisions. The ridges will heal and gradually recede without treatment.
- Bathe and shower as usual. You may wash the incisions gently with mild, unscented soap.
- Use ice packs to reduce swelling and to relieve incisional pain.
- You should wear a support bra both during the day and while you sleep, until your doctor determines that healing is complete.

MEDICATION
- Your doctor may prescribe:
  Pain relievers. Don't take prescription pain medication longer than 4 to 7 days. Use only as much as you need.
  Antibiotics to fight or prevent infection.
- You may use nonprescription drugs, such as acetaminophen, for minor pain. Avoid aspirin.

ACTIVITY
- Resume daily activities and work as soon as possible.
- Avoid vigorous exercise for 6 weeks after surgery.
- Resume driving 1 week after returning home.

DIET—No special diet.

 CALL YOUR DOCTOR IF

- Pain, swelling, redness, drainage or bleeding increases in the surgical area.
- You develop signs of infection, including headache, muscle aches, dizziness or a general ill feeling and fever.
- You experience nausea or vomiting.
- New, unexplained symptoms develop. Drugs used in treatment may produce side effects.

BREAST AUGMENTATION
(Augmentation Mammoplasty)

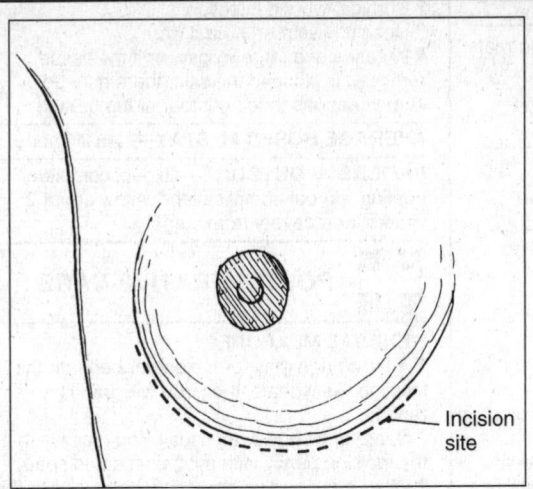

Incisions for the implant may be made under the breast, through the nipple or in the armpit. In this example, it is under the breast line in the chest wall skin.

Incision site

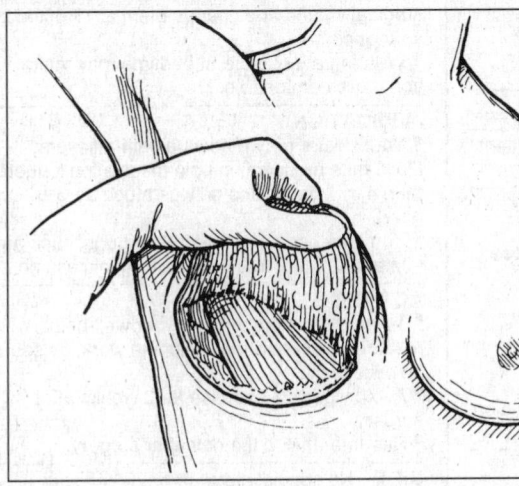

Breast tissue is brought forward by raising muscles from below the breast.

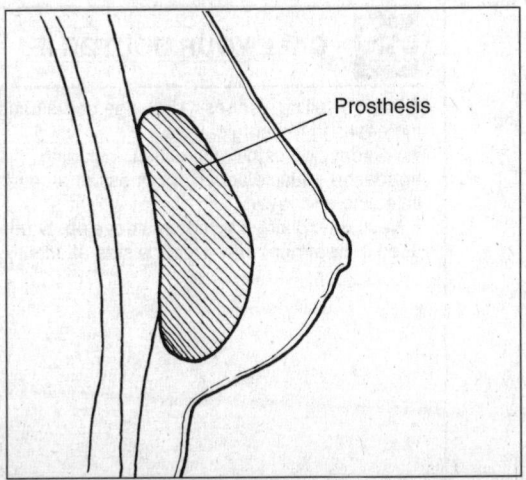

Prosthesis

After the pocket is created, a prosthesis is inserted. The procedure is usually repeated on the other breast.
- Skin is closed with sutures or clips that usually can be removed about 1 week after surgery. A light bandage is usually all that is necessary for a dressing following surgery.

BREAST BIOPSY BY EXCISION

GENERAL INFORMATION

DEFINITION—Removal of suspected abnormal tissue from the breast.

BODY PARTS INVOLVED—Female breast; male breast (rare).

REASONS FOR SURGERY—Clinical or mammographic signs or symptoms that may indicate breast cancer.

SURGICAL RISK INCREASES WITH
- Obesity.
- Stress.
- Smoking.
- Poor nutrition.
- Recent or chronic illness.
- Diabetes mellitus.
- Use of some prescription and nonprescription drugs. Inform your doctor of any drugs, medications, or vitamin and herb supplements you are using or have used in the last month.

WHAT TO EXPECT

WHO OPERATES—General surgeon.

WHERE PERFORMED—Hospital or outpatient surgical facility.

DIAGNOSTIC TESTS
- Before surgery: Blood and urine studies; x-rays of chest; mammogram; ultrasound (see Glossary for both).
- After surgery: Laboratory examination of removed tissue.

ANESTHESIA
- Local anesthesia by injection.
- General anesthesia by injection and inhalation with an airway tube placed in the windpipe.

DESCRIPTION OF OPERATION
- A special wire (the size of a thin guitar string) with a hooked tip may be inserted into the breast to localize the lump or cyst.
- An incision is made over the tissue to be removed. It is often possible to make a very cosmetic incision by cutting at the edge of the areola.
- The suspect tissue is cut free of the surrounding breast tissue and removed.
- Bleeding is controlled with ties or electrocautery.
- The skin is closed with sutures or clips, which usually can be removed about 1 week after surgery.
- The removed tissue will be sent to the pathology laboratory for microscopic examination.

POSSIBLE COMPLICATIONS
- Excessive bleeding.
- Surgical-wound infection.
- Unsightly scar on breast (rare).
- In cases of a large biopsy, or if the tissue removed is close to the skin, there may be some changes to the contour of the breast.

AVERAGE HOSPITAL STAY—Usually none.

PROBABLE OUTCOME—Expect complete healing without complications. Allow about 2 weeks for recovery from surgery.

POSTOPERATIVE CARE

GENERAL MEASURES
- A hard ridge may form along or beneath the incision. As it heals, the ridge will gradually recede.
- Bathe and shower as usual. You may wash the incision gently with mild, unscented soap.
- Wear a supportive bra. Apply bandages to the surgical wound and change them as directed by your doctor.
- Wearing a loose bra at bedtime may make you more comfortable.

MEDICATION
- Your doctor may prescribe pain relievers. Don't take prescription pain medication longer than 4 to 7 days. Use only as much as you need.
- You may use nonprescription drugs, such as acetaminophen, for minor pain. Avoid aspirin.

ACTIVITY
- To help recovery and aid your well-being, resume daily activities, including work, as soon as possible.
- Avoid vigorous exercise for 2 weeks after surgery.
- Resume driving the day after surgery.

DIET—No special diet.

CALL YOUR DOCTOR IF
- Pain, swelling, redness, drainage or bleeding increases in the surgical area.
- You develop signs of infection, including headache, muscle aches, dizziness or a general ill feeling and fever.
- New, unexplained symptoms develop. Drugs used in treatment may produce side effects.

BREAST BIOPSY BY EXCISION

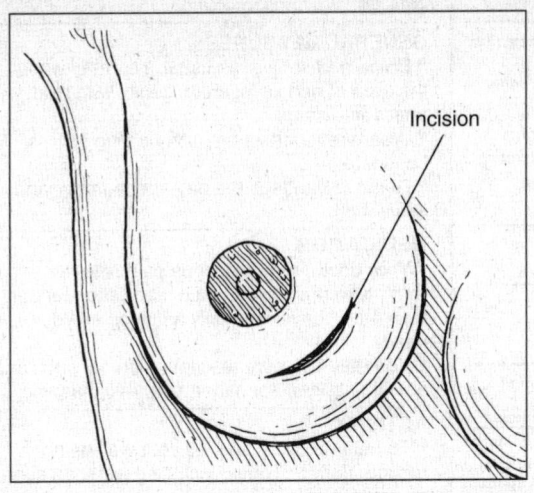

Incision

An illustration of a typical incision over the site of suspected abnormal breast tissue.

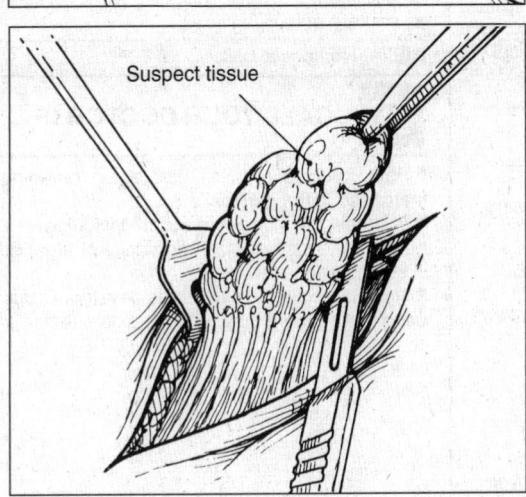

Suspect tissue

The suspect tissue is cut free of the surrounding breast tissue and removed.

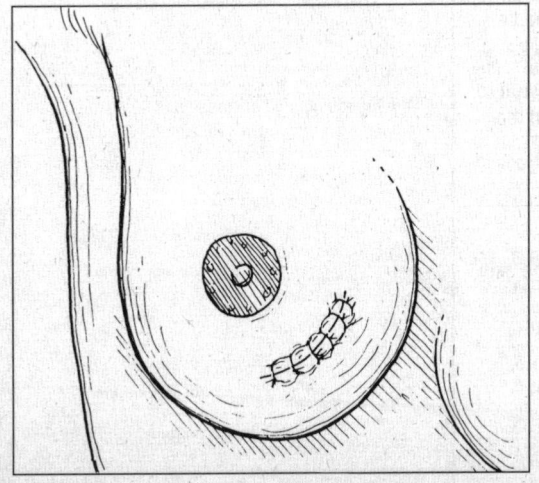

Appearance of the breast after closure of the skin, following tissue removal.

SURGERIES

BREAST BIOPSY BY NEEDLE ASPIRATION

 GENERAL INFORMATION

DEFINITION—Removal of fluid or tissue from one of the female breasts.

BODY PARTS INVOLVED—Breast.

REASONS FOR SURGERY—Diagnosis of a thickening or lump. Needle biopsy is often the best first step for diagnosis of a lump in the breast.

SURGICAL RISK INCREASES WITH—Bleeding disorders.

 WHAT TO EXPECT

WHO OPERATES—Family doctor or general surgeon.

WHERE PERFORMED—Hospital, doctor's office or outpatient surgical facility.

DIAGNOSTIC TESTS
• Before surgery: Medical history and physical examination; ultrasound; mammogram (see Glossary for both).
• After surgery: Laboratory examination of removed fluid or tissue.

ANESTHESIA—Local anesthesia by injection (sometimes). Often, no anesthetic is necessary.

DESCRIPTION OF OPERATION
• A small, hollow needle is inserted into the thickening or lump.
• If the thickening or lump is a cyst, fluid usually can be removed and the cyst will shrink or disappear. This is often considered both therapeutic and diagnostic.
• In some cases, the removed fluid is sent to the laboratory to be examined for abnormal cells.
• If a solid tumor is detected, tissue is removed through the needle for laboratory examination. The tissue is recovered by passing the needle through the suspicious tissue several times, while using a syringe to aspirate as large a sample of cells as possible. The tissue is sent to the laboratory for microscopic examination.
• The needle is withdrawn and pressure is exerted on the site of the biopsy; a bandage is then applied.

POSSIBLE COMPLICATIONS
• Infection in surgical area (rare).
• Collection of blood (hematoma) under the skin where needle was inserted.

AVERAGE HOSPITAL STAY—0 to 1 day.

PROBABLE OUTCOME—Expect complete healing without complications. Allow about 1 week for recovery from surgery.

 POSTOPERATIVE CARE

GENERAL MEASURES
• Bathe and shower as usual. You may wash the area of needle insertion gently with mild, unscented soap.
• Wear a supportive bra until healing is complete.
• Remove bandage the day after surgery and leave it off.

MEDICATION
• Your doctor may prescribe pain relievers. Don't take prescription pain medication longer than 4 to 7 days. Use only as much as you need.
• You may use nonprescription drugs, such as acetaminophen, for minor pain. Avoid aspirin.

ACTIVITY
• To help recovery and aid your well-being, resume daily activities, including work, as soon as you are able.

DIET—No special diet.

 CALL YOUR DOCTOR IF

• Pain, swelling, redness, drainage or bleeding increases in the surgical area.
• You develop signs of infection, including headache, muscle aches, dizziness or a general ill feeling and fever.
• New, unexplained symptoms develop. Drugs used in treatment may produce side effects.

BREAST BIOPSY BY NEEDLE ASPIRATION

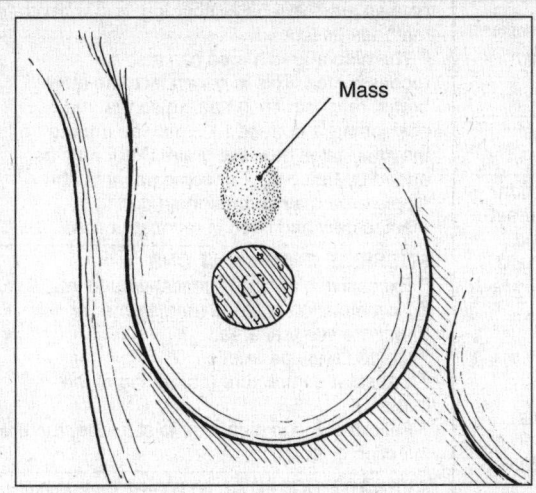

An illustration of a typical mass within the breast.

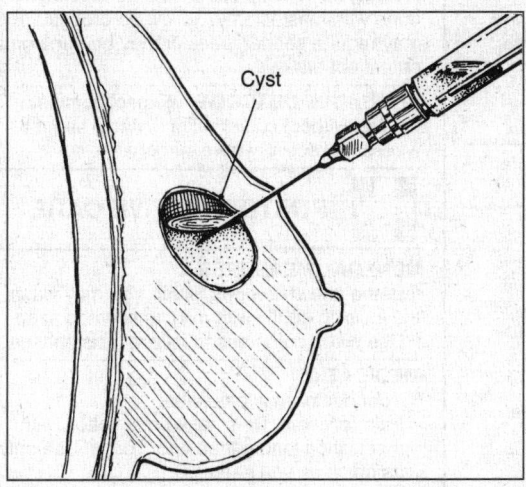

A small, hollow needle is inserted into the thickening or lump. Fluid is aspirated if the lump is a cyst.

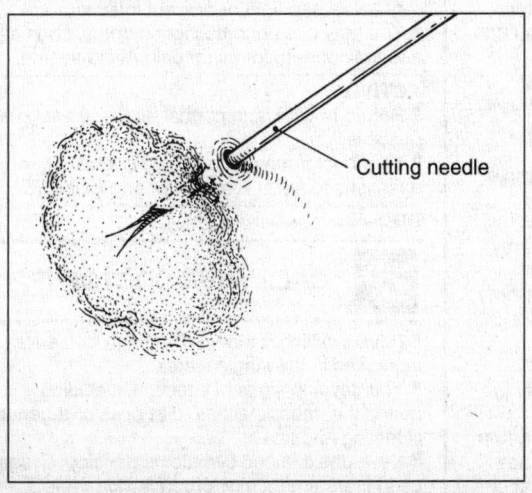

If a solid tumor is detected, tissue is removed through the needle and a laboratory examination is done to determine whether the tissue is benign or malignant.

BREAST RECONSTRUCTION

GENERAL INFORMATION

DEFINITION—Rebuilding the female breast after mastectomy; using an implant or other body tissue.

BODY PARTS INVOLVED—Breasts; chest wall muscles; abdominal wall or back.

REASONS FOR SURGERY—Reconstruction of the breast following a mastectomy for breast cancer is usually done for psychological and cosmetic reasons. It is becoming the standard procedure and, in most areas, is required by law to be covered by medical insurance.

SURGICAL RISK INCREASES WITH
- Obesity; smoking.
- Excess alcohol consumption.
- Recent or chronic illness;diabetes mellitus.
- Previous radiation to the breast.
- Use of some prescription and nonprescription drugs. Inform your doctor of any drugs, medications, or vitamin and herb supplements you are using or have used in the last month.

WHAT TO EXPECT

WHO OPERATES—Plastic surgeon; general surgeon or oncology surgeon (sometimes).

WHERE PERFORMED—Hospital.

DIAGNOSTIC TESTS
- Before surgery: As required for the mastectomy procedure.
- After surgery: As required for follow up of cancer therapy or monitoring.

ANESTHESIA—General anesthesia by injection and inhalation, with an airway tube placed in the windpipe.

DESCRIPTION OF OPERATION
Several options are available and additional methods are undergoing development. You and your surgeon should have a clear understanding of what is to be done during surgery, but the surgeon will need some leeway in case unexpected problems occur.
- During mastectomy: If there is sufficient muscle and skin to cover the implant, a simple silicone or saline implant may be all that is required. If additional muscle and skin is needed, it is brought in (usually from a nearby location on the body) to cover the implant.
- Temporary expander: During the mastectomy or later, a silicone bag with a separate valve is implanted under the skin and muscle. It is inflated at intervals over a 6-week period to expand the skin and muscle. The expander is then replaced by a permanent implant.
- Tissue to form a "new breast" is obtained from the abdominal wall or back. An implant is not necessary. This procedure produces the most

normal and natural breast in appearance and feel, but usually requires more surgery and causes more extensive scarring than with other methods described.
- The nipple-areola area can also be reconstructed. This is generally done after breast reconstruction healing so that the positioning is correct. Skin may be grafted from the inner thigh near the groin. Color may be added by tattooing. For some patients, the nipple area may be preserved during mastectomy and used in reconstruction.

POSSIBLE COMPLICATIONS
- Excessive bleeding; surgical-wound infection.
- Accumulation of blood (hematoma) or fluid under the surgical area.
- Limited shoulder motion.
- Capsular contracture (hardening of the implant).
- Failure of the implant due to slippage, rupture, infection or scarring.

AVERAGE HOSPITAL STAY—1 to 4 days if done with mastectomy. Follow up procedures may require shorter times or may be done on an outpatient basis.

PROBABLE OUTCOME—Expect complete healing without complications. Allow about 6 weeks for recovery from surgery.

POSTOPERATIVE CARE

GENERAL MEASURES
- Bathe and shower as usual. You may wash the incision gently with mild, unscented soap.
- Use warm compress to relieve incisional pain.

MEDICATION
- Your doctor may prescribe:
  Pain relievers. Don't take prescription pain medication longer than 4 to 7 days. Use only as much as you need.
  Antibiotics to fight or prevent infection.
- You may use nonprescription drugs, such as acetaminophen, for minor pain.Avoid aspirin.

ACTIVITY
- Return to work and normal activity as soon as possible.
- Your doctor may recommend special exercises to aid in recovery of arm mobility.

DIET—No special diet.

CALL YOUR DOCTOR IF

- Pain, swelling, redness, drainage or bleeding increases in the surgical area.
- You develop signs of infection, including headache, muscle aches, dizziness or a general ill feeling and fever.
- New, unexplained symptoms develop. Drugs used in treatment may produce side effects.

BREAST RECONSTRUCTION

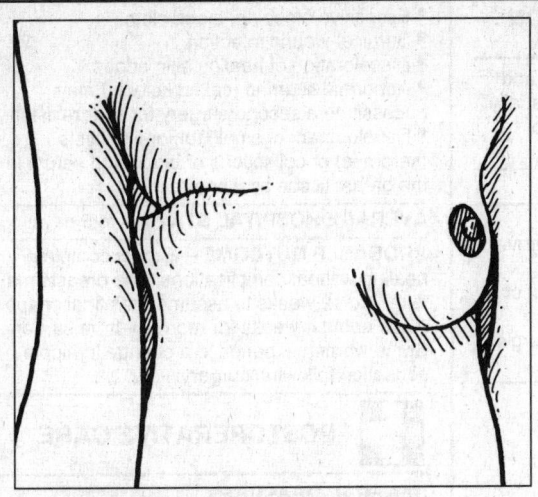

Illustration shows the appearance of right breast after mastectomy.

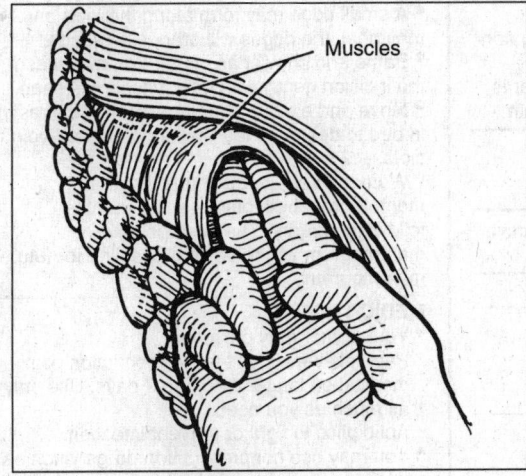

Muscles

A pocket is prepared for an implant.

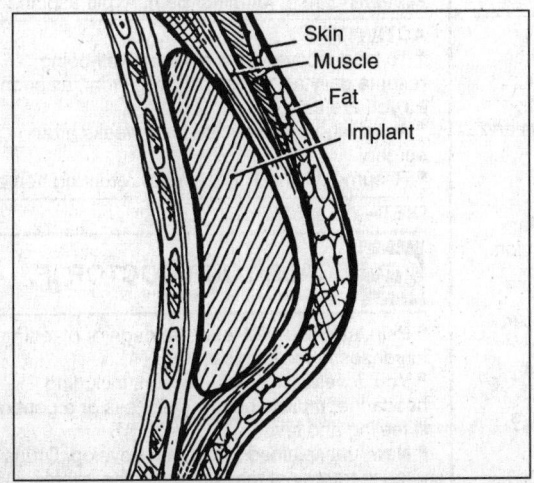

Skin
Muscle
Fat
Implant

Side view of the breast showing the implant in position.

BREAST REDUCTION
(Reduction Mammoplasty)

 GENERAL INFORMATION

DEFINITION—Removal of excess tissue and overlying skin from the female breasts. Usually this surgery also includes reconstruction of breast shape.

BODY PARTS INVOLVED—Breasts.

REASONS FOR SURGERY
- Reduction of overly large breasts to improve appearance and/or emotional well-being.
- Relief of back and neck pain from weight of overly large breasts.
- Reconstruction of a breast to match a surgical change made in the other breast.

SURGICAL RISK INCREASES WITH
- Obesity.
- Smoking.
- Excess alcohol consumption.
- Diabetes mellitus.
- Poor nutrition.
- Use of some prescription and nonprescription drugs. Inform your doctor of any drugs, medications, or vitamin and herb supplements you are using or have used in the last month.

 WHAT TO EXPECT

WHO OPERATES—Plastic and reconstructive surgeon.

WHERE PERFORMED—Hospital.

DIAGNOSTIC TESTS
- Before surgery: Blood and urine studies; mammogram (see Glossary).
- After surgery: Blood studies.

ANESTHESIA—General anesthesia by injection and inhalation with an airway tube placed in the windpipe.

DESCRIPTION OF OPERATION
- The breast is marked where the skin will be removed and where the nipple will be after tissue is removed.
- The skin between the new nipple location and the natural nipple location is incised and removed. The nipple stays attached to underlying tissue.
- Another incision is made below the nipple. Excess tissue is removed through this incision.
- The removed tissue should be sent to a pathology laboratory to be examined and analyzed for any early signs of breast cancer.
- Drains are left in place to prevent fluid or blood from accumulating under the sutures.
- The skin is closed with fine sutures, which usually can be removed about 10 to 14 days after surgery.

POSSIBLE COMPLICATIONS
- Excessive bleeding; blood clots.
- Surgical-wound infection.
- Discoloration of healing skin edges.
- Abnormal scarring (called keloids) may necessitate a second surgery for scar revision.
- Development of small, tumor-like cysts (seromas) or collections of blood and serum in the breast tissue as it heals.

AVERAGE HOSPITAL STAY—4 to 5 days.

PROBABLE OUTCOME—Expect complete healing without complications. The breasts may take 3 to 12 weeks to assume their final shape. Allow about 4 weeks for recovery from surgery. Some women experience a change in nipple sensation following surgery.

 POSTOPERATIVE CARE

GENERAL MEASURES
- A small ridge may form along the incisions. As they heal, the ridges will gradually recede.
- Bathe and shower as usual. You may wash the incision gently with mild, unscented soap.
- Move and elevate your legs often while resting in bed to decrease the likelihood of deep-vein clots.
- Women over age 30 should have a mammogram both before and 6 months following surgery. The postoperative mammogram will serve as a baseline for future mammograms.

MEDICATION
- Your doctor may prescribe:
  Pain relievers. Don't take prescription pain medication longer than 4 to 7 days. Use only as much as you need.
  Antibiotics to fight or prevent infection.
- You may use nonprescription drugs, such as acetaminophen, for minor pain. Avoid aspirin.

ACTIVITY
- To help recovery and aid your well-being, resume daily activities, including work, as soon as you are able.
- Avoid vigorous exercise for 6 weeks after surgery.
- Resume driving 1 month after returning home.

DIET—No special diet.

 CALL YOUR DOCTOR IF

- Pain, swelling, redness, drainage or bleeding increases in the surgical area.
- You develop signs of infection, including headache, muscle aches, dizziness or a general ill feeling and fever.
- New, unexplained symptoms develop. Drugs used in treatment may produce side effects.

BREAST REDUCTION
(Reduction Mammoplasty)

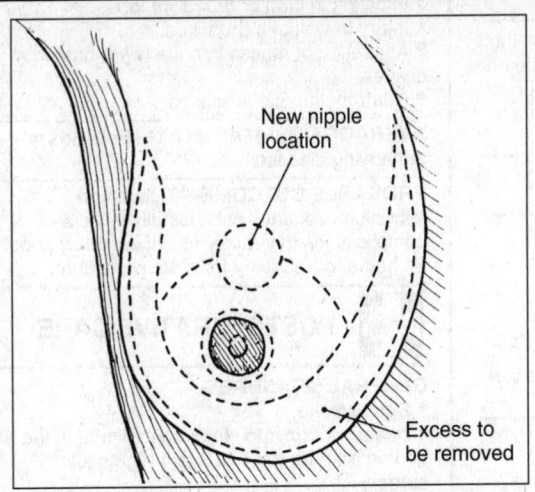

An illustration showing markings on the breast where skin will be removed and the nipple will be placed after the reduction procedure.

New nipple location

Excess to be removed

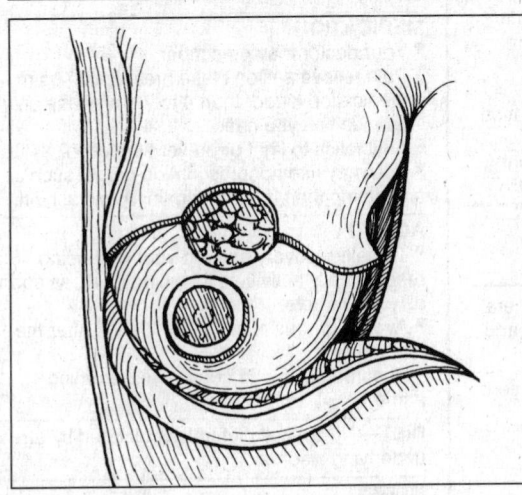

Skin between the new nipple location and the natural nipple location is incised and removed. The nipple stays attached to the underlying tissue.

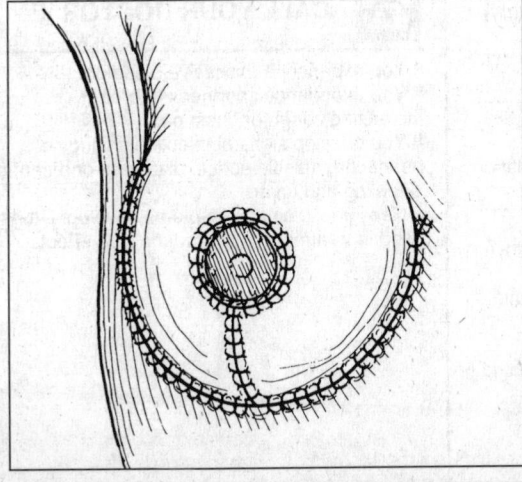

Another incision is made below the nipple. Excess tissue is removed, drains are left in place to prevent collection of fluid, and skin is closed with fine sutures. Sutures are usually removed about 10 to 14 days after surgery.

BRONCHOSCOPY

GENERAL INFORMATION

DEFINITION—Visual examination of the lining of the bronchial tubes and removal of tissue and secretions. The procedure is performed with a flexible bronchoscope, an optical instrument with a lighted tip.

BODY PARTS INVOLVED—Windpipe (trachea); larynx; bronchial tree.

REASONS FOR SURGERY
- Suspected cancer in the bronchial tubes.
- Foreign matter that has been inhaled accidentally.
- Bleeding in the bronchial tubes.
- X-ray studies (bronchograms) to diagnose diseases of the lung, such as bronchiectasis or emphysema.

SURGICAL RISK INCREASES WITH
- Obesity.
- Smoking.
- Recent or chronic illness, especially chronic lung disease.
- Diabetes mellitus.
- Alcoholism.
- Use of some prescription and nonprescription drugs. Inform your doctor of any drugs, medications, or vitamin and herb supplements you are using or have used in the last month.

WHAT TO EXPECT

WHO OPERATES—Thoracic surgeon, general surgeon, pulmonary specialist or ear, nose and throat specialist.

WHERE PERFORMED—Hospital or outpatient surgical facility.

DIAGNOSTIC TESTS
- Before surgery: Blood and urine studies; x-rays of chest; CT scan (see Glossary).
- During surgery: Bronchogram (see Glossary).
- After surgery: Laboratory examination of removed tissue and secretions; x-rays to check for complications.

ANESTHESIA
- Local anesthesia with sedation.
- General anesthesia by injection and inhalation with an airway tube placed in the windpipe.

DESCRIPTION OF OPERATION
- The bronchoscope is inserted in the mouth, past the back of the tongue, into the main bronchial tube and its branches. Supplemental oxygen is supplied during the procedure.
- Foreign matter is removed, if necessary. Tissue is gathered and secretions are collected.
- The bronchoscope is removed.

POSSIBLE COMPLICATIONS
- Excessive bleeding.
- Infection in lung or bronchial tubes.
- Injury to wall of a bronchus.
- Aspiration of mucus into the lower bronchial tissues.
- Heart rhythm disturbances.

AVERAGE HOSPITAL STAY—Depends on underlying disease.

PROBABLE OUTCOME—Tissue and secretions obtained successfully without complications in virtually all cases. Allow about 24 hours for recovery from the procedure.

POSTOPERATIVE CARE

GENERAL MEASURES
- Don't smoke.
- Use a vaporizer to increase moisture in the air you breathe for the first 3 to 4 nights after surgery.

MEDICATION
- Your doctor may prescribe:
  Pain relievers. Don't take prescription pain medication longer than 4 to 7 days. Use only as much as you need.
  Antibiotics to fight or prevent infection.
- You may use nonprescription drugs, such as acetaminophen, for minor pain. Avoid aspirin.

ACTIVITY
- To help recovery and aid your well-being, resume daily activities, including work, as soon as you are able.
- Avoid vigorous exercise for 7 days after the procedure.
- Resume driving 24 hours after returning home.

DIET—No special diet unless dictated by an underlying disorder.

CALL YOUR DOCTOR IF

- You experience excessive bleeding.
- You experience shortness of breath, increasing cough or chest pain.
- You develop signs of infection, including headache, muscle aches, dizziness or a general ill feeling and fever.
- New, unexplained symptoms develop. Drugs used in treatment may produce side effects.

BRONCHOSCOPY

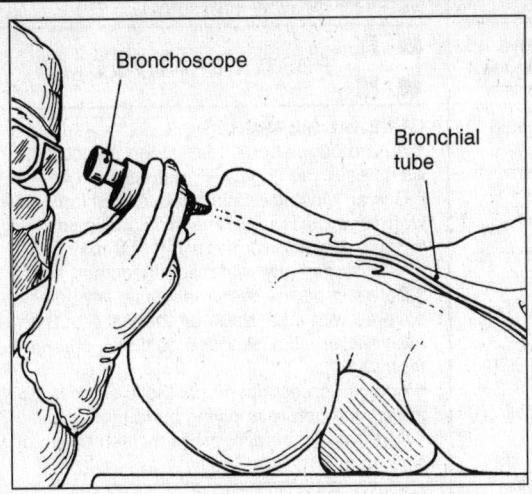

An illustration of the bronchoscope inserted into the mouth past the tongue and into the main bronchial tube and its branches.

Bronchoscope

Bronchial tube

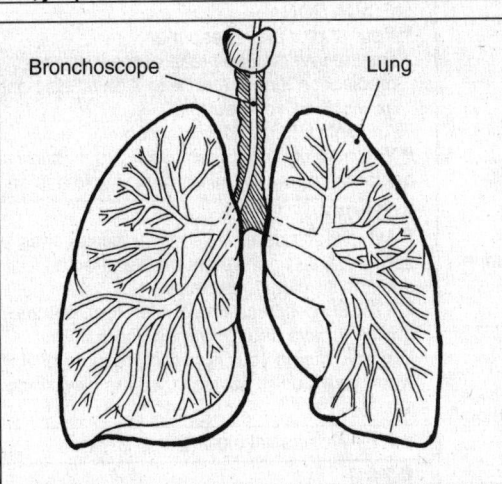

Bronchoscope

Lung

The flexible bronchoscope can be passed into either of the main stem bronchial branches.
- Foreign matter is removed by suction. If necessary, tissue is gathered and secretions are collected to be studied microscopically.

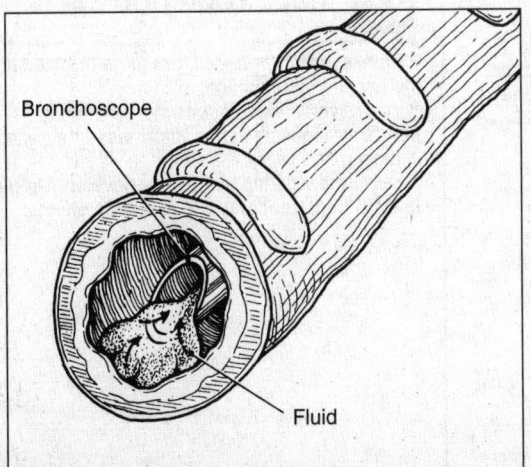

Bronchoscope

Fluid

Fluid being suctioned from the bronchoscope while still in place.

BUNION REMOVAL

GENERAL INFORMATION

DEFINITION—Removal of a bunion, a bony and fibrous outgrowth at the base of the big toe.

BODY PARTS INVOLVED—Foot; joint between the metatarsal bone and big toe; fluid sac that surrounds the joint.

REASONS FOR SURGERY
- Relief of pain.
- Correction of deformity.

SURGICAL RISK INCREASES WITH
- Poor nutrition.
- Recent illness.
- Alcoholism or chronic illness.
- Diabetes mellitus.
- Vascular disease.
- Use of some prescription and nonprescription drugs. Inform your doctor of any drugs, medications, or vitamin and herb supplements you are using or have used in the last month.

WHAT TO EXPECT

WHO OPERATES—General surgeon, orthopedist or podiatrist.

WHERE PERFORMED—Doctor's office, outpatient surgical facility or hospital.

DIAGNOSTIC TESTS
- Before surgery: X-rays of foot; blood and urine studies.
- After surgery: X-rays of foot.

ANESTHESIA
- Local anesthesia by injection.
- Spinal anesthesia by injection.
- General anesthesia by injection and inhalation with an airway tube placed in the windpipe.

DESCRIPTION OF OPERATION
- An incision is made over the bunion.
- The capsule of the joint connecting the metatarsal bone and the big toe is opened.
- A section from the metatarsal bone is cut or filed away and removed. Another small bone (the sesamoid bone) attached to a tendon is removed also.
- Tendons attached to the base of the metatarsal and toe bones are cut. This allows the bones to straighten when healed.
- The skin is closed with sutures, which usually can be removed about 10 days after surgery.

POSSIBLE COMPLICATIONS
- Excessive bleeding.
- Surgical-wound infection.
- Slow healing.

AVERAGE HOSPITAL STAY—0 to 1 day.

PROBABLE OUTCOME—Expect complete healing without complications. Allow about 6 weeks for recovery from surgery.

POSTOPERATIVE CARE

GENERAL MEASURES
- A hard ridge should form along the incision. As it heals, the ridge will gradually recede.
- Use an electric heating pad, a heat lamp or a warm compress to relieve incisional pain.
- Bathe and shower as usual. You may wash the incision gently with mild, unscented soap.
- Between baths, keep the wound dry and covered with a bandage for the first 2 or 3 days after surgery. If a bandage gets wet, change it promptly.
- Apply nonprescription antibiotic ointment to the wound before applying bandages.
- If the wound bleeds, press a clean tissue or cloth to it.

MEDICATION
- Your doctor may prescribe:
  Pain relievers. Don't take prescription pain medication longer than 4 to 7 days. Use only as much as you need.
  Antibiotics to prevent infection.
- You may use nonprescription drugs, such as acetaminophen, for minor pain. Avoid aspirin.

ACTIVITY
- Avoid vigorous exercise for 6 weeks after surgery. Don't put weight on the affected foot until the surgical area heals.
- If the surgery was on your left foot, resume driving 4 days after returning home. If the surgery was on your right foot, resume driving when your doctor advises that it is okay to do so.

DIET—No special diet.

CALL YOUR DOCTOR IF

- Pain, swelling, redness, drainage or bleeding increases in the surgical area.
- You develop signs of infection, including headache, muscle aches, dizziness or a general ill feeling and fever.
- New, unexplained symptoms develop. Drugs used in treatment may produce side effects.

BUNION REMOVAL

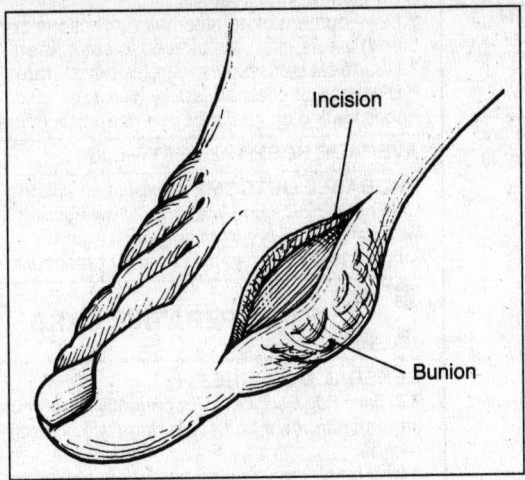

An illustration of a typical bunion. An incision is made over the bunion.

Incision

Bunion

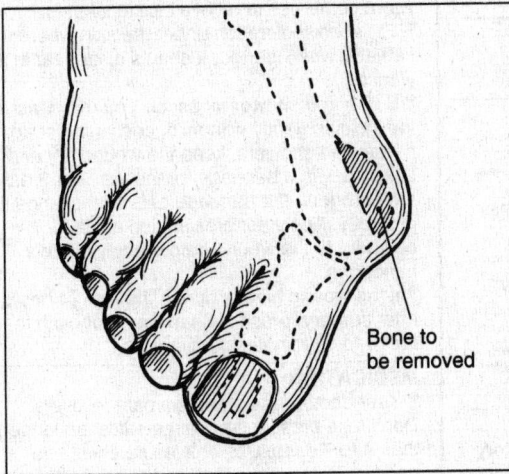

Overgrown section from the metatarsal bone is cut or filed away and removed.

Bone to be removed

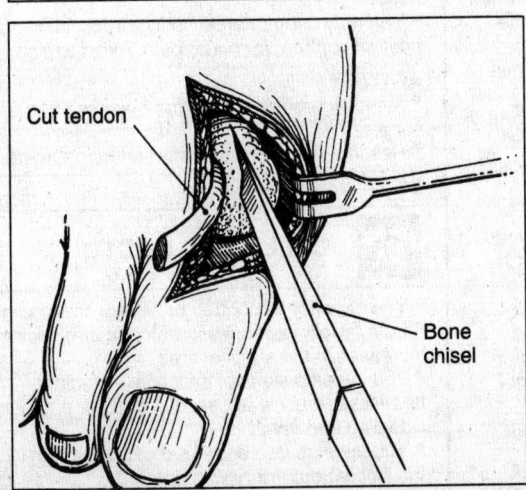

Tendons attached to the base of the metatarsal bone and toe bones are cut to allow bones to straighten when healed.

Cut tendon

Bone chisel

CARDIAC CATHETERIZATION & ANGIOCARDIOGRAPHY

GENERAL INFORMATION

DEFINITION—Diagnostic procedures to examine functions of the heart.

BODY PARTS INVOLVED—Heart muscle and valves; coronary arteries; large artery in arm or leg.

REASONS FOR SURGERY
- Evaluation of chest pain.
- Diagnosis of a congenital heart defect and valvular-heart disease.
- Measurement of the heart muscle's ability to pump blood.
- Identification of narrowing or obstruction in the coronary arteries.

SURGICAL RISK INCREASES WITH
- Stress; obesity; smoking.
- Recent or chronic illness.
- Alcoholism.

WHAT TO EXPECT

WHO OPERATES—Cardiologist.

WHERE PERFORMED—Hospital.

DIAGNOSTIC TESTS
- Before surgery: Blood and urine studies; ECG (see Glossary); chest x-ray.
- During surgery: Intracardiac pressures; cardiac output; cinematography; fluoroscopy; ECG (see Glossary for all).
- After surgery: ECG; blood studies.

ANESTHESIA—Local anesthesia by injection; usually accompanied by sedation.

DESCRIPTION OF OPERATION
- The cardiac catheter is inserted into an artery in the patient's arm or leg. Fluoroscopy provides guidance for the catheter to pass through the artery to the heart.
- Blood-pressure readings are taken, and the heart's ability to pump blood is tested.
- The catheter is guided into the coronary-artery system. Dye is injected through the catheter and into the coronary arteries. Multiple images will be taken to allow identification of any disease in the coronary arteries.
- When all examinations have been completed, the catheter is withdrawn, and the artery into which it was inserted is compressed until bleeding stops. If an arm artery was used, it may need to be repaired. A tight bandage is placed over the entry site for the catheter, and you will be expected to keep that area of your body flat for approximately 6 hours.

POSSIBLE COMPLICATIONS
- Excessive bleeding; blood clot in an artery.
- Reaction to dye (allergy).
- Surgical-wound infection.
- Development of hematomas (collections of blood) where skin was pierced to enter artery.
- Heartbeat disturbance; cardiac arrest (rare).
- Blockage of coronary artery (rare) necessitating immediate open-heart procedure.

AVERAGE HOSPITAL STAY—0 to 1 day.

PROBABLE OUTCOME—Expect complete healing without complications. Allow about 2 weeks for recovery from surgery. Urgent surgery is sometimes indicated by procedure.

POSTOPERATIVE CARE

GENERAL MEASURES
- A hard ridge should form beneath the catheter incision site. As it heals, the ridge will gradually recede.
- Use an electric heating pad, a heat lamp or a warm compress to relieve incisional pain.
- Expect discoloration under the skin where the catheter was inserted. It should disappear in 2 weeks.
- Bathe and shower as usual. You may wash the incision gently with mild, unscented soap.
- Between showers, keep the wound dry and covered with a bandage for the first 2 or 3 days after surgery. If a bandage gets wet, change it promptly. Apply nonprescription antibiotic ointment to the wound before applying new bandages.
- If the wound bleeds during the first 24 hours after surgery, press a clean tissue or cloth to it for 10 to 15 minutes continuously.

MEDICATION
- Your doctor may prescribe pain relievers. Don't take prescription pain medication longer than 4 to 7 days. Use only as much as you need.
- You may use nonprescription drugs, such as acetaminophen, for minor pain. Avoid aspirin.

ACTIVITY
- Avoid vigorous exercise for 2 weeks after surgery.
- Resume driving 2 days after returning home.

DIET—No special diet.

CALL YOUR DOCTOR IF

- You experience sudden or severe chest pain.
- Pain, swelling, redness, drainage or bleeding increases in the surgical area.
- You develop signs of infection, including headache, muscle aches, dizziness or a general ill feeling and fever.
- You develop decreased sensation or pain in the limb where artery was entered.

CARDIAC CATHETERIZATION & ANGIOCARDIOGRAPHY

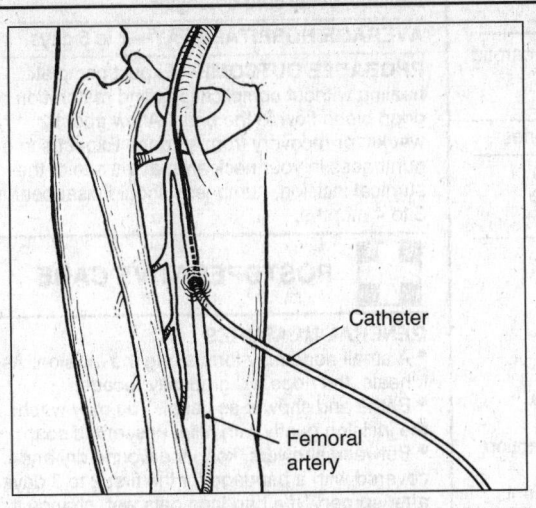

Catheter

Femoral
artery

An illustration of a typical location for catheter insertion in the large artery of the arm. The catheter may also be placed in a large vessel in the leg.
- When the catheter is in place, accurate blood pressure measurements may be made continuously.

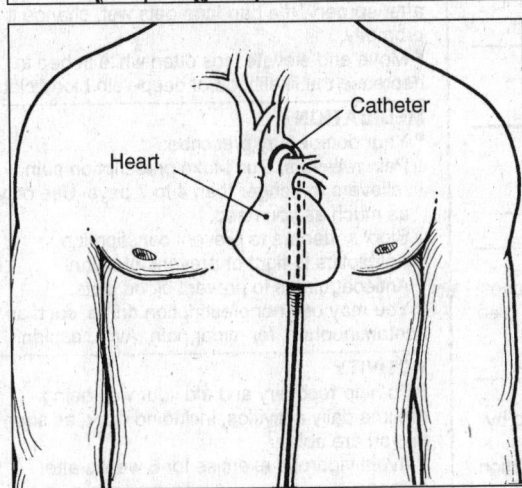

Catheter

Heart

The catheter is guided into the coronary artery system. Pressure readings are made in various chambers of the heart and great blood vessels for later interpretation.

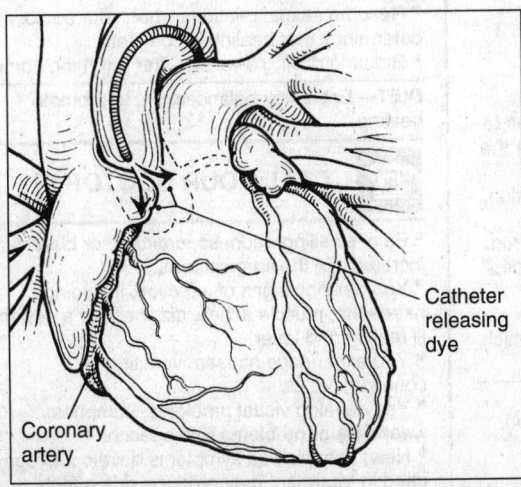

Catheter
releasing
dye

Coronary
artery

Dye is injected through the catheter to fill the coronary arteries to accurately locate any narrowing or obstructions in the coronary artery system.
- When all examinations have been completed, the catheter is withdrawn and the artery it was inserted into is compressed until bleeding stops.

CAROTID ARTERY ENDARTERECTOMY

GENERAL INFORMATION

DEFINITION—Removal of obstruction in carotid (neck) artery usually due to hardening of arteries (arteriosclerosis).

BODY PARTS INVOLVED—Carotid arteries.

REASONS FOR SURGERY—Prevention of stroke and transient ischemic attacks (see Glossary).

SURGICAL RISK INCREASES WITH
- Adults over 60.
- Stress; obesity; smoking.
- Poor nutrition.
- Excess alcohol consumption.
- Recent or chronic illness
- Atherosclerosis; coronary artery disease.
- Diabetes mellitus.
- Use of some prescription and nonprescription drugs. Inform your doctor of any drugs, medications, or vitamin and herb supplements you are using or have used in the last month.

WHAT TO EXPECT

WHO OPERATES—General surgeon, neurosurgeon, cardiovascular surgeon, or peripheral vascular surgeon.

WHERE PERFORMED—Hospital.

DIAGNOSTIC TESTS
- Before surgery: Blood and urine studies; chest x-ray; ECG; arteriograms; CT scan of head (see Glossary for all).
- After surgery: Blood studies.

ANESTHESIA
- Local anesthetic by injection accompanied by sedation.
- General anesthesia by injection and inhalation with an airway tube placed in the windpipe.

DESCRIPTION OF OPERATION
- An incision is made in the neck over the obstruction.
- The obstructed area is isolated. A tube is often placed in the carotid artery and is used to circulate blood around the obstruction while the blockage is being cleared.
- A small incision is made over the obstruction, which is scraped away. The opened area is sometimes patched with a graft fashioned from a vein from another part of the body or a cloth-like material.
- The temporary bypass tube is removed.
- The skin is closed with sutures or clips, which usually can be removed in 2 weeks.

POSSIBLE COMPLICATIONS
- Excessive bleeding; hematoma (blood clot).
- Surgical-wound infection.
- Stroke; heart problems; pneumonia.

- Inadvertent injury to a branch of the nerves to the face, vocal cord or tongue.

AVERAGE HOSPITAL STAY—2 to 5 days.

PROBABLE OUTCOME—Expect complete healing without complications and restoration of good blood flow to the brain. Allow about 2 weeks for recovery from surgery. Expect some numbness in your neck area at the site of the surgical incision; numbness should disappear in 3 to 4 months.

POSTOPERATIVE CARE

GENERAL MEASURES
- A small ridge may form along the incision. As it heals, the ridge will gradually recede.
- Bathe and shower as usual. You may wash the incision gently with mild, unscented soap.
- Between showers, keep the wound dry and covered with a bandage for the first 2 to 3 days after surgery. If a bandage gets wet, change it promptly.
- Move and elevate legs often while in bed to decrease the likelihood of deep-vein blood clots.

MEDICATION
- Your doctor may prescribe:
  Pain relievers. Don't take prescription pain relievers for longer than 4 to 7 days. Use only as much as you need.
  Stool softeners to prevent constipation.
  Antibiotics to fight or prevent infection.
  Anticoagulants to prevent blood clots.
- You may use nonprescription drugs, such as acetaminophen, for minor pain. Avoid aspirin.

ACTIVITY
- To help recovery and aid your well-being, resume daily activities, including work, as soon as you are able.
- Avoid vigorous exercise for 6 weeks after surgery.
- Resume sexual relations when your doctor determines that healing is complete.
- Resume driving 3 weeks after returning home.

DIET—Eat a well-balanced diet to promote healing.

CALL YOUR DOCTOR IF

- Pain, swelling, redness, drainage or bleeding increases in the surgical area.
- You develop signs of infection, including headache, muscle aches, dizziness or a general ill feeling and fever.
- You experience nausea, vomiting or constipation.
- You develop visual problems, numbness, weakness or problems with speech.
- New, unexplained symptoms develop. Drugs used in treatment may produce side effects.

CAROTID ARTERY ENDARTERECTOMY

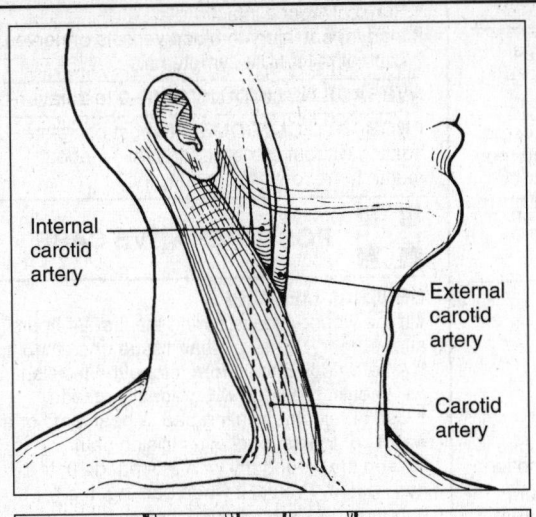

Illustration shows the anatomical locations of the carotid artery, external carotid artery and internal carotid artery.

Internal carotid artery

External carotid artery

Carotid artery

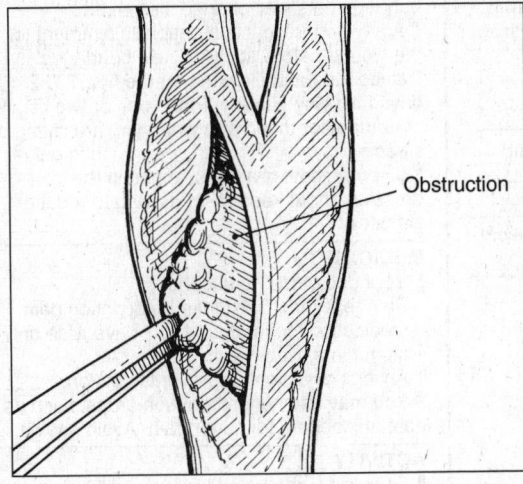

The arterial debris causing the obstruction (which was located by previous special studies) is removed.

Obstruction

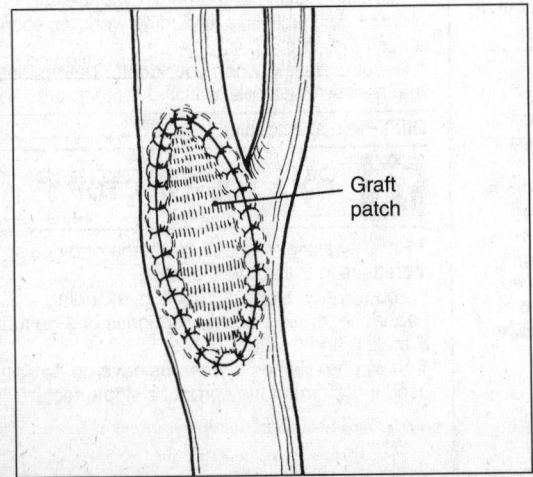

A patch is grafted in place to close the artery that has been cleared of obstruction.

Graft patch

CARPAL-TUNNEL SYNDROME REPAIR

 ## GENERAL INFORMATION

DEFINITION—Cutting the transverse carpal ligament, the fibrous tissue extending across the wrist.

BODY PARTS INVOLVED—Transverse carpal ligament; median nerve and surrounding fibrous tissue; wrist joint.

REASONS FOR SURGERY—Relief of pain or numbness caused by compression of the median nerve.

SURGICAL RISK INCREASES WITH
- Obesity.
- Smoking.
- Poor nutrition.
- Recent or chronic illness.
- Alcoholism.
- Diabetes mellitus.
- Use of some prescription and nonprescription drugs. Inform your doctor of any drugs, medications, or vitamin and herb supplements you are using or have used in the last month.

 ## WHAT TO EXPECT

WHO OPERATES—Hand surgeon, general surgeon, orthopedist or plastic and reconstructive surgeon.

WHERE PERFORMED—Hospital or outpatient surgical facility.

DIAGNOSTIC TESTS
- Before surgery: Blood and urine studies; x-rays of wrist; nerve-conduction tests (see Glossary).
- After surgery: Blood studies.

ANESTHESIA
- Local anesthesia by injection.
- Regional anesthesia by injection.
- General anesthesia by injection and inhalation with an airway tube placed in the windpipe.

DESCRIPTION OF OPERATION
- A tourniquet is applied above the wrist to prevent bleeding in the surgical area.
- An incision is made in the underside of the wrist.
- The transverse carpal ligament is located and cut, releasing the compressed median nerve.
- The skin is closed with fine sutures, which usually can be removed about 10 days after surgery. Absorbable stitches are not removed.
- A bandage is applied, and a splint is used to hold the wrist in position. In some instances, the stitched wound may be left uncovered.

POSSIBLE COMPLICATIONS
- Excessive bleeding.
- Surgical-wound infection.
- Inadvertent injury to blood vessels or nerves.
- Lack of relief from symptoms.

AVERAGE HOSPITAL STAY—0 to 1 day.

PROBABLE OUTCOME—Expect complete healing without complications. Allow about 1 month for recovery from surgery.

 ## POSTOPERATIVE CARE

GENERAL MEASURES
- If the wound bleeds during the first 24 hours after surgery, press a clean tissue or cloth to it.
- A hard ridge should form along the incision. As it heals, the ridge will gradually recede.
- Use an electric heating pad, a heat lamp or a warm compress to relieve incision pain.
- Keep the wound dry with a bandage until it has healed. Protect it when bathing. If a bandage gets wet, change it promptly.
- Apply nonprescription antibiotic ointment to the wound before applying new bandages.
- Keep the hand elevated for the first 1 to 2 days following surgery. Place one or two pillows under the hand and arm when you are sitting or sleeping.
- If your fingers are not wrapped in the dressing, try to keep them moving to reduce stiffness.

MEDICATION
- Your doctor may prescribe:
  Pain relievers. Don't take prescription pain medication longer than 4 to 7 days. Use only as much as you need.
  Antibiotics to fight or prevent infection.
- You may use nonprescription drugs, such as acetaminophen, for minor pain. Avoid aspirin.

ACTIVITY
- To help recovery and aid your well-being, resume daily activities, including work, as soon as you are able.
- Resume driving when your doctor determines that healing is complete.

DIET—No special diet.

 ## CALL YOUR DOCTOR IF

- Pain, swelling, redness, drainage or bleeding increases in the surgical area.
- You develop signs of infection, including headache, muscle aches, dizziness or a general ill feeling and fever.
- New, unexplained symptoms develop. Drugs used in treatment may produce side effects.

CARPAL-TUNNEL SYNDROME REPAIR

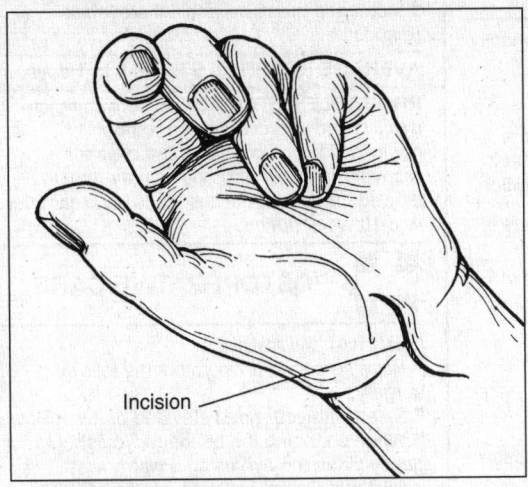

An illustration of the incision site at the wrist area where compression of the median nerve occurs.

Incision

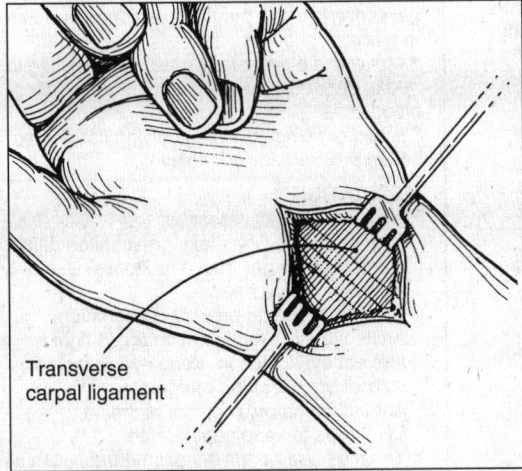

After the skin is incised, the transverse carpal ligament is exposed.

Transverse carpal ligament

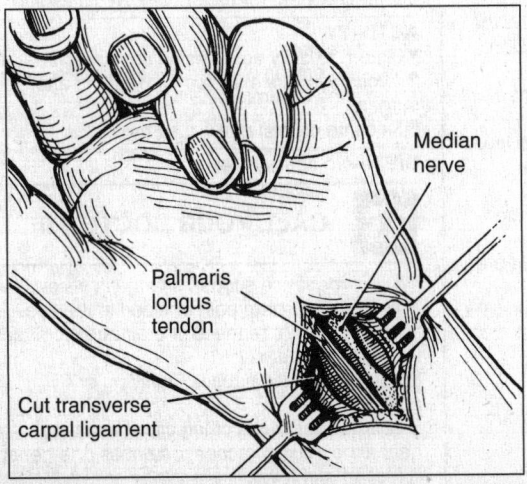

Carpal ligament is located and cut, releasing the compressed median nerve. This usually cures symptoms.

Median nerve

Palmaris longus tendon

Cut transverse carpal ligament

CATARACT EXTRACTION

 GENERAL INFORMATION

DEFINITION—Removal of cataracts, an opacity or clouding of the lens of the eye. This procedure is almost always performed in conjunction with an intraocular (within the eye) lens implant. Several surgical techniques are available; the doctor will choose the one that is most appropriate to your age and eye condition.

BODY PARTS INVOLVED—Eye; cornea; lens; eyelid membrane lining.

REASONS FOR SURGERY—Restoration of normal or near-normal vision.

SURGICAL RISK INCREASES WITH
- Obesity; smoking.
- Newborns and infants.
- Recent or chronic illness.
- Diabetes mellitus.
- Use of some prescription and nonprescription drugs. Inform your doctor of any drugs, medications, or vitamin and herb supplements you are using or have used in the last month.

 WHAT TO EXPECT

WHO OPERATES—Ophthalmologist.

WHERE PERFORMED—Hospital or outpatient facility.

DIAGNOSTIC TESTS
- Before surgery: Blood and urine studies; eye examinations; ultrasound (see Glossary).
- After surgery: Eye examinations.

ANESTHESIA—Local anesthesia by injection. One injection prevents eyelid blinking and another one immobilizes the eyeball.

DESCRIPTION OF OPERATION
- A special instrument is used to hold the eyelids apart.
- A small incision is made in the cornea and the diseased lens is removed through the incision. Often, the lens is first fragmented with ultrasound and the debris is simply suctioned away.
- An artificial lens, known as an intraocular lens, is usually inserted in the eye to replace the discarded lens.
- Few or no stitches are required to close the wound.
- Pilocarpine or atropine eye-drop solutions are placed in the eye to keep the pupil open. Bandages are applied.

POSSIBLE COMPLICATIONS
- Surgical-wound infection.
- Postoperative inflammation.
- Lens capsule thickens causing hazy or cloudy vision.
- Dislocation of intraocular lens implant.

- Astigmatism.
- Retinal detachment.
- Increased pressure within the eyeball (glaucoma).

AVERAGE HOSPITAL STAY—0 to 1 days.

PROBABLE OUTCOME—Expect complete healing and improved vision without complications. Allow about 3-4 days for recovery from surgery. Vision may remain blurred for awhile, but will gradually clear over a 4 to 10 week period.

 POSTOPERATIVE CARE

GENERAL MEASURES
- Have someone drive you home following surgery.
- Sleep with your head elevated on two pillows.
- When changing the bandage, you should gently clean the eye using a warm, wet washcloth. Do not press or rub the eye. The new bandage can then be positioned and taped in place.
- Move and elevate legs often while resting in bed to decrease the likelihood of deep-vein blood clots.
- Avoid bending, straining or lying flat. These cause pressure inside the eye.

MEDICATION
- Your doctor may prescribe:
  Pain relievers. Don't take prescription pain medication longer than 4 to 7 days. Use only as much as you need.
  Stool softeners to prevent constipation.
  Antibiotic eye drops or ointment to fight or prevent eye infection. Keep eye drops cold, but not frozen, in the refrigerator.
  Anti-inflammatory drops or ointment.
  Eye drops to keep pupil dilated.
- You may use nonprescription drugs, such as acetaminophen, for minor pain. Avoid aspirin.

ACTIVITY
- Return to daily activities as soon as possible.
- Avoid vigorous exercise for 6 weeks after surgery.
- Resume driving as advised by doctor.

DIET—No special diet.

 CALL YOUR DOCTOR IF

- You experience sudden change in vision.
- You have a sharp pain or blood in the eye.
- Pain, swelling, redness or drainage increases in the surgical area.
- You experience nausea, vomiting or constipation.
- You develop signs of infection, including headache, muscle aches, dizziness or a general ill feeling and fever.

CATARACT EXTRACTION

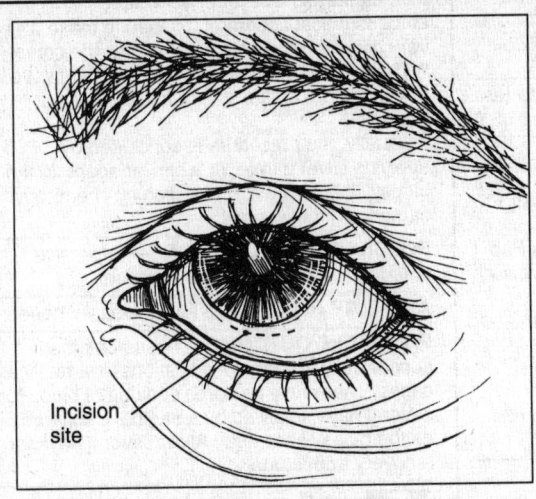

Surgical incision site below the iris.

Incision
site

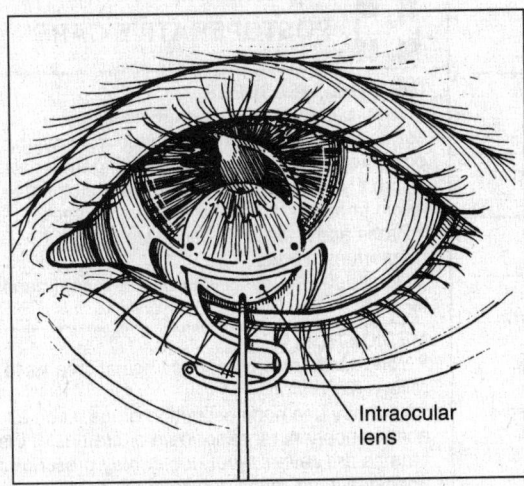

The diseased lens is removed and an
intraocular lens is inserted.

Intraocular
lens

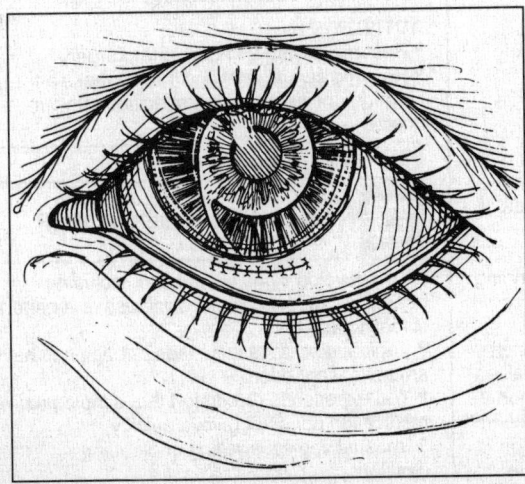

Artificial lens is in place. Incision is
closed with fine sutures.

CERVIX, BIOPSY OF

GENERAL INFORMATION

DEFINITION—Removal of tissue from the cervix (the lower third of the uterus).

BODY PARTS INVOLVED—Cervix; vagina (as route for surgery).

REASONS FOR SURGERY
• Investigation of diseases of the cervix. Laboratory examination of the removed tissue aids in diagnosis.
• Usually follows a visual examination or a Pap smear (see Glossary) of the cervix that revealed a possible abnormality (dysplasia).
• May be done for exploratory purposes for conditions such as infertility.
• Sometimes done as a follow-up in women who have previously been treated for early cervical cancer or dysplasia (atypical cells) of the cervix.

SURGICAL RISK INCREASES WITH
• Previous bleeding disorders.
• Use of drugs such as anticoagulants or aspirin.

WHAT TO EXPECT

WHO OPERATES—Obstetrician-gynecologist, family doctor or general surgeon.

WHERE PERFORMED—Doctor's office or outpatient surgical facility.

DIAGNOSTIC TESTS
• Before surgery: Pap smear (see Glossary); pelvic exam; blood and urine tests.
• During surgery: Your doctor may stain the cervix before removing any sample tissue. Areas that do not hold the stain are the most important ones to examine. The staining is harmless and painless.
• After surgery: Laboratory examination of removed tissue.

ANESTHESIA—Local anesthesia by injection.

DESCRIPTION OF OPERATION
• A speculum is inserted into the vagina to hold it open and to bring the cervix into view.
• Your physician may perform a colposcopic biopsy, in which a slender, optical instrument with a lighted tip is used to pinpoint the areas of the cervix to be biopsied.
• Another instrument is used to gather the tissue. The instrument used will vary, depending on the type of biopsy being performed. In a punch biopsy, the clinician will use a small instrument resembling a paper punch to punch out a small sample of cervical tissue; several punches may be necessary. Another common form of biopsy uses a curette (a thin, metal instrument with a spoon-shaped tip) to scrape tissue from the cervix. Still another technique

that may be used is called LEEP (loop excision electrosurgical procedure). In this procedure, a thin, hand-held wire loop, activated by an electrosurgical generator, is used to make a very precise and uniform cut across the cervix.
• The instruments are removed and the tissue is then sent to a laboratory for microscopic analysis.
• Usually, the procedure is concluded by applying silver nitrate, or a similar agent, to the biopsy sites to prevent bleeding by chemically cauterizing the wounds.

POSSIBLE COMPLICATIONS—Excessive bleeding or surgical-wound infection.

AVERAGE HOSPITAL STAY—Usually none.

PROBABLE OUTCOME—Tissue obtained successfully without complications in virtually all cases. There may be some spotting of blood for several days, followed by a vaginal discharge, as the biopsy sites heal. Allow several days for recovery from surgery.

POSTOPERATIVE CARE

GENERAL MEASURES
• Wear cotton panties or pantyhose with a cotton crotch. Avoid panties made from nylon, polyester, silk or other nonventilating materials.
• Use a sanitary pad to protect your clothing. Avoid tampons, as they may lead to infection.
• Bathe and shower as usual. Use only nonperfumed soap.
• Don't douche unless your doctor recommends it.

MEDICATION
• Your doctor may prescribe vaginal creams to relieve discomfort.
• You may use nonprescription drugs, such as acetaminophen, for minor pain or cramps. If the cramps are severe, your doctor may prescribe additional medication to relieve the pain.

ACTIVITY
• Resume driving 24 hours after surgery.
• Resume sexual relations 1 to 2 weeks after surgery, unless otherwise specified by your doctor.

DIET—No special diet.

CALL YOUR DOCTOR IF

• You develop signs of infection, including headache, muscle aches, dizziness or a general ill feeling and fever.
• Vaginal discharge increases or begins to have an unpleasant odor.
• You experience discomfort that simple pain medication does not relieve quickly.
• Unusual vaginal swelling or bleeding develops.

CERVIX, BIOPSY OF

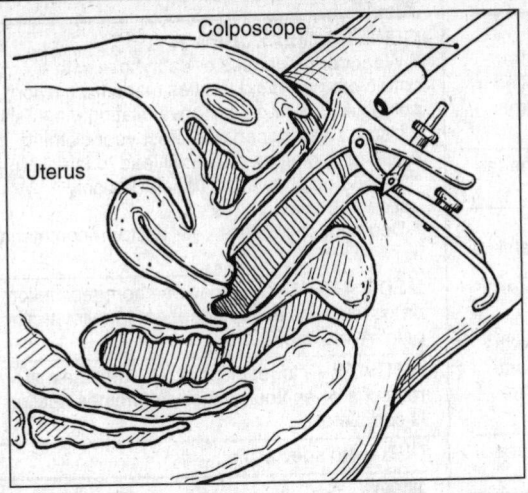

Colposcope

Uterus

Side view of the vagina, cervix and uterus. This illustration shows a speculum inserted into the vagina to stretch it open and expose the cervix (the lower third of the uterus). A colposcope is used to pinpoint the areas to be biopsied.

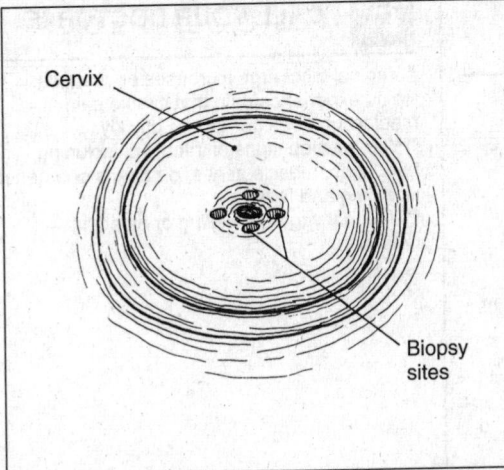

Cervix

Biopsy sites

A closer view of the cervix shows the different sites where biopsies are taken. Biopsy sites are usually chosen on the basis of the appearance of the cervix.

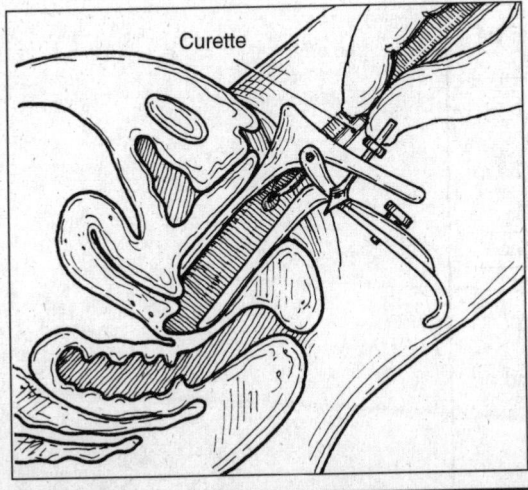

Curette

A curette is inserted and is used to remove small amounts of tissue in the suspected areas of the cervix.

SURGERIES

CERVIX, CRYOSURGERY OF

GENERAL INFORMATION

DEFINITION—Destruction of abnormal (infected or damaged) cells in the cervix, the lower third of the uterus. An instrument called a cryosurgery probe is used to freeze abnormal cells with liquid nitrogen.

BODY PARTS INVOLVED—Cervix; vagina (as route for surgery).

REASONS FOR SURGERY
- Primary treatment of mild to moderate cervical dysplasia (abnormal cell growth).
- Sometimes used to treat severe cervical dysplasia.
- Treatment of benign (noncancerous) growths on the cervix (such as polyps) or genital warts.
- Treatment of cervicitis (inflammation of the cervix).

SURGICAL RISK INCREASES WITH—None expected.

WHAT TO EXPECT

WHO OPERATES—Obstetrician-gynecologist, family doctor or general surgeon.

WHERE PERFORMED—Doctor's office or outpatient surgical facility.

DIAGNOSTIC TESTS
- Before surgery: Pap smear (see Glossary); vaginal exam.
- After surgery: Pap smear in 2 to 3 months.

ANESTHESIA—Usually none.

DESCRIPTION OF OPERATION
- A speculum is inserted into the vagina to hold it open and to bring the cervix into view.
- The cryosurgery probe is held on the affected areas long enough to freeze and destroy abnormal cells.
- The instruments are removed. Discomfort during surgery may vary from one person to the next but should not cause much distress.

POSSIBLE COMPLICATIONS
- Surgical wound infection (rare).
- Cervical stenosis (narrowing).
- Failure of the procedure to destroy all of the cervical dysplasia, particularly with severe dysplasia.

AVERAGE HOSPITAL STAY—Usually none.

PROBABLE OUTCOME—Expect complete healing without complications. You may experience mild uterine cramping and facial flushing. Vaginal discharge is common; discharge may be profuse, foul-smelling, and last for 7 to 10 days or longer. Allow about 3 weeks for recovery from surgery.

POSTOPERATIVE CARE

GENERAL MEASURES
- Wear cotton panties or pantyhose with a cotton crotch. Avoid panties made from nylon, polyester, silk or other nonventilating materials.
- Use a sanitary pad to protect your clothing. Avoid tampons, as they may lead to infection.
- Bathe and shower as usual. Use only unscented soap.
- Don't douche unless your doctor recommends it.

MEDICATION—You may use nonprescription drugs, such as acetaminophen, to relieve minor pain. Avoid aspirin.

ACTIVITY—No restrictions. Resume sexual relations when your doctor determines healing is complete.

DIET—No special diet.

CALL YOUR DOCTOR IF

- Vaginal discharge increases or changes.
- You experience pain that simple pain medication does not relieve quickly.
- You develop signs of infection, including headache, muscle aches, dizziness or a general ill feeling and fever.
- Unusual vaginal swelling or bleeding develops.

CERVIX, CRYOSURGERY OF

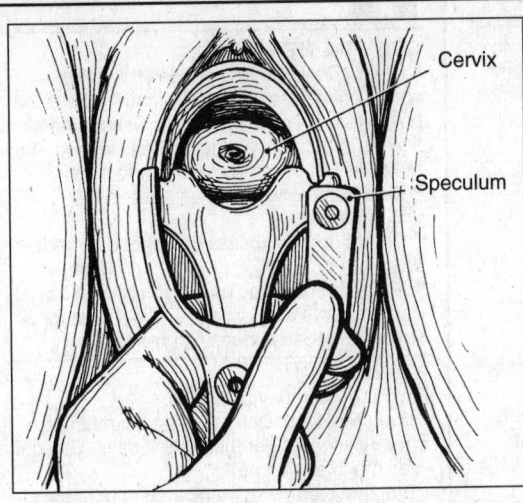

Cervix

Speculum

This view illustrates a female patient with extended legs in stirrups on an examining table to allow examination of the genital area.
• The speculum is inserted into the vagina to stretch it open and expose the cervix.

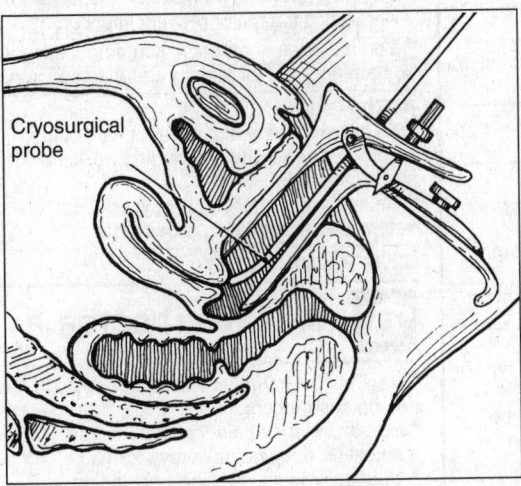

Cryosurgical probe

A side view of the pelvic structures.
• The cryosurgery probe, which has been brought to temperatures well below zero, is held on the affected areas long enough to freeze and destroy the abnormal cervical cells.

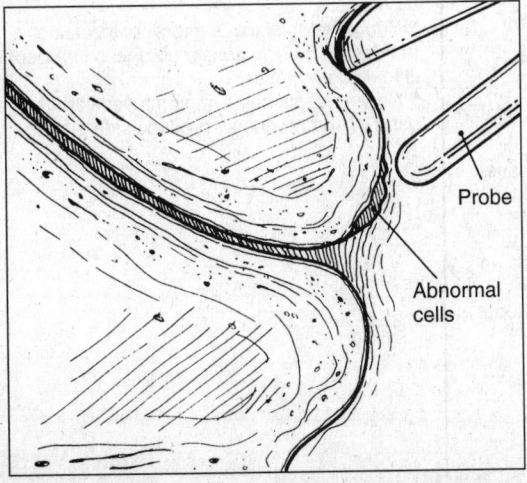

Probe

Abnormal cells

Probe removed after suspicious cells have been destroyed.

SURGERIES

CERVIX, ELECTROCAUTERIZATION OF

 GENERAL INFORMATION

DEFINITION—Destruction of abnormal (infected or damaged) cells in the cervix, in the lower third of the uterus. An instrument called an electrocautery uses electric current to destroy the abnormal tissue.

BODY PARTS INVOLVED—Cervix; vagina (as route for surgery).

REASONS FOR SURGERY
- Presence of abnormal cells in the cervix.
- Inflammation or infection of the cervix.

SURGICAL RISK INCREASES WITH
- Diabetes mellitus.
- Use of some prescription and nonprescription drugs. Inform your doctor of any drugs, medications, or vitamin and herb supplements you are using or have used in the last month.

 WHAT TO EXPECT

WHO OPERATES—Obstetrician-gynecologist, general surgeon or family doctor.

WHERE PERFORMED—Doctor's office or outpatient surgical facility.

DIAGNOSTIC TESTS
- Before surgery: Pap smear (see Glossary); vaginal-discharge study.
- After surgery: Vaginal-discharge study; Pap smear in about 2 months.

ANESTHESIA—Usually none.

DESCRIPTION OF OPERATION
- A speculum is inserted into the vagina to hold it open and to bring the cervix into view.
- The electrocautery probe is inserted into the cervix. The flow of electric current is applied through the probe to destroy abnormal cells. You may experience some mild cramping.
- The instruments are removed. Discomfort after surgery will vary from one person to another, but any pain or cramping should be minor.

POSSIBLE COMPLICATIONS
- Surgical-wound infection.
- Inadvertent damage to normal vaginal tissue.
- Cervical stenosis (narrowing).

AVERAGE HOSPITAL STAY—None

PROBABLE OUTCOME—Healing requires up to 2 months. During this time, you will have a frequent, watery vaginal discharge. Allow about 6 weeks for recovery from surgery.

 POSTOPERATIVE CARE

GENERAL MEASURES
- Wear cotton panties or pantyhose with a cotton crotch. Avoid panties made from nylon, polyester, silk or other nonventilating materials.
- Wear a sanitary pad to protect clothing. Avoid tampons, as they may lead to infection.
- Bathe or shower as usual. Use mild, unscented soap.
- Do not douche unless prescribed by your doctor.
- Following this procedure, you should have a Pap smear (see Glossary) twice a year for 2 years, and then annually thereafter.

MEDICATION
- Your doctor may prescribe:
  Pain relievers. Don't take prescription pain medication longer than 4 to 7 days. Use only as much as you need.
  Vaginal creams or medicated douches.
  Antibiotics to fight or prevent infection.
- You may use nonprescription drugs, such as acetaminophen, for minor pain. Avoid aspirin.

ACTIVITY
- To help recovery and aid your well-being, resume daily activities, including work, as soon as you are able.
- Delay sexual relations until your doctor determines that healing is complete.

DIET—No special diet.

 CALL YOUR DOCTOR IF

- Vaginal discharge increases or begins to have an unpleasant odor.
- You experience pain that simple pain medication does not relieve quickly.
- Unusual vaginal swelling or bleeding develops.
- You develop signs of infection, including headache, muscle aches, dizziness or a general ill feeling and fever.
- New, unexplained symptoms develop. Drugs used in treatment may produce side effects.

CERVIX, ELECTROCAUTERIZATION OF

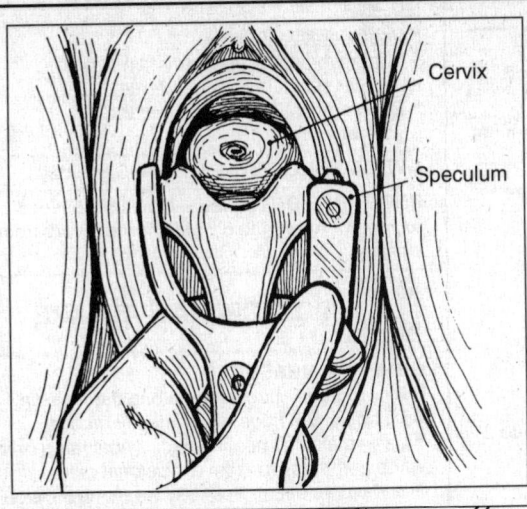

Cervix

Speculum

This view illustrates a female patient with extended legs in stirrups on an examining table to allow examination of the genital area.
- The speculum is inserted into the vagina to stretch it open and expose the cervix.

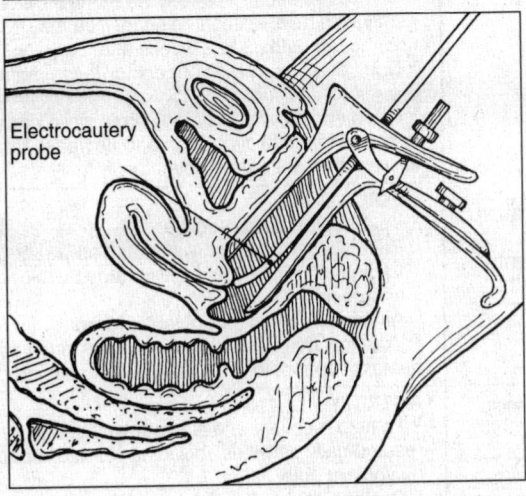

Electrocautery probe

A side view of the pelvic structures showing the speculum in the vagina.
- The electrocautery probe is inserted through the speculum to reach the uterine opening in the cervical area.

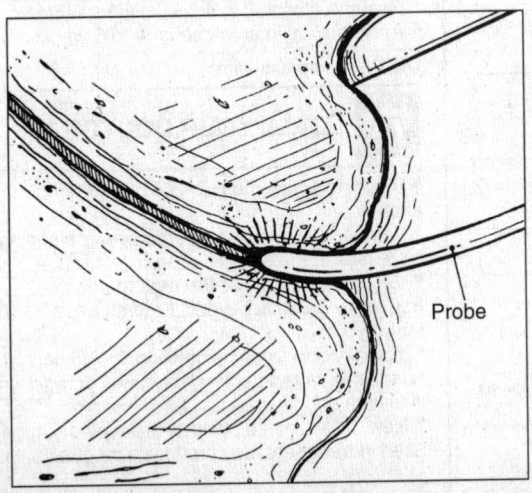

Probe

A view showing the electrocautery probe touching abnormal cervical cells. A flow of electric current is applied through the electrocautery probe to destroy the cells.

CESAREAN SECTION

GENERAL INFORMATION

DEFINITION—Delivery of a baby through an incision in the mother's lower abdominal and uterine walls.

BODY PARTS INVOLVED—Uterus; abdominal wall; placenta; placental membranes; fetus.

REASONS FOR SURGERY—Danger to the mother or baby from one or more of many causes, including:
- Baby's head too large to pass through the birth canal.
- Breech presentation (see Glossary).
- Insufficient contractions of the uterus.
- Abnormal attachment of placenta.
- Severe pre-eclampsia (see Glossary).
- Fetal distress.
- Failure of normal labor in a patient who had a previous cesarean section.
- Acute herpes genitalis infection.

SURGICAL RISK INCREASES WITH
- Obesity; smoking; poor nutrition.
- Excess alcohol consumption.
- Placenta previa with excessive blood loss.
- Pre-eclampsia or eclampsia of pregnancy (see Glossary for both).
- Prior cesarean section.
- Chronic heart or lung disease.
- Use of some prescription and nonprescription drugs. Inform your doctor of any drugs, medications, or vitamin and herb supplements you are using or have used in the last month.

WHAT TO EXPECT

WHO OPERATES—Obstetrician-gynecologist.

WHERE PERFORMED—Hospital.

DIAGNOSTIC TESTS
- Before surgery: Blood and urine studies; sonogram (see Glossary).
- After surgery: Blood and urine studies.

ANESTHESIA
- Local anesthesia by injection
- Spinal anesthesia by injection.
- General anesthesia by injection and inhalation with an airway tube placed in the windpipe (sometimes).

DESCRIPTION OF OPERATION
- An incision is made in the abdomen.
- Another incision is made in the uterus.
- Baby and placenta are removed.
- The uterus is closed and the abdominal contents are replaced. Connective tissue, muscles and skin are closed. The skin is closed with sutures or clips, which usually can be removed 2 to 7 days after surgery.

POSSIBLE COMPLICATIONS
- Excessive bleeding or surgical-wound infection.
- Postoperative anemia.
- Endomyometritis (inflammation of the muscular substance of the uterus).
- Endometritis (inflammation of the endometrium).

AVERAGE HOSPITAL STAY—3 to 5 days.

PROBABLE OUTCOME—No complications expected. Allow 4 to 6 weeks for recovery from surgery.

POSTOPERATIVE CARE

GENERAL MEASURES
- A hard ridge should form along the incision. As it heals, the ridge will gradually recede.
- Use an electric heating pad, a heat lamp or a warm compress to relieve incisional pain.
- Shower as usual. You may wash the incision gently with mild, unscented soap. You may resume tub baths 2 to 3 weeks after surgery.
- Don't douche unless your doctor recommends it.
- Move and elevate your legs often while resting in bed to improve circulation and decrease the likelihood of deep-vein clots.

MEDICATION
- Your doctor may prescribe:
  Pain relievers. Use only as much as you need.
  Vaginal cream, if vaginal discharge develops an unpleasant odor.
  Antibiotics to fight or prevent infection.
- You may use nonprescription drugs, such as acetaminophen, for minor pain. Avoid aspirin.

ACTIVITY
- To help recovery and aid your well-being, resume daily activities, including work, as soon as you are able.
- Resume driving 2 to 4 weeks after surgery.
- Avoid sexual intercourse for 4 to 6 weeks.

DIET—No special diet.

CALL YOUR DOCTOR IF

- Bleeding soaks more than 1 pad or tampon each hour.
- Pain, swelling, redness, drainage or bleeding increases in the surgical area.
- Vaginal discharge or the urge to urinate frequently persists beyond 1 month after surgery.
- You develop signs of infection, including headache, muscle aches, dizziness or a general ill feeling and fever.
- New, unexplained symptoms develop. Drugs used in treatment may produce side effects.

CESAREAN SECTION

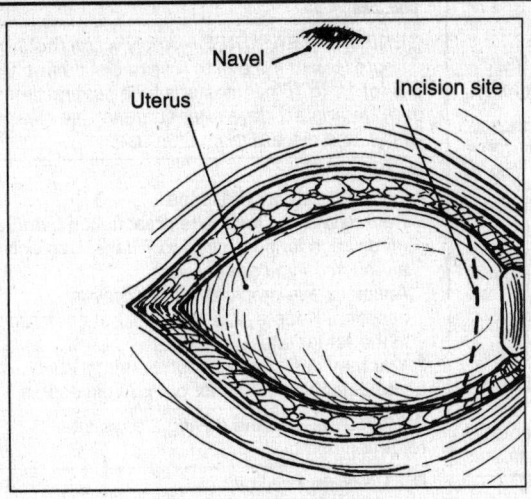

Navel

Uterus

Incision site

An illustration, looking from above, of a patient lying flat on an operating table.
- A vertical incision exposing the uterus, musculature and fatty layer below the skin. Sometimes the incision is a transverse one located just above the area where pubic hair usually ends.

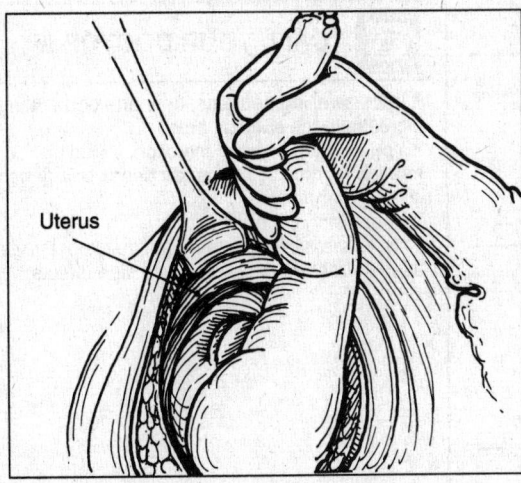

Uterus

Whichever incision site is chosen, it allows exposure of the uterus.
- Another incision is made into the uterus. The baby and the placenta are removed.

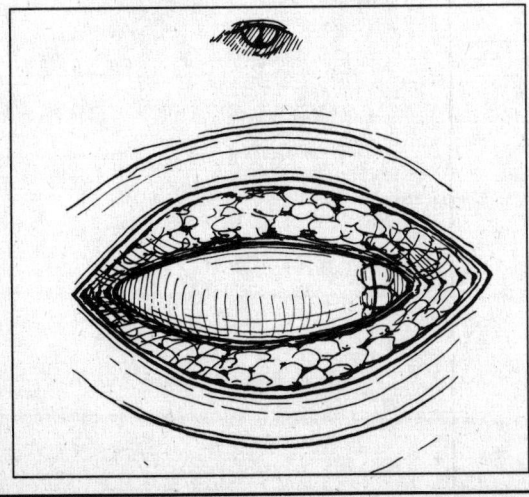

The uterus is closed, followed by closure of connective tissue, muscles and skin of the abdominal wall.

SURGERIES

CHALAZION REMOVAL

 GENERAL INFORMATION

DEFINITION—Removal of a chalazion, a nontender inflammation in the cartilage of the eyelid. Chalazions are caused by a blockage in the meibomian glands (see Glossary).

BODY PARTS INVOLVED—Eyelids (upper or lower); meibomian glands.

REASONS FOR SURGERY—A chalazion is not cancerous or infectious. It is removed to improve appearance or to relieve pressure on an eyeball. Surgery is performed only after simpler treatment has failed.

SURGICAL RISK INCREASES WITH
- Diabetes mellitus.
- Use of some prescription and nonprescription drugs. Inform your doctor of any drugs, medications, or vitamin and herb supplements you are using or have used in the last month.

 WHAT TO EXPECT

WHO OPERATES—Ophthalmologist.

WHERE PERFORMED—Doctor's office or outpatient surgical facility.

DIAGNOSTIC TESTS—Complete eye examination before surgery.

ANESTHESIA—Local anesthesia by injection.

DESCRIPTION OF OPERATION
- The eyelid is turned inside out and held to expose its underside.
- The chalazion is identified.
- An incision is made on the surface of the chalazion.
- The chalazion is cut free and removed.
- The eye is bandaged.

POSSIBLE COMPLICATIONS
- Excessive bleeding.
- Surgical-wound infection.

AVERAGE HOSPITAL STAY—None.

PROBABLE OUTCOME—Expect complete healing without complications. Allow about 1 week for recovery from surgery. Chalazions may recur.

 POSTOPERATIVE CARE

GENERAL MEASURES—Apply warm (not hot) compresses to the eye to relieve discomfort. Do this for 10 to 15 minutes at a time several times daily for about 2 days after surgery. Use clean cloths, and discard them after use.

MEDICATION
- Your doctor may prescribe:
  Pain relievers. Don't take prescription pain medication longer than 4 to 7 days. Use only as much as you need.
  Antibiotic eye drops to fight or prevent infection. Keep eye drops cold, but not frozen, in the refrigerator.
- You may use nonprescription drugs, such as acetaminophen, for minor pain. Avoid aspirin.

ACTIVITY—Resume driving 2 days after returning home.

DIET—No special diet.

 CALL YOUR DOCTOR IF

- Pain, swelling, redness, drainage or bleeding increase in the surgical area.
- You develop signs of infection, including headache, muscle aches, dizziness or a general ill feeling and fever.
- Your vision changes.
- New, unexplained symptoms develop. Drugs used in treatment may produce side effects.

CHALAZION REMOVAL

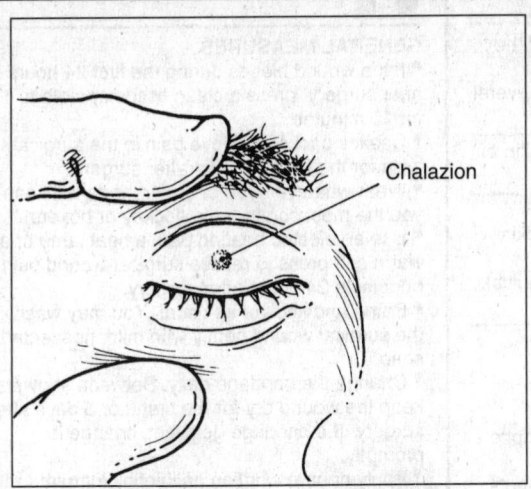

Appearance of the chalazion seen through the eyelid skin.

Chalazion

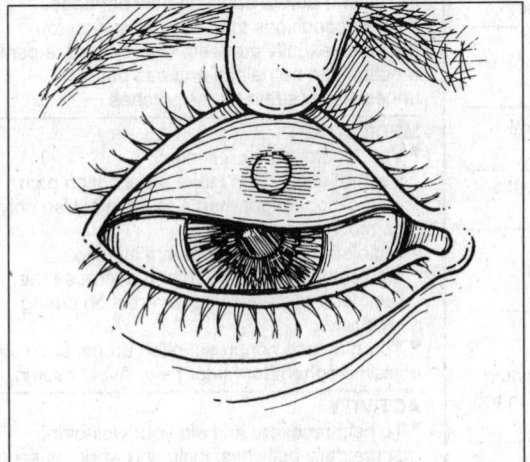

The eyelid is turned inside out and held to expose its underside. The chalazion is identified on the inverted lid.

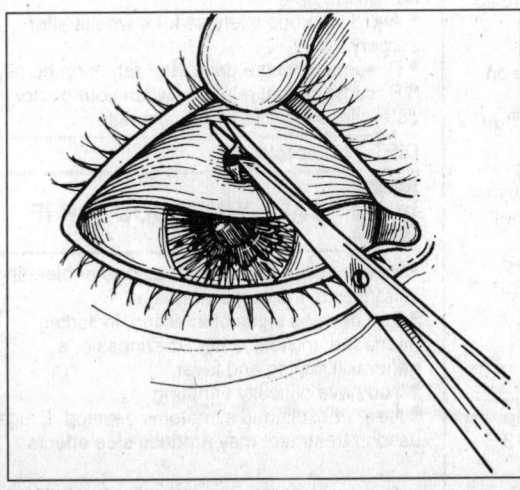

An incision made on the membranous lining of the eyelid allows the chalazion to be cut free and removed.

CIRCUMCISION

 ## GENERAL INFORMATION

DEFINITION—Removal of the foreskin of the penis. This section describes circumcision performed at times other than at birth or several days after birth.

BODY PARTS INVOLVED—Penis; foreskin of the penis.

REASONS FOR SURGERY
- Correction of inability to retract the foreskin completely (phimosis).
- Treatment of infection of the penis (balanitis).
- Urinary tract infection (sometimes).

SURGICAL RISK INCREASES WITH
- Poor nutrition.
- Recent or chronic illness.
- Alcoholism.
- Use of some prescription and nonprescription drugs. Inform your doctor of any drugs, medications, or vitamin and herb supplements you are using or have used in the last month.

 ## WHAT TO EXPECT

WHO OPERATES—Family doctor, general surgeon or urologist.

WHERE PERFORMED—Hospital or outpatient surgical facility.

DIAGNOSTIC TESTS
- Before surgery: Blood and urine studies.
- After surgery: Blood studies.

ANESTHESIA
- Local anesthesia by injection.
- General anesthesia (sometimes) by injection and inhalation with an airway tube placed in the windpipe.

DESCRIPTION OF OPERATION
- The foreskin is carefully retracted from the tip of the penis.
- A clamp is placed under the foreskin.
- The clamped foreskin is slit in two places on the top and bottom of the penis.
- The foreskin between the two slits is cut free and removed.
- The mucous membrane of the foreskin is folded back on itself and sewn to the remaining skin of the penis, usually with sutures that will be absorbed by the body.
- Petroleum jelly and a bandage are applied.

POSSIBLE COMPLICATIONS
- Excessive bleeding
- Surgical-wound infection.

AVERAGE HOSPITAL STAY—0 to 1 day.

PROBABLE OUTCOME—Expect complete healing without complications. Allow about 3 weeks for recovery from surgery.

 ## POSTOPERATIVE CARE

GENERAL MEASURES
- If the wound bleeds during the first 24 hours after surgery, press a clean tissue or cloth to it for 10 minutes.
- Use ice packs to relieve pain in the surgical area for the first 24 hours after surgery.
- Wear whatever type of undershorts will keep you the most comfortable (jockey or boxers).
- Use an electric heating pad, a heat lamp or a warm compress to relieve surgical-wound pain beginning 24 hours after surgery.
- Bathe and shower as usual. You may wash the surgical wound gently with mild, unscented soap.
- Change the bandage daily. Between showers, keep the wound dry for the first 2 or 3 days after surgery. If a bandage gets wet, change it promptly.
- Apply nonprescription antibiotic ointment to the wound before applying new bandages.
- Avoid conditions that may cause you to become sexually aroused. Until healed, a penile erection can be painful and can put unnecessary strain on the stitches.

MEDICATION
- Your doctor may prescribe:
  Pain relievers. Don't take prescription pain medication longer than 4 to 7 days. Use only as much as you need.
  Antibiotics to fight or prevent infection.
  Medications to relax you and decrease the likelihood of developing an erection during recovery.
- You may use nonprescription drugs, such as acetaminophen, for minor pain. Avoid aspirin.

ACTIVITY
- To help recovery and aid your well-being, resume daily activities, including work, as soon as you are able.
- Avoid vigorous exercise for 4 weeks after surgery.
- Resume driving 5 days after returning home.
- Resume sexual relations when your doctor determines that healing is complete.

DIET—No special diet.

 ## CALL YOUR DOCTOR IF

- Pain, swelling, redness, drainage or bleeding increases in the surgical area.
- You develop signs of infection, including headache, muscle aches, dizziness or a general ill feeling and fever.
- You have difficulty urinating.
- New, unexplained symptoms develop. Drugs used in treatment may produce side effects.

CIRCUMCISION

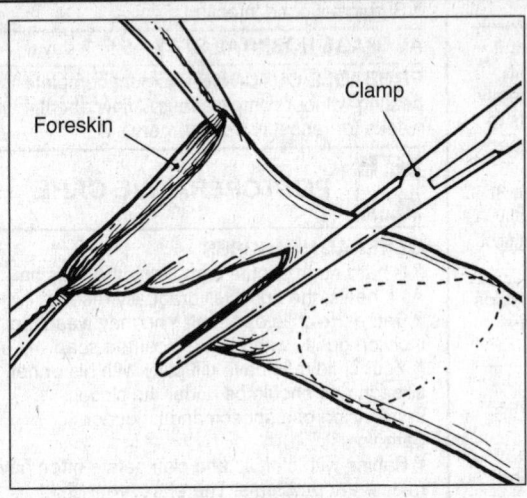

An illustration of the foreskin being carefully retracted and stretched from the tip of the penis with clamps.

Clamp

Foreskin

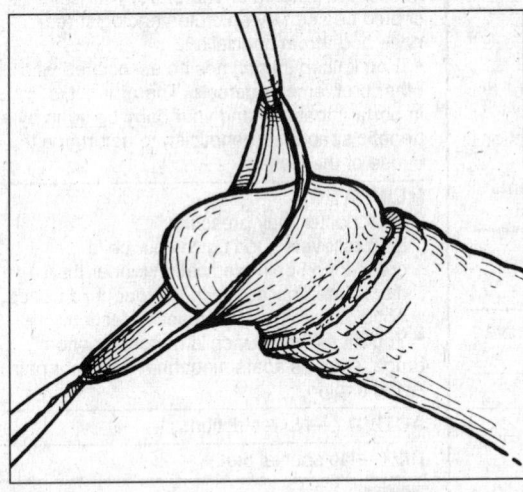

The foreskin between slits is cut free and removed.

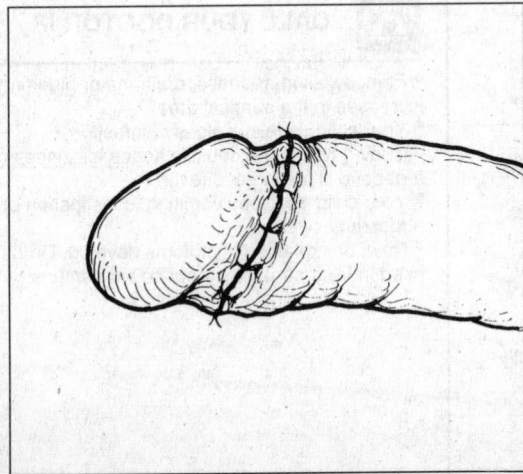

Mucus membrane of foreskin is folded back on itself and sewn to the remaining skin of the penis. Healing is rapid and sutures drop out without painful removal.

SURGERIES

CLEFT LIP REPAIR

 GENERAL INFORMATION

DEFINITION—Repair of a hereditary deformity of the upper lip called a "cleft lip", in which lip, nose and palate structures do not fuse correctly prior to birth. Frequently, this defect extends to the roof of the mouth (palate) and can hamper development of normal speech. Surgery is usually performed when the patient is about 3 months old. If a cleft palate exists, it is usually repaired in a separate surgery when the patient is 12 to 18 months old.

BODY PARTS INVOLVED—Upper lip; muscles surrounding the mouth; membrane lining the mouth; roof of the mouth (palate).

REASONS FOR SURGERY
• Prevention of nursing and feeding problems that can retard normal growth.
• Rearrangement of the distorted tissues to make the lip and palate function normally and appear as normal as possible.

SURGICAL RISK INCREASES WITH
• Other congenital abnormalities.
• Poor nutrition. This often results from inability to nurse properly because of the deformity.
• Use of some prescription and nonprescription drugs. Inform your doctor of any drugs, medications, or vitamin and herb supplements you have given your child in the last month.

 WHAT TO EXPECT

WHO OPERATES—Plastic and reconstructive surgeon.

WHERE PERFORMED—Hospital.

DIAGNOSTIC TESTS
• Before surgery: Blood and urine studies.
• After surgery: Blood studies.

ANESTHESIA
• Local anesthesia by injection.
• General anesthesia by a combination of injection and inhalation with an airway tube placed in the windpipe.

DESCRIPTION OF OPERATION
• The areas are marked where the lip, mouth and palate should be.
• The skin to be relocated is cut free from its underlying tissue. Bleeding is controlled with clamps, medication (epinephrine) or cautery.
• The skin flaps are adjusted to their desired position.
• The muscles and skin edges are reconstructed with fine sutures, which usually can be removed about 7 to 10 days after surgery.

POSSIBLE COMPLICATIONS
• Excessive bleeding.
• Surgical-wound infection.

AVERAGE HOSPITAL STAY—5 to 7 days.

PROBABLE OUTCOME—Expect complete healing without complications. Allow about 4 weeks for recovery from surgery.

 POSTOPERATIVE CARE

GENERAL MEASURES
• A hard ridge should form along the incision. As it heals, the ridge will gradually recede.
• Bathe the child as usual. You may wash the incision gently with mild, unscented soap.
• Your child may have difficulty with his or her speech and should be under the close supervision of a speech and language pathologist.
• Babies with cleft lip and cleft palate often have middle ear problems. Therefore, your child should be seen by an otolaryngologist (ear, nose and throat specialist).
• Cleft lip can sometimes be associated with other problems or defects. Therefore, it is important that you and your baby be seen by a genetic specialist (geneticist) to determine the cause of the cleft lip.

MEDICATION
• Your doctor may prescribe:
Pain relievers. Don't give your child prescription pain medication longer than 4 to 7 days. Use only as much as your child needs. Antibiotics to fight or prevent infection.
• You may give your child nonprescription drugs, such as acetaminophen, for minor pain. Avoid aspirin.

ACTIVITY—No restrictions.

DIET—No special diet.

 CALL YOUR DOCTOR IF

• Pain, swelling, redness, drainage or bleeding increases in the surgical area.
• Your child develops signs of infection, including headache, muscle aches, dizziness or a general ill feeling and fever.
• Your child develops vomiting, constipation or abdominal swelling.
• New, unexplained symptoms develop. Drugs used in treatment may produce side effects.

CLEFT LIP REPAIR

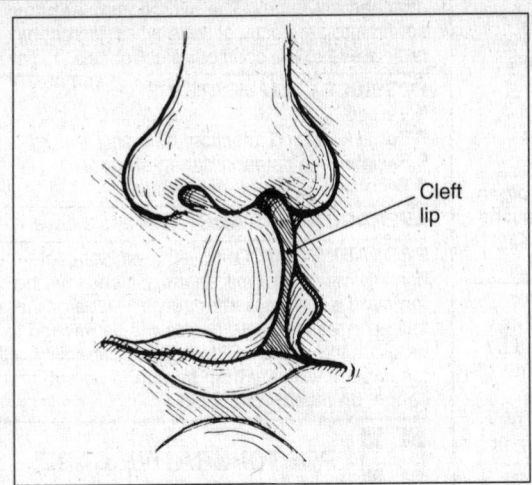

An illustration of mouth and lip skin between the lip and the nose showing the cleft lip deformity.

Cleft lip

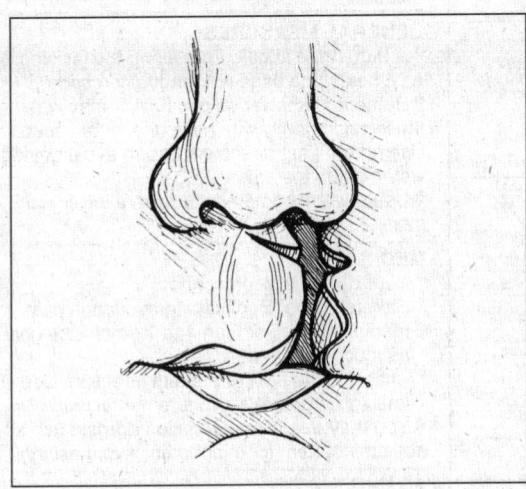

Skin to be relocated is cut free from its underlying tissue.

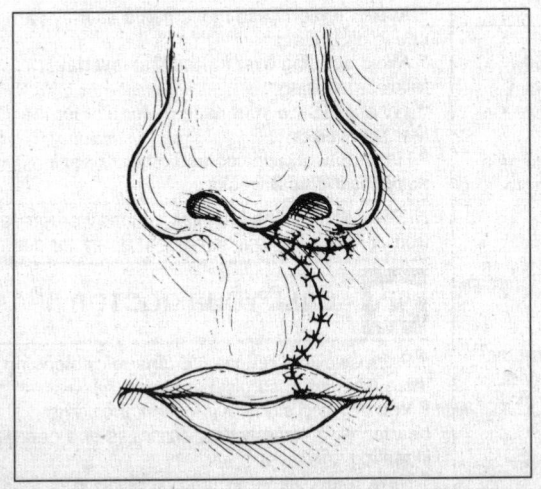

Skin flaps are adjusted to their desired new position and skin edges approximated and sewn.

SURGERIES

COCHLEAR IMPLANT

 GENERAL INFORMATION

DEFINITION—Installation of a microelectronic (tiny electrodes) system designed to improve hearing in some persons with hearing impairments. A cochlear implant consists of 3 parts: a microphone, a microcomputer, and a cochlear electrode.

BODY PARTS INVOLVED—Cochlea (an organ in the inner ear that transforms sound vibrations into nerve impulses for transmission to the brain); skin behind the ear.

REASONS FOR SURGERY—Treatment for profound hearing loss. The sensitive structures within the cochlea may have been damaged by trauma, toxic effect of drugs, or infection. The auditory nerve carrying sound signals to the brain is intact, but it receives no stimulus. The implant provides signals which can be taken up by the auditory nerve. It improves, but cannot restore, normal hearing.

SURGICAL RISK INCREASES WITH
- Recent or chronic illness; diabetes mellitus.
- Use of some prescription and nonprescription drugs. Inform your doctor of any drugs, medications, or vitamin and herb supplements you are using or have used in the last month.

 WHAT TO EXPECT

WHO OPERATES—Ear, nose and throat specialist (otolaryngologist).

WHERE PERFORMED—Hospital.

DIAGNOSTIC TESTS
- Before surgery: Auditory testing.
- After surgery: Auditory testing.

ANESTHESIA—General anesthesia by injection and inhalation, with an airway tube placed in the windpipe.

DESCRIPTION OF OPERATION
- An incision is made behind and slightly above the ear. A burr-type instrument is used to drill a circular hole in the bone for preparation for implanting the internal coil.
- The mastoid bone in the ear is opened to gain access for the electrodes that will be led from the internal coil into the inner ear.
- The internal coil is then positioned in the prepared site and secured with stitches.
- The electrodes are inserted deep in the inner ear.
- Once the surgical wound is healed, an external unit consisting of a stimulator with built-in microphone is provided for wearing behind the ear. It may be attached to eyeglasses or a headband or special magnets between the internal and external components.

- A microcomputer is connected to the microphone by a wire, and is worn in a pouch attached to the belt. The microcomputer turns sound into an electrical code which is sent by radio wave to the cochlear electrodes.

POSSIBLE COMPLICATIONS
- Vertigo.
- Surgical-wound infection; bleeding.
- Facial nerve damage during surgery.
- Technical failure of the implant.

AVERAGE HOSPITAL STAY—2 to 3 days.

PROBABLE OUTCOME—Expect complete healing without complications. Stitches will be removed a few days after surgery. One or more follow up visits to your doctor will be needed to program the implant. The hearing capability with the implant will vary from person to person and cannot be reliably predicted.

 POSTOPERATIVE CARE

GENERAL MEASURES
- A hard ridge should form along the incision. As it heals, the ridge will gradually recede.
- Bathe and shower as usual. You may wash the incision gently with mild, unscented soap. Use an ear plug or shower cap to avoid getting water inside the ear.
- Use a warm compress to relieve incisional pain.

MEDICATION
- Your doctor may prescribe:
  Pain relievers. Don't take prescription pain medication longer than 4 to 7 days. Use only as much as you need.
  Antibiotics to fight or prevent infection. Use antibiotics before any future dental work.
- You may use nonprescription drugs, such as acetaminophen, for minor pain. Avoid aspirin.

ACTIVITY
- Avoid sudden head movements as they can cause dizziness.
- Avoid bending over for the first few days following surgery.
- Try not to blow your nose or sneeze for the first two weeks.
- Resume work, driving and other normal activities in 2 to 3 weeks.

DIET—While in the hospital, you may progress from a liquid diet to a soft diet to a regular diet.

 CALL YOUR DOCTOR IF

- Pain, swelling, redness, drainage or bleeding increases in the surgical area.
- You develop signs of infection, including headache, muscle aches, dizziness or a general ill feeling and fever.
- New, unexplained symptoms develop.

COCHLEAR IMPLANT

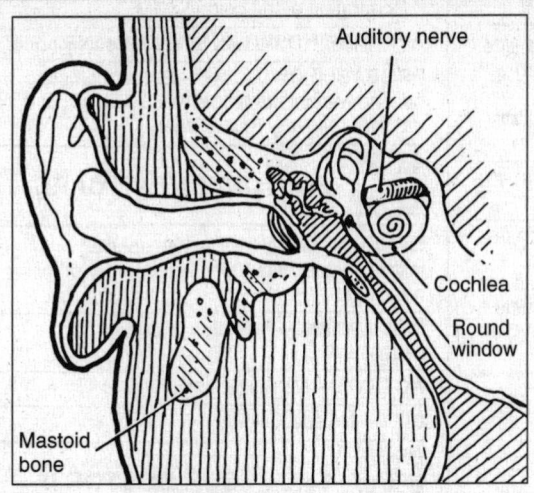

Illustration demonstrating anatomy of the ear where the implant is inserted.

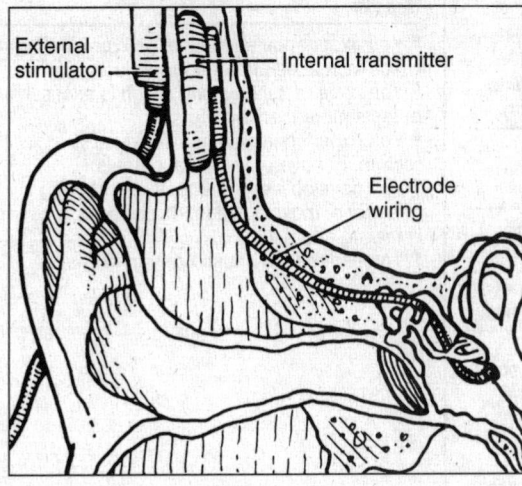

Cochlear implant devices are surgically positioned. Wiring from internal transmitter runs through the middle ear and round window into the cochlea.

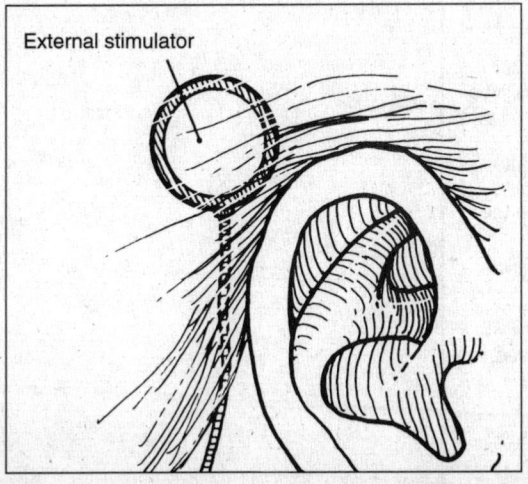

After surgery, the external stimulator is positioned. The illustration shows a wire to the power source.

COLONOSCOPY

GENERAL INFORMATION

DEFINITION—Visual examination of the inside of the rectum and the colon (large intestine) with a fiber-optic scope, in order to identify abnormalities and remove tissue for laboratory examination.

BODY PARTS INVOLVED—Anus; rectum; colon.

REASONS FOR SURGERY—Examination of the rectum and lower intestinal tract for disorders that may include: fissures; fistulas; narrowed sections of the intestine; unexplained blood in stools; benign or cancerous tumors; or precancerous polyps.

SURGICAL RISK INCREASES WITH
- Adults over 60.
- Obesity.
- Smoking.
- Poor nutrition.
- Recent or chronic illness.
- Use of some prescription and nonprescription drugs. Inform your doctor of any drugs, medications, or vitamin and herb supplements you are using or have used in the last month.

WHAT TO EXPECT

WHO OPERATES—General surgeon, family doctor, proctologist or gastroenterologist.

WHERE PERFORMED—Hospital, outpatient surgical facility or well-equipped doctor's office.

DIAGNOSTIC TESTS
- Before surgery: Blood and urine studies; stool examinations; x-rays of lower gastrointestinal tract.
- After surgery: Laboratory examination of removed tissue and other material.

ANESTHESIA—Intravenous sedation.

DESCRIPTION OF OPERATION
- The examination is best accomplished after thorough cleansing of large bowel with laxatives and enemas. Your physician will instruct you on how to cleanse your bowel.
- The colonoscope is lubricated, inserted into the rectum and passed into the colon.
- The colonoscope will be inserted through the full length of the large intestine.
- Affected areas are located, examined or treated. Polyps or tumors are removed for laboratory examination, and other biopsies of the colon wall may also be performed.
- Other necessary minor surgical procedures may be performed. The colonoscope is removed.

POSSIBLE COMPLICATIONS
- Excessive bleeding.
- Perforation of the colon.

AVERAGE HOSPITAL STAY—Usually none.

PROBABLE OUTCOME—Expect complete healing without complications. Allow about 4 days for recovery from surgery.

POSTOPERATIVE CARE

GENERAL MEASURES—No special instructions except those listed under other headings.

MEDICATION—Medicine is usually not necessary.

ACTIVITY—No restrictions.

DIET—No special diet.

CALL YOUR DOCTOR IF

- You experience abdominal pain or bloating which increases after the procedure.
- You have rectal bleeding which is excessive or lasts more than 24 hours.
- You experience pain or swelling in your rectum, or have blood in your stools.
- You develop signs of infection, including headache, muscle aches, dizziness or a general ill feeling and fever.
- You experience nausea or vomiting.

COLONOSCOPY

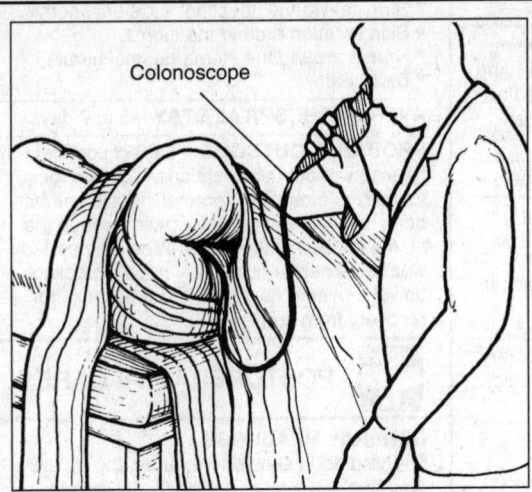

An illustration of a draped patient and the colonoscope inserted into the anal opening and rectum.

Colonoscope

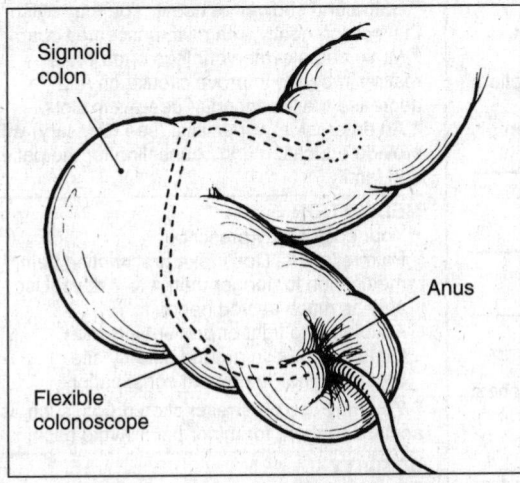

The colonoscope is advanced through the rectum into the sigmoid colon.

Sigmoid colon

Anus

Flexible colonoscope

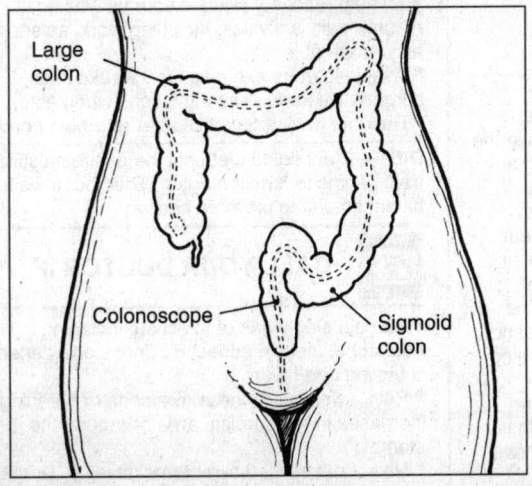

The colonoscope is inserted to the full length of the large intestine. This procedure locates possible affected areas to be examined or treated. Suspicious areas may be biopsied for microscopic examination.

Large colon

Colonoscope

Sigmoid colon

COLOSTOMY

GENERAL INFORMATION

DEFINITION—Creation of an artificial opening between a part of the colon (large intestine) and the surface of the body. All feces will leave the body through this opening, which is called an ostomy or stoma.

BODY PARTS INVOLVED—Large intestine.

REASONS FOR SURGERY
- Injury or infection which has caused perforation and peritonitis (see Glossary).
- Intestinal blockage, usually caused by cancer or scarring from a chronic infection.
- Colon or rectal surgery which weakens an area of the bowel and necessitates a temporary bypass of the colon until the bowel has healed.
- Anal or rectal cancer.

SURGICAL RISK INCREASES WITH
- Stress; obesity; poor nutrition.
- Excess alcohol consumption; smoking.
- Diabetes mellitus.
- Recent illness; chronic illness of the heart, lungs, liver or gastrointestinal tract.
- Use of some prescription and nonprescription drugs. Inform your doctor of any drugs, medications, or vitamin and herb supplements you are using or have used in the last month.

WHAT TO EXPECT

WHO OPERATES—General surgeon; colon-rectal surgeon.

WHERE PERFORMED—Hospital.

DIAGNOSTIC TESTS
- Before surgery: Blood and urine studies; chest and gastrointestinal x-rays; ECG; colonoscopy or sigmoidoscopy (see Glossary for all).
- After surgery: Blood studies.

ANESTHESIA—General anesthesia by injection and inhalation with an airway tube placed in the windpipe.

DESCRIPTION OF OPERATION
- An incision is made in the abdomen. The abdominal muscles are separated to expose the abdominal organs, which are inspected for any undetected disease.
- The colon section that is to be opened is isolated and clamped on both sides, then cut between the clamps. The end of the colon closer to the stomach is brought out of the abdomen and clamped outside the skin. The end farther from the stomach is usually closed, but may be brought out as a separate opening (mucous fistula).
- The abdominal contents are replaced, and muscles are closed around the stoma. Skin is closed with sutures or clips, which usually can be removed in about 1 week.

POSSIBLE COMPLICATIONS
- Excessive bleeding; blood clots.
- Surgical-wound infection; incisional hernia.
- Skin irritation around the stoma.
- Hernia around the stoma (stomal hernia).
- Diarrhea.

AVERAGE HOSPITAL STAY—5 to 7 days.

PROBABLE OUTCOME—Expect complete healing without complications. You can look forward to a relatively normal life, except that bowel movements will now pass through the stoma instead of the rectum. You will need to wear an external colostomy pouch to collect bowel movements. Allow about 6 weeks for recovery from surgery.

POSTOPERATIVE CARE

GENERAL MEASURES
- A hard ridge should form along the incision. As it heals, the ridge will gradually recede.
- Bathe and shower as usual. You may wash the incision gently with mild, unscented soap.
- Move and elevate your legs often while resting in bed to improve circulation and decrease the likelihood of deep-vein clots.
- An enterostomy specialist (see Glossary) will provide education and counseling for the patient and family.

MEDICATION
- Your doctor may prescribe:
  Pain relievers. Don't take prescription pain medication for longer than 4 to 7 days. Use only as much as you need.
  Antibiotics to fight or prevent infection.
  Ointment for skin around ostomy site.
  Stool softener to prevent constipation.
- You may use nonprescription drugs, such as acetaminophen, for minor pain. Avoid aspirin.

ACTIVITY
- To help recovery and aid your well-being, resume daily activities, including work, as soon as you are able.
- Avoid vigorous exercise for 6 weeks after surgery. Resume sexual relations when able.
- Resume driving 3 weeks after returning home.

DIET—Clear liquid diet until the gastrointestinal tract begins to function again. Then eat a well-balanced diet to promote healing.

CALL YOUR DOCTOR IF

- You develop signs of infection, including headache, muscle aches, dizziness or a general ill feeling and fever.
- Pain, swelling, redness, drainage or bleeding increases in the surgical area or around the stoma.
- New, unexplained symptoms develop. Drugs in treatment may produce side effects.

COLOSTOMY

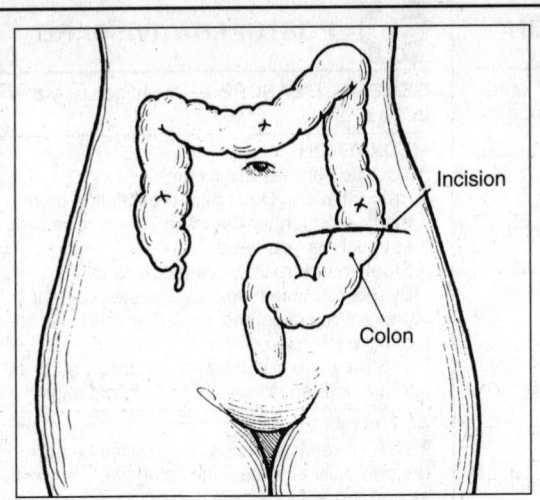

An illustration of the incision site in the left lower abdominal quadrant. The "x's" mark common areas for colon resection.

Incision

Colon

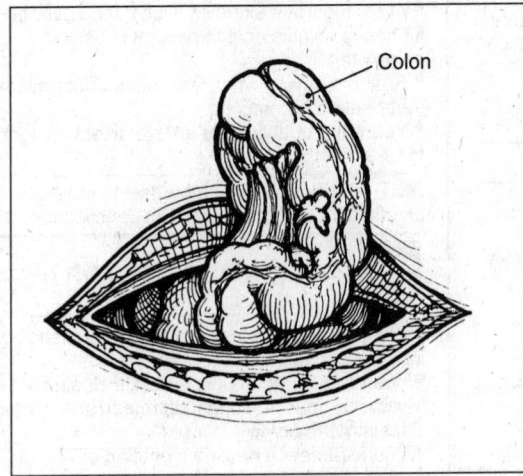

The abdominal muscle is separated to expose the abdominal organs. The colon section to be opened is isolated, clamped on both sides, then cut between the clamps.

Colon

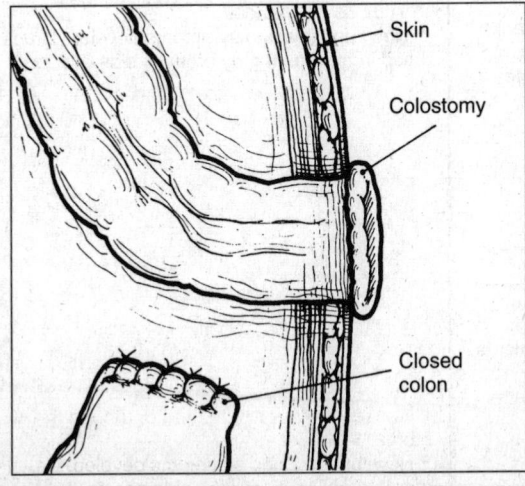

The end of the colon closer to the stomach is brought out of the abdomen and clamped outside the skin. The end farther from the stomach is usually closed, but may also be brought out to the skin.

- After the operation, bowel movements will emerge through the open end of the colostomy, which has been sewn to the skin through an opening in the abdominal wall.

Skin

Colostomy

Closed colon

CORNEA TRANSPLANT
(Keratoplasty)

 GENERAL INFORMATION

DEFINITION—Removing a diseased or injured cornea and replacing it with a healthy cornea from a donor.

BODY PARTS INVOLVED—Cornea (the front part of the eyeball).

REASONS FOR SURGERY—Restoration of vision or prevention of blindness.

SURGICAL RISK INCREASES WITH
• Stress.
• Obesity.
• Smoking.
• Poor nutrition.
• Recent or chronic illness.
• Alcoholism.
• Diabetes mellitus.
• Use of some prescription and nonprescription drugs. Inform your doctor of any drugs, medications, or vitamin and herb supplements you are using or have used in the last month.

 WHAT TO EXPECT

WHO OPERATES—Ophthalmologist.

WHERE PERFORMED—Hospital.

DIAGNOSTIC TESTS
• Before surgery: Blood and urine studies; eye examination.
• After surgery: Eye examination.

ANESTHESIA
• Local anesthesia by injection.
• General anesthesia by injection and inhalation with an airway tube placed in the windpipe.

DESCRIPTION OF OPERATION
• The diseased or injured cornea is cut free with scissors and removed.
• The donor cornea (usually from an eye bank) is grafted into the area with tiny sutures.
• The sutures holding the transplanted cornea are removed when healing has taken place, usually about 3 to 4 weeks after surgery.

POSSIBLE COMPLICATIONS
• Surgical-wound infection.
• Rejection of transplant (rare).
• Secondary glaucoma.

AVERAGE HOSPITAL STAY—2 days.

PROBABLE OUTCOME—Expect complete healing without complications. Allow 3 to 4 weeks for recovery from surgery. Some patients can see better within a day or two of surgery; others may not gain optimum vision for months or even a year or more.

 POSTOPERATIVE CARE

GENERAL MEASURES—Avoid getting water in the eye.

MEDICATION
• Your doctor may prescribe:
  Pain relievers. Don't take prescription pain medication longer than 4 to 7 days. Use only as much as you need.
  Stool softeners to prevent constipation.
  Eyedrops containing a topical steroid to help prevent rejection and an antibiotic to prevent or treat infection.
• You may use nonprescription drugs, such as acetaminophen, for minor pain. Avoid aspirin.

ACTIVITY
• To help recovery and aid your well-being, resume daily activities, including work, as soon as you are able.
• Avoid vigorous exercise. Don't bend over or lift heavy objects until transplant is healed completely.
• Resume driving when your doctor determines that healing is complete.
• You will probably wear an eye shield at night for 2-3 months.

DIET—No special diet. Increase dietary fiber and fluid intake to help prevent constipation.

 CALL YOUR DOCTOR IF

• Pain, swelling, redness, drainage or bleeding increases in the surgical area.
• You develop signs of infection, including headache, muscle aches, dizziness or a general ill feeling and fever.
• You experience nausea, vomiting or constipation.
• Your vision changes.
• New, unexplained symptoms develop. Drugs used in treatment may produce side effects.

CORNEA TRANSPLANT
(Keratoplasty)

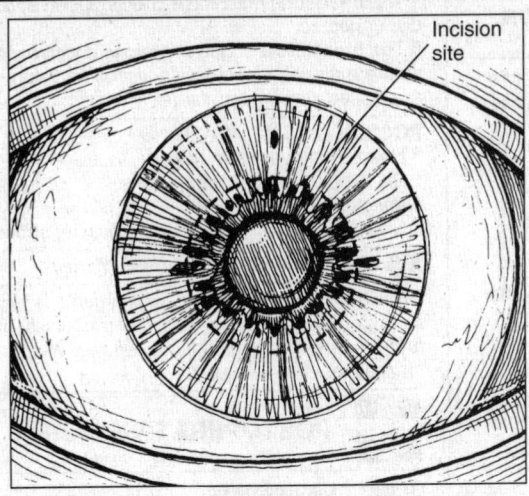

Incision site

An illustration of the incision site and cornea, which covers the pupil of the eye.

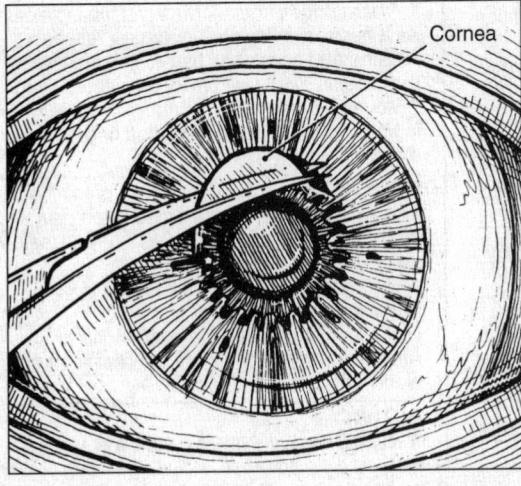

Cornea

Diseased or injured cornea is cut free with scissors and removed.

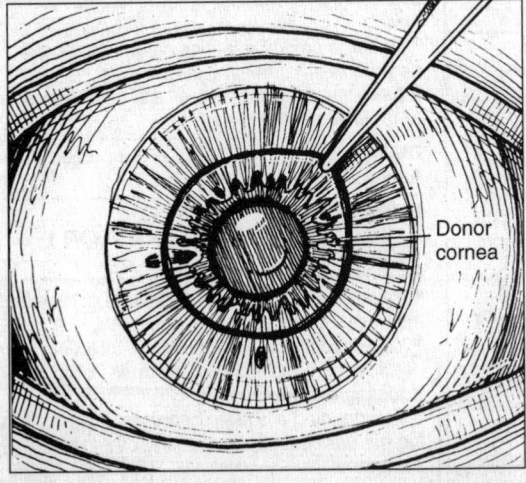

Donor cornea

The donor cornea is fastened into the area with sutures. Sutures can be removed when healing has taken place, usually about 3 to 4 weeks after surgery.

CORONARY ARTERY BYPASS GRAFT
(Heart Bypass)

GENERAL INFORMATION

DEFINITION—Using a section of the patient's leg vein or an artery in the chest wall to bypass a partial or complete blockage in the coronary artery system.

BODY PARTS INVOLVED—Heart; coronary arteries; chest wall; large veins of legs.

REASONS FOR SURGERY
- Angina pectoris.
- Restoration of blood to the heart muscle after a heart attack.
- Prevention of a possible heart attack, if coronary arteries have narrowed.

SURGICAL RISK INCREASES WITH
- Obesity; smoking.
- Recent or chronic illness; diabetes mellitus.
- Chronic obstructive pulmonary disease (COPD); heart failure.
- Use of some prescription and nonprescription drugs. Inform your doctor of any drugs, medications, or vitamin and herb supplements you are using or have used in the last month.

WHAT TO EXPECT

WHO OPERATES—Cardiovascular surgeon.

WHERE PERFORMED—Hospital.

DIAGNOSTIC TESTS
- Before surgery: Blood studies; chest x-ray; cardiac catheterization; ECG; sonogram (see Glossary for all).
- During surgery: ECG; angiograms (see Glossary).
- After surgery: ECG; chest x-ray; sonogram.

ANESTHESIA—General anesthesia by injection and inhalation with an airway tube placed in the windpipe.

DESCRIPTION OF OPERATION
- A section of the patient's large leg vein, or a section of the mammary artery (located in the chest), is removed and set aside to be used as the bypass vein graft.
- An incision is made through the breastbone, and the chest is spread open to expose the heart.
- The heart is stopped with a chemical solution that temporarily paralyzes the heart muscle fibers and the heart's temperature is reduced. Circulation and breathing are then performed by a heart-lung machine.
- The bypass vein graft is sutured in place to allow blood flow to resume beyond the blocked area.
- After reheating the heart, it is given a mild electric shock that causes heartbeat to resume.

- The heart-lung machine is then stopped and disconnected.
- The breastbone edges are rejoined with metal suture material, and muscles, tissue and skin are closed with lighter sutures.

POSSIBLE COMPLICATIONS
- Heart rhythm abnormalities.
- Excessive bleeding; blood clots.
- Infection; kidney failure.
- New area of injury to the heart muscle; stroke.

AVERAGE HOSPITAL STAY—6-10 days.

PROBABLE OUTCOME—Angina pectoris is cured in almost all cases, and the probability of future heart attacks is reduced. Allow 6 weeks for recovery from surgery.

POSTOPERATIVE CARE

GENERAL MEASURES
- A hard ridge should form along the incision. As it heals, the ridge will gradually recede.
- Bathe and shower as usual. You may wash the incision gently with mild, unscented soap.
- Move and elevate legs frequently while resting in bed to decrease the likelihood of deep-vein blood clots.

MEDICATION—Your doctor may prescribe: Pain relievers. Don't take prescription pain medication for longer than 4 to 7 days. Use only as much as you need.
Antiarrhythmics to prevent heartbeat irregularities.
Digitalis to strengthen the heart muscle.
Anticoagulants to decrease the likelihood of blood clots.

ACTIVITY
- To help recovery and aid your well-being, resume daily activities, including driving or work, as soon as your doctor determines that you are able.
- Resume sexual relations when your doctor determines that healing is complete.
- Ask your doctor for advice about an exercise rehabilitation program.

DIET—Low-salt; low-fat; high-fiber (see Appendix for diets).

CALL YOUR DOCTOR IF

- Pain, swelling, redness, drainage or bleeding increases in the surgical area.
- You develop signs of infection, including headache, muscle aches, dizziness or a general ill feeling and fever.
- You develop a cough, heartbeat irregularities, leg pain or constipation; or any other new symptoms.

CORONARY ARTERY BYPASS GRAFT
(Heart Bypass)

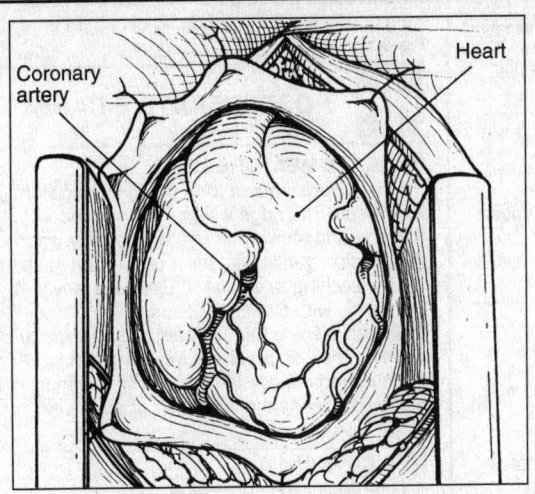

Coronary artery

Heart

An illustration of the heart showing an example of a clogged or occluded coronary artery.

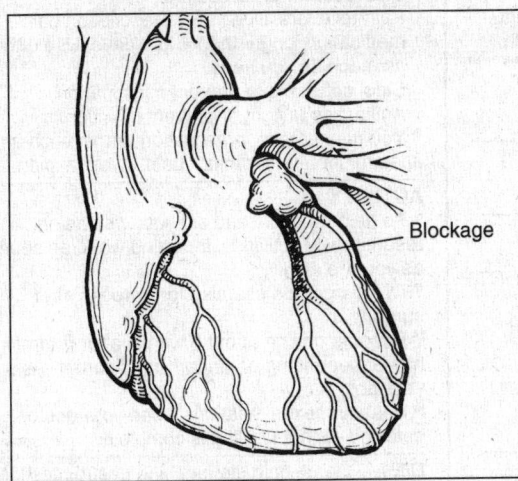

Blockage

The blocked area in this illustration is the left anterior descending coronary artery, a common site for such blockage to occur.

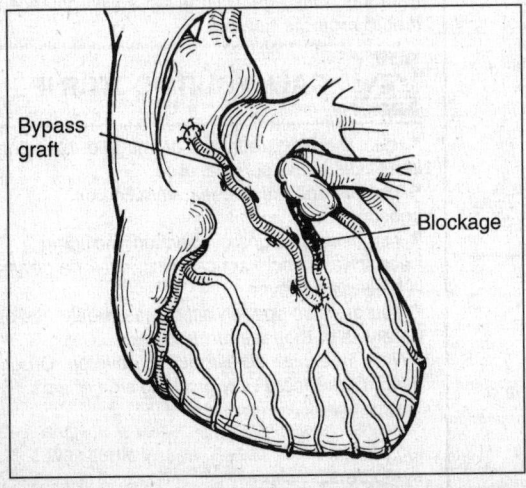

Bypass graft

Blockage

A bypass vein or artery grafted in place allows blood flow to resume beyond the blocked area and thus restore more normal circulation to some of the damaged heart muscle.

SURGERIES

CRANIOTOMY

GENERAL INFORMATION

DEFINITION—Cutting through the skull (cranium) to expose and treat disorders in the brain or associated tissues.

BODY PARTS INVOLVED—Scalp; skull; brain and membrane coverings.

REASONS FOR SURGERY
- Removal of blood clots, aneurysms or tumors.
- Repair of tears in the brain's membrane coverings.
- Drainage of a brain abscess.

SURGICAL RISK INCREASES WITH
- Smoking; excess alcohol consumption.
- Chronic illness.
- Recent illness, especially upper respiratory infection.
- Diabetes mellitus.
- Use of some prescription and nonprescription drugs. Inform your doctor of any drugs, medications, or vitamin and herb supplements you are using or have used in the last month.

WHAT TO EXPECT

WHO OPERATES—Neurosurgeon.

WHERE PERFORMED—Hospital.

DIAGNOSTIC TESTS
- Before surgery: Blood and urine studies; x-rays of skull; MRI; angiogram; EEG; ECG; CT scan (see Glossary for all).
- After surgery: EEG; x-rays of skull; blood studies; CT scan; angiogram (sometimes).

ANESTHESIA—General anesthesia by injection and inhalation with an airway tube placed in the windpipe.

DESCRIPTION OF OPERATION
- A portion of the head area is shaved. An incision is made in the scalp over the area of suspected disorder.
- A flap of bone is cut away from the skull and set aside.
- The disorder is located and treated as necessary.
- The bone flap is replaced.
- The scalp is closed with sutures or clips, which usually can be removed about 1 week after surgery.

POSSIBLE COMPLICATIONS
- Stroke; seizure.
- Excessive bleeding; blood clots.
- Surgical-wound infection.
- Brain damage.
- Swelling of the brain caused by the trauma of surgery.

AVERAGE HOSPITAL STAY—10 to 14 days.

PROBABLE OUTCOME—Expect complete healing of surgical wounds. Allow about 8 weeks for recovery from surgery.

POSTOPERATIVE CARE

GENERAL MEASURES
- A hard ridge should form along the incision. As it heals, the ridge will gradually recede.
- Bathe and shower as usual. You may wash the incision gently with mild, unscented soap.
- After bathing or showering, replace any wet dressings with clean, dry ones.
- Use an electric heating pad, a heat lamp or a warm compress to relieve incisional pain.
- Move and elevate legs often while resting in bed to decrease the likelihood of deep-vein blood clots.

MEDICATION
- Your doctor may prescribe:
  Pain relievers. Don't take prescription pain medication longer than 4 to 7 days. Use only as much as you need.
  Stool softeners to prevent constipation.
  Antibiotics to fight or prevent infection.
- You may use nonprescription drugs, such as acetaminophen, for minor pain. Avoid aspirin.

ACTIVITY
- To help recovery and aid your well-being, resume daily activities, including work, as soon as you are able.
- Avoid vigorous exercise for 6 weeks after surgery.
- Resume driving about 3 weeks after returning home, depending on underlying disorder. Ask your doctor.
- Resume sexual relations when your doctor determines that healing is complete.

DIET—Clear liquid diet until the gastrointestinal tract functions again. Then eat a well-balanced diet to promote healing.

CALL YOUR DOCTOR IF

- Pain, swelling, redness, drainage or bleeding increases in the surgical area.
- You experience nausea, vomiting or constipation.
- You develop signs of infection, including headache, muscle aches, dizziness or a general ill feeling and fever.
- You develop speech difficulties, weakness or paralysis of the face, arms or legs.
- New, unexplained symptoms develop. Drugs used in treatment may produce side effects.

CRANIOTOMY

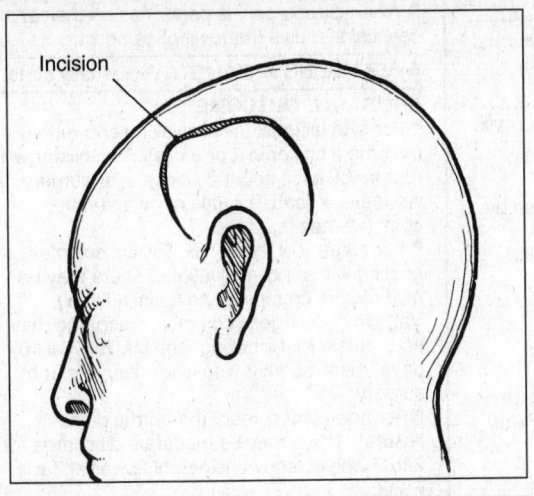

An illustration of a shaved head and a typical incision site on the scalp.

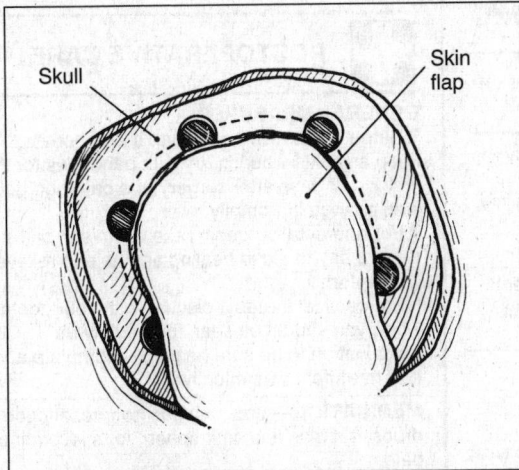

Skin over the scalp is incised, exposing the skull bone, and a flap is formed.

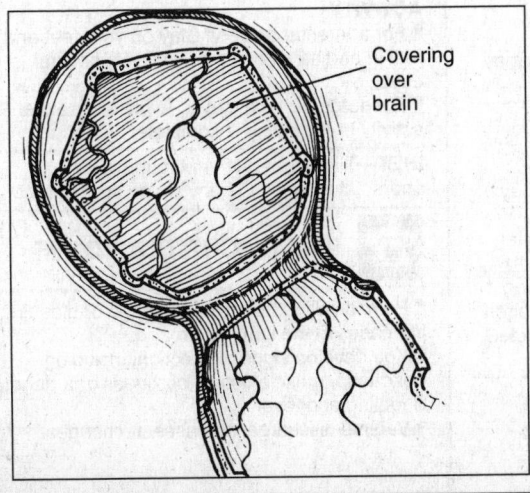

Skin and bone flap are retracted to expose the brain covering where the suspected area of pathology is located.

CRYOSURGERY

 GENERAL INFORMATION

DEFINITION—Thermal destruction of abnormal or diseased tissue by freezing, usually with liquid nitrogen.

BODY PARTS INVOLVED—Skin; anus; cervix.

REASONS FOR SURGERY
- Removal of skin lesions such as acitinic keratoses (precancerous conditions caused by the sun) and warts.
- Treatment of cervicitis (inflammation of the cervix).
- Treatment of mild to moderate cervical dysplasia (abnormal cell growth).
- Sometimes used to treat severe cervical dysplasia.
- Treatment of benign (noncancerous) growths on the cervix (such as polyps) or genital warts.
- Moderate hemorrhoids.
- Anal fissures.

SURGICAL RISK INCREASES WITH—None expected.

 WHAT TO EXPECT

WHO OPERATES—Dermatologist or family doctor (to treat skin lesions); obstetrician-gynecologist (to treat cervicitis or other cervical abnormalities); or general surgeon (for hemorrhoids or fissures).

WHERE PERFORMED—Hospital, outpatient surgical facility, doctor's office or emergency room.

DIAGNOSTIC TESTS
- Before surgery: Blood and urine studies (occasionally).
- After surgery: None expected.

ANESTHESIA—Usually none. For skin lesions, the area to be treated is sometimes anesthetized with an injection of local anesthetic. A general or spinal anesthesia may be used for anorectal lesions.

DESCRIPTION OF OPERATION
- For small skin lesions, liquid nitrogen is applied to a cotton-tipped applicator. The applicator is held to the skin lesions until they are frozen and destroyed.
- For surgery on the cervix or anus, a special probe instrument is used. Liquid nitrogen circulates in the tip of this instrument causing it to become almost as cold as the liquid nitrogen itself. The instrument tip is held on the affected areas until the abnormal tissue is frozen.

POSSIBLE COMPLICATIONS
- Surgical-wound infection (rare).
- Failure of the procedure to destroy all of the abnormal tissue.

- For anorectal surgery: constipation; urinary retention; recurrence of hemorrhoids.
- When cryosurgery is performed on the cervix, cervical stenosis (narrowing) can occur.

AVERAGE HOSPITAL STAY—Usually none.

PROBABLE OUTCOME
- For skin lesions: Initial swelling and redness become a blister in 2 or 3 days. The blister will rupture by itself about 2 weeks after surgery. It will leave a scab, but little or no scar after complete healing.
- For surgery of the cervix: Expect complete healing without complications. There may be mild uterine cramping and facial flushing. Vaginal discharge is common; discharge may be profuse, foul-smelling, and last for 7 to 10 days. Allow about 3 weeks for recovery from surgery.
- For anorectal surgery (hemorrhoids or fissure): There may be moderate discharge for 2 to 3 weeks, and considerable swelling for 1 week.

 POSTOPERATIVE CARE

GENERAL MEASURES
- Bathe and shower as usual. If appropriate, keep any skin wounds dry with bandages for the first 2 or 3 days after surgery. If a bandage gets wet, change it promptly.
- For anorectal surgery: Take warm sitz baths twice a day to aid in healing and help to relieve discomfort.
- For cervical therapy, discuss with your doctor when you should be seen for a follow-up examination to be sure healing is complete and that treatment was effective.

MEDICATION—You may use nonprescription drugs, such as acetaminophen, to relieve minor pain.

ACTIVITY
- For anorectal surgery: Stay off your feet and rest in bed as much as possible for several days.
- For surgery of the cervix: Avoid any sexual activity until healing is complete.

DIET—High-fiber diet or Metamucil for anorectal surgery. Otherwise, no special diet.

 CALL YOUR DOCTOR IF

- Pain, swelling, redness, drainage or bleeding increases in the surgical area.
- You develop signs of infection, including headache, muscle aches, dizziness or a general ill feeling and fever.
- Vaginal discharge increases or changes.

CRYOSURGERY

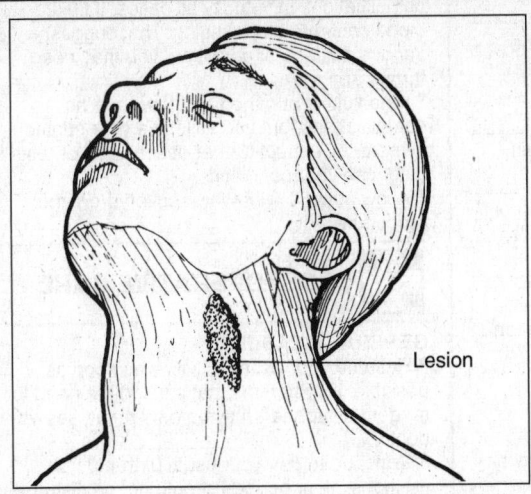

An illustration of a skin lesion on the neck to be treated with cryosurgery (very low temperature).

Lesion

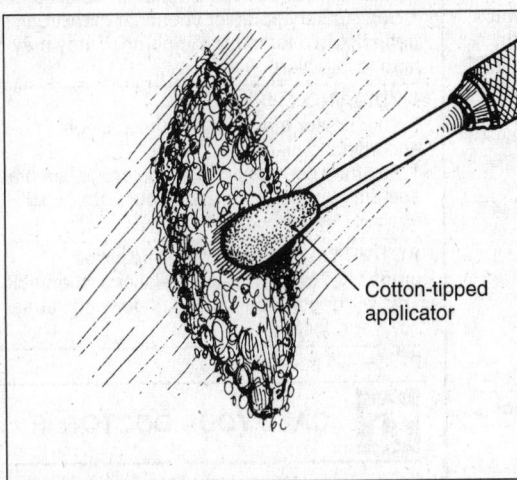

A cotton-tipped applicator that has been dipped in liquid nitrogen is held against the lesion to destroy abnormal cells.

Cotton-tipped applicator

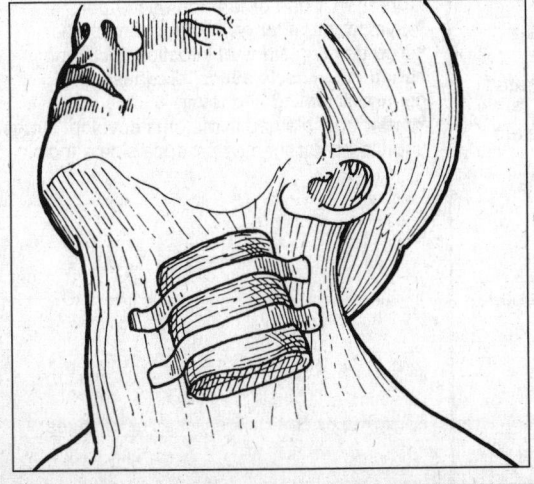

Large treated areas should be covered with bandages until healing is complete.

SURGERIES

CULDOCENTESIS

 GENERAL INFORMATION

DEFINITION—Piercing the "cul-de-sac," the space deep in the vagina behind and under the cervix, in order to obtain a fluid sample for laboratory examination.

BODY PARTS INVOLVED—Vagina; lowest part of pelvis behind the uterus and cervix.

REASONS FOR SURGERY—Investigation of possible ailments in the abdomen and pelvis, including: bleeding inside the lower pelvic cavity; ruptured ectopic pregnancy; ruptured ovarian cyst; ovarian cancer; or pelvic inflammatory disease. Laboratory examination of the removed fluid aids in diagnosis.

SURGICAL RISK INCREASES WITH
- Recent or chronic illness.
- Diabetes mellitus.
- Use of some prescription and nonprescription drugs. Inform your doctor of any drugs, medications, or vitamin and herb supplements you are using or have used in the last month.

 WHAT TO EXPECT

WHO OPERATES—Obstetrician-gynecologist, general surgeon or family doctor.

WHERE PERFORMED—Doctor's office; outpatient surgical facility; or hospital.

DIAGNOSTIC TESTS
- Before surgery: Pap smear; vaginal and abdominal exam; x-rays of lower abdomen.
- After surgery: Laboratory examination of removed fluid.

ANESTHESIA—Local anesthesia by injection.

DESCRIPTION OF OPERATION
- A speculum is inserted into the vagina to hold it open.
- The rear lip of the cervix is raised.
- A local anesthetic is applied to the farthest back portion of the vagina (cul-de-sac).
- The posterior wall of the vagina is penetrated with a needle and syringe.
- Fluid, if present, is aspirated. No sutures are necessary.

POSSIBLE COMPLICATIONS
- Perforation of bladder or bowel (rare).
- Excessive bleeding.
- Surgical-wound infection.

AVERAGE HOSPITAL STAY—Usually none.

PROBABLE OUTCOME
- A fluid sample is obtained successfully without complications in virtually all cases. If fluid or blood confirms other findings that suggest a serious disease or condition, you may need further surgery.
- If no fluid is obtained and there are no complications, but you still have your original symptoms, expect further observation or tests to diagnose your conditions.
- Allow about 1 week for recovery from the procedure.

 POSTOPERATIVE CARE

GENERAL MEASURES
- Resume your usual activities as soon as possible, if symptoms that caused the need for surgery disappear. If symptoms recur, see your doctor.
- Continue to use your usual birth-control methods. Your periods should not be disturbed.
- Use sanitary pads for your next menstrual period. Avoid tampons temporarily; they may lead to infection.

MEDICATION
- Your doctor may prescribe medicines according to diagnosis.
- You may use nonprescription drugs, such as acetaminophen, to relieve minor pain. Avoid aspirin.

ACTIVITY—Resume normal activities gradually. Resume sexual relations when able. This will depend on various underlying causes. Ask your doctor.

DIET—No special diet.

 CALL YOUR DOCTOR IF

- You experience vaginal bleeding that soaks more than 1 pad or tampon each hour.
- Symptoms recur or worsen.
- You develop signs of infection, including headache, muscle aches, dizziness, or a general ill feeling and fever.
- New, unexplained symptoms develop. Drugs used in treatment may produce side effects.

CULDOCENTESIS

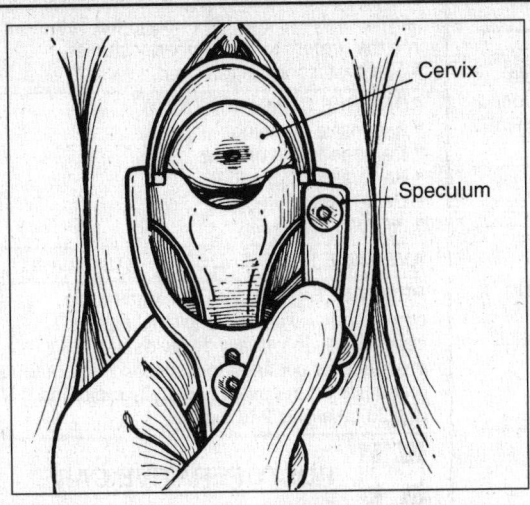

Cervix

Speculum

This view illustrates a female patient with extended legs in stirrups on an examining table to allow examination of the genital area.
- The speculum is inserted into the vagina to stretch it open and expose the cervix.

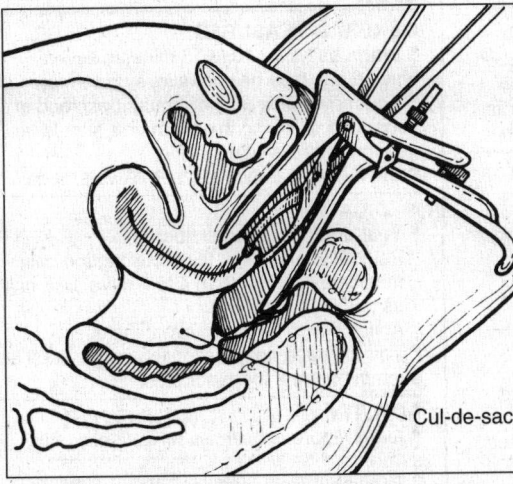

Cul-de-sac

Forceps grasp the rear lip of the cervix to expose the cul-de-sac (the farthest back portion of the vagina).

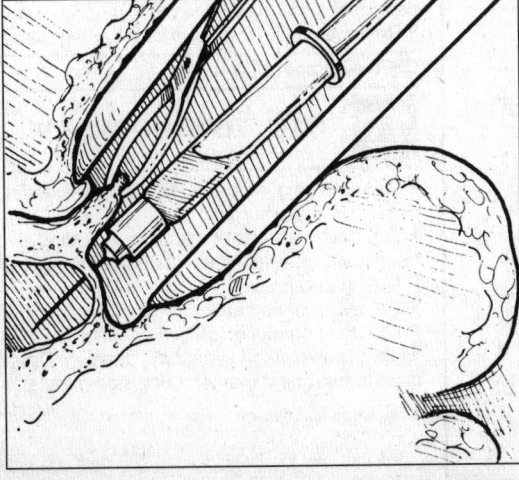

The cul-de-sac is penetrated with needle and syringe. Fluid, if present, is aspirated.

CYSTOSCOPY

GENERAL INFORMATION

DEFINITION—Visual examination of the lower urinary tract and collection of a urine sample from the bladder. The examination is performed with a cystoscope, a thin fiber-optic instrument with a lighted tip.

BODY PARTS INVOLVED—Urethra; bladder; openings into the bladder.

REASONS FOR SURGERY
- Blood in the urine (hematuria).
- Inability to control urination (incontinence).
- Recurrent urinary tract infections.
- Congenital abnormalities of the urinary tract.
- Tumors of the bladder.
- Bladder or kidney stones.
- Tightening of the urethra or the ureters.

SURGICAL RISK INCREASES WITH
- Obesity.
- Smoking.
- Recent or chronic illness.
- Diabetes mellitus.
- Use of some prescription and nonprescription drugs. Inform your doctor of any drugs, medications, or vitamin and herb supplements you are using or have used in the last month.

WHAT TO EXPECT

WHO OPERATES—Urologist.

WHERE PERFORMED—Hospital, doctor's office or outpatient surgical facility.

DIAGNOSTIC TESTS
- Before surgery: Blood and urine studies; x-rays of kidneys, ureters (see Glossary) and bladder; CT scan (see Glossary).
- During surgery: Retrograde pyelograms (see Glossary).
- After surgery: Blood studies.

ANESTHESIA—Spinal anesthesia (sometimes) by injection or injected general anesthesia.

DESCRIPTION OF OPERATION
- The patient urinates before surgery so that urine remaining in the bladder can be measured.
- The cystoscope is lubricated and inserted through the urethra into the bladder. A urine sample is collected.
- Fluid is pumped through the cystoscope to inflate the bladder, which allows visual examination of the entire bladder wall.
- Bladder or kidney stones are removed, if necessary. Tissue samples are gathered and, if necessary, lesions are treated.
- Catheters are passed through the cystoscope and guided to the openings into the ureters. A harmless dye is injected through the catheters into the ureters to perform x-ray studies.
- The cystoscope is removed.

POSSIBLE COMPLICATIONS
- Excessive bleeding.
- Damage to the urethra.
- Perforation of bladder.
- Urinary tract infection.
- Injury to the penis.

AVERAGE HOSPITAL STAY—0 to 3 days.

PROBABLE OUTCOME—Examination completed and urine sample collected successfully in virtually all cases. If the procedure is confined to inspection and manual manipulation, recovery is usually rapid and should take only 2 to 4 days.

POSTOPERATIVE CARE

GENERAL MEASURES
- Warm baths for 10 to 15 minutes several times a day may help to relieve discomfort.
- You may notice a small amount of blood in your urine following the exam; this should last no more than 24 hours.
- Drink eight 8 ounce glasses of water a day.

MEDICATION
- Your doctor may prescribe:
  Pain relievers. Don't take prescription pain medication longer than 4 to 7 days. Use only as much as you need.
  Antibiotics to fight or prevent infection.
- You may use nonprescription drugs, such as acetaminophen, for minor pain.

ACTIVITY
- Avoid vigorous exercise for 2 weeks after surgery.
- Resume sexual relations when your doctor determines that healing is complete.
- Resume driving 2 days after returning home.

DIET—No special diet.

CALL YOUR DOCTOR IF

- Pain, swelling, redness, drainage or bleeding increases in the surgical area.
- You develop signs of infection, including headache, muscle aches, dizziness or a general ill feeling and fever.
- You experience nausea or vomiting.
- You have painful or difficult urination.
- New, unexplained symptoms develop. Drugs used in treatment may produce side effects.

CYSTOSCOPY

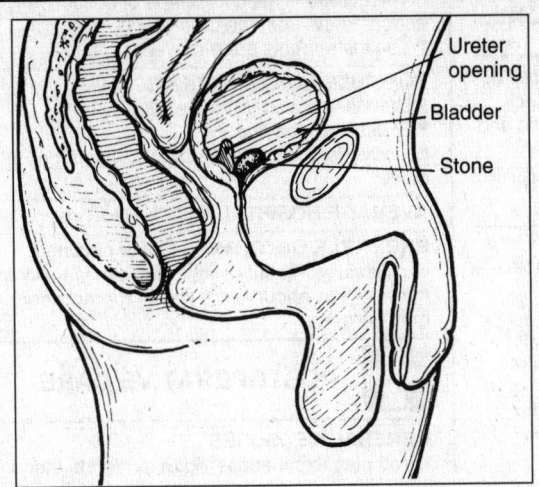

Ureter opening

Bladder

Stone

A cross-section of the male pelvis showing the urethra, bladder and openings into the bladder. A typical stone inside the bladder is illustrated.

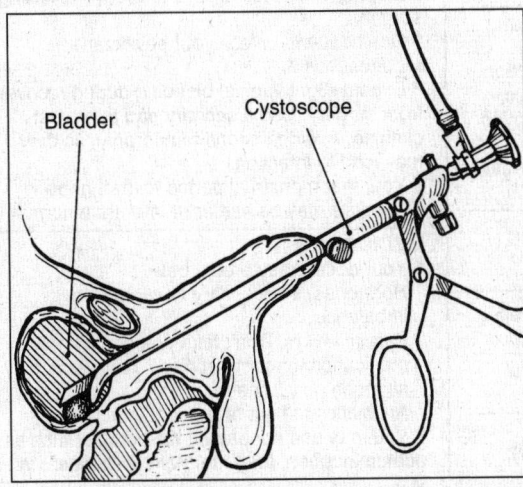

Bladder

Cystoscope

A lubricated cystoscope is inserted through the urethra into the bladder to allow removal of the stone. If needed, a catheter can be passed through the cystoscope.

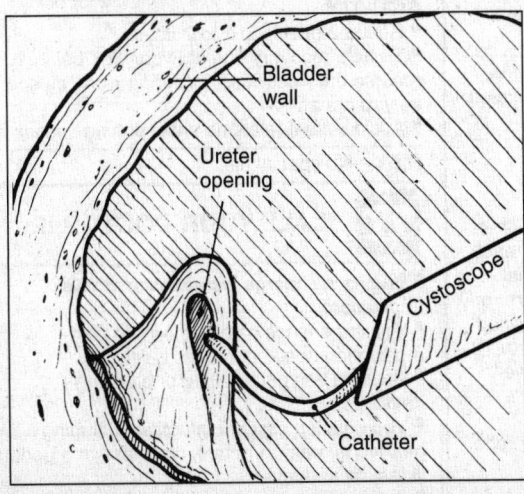

Bladder wall

Ureter opening

Cystoscope

Catheter

A catheter passed through the cystoscope toward the opening of the ureter. The catheter can be passed through the ureteral opening to remove other stones higher in the urinary tract.

SURGERIES

DILATATION AND CURETTAGE OF THE UTERUS (D & C)

GENERAL INFORMATION

DEFINITION—Opening the cervix and scraping the lining (endometrium) and contents of the uterus. The D & C is often both a diagnostic and a therapeutic procedure.

BODY PARTS INVOLVED—Uterus; cervix; vagina (as route for surgery).

REASONS FOR SURGERY
- Diagnosis of abnormal bleeding or possible cancer inside the uterus.
- Incomplete spontaneous miscarriage.
- Treatment of minor diseases of the uterus.
- Prevent or stop hemorrhage or subsequent infection following miscarriage.
- Removal of membranes and placenta after childbirth in cases where they fail to deliver spontaneously (retained placenta).
- Elective abortion during early pregnancy.

SURGICAL RISK INCREASES WITH
- Obesity; smoking; alcoholism.
- Cervical infection or ongoing uterine infection.
- Recent or chronic illness; diabetes mellitus.
- Use of some prescription and nonprescription drugs. Inform your doctor of any drugs, medications, or vitamin and herb supplements you are using or have used in the last month.

WHAT TO EXPECT

WHO OPERATES—Obstetrician-gynecologist, general surgeon or family doctor.

WHERE PERFORMED—Outpatient surgical facility or hospital.

DIAGNOSTIC TESTS
- Before surgery: Pap smear (see Glossary); pregnancy test; blood and hormonal studies.
- After surgery: Blood studies; Pap smear in 2 months.

ANESTHESIA—Local anesthesia by injection, or general anesthesia by injection and inhalation with an airway tube placed in the windpipe.

DESCRIPTION OF OPERATION
- The vagina is cleansed with an antiseptic solution.
- The cervix is carefully opened (dilated), either by inserting a series of tapered metal rods, each with a progressively larger diameter, into the cervical opening at the time of the procedure; or in advance by the use of laminaria (freeze-dried seaweed), which are placed in the cervix 8 to 12 hours prior to surgery. The laminaria will swell and gradually open the cervix to 1 to 2 centimeters.
- A curette is inserted into the uterus. The curette can be a suction device or a looped knife.
- The curette is used to scrape or suction the endometrium from the uterine wall.
- The instruments are removed.

POSSIBLE COMPLICATIONS
- Uterine infection (endometritis).
- Excessive bleeding.
- Inadvertent injury to the uterus, bladder or bowel.

AVERAGE HOSPITAL STAY—0 to 1 day.

PROBABLE OUTCOME—Tissue obtained successfully without complications in virtually all cases. Allow about 4 to 6 weeks for recovery from surgery.

POSTOPERATIVE CARE

GENERAL MEASURES
- You may experience mild to moderate uterine cramping or backache for 2 to 3 days following surgery.
- Don't douche unless your physician recommends it.
- Expect slight vaginal bleeding during recovery from surgery. Use a sanitary pad to protect clothing. Avoid tampons temporarily, as they may lead to infection.
- Your first menstrual period following the procedure may be earlier or later than normal.

MEDICATION
- Your doctor may prescribe:
  Hormones, if necessary to correct an imbalance.
  Pain relievers. Don't take prescription pain medication longer than 4 to 7 days. Use only as much as you need.
  Antibiotics to fight or prevent infection.
- You may use nonprescription drugs, such as acetaminophen, for minor pain. Avoid aspirin.

ACTIVITY
- Resume driving in 1 to 2 days.
- To help recovery and aid your well-being, resume daily activities, including work, as soon as you are able.
- Avoid sexual relations until spotting ceases.

DIET—No special diet.

CALL YOUR DOCTOR IF

- Vaginal discharge increases or smells unpleasant.
- You experience pain that simple pain medication does not relieve quickly.
- Unusual vaginal swelling or bleeding develops.
- You develop signs of infection, including headache, muscle aches, dizziness or a general ill feeling and fever.
- New, unexplained symptoms develop.

DILATATION AND CURETTAGE OF THE UTERUS (D & C)

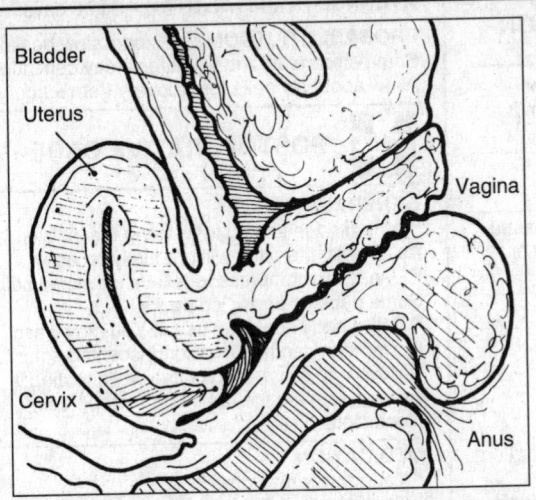

A side view of the female genital area.

Bladder
Uterus
Vagina
Cervix
Anus

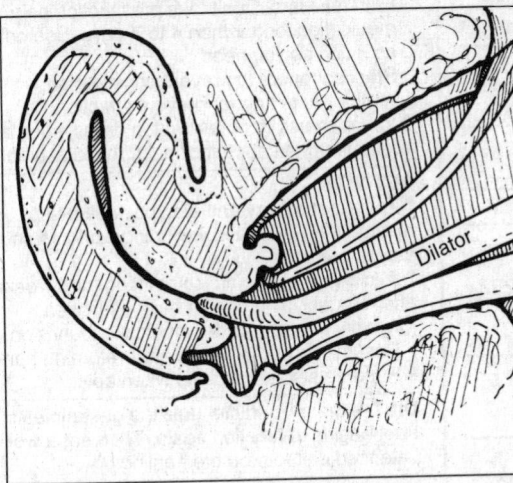

Forceps grasp the anterior portion of the cervix and a dilator is inserted into uterus.

Dilator

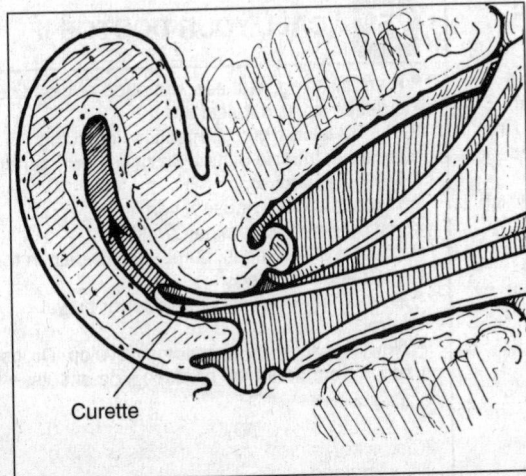

After the cervix has been dilated, a curette is passed into the cavity of the uterus. The curette is used to scrape or suction away the uterine lining for laboratory analysis or therapeutic reasons.

Curette

DISK REMOVAL, RUPTURED
(Laminectomy)

GENERAL INFORMATION

DEFINITION—Removal of part or all of an intervertebral disk that has protruded from its normal position.

BODY PARTS INVOLVED—Spine; intervertebral disk.

REASONS FOR SURGERY—Relief of painful symptoms caused by pressure on nerves or spinal cord.

SURGICAL RISK INCREASES WITH
- Adults over 60.
- Obesity; poor nutrition; smoking.
- Chronic illness, especially back pain or alcoholism.
- Diabetes mellitus.
- Use of some prescription and nonprescription drugs. Inform your doctor of any drugs, medications, or vitamin and herb supplements you are using or have used in the last month.

WHAT TO EXPECT

WHO OPERATES—Neurosurgeon, orthopedist.

WHERE PERFORMED—Hospital.

DIAGNOSTIC TESTS
- Before surgery: Blood and urine studies; x-rays of back and lungs; myelogram; CT scan and/or MRI; ECG (see Glossary for all).
- After surgery: Blood studies; back x-rays.

ANESTHESIA—General anesthesia by injection and inhalation with an airway tube placed in the windpipe.

DESCRIPTION OF OPERATION
- An incision is made over the protruded disk.
- The arches of the spine are cut away and removed to allow visualization of the disk.
- The protruding disk is scooped out.
- Sometimes, the vertebral bone around the affected area is joined together with normal bone taken from your hip area and inserted into the space from which the disk was removed. This procedure is called fusion.
- The skin is closed with sutures or clips, which usually can be removed about 1 week after surgery.

POSSIBLE COMPLICATIONS
- Excessive bleeding; blood clots.
- Surgical-wound infection.
- Injury to nerve roots, which can lead to paralysis.
- Incomplete disk removal.
- Unrelieved or worsened pain.
- Impaired bladder function (rare).

AVERAGE HOSPITAL STAY—2 to 6 days.

PROBABLE OUTCOME—Expect slow healing. Some discomfort and weakness may continue. Allow about 5 weeks for recovery from surgery.

POSTOPERATIVE CARE

GENERAL MEASURES
- A hard ridge should form along the incision. As it heals, the ridge will gradually recede.
- Use warm compress to relieve incisional pain. Some patients prefer ice packs.
- Bathe and shower as usual. You may wash the incision gently with mild, unscented soap.
- Move and elevate legs often while resting in bed to decrease the likelihood of deep-vein blood clots.

MEDICATION
- Your doctor may prescribe:
  Pain relievers. Don't take prescription pain medication longer than 4 to 7 days. Use only as much as you need.
  Stool softeners to prevent constipation.
  Antibiotics to fight or prevent infection.
- You may use nonprescription drugs, such as acetaminophen, for minor pain. Avoid aspirin.

ACTIVITY
- To help recovery and aid your well-being, resume daily activities, including work, as soon as you are able.
- Avoid vigorous exercise or lifting for 6 weeks after surgery. Then begin back exercises (physical therapy) under medical supervision.
- Resume driving 6 weeks after returning home.
- Resume sexual relations when able.

DIET—Clear liquid diet until the gastrointestinal tract begins to function again. Then eat a well-balanced diet to promote healing.

CALL YOUR DOCTOR IF

- Pain, swelling, redness, drainage or bleeding increases in the surgical area.
- You develop signs of infection, including headache, muscle aches, dizziness or a general ill feeling and fever.
- You experience nausea, vomiting, constipation or abdominal swelling.
- You have weakness, numbness or pain in the back, buttocks or legs.
- You experience loss of bladder or bowel control.
- New, unexplained symptoms develop. Drugs used in treatment may produce side effects.

DISK REMOVAL, RUPTURED
(Laminectomy)

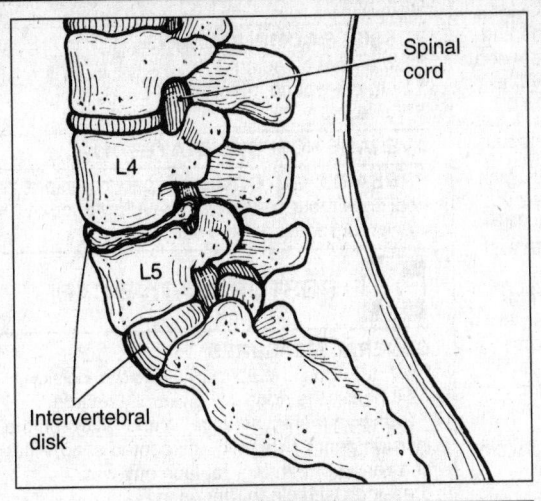

Spinal cord

L4

L5

Intervertebral disk

An illustration of the bony spine, the spinal cord and the protruding intervertebral disk. This example shows the disk separating the 4th and 5th vertebral bodies.

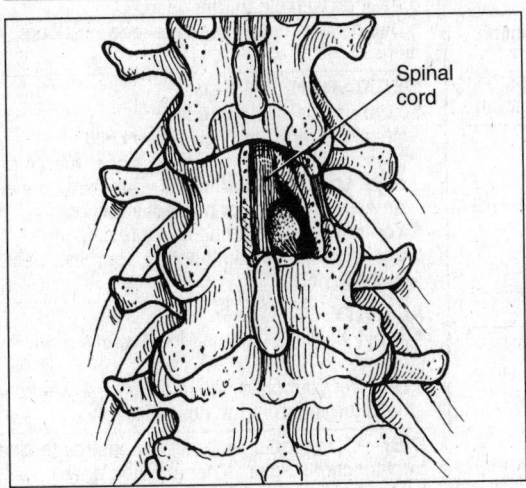

Spinal cord

After the skin has been incised, the arches of the bone are located, cut away and partially or totally removed allowing the protruding disk to be scooped out.

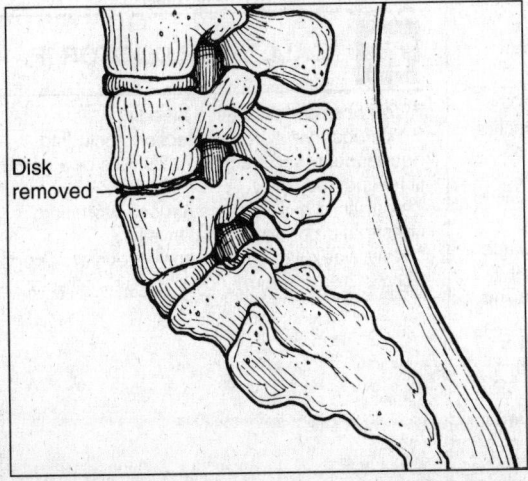

Disk removed

Appearance after the disk has been removed.

SURGERIES

DUCTUS ARTERIOSUS CLOSURE

GENERAL INFORMATION

DEFINITION—Closure of an abnormal opening in the ductus arteriosus, a blood vessel between the heart's aorta and the pulmonary artery that usually closes in the first few days of life.

BODY PARTS INVOLVED—Ductus arteriosus; pulmonary artery; aorta.

REASONS FOR SURGERY—For unknown reasons, closure does not always happen. The surgery is performed so that normal growth and development may occur. If the abnormal opening is large, surgery is performed during the first few days after birth. Otherwise, surgery may be delayed until the child is 1 to 2 years old.

SURGICAL RISK INCREASES WITH
- Preterm infants.
- Obesity.
- Recent or chronic illness.
- Diabetes mellitus.
- Use of some prescription and nonprescription drugs. Inform your doctor of any drugs, medications, or vitamin and herb supplements your child is using or has used in the last month.

WHAT TO EXPECT

WHO OPERATES
- Cardiovascular surgeon.
- Pediatric surgeon.

WHERE PERFORMED—Hospital.

DIAGNOSTIC TESTS
- Before surgery: Blood and urine studies; x-rays of chest; echocardiogram; cardiac catheterization (sometimes); ECG (see Glossary for all).
- During surgery: ECG monitor (see Glossary).
- After surgery: Blood studies.

ANESTHESIA—General anesthesia by injection and inhalation with an airway tube placed in the windpipe.

DESCRIPTION OF OPERATION
- An incision is made in the chest. The muscles are divided and the chest is spread open.
- The lung is deflated to expose the ductus arteriosus.
- The ductus arteriosus is tied tightly or clamped in two places, cut between the clamps and tied. The ends are sewn shut to prevent bleeding from the pulmonary artery or the aorta.
- Tubes are left in place to drain fluid. A catheter is left in place to remove air from the chest so that the lung can reinflate itself within 24 to 48 hours.
- The muscles are sewn together in layers with strong sutures.

- The skin is closed with sutures or clips, which usually can be removed about 1 week after surgery.

POSSIBLE COMPLICATIONS
- Excessive bleeding
- Surgical-wound infection.
- Nerve injury.

AVERAGE HOSPITAL STAY—4 days.

PROBABLE OUTCOME—Expect complete healing without complications. Allow about 4 weeks for recovery from surgery.

POSTOPERATIVE CARE

GENERAL MEASURES
- A hard ridge should form along the incision. As it heals, the ridge will gradually recede.
- Bathe your child as usual. You may wash the incision gently with mild, unscented soap. After showering or bathing, replace any wet dressings with clean, dry ones.
- Use a warm compress to relieve incisional pain.

MEDICATION
- Your doctor may prescribe:
Pain relievers. Don't give your child prescription pain medication longer than 4 to 7 days. Use only as much as your child needs. Antibiotics to fight or prevent infection.
- You may give your child nonprescription drugs, such as acetaminophen, for minor pain. Avoid aspirin.

ACTIVITY
- Avoid vigorous exercise for 6 weeks after surgery.
- Don't let your child ride in a car for 2 weeks after returning from the hospital.

DIET—Clear liquid diet until the gastrointestinal tract functions again. Then provide a well-balanced diet to promote healing.

CALL YOUR DOCTOR IF

- You observe excessive bleeding.
- You observe signs of infection, including headache, muscle aches, dizziness or a general ill feeling and fever.
- Your child experiences nausea, vomiting, constipation or abdominal swelling.
- New, unexplained symptoms develop. Drugs used in treatment may produce side effects.

DUCTUS ARTERIOSUS CLOSURE

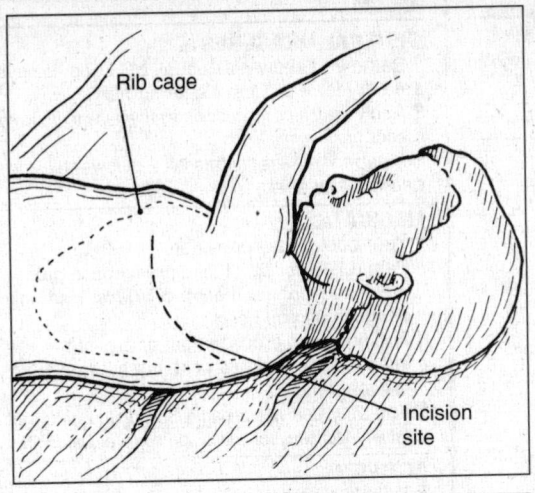

Rib cage

Incision site

An illustration of the surgical site to expose the heart and great blood vessels. The patient is usually placed on the side with arm extended over the head.

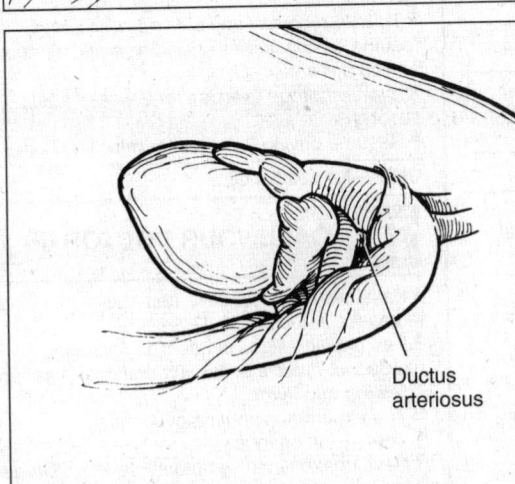

Ductus arteriosus

Shown is the ductus arteriosus, which is a blood vessel between the aorta and the pulmonary artery that usually closes at birth.

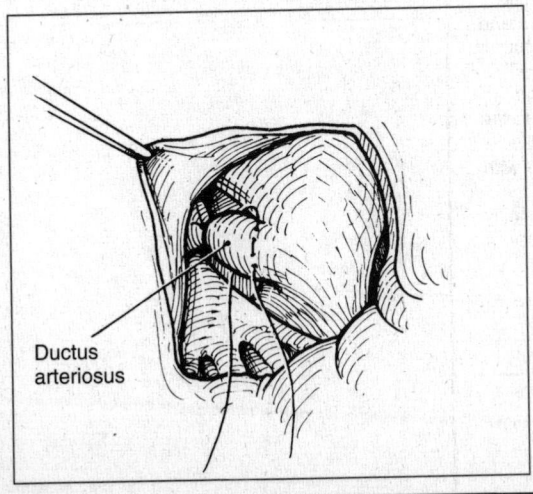

Ductus arteriosus

Ductus arteriosus is tied and ends sewn to prevent bleeding from the pulmonary artery or the aorta.

ECTROPION REPAIR

 GENERAL INFORMATION

DEFINITION—Repair of an ectropion (see Illness section) by removal of excess cartilage in the edge of the eyelid.

BODY PARTS INVOLVED—Lower eyelid.

REASONS FOR SURGERY
- Improved appearance.
- Relief of redness, irritation and discomfort.
- Reduced likelihood of infection in the membrane surrounding the eye.

SURGICAL RISK INCREASES WITH
- Smoking.
- Stress.
- Poor nutrition.
- Recent or chronic illness.
- Alcoholism.
- Diabetes mellitus.
- Use of some prescription and nonprescription drugs. Inform your doctor of any drugs, medications, or vitamin and herb supplements you are using or have used in the last month.

 WHAT TO EXPECT

WHO OPERATES—Ophthalmologist.

WHERE PERFORMED—Hospital, ophthalmologist's office or outpatient surgical facility.

DIAGNOSTIC TESTS
- Before surgery: Blood and urine studies; eye examination.
- After surgery: Eye examination; laboratory examination of removed tissue.

ANESTHESIA—Local anesthesia by injection.

DESCRIPTION OF OPERATION
- An incision is made in the eyelid.
- The cartilage is cut close to the outer eyelid edge. A small wedge of cartilage is cut free and removed. The cartilage is sewn back together with fine sutures.
- Another wedge of cartilage is cut free and removed from the side of the eyelid close to the nose.
- The remaining cartilage is sewn together with fine sutures.
- The skin is closed with sutures, which usually can be removed about 10 days after surgery.

POSSIBLE COMPLICATIONS
- Surgical-wound infection.
- Recurrence.

AVERAGE HOSPITAL STAY—0 to 2 days.

PROBABLE OUTCOME—Expect complete healing without complications. Allow about 2 weeks for recovery from surgery.

 POSTOPERATIVE CARE

GENERAL MEASURES
- Bathe and shower as usual, but keep the eye area dry for 4 to 5 days after surgery.
- Apply warm compresses to the eye to relieve discomfort.
- Sleep for several nights on 2 pillows to decrease swelling.

MEDICATION
- Your doctor may prescribe:
  Pain relievers. Don't take prescription pain medication longer than 4 to 7 days. Use only as much as you need.
  Antibiotic eye drops to fight or prevent infection. Keep drops cold, but not frozen, in the refrigerator.
- You may use nonprescription drugs, such as acetaminophen, for minor pain. Avoid aspirin.

ACTIVITY
- To help recovery and aid your well-being, resume daily activities, including work, as soon as you are able.
- Avoid vigorous exercise for 2 weeks after surgery.
- Resume driving 2 days after returning home.

DIET—No special diet.

 CALL YOUR DOCTOR IF

- Pain, swelling, redness, drainage or bleeding increases in the surgical area.
- You develop signs of infection, including headache, muscle aches, dizziness or a general ill feeling and fever.
- You experience nausea or vomiting.
- Your vision changes.
- New, unexplained symptoms develop. Drugs used in treatment may produce side effects.

ECTROPION REPAIR

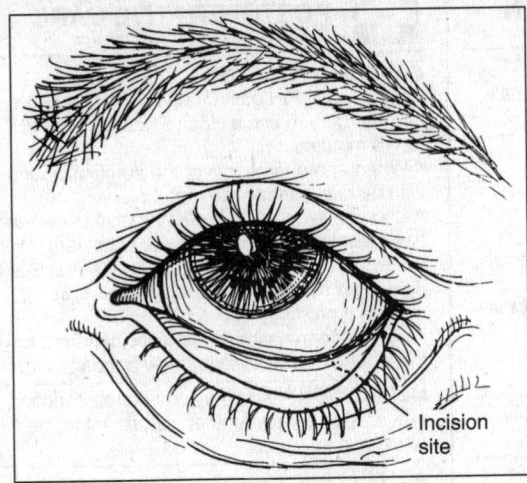

An illustration of the eye, eyelid and typical incision site for ectropion repair.

Incision site

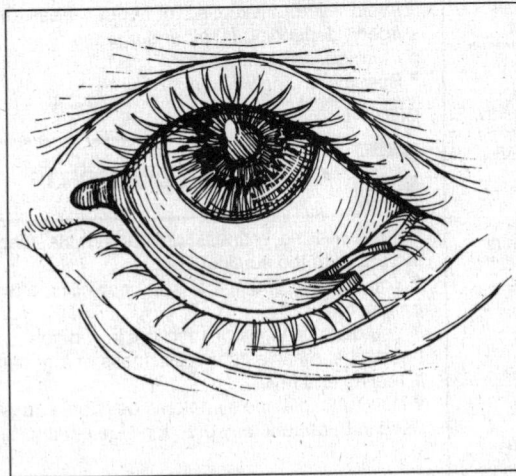

Cartilage is cut close to the outer eyelid edge. A small wedge of cartilage is cut free and removed.

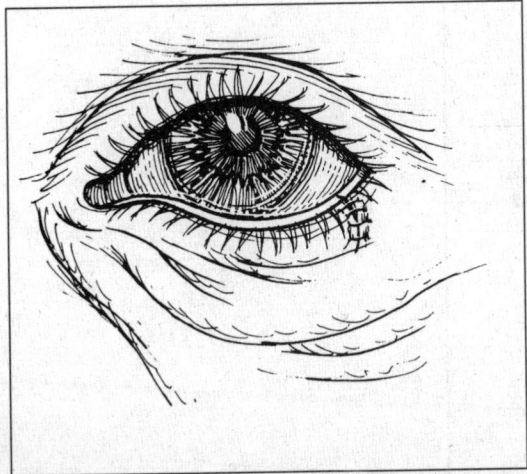

The cartilage is sewn back together and skin closed with small sutures, which are usually removed about 10 days after surgery.

ELECTROCAUTERIZATION
(Electrocoagulation; Electrosurgery; Fulguration)

 GENERAL INFORMATION

DEFINITION—Removal of abnormal or diseased tissue, or control of bleeding in small blood vessels, with controlled electric current.

BODY PARTS INVOLVED—Skin; blood vessels in surgical area.

REASONS FOR SURGERY
* Removal of lesions on the skin.
* Control of bleeding from small blood vessels during other surgeries.
* Stop bleeding from lesions in the lining of the stomach, small intestine or colon during endoscopy.
* Remove lesions in bladder.

SURGICAL RISK INCREASES WITH—None expected.

 WHAT TO EXPECT

WHO OPERATES—Family doctor, urologist, dermatologist, plastic and reconstructive surgeon, gastroenterologist or general surgeon.

WHERE PERFORMED—Hospital, outpatient surgical facility or doctor's office.

DIAGNOSTIC TESTS—Usually none.

ANESTHESIA—Local anesthesia by injection.

DESCRIPTION OF OPERATION—The procedure described here is used for dermatological lesions.
* Usually, a lesion is numbed with local anesthesia, and removed with a curette (see Glossary) or excised.
* Electrocauterization with an electric instrument destroys abnormal tissue that the curette does not remove.

POSSIBLE COMPLICATIONS
* Surgical-wound infection.
* Damage to underlying structure.
* Perforation (in bladder and bowel procedures).

AVERAGE HOSPITAL STAY—Usually none.

PROBABLE OUTCOME—Expect complete healing without complications. The scab will drop off spontaneously and the scar should be small. Allow 2 to 3 weeks for healing and recovery from surgery.

 POSTOPERATIVE CARE

GENERAL MEASURES
* If the wound bleeds during the first 24 hours after surgery, press a clean tissue or cloth to it for 10 minutes.
* When appropriate, cover the surgical wound with a small bandage to protect it.
* Shower as usual. Avoid baths until the wound has completely healed. Between showers, keep the wound dry with a bandage for the first 2 or 3 days after surgery. If a bandage gets wet, change it promptly.
* Apply nonprescription antibiotic ointment to the wound before applying new bandages.

MEDICATION—You may use nonprescription drugs, such as acetaminophen, for minor pain. Avoid aspirin.

ACTIVITY
* Avoid vigorous exercise for about 1 week after surgery, depending on other surgeries performed. Ask your doctor.
* Resume driving when able.

DIET—No special diet.

 CALL YOUR DOCTOR IF

* Pain, swelling, redness, drainage or bleeding increases in the surgical area.
* You develop abdominal pain or swelling after endoscopy.
* You develop signs of infection, including headache, muscle aches, dizziness or a general ill feeling and fever.
* New, unexplained symptoms develop. Drugs used in treatment may produce side effects.

ELECTROCAUTERIZATION
(Electrocoagulation; Electrosurgery; Fulguration)

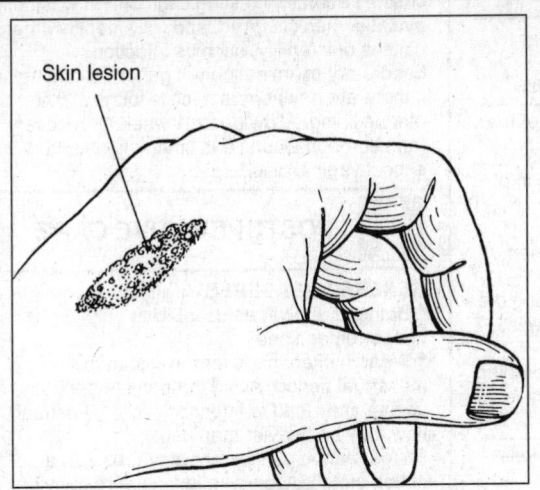

Skin lesion

After local anesthesia, the skin lesion is cleansed thoroughly.
- The location of the skin lesion in this illustration is on the hand and used as an example. The principles and techniques are similar for electrocauterization of skin lesions in other locations.

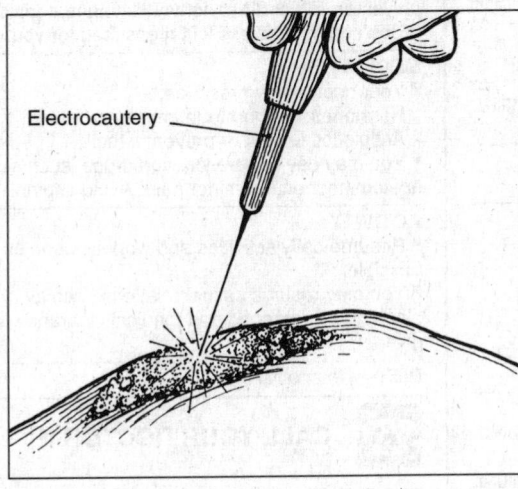

Electrocautery

The electrocautery destroys the cells of the skin lesion and prevents excessive bleeding.

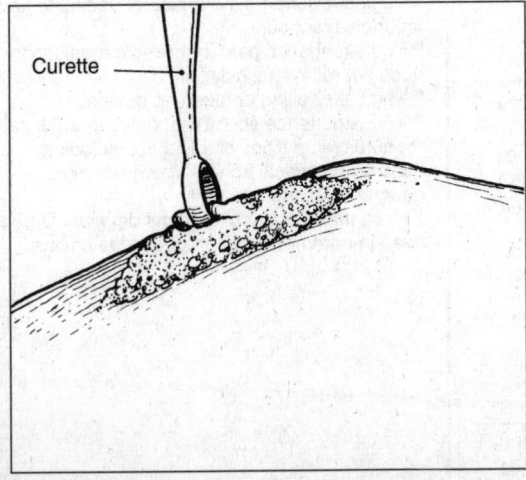

Curette

A curette removes the destroyed tissue. After tissue removal, the electrocautery is once again used to destroy cells at the base of the site where the lesion was removed.

ENDOMETRIAL BIOPSY

GENERAL INFORMATION

DEFINITION—A diagnostic procedure that involves removal of tissue from the endometrium, the inner lining of the uterus.

BODY PARTS INVOLVED—Inner lining of the uterus; vagina (as route for surgery).

REASONS FOR SURGERY—Investigation of bleeding between menstrual periods or postmenopausal bleeding. Also used to investigate infertility. Laboratory examination of the removed tissue aids in diagnosis. If appropriate, the surgery is performed during the last few days of the patient's menstrual cycle. This is the best time to identify possible hormonal problems and, for patients undergoing fertility evaluation, to determine if ovulation is occurring.

SURGICAL RISK INCREASES WITH—None expected.

WHAT TO EXPECT

WHO OPERATES—Obstetrician-gynecologist, general surgeon or family doctor.

WHERE PERFORMED—Doctor's office; outpatient surgical facility; or hospital.

DIAGNOSTIC TESTS
• Before surgery: Pap smear; pregnancy test.
• After surgery: Laboratory examination of removed tissue.

ANESTHESIA—Usually none. Your doctor may prescribe a mild tranquilizer before surgery to calm you.

DESCRIPTION OF OPERATION
• A speculum is inserted into the vagina to hold it open and to bring the cervix into view. In some cases, it is necessary to use a tenaculum, a hooklike instrument that holds and helps stabilize the cervix.
• A small, straw-shaped instrument (or other biopsy instrument) is inserted through the cervix into the uterus. It is gently scraped against the inner lining of the uterus to gather tissue.
• An alternate method involves obtaining the tissue sample with a suction instrument; this procedure is sometimes referred to as vacuum aspiration.
• The instruments are removed. The surgery may cause slight pain, but it should be minor and temporary.

POSSIBLE COMPLICATIONS
• Excessive bleeding.
• Infection of the uterine lining (endometritis).
• Inadvertent injury to the uterus (rare).

AVERAGE HOSPITAL STAY—Usually none.

PROBABLE OUTCOME—Tissue obtained successfully without complications in virtually all cases. Laboratory testing can confirm whether ovulation has occurred, and may identify other causes of infertility, such as infection. Laboratory examination will generally determine if there are any abnormal cells found in the uterine lining. Allow about 1 week for recovery from surgery. During this time, you should expect vaginal discharge.

POSTOPERATIVE CARE

GENERAL MEASURES
• Bathe or shower as usual. Use only nonperfumed soap.
• Wear sanitary pads for the rest of this menstrual period. Avoid tampons temporarily, as they may lead to infection. Your menstrual flow may be heavier than usual.
• Wear cotton panties or pantyhose with a cotton crotch. Avoid panties made from nylon, polyester, silk or other nonventilating materials.
• Don't douche unless it is prescribed for you.

MEDICATION
• Your doctor may prescribe:
  Hormones, if a hormone imbalance exists.
  Antibiotics to fight or prevent infection.
• You may use nonprescription drugs, such as acetaminophen, for minor pain. Avoid aspirin.

ACTIVITY
• Resume daily activities and work as soon as possible.
• You may resume sexual relations once all bleeding has stopped and medical clearance is given.

DIET—No special diet.

CALL YOUR DOCTOR IF

• Vaginal discharge increases or begins to have an unpleasant odor.
• You experience pain that simple medication does not relieve quickly.
• Vaginal swelling or bleeding develops.
• You experience abdominal or lower back pain.
• You develop signs of infection, including headache, muscle aches, dizziness, or a general ill feeling and fever.
• New, unexplained symptoms develop. Drugs used in treatment may produce side effects.

ENDOMETRIAL BIOPSY

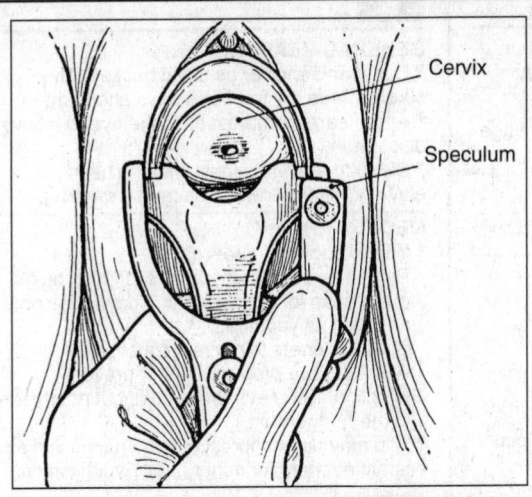

This view illustrates a female patient with extended legs in stirrups on an examining table to allow examination of the genital area.
- The speculum is inserted into the vagina to stretch it open and expose the cervix.

Cervix

Speculum

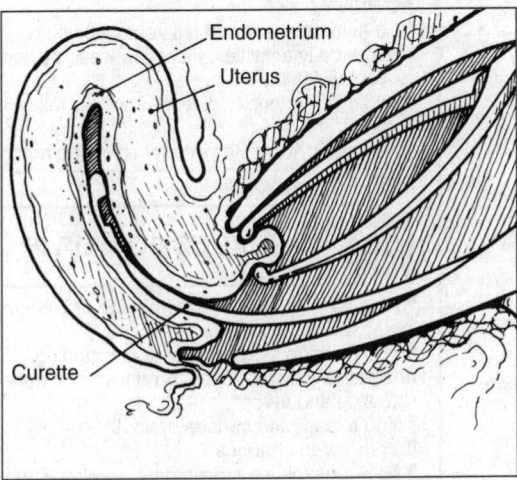

Shown are the uterus, the endometrium (inner lining of the uterus), the operating curette and the forceps holding the upper lip of the cervix to allow introduction of the curette.

Endometrium

Uterus

Curette

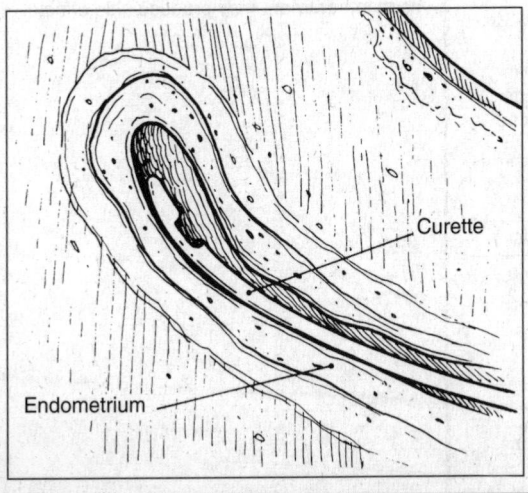

The curette removes a sample of the endometrium. The removed tissue is submitted to the laboratory for study.

Curette

Endometrium

ENTROPION REPAIR

GENERAL INFORMATION

DEFINITION—Shortening of excess tissue in the edge of the eyelid by removal of excess cartilage.

BODY PARTS INVOLVED—Skin and cartilage of the upper eyelid.

REASONS FOR SURGERY
- Improved appearance.
- Relief of redness, irritation and discomfort.

SURGICAL RISK INCREASES WITH
- Stress.
- Smoking.
- Poor nutrition.
- Recent or chronic illness.
- Alcoholism.
- Diabetes mellitus.
- Use of some prescription and nonprescription drugs. Inform your doctor of any drugs, medications, or vitamin and herb supplements you are using or have used in the last month.

WHAT TO EXPECT

WHO OPERATES—Ophthalmologist.

WHERE PERFORMED—Hospital, ophthalmologist's office or outpatient surgical facility.

DIAGNOSTIC TESTS
- Before surgery: Blood and urine studies; eye examination.
- After surgery: Laboratory examination of removed tissue.

ANESTHESIA—Local anesthesia by injection.

DESCRIPTION OF OPERATION
- An incision is made in the eyelid.
- The cartilage is partially cut about midway between the two sides of the eyelid.
- A small amount of the cartilage is cut free of connective tissue and removed.
- The remaining cartilage is closed with silk sutures. The skin is closed over the cartilage with fine sutures that usually can be removed about 10 days after surgery.

POSSIBLE COMPLICATIONS—Surgical-wound infection.

AVERAGE HOSPITAL STAY—1 to 2 days.

PROBABLE OUTCOME—Expect complete healing without complications. Allow about 2 weeks for recovery from surgery.

POSTOPERATIVE CARE

GENERAL MEASURES
- Bathe and shower as usual but keep the surgical area dry for 4 or 5 days after surgery.
- Apply warm compresses to the eye to relieve discomfort.
- Sleep for several nights with the head elevated on 2 pillows to decrease swelling.

MEDICATION
- Your doctor may prescribe:
  Pain relievers. Don't take prescription pain medication longer than 4 to 7 days. Use only as much as you need.
  Stool softeners to prevent constipation.
  Antibiotic eye drops to fight or prevent infection. Keep eye drops cold, but not frozen, in the refrigerator.
- You may use nonprescription drugs, such as acetaminophen, for minor pain. Avoid aspirin.

ACTIVITY
- To help recovery and aid your well-being, resume daily activities, including work, as soon as you are able.
- Avoid vigorous exercise for 2 weeks following surgery.
- Resume driving 2 days after returning home.

DIET—No special diet.

CALL YOUR DOCTOR IF

- Pain, swelling, redness, drainage or bleeding increases in the surgical area.
- You develop signs of infection, including headache, muscle aches, dizziness or a general ill feeling and fever.
- You experience nausea or vomiting.
- Your vision changes.
- New, unexplained symptoms develop. Drugs used in treatment may produce side effects.

ENTROPION REPAIR

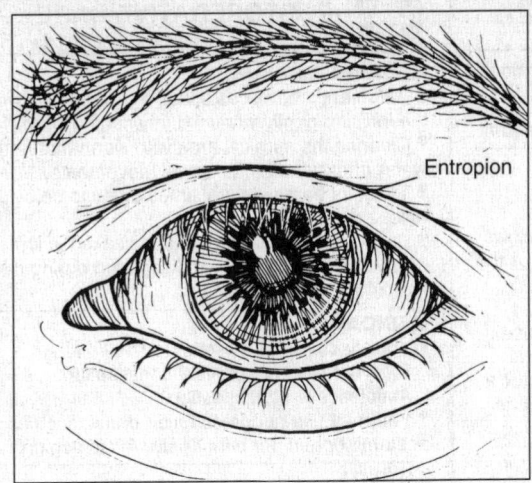

An illustration of excess tissue in the edge of the eyelid.

Entropion

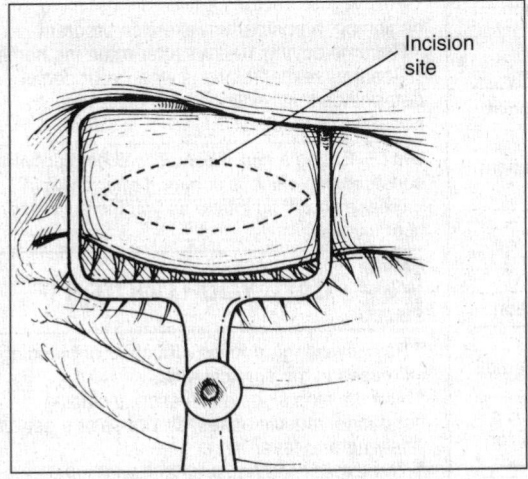

Incision site made in the skin overlying the eyelid.

Incision site

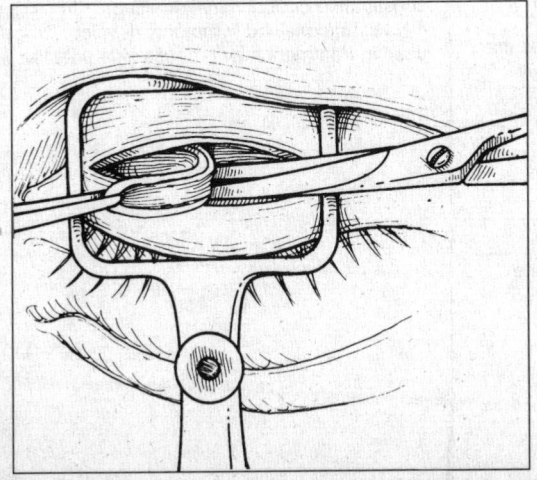

The cartilage in the upper eyelid is cut about midway between the two sides of the eyelid and removed.
• Bleeding is controlled and skin is closed with small sutures, which can be removed in about 10 days following surgery.

EPISIOTOMY
(Perineotomy)

GENERAL INFORMATION

DEFINITION—Surgical incision at the exterior of the vaginal opening to create enlargement.

BODY PARTS INVOLVED—Vagina; perineum.

REASONS FOR SURGERY—Usually performed during childbirth, just before the widest diameter of the baby's head passes through the outlet of the birth canal. This allows easier passage of the baby's head to reduce the potential of damage to the mother's vagina, bladder and rectum. Also helps expedite delivery in the case of forceps or vacuum use, or when there is maternal exhaustion or fetal distress, such as in a case of shoulder dystocia (when the shoulders of the baby get stuck after the head has already delivered).

SURGICAL RISK INCREASES WITH—None expected.

WHAT TO EXPECT

WHO OPERATES—Obstetrician-gynecologist, family doctor or midwife.

WHERE PERFORMED—Hospital or outpatient surgical facility.

DIAGNOSTIC TESTS
• Before surgery: Blood and urine studies.
• After surgery: Blood studies.

ANESTHESIA—Local anesthesia by injection.

DESCRIPTION OF OPERATION
• An incision is made in the perineum (the small area between the vaginal opening and the anus), just before the widest part of the baby's head is to be delivered. The size of the incision depends on how large an opening is required for the baby's head to pass through safely.
• The baby and placenta are delivered.
• The surgical area is repaired with sutures that will be absorbed by the body.

POSSIBLE COMPLICATIONS
• Excessive bleeding
• Surgical-wound infection (rare).
• Inadvertent injury to sphincter or rectum (rare).

AVERAGE HOSPITAL STAY—2 days.

PROBABLE OUTCOME—Expect complete healing without complications. Allow about 6 weeks for recovery from childbirth.

POSTOPERATIVE CARE

GENERAL MEASURES
• Bathe and shower as usual. You may wash the incision gently with mild, unscented soap.
• Cleanse the surgical area with warm (not hot) water after urination or bowel movements.
• Take hot baths several times a day to help relieve discomfort.
• Use ice packs made of gauze soaked in ice-cold witch hazel to relieve discomfort during the first 24 hours after delivery.

MEDICATION
• Your doctor may prescribe:
  Stool softeners to prevent constipation.
  Antibiotics to fight infection.
• You may use nonprescription drugs, such as acetaminophen, for minor pain. Avoid aspirin.

ACTIVITY
• Follow your doctor's advice on resuming, or beginning, a postpartum exercise program.
• Resume driving 10 days after returning home.
• Resume sexual relations when your doctor determines that healing is complete (usually about 3 to 6 weeks).

DIET—Eating a high-fiber diet will help prevent constipation, which is common after childbirth. Increase your fluid intake as you increase your fiber intake.

CALL YOUR DOCTOR IF

• Pain, swelling, redness, drainage or bleeding increases in the surgical area.
• You develop signs of infection, including headache, muscle aches, dizziness or a general ill feeling and fever.
• You experience nausea, vomiting, constipation or abdominal swelling.
• New, unexplained symptoms develop. Drugs used in treatment may produce side effects.

EPISIOTOMY
(Perineotomy)

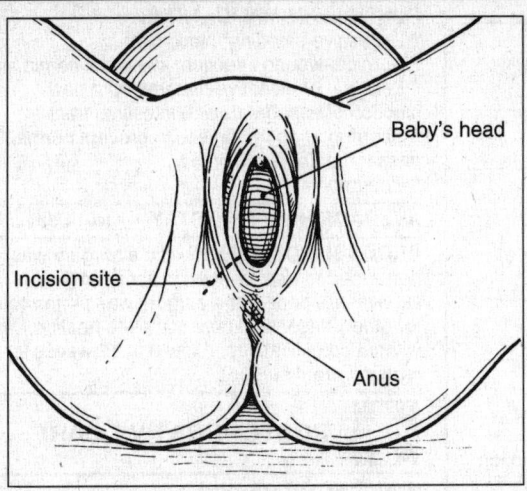

Baby's head

Incision site

Anus

This view illustrates a female patient with extended legs in stirrups on an examining table to allow examination of the genital area.
- The female genital area with a baby's head crowning at the entrance to the vagina and the incision site for the episiotomy.

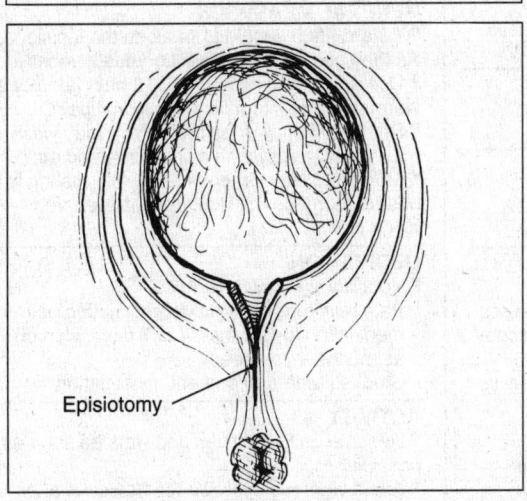

Episiotomy

Incision is made in the perineum just before the widest part of the baby's head is delivered.

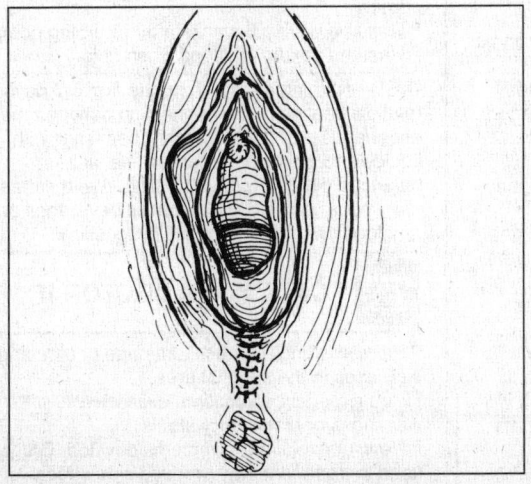

After the baby and placenta have been delivered, the episiotomy site is repaired with absorbable sutures.

ESOPHAGECTOMY

GENERAL INFORMATION

DEFINITION—Removal of part of the esophagus, the tubular passage from the back of the throat to the stomach.

BODY PARTS INVOLVED—Esophagus; stomach; colon (sometimes).

REASONS FOR SURGERY
- Cancer of the esophagus.
- Burns and scarring of the esophagus.
- Opening a closure of the esophagus in a newborn (usually an inherited defect).

SURGICAL RISK INCREASES WITH
- Adults over 60; newborns and infants.
- Obesity; smoking; poor nutrition.
- Excess alcohol consumption.
- Chronic or recent illness, especially pneumonia or diabetes mellitus.
- Use of some prescription and nonprescription drugs. Inform your doctor of any drugs, medications, or vitamin and herb supplements you are using or have used in the last month.

WHAT TO EXPECT

WHO OPERATES—General surgeon or thoracic surgeon.

WHERE PERFORMED—Hospital.

DIAGNOSTIC TESTS
- Before surgery: Blood and urine studies; x-rays of chest and upper gastrointestinal tract; esophagogram; esophagoscopy; bronchoscopy (see Glossary for all).
- After surgery: Blood and urine studies; x-rays of chest and upper gastrointestinal tract.

ANESTHESIA—General anesthesia by injection and inhalation with an airway tube placed in the windpipe.

DESCRIPTION OF OPERATION
- Incisions are made in the abdomen and chest to expose the esophagus.
- The esophagus is isolated and examined.
- Abnormal tissues are removed. If the surgery is performed to treat cancer, nearby lymph glands are also removed.
- The bottom end of the remaining part of the esophagus is joined with the stomach; sometimes the colon is used to bridge the gap.
- The chest and abdomen are closed in layers. The skin is closed with sutures or clips, which usually can be removed about 1 week after surgery.
- During the operation, a thin, plastic tube (called a jejunostomy tube) may be placed in your intestine and brought to the outside. It will be used to provide you with nourishment until you are able to take food by mouth.
- The operation can sometimes be done through an abdominal incision and a small incision at the base of the neck.

POSSIBLE COMPLICATIONS
- Excessive bleeding; blood clots.
- Surgical-wound infection; incisional hernia.
- Leakage of digestive material from new junction of esophagus and intestinal tract.
- Scarring at operation site to prevent normal passage of food and fluids.
- Pneumonia.

AVERAGE HOSPITAL STAY—7 to 14 days.

PROBABLE OUTCOME—If the surgery was performed to treat cancer, chances of 5-year survival are poor. If the surgery was performed for other reasons, expect complete healing without complications. Allow 8 to 12 weeks for recovery from surgery.

POSTOPERATIVE CARE

GENERAL MEASURES
- A hard ridge should form along the incisions. As they heal, the ridges will gradually recede
- Use an electric heating pad, a heat lamp or a warm compress to relieve incisional pain.
- Bathe and shower as usual. You may wash the incision gently with mild, unscented soap.
- Move and elevate legs often while resting in bed to decrease the likelihood of deep-vein blood clots.

MEDICATION
- Your doctor may prescribe:
  Pain relievers. Don't take prescription pain medication longer than 4 to 7 days. Use only as much as you need.
  Stool softeners to prevent constipation.

ACTIVITY
- Resume daily activities and work as soon as possible.
- Avoid vigorous exercise for 12 weeks after surgery.
- Resume driving 3 weeks after returning home.
- Resume sexual relations when able.

DIET—Nothing by mouth for the first 6-7 days to allow healing of the connection between the esophagus and the stomach. Then, start with liquids and gradually progress to a well-balanced diet to promote healing. Avoid coffee, tea, cocoa, cola drinks, alcoholic beverages and any food or spice that cause indigestion.

CALL YOUR DOCTOR IF

- Pain, swelling, redness, drainage or bleeding increases in the surgical area.
- You experience vomiting, excessive weakness or black, tarry stools.
- New, unexplained symptoms develop. Drugs used in treatment may produce side effects.

ESOPHAGECTOMY

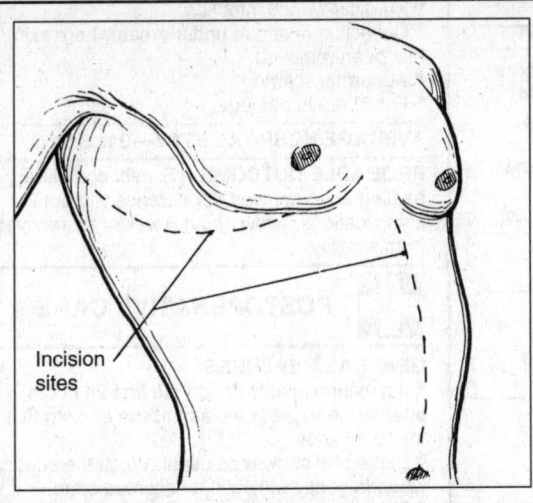

Incision sites

An illustration of the sites where incisions are made in order to expose the esophagus and the stomach.

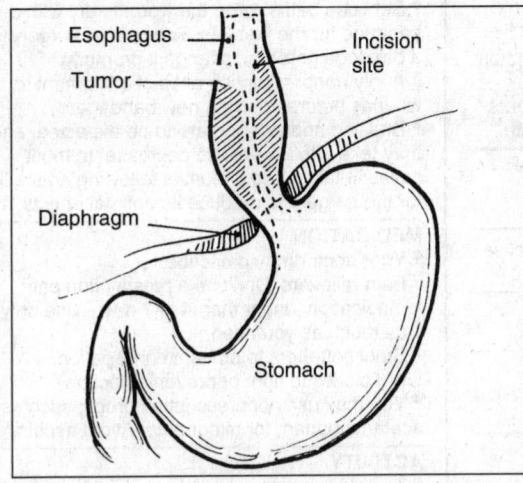

Esophagus

Tumor

Diaphragm

Incision site

Stomach

A portion of the esophagus is removed on both sides of the tumor or other defect.

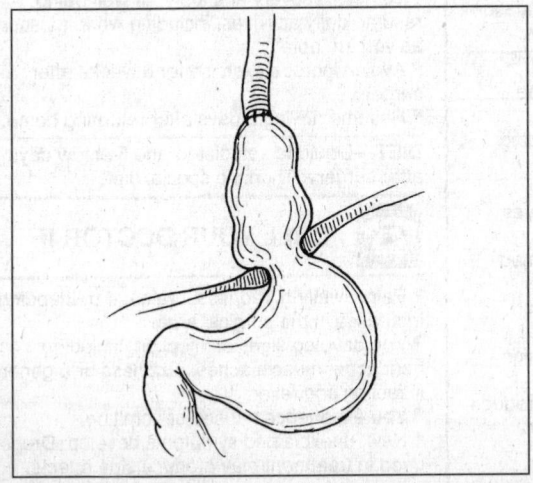

The bottom end of the remaining part of the esophagus is joined with the stomach; sometimes the colon is used to replace the missing portion of the esophagus.

FACE LIFT & BLEPHAROPLASTY

GENERAL INFORMATION

DEFINITION
- Face lift (Rhytidectomy): Removal of excess skin, fat and tissue from the face in order to tighten sagging skin and eliminate wrinkles, jowls, or a double chin.
- Blepharoplasty: Removal of excess fat and skin from around the eyelids to reduce puffiness, bags under the eyes, and wrinkles.

BODY PARTS INVOLVED—Skin and underlying tissue of the face and eyelids.

REASONS FOR SURGERY
- Improved appearance of the face.
- Improved appearance and function of the eyelids.

SURGICAL RISK INCREASES WITH
- Obesity; smoking; stress.
- Poor nutrition.
- Recent or chronic illness.
- Diabetes mellitus.
- Alcoholism.
- Use of some prescription and nonprescription drugs. Inform your doctor of any drugs, medications, or vitamin and herb supplements you are using or have used in the last month.

WHAT TO EXPECT

WHO OPERATES—Plastic and reconstructive surgeon.

WHERE PERFORMED—Doctor's office, outpatient surgical facility or hospital.

DIAGNOSTIC TESTS
- Before surgery: Blood and urine studies.
- After surgery: Blood studies.

ANESTHESIA
- Local anesthesia by injection.
- General anesthesia by injection and inhalation with an airway tube placed in the windpipe.

DESCRIPTION OF OPERATION
- Incisions are made where scarring will be minimal or less visible.
- Care is taken to clamp and tie tiny bleeding vessels during the procedure to prevent collection of scar tissue under the skin.
- Flaps of skin are cut away around the eyes and face. Excess tissue is removed from underlying areas, and excess skin is trimmed away.
- The skin is closed with fine sutures, which usually can be removed about 1 week after surgery. Drains may be placed in the incision and left for several days.
- Bandages and ice packs are applied to reduce swelling and bleeding.

POSSIBLE COMPLICATIONS
- Excessive bleeding; blood clots.
- Surgical-wound infection.
- Collection of serum under areas where skin has been removed.
- Abnormal scarring.
- Facial nerve damage.

AVERAGE HOSPITAL STAY—0 to 3 days.

PROBABLE OUTCOME—Expect complete healing and improved appearance without complications. Allow about 6 weeks for recovery from surgery.

POSTOPERATIVE CARE

GENERAL MEASURES
- If a wound bleeds during the first 24 hours after surgery, press a clean tissue or cloth to it for 10 minutes.
- Bathe and shower as usual. Wash the surgical wounds gently with mild, unscented soap.
- Between baths, keep the wounds dry with a bandage for the first 2 or 3 days after surgery. If a bandage gets wet, change it promptly.
- Apply nonprescription antibiotic ointment to wounds before applying new bandages.
- Bruising and swelling are to be expected, and may take 2 to 3 weeks to decrease. In most cases, it takes 3 to 6 months following a face lift for the surgery to produce its optimal effects.

MEDICATION
- Your doctor may prescribe:
  Pain relievers. Don't take prescription pain medication longer than 4 to 7 days. Use only as much as you need.
  Stool softeners to prevent constipation.
  Antibiotics to fight or prevent infection.
- You may use nonprescription drugs, such as acetaminophen, for minor pain. Avoid aspirin.

ACTIVITY
- To help recovery and aid your well-being, resume daily activities, including work, as soon as you are able.
- Avoid vigorous exercise for 6 weeks after surgery.
- Resume driving 3 days after returning home.

DIET—Liquid to soft diet for the first few days after surgery. Then, no special diet.

CALL YOUR DOCTOR IF

- Pain, swelling, redness, drainage or bleeding increases in the surgical area.
- You develop signs of infection, including headache, muscle aches, dizziness or a general ill feeling and fever.
- You experience nausea or vomiting.
- New, unexplained symptoms develop. Drugs used in treatment may produce side effects.

FACE LIFT & BLEPHAROPLASTY

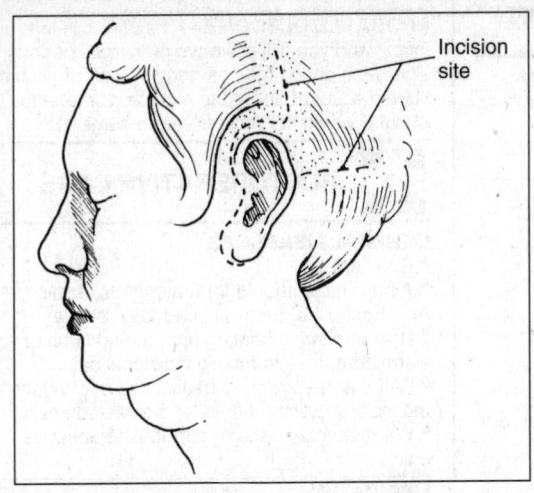

Incision site

Flaps of skin cut away around the eyes and face. Excess tissue is removed from underlying areas and excess skin is trimmed away.

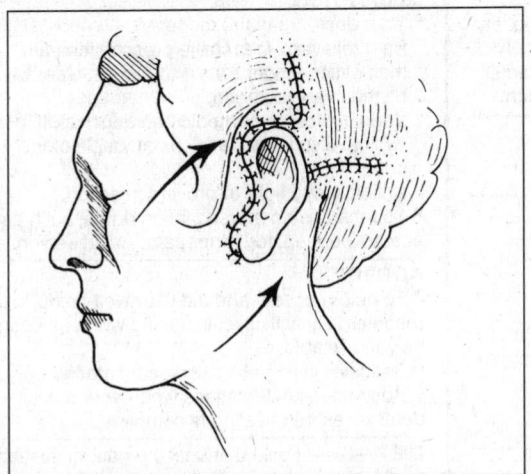

Skin is closed with fine sutures.

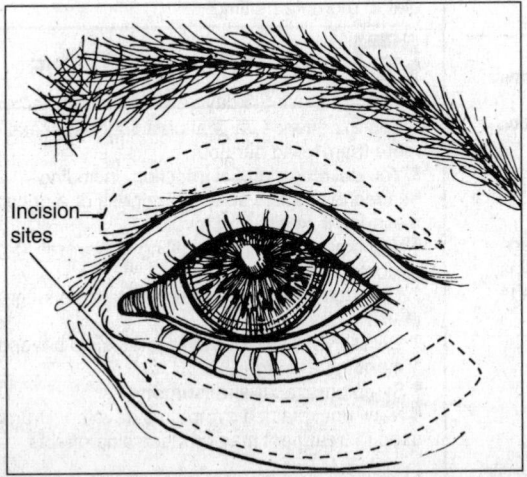

Incision sites

An illustration of excessive tissue surrounding the eye and the incision sites generally used.

FIBROID TUMOR REMOVAL
(Myomectomy)

 GENERAL INFORMATION

DEFINITION—Removal of fibroid tumors (leiomyoma, myoma) from the uterus through an incision in the lower abdomen.

BODY PARTS INVOLVED—Uterus.

REASONS FOR SURGERY
- Pelvic pain or back pain.
- Pressure on the bladder.
- Abnormal uterine bleeding; anemia.
- Difficulty in becoming pregnant.
- Discomfort with sexual intercourse.

SURGICAL RISK INCREASES WITH
- Obesity.
- Smoking.
- Poor nutrition, especially inadequate iron intake that has led to anemia.
- Recent or chronic illness.
- Diabetes mellitus.
- Use of some prescription and nonprescription drugs. Inform your doctor of any drugs, medications, or vitamin and herb supplements you are using or have used in the last month.

 WHAT TO EXPECT

WHO OPERATES—General surgeon or obstetrician-gynecologist.

WHERE PERFORMED—Hospital.

DIAGNOSTIC TESTS
- Before surgery: Blood studies; dilatation and curettage of the uterus (D & C); laparoscopy; x-rays of abdomen; barium-enema x-rays; intravenous pyelogram (see Glossary for all).
- After surgery: Blood studies.

ANESTHESIA—General anesthesia by injection and inhalation with an airway tube placed in the windpipe.

DESCRIPTION OF OPERATION
- One or more incisions are made in the lower abdomen.
- The muscles are separated and connective tissues are cut free to expose the uterus.
- Fibroid tumors are located; each tumor is removed separately, and each excision is repaired.
- The internal structures are closed in layers.
- The skin is closed with sutures or skin clips, which can be removed about 4 to 7 days after surgery.

POSSIBLE COMPLICATIONS
- Excessive bleeding.
- Surgical-wound infection.
- Recurrence of the tumor.
- Perforation of the uterus or bowel during surgery.

AVERAGE HOSPITAL STAY—2 to 3 days.

PROBABLE OUTCOME—The uterus is left intact, and you will still have menstrual periods. Your next period may be heavier than usual but should occur at about the expected time. Allow about 6 weeks for recovery from surgery.

 POSTOPERATIVE CARE

GENERAL MEASURES
- Don't smoke.
- A hard ridge should form along the incision. As it heals, the ridge will gradually recede.
- Use an electric heating pad, a heat lamp or a warm compress to relieve incisional pain.
- Bathe and shower as usual. You may wash the incision gently with mild, unscented soap.
- Wear sanitary pads or tampons to absorb blood.

MEDICATION
- Your doctor may prescribe:
  Pain relievers. Don't take prescription pain medication longer than 4 to 7 days. Use only as much as you need.
  Vaginal creams or medicated douches, if vaginal discharge develops an unpleasant odor.
  Antibiotics to fight or prevent infection.
- You may use nonprescription drugs, such as acetaminophen, for minor pain. Avoid aspirin.

ACTIVITY
- To help recovery and aid your well-being, resume daily activities, including work, as soon as you are able.
- Resume driving about 2 weeks after surgery.
- Resume sexual relations when your doctor determines that healing is complete.

DIET—Clear liquid diet until the gastrointestinal tract functions again. Then eat a well-balanced diet to promote healing.

 CALL YOUR DOCTOR IF

- You experience vaginal bleeding that soaks more than 1 pad per hour.
- You develop signs of infection, including headache, muscle aches, dizziness or a general feeling of ill health and fever.
- You have abdominal swelling or severe abdominal pain.
- The urge to urinate frequently persists longer than 1 month.
- Excessive vaginal discharge persists beyond 1 month after surgery.
- Symptoms recur after surgery.
- New, unexplained symptoms develop. Drugs used in treatment may produce side effects.

FIBROID TUMOR REMOVAL
(Myomectomy)

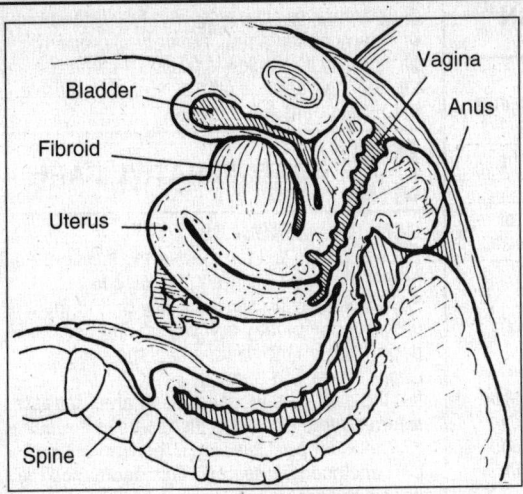

An illustration of the female genital area seen through a cross section.
- In this example, the fibroid tumor is on the front surface of the uterus.

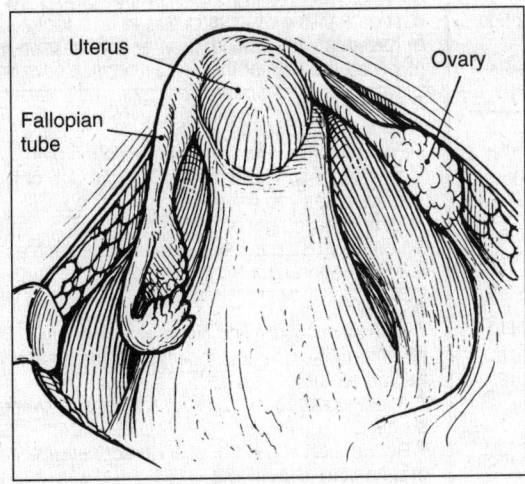

After the skin has been incised and muscles retracted, the uterus and fibroid tumor are visible through the incision site.

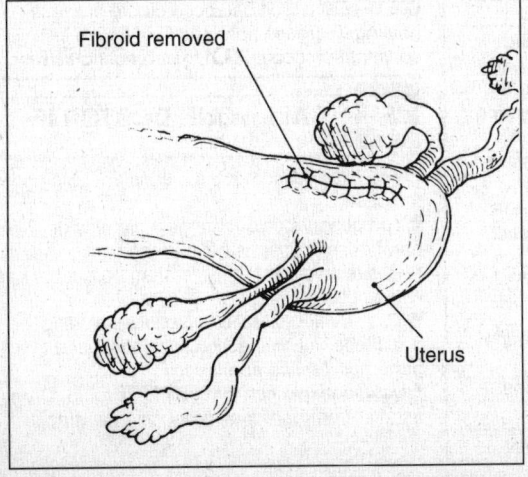

The fibroid tumor is removed and the surgical site is repaired with absorbable sutures.

SURGERIES

FRACTURE REPAIR
(Fracture Reduction)

 GENERAL INFORMATION

DEFINITION—Rejoining ends of a broken bone. The term "broken bone" means the same as "fractured bone."

BODY PARTS INVOLVED—Any bone in the body.

REASONS FOR SURGERY—Restoration of normal position and function of a broken bone.

SURGICAL RISK INCREASES WITH
- Adults over 60.
- Obesity; smoking; poor nutrition; alcoholism.
- Recent or chronic illness.
- Diabetes mellitus.
- Use of some prescription and nonprescription drugs. Inform your doctor of any drugs, medications, or vitamin and herb supplements you are using or have used in the last month.

 WHAT TO EXPECT

WHO OPERATES—Orthopedist, general surgeon or family doctor.

WHERE PERFORMED—Hospital, outpatient surgical facility, doctor's office or emergency room.

DIAGNOSTIC TESTS
- Before surgery: Blood and urine studies; x-ray of affected area.
- During surgery: X-rays.
- After surgery: X-rays through cast or splint to determine if rejoined pieces remain in good position for healing.

ANESTHESIA
- Local anesthesia by injection.
- General anesthesia by injection and inhalation with an airway tube placed in the windpipe.

DESCRIPTION OF OPERATION
- One or more incisions may be made in the skin over the fracture.
- The bone fragments are aligned as close as possible to their normal position without injuring the skin.
- Sometimes, metal pins, screws or plates are used to re-join the areas of the fracture.
- Once the broken ends of bone are "set", the affected part is kept rigid with a plaster cast or splint.

POSSIBLE COMPLICATIONS
- Excessive bleeding.
- Improper alignment or healing of joined bone ends.
- Pressure on nearby nerves; nerve damage.
- Infection.

AVERAGE HOSPITAL STAY—0 to 6 days.

PROBABLE OUTCOME—Children's bones usually heal relatively rapidly. Fractured bones of elderly patients may never heal properly, particularly if nutrition is poor. The time required for healing depends on the type of fracture and the extent of tissue damage.

 POSTOPERATIVE CARE

GENERAL MEASURES
- A hard ridge will form along the incision. As it heals, the ridge will gradually recede.
- Do not allow pressure on any part of the cast until it is completely dry. Drying time varies, depending on the thickness of the cast, temperature and humidity.
- If the cast gets wet and a soft area appears, return to your doctor's office to have it repaired.
- Whenever possible, raise the limb or body part enclosed in the cast. This decreases the possibility of swelling. For example, prop a leg cast on a pillow when in bed, and on a footstool or hassock when sitting; prop an arm cast on a pillow on your chest.

MEDICATION
- Your doctor may prescribe:
  Pain relievers. Don't take prescription pain medication longer than 4 to 7 days. Use only as much as you need.
  Antibiotics to fight or prevent infection.
- You may use nonprescription drugs, such as acetaminophen, for minor pain. Avoid aspirin.

ACTIVITY
- To help recovery and aid your well-being, resume daily activities, including work, as soon as you are able.
- Avoid vigorous exercise for 6 weeks following surgery.
- Resume driving when your doctor determines that healing is complete.

DIET—Eat a well-balanced diet to promote healing. Increase fiber and fluid intake if constipation occurs due to decreased activity.

 CALL YOUR DOCTOR IF

- You experience severe, persistent pain under the cast.
- You observe color change, coldness or numbness in tissues beyond the cast.
- Tissue swelling is greater than before the cast was applied.
- You develop signs of infection, including headache, muscle aches, dizziness, or a general ill feeling and fever.
- New, unexplained symptoms develop. Drugs used in treatment may produce side effects.

FRACTURE REPAIR
(Fracture Reduction)

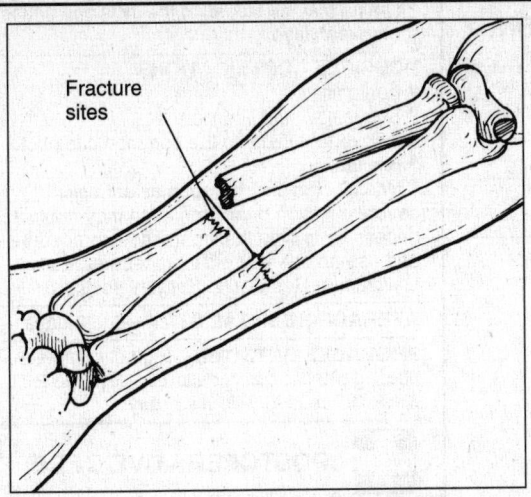

Fracture sites

An illustration of fractures of the forearm bones.

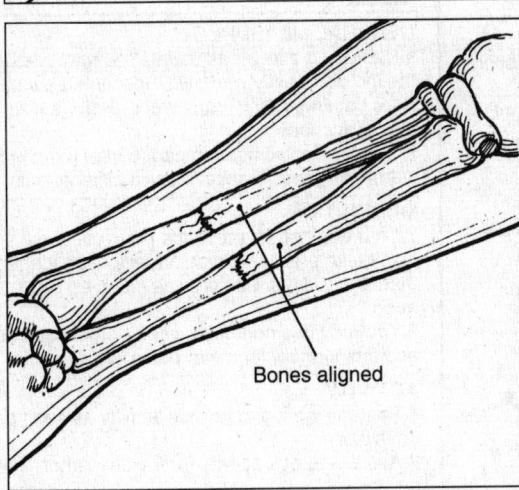

Bones aligned

When possible, the fractured bone ends are aligned by manipulation from the outside. If this cannot be done, the bone fragments can be aligned by surgical procedures to produce the same result.

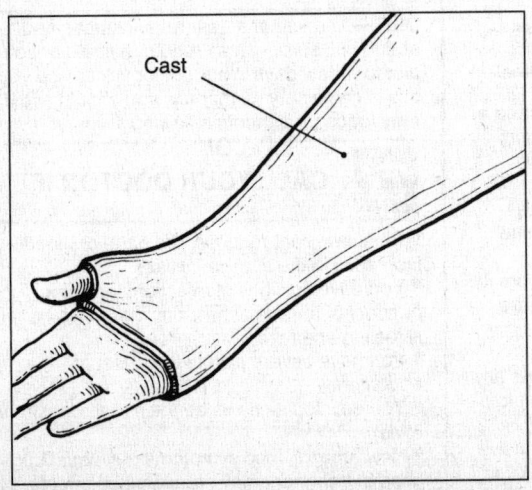

Cast

After the broken ends of bone are joined, the affected part is held in place with a plaster cast or splint.

SURGERIES

GALLBLADDER LAPAROSCOPY
(Laparoscopic Cholecystectomy)

 GENERAL INFORMATION

DEFINITION—Removal of the gallbladder with a laparoscope, a fiber-optic instrument that is used for diagnostic imaging and surgical procedures.

BODY PARTS INVOLVED—Gallbladder; bile ducts; liver.

REASONS FOR SURGERY
- Treatment of gallstones.
- Acute inflammation of the gallbladder.
- Benign and malignant tumors of the gallbladder.
- Chronic gallbladder infection.

SURGICAL RISK INCREASES WITH
- Obesity; smoking.
- Excess alcohol consumption.
- Recent or chronic illness.
- Cirrhosis of the liver.
- Diabetes mellitus.
- Use of some prescription and nonprescription drugs. Inform your doctor of any drugs, medications, or vitamin and herb supplements you are using or have used in the last month.

 WHAT TO EXPECT

WHO OPERATES—General surgeon.

WHERE PERFORMED—Hospital, outpatient surgical facility.

DIAGNOSTIC TESTS
- Before surgery: Blood studies, x-rays, ECG; ultrasound, radionuclide excretion scan (see Glossary for all).
- During surgery: Video screen viewing; x-rays.
- After surgery: X-rays; blood tests.

ANESTHESIA—General anesthesia by injection and inhalation with an airway tube placed in the windpipe.

DESCRIPTION OF OPERATION
- A small incision is made near the navel and a small needle inserted to inflate the abdomen with carbon dioxide to visualize the organs.
- Three small incisions are used to insert instruments to remove the gallbladder. The laparoscope is inserted and used to examine the abdomen visually.
- The gallbladder and the ducts running from it are located and separated, and the ducts are clipped; the gallbladder is cut away and removed.
- The laparoscope and surgical instruments are removed and the carbon dioxide is allowed to escape from the abdomen.
- Small sutures under the skin and an adhesive bandage are used to close the wounds.

- Drains may be placed in the incisions and left for several days.

POSSIBLE COMPLICATIONS
- Peritonitis.
- Surgical wound infection.
- Inadvertent injury to the common bile duct.
- Bile leak.
- Unexpected findings such as adhesions, severe infection or inflammation may make it necessary to stop the laparoscopy procedure and use an open surgical procedure (see Gallbladder Removal in Surgery section).

AVERAGE HOSPITAL STAY—0 to 2 days.

PROBABLE OUTCOME—Expect complete healing without complications. Allow 1 to 2 weeks for recovery from surgery.

 POSTOPERATIVE CARE

GENERAL MEASURES
- Bathe and shower as usual. You may wash the incision gently with mild, unscented soap. After bathing, replace any wet dressings with clean, dry ones.
- Use an electric heating pad, a heat lamp or a warm compress to relieve any incisional pain.

MEDICATION
- Your doctor may prescribe pain relievers. Don't take prescription pain medication longer than 4 to 7 days. Use only as much as you need.
- You may use nonprescription drugs, such as acetaminophen, for minor pain. Avoid aspirin.

ACTIVITY
- Resume work and normal activity as soon as possible.
- Avoid vigorous activity for 6 weeks after surgery.

DIET—The use of a general anesthetic and abdominal surgery may require a liquid or soft diet for a few days. Your doctor will advise you if this is necessary. Generally, you should avoid fatty foods for a month following surgery.

 CALL YOUR DOCTOR IF

- Pain, swelling, redness, drainage or bleeding increases in the surgical areas.
- You develop signs of infection, including headache, muscle aches, dizziness or a general ill feeling and fever.
- You have severe pain in the chest or abdomen.
- You develop signs of jaundice (yellow skin or eyes).
- New, unexplained symptoms develop. Drugs used in treatment may produce side effects.

GALLBLADDER LAPAROSCOPY
(Laparoscopic Cholecystectomy)

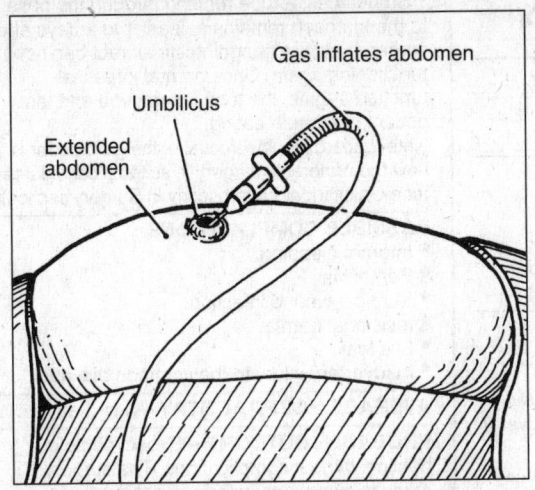

Carbon dioxide is used to inflate the abdomen to separate the organs.

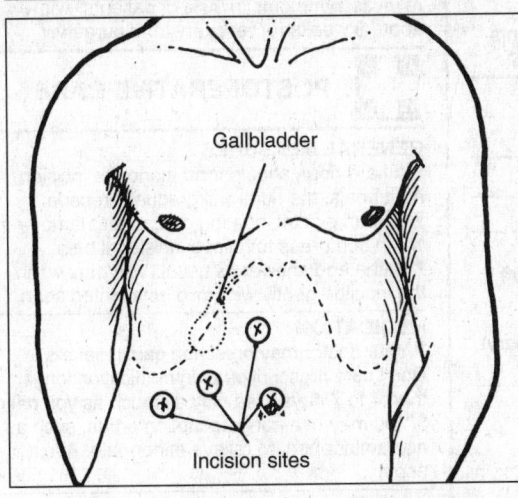

Small incisions are made in the abdomen to allow insertion of the laparoscope.

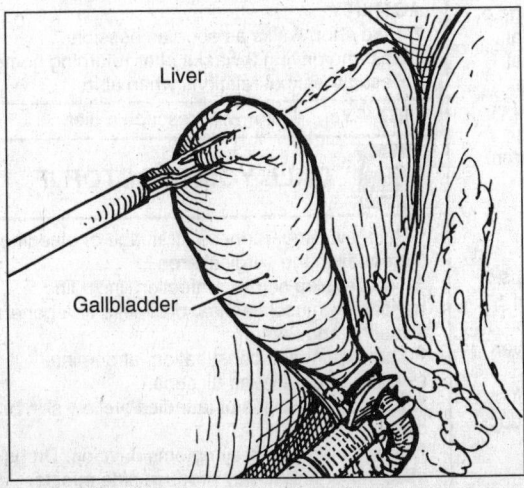

The gallbladder is held in position while the cystic duct is separated and clipped. The gallbladder is cut away and removed.

SURGERIES

GALLBLADDER REMOVAL
(Cholecystectomy, Open)

 GENERAL INFORMATION

DEFINITION—Removal of the gallbladder.

BODY PARTS INVOLVED—Gallbladder; bile ducts.

REASONS FOR SURGERY
- Gallstones.
- Suspected gallbladder tumors.
- Chronic gallbladder infection.
- Sudden, severe infection of the gallbladder that does not respond rapidly to treatment.

SURGICAL RISK INCREASES WITH
- Obesity; smoking.
- Recent or chronic illness.
- Alcoholism; cirrhosis of the liver; diabetes mellitus; heart disease; or chronic obstructive pulmonary disease (COPD).
- Use of some prescription and nonprescription drugs. Inform your doctor of any drugs, medications, or vitamin and herb supplements you are using or have used in the last month.

 WHAT TO EXPECT

WHO OPERATES—General surgeon.

WHERE PERFORMED—Hospital.

DIAGNOSTIC TESTS
- Before surgery: Blood studies; x-rays of the gallbladder; ultrasound; ECG; radionuclide excretion scan (see Glossary for all).
- During surgery: Cholangiogram (see Glossary).
- After surgery: Blood studies.

ANESTHESIA—General anesthesia by injection and inhalation with an airway tube placed in the windpipe.

DESCRIPTION OF OPERATION
- An incision is made under the right rib cage or down the center of the abdomen. Abdominal muscles are separated to expose abdominal organs, which are inspected for undetected disease. Other surgeries may be performed at this time.
- The gallbladder is cut free and removed from under the liver.
- A cholangiogram is done to determine if gallstones are lodged in the bile ducts. If necessary, the gallstones are removed.
- The incision is closed with sutures, skin clips or staples, which usually can be removed about 1 week after surgery. Occasionally, a drainage tube is left in place to drain bile around the liver. If stones are removed from the bile duct, a second tube (T-tube) is placed to drain this duct and allow x-rays to be taken later of the bile duct.

- Sometimes, a tube running through the nose to the stomach remains at least 1 to 2 days after surgery until the gastrointestinal tract begins functioning again. Once normal intestinal function begins, the tube is removed and the patient can begin eating.
Note: Laparoscopic removal of the gallbladder is now the preferable surgery in suitable candidates (see Gallbladder Laparoscopy in Surgery section).

POSSIBLE COMPLICATIONS
- Internal bleeding.
- Peritonitis.
- Surgical-wound infection.
- Incisional hernia.
- Bile leak.
- Inadvertent injury to the common bile duct.

AVERAGE HOSPITAL STAY—3 to 5 days.

PROBABLE OUTCOME—Expect complete healing without complications. The surgery relieves symptoms in 90% of patients. Allow about 3 weeks for recovery from surgery.

 POSTOPERATIVE CARE

GENERAL MEASURES
- A hard ridge should form along the incision. As it heals, the ridge will gradually recede.
- Use an electric heating pad, a heat lamp or a warm compress to relieve incisional pain.
- Bathe and shower as usual. You may wash the incision gently with mild, unscented soap.

MEDICATION
- Your doctor may prescribe pain relievers. Don't take prescription pain medication longer than 4 to 7 days. Use only as much as you need.
- You may use nonprescription drugs, such as acetaminophen, to relieve minor pain. Avoid aspirin.

ACTIVITY
- Take short walks as soon as possible.
- Resume driving 3 weeks after returning home.
- Resume sexual relations when able.

DIET—Your doctor will prescribe a diet.

 CALL YOUR DOCTOR IF

- Pain, swelling, redness, drainage or bleeding increases in the surgical area.
- You develop signs of infection, including headache, muscle aches, dizziness or a general ill feeling and fever.
- You experience constipation, abdominal swelling or unrelieved hiccups.
- You develop signs of jaundice (yellow skin or eyes).
- New, unexplained symptoms develop. Drugs used in treatment may produce side effects.

GALLBLADDER REMOVAL
(Cholecystectomy, Open)

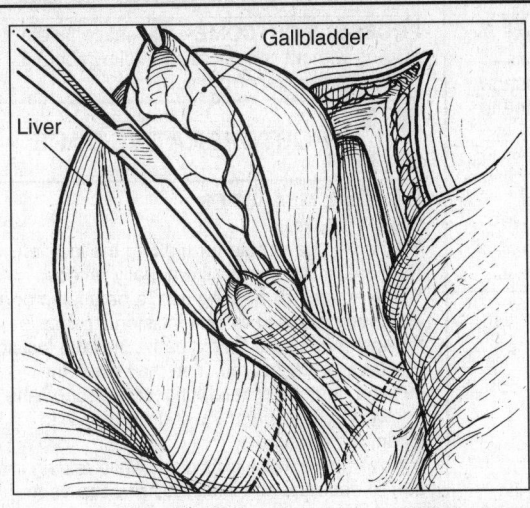

An illustration of the liver and gallbladder located just under the right rib cage. The liver must be retracted upward in order to expose the gallbladder.

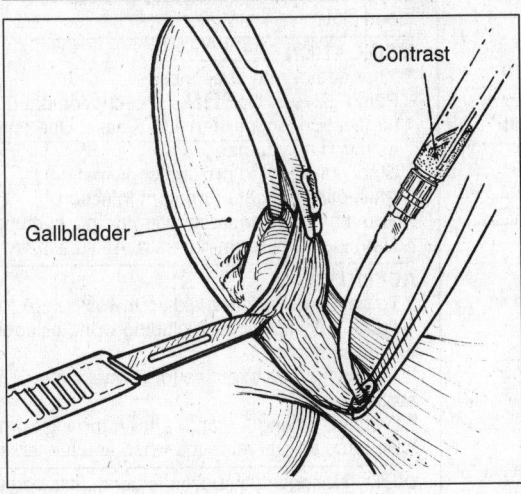

Gallbladder is cut free and removed. Catheter is inserted into bile duct to inject contrast dye for a cholangiography.

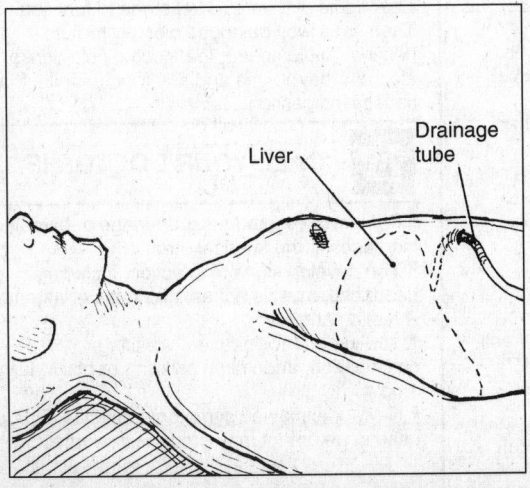

Occasionally, a drainage tube is left in place to drain bile around the liver.

GASTROENTEROSTOMY FOR PYLORIC OBSTRUCTION

GENERAL INFORMATION

DEFINITION—Creation of an artificial passage between the stomach and the small intestine to bypass obstructions caused by ulcer scar tissue.

BODY PARTS INVOLVED—Stomach; duodenum; jejunum (usually).

REASONS FOR SURGERY—Restoration of normal function of the gastrointestinal tract.

SURGICAL RISK INCREASES WITH
- Adults over 60.
- Newborns and infants.
- Stress.
- Obesity.
- Smoking.
- Excess alcohol consumption.
- Poor nutrition.
- Recent or chronic illness.
- Diabetes mellitus.
- Use of some prescription and nonprescription drugs. Inform your doctor of any drugs, medications, or vitamin and herb supplements you are using or have used in the last month.

WHAT TO EXPECT

WHO OPERATES—General surgeon.

WHERE PERFORMED—Hospital.

DIAGNOSTIC TESTS
- Before surgery: Blood and urine studies; gastroscopy; x-rays of upper gastrointestinal tract; serum electrolytes (see Glossary).
- After surgery: Blood and urine studies.

ANESTHESIA—General anesthesia by injection and inhalation with an airway tube placed in the windpipe.

DESCRIPTION OF OPERATION
- An incision is made in the upper abdomen.
- The abdominal muscles are separated to expose the abdominal organs, which are inspected for any undetected disease. Other surgeries may be performed at this time.
- The stomach and jejunum are isolated. A small opening is made in each, and they are joined with sutures at the openings. Usually combined with vagotomy (see in Surgery section) to prevent ulceration of stoma.
- The abdominal muscles are closed with sutures. The skin is closed with sutures or clips, which usually can be removed in about 1 week.

POSSIBLE COMPLICATIONS
- Excessive bleeding.
- Surgical-wound infection.
- Spillage of stomach contents into abdomen.
- Incisional hernia.

AVERAGE HOSPITAL STAY—7 to 10 days.

PROBABLE OUTCOME—Expect complete healing without complications. Allow about 6 weeks for recovery from surgery.

POSTOPERATIVE CARE

GENERAL MEASURES
- Don't smoke.
- A hard ridge should form along the incision. As it heals, the ridge will gradually recede.
- Use an electric heating pad, a heat lamp or a warm compress to relieve incisional pain.
- Shower as usual. Avoid baths until the incision has completely healed. You may wash the incision gently with mild, unscented soap. After showering, replace any wet dressings with clean, dry ones.
- Move and elevate legs often while resting in bed to decrease the likelihood of deep-vein blood clots.

MEDICATION
- Your doctor may prescribe:
  Pain relievers. Don't take prescription pain medication longer than 4 to 7 days. Use only as much as you need.
  Stool softeners to prevent constipation.
  Antibiotics to fight or prevent infection.
- You may use nonprescription drugs, such as acetaminophen, for minor pain. Avoid aspirin.

ACTIVITY
- To help recovery and aid your well-being, resume daily activities, including work, as soon as you are able.
- Avoid vigorous exercise for 6 weeks after surgery.
- Resume driving 1 month after returning home.
- Resume sexual relations when you feel able.

DIET—Nasogastric suction is used; followed by clear liquid diet until bowel starts to function. Then eat a well-balanced diet to promote healing. Avoid coffee, tea, cocoa, cola drinks, alcoholic beverages and any food or spice that causes indigestion.

CALL YOUR DOCTOR IF

- Pain, swelling, redness, drainage or bleeding increases in the surgical area.
- You develop signs of infection, including headache, muscle aches, dizziness or a general ill feeling and fever.
- You experience nausea, vomiting, constipation, abdominal swelling or black, tarry stools.
- New, unexplained symptoms develop. Drugs used in treatment may produce side effects.

GASTROENTEROSTOMY FOR PYLORIC OBSTRUCTION

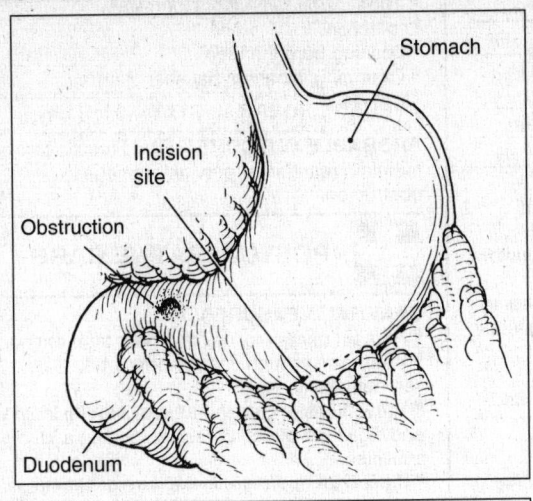

An illustration of a typical obstruction site in the lower end of the stomach, just before the duodenum (beginning of the first part of the intestine).

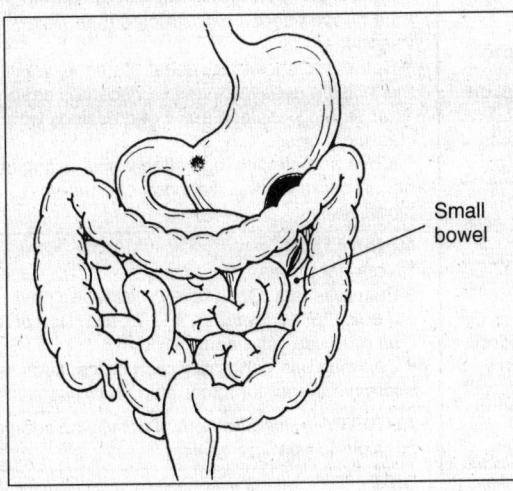

After the stomach and a small loop of small intestine are isolated, an opening is made in each.

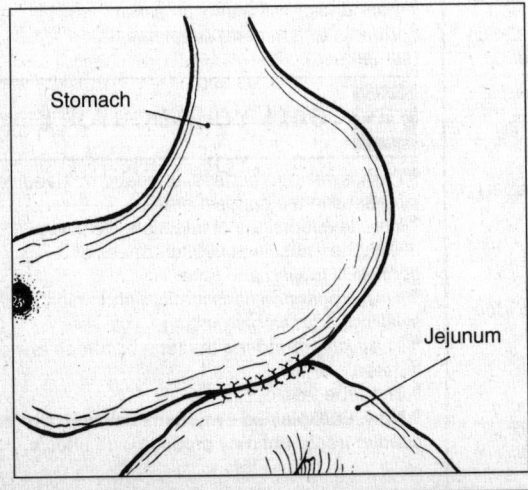

The cut end of the stomach is then joined with the surgically opened part of the jejunum, once again establishing a clear channel for the passage of food and fluids.

SURGERIES

GASTROSTOMY

 GENERAL INFORMATION

DEFINITION—Making a surgical opening into the stomach for placement of a feeding or drainage tube.

BODY PARTS INVOLVED—Stomach; skin; structures of the abdominal wall.

REASONS FOR SURGERY
- Prevention of pneumonia in patients with swallowing disorders.
- Provide nutrition to those who cannot swallow.
- Blockage of esophagus.
- To provide access to the stomach for feeding or drainage of stomach contents. It is frequently used in patients who cannot or will not eat adequate amounts of food, or to drain the stomach when prolonged drainage is required.

SURGICAL RISK INCREASES WITH
- Obesity; poor nutrition.
- Recent or chronic illness, especially chronic lung disease.
- Diabetes mellitus.
- Excess alcohol consumption.
- Use of some prescription and nonprescription drugs. Inform your doctor of any drugs, medications, or vitamin and herb supplements you are using or have used in the last month.

 WHAT TO EXPECT

WHO OPERATES—General surgeon or gastroenterologist.

WHERE PERFORMED—Hospital or outpatient surgical facility.

DIAGNOSTIC TESTS—Before surgery: Blood and urine studies; x-rays of gastrointestinal tract; endoscopy (see Glossary).

ANESTHESIA
- Local anesthesia by injection.
- General anesthesia by injection and inhalation with an airway tube placed in the windpipe.

DESCRIPTION OF OPERATION
- An incision is made in the abdominal wall.
- The stomach is isolated and an opening is made into it.
- The tube (usually polyvinylchloride or rubber) is secured by sutures around it to hold it in place.
- The other end of the tube is pulled to the outside through the incision site.
- The abdominal incision is closed and the tube is stitched to the skin.
- The procedure may also be accomplished with gastroscopy (see Gastrostomy, Percutaneous Endoscopic in Surgery section).

POSSIBLE COMPLICATIONS
- Skin irritation around the gastrostomy tube.
- Tube dislodgement or clogging.
- Infection.
- Leaking from the tube.
- Cramping; bloating; nausea; diarrhea.

AVERAGE HOSPITAL STAY—0 to 1 day.

PROBABLE OUTCOME—Good results to maintain nutrition or provide drainage if obstructed.

 POSTOPERATIVE CARE

GENERAL MEASURES
- Remain upright for 1/2 to 1 hour after eating.
- Keep skin around gastrostomy tube scrupulously clean.
- Prevent dislodging the tube by careful taping and vigilance during dressing, feeding and activities.
- If used for drainage, make sure gastrostomy tube doesn't become obstructed (use water irrigations).
- Bathe and shower as usual. You may wash the incision gently with mild, unscented soap. After bathing, replace any wet dressings with clean, dry ones.
- Move and elevate legs often while resting in bed to decrease the likelihood of deep-vein blood clots.

MEDICATION
- Your doctor may prescribe:
  Pain relievers. Don't take prescription pain medication longer than 4 to 7 days. Use only as much as you need.
- You may use nonprescription drugs, such as acetaminophen, for minor pain. Avoid aspirin.

ACTIVITY—Resume normal activity as soon as possible to promote healing.

DIET
- Your doctor will prescribe a diet.
- Vitamin and mineral supplements (sometimes).

 CALL YOUR DOCTOR IF

- Pain, swelling, redness, drainage or bleeding increases in the surgical area.
- You develop signs of infection, including headache, muscle aches, dizziness or a general ill feeling and fever.
- You experience constipation, abdominal swelling, nausea or vomiting.
- The skin around the the tube becomes raw or irritated.
- The tube falls out.
- New, unexplained symptoms develop. Drugs used in treatment may produce side effects.

GASTROSTOMY

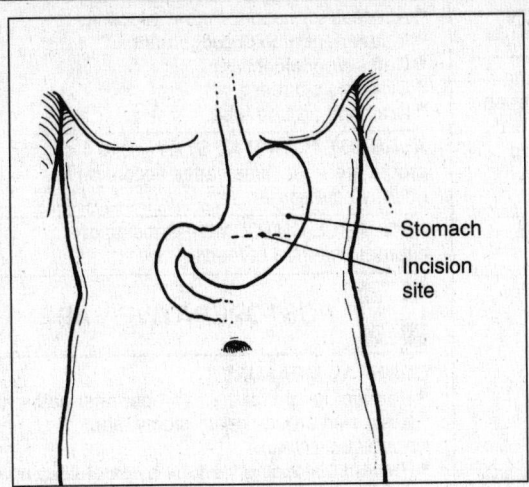

An illustration of the abdomen with proposed incision site for gastrostomy.

Stomach

Incision site

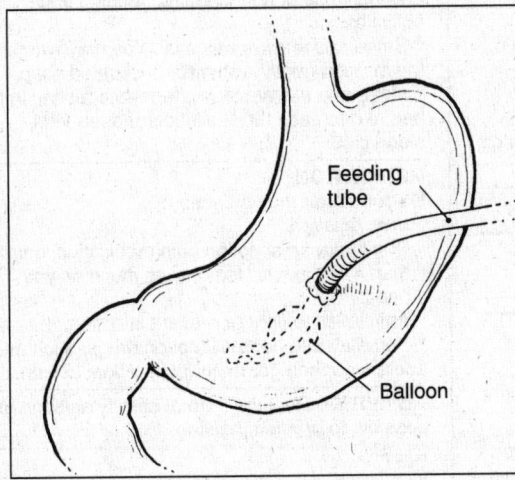

After the stomach has been located, a small opening is made into it and the stomach tube is pushed into the cavity of the stomach. The tube is secured by a balloon within the stomach.

Feeding tube

Balloon

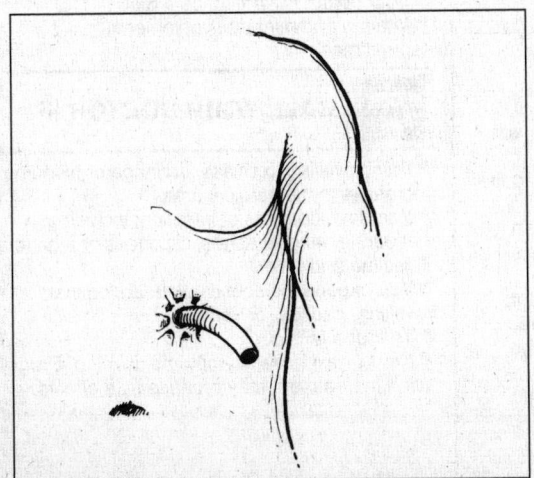

The other end of the tube is pulled to the outside through a separate small incision.

GASTROSTOMY, PERCUTANEOUS ENDOSCOPIC (P.E.G. Procedure)

 GENERAL INFORMATION

DEFINITION—Surgical technique for placing a feeding tube without having to perform an open laparotomy (operation on the abdomen). This procedure is less costly and time consuming than a surgical gastrostomy (see in Surgery section).

BODY PARTS INVOLVED—Stomach; skin; structures of the abdominal wall.

REASONS FOR SURGERY
- To provide nutrition for those who cannot swallow.
- To provide nutrition to those who cannot or will not eat adequate amounts of food.
- Blockage of esophagus.
- Prevention of pneumonia in patients with swallowing disorders.

SURGICAL RISK INCREASES WITH
- Stress; obesity; poor nutrition.
- Recent or chronic illness, especially chronic lung disease.
- Diabetes mellitus.
- Excess alcohol consumption.
- Use of some prescription and nonprescription drugs. Inform your doctor of any drugs, medications, or vitamin and herb supplements you are using or have used in the last month.

 WHAT TO EXPECT

WHO OPERATES—General surgeon or gastroenterologist.

WHERE PERFORMED—Hospital or outpatient surgical facility.

DIAGNOSTIC TESTS—Before surgery: Blood and urine studies; x-rays of gastrointestinal tract.

ANESTHESIA—Local anesthesia (usually lidocaine spray).

DESCRIPTION OF OPERATION
- The endoscopist anesthetizes the throat with lidocaine or other local anesthesia.
- The endoscopist passes the endoscope to the appropriate point in the stomach.
- A small incision is made in the skin and an intravenous cannula is pushed through the skin into the stomach.
- A string is passed into the stomach through the cannula; the string is grasped inside the stomach and is brought back out through the mouth.
- The gastrostomy tube is tied to the string, then pulled back into the stomach and out through the abdominal wall.
- The gastrostomy tube is then fixed to the abdominal wall.

POSSIBLE COMPLICATIONS
- Abscess formation; wound infection.
- Inadvertent tube dislodgement.
- Catheter malfunction.
- Clogging of tube.
- Drainage around tube.

AVERAGE HOSPITAL STAY—0 to 1 day for procedure. Total time varies according to underlying disorder.

PROBABLE OUTCOME—Satisfactory alternate method of feeding.

 POSTOPERATIVE CARE

GENERAL MEASURES
- Remain upright for 1/2 to 1 hour after eating.
- Keep skin around gastrostomy tube scrupulously clean.
- Prevent dislodging the tube by careful taping and vigilance during dressing, feeding and activities.
- Bathe and shower as usual. You may wash the incision gently with mild, unscented soap.
- Move and elevate legs often while resting in to bed to decrease the likelihood of deep-vein blood clots.

MEDICATION
- Your doctor may prescribe:
  Pain relievers.
  Don't take prescription pain medication longer than 4 to 7 days. Use only as much as you need.
  Antibiotics to fight or prevent infection.
- You may use nonprescription drugs, such as acetaminophen, for minor pain. Avoid aspirin.

ACTIVITY—Resume normal activity as soon as possible to promote healing.

DIET
- Your doctor will prescribe a diet.
- Vitamin and mineral supplements (sometimes).

 CALL YOUR DOCTOR IF

- Pain, swelling, redness, drainage or bleeding increases in the surgical area.
- You develop signs of infection, including headache, muscle aches, dizziness or a general ill feeling and fever.
- You experience constipation, abdominal swelling, nausea, or vomiting.
- The tube falls out.
- New, unexplained symptoms develop. Drugs used in treatment may produce side effects.

GASTROSTOMY, PERCUTANEOUS ENDOSCOPIC (P.E.G. Procedure)

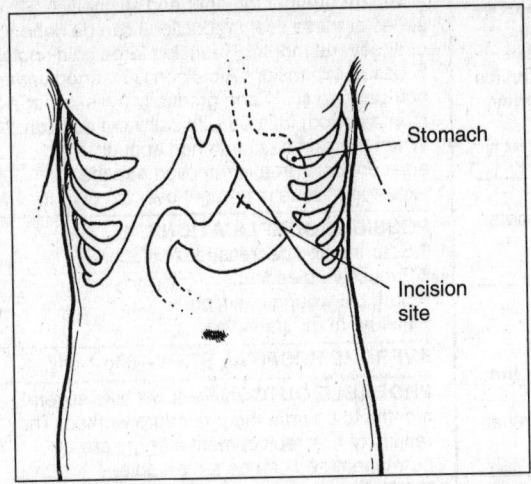

An illustration of the incision site in the abdomen over the position in the stomach chosen for the gastrostomy.

Stomach

Incision site

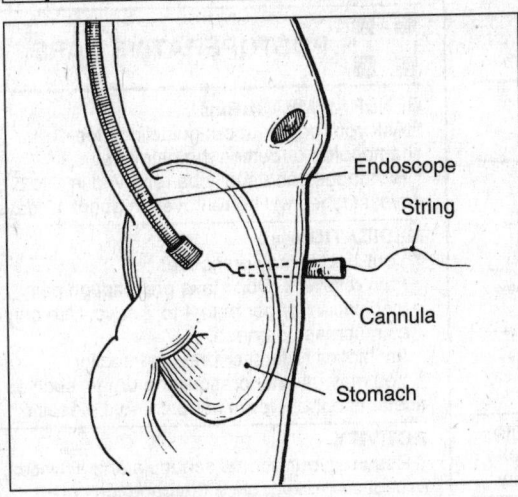

Shown are the endoscope at the upper end of the stomach and a tube inside the endoscope. The doctor makes a small incision into the skin and pushes an intravenous cannula through the skin into the stomach.

Endoscope

String

Cannula

Stomach

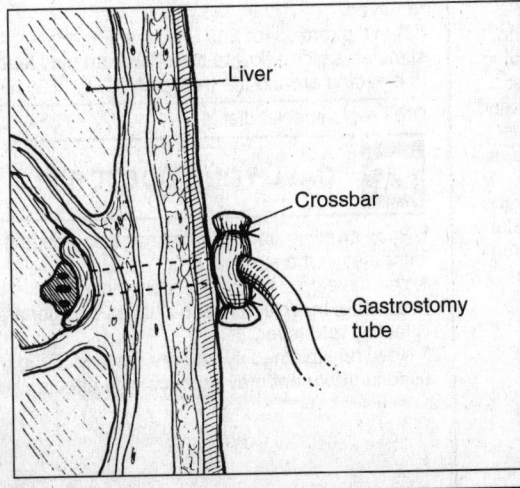

Final appearance with the feeding tube in place. The external end of the feeding tube is clamped to provide access for feeding in the future (not illustrated).

Liver

Crossbar

Gastrostomy tube

HAIR TRANSPLANT

GENERAL INFORMATION

DEFINITION—Relocating hair-bearing skin, usually from the back of the head to the front. Multiple procedures are necessary with intervals in between, so that the total time involved may be 18 months or more.

BODY PARTS INVOLVED—Hair and scalp.

REASONS FOR SURGERY—To correct markedly receding hairlines or large bald spots caused by pattern baldness (see in Illness section), an inherited trait.

SURGICAL RISK INCREASES WITH
- Smoking.
- Recent or chronic illness; diabetes mellitus.
- Poor quality hair on the back and sides of the head.
- Hair transplants that are performed before hair loss has come to a standstill.
- Use of some prescription and nonprescription drugs. Inform your doctor of any drugs, medications, or vitamin and herb supplements you are using or have used in the last month.

WHAT TO EXPECT

WHO OPERATES—Plastic surgeon; other doctor with special training (sometimes).

WHERE PERFORMED—Doctor's office, outpatient surgical facility, special hair-transplant clinic or hospital (for more complex procedures).

DIAGNOSTIC TESTS
- Before surgery: Physical examination.
- After surgery: None required.

ANESTHESIA—Local anesthetic injected into both the donor and recipient sites. In complex procedures, more sedation may be necessary.

DESCRIPTION OF OPERATION—Several procedures are available. You and your doctor will decide the most appropriate one depending on the degree and location of your baldness.
- Punch grafts (plugs): A round graft is punched out of a donor site and fitted into a hole in the bald area. Each punch contains about 15 hairs plus skin and fatty tissue.
- Mini-plugs: About half the size of punch grafts and used to fill in spaces between larger grafts.
- Micro-plugs: Made by splitting one large plug into 4 to fill in spaces. Adds a more irregular natural look to hairline.
- Strip grafts: Similar to punch grafts except the graft is long and thin. May be used to finish hairline once plugs have filled in bald spot.
- Flaps: A flap of hair on the back or side is cut out and swiveled onto the bald spot. The cut edges of the donor site are brought together and stitched closed.

- Scalp reduction: An area of bald skin (2 inches by six inches) is cut out and the two sides are brought together and stitched. A series of these scalp reductions can be done over several months, reducing large bald spots.
- Tissue expansion: A balloon is inserted under hair-bearing scalp and gradually (weekly, for a 2 month period) inflated with saltwater solution. When the skin has stretched enough, the adjacent bald area is removed and the expanded tissue is brought over to cover it.

POSSIBLE COMPLICATIONS
- Scarring and decreased circulation.
- Excessive bleeding.
- Surgical-wound infection.
- Failure of the transplant.

AVERAGE HOSPITAL STAY—0 to 1 day.

PROBABLE OUTCOME—It will take several months to be sure the procedure worked. The results of hair replacement surgery are permanent and can be remarkable.

POSTOPERATIVE CARE

GENERAL MEASURES
- Ask your doctor about guidelines for shampooing or getting the hair wet.
- Bandages can usually be removed in 2 to 5 days; stitches will be removed in about 10 days.

MEDICATION
- Your doctor may prescribe:
  Pain relievers. Don't take prescription pain medication longer than 4 to 7 days. Use only as much as you need.
  Antibiotics to fight or prevent infection.
- You may use nonprescription drugs, such as acetaminophen, for minor pain. Avoid aspirin.

ACTIVITY
- Resume your normal schedule and activities, except swimming, once the bandages are removed.
- Avoid exercise for 2 to 3 weeks. Exercise stimulates blood flow to the scalp and may lead to bleeding around the transplants.

DIET—No special diet.

CALL YOUR DOCTOR IF

- Pain, swelling, redness, drainage or bleeding increases in the surgical area.
- You develop signs of infection, including headache, muscle aches, dizziness or a general ill feeling and fever.
- New, unexplained symptoms develop. Drugs used in treatment may produce side effects.

HAIR TRANSPLANT

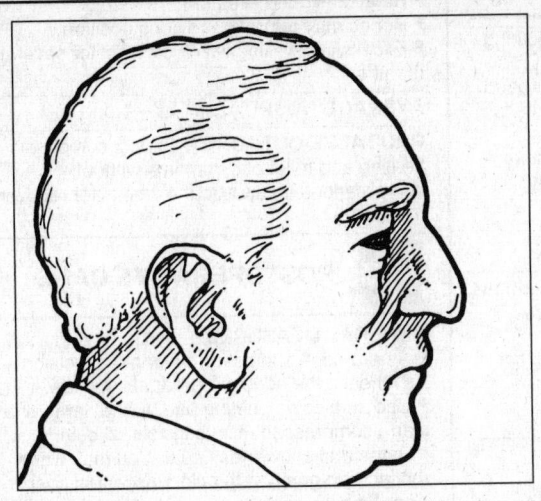

The surgical area before a plug transplant.

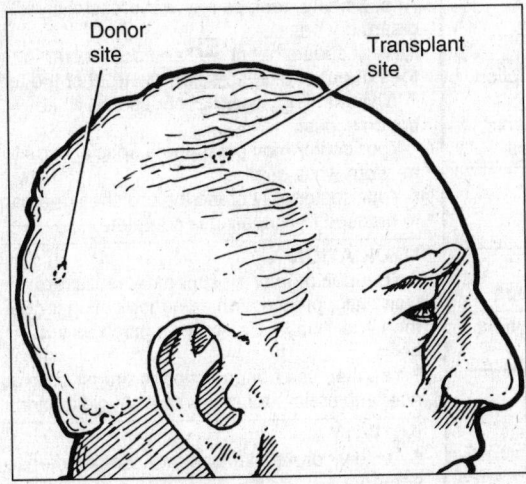

Donor site

Transplant site

A round plug is removed from a donor site and prepared for insertion into the transplant site.

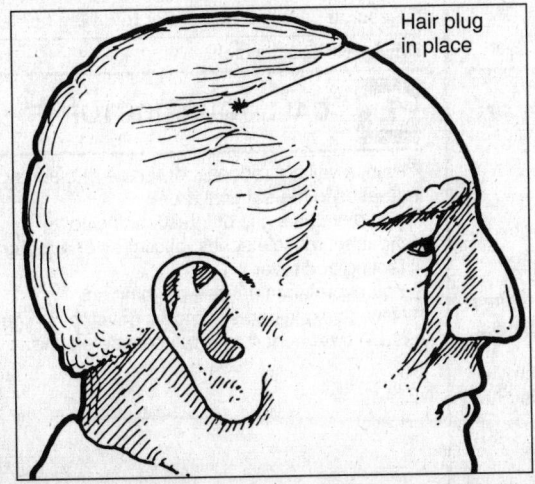

Hair plug in place

Hair plug is in place.

HAMMERTOE CORRECTION

GENERAL INFORMATION

DEFINITION—Removal of tendons and joining of middle joints in the toes to correct hammertoe, a deformity in which the toes bend downward. This causes the tops of the toes to become callused from rubbing against the inside of shoes. Hammertoe probably results from wearing shoes that do not fit properly, especially high-heeled shoes that place pressure on the front part of the foot and compress the smaller toes together tightly.

BODY PARTS INVOLVED—All toes except the big toes; tendons, blood vessels and nerves connected to these toes; overlying skin.

REASONS FOR SURGERY
- Relief of painful calluses.
- Prevention of permanent deformity.

SURGICAL RISK INCREASES WITH
- Obesity.
- Smoking.
- Excess alcohol consumption.
- Diabetes mellitus.
- Use of some prescription and nonprescription drugs. Inform your doctor of any drugs, medications, or vitamin and herb supplements you are using or have used in the last month.

WHAT TO EXPECT

WHO OPERATES—General surgeon (sometimes), podiatrist or orthopedic surgeon.

WHERE PERFORMED—Hospital or outpatient surgical facility.

DIAGNOSTIC TESTS
- Before surgery: Blood and urine studies; x-rays of feet.
- After surgery: Blood studies.

ANESTHESIA
- Local anesthesia by injection.
- Regional anesthesia by injection.

DESCRIPTION OF OPERATION
- After local anesthesia is injected, a tourniquet is applied above the ankle to keep the surgical area from bleeding.
- An incision is made through the skin.
- The tendons that attach to the toes are located, cut free of connective tissue to foot bones, and realigned so that they no longer bend downward.
- The middle joints of the affected toes are often connected together permanently with fine pins and wire sutures.
- The skin is closed with fine sutures, which usually can be removed about 7 to 10 days after surgery.
- A dressing is placed over the toes to help maintain their new position.

POSSIBLE COMPLICATIONS
- Excessive bleeding.
- Surgical-wound infection.
- Bones may return to previous position.
- Excessive swelling which can last for several months.

AVERAGE HOSPITAL STAY—None.

PROBABLE OUTCOME—Expect complete healing and relief of symptoms without complications. Allow about 4 weeks for recovery from surgery.

POSTOPERATIVE CARE

GENERAL MEASURES
- A hard ridge should form along the incision. As it heals, the ridge will gradually recede.
- Use an electric heating pad, a heat lamp or a warm compress to relieve incisional pain.
- Bathe and shower as usual. You may wash the incision gently with mild, unscented soap. After bathing, replace any wet dressings with clean, dry ones.
- Wear shoes that fit well and do not cramp the toes or put undue stress on the front of the foot.
- While healing, wear flat shoes and white cotton socks.
- Your doctor may prescribe a special shoe to be worn while healing.
- Your doctor may prescribe crutches or a cane to be used until healing is complete.

MEDICATION
- Your doctor may prescribe pain relievers. Don't take prescription pain medication longer than 4 to 7 days. Use only as much as you need.
- You may use nonprescription drugs, such as acetaminophen, for minor pain. Avoid aspirin.

ACTIVITY
- Avoid vigorous exercise for 6 weeks after surgery.
- Resume driving 1 week after returning home.

DIET—No special diet.

CALL YOUR DOCTOR IF

- Pain, swelling, redness, drainage or bleeding increases in the surgical area.
- You develop signs of infection, including headache, muscle aches, dizziness or a general ill feeling and fever.
- You experience nausea or vomiting.
- New, unexplained symptoms develop. Drugs used in treatment may produce side effects.

HAMMERTOE CORRECTION

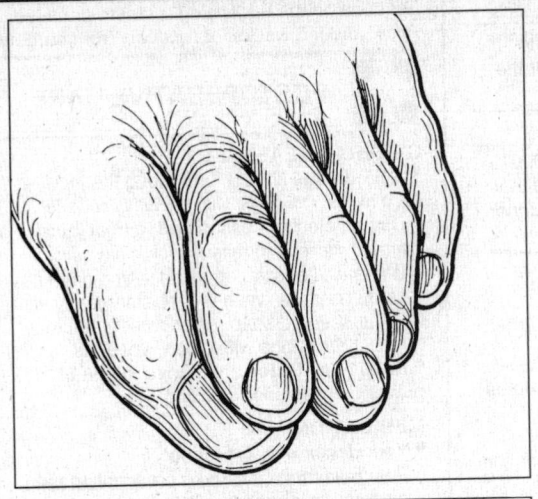

An illustration of a typical hammer toe (a deformity in which the toes bend downward).

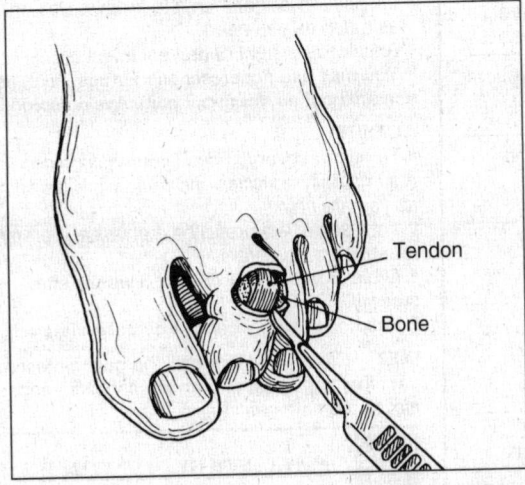

After local anesthesia is injected, tendons are located and divided so toes no longer bend downward.

Tendon

Bone

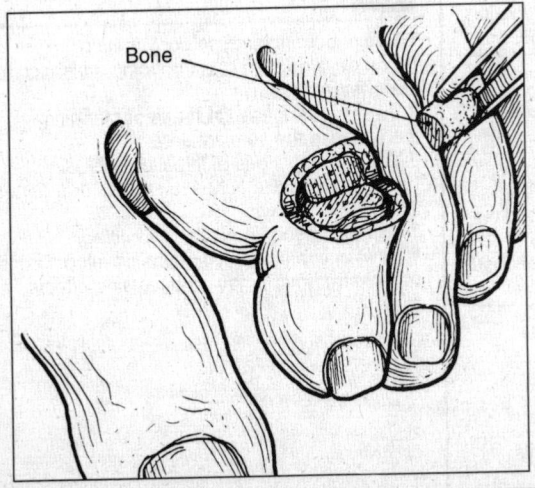

The portion of bone is removed and toes can return to normal shape.

Bone

HAND SURGERY

 GENERAL INFORMATION

DEFINITION—Any operation performed to restore or preserve the normal function of the hand.

BODY PARTS INVOLVED—Hand.

REASONS FOR SURGERY—Preservation or restoration of normal function of the hand that has been lost or impaired by disease, injury,or malformation.

SURGICAL RISK INCREASES WITH
• Obesity.
• Smoking.
• Poor nutrition.
• Excess alcohol consumption.
• Recent or chronic illness, especially diabetes mellitus, peripheral vascular disease and arthritis.
• Use of some prescription and nonprescription drugs. Inform your doctor of any drugs, medications, or vitamin and herb supplements you are using or have used in the last month.

 WHAT TO EXPECT

WHO OPERATES—General surgeon, hand surgeon, plastic surgeon, or orthopedic surgeon.

WHERE PERFORMED—Doctor's office, outpatient surgical facility, hospital or emergency room.

DIAGNOSTIC TESTS
• Before surgery: Blood and urine studies; x-rays of hands.
• After surgery: Blood studies.

ANESTHESIA
• Local anesthesia (sometimes) by injection.
• Regional anesthesia by injection.
• General anesthesia by injection and inhalation with an airway tube placed in the windpipe.

DESCRIPTION OF OPERATION
• The arm of the affected hand is elevated and wrapped with a blood-pressure cuff inflated to higher than normal blood pressure. This prevents the surgical area from bleeding.
• The surgery is performed carefully, but as quickly as possible. The procedures depend on the injury or disease in the hand.
• The wound is covered with gauze and padded dressings.

POSSIBLE COMPLICATIONS
• Excessive bleeding.
• Surgical-wound infection.
• Nerve damage.
• Scarring of tendons which limits motion.

AVERAGE HOSPITAL STAY—0 to 2 days.

PROBABLE OUTCOME—Expect complete healing of surgical wound. Success of surgery depends on the underlying problem or cause. Allow about 3 weeks for recovery from surgery.

 POSTOPERATIVE CARE

GENERAL MEASURES
• A hard ridge should form along the incision. As it heals, the ridge will gradually recede.
• Use an electric heating pad, a heat lamp or a warm compress to relieve incisional pain.
• Bathe and shower as usual, if you don't have a cast. You may wash the incision gently with mild, unscented soap. After bathing, replace any wet dressings with clean, dry ones.
• Keep the affected arm above the heart to prevent or decrease swelling.

MEDICATION
• Your doctor may prescribe:
  Pain relievers. Don't take prescription pain medication longer than 4 to 7 days. Use only as much as you need.
  Antibiotics to fight or prevent infection.
• You may use nonprescription drugs, such as acetaminophen, for minor pain. Avoid aspirin.

ACTIVITY
• To help recovery and aid your well-being, resume daily activities, including work, as soon as you are able.
• Your doctor will prescribe a physical therapy rehabilitation program.
• Avoid vigorous exercise for 3 weeks after surgery.
• Resume driving when the hand has healed.

DIET—Clear liquid diet until the gastrointestinal tract functions again. Then eat a well-balanced diet to promote healing.

 CALL YOUR DOCTOR IF

• You experience nausea or vomiting.
• You develop pain or a throbbing sensation in the affected hand.
• Swelling, redness, drainage or bleeding increases in the surgical area.
• You develop signs of infection, including headache, muscle aches, dizziness or a general ill feeling and fever.
• You experience nausea or vomiting.
• New, unexplained symptoms develop. Drugs used in treatment may produce side effects.

HAND SURGERY

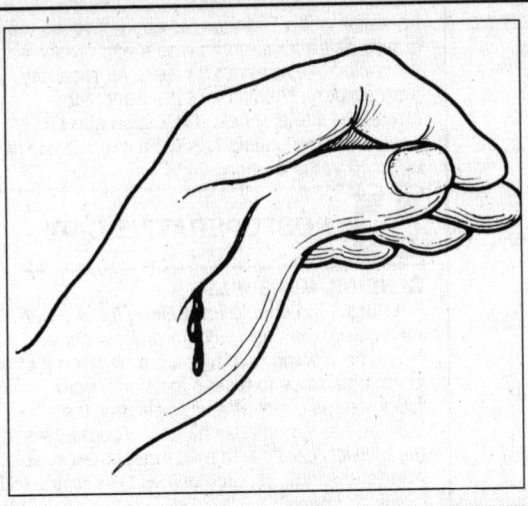

A typical hand injury with a deep laceration.
- Hand injuries may include severed nerves or blood vessels, severed or injured tendons or connective tissue, or amputated fingers.

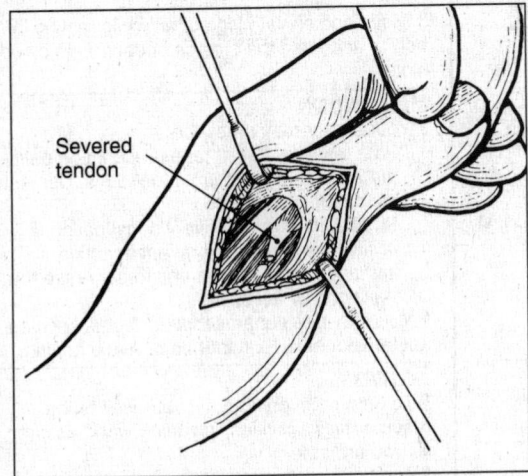

Severed tendon

The ragged injury is made into a clean surgical incision and muscles and connective tissue retracted for exposure. A severed tendon can be seen and repaired.

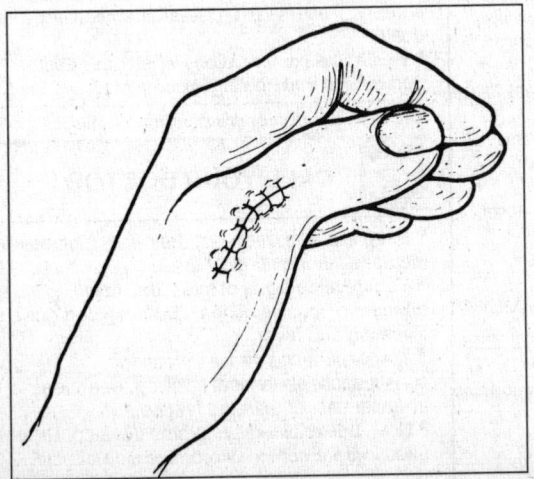

Skin is carefully closed after repair to the injured hand tissue. The hand and forearm are usually kept rigid with a plaster cast or splint.

HEART TRANSPLANTATION

 GENERAL INFORMATION

DEFINITION—Replacement of a diseased heart with a healthy heart.

BODY PARTS INVOLVED—Diseased or abnormal heart; healthy heart from donor.

REASONS FOR SURGERY
- Heart failure from coronary artery disease.
- Heart failure from cardiomyopathy.
- Valvular heart disease with congestive heart failure.
- Heart failure from severe congenital heart disease.

SURGICAL RISK INCREASES WITH
- Adults over 60; obesity; poor nutrition.
- Recent or chronic illness; diabetes mellitus.
- Alcoholism; smoking.
- Use of some prescription and nonprescription drugs. Inform your doctor of any drugs, medications, or vitamin and herb supplements you are using or have used in the last month.

 WHAT TO EXPECT

WHO OPERATES—Cardiovascular surgeon.

WHERE PERFORMED—Hospital.

DIAGNOSTIC TESTS
- Before surgery: Blood and urine studies; chest x-ray; studies of the immune system; ECG; cardiac catheterization; ultrasound (see Glossary for all).
- During surgery: Cardiac monitoring.
- After surgery: Blood studies; ECG.

ANESTHESIA—General anesthesia by injection and inhalation with an airway tube placed in the windpipe.

DESCRIPTION OF OPERATION
- A healthy heart is obtained from a donor who has died from disease other than heart disease, HIV, or hepatitis (see Glossary for both); or accident.
- An incision is made in the recipient's chest to expose the heart.
- A heart-lung machine sustains life while the diseased heart is cut free and removed, and until the donor heart has been transplanted.
- The donor heart is sewn into place. The aorta, pulmonary artery, superior vena cava and inferior vena cava are connected to the new heart.
- The skin is closed with sutures or clips, which are removed about 1 week after surgery.

POSSIBLE COMPLICATIONS
- Excessive bleeding; surgical-wound infection.
- Life-threatening general infections.
- Rejection of the transplanted heart.
- Cancer which develops as an adverse effect of immunosuppressant drugs.

AVERAGE HOSPITAL STAY—10 to 21 days.

PROBABLE OUTCOME—A successful transplantation prolongs life and improves the quality of life for patients who might otherwise have died. Allow about 6 weeks for recovery from surgery. Rejection of the transplant remains a life-long risk. If rejection can be controlled, the patient has a life expectancy of up to 10 years or more.

 POSTOPERATIVE CARE

GENERAL MEASURES
- A hard ridge should form along the incision. As it heals, the ridge will gradually recede.
- Use an electric heating pad, a heat lamp or a warm compress to relieve incisional pain.
- Shower as usual. Avoid baths until the incision has completely healed. You may wash the incision gently with mild, unscented soap. After showering, replace any wet dressings with clean, dry ones.
- Move and elevate legs often while resting in bed to decrease the chance of deep-vein blood clots.

MEDICATION
- Your doctor may prescribe:
  Pain relievers. Don't take prescription pain medication longer than 4 to 7 days. Use only as much as you need.
  Stool softeners to prevent constipation.
  Antibiotics to fight or prevent infection.
  Immunosuppressant drugs to decrease the likelihood of rejection.
- You may use nonprescription drugs, such as acetaminophen, for minor pain. Avoid aspirin.

ACTIVITY
- To help recovery and aid your well-being, resume daily activities, including work, as soon as you are able.
- Avoid vigorous exercise for 6 weeks after surgery. Resume exercise after consulting your doctor.
- Resume sexual relations when your doctor determines that healing is complete.

DIET—Your doctor will prescribe a diet.

 CALL YOUR DOCTOR IF

- Pain, swelling, redness, drainage or bleeding increases in the surgical area.
- You develop signs of infection, including headache, muscle aches, dizziness or a general ill feeling and fever.
- You experience nausea, vomiting, constipation, abdominal swelling, heartbeat irregularities, or extreme fatigue.
- New, unexplained symptoms develop. Drugs used in treatment may produce side effects.

HEART TRANSPLANTATION

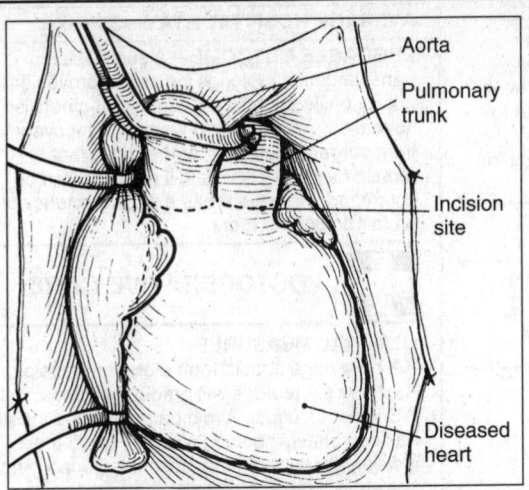

Aorta

Pulmonary trunk

Incision site

Diseased heart

An illustration of a diseased heart. The major blood vessels into and away from the heart are clamped and incision sites for the heart transplant indicated.

- A heart-lung machine sustains life while the diseased heart is cut free and removed, and until the donor heart has been transplanted.

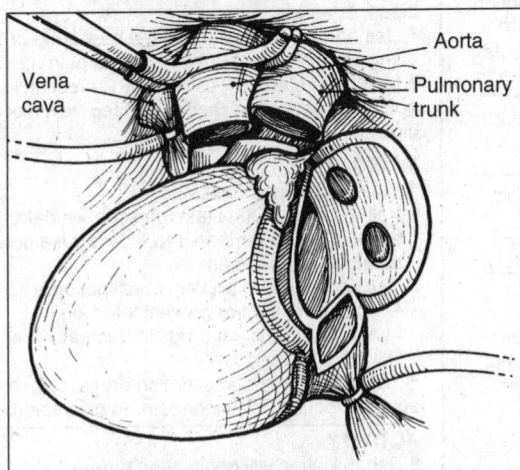

Aorta

Pulmonary trunk

Vena cava

After major vessels have been severed, the diseased heart is now ready to be removed from the chest and discarded.

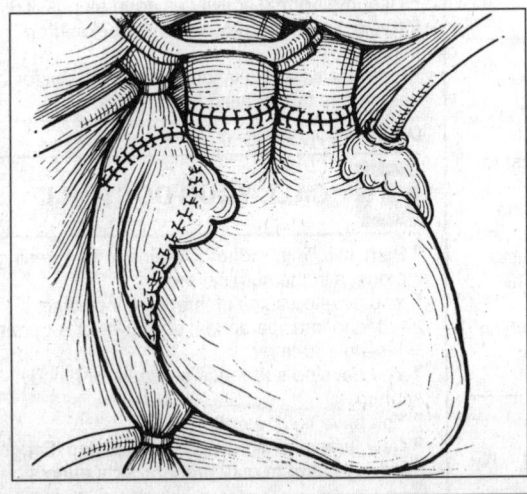

The donor heart is sewn in place. The aorta, pulmonary arteries, superior vena cava and inferior vena cava are connected to the new heart.

- The donor heart, which had been kept motionless by cooling, is now stimulated to resume beating with warming and a weak electrical current.

SURGERIES

HEART-LUNG TRANSPLANTATION

 GENERAL INFORMATION

DEFINITION—Replacement of poorly functioning lungs and a damaged or healthy heart with donor organs. If the recipient's heart is normal, it may be extracted and donated to another patient in need of a heart transplantation only (see Heart Transplantation in Surgery section).

BODY PARTS INVOLVED—Lungs, heart, trachea and blood vessels.

REASONS FOR SURGERY—Chronic lung disorders such as pulmonary hypertension, emphysema, cystic fibrosis and other lung conditions causing pulmonary fibrosis.

SURGICAL RISK INCREASES WITH
- Adults over 60; obesity; poor nutrition.
- Recent or chronic illness.
- Alcoholism; smoking.
- Diabetes mellitus.
- Use of some prescription and nonprescription drugs. Inform your doctor of any drugs, medications, or vitamin and herb supplements you are using or have used in the last month.

 WHAT TO EXPECT

WHO OPERATES—Cardiovascular surgeon, thoracic surgeon.

WHERE PERFORMED—Hospital.

DIAGNOSTIC TESTS
- Before surgery: Blood and urine studies; studies of the immune system; ECG; cardiac catheterization; echocardiography, ultrasound; biopsy; pulmonary angiography; lung function studies (see Glossary for all).
- During surgery: Cardiac monitoring (see Glossary).
- After surgery: Repeat of some tests for monitoring of the new organs.

ANESTHESIA—General anesthesia by injection and inhalation, with an airway tube placed in the windpipe.

DESCRIPTION OF OPERATION
- An incision is made in the recipient's chest to expose the heart and lungs.
- A heart-lung machine sustains life while the diseased organs are cut free and removed, and until the donor organs have been transplanted.
- The donor organs are sewn into place. The new lungs are connected to the trachea.
- The skin is closed with sutures or clips, which usually can be removed about 1 week after surgery.

POSSIBLE COMPLICATIONS
- Excessive bleeding; blood clots.
- Surgical-wound infection.

- Life-threatening general infections.
- Rejection of transplanted organs.

AVERAGE HOSPITAL STAY—3 weeks.

PROBABLE OUTCOME—A successful transplantation prolongs life and improves the quality of life for patients who might otherwise have died. Allow about 6 weeks for recovery from surgery. Rejection of the transplant remains a risk indefinitely. If rejection can be controlled, the patient has a life expectancy of up to 10 years or more.

 POSTOPERATIVE CARE

GENERAL MEASURES
- A hard ridge should form along the incision. As it heals, the ridge will gradually recede.
- Shower as usual. Avoid baths until the incision has completely healed. You may wash the incision gently with mild, unscented soap. After showering, replace any wet dressings with clean, dry ones.
- Use an electric heating pad, a heat lamp or a warm compress to relieve incisional pain.
- Move and elevate legs often while resting in bed to decrease the chance of deep-vein blood clots.

MEDICATION
- Your doctor may prescribe:
  Pain relievers. Don't take prescription pain medication longer than 4 to 7 days. Use only as much as you need.
  Stool softeners to prevent constipation.
  Antibiotics to fight or prevent infection.
  Immunosuppressant drugs to decrease the likelihood of rejection.
- You may use nonprescription drugs, such as acetaminophen, for minor pain. Avoid aspirin.

ACTIVITY
- Rehabilitation will begin after surgery.
- Resume normal activity as soon as possible.
- Avoid vigorous exercise for 6 weeks after surgery.
- Resume sexual relations when your doctor determines that healing is complete.

DIET—Your doctor will prescribe a diet.

 CALL YOUR DOCTOR IF

- Pain, swelling, redness, drainage or bleeding increases in the surgical area.
- You develop signs of infection, including headache, muscle aches, dizziness or a general ill feeling and fever.
- You develop shortness of breath or bloody sputum.
- You have fluid retention.
- New, unexplained symptoms develop. Drugs used in treatment may produce side effects.

HEART-LUNG TRANSPLANTATION

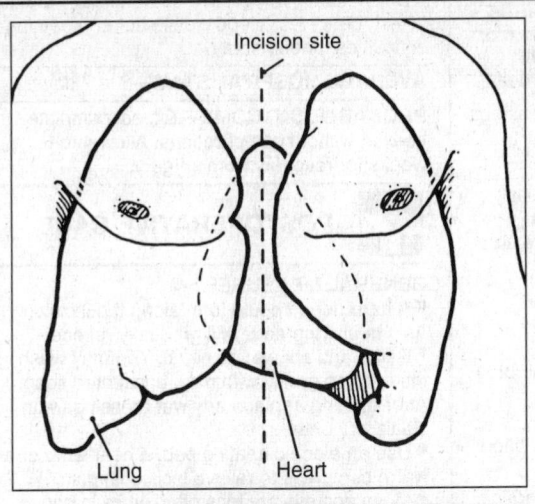

Illustration demonstrating surgical anatomy. Mid-line incision is made and recipient's heart and lungs are exposed.

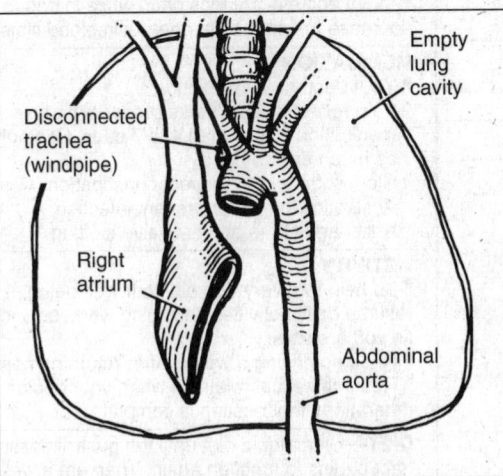

Recipient's heart and lungs are removed, leaving an empty cavity where new organs will be attached.

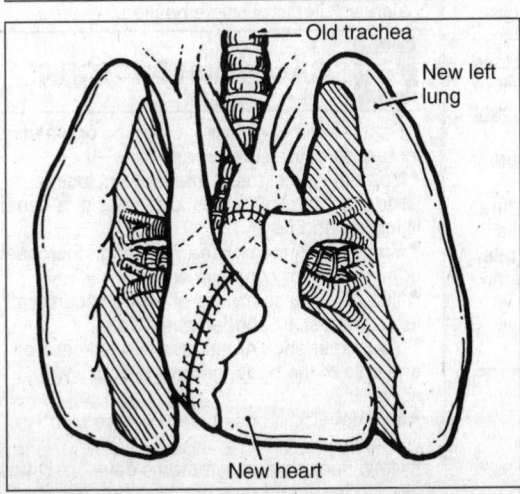

Donor's heart and lungs are sewn into position. The surgical site is examined for any leaks prior to closing of the chest.

HEART VALVE REPLACEMENT

 GENERAL INFORMATION

DEFINITION—Replacement of one or more diseased heart valves with porcine (derived from swine) or artificial valves.

BODY PARTS INVOLVED—Valves that separate major sections of the heart.

REASONS FOR SURGERY—Prevention of complications resulting from valvular heart disease, especially congestive heart failure and bacterial endocarditis.

SURGICAL RISK INCREASES WITH
• Adults over 60.
• Obesity; smoking; poor nutrition.
• Recent illness such as acute upper respiratory infection.
• Alcoholism or chronic illness.
• Use of some prescription and nonprescription drugs. Inform your doctor of any drugs, medications, or vitamin and herb supplements you are using or have used in the last month.

 WHAT TO EXPECT

WHO OPERATES—Cardiovascular surgeon.

WHERE PERFORMED—Hospital.

DIAGNOSTIC TESTS
• Before surgery: Blood and urine studies; x-rays of chest; ECG; cardiac catheterization (see Glossary for both).
• During surgery: ECG monitor.
• After surgery: Blood studies; ECG.

ANESTHESIA—General anesthesia by injection and inhalation with an airway tube placed in the windpipe.

DESCRIPTION OF OPERATION
• An incision is made in the chest, and the breastbone is divided. The chest is opened to expose the heart.
• A heart-lung machine circulates enough blood to sustain life throughout the surgical procedure.
• The diseased heart valves are located through delicate incisions made in the heart.
• Diseased valves are removed and replaced with artificial or porcine valves.
• The incisions in the heart are closed with fine sutures, and the chest cavity is reconstructed with wire sutures. The skin is closed with lighter sutures or clips, which usually can be removed about 1 week after surgery.
• Drains may be left in place for several days following the surgery.

POSSIBLE COMPLICATIONS
• Excessive bleeding; blood clots.
• Surgical-wound infection.
• Failure of the heart to resume normal heartbeat (rare).
• Clotting or infection of valve.

• Kidney damage or kidney failure.
• Heart attack; congestive heart failure; cardiac arrest; deep-vein blood clots; stroke; breathing difficulties; pneumonia.

AVERAGE HOSPITAL STAY—5 to 7 days.

PROBABLE OUTCOME—Expect complete healing without complications. Allow 4 to 6 weeks for recovery from surgery.

 POSTOPERATIVE CARE

GENERAL MEASURES
• A hard ridge should form along the incision. As it heals, the ridge will gradually recede.
• Bathe and shower as usual. You may wash the incision gently with mild, unscented soap. After bathing, replace any wet dressings with clean, dry ones.
• Use an electric heating pad, a heat lamp or a warm compress to relieve incisional pain.
• Move and elevate legs often while in bed to decrease the chance of deep-vein blood clots.

MEDICATION
• Your doctor may prescribe:
  Pain relievers. Don't take prescription pain medication longer than 4 to 7 days. Use only as much as you need.
  Stool softeners to prevent constipation.
  Antibiotics to fight or prevent infection.
  Anticoagulant to prevent valve clotting.

ACTIVITY
• To help recovery and aid your well-being, resume daily activities, including work, as soon as you are able.
• Resume driving 5 weeks after returning home.
• Resume sexual relations when your doctor determines that healing is complete.

DIET—Clear liquid diet until the gastrointestinal tract begins to function again. Then eat a well-balanced diet to promote healing.

 CALL YOUR DOCTOR IF

• Pain, swelling, redness, drainage or bleeding increases in the surgical area.
• You develop signs of infection, including headache, muscle aches, dizziness or a general ill feeling and fever.
• You experience nausea, vomiting, decreased urine output, or constipation.
• You develop shortness of breath, heartbeat irregularities, or sudden chest pain.
• You experience numbness or weakness on one side of the body, or have difficulty with speech.
• You develop a nose bleed or have blood in your urine.
• New, unexplained symptoms develop. Drugs used in treatment may produce side effects.

HEART VALVE REPLACEMENT

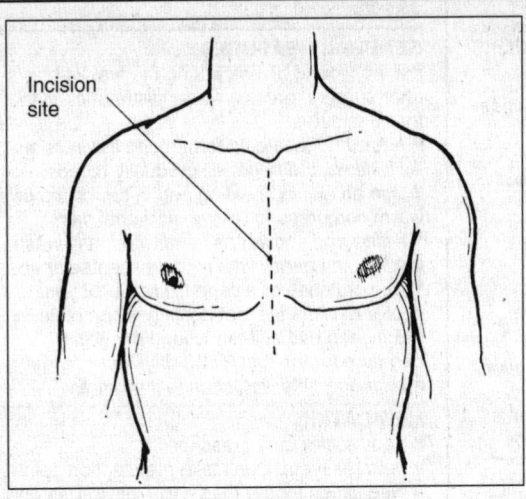

Incision site

An illustration of the incision site over the breast bone, which will be spread to allow exposure of the heart.
- A heart-lung machine circulates enough blood to sustain life throughout the surgical procedure.

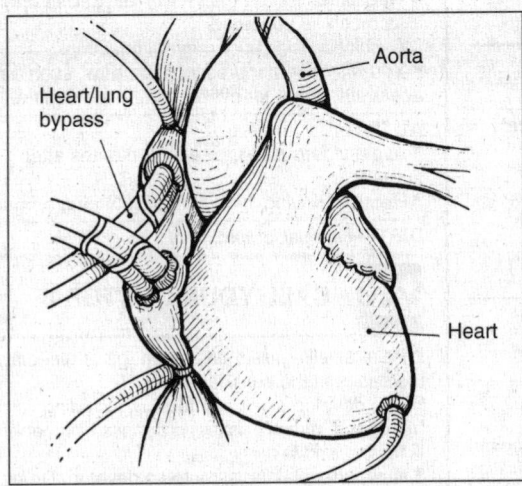

Aorta

Heart/lung bypass

Heart

The diseased heart valves are located through delicate incisions made in the heart.

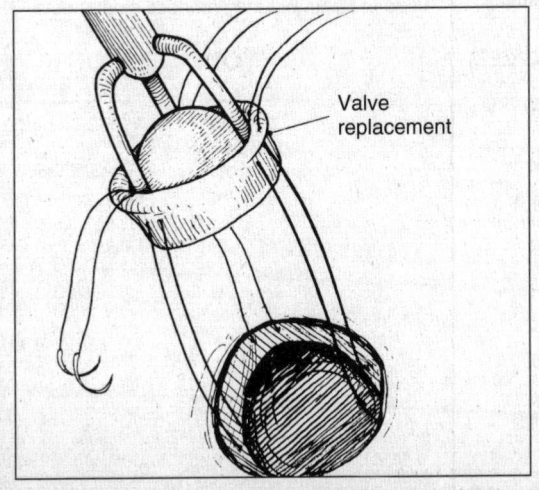

Valve replacement

Diseased valves are removed and replaced with artificial or porcine valves.
- The incisions made in the heart are closed with fine sutures. The chest cavity is reconstructed with wire sutures in the chest muscle and breast bone.

SURGERIES

HEEL SPUR REMOVAL

 GENERAL INFORMATION

DEFINITION—Removal of a heel spur, a sharp outgrowth on the bone of the heel.

BODY PARTS INVOLVED—Bottom of the heel bone.

REASONS FOR SURGERY—Relief of pain.

SURGICAL RISK INCREASES WITH
- Obesity.
- Smoking.
- Poor nutrition.
- Excess alcohol consumption.
- Recent or chronic illness.
- Diabetes mellitus.
- Use of some prescription and nonprescription drugs. Inform your doctor of any drugs, medications, or vitamin and herb supplements you are using or have used in the last month.

 WHAT TO EXPECT

WHO OPERATES—General surgeon, orthopedist or podiatrist.

WHERE PERFORMED—Outpatient surgical facility or doctor's office.

DIAGNOSTIC TESTS
- Before surgery: Blood and urine studies; x-rays of both feet.
- After surgery: Blood studies; laboratory examination of removed tissue.

ANESTHESIA
- Local anesthesia by injection.
- Spinal anesthesia by injection.

DESCRIPTION OF OPERATION
- An incision is made over the spur.
- The spur is cut free and removed with special instruments.
- The skin is closed with sutures, which usually can be removed about 10 to 14 days after surgery.

POSSIBLE COMPLICATIONS
- Excessive bleeding.
- Surgical-wound infection.

AVERAGE HOSPITAL STAY—Usually none.

PROBABLE OUTCOME—Expect complete healing without complications. Allow about 6 weeks for recovery from surgery.

 POSTOPERATIVE CARE

GENERAL MEASURES
- If the wound bleeds during the first 24 hours after surgery, press a clean tissue or cloth to it for 10 minutes.
- A hard ridge should form along the incision. As it heals, the ridge will gradually recede.
- Use an electric heating pad, a heat lamp or a warm compress to relieve incisional pain.
- Bathe and shower as usual. You may wash the incision gently with mild, unscented soap.
- Use crutches or a cane to walk until your doctor determines that healing is complete.
- Between baths, keep wound dry with a bandage for the first 2 or 3 days after surgery. If a bandage gets wet, change it promptly.

MEDICATION
- Your doctor may prescribe:
  Pain relievers. Don't take prescription pain medication longer than 4 to 7 days. Use only as much as you need.
  Antibiotics to fight or prevent infection.
- You may use nonprescription drugs, such as acetaminophen, for minor pain. Avoid aspirin.

ACTIVITY
- Avoid vigorous exercise for 3 months after surgery.
- Resume driving 1 week after returning home.

DIET—No special diet.

 CALL YOUR DOCTOR IF

- Pain, swelling, redness, drainage or bleeding increases in the surgical area.
- You develop signs of infection, including headache, muscle aches, dizziness or a general ill feeling and fever.
- New, unexplained symptoms develop. Drugs used in treatment may produce side effects.

HEEL SPUR REMOVAL

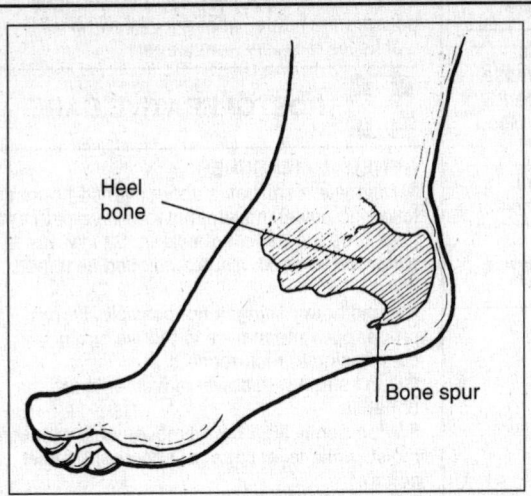

An illustration of a typical bone spur on the heel bone.

Heel bone

Bone spur

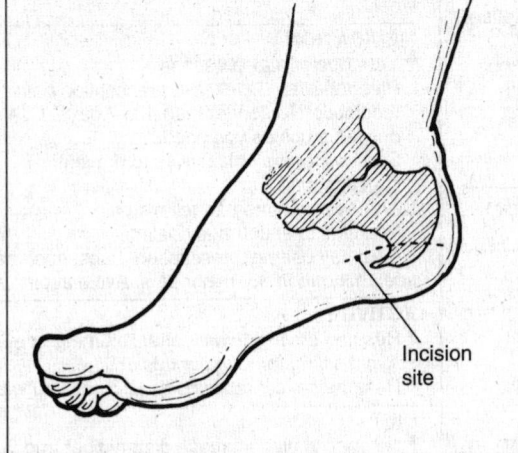

A typical incision site to enable removal of the bone spur, which is cut free and removed with special instruments.

Incision site

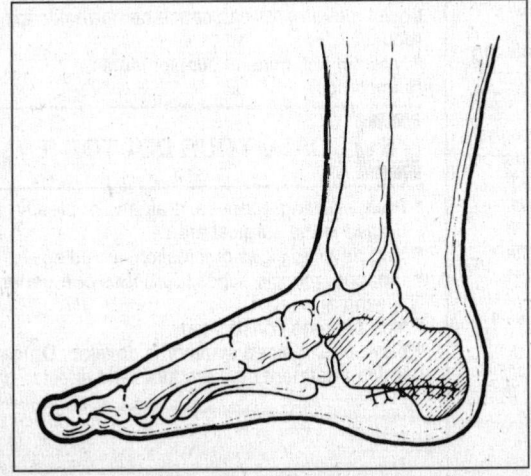

Skin is closed with sutures, which can usually be removed about 10 to 14 days after surgery.

HEMORRHOID BANDING

GENERAL INFORMATION

DEFINITION—Destruction of hemorrhoids (varicose veins that occur inside or outside the anus) by a technique that uses a rubber band over the stalk of the hemorrhoid to cut off blood flow.

BODY PARTS INVOLVED—Anus; rectum; dilated veins in anus and rectum (hemorrhoids).

REASONS FOR SURGERY
- Pain, excessive bleeding, itching or prolapse of dilated veins in the rectum and anus.

SURGICAL RISK INCREASES WITH
- Obesity.
- Smoking.
- Poor nutrition.
- Adults over 60.
- Excess alcohol consumption.
- Recent or chronic illness.
- Diabetes mellitus.
- Inflammatory bowel disease.
- Use of some prescription and nonprescription drugs. Inform your doctor of any drugs, medications, or vitamin and herb supplements you are using or have used in the last month.

WHAT TO EXPECT

WHO OPERATES—Proctologist, colon-rectal surgeon or general surgeon.

WHERE PERFORMED—Doctor's office, hospital or outpatient surgical facility.

DIAGNOSTIC TESTS
- Before surgery: Blood and urine studies; anoscopy; sigmoidoscopy (see Glossary for both).
- After surgery: Blood studies.

ANESTHESIA
- Local anesthesia by injection.
- Spinal anesthesia by injection.
- General anesthesia by injection and inhalation with an airway tube placed in the windpipe.

DESCRIPTION OF OPERATION
- The doctor inserts several fingers to dilate the anal muscles. Sometimes anal muscles must be dilated vigorously to expose the hemorrhoids.
- The hemorrhoid is visualized and grasped with a special instrument.
- A small rubber band is slipped over the stalk of the hemorrhoid to bind it and cut off blood flow.

POSSIBLE COMPLICATIONS
- Excessive bleeding.
- Surgical-wound infection.
- Severe pain, especially with bowel movements.
- Urinary retention.

AVERAGE HOSPITAL STAY—0 to 1 day.

PROBABLE OUTCOME—Curable in most patients, no matter what age. Allow about 2 weeks for recovery from surgery.

POSTOPERATIVE CARE

GENERAL MEASURES
- Take warm sitz baths about every 4 hours and following bowel movements to relieve pain and help keep the rectal area clean. Sit in warm water for 10 to 20 minutes as often as it feels good.
- Avoid heavy lifting. If not possible, learn proper body mechanics to reduce strain contributing to recurrence.
- Don't strain with bowel movements or urination.
- Wipe gently after bowel movements with soft, moist, white toilet paper or absorbent, moist cotton.
- Expect drainage from the rectum for 2 to 3 weeks.

MEDICATION
- Your doctor may prescribe:
  Pain relievers. Don't take prescription pain medication for longer than 4 to 7 days. Use only as much as you need.
  Stool softeners or laxatives to prevent constipation.
  Analgesic ointment to relieve pain.
  Vitamins to encourage healing.
- You may use nonprescription drugs, such as acetaminophen, for minor pain. Avoid aspirin.

ACTIVITY
- Resume driving 1 week after returning home.
- Avoid sitting for long periods of time.
- Resume sexual relations as soon as you wish.

DIET
- No special diet. Increase dietary fiber and fluid intake to prevent constipation. Straining during bowel movements can cause hemorrhoids to recur.
- Vitamin and mineral supplements (sometimes).

CALL YOUR DOCTOR IF

- Pain, swelling, redness, drainage or bleeding increase in the surgical area.
- You develop signs of infection, including headache, muscle aches, dizziness or a general ill feeling and fever.
- You become constipated
- New, unexplained symptoms develop. Drugs used in treatment may produce side effects.

HEMORRHOID BANDING

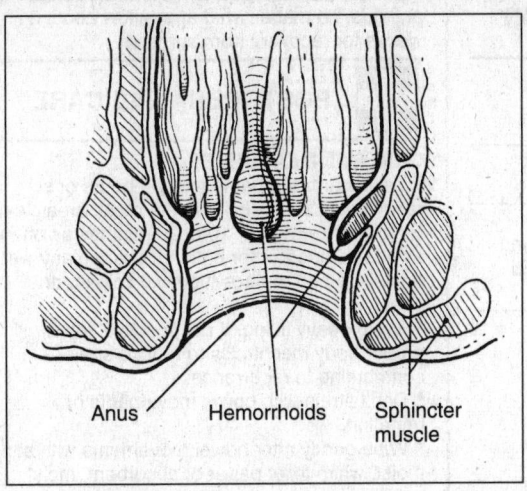

An illustration of a cross-sectional view of the region of the body containing the anus, the sphincter muscle of the anus and a view of an internal hemorrhoid just inside the anus.

Anus   Hemorrhoids   Sphincter muscle

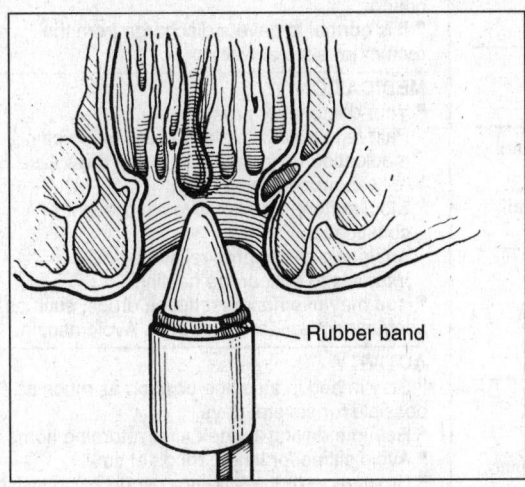

The hemorrhoid is found and grasped with a special instrument.

Rubber band

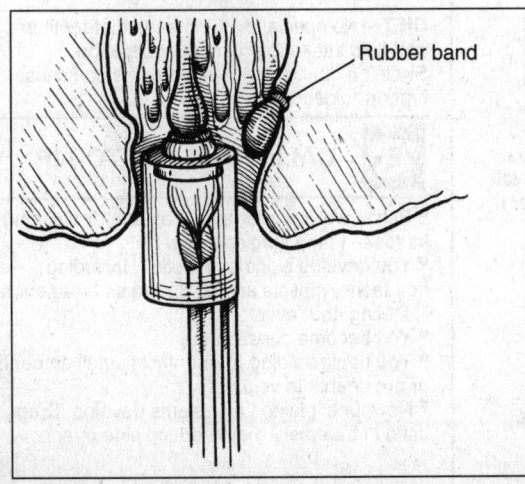

A small rubber band is slipped over the stalk of the hemorrhoid to bind it and cut off the blood flow.

Rubber band

SURGERIES

HEMORRHOID REMOVAL
(Hemorrhoidectomy)

GENERAL INFORMATION

DEFINITION—Removal of hemorrhoids (varicose veins that occur inside or on the outside of the anus).

BODY PARTS INVOLVED—Dilated veins around the anus or just inside the rectum.

REASONS FOR SURGERY
- Relief of excessive itching, pain or bleeding.
- Relief of a painful thrombosed hemorrhoid (hemorrhoid containing a blood clot).

SURGICAL RISK INCREASES WITH
- Adults over 60.
- Obesity.
- Smoking.
- Poor nutrition.
- Excess alcohol consumption.
- Chronic illness.
- Inflammatory bowel disease.
- Bleeding problems.

WHAT TO EXPECT

WHO OPERATES—Proctologist, colon-rectal surgeon or general surgeon.

WHERE PERFORMED—Outpatient surgical facility or hospital.

DIAGNOSTIC TESTS
- Before surgery: Blood and urine studies; anoscopy: sigmoidoscopy (see Glossary for both).
- After surgery: Blood studies.

ANESTHESIA
- Local anesthesia by injection.
- Spinal anesthesia by injection.
- General anesthesia by injection and inhalation with an airway tube placed in the windpipe.

DESCRIPTION OF OPERATION
- The dilated veins from around the anus and inside the rectum are cut free and removed, with care taken not to damage the sphincter muscle. Sometimes anal muscles must be dilated vigorously to expose the hemorrhoids.
- The surgical area may be sewn closed or left open, and medicated gauze is used to cover it.

POSSIBLE COMPLICATIONS
- Excessive bleeding.
- Surgical-wound infection.
- Urinary retention (common).
- Stricture of anus.
- Severe pain, especially with bowel movements.

AVERAGE HOSPITAL STAY—2 to 3 days.

PROBABLE OUTCOME—Curable in most patients, no matter what age. Allow about 3 weeks for recovery from surgery.

POSTOPERATIVE CARE

GENERAL MEASURES
- Take warm sitz baths every 4 hours or so relieve pain and help keep the rectal area clean. Sit in warm water for 10 to 20 minutes as often as it feels good. After bathing, change any wet dressings and replace them with clean, dry ones.
- Avoid heavy lifting. If not possible, learn proper body mechanics to reduce strain contributing to recurrence.
- Don't strain with bowel movements or urination.
- Wipe gently after bowel movements with soft, moist, white toilet paper or absorbent, moist cotton.
- It is normal to have a discharge from the rectum for several weeks.

MEDICATION
- Your doctor may prescribe:
  Pain relievers. Don't take prescription pain medication for longer than 4 to 7 days. Use only as much as you need.
  Stool softeners or laxatives to prevent constipation.
  Analgesic ointment to relieve pain.
  Vitamins to encourage healing.
- You may use nonprescription drugs, such as acetaminophen, for minor pain. Avoid aspirin.

ACTIVITY
- Stay in bed in a supine position as much as possible for several days.
- Resume driving 1 week after returning home.
- Avoid sitting for long periods of time.
- Resume sexual relations as soon as you wish.

DIET—No special diet. Increase dietary fiber and fluid intake to prevent constipation. Straining during bowel movements can cause hemorrhoids to recur.

CALL YOUR DOCTOR IF

- Pain, swelling, redness, drainage or bleeding increase in the surgical area.
- You develop signs of infection, including headache, muscle aches, dizziness or a general ill feeling and fever.
- You become constipated.
- You begin voiding frequently in small amounts or are unable to void.
- New, unexplained symptoms develop. Drugs used in treatment may produce side effects.

HEMORRHOID REMOVAL
(Hemorrhoidectomy)

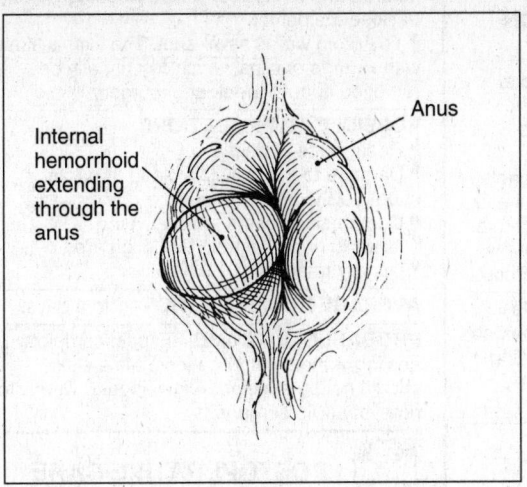

An illustration of a typical internal hemorrhoid arising from inside the anus and extending through the anal opening.

Internal hemorrhoid extending through the anus

Anus

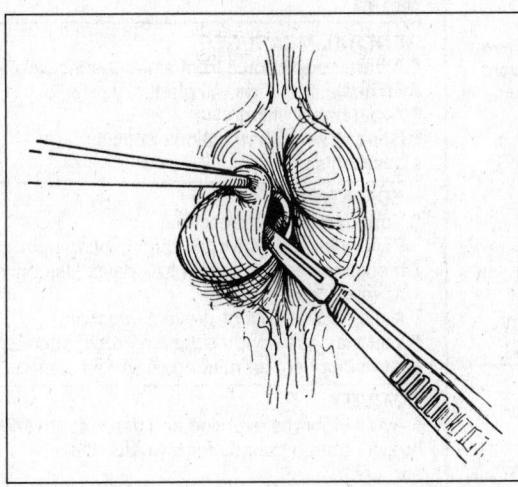

Dilated veins around the anus and inside the rectum are cut free and removed, with care taken not to damage the sphincter muscles.

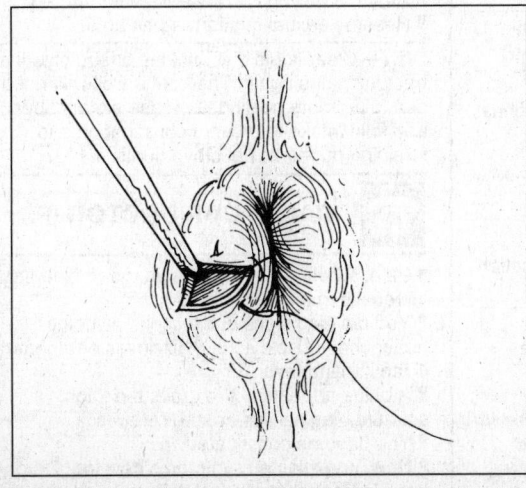

The surgical area is sewn closed or left open and medicated gauze is used to cover.

SURGERIES

HERNIA REPAIR, FEMORAL
(Femoral Herniorrhaphy)

 GENERAL INFORMATION

DEFINITION—Closing or repairing a femoral hernia, an internal defect or weakness in the muscles of the abdominal wall. Sometimes, some fatty tissue or an intestine protrudes through the hernia defect, causing a noticeable bulge. If the intestine becomes trapped in the hernia defect, it is called an incarcerated hernia. If the intestine's blood supply is blocked by the hernia defect, it is called a strangulated hernia.

BODY PARTS INVOLVED—Groin (muscles and ligaments inside the lower abdomen next to the genitals); abdominal muscles; the opening allowing the femoral artery to pass from the abdomen to the leg.

REASONS FOR SURGERY
- Incarcerated hernia. This is an emergency!
- Strangulated hernia. This is an emergency!
- Uncomplicated hernia. Most surgeons recommend operating on a femoral hernia, even if no symptoms are present, in order to prevent the serious complications of incarceration or strangulation.

SURGICAL RISK INCREASES WITH
- Adults over 60; obesity; smoking.
- Excess alcohol consumption.
- Recent or chronic illness, especially chronic lung disease or diabetes mellitus.
- Use of some prescription and nonprescription drugs. Inform your doctor of any drugs, medications, or vitamin and herb supplements you are using or have used in the last month.

 WHAT TO EXPECT

WHO OPERATES—General surgeon or urologist.

WHERE PERFORMED—Hospital or outpatient surgical facility.

DIAGNOSTIC TESTS
- Before surgery: Blood and urine studies; chest x-ray: ECG (see Glossary).
- After surgery: Blood studies.

ANESTHESIA
- Spinal anesthesia by injection.
- Local anesthesia by injection.
- General anesthesia by injection and inhalation with an airway tube placed in the windpipe.

DESCRIPTION OF OPERATION
- An incision is made in the groin area. The muscles and tissue are separated and the hernia sac is opened.
- The contents of the hernia sac are replaced in the abdominal cavity. The neck of the sac is sutured and a "plug" of plastic webbing is used to close the defect.
- The groin wall is sewn shut. The skin is closed with sutures or clips, which can usually be removed about 1 week after surgery.

POSSIBLE COMPLICATIONS
- Recurrence of hernia.
- Damage to the testicle's blood or nerve supply, if the patient is male.
- Compression of the femoral vein.
- Injury to nerve to groin and thigh area.
- Urinary retention.

AVERAGE HOSPITAL STAY—1 to 4 days.

PROBABLE OUTCOME—Expect complete healing without complications. Male virility should not be affected. Allow about 6 weeks for recovery from surgery.

 POSTOPERATIVE CARE

GENERAL MEASURES
- A hard ridge should form along the incision. As it heals, the ridge will gradually recede.
- Avoid heavy lifting.
- Don't strain with urination or bowel movements.

MEDICATION
- Your doctor may prescribe:
  Pain relievers. Don't take prescription pain medication longer than 4 to 7 days. Use only as much as you need.
  Antibiotics to fight or prevent infection.
- You may use nonprescription drugs, such as acetaminophen, for minor pain. Avoid aspirin.

ACTIVITY
- Avoid vigorous exercise and don't lift anything heavier than 5 pounds for 6 weeks after surgery.
- Resume driving 3 to 4 weeks after surgery.
- Resume sexual relations when able.

DIET—Clear liquid diet until the gastrointestinal tract functions again. Then eat a well-balanced diet to promote healing. Increase dietary fiber and fluid intake to prevent constipation and straining during bowel movements.

 CALL YOUR DOCTOR IF

- Pain, swelling, redness, drainage or bleeding increases in the surgical area.
- You develop signs of infection, including headache, muscle aches, dizziness or a general ill feeling and fever.
- A bulge appears in the groin, the thigh, scrotum, vaginal lips or surgical area.
- You become constipated.
- New, unexplained symptoms develop. Drugs used in treatment may produce side effects.

HERNIA REPAIR, FEMORAL
(Femoral Herniorrhaphy)

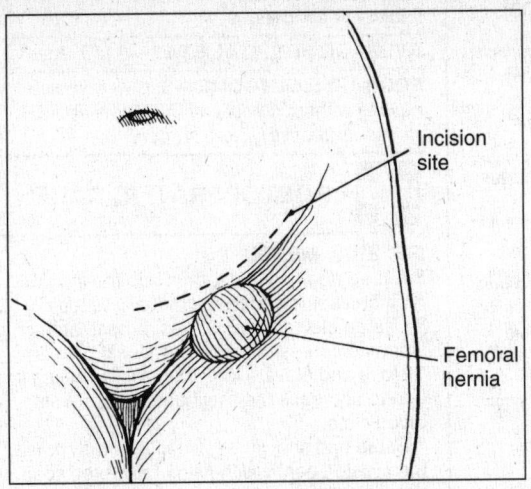

An illustration of a typical femoral hernia located in the groin.

Incision site

Femoral hernia

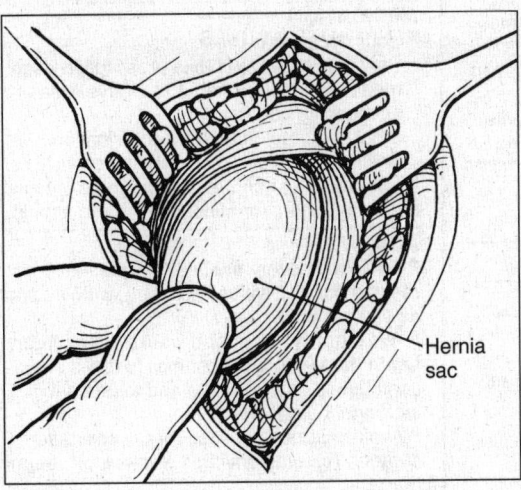

Skin has been incised and the muscles retracted disclosing the hernia sac.
- Contents of the hernia sac are replaced in the abdominal cavity.
- Muscles and fascia are used to cover the defect that allowed the hernia to protrude.
- Sometimes a plug of mesh or patch of mesh is used to bolster the defect.

Hernia sac

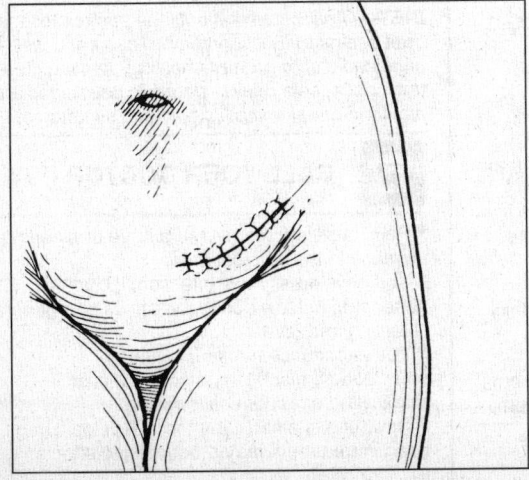

Muscle layers are sewn together followed by skin closure with sutures or clips, which can usually be removed about 1 week after surgery.

SURGERIES

HERNIA REPAIR, HIATAL
(Hiatal Herniorrhaphy)

 GENERAL INFORMATION

DEFINITION—Closure of a hiatal hernia, an abnormal weakness or opening in the diaphragm, where the esophagus enters the abdomen.

BODY PARTS INVOLVED—Lower esophagus; diaphragm; upper part of stomach.

REASONS FOR SURGERY
- Relief of painful symptoms.
- Prevent the stomach from shifting upward into the chest cavity.
- Prevent the stomach from spilling digestive acid into the esophagus, causing infection, pain and scarring.

SURGICAL RISK INCREASES WITH
- Adults over 60; newborns and infants.
- Obesity or poor nutrition.
- Smoking, alcoholism.
- Recent or chronic illness, especially diabetes mellitus or chronic lung disease.
- Use of some prescription and nonprescription drugs. Inform your doctor of any drugs, medications, or vitamin and herb supplements you are using or have used in the last month.

 WHAT TO EXPECT

WHO OPERATES—General surgeon.

WHERE PERFORMED—Hospital.

DIAGNOSTIC TESTS
- Before surgery: Blood and urine studies; x-rays of chest and upper gastrointestinal tract; ECG; endoscopy (see Glossary for both).
- After surgery: Blood studies.

ANESTHESIA—General anesthesia by injection and inhalation with an airway tube placed in the windpipe.

DESCRIPTION OF OPERATION
- An incision is made in the abdomen or the chest.
- The hernia in the diaphragm is located and, in some cases, closed with sutures.
- The top of the stomach is wrapped around the lower part of the esophagus and sutured in place.
- Sometimes, the vagus nerve is removed to reduce the amount of acid the stomach produces.
- The skin is closed with sutures or clips, which usually can be removed about 1 week after surgery.
- Laparoscopic repair is now available for some patients (see Laparoscopy in Surgery section).

POSSIBLE COMPLICATIONS—Excessive bleeding or surgical-wound infection.

- Incisional hernia.
- Injury to esophagus.

AVERAGE HOSPITAL STAY—5 to 7 days.

PROBABLE OUTCOME—Expect complete healing without complications. Allow about 6 weeks for recovery from surgery.

 POSTOPERATIVE CARE

GENERAL MEASURES
- A hard ridge should form along the incision. As it heals, the ridge will gradually recede.
- Use an electric heating pad, a heat lamp or a warm compress to relieve incisional pain.
- Move and elevate legs often while resting in bed to decrease the likelihood of deep-vein blood clots.
- Bathe and shower as usual. You may wash the incision gently with mild, unscented soap.

MEDICATION
- Your doctor may prescribe:
  Pain relievers. Don't take prescription pain medication longer than 4 to 7 days. Use only as much as you need.
  Stool softeners to prevent constipation.
  Antibiotics to fight or prevent infection.
- You may use nonprescription drugs, such as acetaminophen, for minor pain. Avoid aspirin.

ACTIVITY
- To help recovery and aid your well-being, resume daily activities, including work, as soon as you are able.
- Avoid heavy lifting for 6 weeks after surgery. Learn proper body mechanics to avoid strain contributing to recurrence and to prevent incisional hernia.
- Avoid vigorous exercise for 6 weeks after surgery. Resume driving 4 weeks after returning home.

DIET—Clear liquid diet until the gastrointestinal tract begins to function again. Then eat a well-balanced diet to promote healing. Avoid coffee, tea, cocoa, cola drinks, alcoholic beverages and any food or spice that aggravates symptoms.

 CALL YOUR DOCTOR IF

- Pain, swelling, redness, drainage or bleeding increase in the surgical area.
- You develop signs of infection, including headache, muscle aches, dizziness or a general ill feeling and fever.
- You experience nausea, vomiting, constipation, black tarry stools, difficulty in swallowing or abdominal swelling.
- New, unexplained symptoms develop. Drugs used in treatment may produce side effects.

HERNIA REPAIR, HIATAL
(Hiatal Herniorrhaphy)

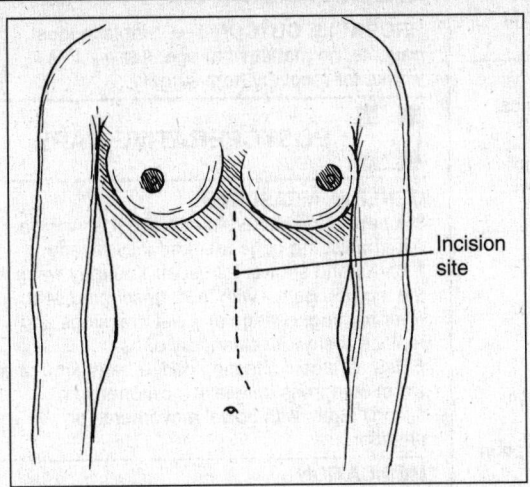

An illustration of a typical incision site to allow exposure of the lower end of the esophagus, the upper end of the stomach, and the diaphragm (a large muscle that separates the chest from the abdominal cavity).

Incision site

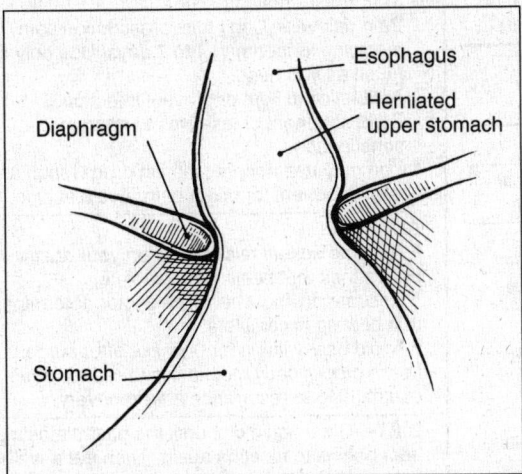

The herniated upper stomach through the widened opening in the diaphragm.

Esophagus

Herniated upper stomach

Diaphragm

Stomach

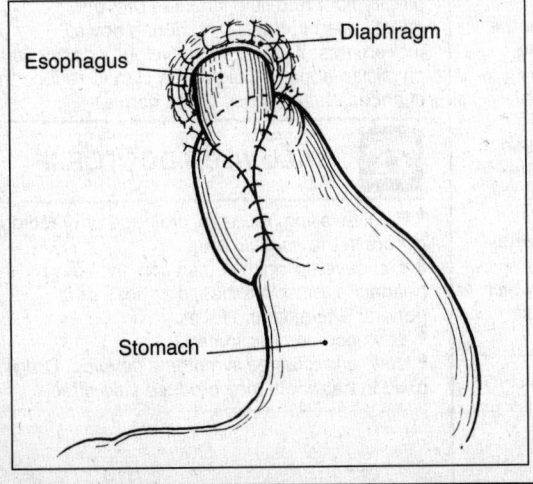

The top of the stomach is wrapped around the lower part of the esophagus and sutured in place.

Diaphragm

Esophagus

Stomach

HERNIA REPAIR, INCISIONAL
(Incisional Herniorrhaphy)

 GENERAL INFORMATION

DEFINITION—Repair of a defect in the abdominal wall created by a previous surgical incision.

BODY PARTS INVOLVED—Abdomen and intestines where previous surgery has been performed.

REASONS FOR SURGERY
- Possible strangulation of bowel.
- Painful lump in the abdomen.

SURGICAL RISK INCREASES WITH
- Obesity; poor nutrition.
- Excess alcohol consumption; smoking.
- Recent or chronic illness, especially chronic lung disease or diabetes mellitus.
- Use of some prescription and nonprescription drugs. Inform your doctor of any drugs, medications, or vitamin and herb supplements you are using or have used in the last month.

 WHAT TO EXPECT

WHO OPERATES—General surgeon.

WHERE PERFORMED—Outpatient surgical facility or hospital.

DIAGNOSTIC TESTS
- Before surgery: Blood and urine studies; x-rays of the abdomen and chest; ECG (see Glossary).
- After surgery: Blood studies.

ANESTHESIA
- Local anesthesia by injection.
- Spinal anesthesia by injection.
- General anesthesia by injection and inhalation with an airway tube placed in the windpipe.

DESCRIPTION OF OPERATION
- An incision is made in the abdomen over the defect. The area is examined for protruding intestine.
- The intestine is replaced in the abdominal cavity. Frequently, plastic mesh is used to strengthen the repair. The mesh can be used to cover the defect in the abdominal wall or the muscles can be closed and the mesh used to reinforce them.
- A drain is sometimes left in place for several days.
- The skin is closed with sutures or clips, which usually can be removed about 1 week after surgery.

POSSIBLE COMPLICATIONS
- Surgical-wound infection.
- Inadvertent injury to intestinal tract.
- Bowel obstruction.
- Recurrent hernia.

AVERAGE HOSPITAL STAY—0 to 4 days.

PROBABLE OUTCOME—Curable in most patients, no matter what age. Allow 2 to 4 weeks for recovery from surgery.

 POSTOPERATIVE CARE

GENERAL MEASURES
- A hard ridge should form along the incision. As it heals, the ridge will gradually recede.
- Bathe and shower as usual. You may wash the incision gently with mild, unscented soap. After bathing, change any wet dressings and replace them with clean, dry ones.
- Use an electric heating pad, a heat lamp or a warm compress to relieve incisional pain.
- Don't strain with bowel movements or urination.

MEDICATION
- Your doctor may prescribe:
  Pain relievers. Don't take prescription pain medicine longer than 4 to 7 days. Use only as much as you need.
  Antibiotics to fight or prevent infection.
  Stool softeners or laxatives to prevent constipation.
- You may use nonprescription drugs, such as acetaminophen, for minor pain. Avoid aspirin.

ACTIVITY
- Resume sexual relations when your doctor determines that healing is complete.
- Resume driving when your doctor determines that healing is complete.
- Avoid heavy lifting for 6 weeks after surgery. Learn proper body mechanics to reduce strain contributing to recurrence after recovery.

DIET—Clear liquid diet until the gastrointestinal tract begins to function again. Then eat a well-balanced diet to promote healing. Increase dietary fiber and fluid intake to prevent constipation and straining during bowel movements. If you are overweight, consult your physician about a weight loss plan to reduce the chances of recurrence of the hernia.

 CALL YOUR DOCTOR IF

- Pain, swelling, redness, drainage or bleeding occurs in the surgical area.
- You develop signs of infection, including headache, muscle aches, dizziness or a general ill feeling and fever.
- You become constipated.
- New, unexplained symptoms develop. Drugs used in treatment may produce side effects.

HERNIA REPAIR, INCISIONAL
(Incisional Herniorrhaphy)

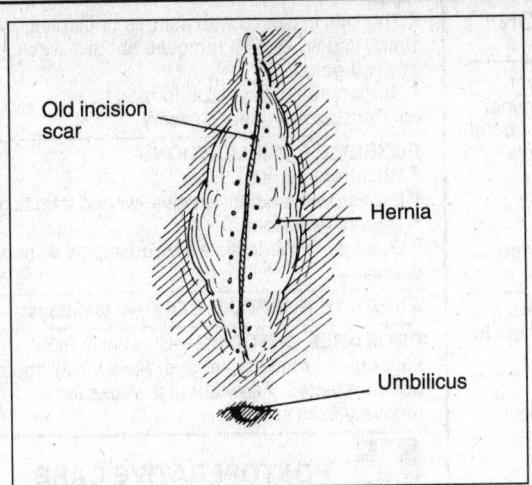

Old incision scar

Hernia

Umbilicus

An illustration of an incisional hernia in the abdominal wall protruding through an old incision scar.

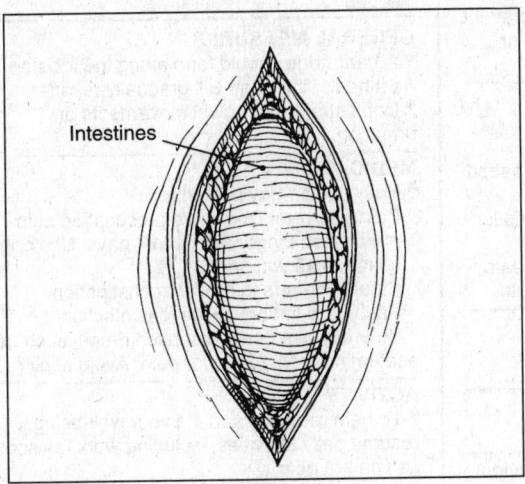

Intestines

Abdominal muscles retracted to reveal intestines pushing through the abdominal muscles.

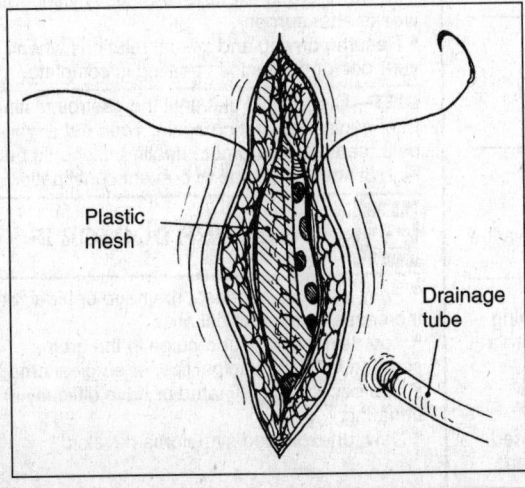

Plastic mesh

Drainage tube

The intestine is replaced in the abdominal cavity. Frequently a plastic mesh is used to strengthen the repair.

SURGERIES

HERNIA REPAIR, INGUINAL
(Inguinal Herniorrhaphy)

 GENERAL INFORMATION

DEFINITION—Closing or repairing a defect (opening) in the muscle layer of the abdominal wall in the inguinal (groin) area. If bowel or other abdominal contents are caught in the hernia and cannot be pushed back, it is called an incarcerated hernia. If the opening is so tight that it has cut off the blood supply to the incarcerated tissue, it is called a strangulated hernia.

BODY PARTS INVOLVED—Groin muscles and ligaments inside the lower abdomen next to the genitals; abdominal muscles.

REASONS FOR SURGERY
- Incarcerated hernia: This is an emergency!
- Strangulated hernia: This is an emergency!
- Uncomplicated hernia: Most doctors recommend operating on a hernia even if no hernia symptoms are present in order to prevent the serious complications of incarceration or strangulation.

SURGICAL RISK INCREASES WITH
- Adults over 60; newborns and infants.
- Excess alcohol consumption; smoking.
- Chronic lung disease, prostatism, constipation or family history of hernias.
- Use of some prescription and nonprescription drugs. Inform your doctor of any drugs, medications, or vitamin and herb supplements you are using or have used in the last month.

 WHAT TO EXPECT

WHO OPERATES—General surgeon or urologist.

WHERE PERFORMED—Hospital or outpatient surgical facility.

DIAGNOSTIC TESTS
- Before surgery: Blood and urine studies; x-rays of abdomen and chest; ECG (see Glossary).
- After surgery: Blood studies.

ANESTHESIA
- Spinal anesthesia by injection.
- Local anesthesia by injection.
- General anesthesia by injection and inhalation with an airway tube placed in the windpipe.

DESCRIPTION OF OPERATION
- There are various techniques for performing this surgery. Described here is an open hernia repair:
- An incision is made in the abdomen. The abdominal muscles are separated.
- The hernia is located and repaired or closed.
- A plastic mesh is often used to reinforce the repair.
- The skin is closed with sutures or staples, which usually can be removed about 1 week after surgery.
- Surgery may also be performed laparoscopically (see Glossary).

POSSIBLE COMPLICATIONS
- Recurrent hernia.
- Excessive bleeding; surgical-wound infection.
- Urinary retention.
- Damage to the testicle's blood supply or nerve supply.

AVERAGE HOSPITAL STAY—0 to 4 days.

PROBABLE OUTCOME—Curable in most patients, no matter what age. Male virility should not be affected. Allow about 6 weeks for recovery from surgery.

 POSTOPERATIVE CARE

GENERAL MEASURES
- A hard ridge should form along the incision. As it heals, the ridge will gradually recede.
- Don't strain with bowel movements or urination.

MEDICATION
- Your doctor may prescribe:
  Pain relievers. Don't take prescription pain medication longer than 4 to 7 days. Use only as much as you need.
  Stool softeners to prevent constipation.
  Antibiotics to fight or prevent infection.
- You may use nonprescription drugs, such as acetaminophen, for minor pain. Avoid aspirin.

ACTIVITY
- To help recovery and aid your well-being, resume daily activities, including work, as soon as you are able.
- Avoid vigorous exercise and heavy lifting for 6 weeks after surgery.
- Resume driving and sexual relations when your doctor determines healing is complete.

DIET—Clear liquid diet until the gastrointestinal tract begins to function again. Then eat a well-balanced diet to promote healing. It should be high in fiber and fluids to prevent constipation.

 CALL YOUR DOCTOR IF

- Pain, swelling, redness, drainage or bleeding increases in the surgical area.
- You develop pain or a bulge in the groin, scrotum, testicle, vaginal lips, or surgical area.
- You become constipated or have difficulty in urinating.
- New, unexplained symptoms develop.

HERNIA REPAIR, INGUINAL
(Inguinal Herniorrhaphy)

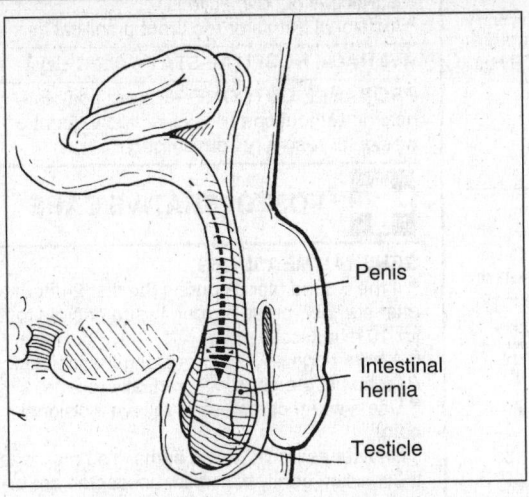

A side view of the male pelvic region.
- A typical inguinal hernia in which a loop of intestine has dropped down into the scrotum.

Penis

Intestinal hernia

Testicle

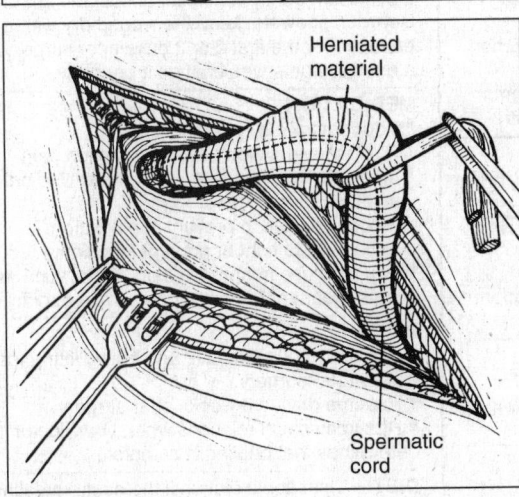

Herniated material

Spermatic cord

The hernia is located and repaired or closed, being careful not to injure the spermatic cord.

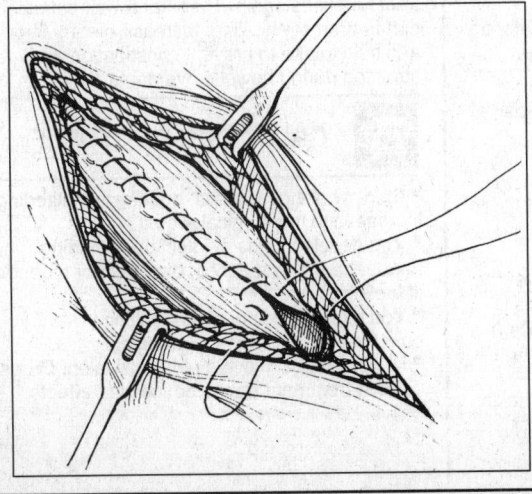

Sometimes, if the hernia is large enough to warrant more than natural tissue, a fine mesh gauze patch may be sewn in place to prevent abdominal contents from causing a recurrent hernia.

HERNIA REPAIR, UMBILICAL

 GENERAL INFORMATION

DEFINITION—Closure of an umbilical hernia, a weakening in the muscles around the umbilicus (navel) that allows abdominal contents to protrude prominently.

BODY PARTS INVOLVED—Abdominal muscular wall around the navel.

REASONS FOR SURGERY
- Improved appearance.
- Relief of pain.
- Prevention of incarceration or strangulation of the intestines (see Hernia Repair, Inguinal in Surgery section).

SURGICAL RISK INCREASES WITH
- Newborns and infants.
- Obesity; poor nutrition.
- Smoking; alcoholism.
- Recent or chronic illness, especially chronic lung disease.
- Diabetes mellitus.
- Use of some prescription and nonprescription drugs. Inform your doctor of any drugs, medications, or vitamin and herb supplements you are using or have used in the last month.

 WHAT TO EXPECT

WHO OPERATES—General surgeon or pediatric surgeon.

WHERE PERFORMED—Hospital or outpatient surgical facility.

DIAGNOSTIC TESTS
- Before surgery: Blood and urine studies; abdominal and chest x-rays; ECG (see Glossary).
- After surgery: Blood studies.

ANESTHESIA
- Local anesthesia by injection.
- Spinal anesthesia by injection.
- General anesthesia by injection and inhalation with an airway tube placed in the windpipe.

DESCRIPTION OF OPERATION
- An incision is made slightly above or below the navel.
- Sometimes, an incision is made in the peritoneum to open the peritoneal cavity. The contents of the hernia sac are located and replaced in the abdominal cavity. The peritoneum is closed.
- The large abdominal muscle is pulled over the defect. The membrane covering the muscle is overlapped and tied to close the defect. When the hernia is large, plastic mesh is sometimes used to cover the defect.
- The skin is closed with sutures or clips, which usually can be removed about 10 days after surgery.

POSSIBLE COMPLICATIONS
- Excessive bleeding.
- Surgical-wound infection.
- Incisional hernia or recurrent umbilical hernia.

AVERAGE HOSPITAL STAY—0 to 1 day.

PROBABLE OUTCOME—Expect complete healing without complications. Allow about 3 weeks for recovery from surgery.

 POSTOPERATIVE CARE

GENERAL MEASURES
- If the wound bleeds during the first 24 hours after surgery, press a clean tissue or cloth to it for 10 minutes.
- A hard ridge should form along the incision. As it heals, the ridge will gradually recede.
- Use a warm compress to relieve incisional pain.
- Shower as usual. Avoid baths. You may wash the incision gently with mild, unscented soap. Between showers, keep the wound dry with a bandage for the first 2 or 3 days after surgery. If a bandage gets wet, change it promptly.

MEDICATION
- Your doctor may prescribe:
  Pain relievers. Don't use prescription pain medication longer than 4 to 7 days. Use only as much as you need.
  Stool softeners to prevent constipation.
  Antibiotics to fight or prevent infection.
- You may use nonprescription drugs, such as acetaminophen, for minor pain. Avoid aspirin.

ACTIVITY
- Avoid vigorous exercise and heavy lifting for 6 weeks after surgery.
- Resume driving 3 weeks after surgery.
- Resume sexual relations when your doctor determines that healing is complete.

DIET—Clear liquid diet until the gastrointestinal tract functions again. Then eat a well-balanced diet to promote healing. Increase dietary fiber and fluid intake to prevent constipation and straining during bowel movements.

 CALL YOUR DOCTOR IF

- Pain, swelling, redness, drainage or bleeding increases in the surgical area.
- You develop signs of infection, including headache, muscle aches, dizziness or a general ill feeling and fever.
- You experience nausea, vomiting, constipation or abdominal swelling.
- New, unexplained symptoms develop. Drugs used in treatment may produce side effects.

HERNIA REPAIR, UMBILICAL

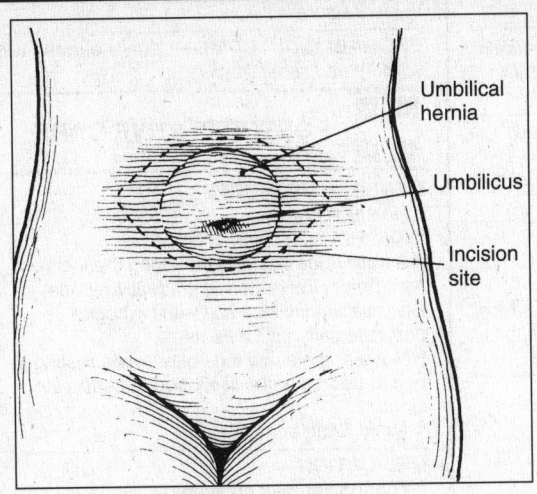

An illustration of a typical umbilical (navel) hernia and the incision site for the hernia repair.

Umbilical hernia

Umbilicus

Incision site

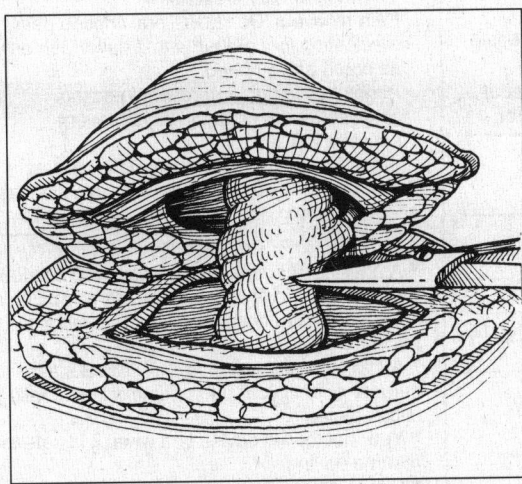

The incision is extended into the peritoneum to open the cavity.
- Contents of the hernia sac are located and replaced in the abdominal cavity.

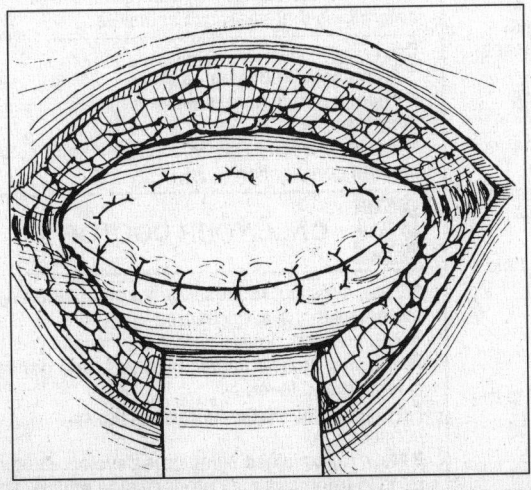

The peritoneum is closed. The large abdominal muscles will be pulled over the defect, then muscle layers and skin will be closed.

HIP NAILING FOR HIP FRACTURE

GENERAL INFORMATION

DEFINITION—A surgical procedure to reattach the broken fragments of the fractured femur near the hip.

BODY PARTS INVOLVED—The head and neck of the femur and the acetabulum (the socket of the pelvis that receives the femur to form the hip joint).

REASONS FOR SURGERY
- To make early movement of the hip joint possible after fracture.
- To prevent prolonged bed confinement, which is usually dangerous in the elderly age group when hip fractures become more common.

SURGICAL RISK INCREASES WITH
- Adults over 60; obesity; poor nutrition.
- Smoking.
- Excess alcohol consumption.
- Recent or chronic illness.
- Diabetes mellitus.
- Use of some prescription and nonprescription drugs. Inform your doctor of any drugs, medications, or vitamin and herb supplements you are using or have used in the last month.

WHAT TO EXPECT

WHO OPERATES—Orthopedic surgeon; general surgeon (sometimes).

WHERE PERFORMED—Hospital.

DIAGNOSTIC TESTS—Before surgery: Blood and urine studies; x-rays of hip and lung.

ANESTHESIA—General anesthesia by injection and inhalation with an airway tube placed in the windpipe.

DESCRIPTION OF OPERATION
- After anesthesia, the area adjacent to the fractured hip is cleaned, shaven and draped.
- An incision is made at a point allowing access to the fractured parts.
- The broken fragments are realigned under direct vision.
- Plates are fitted to hold the nail to be inserted into the fractured fragments.
- The nail is hammered into the broken parts to hold them together and give strength to the injured area of the bone.
- The plate is attached to healthy bone to hold the nail in place.

POSSIBLE COMPLICATIONS
- Surgical-wound infection.
- Excessive bleeding.
- Blood clots breaking loose and traveling to the lungs (pulmonary embolism).
- Refracture at the hip.

AVERAGE HOSPITAL STAY—4 to 7 days, depending on the condition of the patient prior to hip fracture.

PROBABLE OUTCOME—Usually curable with surgery and rehabilitation.

POSTOPERATIVE CARE

GENERAL MEASURES
- No smoking.
- Keep incision clean and dry.
- A hard ridge should form along the incision. As it heals, the ridge will gradually recede. Cleanse the incision site with hydrogen peroxide daily until it heals.
- Move and elevate legs often while resting in bed to decrease the likelihood of deep-vein blood clots.
- Avoid lifting heavy objects.

MEDICATION
- Your doctor may prescribe:
  Pain relievers. Don't take prescription pain medication longer than 4 to 7 days. Use only as much as you need.
  Antibiotics to fight or prevent infection.
  Stool softeners or laxatives to prevent constipation.
  Blood thinners to help prevent blood clots.
- You may use nonprescription drugs, such as acetaminophen, for minor pain. Avoid aspirin.

ACTIVITY
- A physical therapy program will be prescribed by your doctor. Usually you will start by using a walker, then crutches, followed by a cane if necessary.
- Avoid vigorous exercise for 12 weeks after surgery or until your doctor determines healing is complete.
- Your doctor will advise you when it is safe to resume driving.
- Resume sexual activity when your doctor determines that healing is complete.

DIET
- As prescribed by your doctor.
- Vitamin and mineral supplements (sometimes).
- Increase dietary fiber and fluid intake to help prevent constipation.

CALL YOUR DOCTOR IF

- Pain, swelling, redness, drainage or bleeding increases in the surgical area.
- You develop signs of infection, including headache, muscle aches, dizziness or a general ill feeling and fever.
- You experience nausea, vomiting, or constipation.
- New, unexplained symptoms develop. Drugs used in treatment may produce side effects.

HIP NAILING FOR HIP FRACTURE

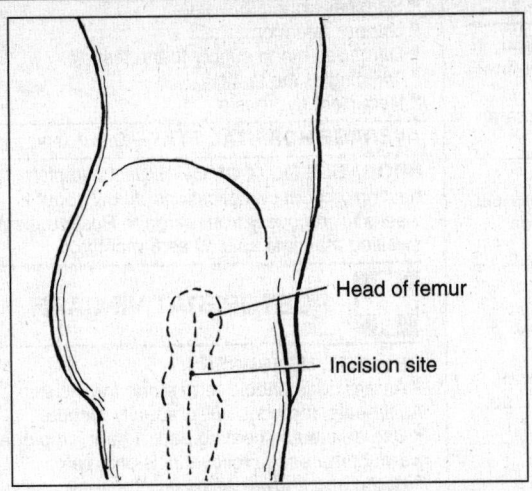

An illustration of an incision made over the affected hip showing the head of the femur that is fractured.

- Head of femur
- Incision site

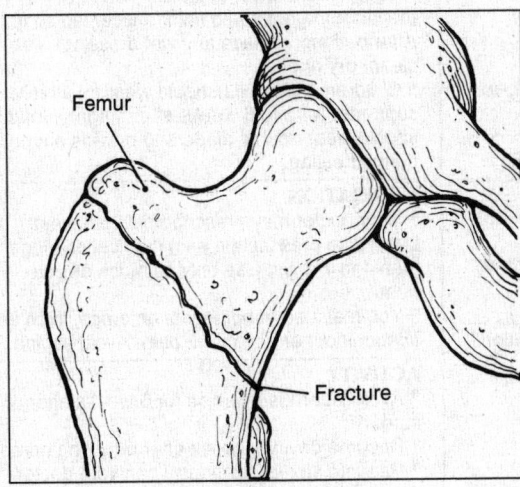

A closer view of the fractured femur.

- Femur
- Fracture

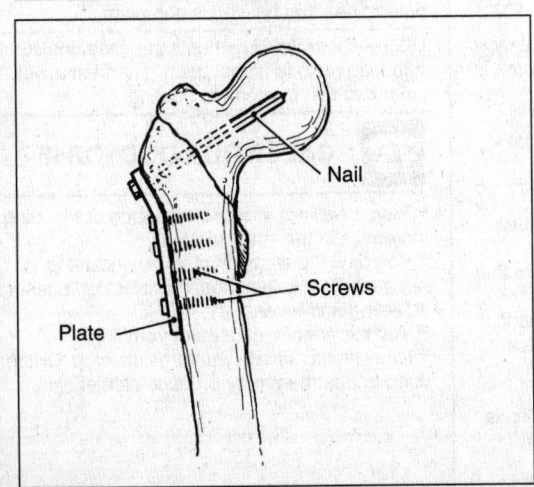

The bone fragments are realigned, and a plate, which is attached to healthy bone by a number of screws, is used to hold the nail in place. The nail is hammered into the broken parts of the femur, giving strength to the broken area of the bone.

- Nail
- Screws
- Plate

HYDROCELECTOMY

GENERAL INFORMATION

DEFINITION—Removal of a hydrocele, fluid that has collected in a small sac usually on the testicle or in the membrane covering the testicle. Hydroceles frequently occur in infants, but may also occur in adults.

BODY PARTS INVOLVED—Scrotum; spermatic cord; membrane covering the testicle (tunica vaginalis); blood vessels and nerves connected to the scrotum.

REASONS FOR SURGERY
- In infants: completion of the repair of a congenital inguinal hernia, which frequently accompanies a congenital hydrocele.
- In adults: removal of an uncomfortable and unsightly scrotal cyst that may conceal a tumor in the testicle.

SURGICAL RISK INCREASES WITH
- Obesity; poor nutrition.
- Smoking; alcoholism.
- Chronic or recent illness.
- Diabetes mellitus.
- Use of some prescription and nonprescription drugs. Inform your doctor of any drugs, medications, or vitamin and herb supplements you are using or have used in the last month.

WHAT TO EXPECT

WHO OPERATES—General surgeon or urologist.

WHERE PERFORMED—Hospital or outpatient surgical facility.

DIAGNOSTIC TESTS
- Before surgery: Blood and urine studies; ultrasound (see Glossary).
- After surgery: Usually none.

ANESTHESIA
- General anesthesia by injection and inhalation with an airway tube placed in the windpipe in infants.
- Local anesthesia by injection.
- Spinal anesthesia by injection (sometimes) in older children and adults.

DESCRIPTION OF OPERATION
- An incision is made in the scrotum over the testicle.
- The hydrocele is located and cut free from the scrotal contents.
- The hydrocele is incised, and the fluid inside it is drained. The skin edges of the hydrocele are tucked under and sewn together to prevent refilling.
- The scrotal contents are replaced. The skin is closed with fine suture material that will be absorbed by the body.

POSSIBLE COMPLICATIONS
- Excessive bleeding.
- Surgical-wound infection.
- Urinary retention.
- Damaged blood supply to the testicle.
- Twisting of the testicle.
- Recurrent hydrocele.

AVERAGE HOSPITAL STAY—0 to 1 day.

PROBABLE OUTCOME—Expect complete healing without complications. Allow about 2 weeks for recovery from surgery. Post-surgical swelling may last as long as 6 months.

POSTOPERATIVE CARE

GENERAL MEASURES
- A hard ridge should form along the incision. As it heals, the ridge will gradually recede.
- Use an electric heating pad, a heat lamp or a warm compress to relieve incisional pain.
- Bathe and shower as usual. You may wash the incision gently with mild, unscented soap. After bathing, replace any wet dressings with clean, dry ones.
- Children and adults should wear an athletic supporter for 3 to 6 weeks after surgery. Infants should wear double diapers to provide support during healing.

MEDICATION
- Your doctor may prescribe pain relievers. Don't take prescription pain medication longer than 4 to 7 days. Use only as much as you need.
- You may use nonprescription drugs, such as acetaminophen, for minor pain. Avoid aspirin.

ACTIVITY
- Avoid vigorous exercise for 6 weeks after surgery.
- Resume driving 1 week after returning home.
- Resume sexual relations when your doctor determines that healing is complete.

DIET—Clear liquid diet until the gastrointestinal tract begins to function again. Then eat a well-balanced diet to promote healing.

CALL YOUR DOCTOR IF
- Pain, swelling, redness, drainage or bleeding increases in the surgical area.
- You develop signs of infection, including headache, muscle aches, dizziness or a general ill feeling and fever.
- You experience nausea or vomiting.
- New, unexplained symptoms develop. Drugs used in treatment may produce side effects.

HYDROCELECTOMY

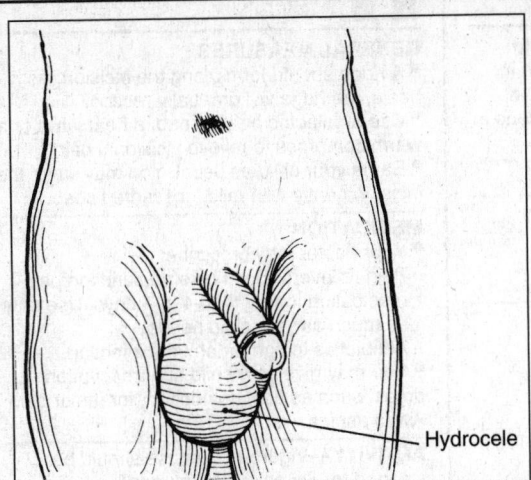

An illustration of a typical hydrocele distending one portion of the scrotum.

Hydrocele

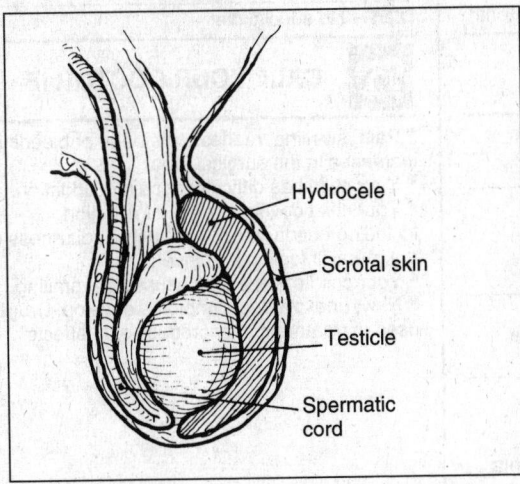

A hydrocele and surrounding tissues including the spermatic cord, testicle and scrotum.

Hydrocele

Scrotal skin

Testicle

Spermatic cord

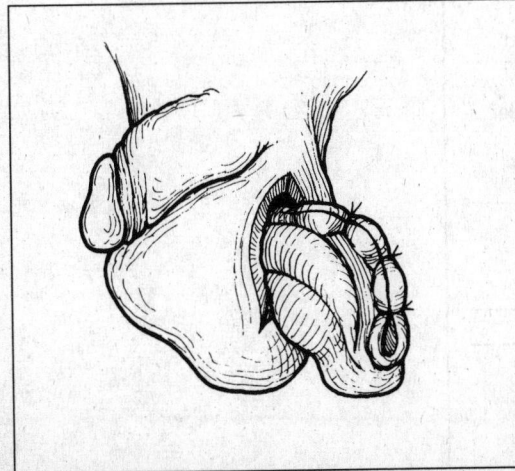

After the hydrocele has been incised and the fluid inside drained, the edges of the hydrocele are tucked under and sewn together to prevent refilling.
  • The scrotal contents are then replaced and the skin closed with fine absorbable sutures that need not be removed.

HYPOSPADIAS REPAIR & URETHROPLASTY

 GENERAL INFORMATION

DEFINITION—Creation of a new urethra to correct hypospadias, a congenital disorder in which the urethra opening is in an abnormal location on the penis. Surgery is usually done in infancy or early childhood.

BODY PARTS INVOLVED—Urethra.

REASONS FOR SURGERY
- Prevention of urinary-tract infections.
- Establishment of sexual function.
- Correction of abnormal urination patterns.

SURGICAL RISK INCREASES WITH
- Obesity.
- Poor nutrition.
- Recent or chronic illness.
- Diabetes mellitus.
- Use of some prescription and nonprescription drugs. Inform your doctor of any drugs, medications, or vitamin and herb supplements your child is using or has used in the last month.

 WHAT TO EXPECT

WHO OPERATES—Urologist.

WHERE PERFORMED—Hospital.

DIAGNOSTIC TESTS
- Before surgery: Blood and urine studies.
- After surgery: Blood studies; laboratory examination of removed tissue.

ANESTHESIA—General anesthesia by injection and inhalation, with an airway tube placed in the windpipe.

DESCRIPTION OF OPERATION
- An incision is made over the abnormal opening of the urethra.
- An instrument is passed through the urethra and extended along its full length. Abnormal scar tissue is cut free and removed. A new urethra is fashioned from existing tissue and sewn around a catheter, which will remain in place until healing is complete.
- After healing, the catheter is removed under anesthesia.
- The skin is closed with sutures that will be absorbed by the body.

POSSIBLE COMPLICATIONS
- Excessive bleeding.
- Surgical-wound infection.
- Scarring of urethra.

AVERAGE HOSPITAL STAY—2-7 days.

PROBABLE OUTCOME—Expect complete healing without complications. Allow about 3 months for recovery from surgery.

 POSTOPERATIVE CARE

GENERAL MEASURES
- A ridge should form along the incision. As it heals, the ridge will gradually recede.
- Use an electric heating pad, a heat lamp or a warm compress to relieve incisional pain.
- Bathe your child as usual. You may wash the incision gently with mild, unscented soap.

MEDICATION
- Your doctor may prescribe:
  Pain relievers. Don't take prescription pain medication longer than 4 to 7 days. Use only as much as your child needs.
  Antibiotics to fight or prevent infection.
- You may give your child nonprescription drugs, such as acetaminophen, for minor pain. Avoid aspirin.

ACTIVITY—Vigorous exercise should be avoided for 6 weeks after surgery.

DIET—No special diet.

 CALL YOUR DOCTOR IF

- Pain, swelling, redness, drainage or bleeding increases in the surgical area.
- Your child has difficulty or pain in urination.
- Your child develops signs of infection, including headache, muscle aches, dizziness or a general ill feeling and fever.
- Your child experiences nausea or vomiting.
- New, unexplained symptoms develop. Drugs used in treatment may produce side effects.

HYPOSPADIAS REPAIR & URETHROPLASTY

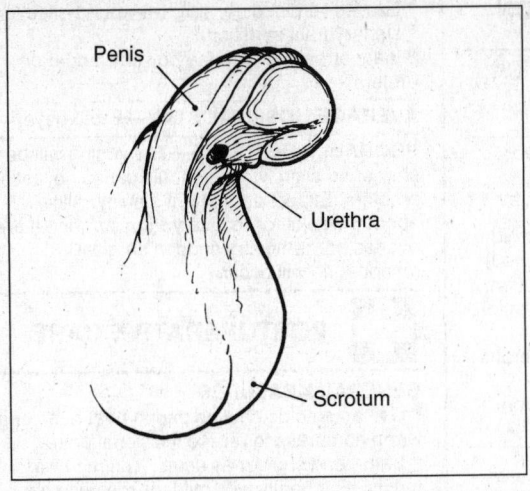

Penis

Urethra

Scrotum

A typical hypospadias with opening of the urethra under the head of the penis.
  • Openings of the urethra may occur in various other places on the penis other than its normal opening.

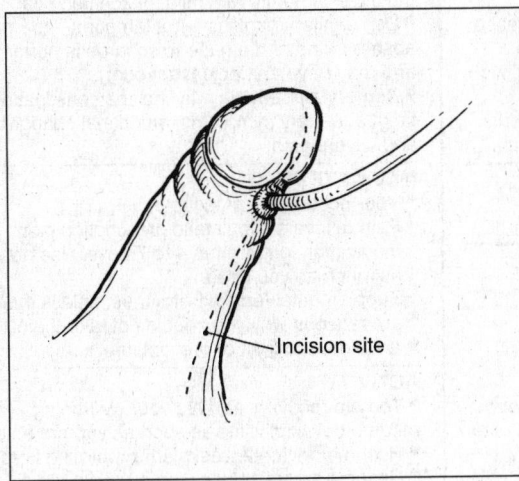

Incision site

An instrument is placed through the urethra and is extended along its full length. Abnormal scar tissue is cut free and removed.
  • A new urethra is fashioned from existing tissue and sewn around a catheter which will remain in place until healing is complete.

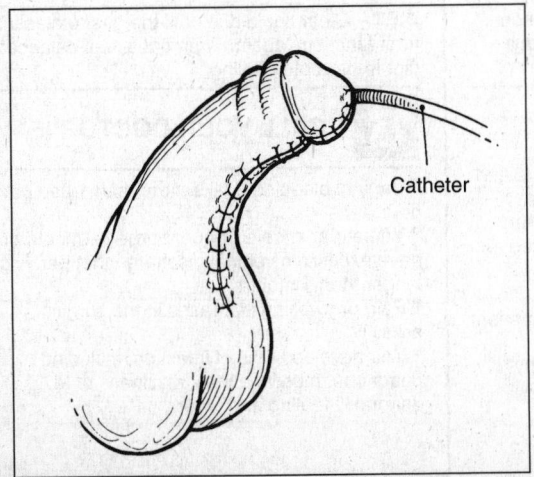

Catheter

After healing, the catheter is removed under anesthesia.

HYSTERECTOMY (ABDOMINAL) WITH SALPINGO-OOPHORECTOMY

 GENERAL INFORMATION

DEFINITION—Removal of the uterus, cervix, and often the fallopian tubes and ovaries, through an incision in the abdomen.

BODY PARTS INVOLVED—Uterus; cervix; fallopian tubes; ovaries; vagina.

REASONS FOR SURGERY
- Uterus: Cancer or suspected cancer; fibroid tumors; chronic bleeding; prolapsed (dropped) uterus; endometriosis; chronic pelvic infection; severe menstrual pain; or voluntary sterilization.
- Fallopian tubes and ovaries: Cancer or suspected cancer of the ovaries; precancerous or twisted ovarian cysts; ovarian pregnancy; ovarian abscess; damage to the ovaries from severe endometriosis.

SURGICAL RISK INCREASES WITH
- Obesity; smoking.
- Iron-deficiency anemia; heart or lung disease; or diabetes mellitus.
- Use of some prescription and nonprescription drugs. Inform your doctor of any drugs, medications, or vitamin and herb supplements you are using or have used in the last month.

 WHAT TO EXPECT

WHO OPERATES—General surgeon or obstetrician-gynecologist.

WHERE PERFORMED—Hospital.

DIAGNOSTIC TESTS
- Before surgery: Blood and urine studies; x-rays of abdomen and kidneys; dilatation and curettage of the uterus (D & C); ultrasound (see Glossary for both).
- After surgery: Blood studies.

ANESTHESIA—Spinal anesthesia or general anesthesia by injection and inhalation with an airway tube placed in the windpipe.

DESCRIPTION OF OPERATION
- An incision is made in the abdomen.
- The abdominal organs are examined.
- In a simple hysterectomy, only the uterus and cervix are removed, along with any visible tumors. In a total hysterectomy, the fallopian tubes and ovaries are cut free and removed as well (salpingo-oophorectomy).
- Any stretched ligaments are repaired.
- The vagina is closed with sutures at its deeper end; the surgical wound is closed.
- The procedure may also be performed by laparoscopy (see in Surgery section).

POSSIBLE COMPLICATIONS
- Excessive bleeding; surgical-wound infection.
- Urinary tract infection.
- Inadvertent injury to the bowel, bladder or ureters.

AVERAGE HOSPITAL STAY—2 to 5 days.

PROBABLE OUTCOME—The vagina will be shortened slightly. This should cause no lasting problem. Expect permanent sterility. Allow about 6 weeks for recovery from surgery. If the ovaries are removed, sudden surgical menopause will occur.

 POSTOPERATIVE CARE

GENERAL MEASURES
- Use an electric heating pad, a heat lamp or a warm compress to relieve incisional pain.
- Bathe and shower as usual. You may wash the incision gently with mild, unscented soap.
- Use sanitary napkins—not tampons—to absorb blood or drainage (discharge is normal, and may have an unpleasant odor).
- Surgery aftereffects may include constipation, fatigue, urinary symptoms, emotional changes and weight gain.

MEDICATION
- Your doctor may prescribe:
  Pain relievers. Don't take prescription pain medication longer than 4 to 7 days. Use only as much as you need.
  Supplemental female hormones, unless there are reasons why you should not take them.
- Antibiotics to fight or prevent infection.

ACTIVITY
- To help recovery and aid your well-being, resume daily activities as soon as you are able.
- Resume driving 2 weeks after returning home.
- Resume sexual relations in 4 to 6 weeks.

DIET—Clear liquid diet until the gastrointestinal tract functions again. Then eat a well-balanced diet to promote healing.

 CALL YOUR DOCTOR IF

- Vaginal bleeding soaks more than 1 pad per hour.
- You experience a frequent urge to urinate or have excessive vaginal discharge that persists longer than 1 month.
- Pain or swelling increases in the surgical area.
- You develop signs of infection, including headache, muscle aches, dizziness or a general ill feeling and fever.

HYSTERECTOMY (ABDOMINAL) WITH SALPINGO-OOPHORECTOMY

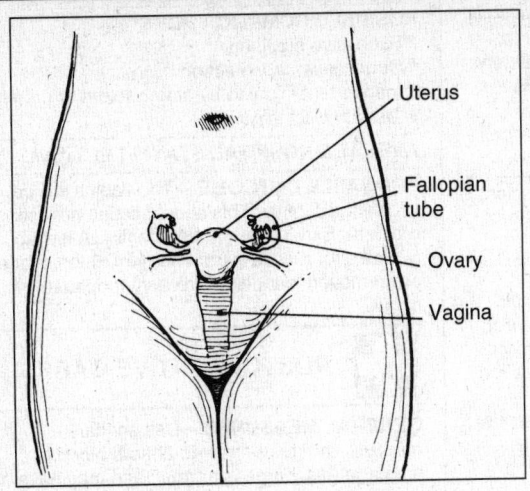

Uterus

Fallopian tube

Ovary

Vagina

Shown are parts of the female reproductive tract including the uterus, fallopian tubes, ovaries and vagina.

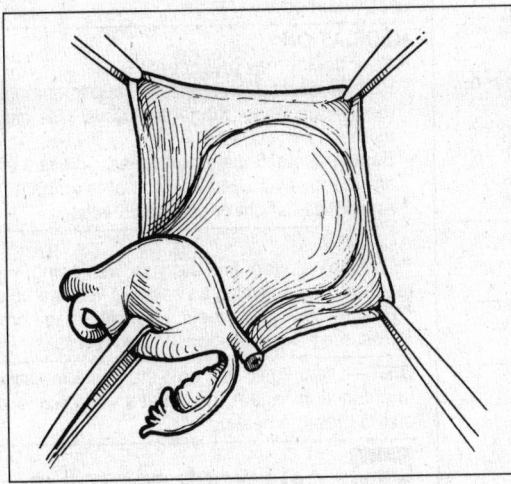

After an incision (either vertical or transverse) has been made in the lower abdomen and the muscles retracted, the uterus, cervix, fallopian tubes and ovaries are cut free and removed.

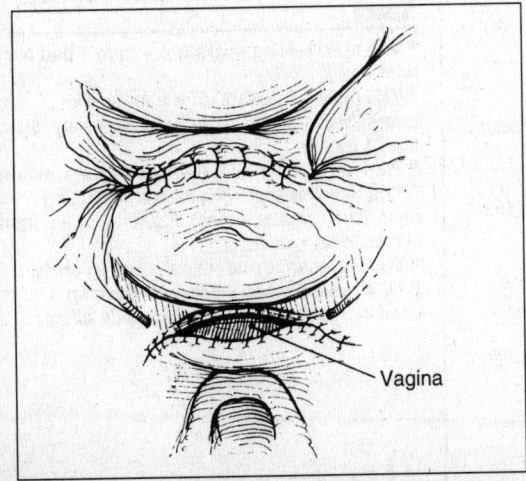

The vagina is closed with sutures.
• The abdominal wall is closed in layers and the skin is closed with sutures that usually can be removed in 10 to 14 days (not illustrated).

Vagina

SURGERIES

HYSTERECTOMY (VAGINAL)

GENERAL INFORMATION

DEFINITION—Removal of the uterus, cervix, fallopian tubes and ovaries through an incision in the deepest recesses of the vagina. This surgery is frequently accompanied by reconstructive surgery (colporrhaphy), to repair weakened bladder and rectal muscles.

BODY PARTS INVOLVED—Bladder muscles; rectal muscles; uterus; cervix; fallopian tubes; ovaries; vagina.

REASONS FOR SURGERY
- Uterus: Cancer or suspected cancer; fibroid tumors; chronic bleeding; prolapsed (dropped) uterus; endometriosis; chronic pelvic infection; severe menstrual pain; or voluntary sterilization.
- Fallopian tubes and ovaries: Cancer or suspected cancer of the ovaries; precancerous or twisted ovarian cysts; ovarian pregnancy; ovarian abscess; damage to the ovaries from severe endometriosis.

SURGICAL RISK INCREASES WITH
- Obesity; smoking.
- Iron-deficiency anemia; heart or lung disease; or diabetes mellitus.
- Use of some prescription and nonprescription drugs. Inform your doctor of any drugs, medications, or vitamin and herb supplements you are using or have used in the last month.

WHAT TO EXPECT

WHO OPERATES—General surgeon or obstetrician-gynecologist.

WHERE PERFORMED—Hospital.

DIAGNOSTIC TESTS
- Before surgery: Blood and urine studies; x-rays of abdomen and kidneys; dilatation and curettage of the uterus (D & C); ultrasound (see Glossary for both).
- After surgery: Blood studies.

ANESTHESIA
- Spinal anesthesia by injection.
- General anesthesia by injection and inhalation with an airway tube placed in the windpipe.

DESCRIPTION OF OPERATION
- The vaginal walls are carefully separated from the bladder muscles and rectal muscles.
- The deepest recesses of the vagina are opened. The cervix and uterus are cut free and removed. The rear part of the vagina is closed with sutures.
- The bladder muscles and rectal muscles are sewn into their proper position. Supporting tissue is repaired.
- A small foley catheter may be in the bladder for several days.

- The procedure may also be performed by laparoscopy (see in Surgery section).

POSSIBLE COMPLICATIONS
- Excessive bleeding.
- Surgical-wound infection.
- Inadvertent injury to bladder, rectum or ureters.
- Urinary tract infection.

AVERAGE HOSPITAL STAY—1 to 3 days.

PROBABLE OUTCOME—The vagina will be shortened slightly. This should cause no lasting problem. Expect permanent sterility. Allow about 6 weeks for recovery from surgery. If the ovaries are removed, sudden surgical menopause will occur.

POSTOPERATIVE CARE

GENERAL MEASURES—Use sanitary napkins—not tampons—to absorb blood or drainage (discharge is normal, and may have an unpleasant odor).

MEDICATION
- Your doctor may prescribe:
  Pain relievers. Don't take prescription pain medication longer than 4 to 7 days. Use only as much as you need.
  Supplemental female hormones, unless there are reasons why you should not take them.
- Antibiotics to fight or prevent infection.

ACTIVITY
- To help recovery and aid your well-being, resume daily activities as soon as you are able.
- Resume driving 2 weeks after returning home.
- Resume sexual relations in 4 to 6 weeks.

DIET—Clear liquid diet until the gastrointestinal tract functions again. Then eat a well-balanced diet to promote healing.

CALL YOUR DOCTOR IF

- Vaginal bleeding soaks more than 1 pad per hour.
- You have a frequent urge to urinate or excessive vaginal discharge that persists longer than 1 month.
- Pain or swelling increases in the surgical area.
- You develop signs of infection, including headache, muscle aches, dizziness or a general ill feeling and fever.
- You experience abdominal swelling or pain.
- New, unexplained symptoms develop. Drugs used in treatment may produce side effects.

HYSTERECTOMY (VAGINAL)

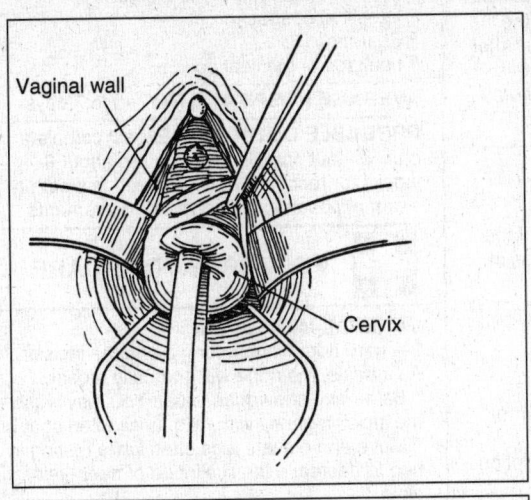

Vaginal wall

Cervix

This view illustrates a female patient with extended legs in stirrups on an examining table to allow examination of the genital area.
- An illustration of the vagina and cervix showing the first incision made to separate the cervix from the lowest layers of the bladder.

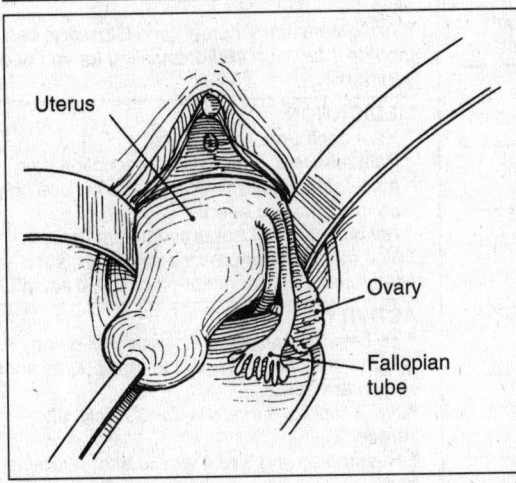

Uterus

Ovary

Fallopian tube

The deepest recesses of the vagina are opened. The cervix, uterus, fallopian tubes and ovaries are cut free and removed. The bladder is repaired (not illustrated).

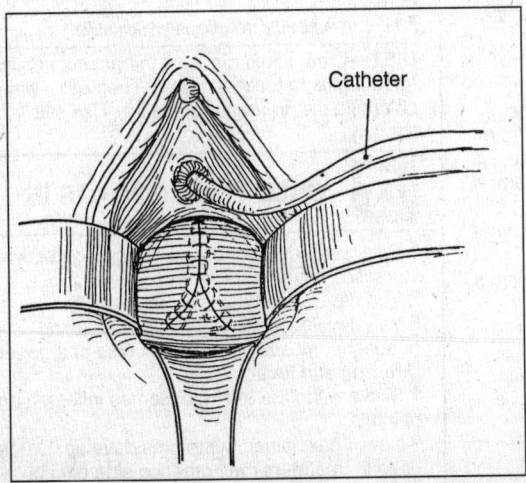

Catheter

A small catheter is left in the bladder to remain there 7 to 10 days while muscles of the bladder heal.

ILEOSTOMY

GENERAL INFORMATION

DEFINITION—Creation of an opening in the ileum, the lower part of the small intestine. After surgery, all feces leave the body through this opening, which is called an "ostomy" or "stoma."

BODY PARTS INVOLVED—Ileum; cecum.

REASONS FOR SURGERY
- Ulcerative colitis.
- Colon cancer.
- Colon surgery which weakens an area of the colon and necessitates a temporary bypass of the intestine until the colon has healed.

SURGICAL RISK INCREASES WITH
- Adults over 60; newborns and infants.
- Obesity; smoking; poor nutrition.
- Excess alcohol consumption.
- Recent or chronic illness, especially heart or lung disease or diabetes mellitus.
- Use of some prescription and nonprescription drugs. Inform your doctor of any drugs, medications, or vitamin and herb supplements you are using or have used in the last month.

WHAT TO EXPECT

WHO OPERATES—General surgeon; colon-rectal surgeon.

WHERE PERFORMED—Hospital.

DIAGNOSTIC TESTS
- Before surgery: Blood and urine studies; x-rays; ECG; sigmoidoscopy; colonoscopy (see Glossary for all).
- After surgery: Blood and urine studies.

ANESTHESIA—General anesthesia by injection and inhalation with an airway tube placed in the windpipe.

DESCRIPTION OF OPERATION
- An incision is made in the abdomen over the diseased intestinal tract.
- The muscles of the abdominal wall are separated to expose the abdominal organs, which are inspected for undetected disease. Other surgeries may be performed at this time.
- The ileum is clamped on both sides of the area to be opened and cut between the clamps. The part closer to the stomach is brought through another small incision in the abdominal wall to accept the stoma.
- The part of the intestinal tract below the ileum, usually around the diseased part of the intestine, is closed with sutures or is removed with the diseased colon. The abdominal contents are replaced. The muscles and skin are closed with sutures, which usually can be removed about 1 week after surgery.

POSSIBLE COMPLICATIONS
- Excessive bleeding.

- Surgical-wound infection; abscess.
- Incisional hernia.
- Skin irritation around the stoma.
- Intestinal obstruction.
- Scarring.
- Leakage of the ileal pouch.

AVERAGE HOSPITAL STAY—5 to 7 days.

PROBABLE OUTCOME—Expect complete cure without complications. Allow about 6 weeks for recovery. You will need to wear an external pouch to collect bowel movements.

POSTOPERATIVE CARE

GENERAL MEASURES
- A hard ridge should form along the incision. As it heals, the ridge will gradually recede.
- Bathe and shower as usual. You may wash the incision gently with mild, unscented soap.
- Move and elevate legs often while resting in bed to decrease the likelihood of deep-vein clots.
- An "enterostomy nurse" (see Glossary) can provide education and counseling for you and your family.

MEDICATION
- Your doctor may prescribe:
  Pain relievers. Don't take prescription pain medication longer than 4 to 7 days. Use only as much as you need.
  Antibiotics to fight or prevent infection.
- You may use nonprescription drugs, such as acetaminophen, for minor pain. Avoid aspirin.

ACTIVITY
- To help recovery and aid your well-being, resume daily activities, including work, as soon as you are able.
- Avoid vigorous exercise for 6 weeks after surgery.
- Resume driving 3 to 4 weeks after returning home.
- Resume sexual relations when able.

DIET—Clear liquid diet until the gastrointestinal tract begins to function again. Then eat a well-balanced diet to promote healing. Use salt liberally.

CALL YOUR DOCTOR IF

- Pain, swelling, redness, drainage or bleeding increases in the surgical area.
- You have abdominal swelling or pain.
- You develop signs of infection, including headache, muscle aches, dizziness or a general ill feeling and fever.
- Skin around the stoma becomes inflamed and painful.
- New, unexplained symptoms develop. Drugs used in treatment may produce side effects.

ILEOSTOMY

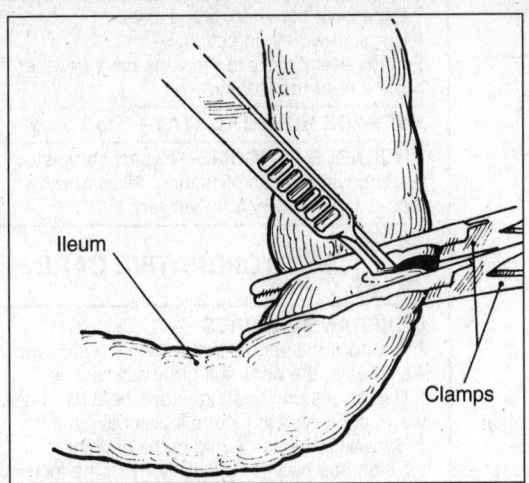

The muscles of the abdominal wall are separated to expose the abdominal organs, which are inspected for disease (not illustrated). The ileum is clamped on both sides of the area to be opened and cut between the clamps.

Ileum

Clamps

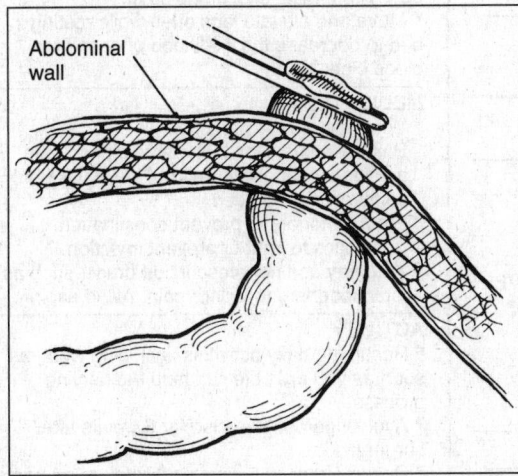

The part closer to the stomach is brought through another small incision in the abdominal wall to accept the stoma.
- The part of the intestinal tract below the ileum, usually around the diseased part of the intestine, is closed with sutures. The abdominal contents are replaced.

Abdominal wall

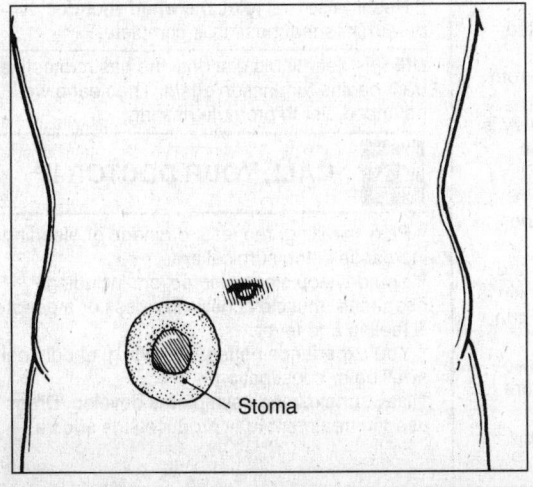

The stoma is shown in a frequently used location extending through the abdominal wall. After surgery, fecal contents will pass into an ileostomy bag.

Stoma

SURGERIES

KIDNEY REMOVAL
(Nephrectomy)

 ## GENERAL INFORMATION

DEFINITION—Removal of a kidney.

BODY PARTS INVOLVED—Kidney; blood vessels connected to kidney; ureter.

REASONS FOR SURGERY
- Cancer or suspected cancer of the kidney.
- Severe kidney trauma.
- Dysfunctional kidney due to infection.

SURGICAL RISK INCREASES WITH
- Adults over 60; newborns and infants.
- Obesity; poor nutrition.
- Smoking; alcoholism.
- Recent or chronic illness.
- Diabetes mellitus.
- Use of some prescription and nonprescription drugs. Inform your doctor of any drugs, medications, or vitamin and herb supplements you are using or have used in the last month.

 ## WHAT TO EXPECT

WHO OPERATES—General surgeon or urologist.

WHERE PERFORMED—Hospital.

DIAGNOSTIC TESTS
- Before surgery: Blood and urine studies; x-rays of kidneys, lower gastrointestinal tract and chest ; ECG; ultrasound; cystoscopy; IVP; MRI; CT scan (see Glossary for all).
- After surgery: Blood studies.

ANESTHESIA—General anesthesia by injection and inhalation with an airway tube placed in the windpipe.

DESCRIPTION OF OPERATION
- An incision is made, usually in the left or right flank, but sometimes in the abdomen.
- The vein leading from the kidney is located, isolated and tied.
- The ureter is located, tied and cut away from the kidney.
- The artery that supplies blood to the kidney is clamped in two places and cut between the clamps.
- The kidney is freed of adhesions or adjoining connective tissue and removed; surrounding lymph nodes may also be removed.
- All disconnected blood vessels are tied, and the muscles are closed with sutures. The skin is closed with sutures or clips, which usually can be removed in about 1 week after surgery.
- A urinary catheter (Foley) will be left in place for several days to make it easier to measure the amount of urine you are producing.
- Surgery may also be done by laparoscopy (see in Surgery section).

POSSIBLE COMPLICATIONS
- Excessive bleeding; blood clots.
- Surgical-wound infection.
- Inadvertent injury to the vena cava or other organs near the kidney.

AVERAGE HOSPITAL STAY—3 to 5 days.

PROBABLE OUTCOME—Expect complete healing without complications. Allow about 4 weeks for recovery from surgery.

 ## POSTOPERATIVE CARE

GENERAL MEASURES
- A hard ridge should form along the incision. As it heals, the ridge will gradually recede.
- Use an electric heating pad, a heat lamp or a warm compress to relieve incisional pain.
- Shower as usual. Avoid baths until the incision has healed. You may wash the incision gently with mild, unscented soap.
- Move and elevate legs often while resting in bed to decrease the likelihood of deep-vein blood clots.

MEDICATION
- Your doctor may prescribe:
  Pain relievers. Don't take prescription pain medication longer than 4 to 7 days. Use only as much as you need.
  Stool softeners to prevent constipation.
  Antibiotics to fight or prevent infection.
- You may use nonprescription drugs, such as acetaminophen, for minor pain. Avoid aspirin.

ACTIVITY
- Resuming daily activities, including work, as soon as you are able can help the healing process.
- Avoid vigorous exercise for 6 weeks after surgery.
- Resume driving 5 weeks after returning home.
- Resume sexual relations when your doctor determines that healing is complete.

DIET—Clear liquid diet until the gastrointestinal tract begins to function again. Then eat a well-balanced diet to promote healing.

 ## CALL YOUR DOCTOR IF

- Pain, swelling, redness, drainage or bleeding increases in the surgical area.
- You develop signs of infection, including headache, muscle aches, dizziness or a general ill feeling and fever.
- You experience nausea, vomiting, abdominal swelling or constipation.
- New, unexplained symptoms develop. Drugs used in treatment may produce side effects.

KIDNEY REMOVAL
(Nephrectomy)

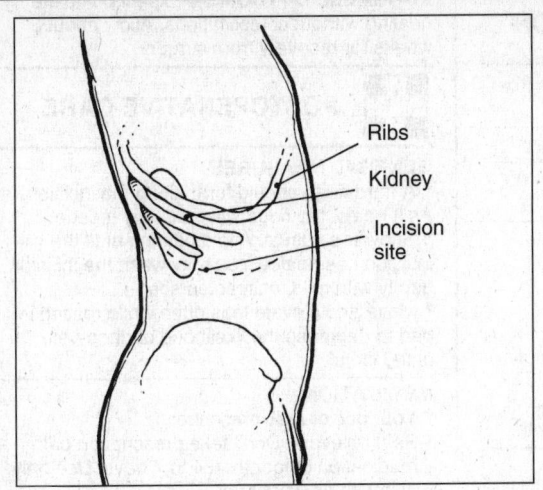

The usual incision for kidney removal in the flank below the last rib.

Ribs

Kidney

Incision site

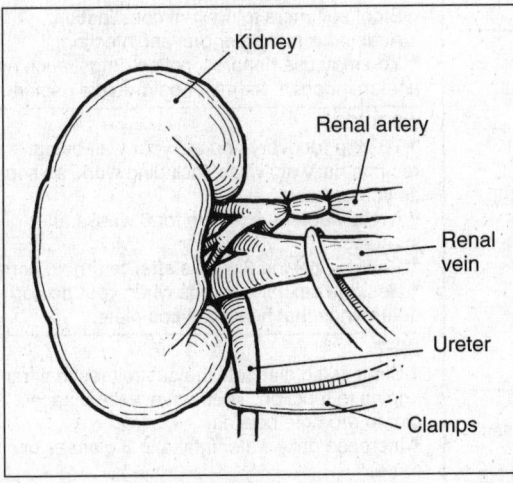

The vein leading from the kidney is located, isolated and tied.
- The ureter is located, tied and cut away from the kidney.
- The artery that supplies blood to the kidney is clamped in 2 places and cut between the clamps.
- The kidney is removed.

Kidney

Renal artery

Renal vein

Ureter

Clamps

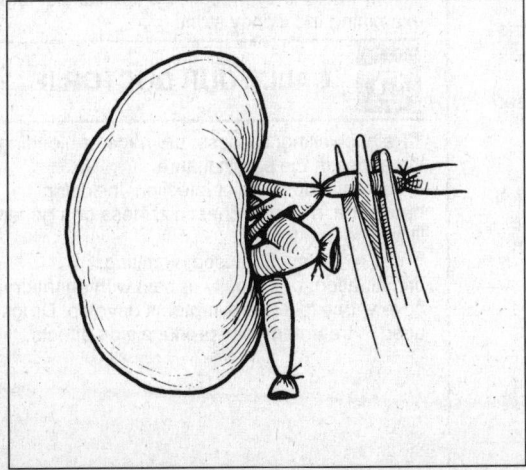

All disconnected blood vessels are tied. The abdominal muscles are closed (not illustrated).

SURGERIES

KIDNEY STONE REMOVAL
(Ureterolithotomy)

 GENERAL INFORMATION

DEFINITION—Removal of a kidney stone from one of the ureters.

BODY PARTS INVOLVED—Ureter; kidney.

REASONS FOR SURGERY—Restoration of normal urine flow in the ureter.

SURGICAL RISK INCREASES WITH
- Obesity; smoking; alcoholism.
- Poor nutrition.
- Recent or chronic illness.
- Diabetes mellitus.
- Use of some prescription and nonprescription drugs. Inform your doctor of any drugs, medications, or vitamin and herb supplements you are using or have used in the last month.

 WHAT TO EXPECT

WHO OPERATES—Urologist or general surgeon.

WHERE PERFORMED—Hospital.

DIAGNOSTIC TESTS
- Before surgery: Blood and urine studies; x-rays of chest; ECG; intravenous pyelogram; ultrasound: CT scan (see Glossary for all).
- During surgery: Retrograde pyelogram (see Glossary).
- After surgery: Blood studies; urine tests.

ANESTHESIA—General anesthesia by injection and inhalation with an airway tube placed in the windpipe.

DESCRIPTION OF OPERATION
- An incision is made in the flank. The muscles are separated and the ureter is exposed.
- A small incision is made in the ureter. The kidney stone is pulled free and removed.
- A tube is left in the wound for drainage, and a tube is inserted in the ureter to restore urine flow. This tube is removed after healing.
- Muscle layers are closed. The skin is closed with sutures or clips, which usually can be removed about 1 week after surgery.
- Some kidney stones may also be removed with lithotripsy (see in Surgery section), which involves the use of shockwaves to crush the stone so that it can be passed from the body with your urine.

POSSIBLE COMPLICATIONS
- Excessive bleeding.
- Surgical-wound infection.
- Urine leakage.
- Scarring at operative site causing obstruction or partial obstruction.

AVERAGE HOSPITAL STAY—4 to 5 days.

PROBABLE OUTCOME—Expect complete healing without complications. Allow about 2 weeks for recovery from surgery.

 POSTOPERATIVE CARE

GENERAL MEASURES
- A hard ridge should form along the incision. As it heals, the ridge will gradually recede.
- Shower as usual. Avoid bathing until the incision has healed You may wash the incision gently with mild, unscented soap.
- Move and elevate legs often while resting in bed to decrease the likelihood of deep-vein blood clots.

MEDICATION
- Your doctor may prescribe:
  Pain relievers. Don't take prescription pain medication longer than 4 to 7 days. Use only as much as you need.
  Stool softeners to prevent constipation.
  Antibiotics to fight or prevent infection.
- You may use nonprescription drugs, such as acetaminophen, for minor pain. Avoid aspirin.

ACTIVITY
- To help recovery and aid your well-being, resume daily activities, including work, as soon as you are able.
- Avoid vigorous exercise for 6 weeks after surgery.
- Resume driving 2 weeks after returning home.
- Resume sexual relations when your doctor determines that healing is complete.

DIET
- Clear liquid diet until the gastrointestinal tract begins to function. Then eat a well-balanced diet to promote healing.
- Increase daily water intake to 8 glasses or more.
- Your doctor may prescribe a special diet after examining the kidney stone.

 CALL YOUR DOCTOR IF

- Pain, swelling, redness, drainage or bleeding increases in the surgical area.
- You develop signs of infection, including headache, muscle aches, dizziness or a general ill feeling and fever.
- You experience nausea, vomiting, constipation, or difficulty or pain with urination.
- New, unexplained symptoms develop. Drugs used in treatment may produce side effects.

KIDNEY STONE REMOVAL
(Ureterolithotomy)

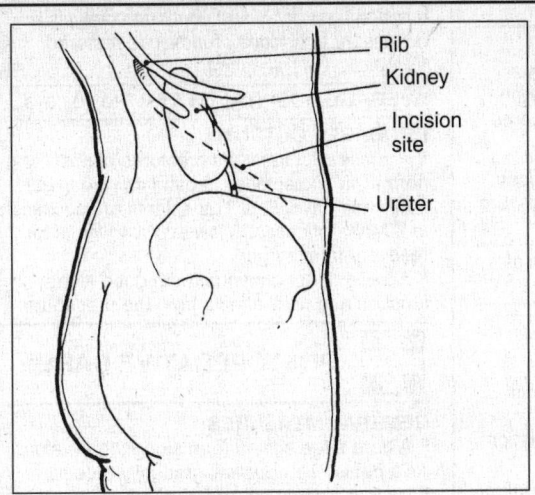

Incision site on the skin in the flank under the last rib.

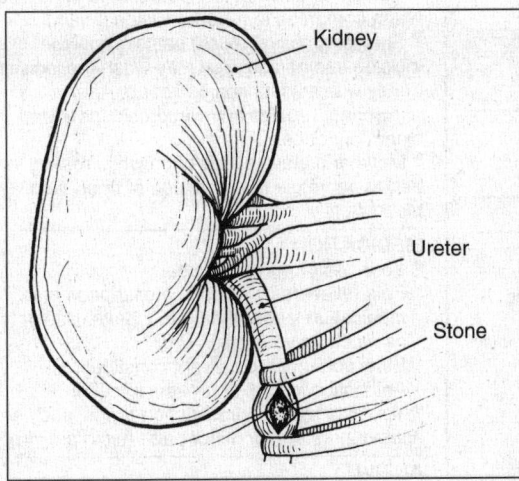

After a small incision has been made in the ureter, the kidney stone is pulled free and removed.

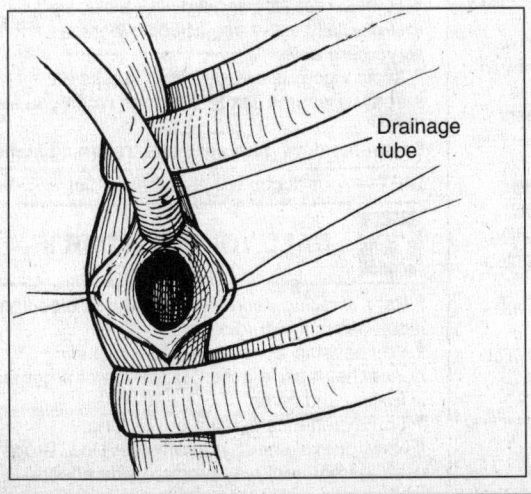

A tube is inserted for drainage. The tissues under the skin are closed with large absorbable sutures. The skin is closed with sutures or clips that usually can be removed about 1 week after surgery.

SURGERIES

KIDNEY TRANSPLANTATION

 GENERAL INFORMATION

DEFINITION—Replacement of a diseased kidney with a healthy kidney obtained from a healthy donor with compatible immunological characteristics. The donated kidney may come from a living relative or deceased donor.

BODY PARTS INVOLVED—Diseased kidney; healthy donor kidney; blood vessels to and from the kidney; ureters.

REASONS FOR SURGERY—Restoration of normal kidney function.

SURGICAL RISK INCREASES WITH
- Adults over 60.
- Obesity; poor nutrition.
- Recent or chronic illness; diabetes mellitus.
- Alcoholism; smoking.
- Use of some prescription and nonprescription drugs. Inform your doctor of any drugs, medications, or vitamin and herb supplements you are using or have used in the last month.

 WHAT TO EXPECT

WHO OPERATES—General surgeon or urologist with transplant experience and training.

WHERE PERFORMED—Hospital.

DIAGNOSTIC TESTS
- Before surgery: Blood and urine studies; x-rays of kidneys; ECG; CT scan; ultrasound.
- After surgery: Blood studies.

ANESTHESIA—General anesthesia by injection and inhalation with an airway tube placed in the windpipe.

DESCRIPTION OF OPERATION
- The diseased kidney from the recipient may be removed several weeks in advance. During this time, dialysis (see Glossary) provides artificial kidney function.
- Often, the recipients kidneys are not removed; they are left in place and the donor kidney is placed in the lower right part of the abdomen.
- A kidney is removed from the donor, then chilled and preserved for up to 12 hours.
- An incision is made in the abdomen of the recipient. The abdominal cavity is examined. The new kidney is placed and sewn in position.
- The blood vessels and ureters are connected to the new kidney.
- The peritoneum and abdominal muscles are closed.
- The skin is closed with sutures or clips, which usually can be removed about 1 week after surgery.

POSSIBLE COMPLICATIONS
- Excessive bleeding.
- Surgical-wound infection.
- Ureter leak; blockage of ureter.
- Occasionally, the new kidney does not function right away and continued dialysis is necessary until kidney function is restored.
- Rejection of transplant.

AVERAGE HOSPITAL STAY—7 to 10 days.

PROBABLE OUTCOME
- A successful transplant restores almost normal life expectancy in patients who might otherwise have died. Transplants are successful in 70-80% of cases. Allow about 4 weeks for recovery from surgery.
- A living donor continues with good kidney function and no ill effects from the procedure.

 POSTOPERATIVE CARE

GENERAL MEASURES
- A hard ridge should form along the incision. As it heals, the ridge will gradually recede.
- Use an electric heating pad, a heat lamp or a warm compress to relieve incisional pain.
- Shower as usual. Avoid bathing until the incision has healed. You may wash the incision gently with mild, unscented soap. After showering, replace any wet dressings with clean, dry ones.
- Move and elevate legs often while resting in bed to decrease the likelihood of deep-vein blood clots.

MEDICATION
- Your doctor may prescribe:
  Pain relievers. Don't take prescription pain medication longer than 4 to 7 days. Use only as much as you need.
  Stool softeners to prevent constipation.
  Antibiotics to fight or prevent infection.
- You may use nonprescription drugs, such as acetaminophen, for minor pain. Avoid aspirin.

ACTIVITY
- To help recovery and aid your well-being, resume daily activities, including work, as soon as you are able.
- Avoid vigorous exercise for 6 weeks after surgery. Resume sexual relations when you feel able.
- Resume driving 2 weeks after returning home.

DIET—Your doctor will prescribe a diet.

 CALL YOUR DOCTOR IF

- Pain, swelling, redness, drainage or bleeding increases in the surgical area.
- You develop signs of infection, including headache, muscle aches, dizziness or a general ill feeling and fever.
- You experience nausea or vomiting.
- New, unexplained symptoms develop. Drugs used in treatment may produce side effects.

KIDNEY TRANSPLANTATION

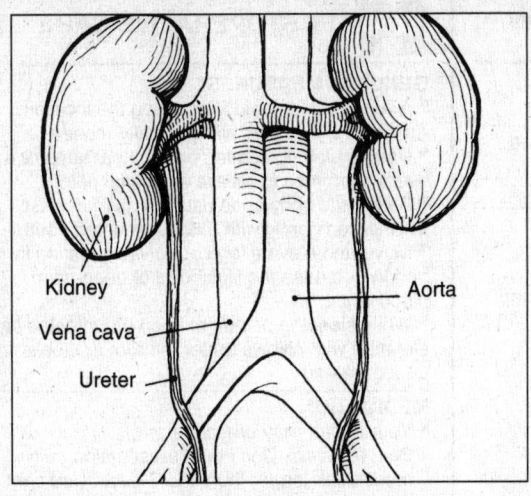

Shown are the kidneys and the adjoining body structures involved in the transplantation.

Kidney

Vena cava

Ureter

Aorta

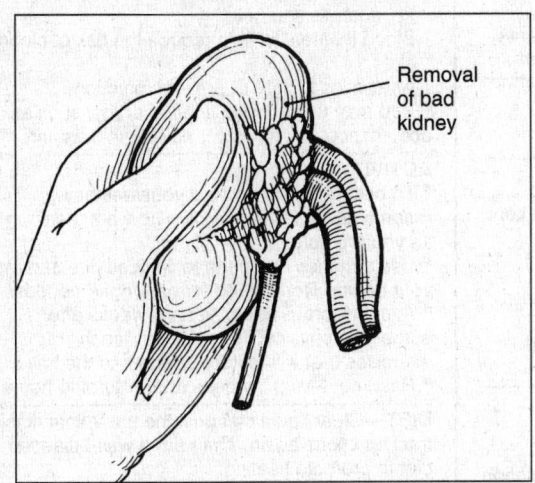

Removal of bad kidney

A kidney is removed from the donor, chilled and preserved for up to 12 hours.

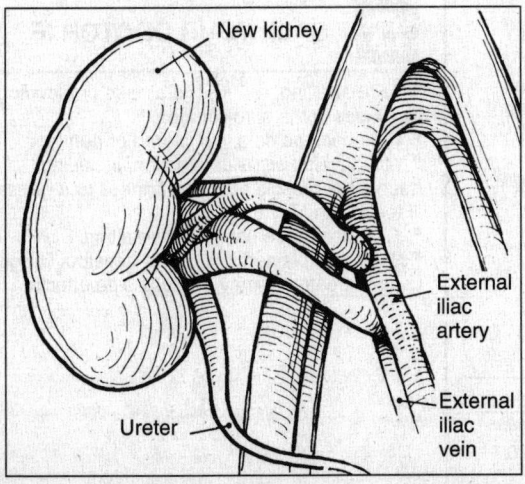

New kidney

New kidney is placed and sewn into position. The blood vessels and ureters are connected to the new kidney.
- The abdominal muscles and skin are closed in layers (not illustrated).

External iliac artery

External iliac vein

Ureter

KNEECAP REMOVAL (Patellectomy)

 GENERAL INFORMATION

DEFINITION—Removal of the kneecap (patella).

BODY PARTS INVOLVED—Kneecap; knee joint; muscles and ligaments attached to kneecap.

REASONS FOR SURGERY
- Fracture of the kneecap.
- Recurrent dislocations of the kneecap.
- Painful degenerative arthritis in the kneecap.

SURGICAL RISK INCREASES WITH
- Obesity.
- Smoking.
- Poor nutrition.
- Recent or chronic illness.
- Diabetes mellitus.
- Use of some prescription and nonprescription drugs. Inform your doctor of any drugs, medications, or vitamin and herb supplements you are using or have used in the last month.

 WHAT TO EXPECT

WHO OPERATES—Orthopedist.

WHERE PERFORMED—Hospital or outpatient surgical facility.

DIAGNOSTIC TESTS
- Before surgery: Blood and urine studies; x-rays of both knees.
- After surgery: Blood studies; x-rays of the affected knee.

ANESTHESIA
- Local anesthesia by injection.
- Spinal anesthesia by injection.
- General anesthesia by injection and inhalation with an airway tube placed in the windpipe.

DESCRIPTION OF OPERATION
- An incision is made around the kneecap.
- The muscles and tendons attached to the kneecap are cut, and the kneecap is removed.
- The muscles are sewn back together with strong suture material.
- The skin is closed with sutures or clips, which usually can be removed about 1 week after surgery.

POSSIBLE COMPLICATIONS
- Excessive bleeding.
- Surgical-wound infection.
- Blood clots which can break loose and traveling to the lung.

AVERAGE HOSPITAL STAY—3 to 6 days.

PROBABLE OUTCOME—Expect complete healing without complications. Allow about 6 weeks for recovery from surgery.

 POSTOPERATIVE CARE

GENERAL MEASURES
- A hard ridge should form along the incision. As it heals, the ridge will gradually recede.
- Use an electric heating pad, a heat lamp or a warm compress to relieve incisional pain.
- Bathe and shower as usual. You may wash the incision gently with mild, unscented soap.
- Move and elevate legs often while resting in bed to decrease the likelihood of deep-vein blood clots.
- While sleeping or sitting, keep the affected leg elevated with pillows under the foot or blocks under the bed.

MEDICATION
- Your doctor may prescribe:
  Pain relievers. Don't take prescription pain medication longer than 4 to 7 days. Use only as much as you need.
  Blood thinners to help reduce the risk of blood clots.
  Antibiotics to fight or prevent infection.
- You may use nonprescription drugs, such as acetaminophen, for minor pain. Avoid aspirin.

ACTIVITY
- To help recovery and aid your well-being, resume daily activities, including work, as soon as you are able.
- Use crutches or a cane to walk as directed by your doctor. Don't stand for prolonged periods.
- Avoid vigorous exercise for 6 weeks after surgery. A physical therapist can teach you exercises that will restore strength to the knee.
- Resume driving 3 weeks after returning home.

DIET—Clear liquid diet until the gastrointestinal tract functions again. Then eat a well-balanced diet to promote healing.

 CALL YOUR DOCTOR IF

- Pain, swelling, redness, drainage or bleeding increases in the surgical area.
- Toes become cold, discolored or numb.
- You develop signs of infection, including headache, muscle aches, dizziness or a general ill feeling and fever.
- You experience nausea or vomiting.
- New, unexplained symptoms develop. Drugs used in treatment may produce side effects.

KNEECAP REMOVAL
(Patellectomy)

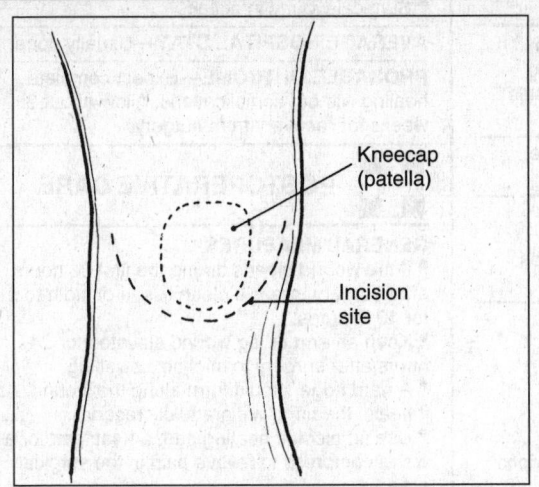

The kneecap and the proposed incision site for kneecap removal.

Kneecap (patella)

Incision site

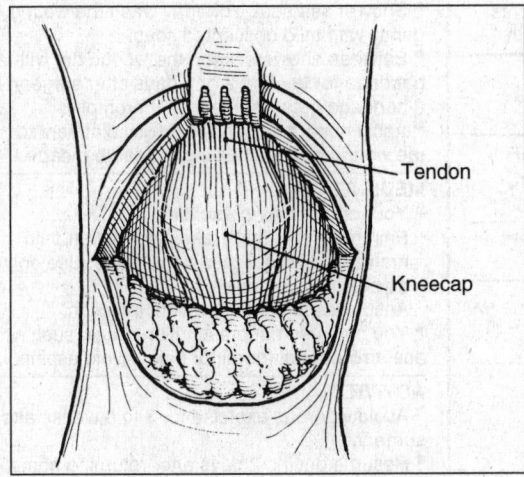

Muscles and tendons attached to the kneecap are cut and the kneecap is removed.

Tendon

Kneecap

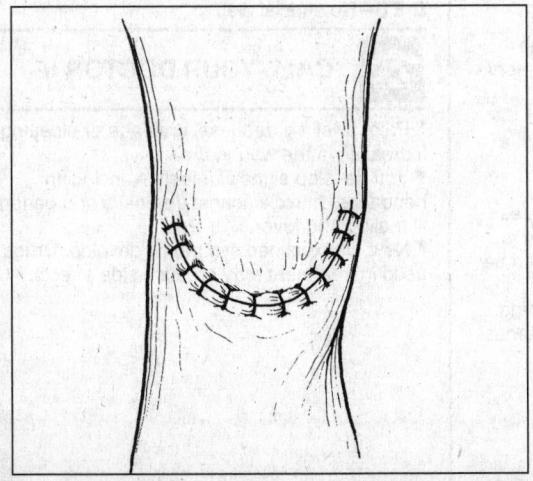

The muscles are sewn back together with strong suture material and the skin is closed with sutures or clips that usually can be removed about 1 week after surgery.

LACERATION REPAIR

GENERAL INFORMATION

DEFINITION—Repair of lacerations (open wounds in the skin extending to underlying tissue and sometimes muscle, blood vessels and nerves).

BODY PARTS INVOLVED—Skin; muscle; connective tissue.

REASONS FOR SURGERY
- Prevention of bleeding and infection.
- Examination to identify underlying injuries.
- Closure of the skin to hasten healing.

SURGICAL RISK INCREASES WITH
- Obesity.
- Smoking.
- Poor nutrition.
- Recent or chronic illness.
- Diabetes mellitus.
- Use of some prescription and nonprescription drugs. Inform your doctor of any drugs, medications, or vitamin and herb supplements you are using or have used in the last month.

WHAT TO EXPECT

WHO OPERATES—Family doctor, general surgeon, plastic and reconstructive surgeon, orthopedist or hand surgeon.

WHERE PERFORMED—Hospital, outpatient surgical facility or emergency room.

DIAGNOSTIC TESTS
- Before surgery: Blood and urine studies.
- After surgery: Blood studies.

ANESTHESIA
- Local anesthesia by injection.
- General anesthesia by a combination of injection and inhalation with an airway tube placed in the windpipe.

DESCRIPTION OF OPERATION
- The wound is cleansed and irrigated. The wound is inspected for possible tendon or nerve injury.
- The skin edges are examined. Shredded tissue and debris are removed. Sometimes, a ragged edge is trimmed for better cosmetic results.
- The underlying tissue is closed with sutures that will be absorbed by the body. The skin is closed with small sutures, which usually can be removed about 1 week after surgery.
- A bandage may be used to control bleeding.
- You may need an injection to prevent tetanus. Ask your doctor.

POSSIBLE COMPLICATIONS
- Excessive bleeding.
- Surgical-wound infection.

AVERAGE HOSPITAL STAY—Usually none.

PROBABLE OUTCOME—Expect complete healing without complications. Allow about 3 weeks for recovery from surgery.

POSTOPERATIVE CARE

GENERAL MEASURES
- If the wound bleeds during the first 24 hours after surgery, press a clean tissue or cloth to it for 10 minutes.
- Keep an arm or leg wound elevated for 24 hours after surgery to minimize swelling.
- A hard ridge should form along the wound. As it heals, the ridge will gradually recede.
- Use an electric heating pad, a heat lamp or a warm compress to relieve pain in the surgical area.
- Shower as usual. You may wash the wound gently with mild unscented soap.
- Between showers, keep the wound dry with a bandage for the first 2 or 3 days after surgery. If a bandage gets wet, change it promptly.
- Apply nonprescription antibiotic ointment to the wound before applying a clean bandage.

MEDICATION
- Your doctor may prescribe:
  Pain relievers. Don't take prescription pain medication longer than 4 to 7 days. Use only as much as you need.
  Antibiotics to fight or prevent infection.
- You may use nonprescription drugs, such as acetaminophen, for minor pain. Avoid aspirin.

ACTIVITY
- Avoid vigorous exercise for 3 to 6 weeks after surgery.
- Resume driving 2 days after returning home.

DIET—No special diet.

CALL YOUR DOCTOR IF

- Pain, swelling, redness, drainage or bleeding increases in the wound area.
- You develop signs of infection, including headache, muscle aches, dizziness or a general ill feeling and fever.
- New, unexplained symptoms develop. Drugs used in treatment may produce side effects.

LACERATION REPAIR

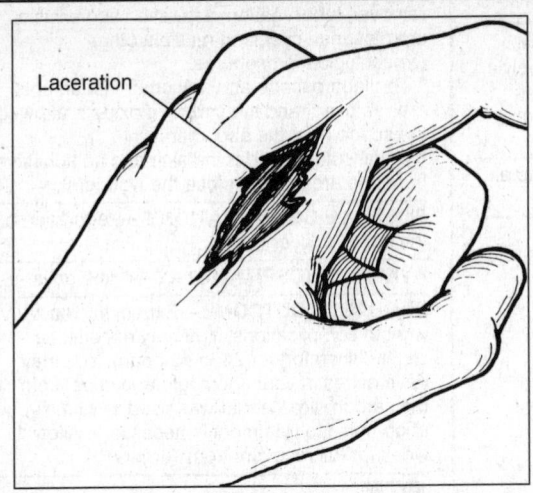

Laceration

A typical laceration on the side of the hand and finger.

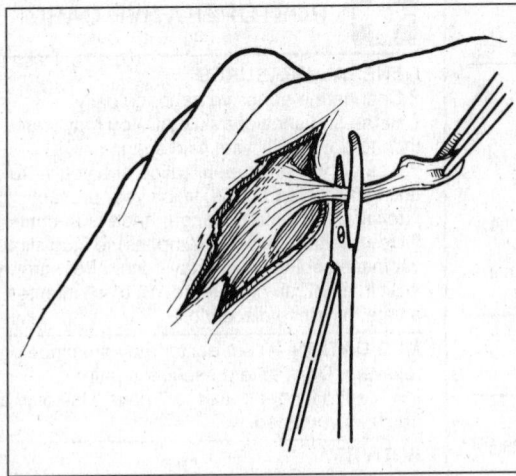

Shredded tissue and debris are removed. Sometimes a ragged edge of skin is trimmed for better cosmetic results.

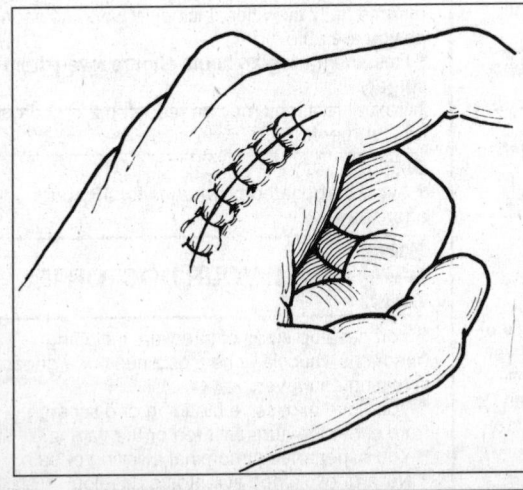

The underlying tissue is closed with sutures that will be absorbed by the body. Skin is closed with small sutures that usually can be removed about 1 week after surgery.

LAPAROSCOPY

GENERAL INFORMATION

DEFINITION—Procedure that allows visual examination and some treatments of the pelvic and abdominal organs. The procedure is performed with a laparoscope, a fiber-optic instrument.

BODY PARTS INVOLVED—Abdomen and all its contents.

REASONS FOR SURGERY
- Evaluation and treatment of infertility in women.
- Evaluation of known or suspected endometriosis.
- Complications from pelvic disease.
- Masses or cysts in the pelvis.
- Undiagnosed pelvic or abdominal pain.
- Fibroid tumors of the uterus.
- Hysterectomy; voluntary sterilization.
- Diagnosis and treatment of an ectopic pregnancy (see Glossary).
- Diagnosis and treatment for a variety of abdominal disorders.

SURGICAL RISK INCREASES WITH
- Obesity; smoking; heart or lung disease.
- Advanced pregnancy.
- Previous abdominal surgery for intra-abdominal infections (such as ruptured appendicitis); previous bowel surgery.
- Use of some prescription and nonprescription drugs. Inform your doctor of any drugs, medications, or vitamin and herb supplements you are using or have used in the last month.

WHAT TO EXPECT

WHO OPERATES—General surgeon, obstetrician-gynecologist, gastroenterologist, or specially trained family doctors.

WHERE PERFORMED—Outpatient surgical facility or hospital.

DIAGNOSTIC TESTS—Before surgery: Blood studies.

ANESTHESIA
- General anesthesia by injection and inhalation with an airway tube placed in the windpipe.
- Local anesthesia (sometimes).

DESCRIPTION OF OPERATION
- A small incision is made in or below the patient's navel. A needle is inserted to inflate the abdomen with carbon dioxide.
- The operating table is tilted to allow the bowel and carbon dioxide to float up toward the chest. The laparoscope is then inserted through the incision and is used to examine the abdomen visually. Occasionally, other small incisions are made in order to insert other surgical instruments.

- The laparoscope is can also be used to used to perform surgeries, including gallbladder removal, tubal ligation, aspiration and excision of an ovarian cyst, and multiple other gynecological procedures.
- The laparoscope and any other instruments are removed, and the carbon dioxide is allowed to escape from the abdomen.
- Small sutures under the skin and an adhesive bandage are used to close the wound(s).

POSSIBLE COMPLICATIONS—Perforation of the bowel or liver (rare).

AVERAGE HOSPITAL STAY—0 to 2 days.

PROBABLE OUTCOME—Expect full recovery without complications. You may experience slight discomfort for 24 to 48 hours. You may have aches in your shoulders and chest from the carbon dioxide that was used to inflate your abdomen. No treatment is necessary. Allow 1 week for full recovery from surgery.

POSTOPERATIVE CARE

GENERAL MEASURES
- Change the adhesive bandage daily.
- Bathe and shower as usual. You may wash the incision gently with mild soap.
- If surgery was for sterilization and you were taking birth-control pills, finish your present package; then you no longer need birth-control.
- Use sanitary pad (not tampons) to stop slight vaginal bleeding which may occur after surgery.
- Sit in a hot tub of water for 10 to 15 minutes at a time to relieve discomfort.

MEDICATION—Your doctor may prescribe pain relievers. Don't take prescription pain medication longer than 4 to 7 days. Use only as much as you need.

ACTIVITY
- To help recovery and aid your well-being, resume daily activities, including work, as soon as you are able.
- Resume driving 24 hours after recovery from surgery.
- Sexual relations may be resumed 2 or 3 days after surgery.

DIET
- Avoid carbonated beverages for 48 hours after surgery.

CALL YOUR DOCTOR IF

- You develop signs of infection, including headache, muscle aches, dizziness or a general ill feeling and fever.
- You have excessive bleeding or discharge from either the surgical area or the vagina.
- You experience abdominal swelling or pain.
- New, unexplained symptoms develop.

LAPAROSCOPY

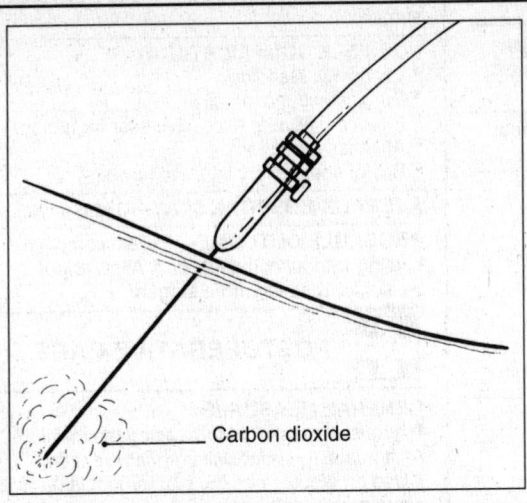

A hollow needle is inserted through the abdominal wall to inflate the abdomen with carbon dioxide.
- The operating table is tilted to allow the bowel and carbon dioxide to flow upward toward the chest.

Carbon dioxide

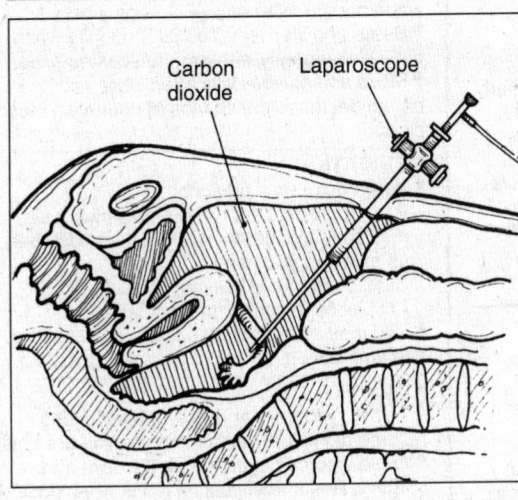

The laparoscope is inserted through the incision area to allow examination of the abdominal contents under direct vision.

Carbon dioxide

Laparoscope

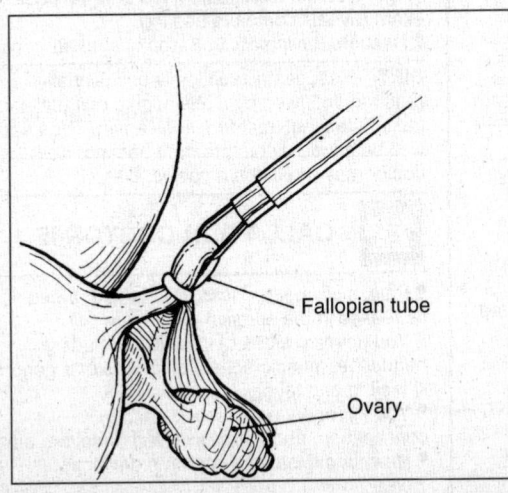

The laparoscope may be used to provide passage of other instruments for doctors to perform surgical procedures if necessary.
- After the laparoscope is removed, carbon dioxide is allowed to escape from the abdomen. The small amount remaining will be readily absorbed by the body.
- Sutures under the skin and adhesive bandages are used to close the wound (not illustrated).

Fallopian tube

Ovary

LAPAROTOMY

 GENERAL INFORMATION

DEFINITION—Exploratory abdominal surgery to identify, diagnose, or treat a variety of conditions.

BODY PARTS INVOLVED—Skin; abdominal muscles; peritoneum; abdominal organs.

REASONS FOR SURGERY
- Diagnostic examination of the abdominal organs.
- Collection of tissue samples for diagnosis.
- Closure of hernias in the abdominal wall.
- Repair or removal of abnormal tissue.
- Removal of diseased organs.
- Correction of unsightly or disfiguring abnormalities.

SURGICAL RISK INCREASES WITH
- Stress; obesity; smoking.
- Excess alcohol consumption.
- Poor nutrition.
- Recent acute respiratory infection.
- Chronic illness.
- Diabetes mellitus.
- History of prior abdominal surgery, particularly if it occurred at the site of the current surgery.
- Use of some prescription and nonprescription drugs. Inform your doctor of any drugs, medications, or vitamin and herb supplements you are using or have used in the last month.

 WHAT TO EXPECT

WHO OPERATES—General surgeon or obstetrician-gynecologist.

WHERE PERFORMED—Hospital.

DIAGNOSTIC TESTS
- Before surgery: Blood and urine studies; x-rays of kidneys and chest; ECG; ultrasound; MRI; CT scan; laparoscopy (see Glossary for all).
- After surgery: Blood studies.

ANESTHESIA—Spinal or general anesthesia by injection and inhalation with an airway tube placed in the windpipe.

DESCRIPTION OF OPERATION
- An incision is made in the abdomen. The abdominal muscles are separated, and the peritoneum (see Glossary) is opened.
- Blood vessels cut during the surgery are clamped and tied. Wound edges are retracted with a special instrument.
- Fluid in the abdominal cavity is often removed for laboratory examination.
- The abdominal organs are examined. Other surgeries may be performed at this time.
- Samples of suspicious tissue are gathered or diseased areas are treated.
- The peritoneum is closed, and the muscles are reconstructed with heavy sutures.

- The skin is closed with sutures or clips, which usually can be removed about 3 to 7 days after surgery.

POSSIBLE COMPLICATIONS
- Excessive bleeding.
- Surgical-wound infection.
- Incisional hernia; excessive scar formation.
- Abscess formation.
- Bowel obstruction; injury to bowel.

AVERAGE HOSPITAL STAY—3 to 5 days.

PROBABLE OUTCOME—Expect complete healing without complications. Allow about 4 weeks for recovery from surgery.

 POSTOPERATIVE CARE

GENERAL MEASURES
- A hard ridge should form along the incision. As it heals, the ridge will gradually recede.
- Use an electric heating pad, a heat lamp or a warm compress to relieve incisional pain.
- Bathe and shower as usual. You may wash the incision gently with mild, unscented soap.
- Move and elevate legs often while resting in bed to decrease the chance of deep-vein blood clots.

MEDICATION
- Your doctor may prescribe:
  Pain relievers. Don't take prescription pain medication longer than 4 to 7 days. Use only as much as you need.
  Stool softeners to prevent constipation.
  Antibiotics to fight or prevent infection.
- You may use nonprescription drugs, such as acetaminophen, for minor pain. Avoid aspirin.

ACTIVITY
- To help recovery and aid your well-being, resume daily activities as soon as you are able.
- Avoid vigorous exercise for 6 weeks after surgery. Resume sexual relations when doctor's exam reveals complete healing.
- Resume driving about 3 weeks after surgery.

DIET—Nasogastric suction is occasionally required, followed by a clear liquid diet until the gastrointestinal tract functions again. Then eat a well-balanced diet to promote healing. Your doctor may prescribe a special diet.

 CALL YOUR DOCTOR IF

- Pain, swelling, redness, drainage or bleeding increases in the surgical area.
- You develop signs of infection, including headache, muscle aches, dizziness or a general ill feeling and fever.
- You experience nausea, vomiting, constipation, abdominal swelling or severe pain.
- New, unexplained symptoms develop.

LAPAROTOMY

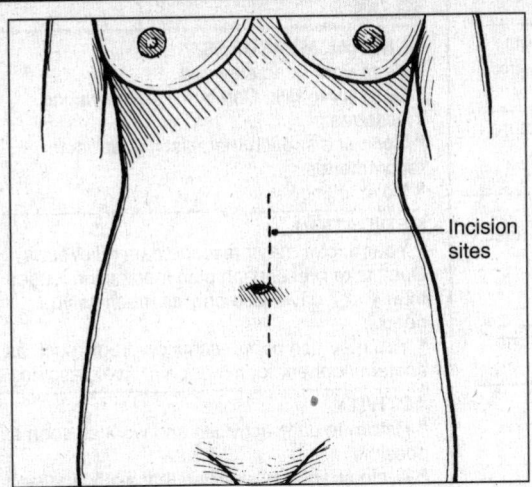

Incision sites

The incision site frequently used for a laparotomy (any opening made into the abdomen).

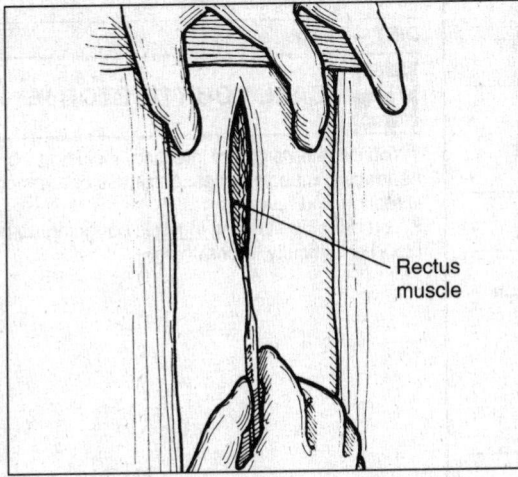

Rectus muscle

Wound edges are retracted with special instruments.
- Fluid in the abdominal cavity is often removed for laboratory examination.
- The abdominal organs are examined.
- Samples of suspicious tissue are gathered or diseased areas are treated (not illustrated).

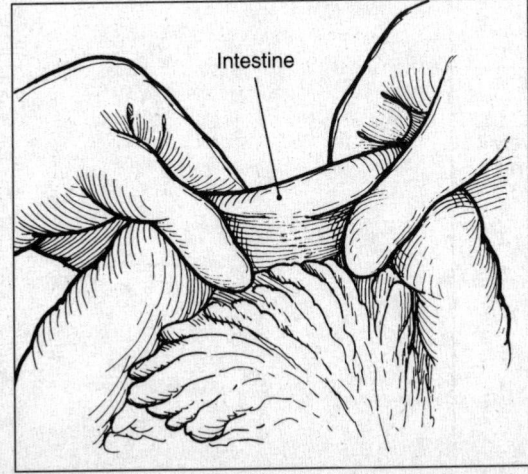

Intestine

After inspection of all abdominal contents (the intestine is examined here between the surgeon's fingers), the abdominal contents are replaced into normal position. The muscles are closed, and the skin is closed with sutures that can be removed after 3 to 7 days.

LARYNGOSCOPY

GENERAL INFORMATION

DEFINITION—Procedure that allows visual examination and some treatment of the larynx (voice box).

BODY PARTS INVOLVED—Larynx, structure at the top of the windpipe that controls the voice.

REASONS FOR SURGERY
- To remove laryngeal polyps, singer's nodules and other benign growths.
- To remove enough tissue to biopsy.
- To assess vocal cord mobility.

SURGICAL RISK INCREASES WITH—None expected.

WHAT TO EXPECT

WHO OPERATES—Ear, nose and throat specialist (otolaryngologist).

WHERE PERFORMED—Hospital, outpatient surgical facility or doctor's office.

DIAGNOSTIC TESTS
- Before surgery: None.
- After surgery: Microscopic examination of removed tissue.

ANESTHESIA—Local anesthesia spray or general anesthesia.

DESCRIPTION OF OPERATION
- A fiberoptic laryngoscope is passed through the mouth and pharynx to extend to the larynx (voice-box).
- The larynx is examined visually by the operator.
- Specimens may be removed by snare to study for nodules, polyps or malignant changes.

POSSIBLE COMPLICATIONS
- Excessive bleeding.
- Swelling of tissues in the neck.
- Laryngospasm (closing of larynx).

AVERAGE HOSPITAL STAY—Usually no more than 1 day.

PROBABLE OUTCOME—Complete recovery if growth is benign. If growth is malignant, larynx removal may be necessary (see in Surgery section).

POSTOPERATIVE CARE

GENERAL MEASURES
- Keep your head elevated.
- Don't try to talk. Communicate by writing messages.
- Consult a speech therapist if your doctor recommends.
- No smoking.

MEDICATION
- Your doctor may prescribe pain relievers. Don't take prescription pain medication longer than 4 to 7 days. Use only as much as you need.
- You may use nonprescription drugs, such as acetaminophen, for minor pain. Avoid aspirin.

ACTIVITY
- Return to daily activities and work as soon as possible.
- Avoid strenuous exercise that would cause heavy breathing for several days.

DIET—No special diet.

CALL YOUR DOCTOR IF

- You develop signs of infection, including headache, muscle aches, dizziness or a general ill feeling and fever.
- You develop swelling in neck, coughing up of blood or difficulty in breathing.

LARYNGOSCOPY

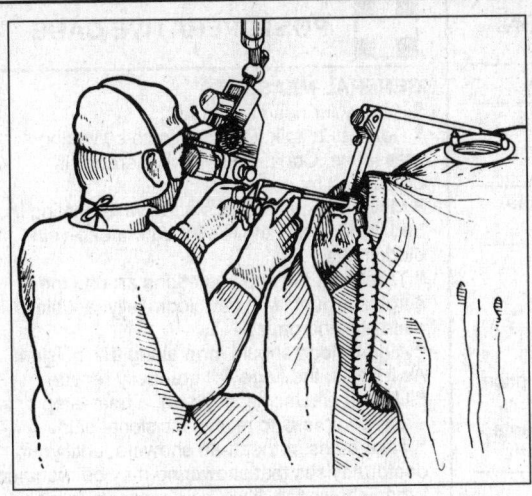

An illustration of the patient lying on his back. Instrumentation is in place and a fiber optic laryngoscope is passed through the mouth and pharynx to extend to the larynx.

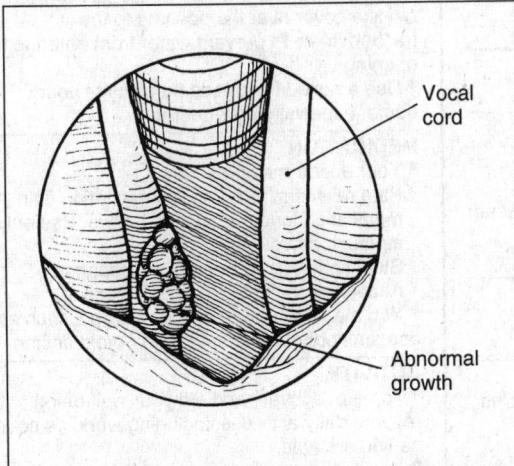

An illustration of an abnormal growth on the patient's vocal cord.

Vocal cord

Abnormal growth

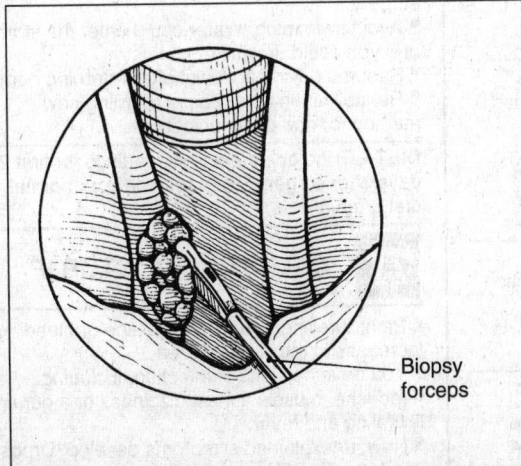

Tissue specimens are removed with biopsy forceps to study for nodules, polyps or malignant changes.

Biopsy forceps

LARYNX REMOVAL
(Laryngectomy)

 GENERAL INFORMATION

DEFINITION—Removal of the larynx.

BODY PARTS INVOLVED—Larynx (voice box); organ at the top of the windpipe that controls the voice.

REASONS FOR SURGERY—Cancer of the larynx.

SURGICAL RISK INCREASES WITH
- Adults over 60.
- Obesity; smoking; stress; poor nutrition.
- Recent or chronic illness; alcoholism.
- Diabetes mellitus.
- Use of some prescription and nonprescription drugs. Inform your doctor of any drugs, medications, or vitamin and herb supplements you are using or have used in the last month.

 WHAT TO EXPECT

WHO OPERATES—Ear, nose and throat specialist (otolaryngologist).

WHERE PERFORMED—Hospital.

DIAGNOSTIC TESTS
- Before surgery: Blood and urine studies; laryngoscopy (see in Surgery section); CT scan; MRI; ECG (see Glossary for all).
- After surgery: Blood studies.

ANESTHESIA—General anesthesia by injection and inhalation with an airway tube placed in the windpipe.

DESCRIPTION OF OPERATION
- An incision is made in the neck. The muscles that attach the larynx to the windpipe are divided.
- The blood vessels and nerves that supply the larynx are located and cut.
- The larynx is cut free and removed with surrounding lymph node tissue (e.g., neck dissection) if indicated.
- A tracheostomy tube (see Glossary) is fitted and positioned.
- The muscles and skin edges are closed around the tube with sutures or clips, which usually can be removed about 1 week after surgery.

POSSIBLE COMPLICATIONS
- Excessive bleeding; surgical-wound infection.
- Inadvertent injury to the esophagus or trachea.
- Difficulty swallowing (usually temporary).

AVERAGE HOSPITAL STAY—5 to 7 days.

PROBABLE OUTCOME—Expect complete healing of the surgical wound. Allow about 4 weeks for recovery from surgery.

 POSTOPERATIVE CARE

GENERAL MEASURES
- Keep your head elevated.
- Don't try to talk. Communicate by writing messages. Consult a speech therapist if prescribed by doctor.
- Move and elevate legs often while resting in bed to decrease the likelihood of deep-vein blood clots.
- Treat crusting and secretions around the surgical wound with petroleum jelly, antibiotic ointment and gauze.
- A hard ridge should form along the incision. As it heals, the ridge will gradually recede.
- Use an electric heating pad, a heat lamp or a warm compress to relieve incisional pain.
- Take baths, rather than showers, until your doctor advises that showering may be resumed. When showering, it will be necessary to wear a bib-like cover over the opening to the tracheostomy to prevent water from entering the opening.
- Use a humidifier to add humidity to your home, especially your bedroom.

MEDICATION
- Your doctor may prescribe:
  Pain relievers. Don't take prescription pain medication longer than 4 to 7 days. Use only as much as you need.
  Stool softeners to prevent constipation.
  Antibiotics to fight or prevent infection.
- You may use nonprescription drugs, such as acetaminophen, for minor pain. Avoid aspirin.

ACTIVITY
- To help recovery and aid your well-being, resume daily activities, including work, as soon as you are able.
- Avoid vigorous exercise for 6 weeks after surgery.
- Avoid swimming. Water could enter the stoma and you could drown.
- Resume driving 2 weeks after returning home.
- Rehabilitation may require learning new method for oral communication.

DIET—Tube or intravenous feedings for first 2 days after surgery. Then resume your normal diet gradually.

 CALL YOUR DOCTOR IF

- Pain, swelling, redness, drainage or bleeding increases in the surgical area.
- You develop signs of infection, including headache, muscle aches, dizziness or a general ill feeling and fever.
- New, unexplained symptoms develop. Drugs used in treatment may produce side effects.

LARYNX REMOVAL
(Laryngectomy)

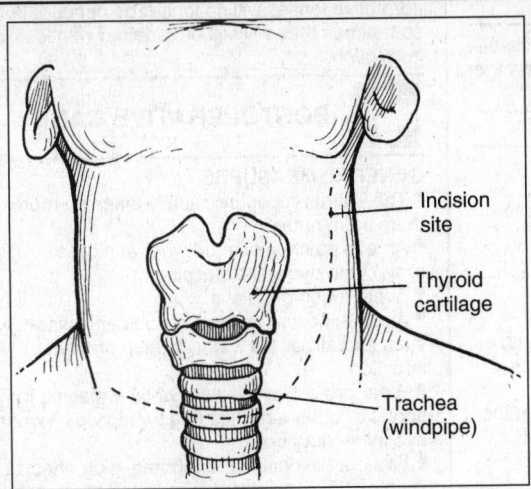

Structures in the neck. The larynx (voice box) is at the top of the windpipe.

Incision site

Thyroid cartilage

Trachea (windpipe)

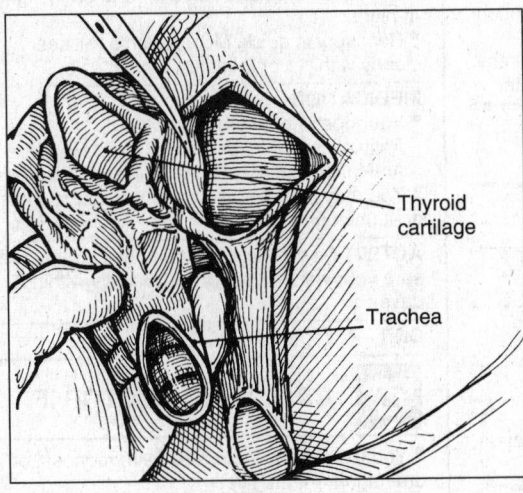

After an incision has been made in the neck, the muscles that attach the larynx to the windpipe are divided.
- The larynx has been cut free and removed

Thyroid cartilage

Trachea

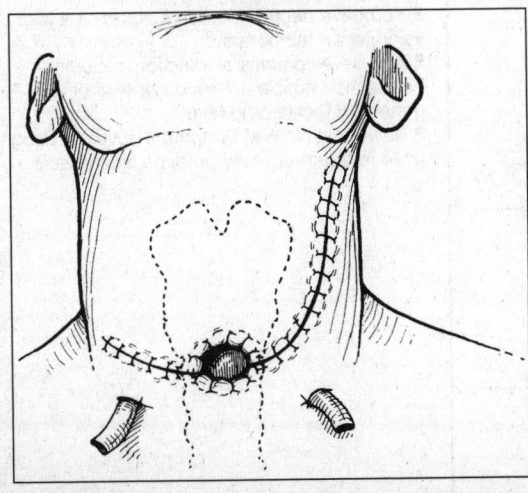

The trachea is sutured to the skin, allowing for a permanent tracheostomy. The muscle and skin edges are closed around the tube with sutures or clips that usually can be removed about 1 week after surgery.

LASER IN-SITU KERATOMILEUSIS (LASIK)

 ## GENERAL INFORMATION

DEFINITION—Removal of a thin layer of tissue from the center of the cornea in order to change the shape of the cornea and improve vision.

BODY PARTS INVOLVED—Cornea.

REASONS FOR SURGERY—To improve vision in patients with nearsightedness, farsightedness or astigmatism. The goal is to eliminate the need for corrective lenses (glasses or contacts).

SURGICAL RISK INCREASES WITH
- Vascular disease; autoimmune disease.
- Progressive myopia, hyperopia, or amblyopia (lazy eye).
- Women who are pregnant, nursing, or planning on becoming pregnant within 6 months.
- Active or recurrent eye disease, especially glaucoma.
- Diabetes mellitus.
- Use of some prescription and nonprescription drugs. Inform your doctor of any drugs, medications, or vitamin and herb supplements you are using or have used in the last month.

 ## WHAT TO EXPECT

WHO OPERATES—Specially trained ophthalmologist.

WHERE PERFORMED—Doctor's office or outpatient surgical facility.

DIAGNOSTIC TESTS—Eye examination to determine degree of correction required.

ANESTHESIA—Topical anesthesia.

DESCRIPTION OF OPERATION
- The surgery involves folding back a thin layer of the outer corneal tissue.
- A thin layer of internal corneal tissue is then removed with the excimer laser. This causes the center of the cornea to flatten (for nearsightedness) or steepen (for farsightedness) or become more rounded (for astigmatism).
- Following removal of the tissue, the flap is replaced. It will usually adhere back in place without the need for sutures.

POSSIBLE COMPLICATIONS
- Infection.
- Difference in power between the two eyes.
- Double vision; hazy vision.
- Increased or decreased sensitivity to light.
- Loss of vision (rare).
- Over or under correction.

AVERAGE HOSPITAL STAY—None.

PROBABLE OUTCOME—Expect complete healing without complications. Usually, corrective lenses will no longer be needed, but sometimes they will still be required with less correction.

 ## POSTOPERATIVE CARE

GENERAL MEASURES
- The entire procedure usually takes no more tham 15 minutes.
- An eye patch should be worn at night to protect the eye while sleeping.
- Avoid rubbing the eye.
- Avoid exposing the eye to nonsterile water, such as bath or tap water, to help prevent infection.
- Wear protective eyewear while engaging in sports or other activities (e.g., shop work) where eye injury may occur.
- You may experience temporary side effects such as dry eyes and halos around bright lights at night.
- Recovery is quick. Most patients will see clearly within 1 or 2 days.

MEDICATION
- Your doctor may prescribe:
  Antibiotics to fight or prevent infection.
  Anti-inflammatory and moisturizing eye drops.
- You may use nonprescription drugs, such as acetaminophen, for minor pain. Avoid aspirin.

ACTIVITY—Resume driving only after you are sure your vision is adequate (usually within 2 days).

DIET—No special diet.

 ## CALL YOUR DOCTOR IF

- You experience increased pain, redness, or drainage from the eye.
- You have decreased visual acuity or a loss of vsion, even temporarily.
- You develop signs of infection, including headache, muscle aches, dizziness, or a general ill feeling and fever.
- New, unexplained symptoms develop. Drugs used in treatment may produce side effects.

LASER IN-SITU KERATOMILEUSIS (LASIK)

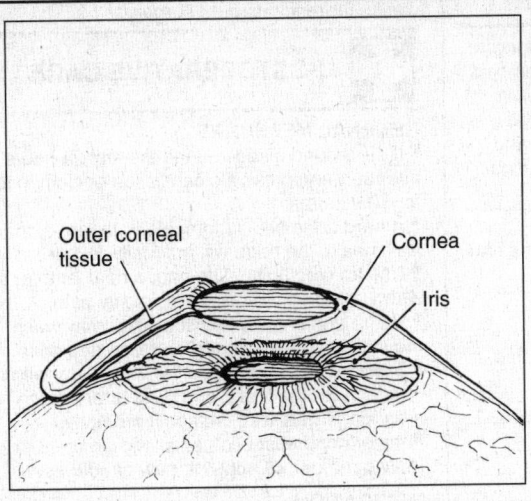

An illustration of the eye, showing a thin layer of outer corneal tissue which has been cut and folded back.

Outer corneal tissue

Cornea

Iris

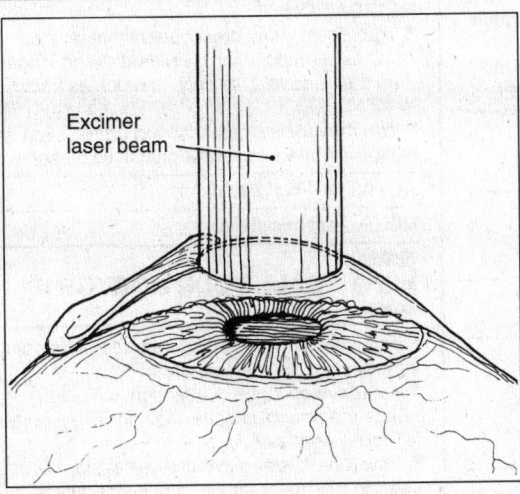

A thin layer of internal corneal tissue is then removed with an excimer laser.

- The laser beam can be used to change the shape of the cornea in a number of ways, depending on the type of refractive error which is affecting the patient's vision.

Excimer laser beam

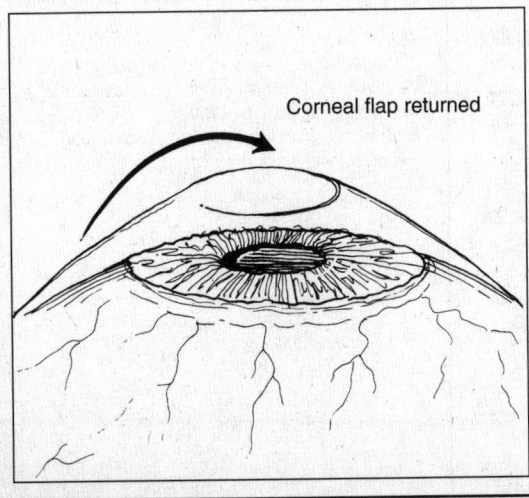

Following removal of the tissue, the flap is replaced. It will usually adhere back in place without the need for sutures.

Corneal flap returned

LIPOMA REMOVAL

GENERAL INFORMATION

DEFINITION—Removal of a lipoma (benign, fatty tumor). Lipomas vary in size. A lipoma can be pea-sized or larger than a grapefruit. Lipomas can be found anywhere on the body, but are most commonly found in the front and back of the chest and abdomen, or in the legs and arms.

BODY PARTS INVOLVED—Skin and underlying tissue, usually on the back, arms and legs.

REASONS FOR SURGERY
• Improved appearance.
• If lipoma is bothersome, e.g., at the belt-line.
• Diagnosis of lipoma is not certain.
• Prevention of cancer (rare).

SURGICAL RISK INCREASES WITH
• Recent or chronic illness.
• Diabetes mellitus.
• Use of some prescription and nonprescription drugs. Inform your doctor of any drugs, medications, or vitamin and herb supplements you are using or have used in the last month.

WHAT TO EXPECT

WHO OPERATES—Family doctor, general surgeon, dermatologist or plastic and reconstructive surgeon.

WHERE PERFORMED—Doctor's office or outpatient surgical facility.

DIAGNOSTIC TESTS
• Before surgery: Blood and urine studies; ultrasound; CT scan (see Glossary for both).
• After surgery: Laboratory examination of removed tissue.

ANESTHESIA
• Local anesthesia by injection.
• General anesthesia by injection and inhalation with an airway tube placed in the windpipe (for larger lipomas).

DESCRIPTION OF OPERATION
• An incision is made over the lipoma.
• The lipoma is cut free from surrounding connective tissue and removed.
• The skin is closed with sutures or clips, which usually can be removed about 1 week after surgery.
• Lipomas can also be removed by liposuction (see in Surgery section).

POSSIBLE COMPLICATIONS
• Excessive bleeding.
• Surgical-wound infection.

AVERAGE HOSPITAL STAY—None.

PROBABLE OUTCOME—Expect complete healing without complications. Allow about 3 weeks for recovery from surgery.

POSTOPERATIVE CARE

GENERAL MEASURES
• If the wound bleeds during the first 24 hours after surgery, press a clean tissue or cloth to it for 10 minutes.
• A hard ridge should form along the incision. As it heals, the ridge will gradually recede.
• Use an electric heating pad, a heat lamp or a warm compress to relieve incisional pain.
• Bathe and shower as usual. You may wash the incision gently with mild, unscented soap.
• Between showers, keep the wound dry with a bandage for the first 2 or 3 days after surgery. If a bandage gets wet, change it promptly.
• Apply nonprescription antibiotic ointment to the wound before applying new bandages.

MEDICATION
• Your doctor may prescribe pain relievers. Don't take prescription pain medication longer than 4 to 7 days. Use only as much as you need.
• You may use nonprescription drugs, such as acetaminophen, for minor pain. Avoid aspirin.

ACTIVITY—No restrictions.

DIET—No special diet.

CALL YOUR DOCTOR IF

• Pain, swelling, redness, drainage or bleeding increases in the surgical area.
• You develop signs of infection, including headache, muscle aches, dizziness or a general ill feeling and fever.
• New, unexplained symptoms develop. Drugs used in treatment may produce side effects.

LIPOMA REMOVAL

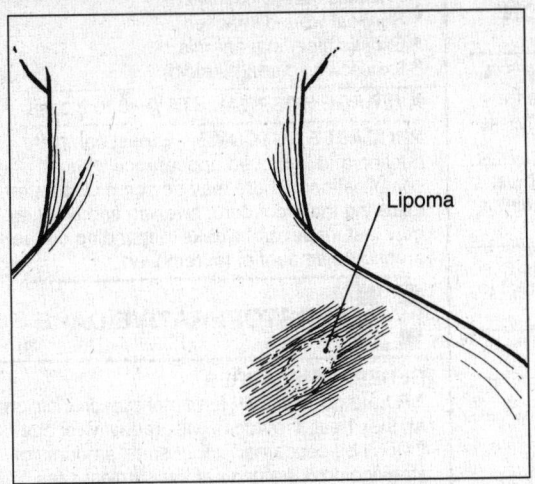

A typical lipoma situated just under the skin. Lipomas may be found in scattered locations over the entire body.

Lipoma

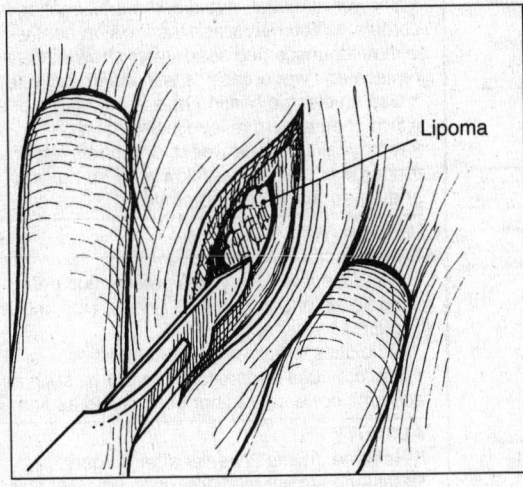

The lipoma is cut free from surrounding connective tissue and removed.

Lipoma

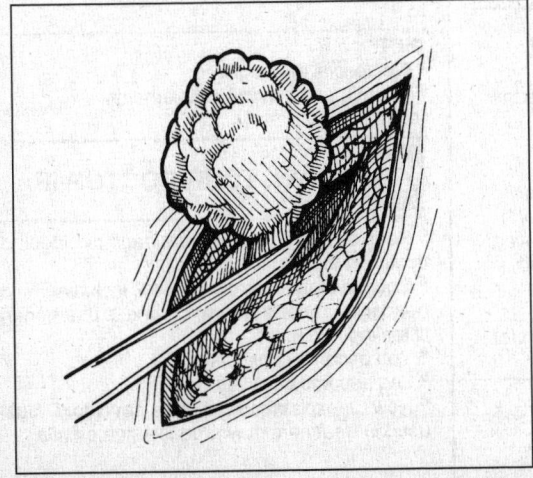

After the lipoma has been excised, the skin is closed with sutures or clips, which usually can be removed about 1 week after surgery (not illustrated).

LIPOSUCTION
(Suction Lipectomy)

GENERAL INFORMATION

DEFINITION—A surgical technique using suction equipment to permanently remove fat deposits, usually from the thighs, hips, buttocks, abdomen or chin.

BODY PARTS INVOLVED—Thighs and hips; buttocks; fat cells of the abdominal wall; chin or other small areas.

REASONS FOR SURGERY—Cosmetic improvement of fat deposits that are resistant to diet and/or exercise.

SURGICAL RISK INCREASES WITH
- Extreme obesity; smoking.
- Recent or chronic illness.
- Diabetes mellitus.
- Excess alcohol consumption.
- History of phlebitis.
- Use of some prescription and nonprescription drugs. Inform your doctor of any drugs, medications, or vitamin and herb supplements you are using or have used in the last month.

WHAT TO EXPECT

WHO OPERATES—Plastic surgeon.

WHERE PERFORMED—Outpatient surgical facility, hospital or doctor's office.

DIAGNOSTIC TESTS
- Before surgery: Blood and urine studies.
- After surgery: Blood and urine studies.

ANESTHESIA
- Local anesthesia and sedation for small areas.
- General anesthesia by injection and inhalation with an airway tube placed in the windpipe is usually used for larger areas of fat.

DESCRIPTION OF OPERATION
- The plastic surgeon marks areas to be operated on.
- Incisions (about 1/4 inch each) are made in suction areas.
- A suction tube, with one end attached to suction equipment, is repeatedly pushed through the incision into the excess fat and moved back and forth (20 to 30 times at each site) until the desired amount of fat is removed.
- Each incision is stapled or stitched closed, and a pressure dressing is placed over the wounds.
- Drains may be left in place under the skin for several days following surgery.

POSSIBLE COMPLICATIONS
- Nerve damage.
- Resuctioning in some areas may be necessary.
- Phlebitis (see Glossary).
- Surgical wound infection.
- Excess bleeding; anemia.
- Excessive scarring (keloid).

AVERAGE HOSPITAL STAY—0 to 2 days.

PROBABLE OUTCOME—Expect complete healing and improved appearance without complications. There may be some discomfort following the procedure; swelling and bruising may last for several weeks, depending on the areas and amount of fat removed.

POSTOPERATIVE CARE

GENERAL MEASURES
- A hard ridge should form along each incision. As they heal, the ridges will gradually recede.
- Don't be concerned about small amounts of straw-colored drainage at the surgical sites.
- Shower as usual. Avoid baths until healing is complete. You may wash the incision gently with mild, unscented soap. After showering, replace any wet dressings with clean, dry ones.
- Use an electric heating pad, a heat lamp or a warm compress to relieve incisional pain.
- It may take several weeks or months for tenderness to subside. Allow time for healing and for appearance to improve.

MEDICATION
- Your doctor may prescribe:
  Pain relievers. Don't take prescription pain medicine longer than 4 to 7 days. Use only as much as you need.
  Antibiotics to fight or prevent infection.
- You may use nonprescription drugs, such as acetaminophen, for minor pain. Avoid aspirin.

ACTIVITY
- Resume driving 2 weeks after surgery.
- Resume sexual relations when you feel able to.

DIET
- No special diet required.
- Vitamin and mineral supplements (sometimes).

CALL YOUR DOCTOR IF

- Pain, swelling, redness, drainage or bleeding occurs in the surgical area.
- You develop signs of infection, including headache, muscle aches, dizziness or a general ill feeling and fever.
- You become constipated.
- Leg becomes swollen or painful.
- New, unexplained symptoms develop. Drugs used in treatment may produce side effects.

LIPOSUCTION
(Suction Lipectomy)

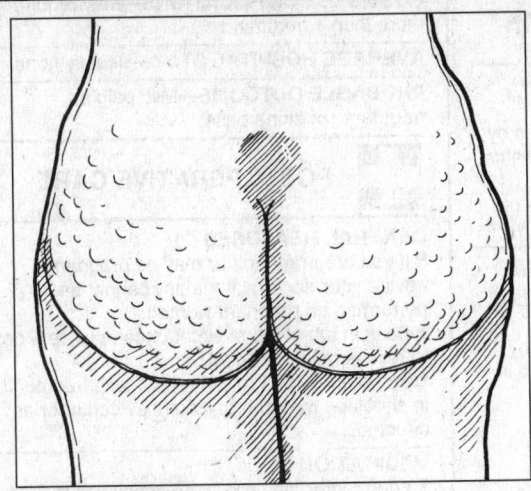

An illustration of fatty deposits under the skin in the buttocks area.

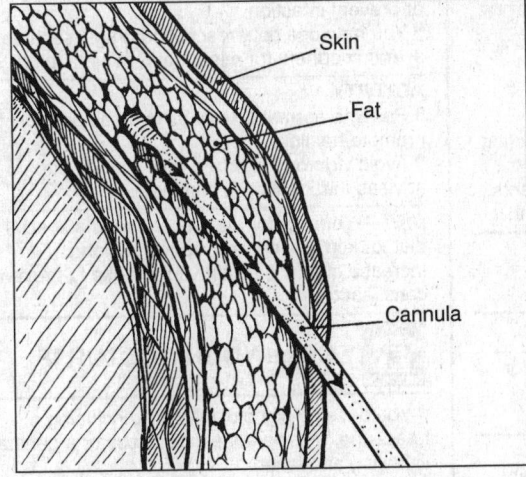

Skin

Fat

Cannula

Approximate 1 inch incisions are made in suction areas and a suction tube with one end attached to suction equipment is pushed through the incision into the excess fat and moved back and forth repeatedly.

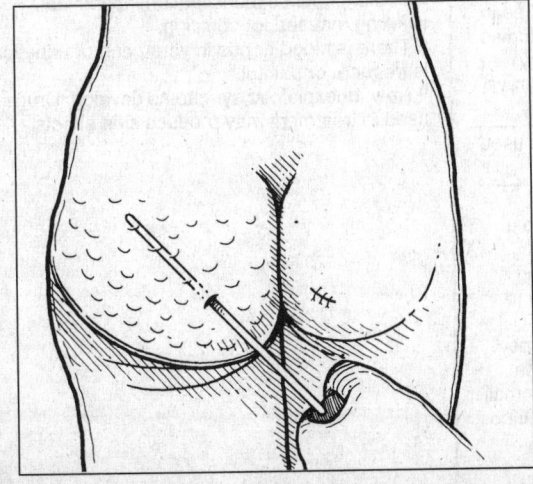

Liposuction complete on the patient's right side and progressing to the left side.

LITHOTRIPSY
(Shock Wave Treatment for Kidney Stones)

 GENERAL INFORMATION

DEFINITION—A technique to crush kidney stones inside the body without a surgical incision. These stones are too large to pass by normal elimination. Seventy percent of patients pass stones spontaneously; 30% require urological treatment. This technique is one of the available treatments.

BODY PARTS INVOLVED—Kidney; ureter; bladder.

REASONS FOR SURGERY
- Kidney stones that are too large to pass by normal elimination. They are usually lodged in the kidney or upper third of the ureter.
- Relieve blocked urine flow.
- Decrease chance of infection.
- Relieve pain from kidney stone.
- Decrease chance of damage to kidney.

SURGICAL RISK INCREASES WITH
- Poor heart or respiratory function.
- Presence of a cardiac pacemaker.
- Pregnancy.
- Bleeding disorders.
- Use of some prescription and nonprescription drugs. Inform your doctor of any drugs, medications, or vitamin and herb supplements you are using or have used in the last month.

 WHAT TO EXPECT

WHO OPERATES—Urologist.

WHERE PERFORMED—A special center for lithotripsy. Usually in an outpatient surgical facility of a regional referral center.

DIAGNOSTIC TESTS
- Before surgery: Cystoscopy (see in Surgery section), x-rays of kidneys; ultrasound; CT scan (see Glossary for both); blood and urine studies.
- During surgery: Ultrasound (see Glossary).
- After surgery: Blood and urine studies, x-rays, ultrasound (see Glossary).

ANESTHESIA—Usually none. Sedation is used in most cases.

DESCRIPTION OF OPERATION
- For one method, the patient rests in a tub of warm water after being sedated.
- Another method avoids the water by using a membrane coupling device applied directly to the skin overlying the kidney.
- The lithotripsy unit sends out high frequency sound waves directed toward the stone. The shock waves pulverize the stones and the small particles then pass spontaneously in your urine over 2-5 days.

POSSIBLE COMPLICATIONS—May require more than 1 treatment.

AVERAGE HOSPITAL STAY—Usually none.

PROBABLE OUTCOME—Mild pain as fragments of stone pass.

 POSTOPERATIVE CARE

GENERAL MEASURES
- If you are pregnant, or may be pregnant, advise your doctor. Lithotripsy cannot be performed on pregnant women.
- Soak in tub of warm water once or twice a day to relieve mild back pain.
- Strain urine for 1 to 2 weeks. Place fragments in envelope to return to lithotripsy center or as directed.

MEDICATION
- Your doctor may prescribe antibiotics to fight or prevent infection.
- You may use nonprescription drugs, such as acetaminophen, for minor pain. Avoid aspirin.

ACTIVITY
- Resume normal activity as soon as possible to promote healing.
- Avoid vigorous exercise until your doctor advises that healing is complete.

DIET—Your doctor may recommend a special diet to help prevent recurrence of stones. Increase dietary fiber and fluid intake to prevent constipation.

 CALL YOUR DOCTOR IF

- You develop signs of infection, including headache, muscle aches, dizziness or a general ill feeling and fever.
- You experience, constipation, abdominal swelling, nausea, or vomiting.
- There is blood or pus in your urine or urination is frequent or painful.
- New, unexplained symptoms develop. Drugs used in treatment may produce side effects.

LITHOTRIPSY
(Shock Wave Treatment for Kidney Stones)

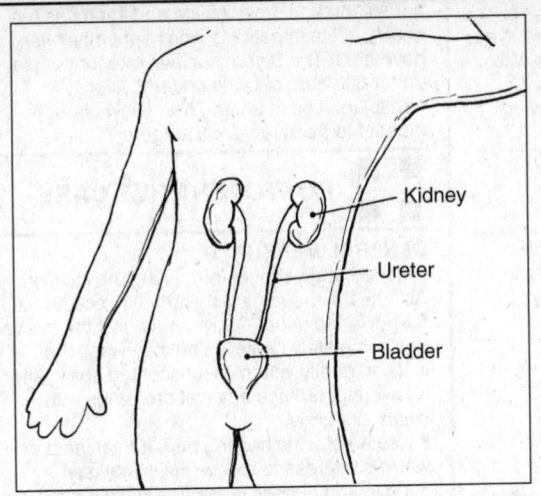

An illustration of the urinary tract.

Kidney

Ureter

Bladder

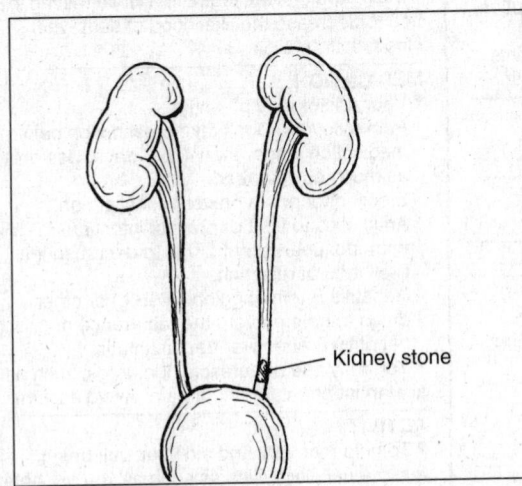

A stone is shown in the ureter leading from the left kidney.

Kidney stone

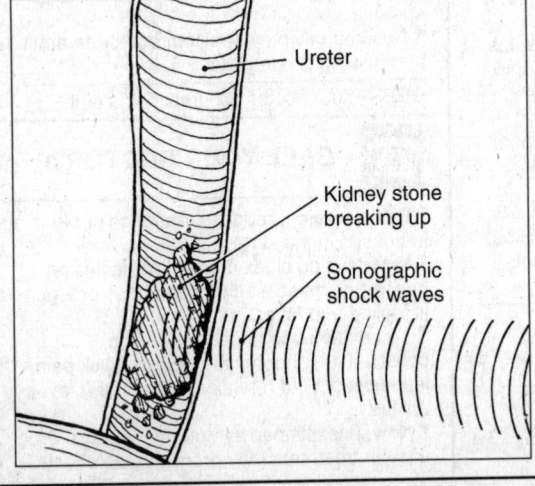

The lithotripsy unit turns out high frequency sound waves directed toward the stone. The shock waves pulverize the stone into small particles which then pass spontaneously in the patient's urine.

Ureter

Kidney stone breaking up

Sonographic shock waves

LIVER TRANSPLANTATION

GENERAL INFORMATION

DEFINITION—Replacement of a diseased liver with a healthy liver obtained from a donor with compatible immunological characteristics. In some cases, a segment of the liver of a living, related donor may be used.

BODY PARTS INVOLVED—Diseased or abnormal liver; healthy donor liver; blood vessels and bile ducts connected to liver.

REASONS FOR SURGERY—End-stage liver failure from liver cancer or other liver disease, such as chronic hepatitis or primary biliary cirrhosis (see Glossary for both).

SURGICAL RISK INCREASES WITH
- Adults over 60; infants.
- Obesity; smoking; stress.
- Excess alcohol consumption.
- Poor nutrition.
- Recent or chronic illness; diabetes mellitus.
- Use of some prescription and nonprescription drugs. Inform your doctor of any drugs, medications, or vitamin and herb supplements you are using or have used in the last month.

WHAT TO EXPECT

WHO OPERATES—General surgeon with transplant experience and training.

WHERE PERFORMED—Hospital.

DIAGNOSTIC TESTS
- Before surgery: Immune-system and liver-matching procedures; studies of body systems.
- After surgery: Blood studies.

ANESTHESIA—General anesthesia by injection and inhalation with an airway tube placed in the windpipe.

DESCRIPTION OF OPERATION
- Liver is removed from donor, then chilled and preserved until surgery.
- An incision is made under the recipient's ribs. The abdominal muscles are separated or split, and the peritoneal cavity is opened.
- The liver and its bile ducts are isolated.
- The liver is cut free and removed. The donor liver is positioned and sewn in place. Blood vessels and bile ducts are connected.
- The peritoneum and abdominal muscles are closed. The skin is closed with sutures or clips, which usually can be removed about 1 week after surgery.

POSSIBLE COMPLICATIONS
- Excessive bleeding.
- Surgical-wound infection.
- Rejection of transplant.
- Bile-duct obstruction.
- Recurrence of hepatitis B or C in the new, previously healthy liver.

AVERAGE HOSPITAL STAY—3 weeks.

PROBABLE OUTCOME—A successful transplantation prolongs life and improves the quality of life in patients who might otherwise have died. The 5-year survival rate for people under 60 years old who undergo liver transplantation is about 75%. Allow about 6 months for recovery from surgery.

POSTOPERATIVE CARE

GENERAL MEASURES
- A hard ridge should form along the incision. As it heals, the ridge will gradually recede.
- Shower as usual. Avoid baths until the incision has completely healed. You may wash the incision gently with mild, unscented soap. After showering, replace any wet dressings with clean, dry ones.
- Use an electric heating pad, a heat lamp or a warm compress to relieve incisional pain.
- Move and elevate legs often while resting in bed to decrease the likelihood of deep-vein blood clots.

MEDICATION
- Your doctor may prescribe:
  Pain relievers. Don't take prescription pain medication longer than 4 to 7 days. Use only as much as you need.
  Stool softeners to prevent constipation.
  Antibiotics to fight or prevent infection.
  Immunosuppressant drugs to decrease the likelihood of rejection.
  Hepatitis B immunoglobin (HBIg) or other drugs to help prevent the recurrence of hepatitis B after liver transplantation.
- You may use nonprescription drugs, such as acetaminophen, for minor pain. Avoid aspirin.

ACTIVITY
- To help recovery and aid your well-being, resume daily activities as soon as you are able.
- Avoid vigorous exercise for 6 weeks after surgery.
- Resume driving when your doctor determines that healing is complete.

DIET—Your doctor will prescribe a diet.

CALL YOUR DOCTOR IF

- Pain, swelling, redness, drainage or bleeding increases in the surgical area.
- You develop signs of infection, including headache, muscle aches, dizziness or a general ill feeling and fever.
- You experience nausea, vomiting, constipation, abdominal swelling, back pain, jaundice; or fluid retention in abdomen, eyes or ankles.
- New, unexplained symptoms develop. Drugs used in treatment may produce side effects.

LIVER TRANSPLANTATION

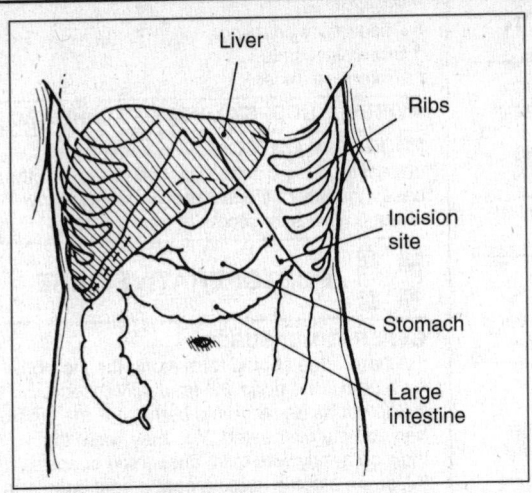

An illustration of the liver showing its anatomical relationship to other parts of the chest and abdomen.

Liver

Ribs

Incision site

Stomach

Large intestine

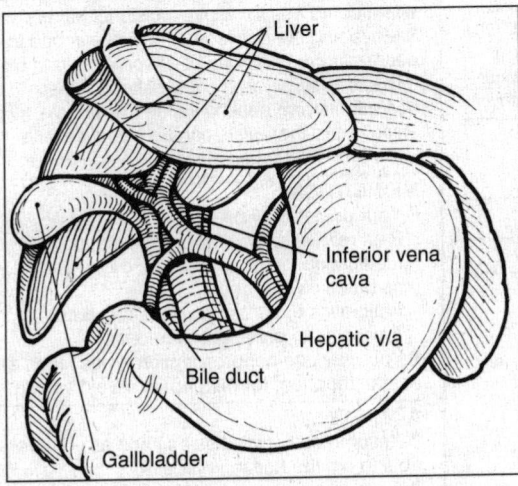

The liver and its bile ducts are isolated, cut free and removed.

Liver

Inferior vena cava

Hepatic v/a

Bile duct

Gallbladder

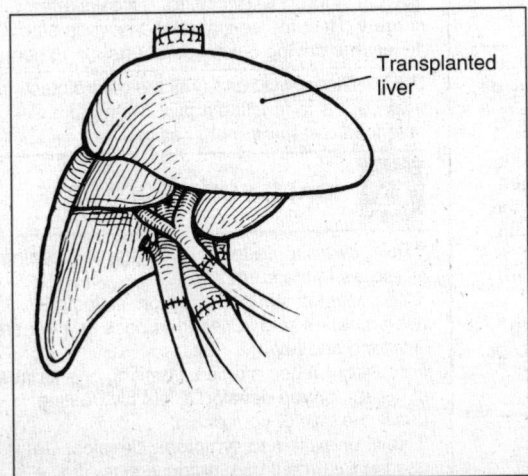

The donor liver is positioned and sewn into place. Blood vessels and bile ducts are connected.

Transplanted liver

LUNG RESECTION
(Lobectomy; Pneumonectomy)

GENERAL INFORMATION

DEFINITION—Removal of tissue from the lungs. If part of a lung (usually called a lobe) is removed, the surgery is called lobectomy. If the entire lung is removed, the surgery is called pneumonectomy.

BODY PARTS INVOLVED—Lung; bronchial tubes; blood vessels in chest; ribs.

REASONS FOR SURGERY
- Cancer or suspected cancer of the lung.
- Diseased lobes of the lung caused by several chronic conditions, especially bronchiectasis.

SURGICAL RISK INCREASES WITH
- Adults over 60; obesity; poor nutrition.
- Excess alcohol consumption; smoking.
- Recent illness, especially upper-respiratory infection.
- Chronic illness, especially diabetes mellitus.
- Use of some prescription and nonprescription drugs. Inform your doctor of any drugs, medications, or vitamin and herb supplements you are using or have used in the last month.

WHAT TO EXPECT

WHO OPERATES—Thoracic surgeon.

WHERE PERFORMED—Hospital.

DIAGNOSTIC TESTS
- Before surgery: Blood and urine studies; x-rays of chest and lungs; ECG; CT scan; bronchoscopy (see Glossary for all); pulmonary function studies.
- During surgery: ECG monitor.
- After surgery: Blood studies.

ANESTHESIA—General anesthesia by injection and inhalation with an airway tube placed in the windpipe.

DESCRIPTION OF OPERATION
- An incision is made in the chest. A rib may be removed for better exposure to the lungs.
- The blood supply to the diseased area is isolated and tied off.
- The diseased area is located and examined. The growth, the lobe in which it appears or the entire lung is cut free and removed along with lymph nodes in the area (if appropriate).
- A tube is inserted to drain fluid and air from the surgical area.
- The muscles are reconstructed with strong sutures. The skin is closed with sutures or clips, which usually can be removed about 1 week after surgery.

POSSIBLE COMPLICATIONS
- Excessive bleeding.
- Surgical-wound infection.
- Pneumonia.
- Respiratory crippling.
- Bronchial fistula.
- Prolonged air leak.

AVERAGE HOSPITAL STAY—7 to 10 days.

PROBABLE OUTCOME—In some cases, underlying lung disease may be cured. In other cases, quality of life may be improved. Allow about 6 weeks for recovery from surgery.

POSTOPERATIVE CARE

GENERAL MEASURES
- A hard ridge should form along the incision. As it heals, the ridge will gradually recede.
- Shower as usual. Avoid baths until the incision has completely healed. You may wash the incision gently with mild, unscented soap.
- Use an electric heating pad, a heat lamp or a warm compress to relieve incisional pain.
- Move and elevate legs often while in bed to decrease the likelihood of deep-vein blood clots.
- Breathe deeply and cough often to keep secretions from pooling inside the lungs. Respiratory therapists can help you learn to keep bronchial tubes clear. Ask your doctor.

MEDICATION
- Your doctor may prescribe:
  Pain relievers. Don't take prescription pain medication longer than 4 to 7 days. Use only as much as you need.
  Antibiotics to fight or prevent infection.
  A vaccine to prevent pneumonia.
- You may use nonprescription drugs, such as acetaminophen, for minor pain. Avoid aspirin.

ACTIVITY
- Resume daily activities as soon as you are able to aid the healing process.
- Avoid vigorous exercise for 6 weeks after surgery. Resume sexual relations when able.
- Resume driving 5 weeks after returning home.

DIET—Clear liquid diet until the gastrointestinal tract begins to function again. Then eat a well-balanced diet to promote healing.

CALL YOUR DOCTOR IF

- Pain, swelling, redness, drainage or bleeding increases in the surgical area.
- You develop signs of infection, including headache, muscle aches, dizziness or a general ill feeling and fever.
- You experience nausea, vomiting or shortness of breath, or you develop a "bubbly" feeling under the skin of your chest.
- New, unexplained symptoms develop. Drugs used in treatment may produce side effects.

LUNG RESECTION
(Lobectomy; Pneumonectomy)

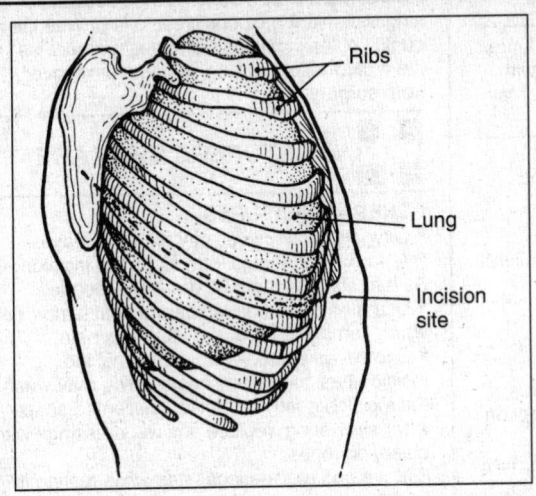

Ribs

Lung

Incision
site

An illustration showing the usual incision site across the chest.

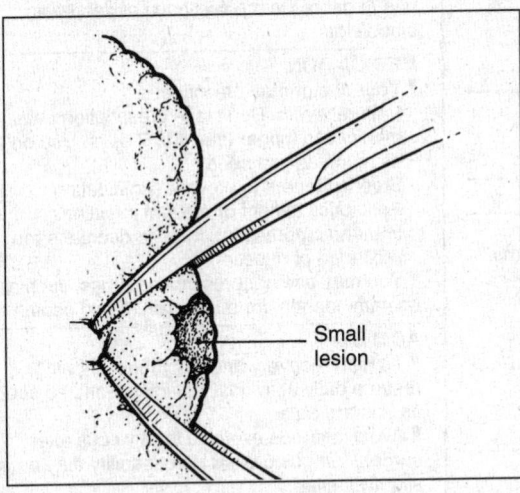

Small
lesion

The diseased area on the lung is located and examined. The tumor, the lobe in which it appears, or the entire lung may be cut free and removed.

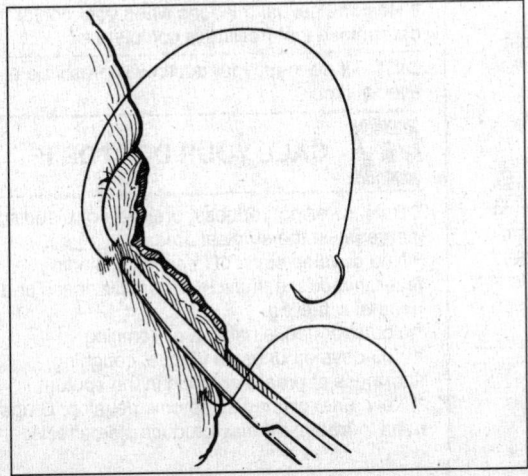

Muscles of the chest wall are reconstructed with strong sutures. A tube is usually left in place to drain fluid and air from the surgical area and to help the lung reinflate following surgery.

SURGERIES

LUNG TRANSPLANTATION

GENERAL INFORMATION

DEFINITION—Replacement of diseased lungs with healthy lungs obtained from a donor with compatible immunological characteristics. May involve one or both lungs.

BODY PARTS INVOLVED—Diseased or abnormal lungs; healthy donor lungs; blood vessels and bronchial tubes to the lungs.

REASONS FOR SURGERY—Pulmonary hypertension (see Glossary); respiratory failure; cystic fibrosis; bronchiectasis.

SURGICAL RISK INCREASES WITH
- Adults over 60; obesity; smoking; stress.
- Poor nutrition; alcoholism.
- Recent or chronic illness; diabetes mellitus.
- Use of some prescription and nonprescription drugs. Inform your doctor of any drugs, medications, or vitamin and herb supplements you are using or have used in the last month.

WHAT TO EXPECT

WHO OPERATES—Thoracic surgeon or cardiovascular surgeon with transplant experience and training.

WHERE PERFORMED—Hospital.

DIAGNOSTIC TESTS
- Before surgery: Evaluation of body systems, especially the respiratory system; immune-system and lung-matching procedures.
- During surgery: Cardiac monitor.
- After surgery: Blood studies.

ANESTHESIA—General anesthesia by injection and inhalation with an airway tube placed in the windpipe.

DESCRIPTION OF OPERATION
- Healthy lungs are removed from the donor, chilled and preserved up to 12 hours.
- An incision is made in the recipient's chest and the chest is spread apart.
- The heart-lung machine (see Glossary) sustains life during surgery.
- The lungs are cut free of the connecting bronchial tubes and blood vessels and removed.
- The donor lungs are positioned and sewn in place. Blood vessels and bronchial tubes are connected. Chest tubes remain for drainage.
- The chest muscles are closed. The skin is closed with sutures or clips, which usually can be removed about 1 week after surgery.

POSSIBLE COMPLICATIONS
- Excessive bleeding.
- Surgical-wound infection.
- Pneumonia.
- Rejection of transplanted lung.

AVERAGE HOSPITAL STAY—3 weeks.

PROBABLE OUTCOME—When successful, a lung transplant prolongs life and improves the quality of life in patients who might otherwise have died. Allow about 6 months for recovery from surgery.

POSTOPERATIVE CARE

GENERAL MEASURES
- Oxygen will be necessary for 1 to 7 days.
- A hard ridge should form along the incision. As it heals, the ridge will gradually recede.
- Use an electric heating pad, a heat lamp or a warm compress to relieve incisional pain.
- Shower as usual. Avoid baths until the incision has completely healed. You may wash the incision gently with mild, unscented soap. After showering, replace any wet dressings with clean, dry ones.
- Move and elevate legs often while resting in bed to decrease the likelihood of deep-vein blood clots.

MEDICATION
- Your doctor may prescribe:
  Pain relievers. Don't take prescription pain medication longer than 4 to 7 days. Use only as much as you need.
  Stool softeners to prevent constipation.
  Antibiotics to fight or prevent infection.
  Immunosuppressant drugs to decrease the likelihood of rejection.
- You may use nonprescription drugs, such as acetaminophen, for minor pain. Avoid aspirin.

ACTIVITY
- To help recovery and aid your well-being, resume daily activities, including work, as soon as you are able.
- Avoid vigorous exercise for 6 weeks after surgery. Ongoing exercise capability may be slightly limited.
- Resume sexual relations when your doctor determines that healing is complete.

DIET—If needed, your doctor will prescribe a special diet.

CALL YOUR DOCTOR IF

- Pain, swelling, redness, drainage or bleeding increases in the surgical area.
- You develop signs of infection, including fever, headache, muscle aches, dizziness or a general ill feeling.
- You experience nausea or vomiting.
- You develop unusual fatigue, coughing, shortness of breath or blood in the sputum.
- New, unexplained symptoms develop. Drugs used in treatment may produce side effects.

LUNG TRANSPLANTATION

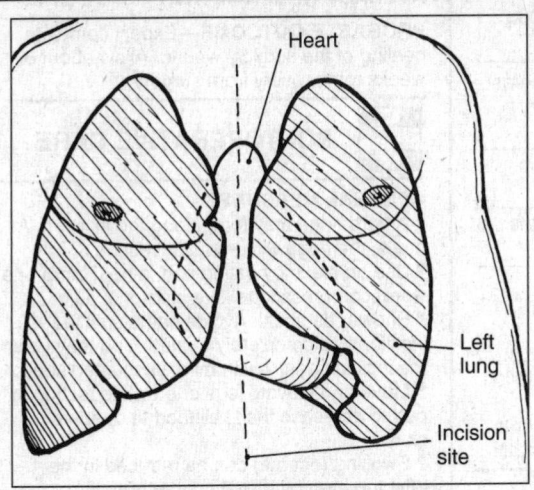

Heart

Left
lung

Incision
site

An illustration of the incision site, the chest and underlying heart and lung.

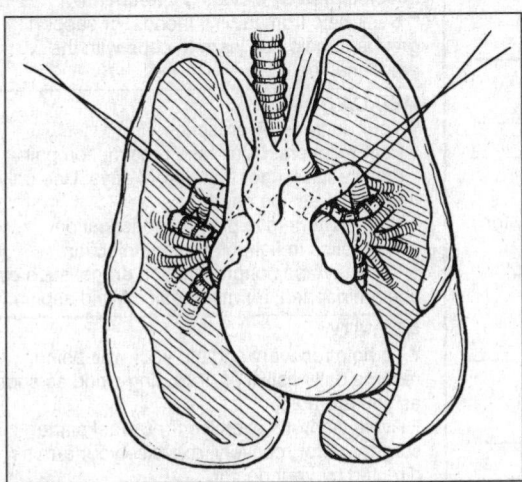

A heart-lung machine sustains life during surgery. The recipient's lungs are cut free of connecting bronchial tubes and blood vessels and removed.

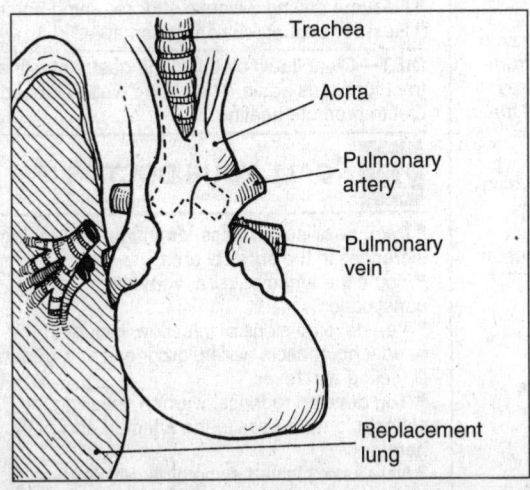

Trachea

Aorta

Pulmonary
artery

Pulmonary
vein

Replacement
lung

The replacement lungs are positioned and sewn in place. Blood vessels and bronchial tubes are connected, chest tubes remain for drainage.
* The chest muscles are closed and the skin is closed with sutures or clips, which usually can be removed about 1 week after surgery (not illustrated).

MASTECTOMY, MODIFIED RADICAL
(Total Mastectomy)

GENERAL INFORMATION

DEFINITION—Complete removal of the breast, including the nipple, and removal of axillary nodes.

BODY PARTS INVOLVED—Breast; lymph glands.

REASONS FOR SURGERY—Cancer of the breast.

SURGICAL RISK INCREASES WITH
- Obesity or poor nutrition.
- Smoking; stress; adults over 60.
- Recent or chronic illness; diabetes mellitus.
- Use of some prescription and nonprescription drugs. Inform your doctor of any drugs, medications, or vitamin and herb supplements you are using or have used in the last month.

WHAT TO EXPECT

WHO OPERATES—General surgeon or oncological surgeon.

WHERE PERFORMED—Hospital.

DIAGNOSTIC TESTS
- Before surgery: Blood and urine studies; mammogram; needle biopsy (see Glossary for both).
- During surgery: Laboratory examination of removed tissue by frozen section.
- After surgery: Blood studies; laboratory examination of removed tissue.

ANESTHESIA—General anesthesia by injection and inhalation with an airway tube placed in the windpipe.

DESCRIPTION OF OPERATION
- An incision is made encompassing the entire breast.
- The underlying tissue is cut free and removed in one piece, along with the lymph glands from the armpit. Bleeding is controlled with sutures and electrocauterization. A tube is inserted for drainage, and will be left in place for 1 to 2 weeks.
- The skin is closed with sutures or clips, which usually can be removed about 1 week after surgery.
- See Breast Reconstruction in Surgery section.

POSSIBLE COMPLICATIONS
- Excessive bleeding.
- Surgical-wound infection.
- Depression.
- Accumulation of blood or serum under the skin in the surgical area.
- Limited shoulder motion; nerve damage.
- Lymphedema (see Glossary).
- Skin loss over mastectomy site.

AVERAGE HOSPITAL STAY—0 to 2 days.

PROBABLE OUTCOME—Expect complete healing of the surgical wound. Allow about 6 weeks for recovery from surgery.

POSTOPERATIVE CARE

GENERAL MEASURES
- A hard ridge may form along the incision. As it heals, the ridge will gradually recede.
- Use an electric heating pad, a heat lamp or a warm compress to relieve incisional pain.
- Shower as usual. Avoids baths until the incision has completely healed. You may wash the incision gently with mild, unscented soap.
- Move and elevate legs often while resting in bed to decrease the likelihood of deep-vein clots.
- Swelling (edema) can be reduced in the affected area by elevating it frequently.
- Seek help from family, friends, or support groups to help you learn to cope with the emotional feelings.

MEDICATION
- Your doctor may prescribe:
  Pain relievers. Don't take prescription pain medication longer than 4 to 7 days. Use only as much as you need.
  Stool softeners to prevent constipation.
  Antibiotics to fight or prevent infection.
- You may use nonprescription drugs, such as acetaminophen, for minor pain. Avoid aspirin.

ACTIVITY
- To help recovery and aid your well-being, resume daily activities, including work, as soon as you are able.
- Avoid vigorous exercise for 6 weeks after surgery. After recovery, exercise your arm as directed by your doctor.
- Resume driving 2 weeks after returning home.
- Resume sexual relations when able.

DIET—Clear liquid diet until the gastrointestinal tract functions again. Then eat a well-balanced diet to promote healing.

CALL YOUR DOCTOR IF

- Pain, swelling, redness, drainage or bleeding increases in the surgical area.
- You experience nausea, vomiting or constipation.
- You develop signs of infection, including headache, muscle aches, dizziness or a general ill feeling and fever.
- You develop redness, warmth, swelling, stiffness or hardness in the affected arm or hand.
- New, unexplained symptoms develop.

MASTECTOMY, MODIFIED RADICAL
(Total Mastectomy)

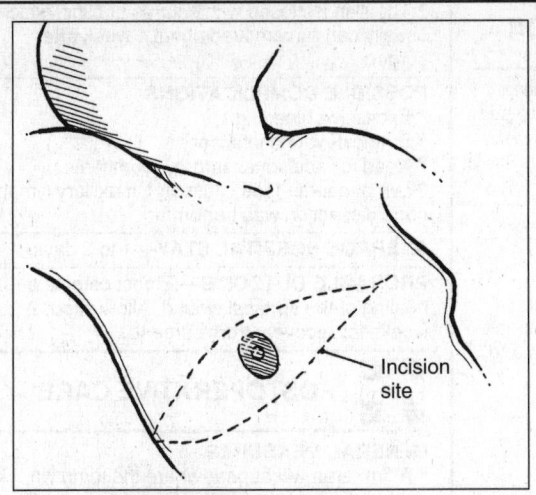

The usual site and elliptical form of the incision to remove the breast and underlying tissue.

Incision site

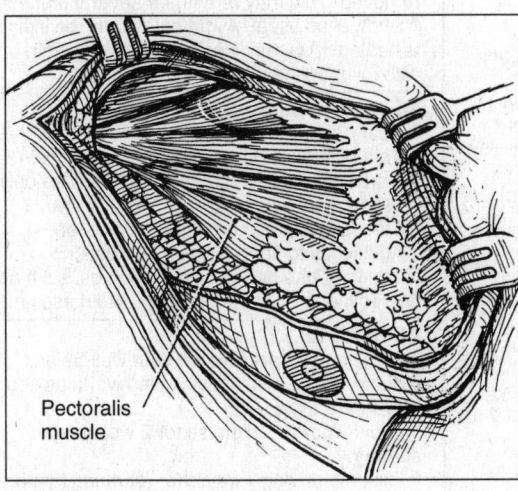

Underlying breast tissue is cut free and removed in one block with lymph glands from the armpit. The underlying muscle is left in place.

Pectoralis muscle

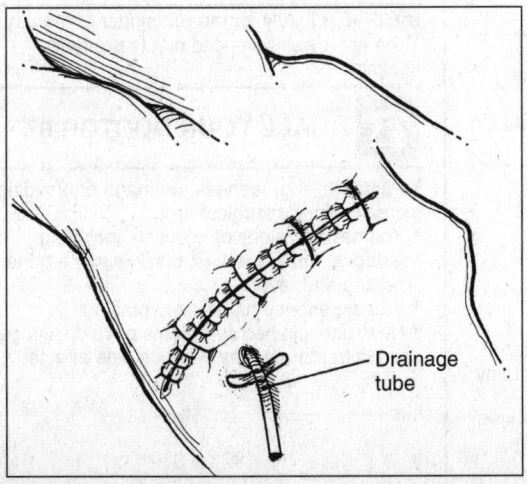

A tube is inserted for drainage. The tissues under the skin are closed with large, absorbable sutures. The skin is closed with sutures or clips that usually can be removed about 1 week after surgery.

Drainage tube

MASTECTOMY, PARTIAL (Lumpectomy)

GENERAL INFORMATION

DEFINITION—Removal of a lump from the female breast that is known or suspected to be cancerous. Lumpectomy is the least invasive procedure for breast cancer surgery, and is the most likely to leave the breast looking normal.

BODY PARTS INVOLVED—Breast.

REASONS FOR SURGERY—Cancer or suspected cancer of the breast. There is frequently more than one option for surgical treatment. Be sure you understand the rationale for any recommended procedure, the risks and benefits involved, as well as any possible alternative treatments.

SURGICAL RISK INCREASES WITH
- Obesity; smoking; stress.
- Poor nutrition.
- Recent or chronic illness.
- Diabetes mellitus.
- Use of some prescription and nonprescription drugs. Inform your doctor of any drugs, medications, or vitamin and herb supplements you are using or have used in the last month.

WHAT TO EXPECT

WHO OPERATES—General surgeon or oncological surgeon.

WHERE PERFORMED—Hospital.

DIAGNOSTIC TESTS
- Before surgery: Blood and urine studies; x-rays of chest; mammograms (see Glossary).
- During surgery: Laboratory examination of the removed lump by a pathologist.
- After surgery: Blood studies; laboratory examination of removed tissue; sometimes bone scans.

ANESTHESIA
- Local anesthesia by injection, accompanied by sedation.
- General anesthesia by injection and inhalation with an airway tube placed in the windpipe.

DESCRIPTION OF OPERATION
- An incision is made over the lump to be removed.
- The lump and a small surrounding area of normal tissue are cut free and removed. Bleeding is controlled with ties and electrocauterization.
- It is frequently necessary to perform axillary node dissection in conjunction with lumpectomy. If lymph node dissection is necessary, a separate incision in the axilla (under the armpit) is made to sample or significantly remove the axillary lymph nodes.

- The skin is closed with sutures or clips, which usually can be removed about 1 week after surgery.

POSSIBLE COMPLICATIONS
- Excessive bleeding.
- Surgical-wound infection.
- Need for additional surgery (sometimes).
- Lymphedema (see Glossary), if axillary lymph node dissection was performed.

AVERAGE HOSPITAL STAY—1 to 2 days.

PROBABLE OUTCOME—Expect complete healing of the surgical wound. Allow about 2 weeks for recovery from surgery.

POSTOPERATIVE CARE

GENERAL MEASURES
- A firm area will appear where the lump was removed. This may remain for several months.
- Shower as usual. Avoid baths until the incision is healed. You may wash the incision gently with mild, unscented soap.

MEDICATION
- Your doctor may prescribe:
  Pain relievers. Don't take prescription pain medication longer than 4 to 7 days. Use only as much as you need.
  Stool softeners to prevent constipation.
  Antibiotics to fight or prevent infection.
- You may use nonprescription drugs, such as acetaminophen, for minor pain. Avoid aspirin.

ACTIVITY
- To help recovery and aid your well-being, resume daily activities, including work, as soon as you are able.
- Avoid vigorous exercise for 2 weeks after surgery.
- Resume driving 1 day after returning home.

DIET—Eat lightly for the remainder of the day. Then eat a well-balanced diet to promote healing.

CALL YOUR DOCTOR IF

- Pain, swelling, redness, drainage or bleeding increases in the surgical area.
- You develop signs of infection, including headache, muscle aches, dizziness or a general ill feeling and fever.
- You experience nausea or vomiting.
- New, unexplained symptoms develop. Drugs used in treatment may produce side effects.

MASTECTOMY, PARTIAL
(Lumpectomy)

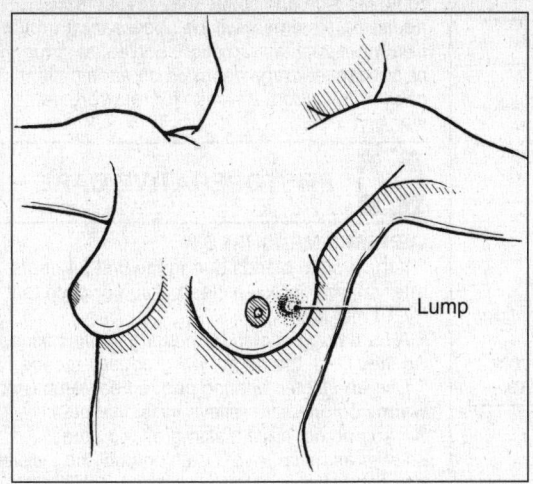

A breast lump in a typical location.

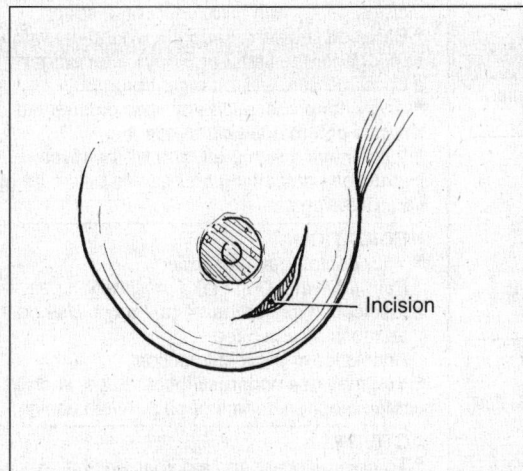

After the skin has been incised, the lump and a small surrounding area of normal tissue are cut free.

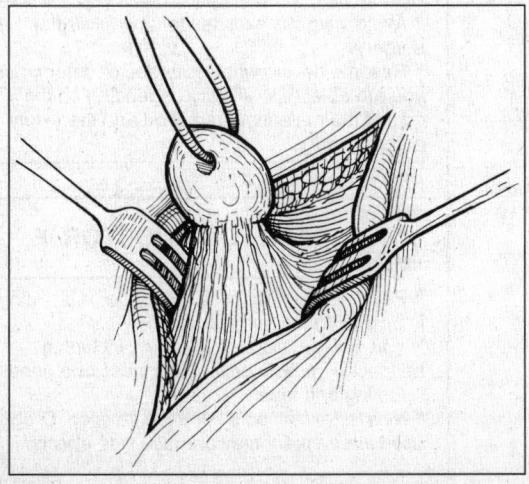

The lump is removed. Afterwards, the remaining breast is carefully palpated for any additional suspicious areas or suspicious lymph nodes.

SURGERIES

MELANOMA REMOVAL

GENERAL INFORMATION

DEFINITION—Removal of any lesion on the skin that might be malignant melanoma, the most dangerous form of skin cancer.

BODY PARTS INVOLVED—Skin.

REASONS FOR SURGERY—Treatment of malignant melanoma.

SURGICAL RISK INCREASES WITH
- Obesity; smoking; poor nutrition.
- Recent or chronic illness.
- Diabetes mellitus.
- Use of some prescription and nonprescription drugs. Inform your doctor of any drugs, medications, or vitamin and herb supplements you are using or have used in the last month.

WHAT TO EXPECT

WHO OPERATES—General surgeon, dermatologist or plastic and reconstructive surgeon.

WHERE PERFORMED—Hospital or outpatient surgical facility.

DIAGNOSTIC TESTS
- Before surgery: Blood and urine studies.
- During surgery: Microscopic examination of skin margins to determine how much skin to remove.
- After surgery: Laboratory examination of removed tissue. Possibly, CT scan; MRI; bone scans; PET scan (see Glossary for all).

ANESTHESIA
- Local anesthesia by injection.
- General anesthesia by injection and inhalation with an airway tube placed in the windpipe.

DESCRIPTION OF OPERATION
- Surgery is directed primarily toward cure and secondarily toward preservation of normal appearance.
- The tumor is removed along with a surrounding portion of normal, healthy skin to ensure complete removal of all cancer cells.
- Skin grafts (see in Surgery section) are frequently needed to close large skin defects.
- The skin is closed with fine suture material or clips, which usually can be removed about 10 days after surgery.

POSSIBLE COMPLICATIONS
- Surgical-wound infection.
- Excessive bleeding.
- Residual cancer due to not removing enough diseased skin.

AVERAGE HOSPITAL STAY—0 to 2 days.

PROBABLE OUTCOME—Expect complete healing of the surgical wounds. Examination of removed skin and tissue may reveal that additional treatment will be necessary. Further treatment such as radiation, additional surgery, or anticancer drugs depends on each patient's case. Allow about 2 weeks for recovery from surgery.

POSTOPERATIVE CARE

GENERAL MEASURES
- If the wound bleeds during the first 24 hours after surgery, press a clean tissue or cloth to it for 10 minutes.
- A hard ridge should form along the incisions. As they heal, the ridges will gradually recede.
- Use an electric heating pad, a heat lamp or a warm compress, to relieve incisional pain.
- If you do not have a skin graft, you may shower as usual. Avoid bathing until the incision has completely healed. You may wash the incision gently with mild, unscented soap.
- Between showers, keep the wound dry with a bandage for the first 2 or 3 days after surgery. If a bandage gets wet, change it promptly.
- Apply nonprescription antibiotic ointment to wounds before applying bandages.
- If you have a skin graft, you will be given instructions on bathing and how to take care of your dressings.

MEDICATION
- Your doctor may prescribe:
  Pain relievers. Don't take prescription pain medication longer than 4 to 7 days. Use only as much as you need.
  Antibiotics to prevent infection.
- You may use nonprescription drugs, such as acetaminophen, for minor pain. Avoid aspirin.

ACTIVITY
- To help recovery and aid your well-being, resume daily activities as soon as you are able.
- Avoid vigorous exercise for 2 weeks after surgery.
- Resume driving when your doctor determines you are able; this will vary depending on the size of the melanoma removed and the extent of the surgery.

DIET—No special diet.

CALL YOUR DOCTOR IF

- Pain, swelling, redness, drainage or bleeding increases in the surgical area.
- You develop signs of infection, including headache, muscle aches, dizziness or a general ill feeling and fever.
- New, unexplained symptoms develop. Drugs used in treatment may produce side effects.

MELANOMA REMOVAL

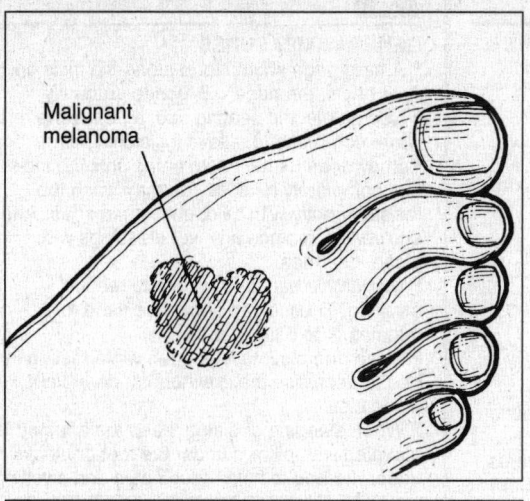

Malignant melanoma

A large lesion on the skin, in this case, on the top of the foot at the base of the toes.
- Melanomas may also appear on other skin locations.

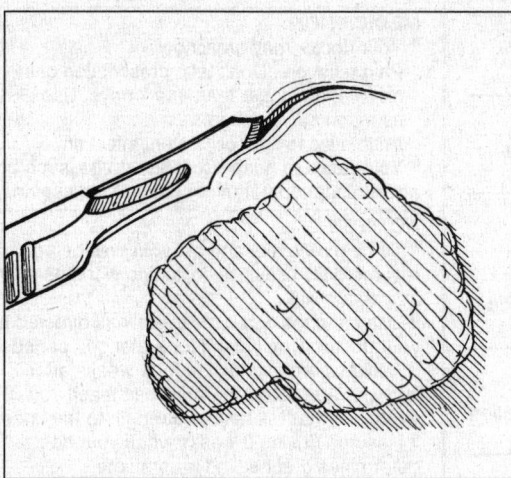

The tumor is removed along with the surrounding portion of normal, healthy skin (usually 2-3 centimeters) to ensure complete removal of all cancerous cells.

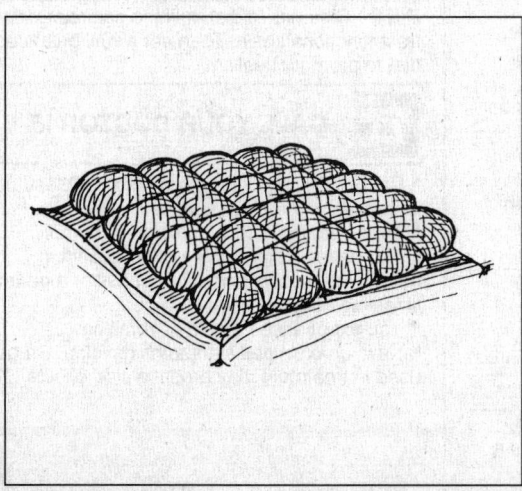

If possible, the skin is closed without grafting, but frequently a skin graft from another site must be used to completely close large lesion sites.
- Sutures used for closure or for skin grafting can usually be removed about 10 days after surgery.

MENISCECTOMY

GENERAL INFORMATION

DEFINITION—Removal of torn cartilage in the knee.

BODY PARTS INVOLVED—Knee and all its parts.

REASONS FOR SURGERY
• Prevention of permanent damage to the knee joint.
• Stop "locking" of knee joint.
• Relieve pain and swelling of knee.

SURGICAL RISK INCREASES WITH
• Obesity.
• Smoking.
• Recent or chronic illness.
• Diabetes mellitus.
• Use of some prescription and nonprescription drugs. Inform your doctor of any drugs, medications, or vitamin and herb supplements you are using or have used in the last month.

WHAT TO EXPECT

WHO OPERATES—Orthopedist.

WHERE PERFORMED—Hospital or outpatient surgical facility.

DIAGNOSTIC TESTS
• Before surgery: Blood and urine studies; x-rays of both knees; MRI; arthrogram (see Glossary for both).
• After surgery: X-rays of affected knee; blood studies.

ANESTHESIA
• Spinal anesthesia by injection.
• General anesthesia by injection and inhalation with an airway tube placed in the windpipe.

DESCRIPTION OF OPERATION
• The affected area can be approached by arthroscopy (see Glossary) or by incision into the knee joint. Either approach exposes the injured cartilage.
• If the torn cartilage can be repaired, it will be sutured. Or, if the torn cartilage cannot be repaired, the torn portion will be removed. Any injured ligaments are sewn together.
• The skin is closed with sutures or clips, which usually can be removed about 1 week after surgery.

POSSIBLE COMPLICATIONS
• Excessive bleeding; blood clots.
• Surgical-wound infection.
• Weakened knee joint and subsequent arthritis.

AVERAGE HOSPITAL STAY—0 to 2 days.

PROBABLE OUTCOME—Expect complete recovery without complications. Allow about 6 weeks for recovery from surgery.

POSTOPERATIVE CARE

GENERAL MEASURES
• A hard ridge should form along the incision. As it heals, the ridge will recede gradually.
• Use an electric heating pad, a heat lamp or a warm compress to relieve incisional pain.
• Shower as usual. Avoid baths until the incision has completely healed. You may wash the incision gently with mild, unscented soap. After showering, replace any wet dressings with clean, dry ones.
• Use an ice bag on the knee to reduce swelling. The ice bag should be used for 20 minutes, 4 to 5 times a day.
• Move and elevate legs often while resting in bed to decrease the likelihood of deep-vein blood clots.
• When sleeping or sitting, keep the affected leg elevated with pillows under the foot or blocks under the bed to help reduce pain and swelling.

MEDICATION
• Your doctor may prescribe:
  Pain relievers. Don't take prescription pain medication longer than 4 to 7 days. Use only as much as you need.
  Antibiotics to fight or prevent infection.
• You may use nonprescription drugs, such as acetaminophen, for minor pain. Avoid aspirin.

ACTIVITY
• To help recovery and aid your well-being, resume daily activities, including work, as soon as you are able.
• Use crutches or a cane to walk as directed by your doctor. Don't stand for prolonged periods.
• Avoid vigorous exercise for 4 weeks after surgery. A physical therapist can teach you exercises that will restore strength to the knee.
• Resume driving 3 weeks when your doctor determines that healing is complete.

DIET—Clear liquid diet until the gastrointestinal tract functions again. Then eat a well-balanced diet to promote healing.

CALL YOUR DOCTOR IF

• Pain, swelling, redness, drainage or bleeding increases in the surgical area.
• Toes become cold, discolored or numb.
• You develop signs of infection, including headache, muscle aches, dizziness or a general ill feeling and fever.
• You experience nausea or vomiting.
• New, unexplained symptoms develop. Drugs used in treatment may produce side effects.

MENISCECTOMY

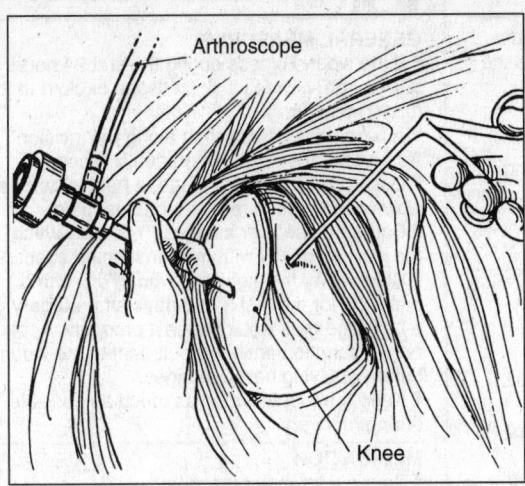

An arthroscope inserted into a knee joint. The illustration shows surgical drapes around the joint.

Arthroscope

Knee

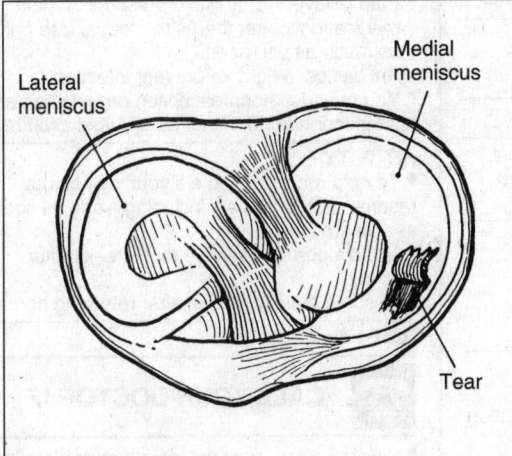

The surgeon can visualize through the arthroscope any tear in either meniscus.

Lateral meniscus

Medial meniscus

Tear

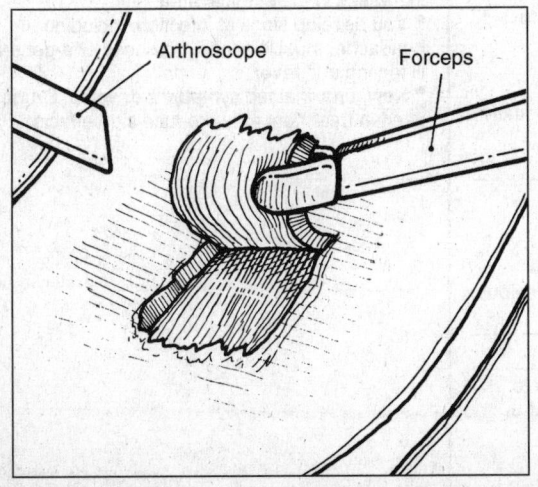

The torn meniscus is removed with forceps and extracted through the opening in the skin.
- Skin is closed with sutures or clips that usually can be removed about 1 week after surgery (not illustrated).

Arthroscope

Forceps

SURGERIES

MORTON'S NEUROMA REMOVAL

 ## GENERAL INFORMATION

DEFINITION—Removal of Morton's neuroma, a small benign tumor in the nerve that serves the toes. Its cause is unknown and it produces severe pain.

BODY PARTS INVOLVED—A small tumor between the 2nd and 3rd toes or the 3rd and 4th toes. It may occur in either or both feet.

REASONS FOR SURGERY—Relief of pain caused by the neuroma.

SURGICAL RISK INCREASES WITH
- Obesity.
- Smoking.
- Poor nutrition.
- Recent or chronic illness.
- Diabetes mellitus.
- Use of some prescription and nonprescription drugs. Inform your doctor of any drugs, medications, or vitamin and herb supplements you are using or have used in the last month.

 ## WHAT TO EXPECT

WHO OPERATES—Orthopedist, podiatrist.

WHERE PERFORMED—Hospital, outpatient surgical facility, doctor's office or emergency room.

DIAGNOSTIC TESTS
- Before surgery: Blood and urine studies; x-rays of the foot.
- After surgery: Laboratory examination of removed tissue.

ANESTHESIA
- Local anesthesia by injection.
- General anesthesia by injection and inhalation with an airway tube placed in the throat.

DESCRIPTION OF OPERATION
- A tourniquet is wrapped around the leg to decrease bleeding in the surgical area.
- The neuroma is located, cut free from surrounding tissue and removed.
- The skin is closed with sutures, which usually can be removed about 10 to 14 days after surgery. The tourniquet is removed.

POSSIBLE COMPLICATIONS
- Excessive bleeding.
- Surgical-wound infection.
- Numbness in toes due to cut nerve (less bothersome for many patients than the previous pain caused by the neuroma).

AVERAGE HOSPITAL STAY—0 to 1 day.

PROBABLE OUTCOME—Expect complete healing without complications. Allow about 3 weeks for recovery from surgery.

 ## POSTOPERATIVE CARE

GENERAL MEASURES
- If the wound bleeds during the first 24 hours after surgery, press a clean tissue or cloth to it for 10 minutes.
- A hard ridge should form along the incision. As it heals, the ridge will gradually recede.
- Use an electric heating pad, a heat lamp or a warm compress to relieve incisional pain.
- Bathe and shower as usual. You may wash the incision gently with mild unscented soap.
- Between baths, keep the wound dry with a bandage for the first 2 or 3 days after surgery. If a bandage gets wet, change it promptly. Apply nonprescription antibiotic ointment to the wound before applying new bandages.
- Keep the foot elevated as much as possible during recovery.

MEDICATION
- Your doctor may prescribe:
  Pain relievers. Don't take prescription pain medication longer than 4 to 7 days. Use only as much as you need.
  Antibiotics to fight or prevent infection.
- You may use nonprescription drugs, such as acetaminophen, for minor pain. Avoid aspirin.

ACTIVITY
- To help recovery and aid your well-being, resume daily activities, including work, as soon as you are able.
- Avoid vigorous exercise for 6 weeks after surgery.
- Resume driving 1 week after returning home.

DIET—No special diet.

 ## CALL YOUR DOCTOR IF

- Pain, swelling, redness, drainage or bleeding increases in the surgical area.
- You develop signs of infection, including headache, muscle aches, dizziness or a general ill feeling and fever.
- New, unexplained symptoms develop. Drugs used in treatment may produce side effects.

MORTON'S NEUROMA REMOVAL

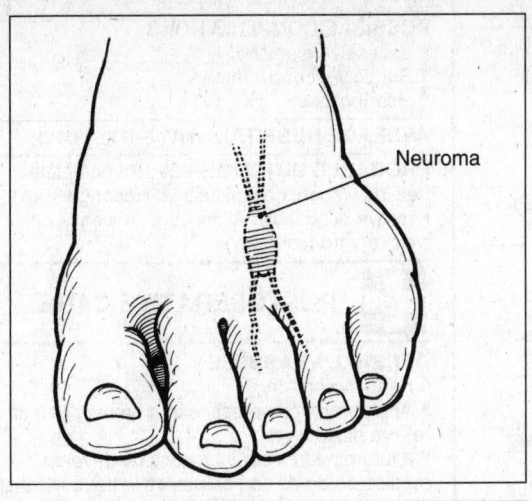

A typical location between the 3rd and 4th toes for a Morton's neuroma (a small benign tumor of nerve tissue).

Neuroma

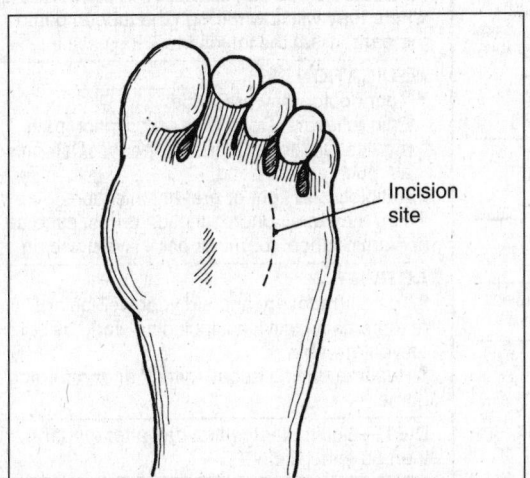

After a tourniquet has been wrapped around the leg to decrease bleeding in the surgical area, an incision is made through the skin.

Incision site

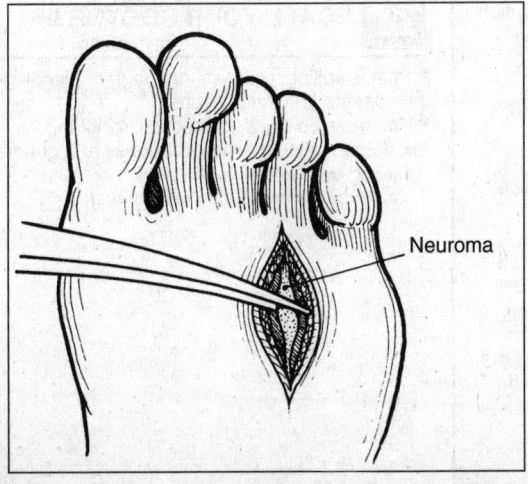

The neuroma is located, cut free from the surrounding tissue and removed.
- After removal, skin is closed with sutures that usually can be removed about 10 to 14 days after surgery (not illustrated).
- The tourniquet is removed to allow normal circulation to the leg and foot (not illustrated).

Neuroma

SURGERIES

MYRINGOTOMY

GENERAL INFORMATION

DEFINITION—Opening the eardrum (tympanic membrane) to remove fluid in the middle ear. This fluid consists of blood, pus, water and debris, and usually collects because of infection or allergy. Frequently, a small tube is inserted in the middle ear to maintain drainage.

BODY PARTS INVOLVED—Eardrum; middle ear; external ear canal (route for surgery).

REASONS FOR SURGERY
- Relief of pain caused by pressure.
- Prevent recurrent infections.
- Prevention of temporary or permanent hearing loss.

SURGICAL RISK INCREASES WITH
- Smoking.
- Recent illness, especially upper-respiratory infection.
- Chronic illness, especially diabetes mellitus.
- Previous perforation of the eardrum.
- Use of some prescription and nonprescription drugs. Inform your doctor of any drugs, medications, or vitamin and herb supplements you are using or have used in the last month.

WHAT TO EXPECT

WHO OPERATES—Ear, nose and throat specialist (otolaryngologist).

WHERE PERFORMED—Hospital or outpatient surgical facility.

DIAGNOSTIC TESTS
- Before surgery: Blood and urine studies; hearing tests; tympanogram (see Glossary).
- After surgery: Blood studies; hearing tests.

ANESTHESIA
- Local anesthesia by topical application.
- General anesthesia by injection and inhalation with an airway tube placed in the windpipe.

DESCRIPTION OF OPERATION
- An instrument called an ear speculum is placed in the external ear canal, and the operative microscope is positioned.
- An tiny incision is made around the eardrum, with care taken not to injure the small bones in the middle ear.
- The fluid is drained, and a tiny small tube (about the size of a grain of rice) is usually left in place to continue drainage.
- No sutures are placed in the eardrum. It will heal by itself, if infection is minimal or absent.
- The tube will prevent premature closure of the eardrum and allow the middle ear to heal. The tube will usually fall out by itself in 6 to 12 months. Occasionally, it will need to be surgically removed.

- The procedure is often repeated in the other ear.

POSSIBLE COMPLICATIONS
- Excessive bleeding.
- Surgical-wound infection.
- Hearing loss.

AVERAGE HOSPITAL STAY—0 to 1 day.

PROBABLE OUTCOME—Expect complete healing without complications. Hearing should improve noticeably. Allow about 4 weeks for recovery from surgery.

POSTOPERATIVE CARE

GENERAL MEASURES
- Keep the ear dry.
- Apply warm compresses or a heating pad to relieve discomfort.
- If future middle ear infections do develop, medicated drops can be placed in the ear canal where they will flow through the tube and into the ear to treat the infection.

MEDICATION
- Your doctor may prescribe:
  Pain relievers. Don't take prescription pain medication longer than 4 to 7 days. Use only as much as you need.
  Antibiotics to fight or prevent infection.
- You may use nonprescription drugs, such as acetaminophen, for minor pain. Avoid aspirin.

ACTIVITY
- To help recovery and aid your well-being, resume daily activities, including work, as soon as you are able.
- Resume driving about 1 week after returning home.

DIET—Liquid diet the first day after surgery, then no special diet.

CALL YOUR DOCTOR IF

- Pain, swelling, redness, drainage or bleeding increases in the surgical area.
- You develop signs of infection, including headache, muscle aches, dizziness or a general ill feeling and fever.
- You experience nausea or vomiting.

MYRINGOTOMY

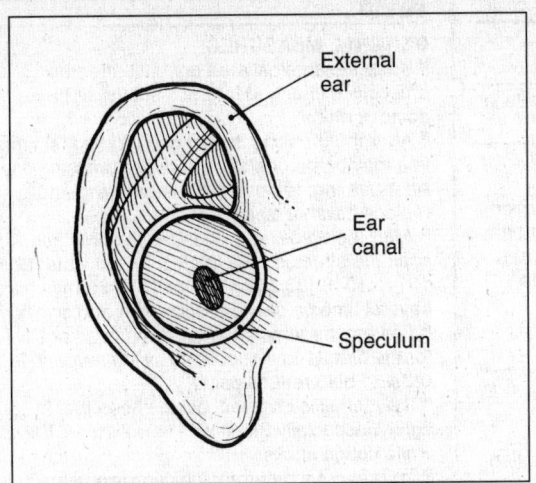

External
ear

Ear
canal

Speculum

An illustration of parts of the ear, including cartilage and skin of the external ear. The ear canal, which goes from the outside inward to reach the eardrum, can be seen through a speculum inserted into the ear canal.

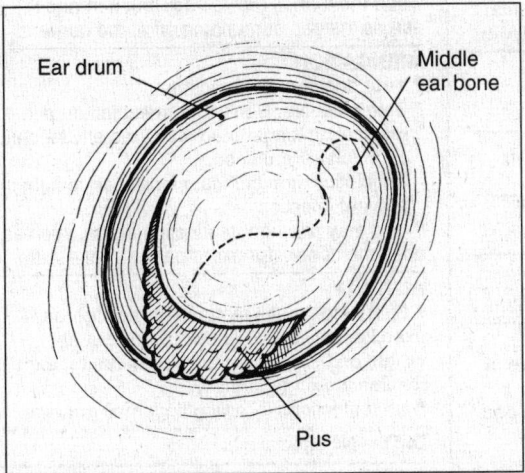

Ear drum

Middle
ear bone

Pus

A tiny incision is made in a low section of the eardrum allowing fluid to drain.

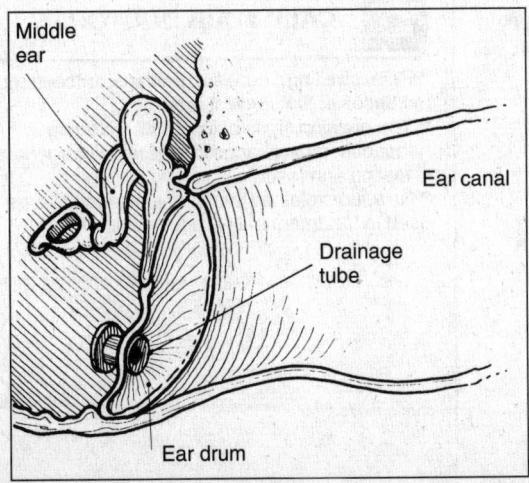

Middle
ear

Ear canal

Drainage
tube

Ear drum

A drainage tube is usually left in place to continue drainage.
- No sutures are placed in the eardrum; it will heal by itself if infection is minimal or absent.
- The tubes will prevent premature closure of the eardrum and allow the middle ear to heal. Usually the tubes will come out by themselves 6 to 12 months following surgery.

SURGERIES

NAIL REMOVAL

 ## GENERAL INFORMATION

DEFINITION—Removal of part or all of a toenail or fingernail.

BODY PARTS INVOLVED—Toenail, usually in the big toe; any fingernail.

REASONS FOR SURGERY
- Relief of painful symptoms of an ingrown toenail or fingernail, with or without an infection.
- Nails may be removed due to injury (with part of the nail torn away); splinters that cannot be removed without removing the nail; or warts under the nail.
- Nail infection (usually fungus).
- Correction of abnormal nail growth.

SURGICAL RISK INCREASES WITH
- Poor circulation in extremities.
- Diabetes mellitus.
- Use of some prescription and nonprescription drugs. Inform your doctor of any drugs, medications, or vitamin and herb supplements you are using or have used in the last month.

 ## WHAT TO EXPECT

WHO OPERATES—General surgeon, family doctor, dermatologist or podiatrist.

WHERE PERFORMED—Doctor's office or outpatient surgical facility.

DIAGNOSTIC TESTS—None required.

ANESTHESIA—Local anesthesia by injection.

DESCRIPTION OF OPERATION
- A section of skin is cut on the affected side of the toe.
- Part or all of the nail is pulled up along its bed and cut free of its underlying tissue.
- The nail bed along the affected side is scraped.
- A special nonstick bandage is applied tightly to prevent bleeding. Usually, no sutures are needed.

POSSIBLE COMPLICATIONS
- Excessive bleeding.
- Surgical-wound infection.

AVERAGE HOSPITAL STAY—None.

PROBABLE OUTCOME—Expect complete healing without complications. Allow about 3 weeks for recovery from surgery. The nail should eventually grow back.

 ## POSTOPERATIVE CARE

GENERAL MEASURES
- Keep the surgical area dry until after the dressing is changed for the first time at the doctor's office.
- After the dressing is changed for the first time, you may bathe or shower with the dressing on. After bathing, remove the wet dressing and replace it with a clean, dry one.
- After the dressing is changed the first time, soak the affected area in plain or salt water at 101 to 104F (38.3 to 40C) for 10 to 20 minutes several times a day to reduce pain and swelling.
- Elevate the affected area as much as possible for the first 24 to 48 hours following surgery, in order to help reduce pain.
- If a toenail is involved, avoid shoes that fit tightly, especially those with narrow toes. Wear white cotton socks.
- To prevent a recurrence of ingrown toenail, when the toenail grows back, cut it straight across instead of rounding off at the corners.

MEDICATION
- Your doctor may prescribe:
  Pain relievers. Don't take prescription pain medication longer than 4 to 7 days. Use only as much as you need.
  Antibiotics or antifungal medication to fight or prevent infection.
- You may use nonprescription drugs, such as acetaminophen, for minor pain. Avoid aspirin.

ACTIVITY
- Following toenail removal, avoid vigorous exercise until the nail heals. Don't put any weight on the affected foot for 24 hours, then resume walking gradually.
- No restrictions following fingernail removal.

DIET—No special diet.

 ## CALL YOUR DOCTOR IF

- Pain, swelling, redness, drainage or bleeding increases in the surgical area.
- You develop signs of infection, including headache, muscle aches, dizziness or a general ill feeling and fever.
- New, unexplained symptoms develop. Drugs used in treatment may produce side effects.

NAIL REMOVAL

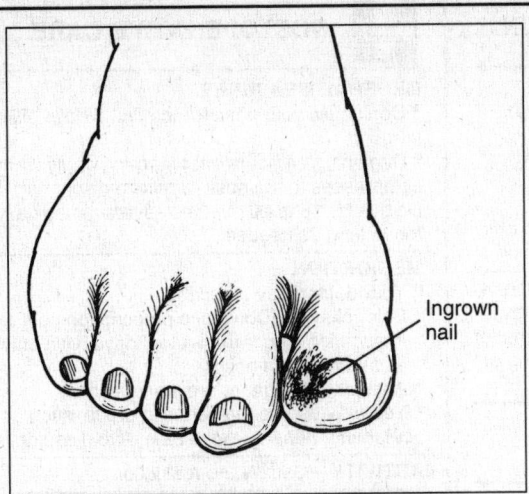

An ingrown toenail in the great toe.

Ingrown
nail

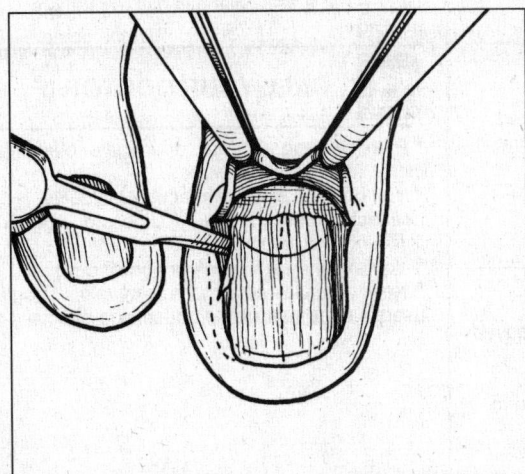

A section of the skin is cut on the affected side of the toe.
- Part or all of the nail is pulled up along its bed and cut free of its underlying tissue.

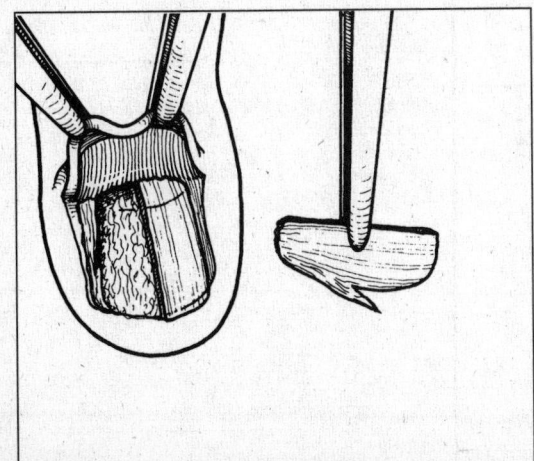

The toenail is removed and the nailbed along the affected side is scraped to prevent recurrence, if possible. The nailbed hardens slowly. A new nail usually grows to replace the removed one.

NASAL POLYPS REMOVAL
(Nasal Polypectomy)

 GENERAL INFORMATION

DEFINITION—Removal of nasal polyps, accumulations of fluid under the membrane lining inside the nose.

BODY PARTS INVOLVED—Nose and its membrane lining.

REASONS FOR SURGERY—Restoration of normal breathing.

SURGICAL RISK INCREASES WITH—Use of some prescription and nonprescription drugs. Inform your doctor of any drugs, medications, or vitamin and herb supplements you are using or have used in the last month.

 WHAT TO EXPECT

WHO OPERATES—Ear, nose and throat specialist (otolaryngologist).

WHERE PERFORMED—Doctor's office, hospital or outpatient surgical facility.

DIAGNOSTIC TESTS—Often, none required. Sometimes, blood and urine studies are done before surgery.

ANESTHESIA
- Local anesthesia by topical application.
- Local anesthesia by injection.

DESCRIPTION OF OPERATION
- The nose is held open with a speculum.
- The polyps are located, clamped and removed with a wire loop.
- Bleeding is controlled with electrocautery.
- Petroleum jelly and gauze may be applied to the surgical area to prevent bleeding. Your doctor will remove this dressing, usually 3 to 4 days after surgery.

POSSIBLE COMPLICATIONS
- Excessive bleeding.
- Surgical-wound infection.

AVERAGE HOSPITAL STAY—0 to 1 day.

PROBABLE OUTCOME—Expect complete healing without complications. Allow about 2 weeks for recovery from surgery.

 POSTOPERATIVE CARE

GENERAL MEASURES
- Don't blow your nose for the first 3 days after surgery.
- Beginning 24 hours after surgery, apply warm compresses to the nose to relieve discomfort. Do this for 15 to 20 minutes several times daily, for as long as needed.

MEDICATION
- Your doctor may prescribe:
  Pain relievers. Don't take prescription pain medication longer than 4 to 7 days. Use only as much as you need.
  Antibiotics to fight or prevent infection.
- You may use nonprescription drugs, such as acetaminophen, to relieve pain. Avoid aspirin.

ACTIVITY—Usually, no restrictions.

DIET—Eat a well-balanced diet to promote healing.

 CALL YOUR DOCTOR IF

- Pain, swelling, redness, drainage or bleeding increase in the surgical area.
- You develop signs of infection, including headache, muscle aches, dizziness or a general ill feeling and fever.
- You experience nausea or vomiting.
- New, unexplained symptoms develop. Drugs used in treatment may produce side effects.

NASAL POLYPS REMOVAL
(Nasal Polypectomy)

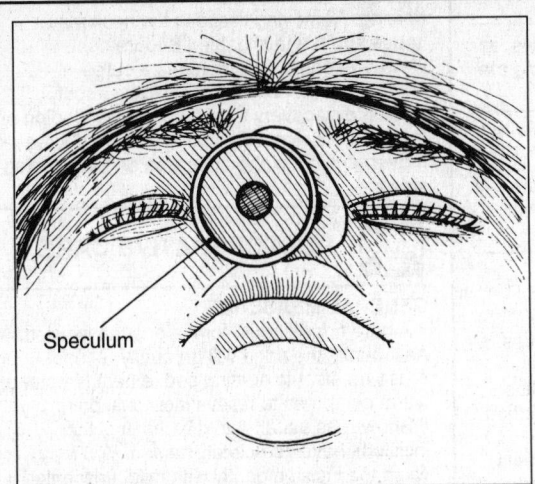

A speculum is used to visualize polyps inside the nose.

Speculum

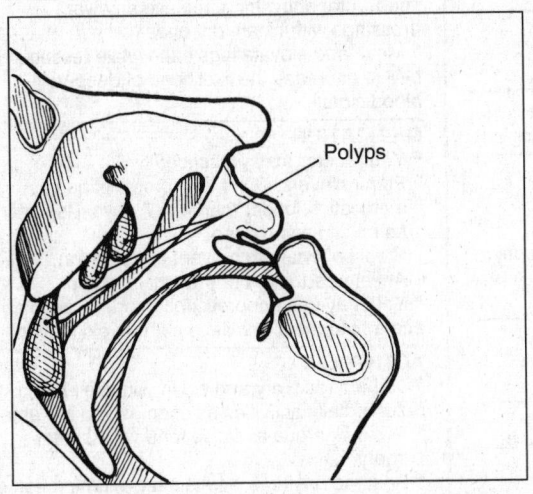

With the speculum in place, the polyps are visually located by the operator.

Polyps

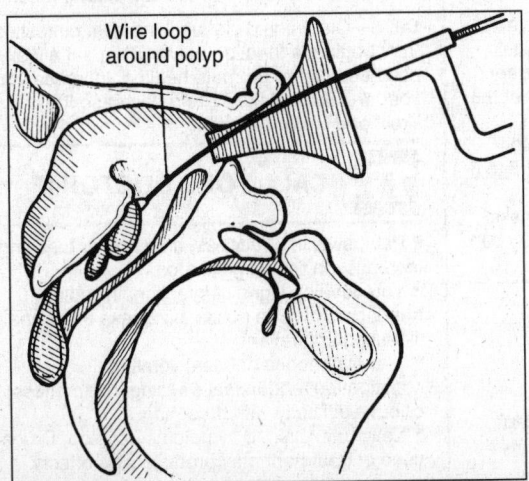

Wire loop around polyp

The polyps are clamped and removed with a wire snare.
- Following surgery, the nose is generally packed with petroleum jelly and gauze to prevent bleeding. This pack will be removed at a later time by your doctor.

NECK, RADICAL DISSECTION OF

 GENERAL INFORMATION

DEFINITION—Removal of the lymph nodes, a large muscle, and some of the nerves along the side of the neck.

BODY PARTS INVOLVED—Neck muscles; lymph glands; windpipe.

REASONS FOR SURGERY—Cancer in the oral cavity or neck, which will spread to other parts of the body if not removed.

SURGICAL RISK INCREASES WITH
- Adults over 60; obesity; smoking.
- Poor nutrition.
- Recent illness, especially respiratory illness.
- Alcoholism.
- Chronic illness, especially diabetes mellitus.
- Use of some prescription and nonprescription drugs. Inform your doctor of any drugs, medications, or vitamin and herb supplements you are using or have used in the last month.

 WHAT TO EXPECT

WHO OPERATES—Ear, nose and throat specialist or general surgeon (otolaryngologist).

WHERE PERFORMED—Hospital.

DIAGNOSTIC TESTS
- Before surgery: Blood and urine studies; x-rays of chest; ECG; CT scan; needle biopsy; open biopsy (see Glossary for all).
- After surgery: Blood studies.

ANESTHESIA—General anesthesia by injection and inhalation with an airway tube placed in the windpipe.

DESCRIPTION OF OPERATION
- An incision shaped like an "H" is made in the neck. Skin flaps are separated from the underlying tissue.
- The lymph glands, muscles, jugular vein and connective tissue are cut free and removed.
- Sometimes, a tracheostomy (see in Surgery section) is performed. In other cases, part of the jaw and tongue are also removed.
- Tubes are left in the surgical area to drain secretions; the tubes are usually removed 3 to 5 days following surgery.
- The connective tissue is closed, and the skin is closed with sutures or clips, which usually can be removed about 1 week after surgery.

POSSIBLE COMPLICATIONS
- Excessive bleeding.
- Surgical-wound infection.
- Restricted breathing.
- Permanent weakness of lower lip.
- Inadvertent injury to the large blood vessels and nerves in the neck, tip of the lung, thoracic duct or laryngeal nerve.

AVERAGE HOSPITAL STAY—3 to 5 days.

PROBABLE OUTCOME—Expect complete healing. Removing tissue in the neck may cause some unavoidable disfigurement. However, some cancers can be cured completely with this surgery. Allow about 4 weeks for recovery from surgery. Depending on the muscles removed, you may have decreased movement in the shoulder area on the affected side.

 POSTOPERATIVE CARE

GENERAL MEASURES
- A hard ridge should form along the incision. As it heals, the ridge will gradually recede.
- Use an electric heating pad, a heat lamp or a warm compress to relieve incisional pain.
- Shower as usual. Avoid baths until the incisions have completely healed. You may wash the incision gently with mild, unscented soap. After showering, replace any wet dressings with clean, dry ones.
- Move and elevate legs often while resting in bed to decrease the likelihood of deep-vein blood clots.

MEDICATION
- Your doctor may prescribe:
  Pain relievers. Don't take prescription pain medication longer than 4 to 7 days. Use only as much as you need.
  Stool softeners to prevent constipation.
  Antibiotics to fight or prevent infection.
- You may use nonprescription drugs, such as acetaminophen, to relieve pain. Avoid aspirin.

ACTIVITY
- To help recovery and aid in your well-being, resume daily activities as soon as you are able.
- Avoid vigorous exercise for 6 weeks after surgery.
- Resume driving 5 weeks after returning home.

DIET—Clear liquid diet until the gastrointestinal tract begins to function again. Then eat a well-balanced diet to promote healing. Increase your fiber and fluid intake to help decrease the likelihood of constipation.

 CALL YOUR DOCTOR IF

- Pain, swelling, redness, drainage or bleeding increases in the surgical area.
- You develop signs of infection, including headache, muscle aches, dizziness or a general ill feeling and fever.
- You experience nausea; vomiting; constipation; abdominal swelling; hoarseness; or have difficulty with breathing.
- New, unexplained symptoms develop. Drugs used in treatment may produce side effects.

NECK, RADICAL DISSECTION OF

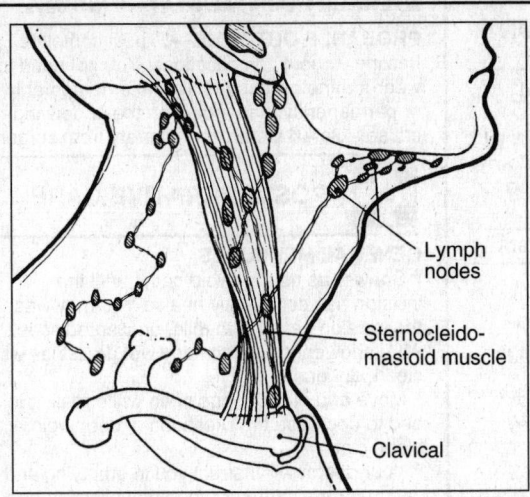

The lymph nodes, muscle and bone in the neck.

Lymph nodes

Sternocleido-mastoid muscle

Clavical

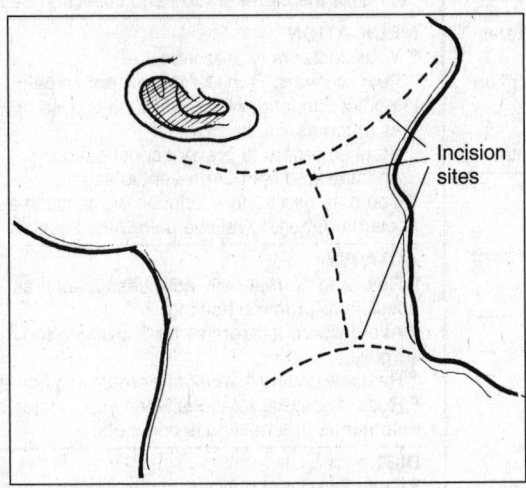

An illustration of the usual incision sites for radical neck dissection.

Incision sites

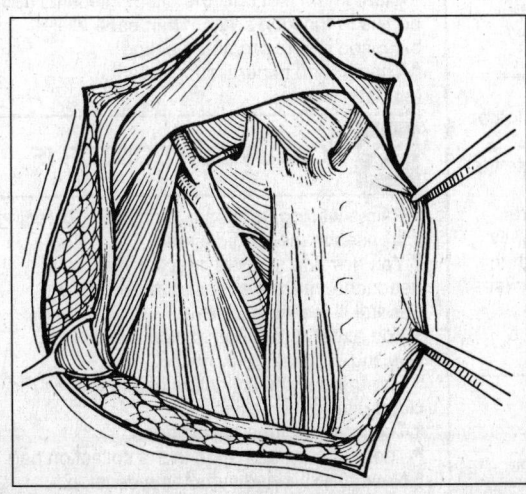

The lymph glands, muscles and connective tissue are cut free and removed.
- Sometimes a tracheostomy is performed to allow free passage of air following surgery.
- Tubes are left in the surgical area to drain secretions (not illustrated).
- The connective tissues are closed and the skin is closed with sutures or clips, which usually can be removed about 1 week after surgery (not illustrated).

NEPHROSTOMY, PERCUTANEOUS
(Nephrolithotomy, Percutaneous)

 GENERAL INFORMATION

DEFINITION—Creating a puncture wound through the skin and muscles of the back directly into the collecting system of the kidney (where urine is collected before traveling down the ureter to the bladder) and placing a tube for access or drainage.

BODY PARTS INVOLVED—Kidney; ureter.

REASONS FOR SURGERY
• To create an opening into the kidney to maintain temporary or permanent urinary drainage when there is a temporary blockage downstream toward the bladder.
• To provide access to remove or break up stones in the collecting system of the kidney.

SURGICAL RISK INCREASES WITH
• Adults over 60; newborns and infants.
• Obesity; smoking; poor nutrition.
• Recent or chronic illness, especially diabetes mellitus or alcoholism.
• Use of some prescription and nonprescription drugs. Inform your doctor of any drugs, medications, or vitamin and herb supplements you are using or have used in the last month.

 WHAT TO EXPECT

WHO OPERATES—General surgeon or urologist.

WHERE PERFORMED—Hospital.

DIAGNOSTIC TESTS
• Before surgery: Blood and urine studies; ultrasound; CT scan; IVP; cystoscopy (see Glossary for all).
• After surgery: Blood and urine studies.

ANESTHESIA—General anesthesia by injection and inhalation with an airway tube placed in the windpipe.

DESCRIPTION OF OPERATION
• An small incision is made, usually in the left or right flank, but sometimes in the abdomen.
• A special needle-like device is passed into the kidney.
• A catheter is passed through the puncture wound into the collecting system of the kidney.
• Stone removal may be accomplished with this procedure, or by pulverization by lithotripsy (see in Surgery section).
• Urine produced by this kidney reaches the outside through the catheter.

POSSIBLE COMPLICATIONS
• Excessive bleeding; blood clots.
• Surgical-wound infection.
• Inadvertent injury to the vena cava or other organs near the kidney.

AVERAGE HOSPITAL STAY—0 to 3 days.

PROBABLE OUTCOME—Expect complete healing without complications. You will need to wear a urine collection bag, either temporarily or permanently, depending on the underlying cause. Allow 4 weeks for recovery from surgery.

 POSTOPERATIVE CARE

GENERAL MEASURES
• Shower as usual. Avoid baths until the incision has completely healed You may wash the incision gently with mild, unscented soap. After showering, replace any wet dressings with clean, dry ones.
• Move and elevate legs often while resting in bed to decrease the likelihood of deep-vein blood clots.
• Your doctor will instruct you in emptying and caring for the catheter tube and collection bag.

MEDICATION
• Your doctor may prescribe:
  Pain relievers. Don't take prescription pain medication longer than 4 to 7 days. Use only as much as you need.
  Stool softeners to prevent constipation.
  Antibiotics to fight or prevent infection.
• You may use nonprescription drugs, such as acetaminophen, to relieve pain. Avoid aspirin.

ACTIVITY
• Return to normal daily activities as soon as possible to promote healing.
• Avoid vigorous exercise for 2 weeks after surgery.
• Resume driving 1 week after returning home.
• Resume sexual relations when your doctor determines that healing is complete.

DIET
• Clear liquid diet until the gastrointestinal tract begins to function again. Then eat a well-balanced diet to promote healing.
• Vitamin and mineral supplements (sometimes).

 CALL YOUR DOCTOR IF

• Pain, swelling, redness, drainage or bleeding increases in the surgical area.
• You develop signs of infection, including headache, muscle aches, dizziness or a general ill feeling and fever.
• You experience constipation, abdominal swelling, nausea, or vomiting.
• The urine in the collection bag becomes red, cloudy, or foul-smelling.
• The catheter tube is dislodged.
• There is very little urine in the collection bag.
• New, unexplained symptoms develop.

NEPHROSTOMY, PERCUTANEOUS
(Nephrolithotomy, Percutaneous)

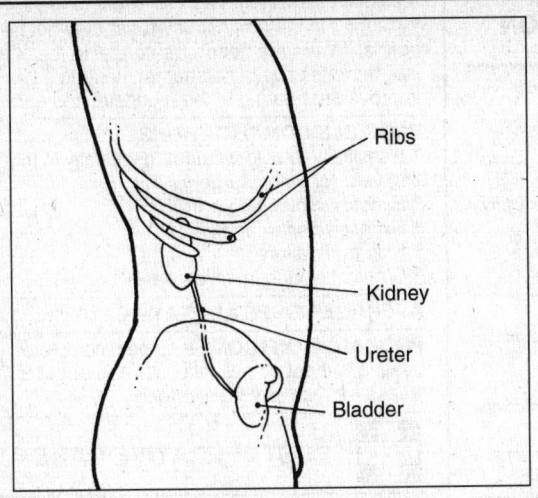

An illustration of a patient's right flank showing the kidney and surrounding structures.

Ribs

Kidney

Ureter

Bladder

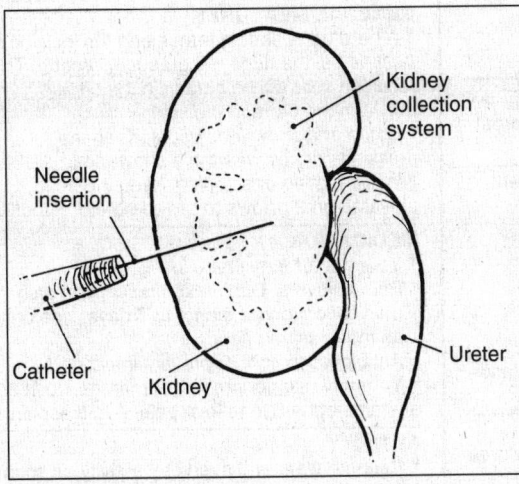

A special needle-like device is passed into the kidney. A catheter is passed through the puncture wound and into the collecting system of the kidney.

Kidney collection system

Needle insertion

Catheter

Kidney

Ureter

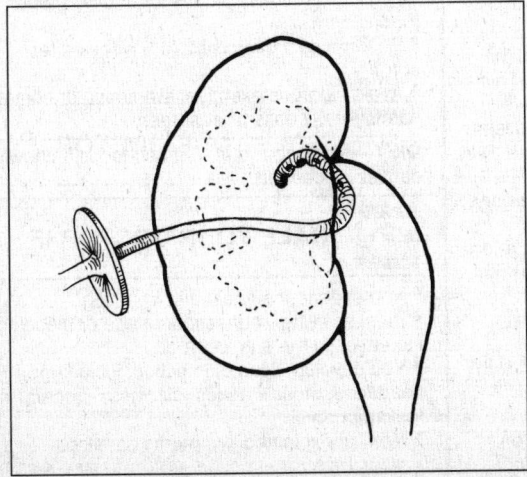

Urine produced by this kidney reaches the outside through the catheter.

SURGERIES

OTOPLASTY
(Ear Plastic Surgery)

GENERAL INFORMATION

DEFINITION—Cosmetic or reconstructive surgery on the outer ear.

BODY PARTS INVOLVED—Ears.

REASONS FOR SURGERY
- Improve appearance of the outer ear (usually to flatten protruding ears).
- To construct or repair a missing or badly damaged ear.

SURGICAL RISK INCREASES WITH
- Previous severe ear injury such as burn or extensive laceration.
- Diabetes mellitus.
- Use of some prescription and nonprescription drugs. Inform your doctor of any drugs, medications, or vitamin and herb supplements you are using or have used in the last month.

WHAT TO EXPECT

WHO OPERATES—Plastic surgeon, reconstructive surgeon, or ear, nose and throat specialist.

WHERE PERFORMED—Hospital; outpatient facility, well-equipped doctor's office.

DIAGNOSTIC TESTS
- Before surgery: Blood and urine studies.
- After surgery: Usually none necessary.

ANESTHESIA
- Local anesthesia by injection.
- General anesthesia by injection and inhalation with an airway tube placed in the windpipe.

DESCRIPTION OF OPERATION
To flatten protruding ears (several procedures are available, one is described here):
- A flap of skin is removed from the back of each ear.
- The underlying cartilage is remolded and the two edges of the wound stitched together. This brings the ear closer to the head.
- Bulky dressings are applied to the ear and left on for a few days. They are replaced by a headband that is worn for several weeks. Stitches are removed about a week after surgery.
For a missing or badly damaged ear:
- The procedure is extensive and complex and normally involves more than one operation with long intervals of healing in-between.
- A piece of rib cartilage is removed and sculptured to resemble a normal ear.
- The cartilage is transferred to a pocket of skin at the site where the ear will be located. Sometimes a skin graft is necessary.
- Dressings are applied to the ear and left on for 10-14 days until healing is completed and

the stitches are removed.
- Hearing in the reconstructed ear may not be normal. When the hearing is normal in the other ear, there is usually no attempt made to improve the hearing in the reconstructed ear.

POSSIBLE COMPLICATIONS
- Sensitivity to cold weather, especially in the first year following surgery.
- Excessive bleeding (rare).
- Excessive scarring (keloid).
- Skin graft failure.
- Surgical wound infection (rare).

AVERAGE HOSPITAL STAY—0 to 1 day.

PROBABLE OUTCOME—Expect complete healing without complications. Allow about 2 weeks for recovery from surgery.

POSTOPERATIVE CARE

GENERAL MEASURES
- A hard ridge should form along the incision. As it heals, the ridge will gradually recede. The resulting scar will be hidden in the crease between the ear and the scalp.
- Bathe and shower as usual. Keep the dressings dry by wearing a shower cap.
- While resting or sleeping, keep the head elevated on 2 pillows to provide greater comfort.

MEDICATION
- Your doctor may prescribe:
  Pain relievers. Don't take prescription pain medication longer than 4 to 7 days. Use only as much as you need.
  Antibiotics to fight or prevent infection.
- You may use nonprescription drugs, such as acetaminophen, to relieve pain. Avoid aspirin.

ACTIVITY
- Resume work and everyday activity as soon as possible (usually 5 days for adults, 1 week for children).
- Resume mild exercise 2 to 3 weeks after surgery.
- Avoid vigorous exercise, swimming or contact sports for 6 weeks after surgery.

DIET—No special diet. Eat soft foods if chewing causes discomfort.

CALL YOUR DOCTOR IF

- You experience nausea or vomiting.
- Pain, swelling, redness, drainage or bleeding increases in the surgical area.
- You develop signs of infection, including headache, muscle aches, dizziness, general ill feeling or fever.
- New, unexplained symptoms develop.

OTOPLASTY
(Ear Plastic Surgery)

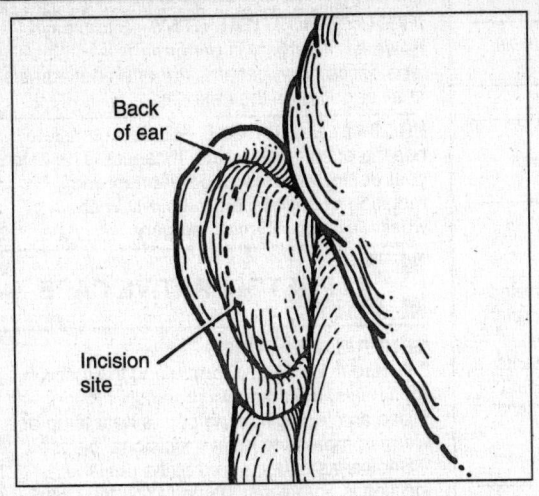

Back
of ear

Incision
site

Anatomy and incision site on the
back of the ear are identified and
marked prior to surgery.

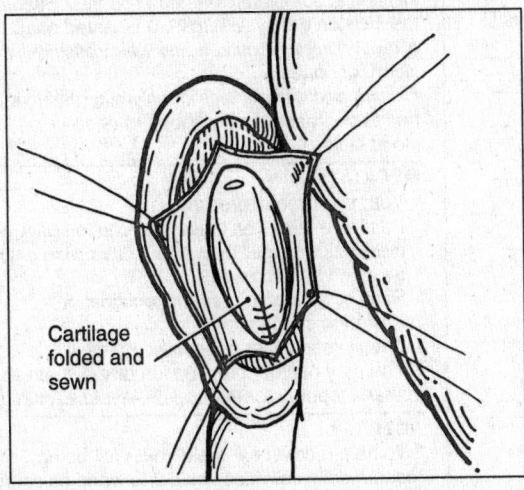

Cartilage
folded and
sewn

Skin is opened revealing underlying
cartilage, which is remolded to bring
ear closer to the head.

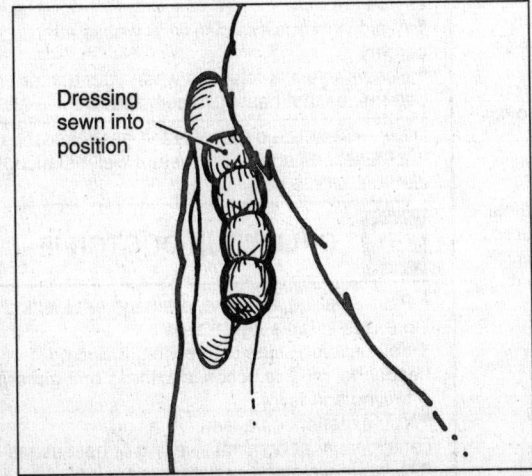

Dressing
sewn into
position

Skin is sewn closed and a dressing is
applied.

OVARIAN CYST OR TUMOR REMOVAL

GENERAL INFORMATION

DEFINITION—Removal of cysts or tumors on an ovary.

BODY PARTS INVOLVED—Ovary, pelvis.

REASONS FOR SURGERY
- Cancer or suspected cancer in the ovaries.
- Rupture or twisting of an ovarian cyst.

SURGICAL RISK INCREASES WITH
- Adults over 60; stress; obesity.
- Poor nutrition; alcoholism; smoking.
- Recent or chronic illness, especially diabetes.
- Use of some prescription and nonprescription drugs. Inform your doctor of any drugs, medications, or vitamin and herb supplements you are using or have used in the last month.

WHAT TO EXPECT

WHO OPERATES—Obstetrician-gynecologist or general surgeon.

WHERE PERFORMED—Hospital.

DIAGNOSTIC TESTS
- Before surgery: Blood and urine studies; CT scan of pelvic organs; laparoscopy or culdoscopy; ultrasound; x-rays of chest, lower abdomen and lower intestinal tract; culdocentesis (see Glossary for all).
- During surgery: Laboratory examination of removed tissue by frozen section (see Glossary).
- After surgery: Blood studies.

ANESTHESIA—General anesthesia by injection and inhalation with an airway tube placed in the windpipe.

DESCRIPTION OF OPERATION
- An incision is made in the abdomen. The abdominal muscles are separated and the peritoneum is opened.
- Blood vessels supplying the ovaries are located, clamped and tied.
- The tumor or cyst in the ovary is located, cut free and removed or the cyst may be destroyed by electrocauterization (see Glossary).
- If examination reveals signs of cancer, the ovary is removed.
- The peritoneum is closed, and the abdominal muscles are sewn together with heavy sutures.
- The skin is closed with sutures or clips, which usually can be removed 10 days after surgery.
- This surgery, under many conditions, can be performed laparoscopically (see Glossary). Your doctor can determine which approach is best for your circumstances.

POSSIBLE COMPLICATIONS
- Excessive bleeding.
- Surgical-wound infection.
- Recurrent cancer.
- Excessive scarring (keloid).

AVERAGE HOSPITAL STAY—3 to 5 days. However, if surgery is performed laparoscopically, patients are often not admitted at all or go home the next day.

PROBABLE OUTCOME—Expect complete healing of surgical wound. If cancer is detected, your doctor will prescribe treatment with radiation or anticancer drugs. Allow about 4 weeks for recovery from surgery.

POSTOPERATIVE CARE

GENERAL MEASURES
- A hard ridge should form along the incision. As it heals, the ridge will gradually recede.
- Use an electric heating pad, a heat lamp or a warm compress to relieve incisional pain.
- Shower as usual. Avoid baths until the incision is completely healed. You may wash the incision gently with mild, unscented soap. After showering, replace any wet dressings with clean, dry ones.
- Move and elevate legs often while resting in bed to decrease the likelihood of deep-vein blood clots.

MEDICATION
- Your doctor may prescribe:
  Pain relievers. Don't take prescription pain medication longer than 4 to 7 days. Use only as much as you need.
  Stool softeners to prevent constipation.
  Hormone supplements.
  Antibiotics to fight or prevent infection.
- You may use nonprescription drugs, such as acetaminophen, for minor pain. Avoid aspirin.

ACTIVITY
- To help recovery and aid your well-being, resume daily activities, including work, as soon as you are able.
- Avoid vigorous exercise for 6 weeks after surgery.
- Resume sexual relations when your doctor determines that healing is complete.

DIET—Clear liquid diet until the gastrointestinal tract functions again. Then eat a well-balanced diet to promote healing.

CALL YOUR DOCTOR IF

- Pain, swelling, redness, drainage or bleeding increases in the surgical area.
- You develop signs of infection, including headache, muscle aches, dizziness or a general ill feeling and fever.
- You experience nausea, vomiting, constipation, abdominal swelling or hot flashes.
- New, unexplained symptoms develop.

OVARIAN CYST OR TUMOR REMOVAL

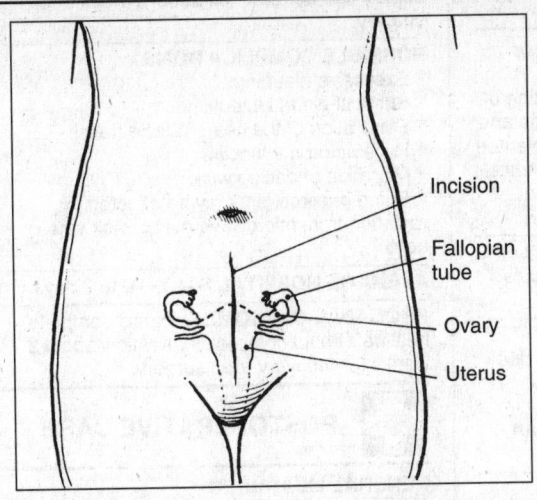

The organs of the female reproductive tract and the usual abdominal incision for this surgical procedure.

Incision

Fallopian tube

Ovary

Uterus

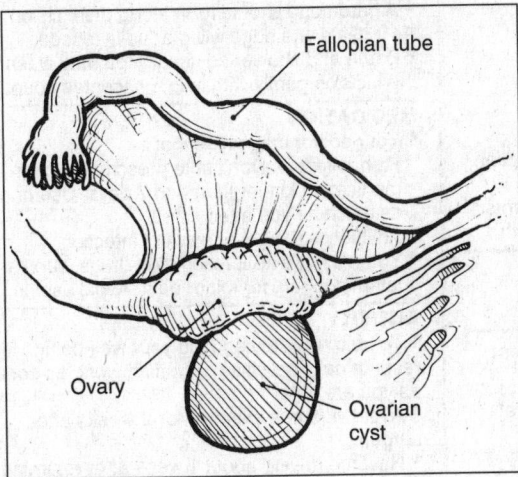

After the incision has been made through the skin and underlying tissue, the tumor or cyst in the ovary is located, cut free and removed.
- If cancer is identified, a wider removal of tissue is indicated.

Fallopian tube

Ovary

Ovarian cyst

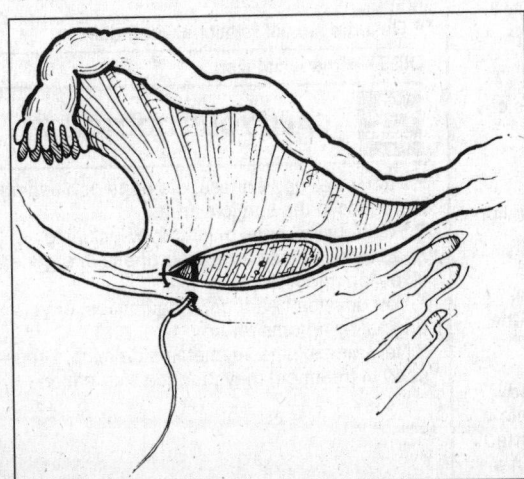

The bed of the ovarian cyst or tumor is sutured closed to prevent bleeding and adhesions.
- The peritoneum is closed. The abdominal muscles are sewn together with heavy sutures and the skin is closed with sutures or clips, which usually can be removed about 10 days after surgery (not illustrated).

SURGERIES

PACEMAKER IMPLANTATION

 GENERAL INFORMATION

DEFINITION—Placement of a temporary or permanent pacemaker into the chest wall. A pacemaker is an electronic device consisting of an electrode connected to the heart muscle and a regulatory device and power source implanted under the skin. It provides regular, mild electric shocks that stimulate the heart muscle and maintain normal heartbeat.

BODY PARTS INVOLVED—Veins in neck or under collarbone; tissue under the skin below the collarbone; heart.

REASONS FOR SURGERY
- Regulation of heartbeat that has slowed due to heart disease.
- Treatment of heart block.
- Following cardiac surgery to regulate heart rate.

SURGICAL RISK INCREASES WITH
- Adults over 60.
- Obesity.
- Smoking.
- Excess alcohol consumption.
- Recent or chronic illness.
- Diabetes mellitus.
- Use of some prescription and nonprescription drugs. Inform your doctor of any drugs, medications, or vitamin and herb supplements you are using or have used in the last month.

 WHAT TO EXPECT

WHO OPERATES—Cardiovascular surgeon, cardiologist (sometimes).

WHERE PERFORMED—Outpatient surgical facility or hospital.

DIAGNOSTIC TESTS
- Before surgery: Blood and urine studies; x-rays of chest; ECG (see Glossary).
- During surgery: ECG; fluoroscopy (see Glossary for both).
- After surgery: ECG (see Glossary); x-rays of chest.

ANESTHESIA
- Local anesthesia by injection.
- General anesthesia by injection and inhalation with an airway tube placed in the windpipe.

DESCRIPTION OF OPERATION
- A needle is inserted in a vein under the collarbone. An electrode is passed through the vein into the heart. The implantation site is confirmed.
- The electrode is attached to the power and regulating units. A small incision is made below the collarbone, and the entire device is inserted into the incision and placed under the skin in a pouch created from tissue.

- The skin is closed with suture material, which usually can be removed about 1 week after surgery.

POSSIBLE COMPLICATIONS
- Excessive bleeding.
- Surgical-wound infection.
- Perforation of the heart muscle (rare).
- Pacemaker malfunction.
- Migration of pacing wire.
- Some pacemakers may be affected by radiation from microwave ovens. Ask your doctor.

AVERAGE HOSPITAL STAY—0 to 2 days.

PROBABLE OUTCOME—Expect complete healing without complications. Allow about 2 weeks for recovery from surgery.

 POSTOPERATIVE CARE

GENERAL MEASURES
- A hard ridge should form along the incision. As it heals, the ridge will gradually recede.
- Bathe and shower as usual. You may wash the incision gently with mild, unscented soap.

MEDICATION
- Your doctor may prescribe:
  Pain relievers. Don't take prescription pain medication longer than 4 to 7 days. Use only as much as you need.
  Antibiotics to fight or prevent infection.
- You may use nonprescription drugs, such as acetaminophen, for minor pain. Avoid aspirin.

ACTIVITY
- To help recovery and aid your well-being, resume daily activities, including work, as soon as you are able.
- Avoid vigorous exercise for 2 weeks after surgery.
- Resume driving about 1 week after returning home.
- Resume sexual relations when able.

DIET—No special diet.

 CALL YOUR DOCTOR IF

- Pain, swelling, redness, drainage or bleeding increases in the surgical area.
- You develop signs of infection, including headache, muscle aches, dizziness or a general ill feeling and fever.
- You develop heartbeat irregularities, or your original symptoms return.
- New, unexplained symptoms develop. Drugs used in treatment may produce side effects.

PACEMAKER IMPLANTATION

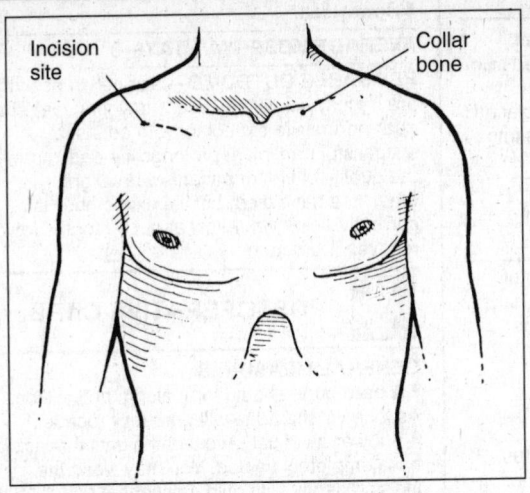

An illustration of the chest, collarbone and incision site generally used for pacemaker insertion.

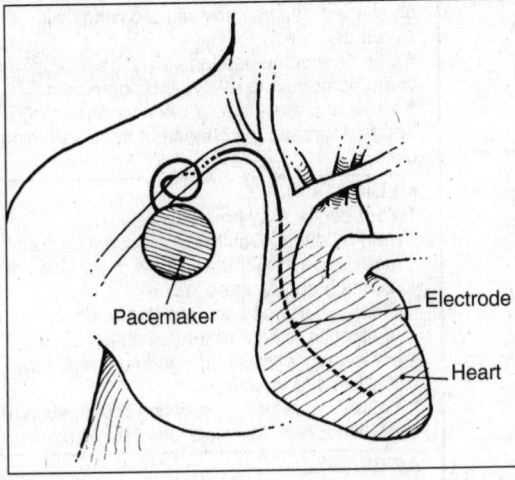

An electrode is passed through a vein near the incision site, which ends inside the heart cavity.
- The electrode is attached to the power and regulating units. The entire device is inserted under the skin into a pouch created from tissue under the collarbone.

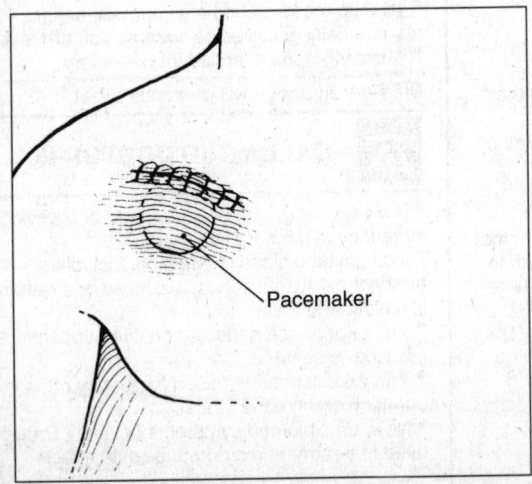

The pacemaker in place. The skin has been closed with sutures that usually can be removed about 1 week after surgery.

PANCREAS TRANSPLANTATION

 GENERAL INFORMATION

DEFINITION—Replacement of a diseased pancreas with a healthy pancreas obtained from a donor with compatible immunological characteristics. The duodenum is also replaced to allow drainage of pancreatic secretions into the gastrointestinal tract.

BODY PARTS INVOLVED—Diseased or abnormal pancreas and duodenum; healthy donor pancreas and duodenum.

REASONS FOR SURGERY—Prevention of complications of severe diabetes mellitus, such as kidney failure and damage to the retinas.

SURGICAL RISK INCREASES WITH
- Obesity; smoking; stress.
- Poor nutrition.
- Excess alcohol consumption.
- Recent or chronic illness; diabetes mellitus.
- Use of some prescription and nonprescription drugs. Inform your doctor of any drugs, medications, or vitamin and herb supplements you are using or have used in the last month.

 WHAT TO EXPECT

WHO OPERATES—General surgeon.

WHERE PERFORMED—Hospital.

DIAGNOSTIC TESTS
- Before surgery: Evaluation of all body systems; immune-system and pancreas matching procedures.
- After surgery: Blood studies.

ANESTHESIA—General anesthesia by injection and inhalation with an airway tube placed in the windpipe.

DESCRIPTION OF OPERATION
- The pancreas is removed from the donor, chilled and preserved up to 12 hours until surgery.
- An incision is made under the ribs.
- The abdominal muscles are divided and the peritoneal cavity is entered.
- The pancreas and duodenum are cut free and removed.
- The donor pancreas and duodenum are positioned and connected to blood vessels.
- Sometimes, only the cells of the pancreas that produce insulin (islet cells) are transplanted. In some patients, this is all that is necessary to re-establish normal function.
- The peritoneum and muscles are closed. The skin is closed with sutures or clips, which usually can be removed in 1 week.

POSSIBLE COMPLICATIONS
- Excessive bleeding.
- Surgical-wound infection.
- Rejection of transplant.
- Development of a pancreatic fistula.
- Bowel leak.

AVERAGE HOSPITAL STAY—3 weeks.

PROBABLE OUTCOME—Islet-cell transplants are usually successful in giving young diabetics near-normal life expectancy. In adults, a successful transplant prolongs life and improves the quality of life for patients who might otherwise have died, but life expectancy is currently unknown. Allow about 6 months for recovery from surgery.

 POSTOPERATIVE CARE

GENERAL MEASURES
- A hard ridge should form along the incision. As it heals, the ridge will gradually recede.
- Shower as usual. Avoid baths until the incision has completely healed. You may wash the incision gently with mild, unscented soap. After showering, replace any wet dressings with clean, dry ones.
- Use an electric heating pad, a heat lamp or a warm compress to relieve incisional pain.
- Move and elevate legs often while resting in bed to decrease the chance of deep-vein blood clots.

MEDICATION
- Your doctor may prescribe:
  Pain relievers. Don't take prescription pain medication longer than 4 to 7 days. Use only as much as you need.
  Stool softeners to prevent constipation.
  Antibiotics to fight or prevent infection.
  Immunosuppressant drugs to decrease the likelihood of rejection.
- You may use nonprescription drugs, such as acetaminophen, for minor pain. Avoid aspirin.

ACTIVITY
- To help recovery and aid your well-being, resume daily activities as soon as you are able.
- Avoid vigorous exercise for 6 months.

DIET—You doctor will prescribe a diet.

 CALL YOUR DOCTOR IF

- Pain, swelling, redness, drainage or bleeding increases in the surgical area.
- You develop signs of infection, including headache, muscle aches, dizziness or a general ill feeling and fever.
- You experience nausea, vomiting, abdominal swelling or constipation.
- You experience increased frequency of urination or increased thirst.
- New, unexplained symptoms develop. Drugs used in treatment may produce side effects.

PANCREAS TRANSPLANTATION

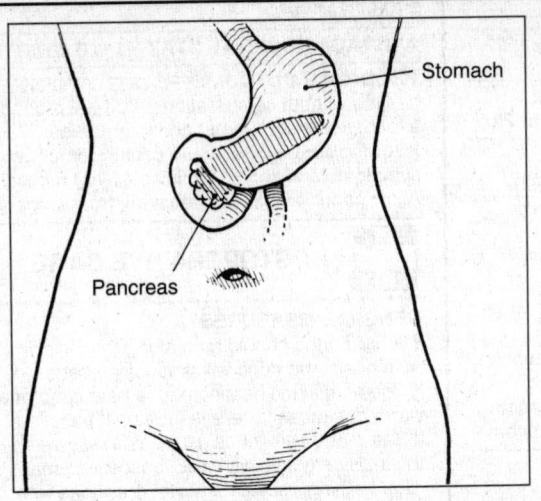

An illustration of the normal location and anatomy of the pancreas.

Stomach

Pancreas

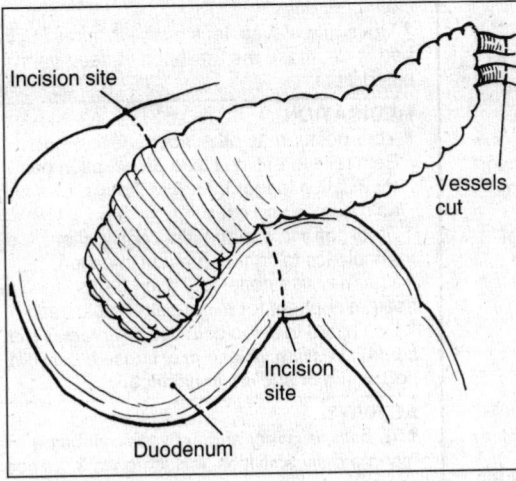

The diseased pancreas and the duodenum are cut free and removed.

Incision site

Vessels cut

Incision site

Duodenum

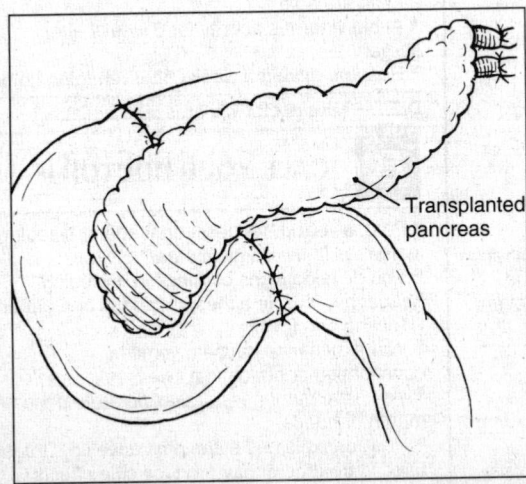

The donor pancreas and duodenum are positioned and connected to the blood vessels.
• Following transplant, muscles and skin are closed with sutures or clips that usually can be removed about 1 week after surgery (not illustrated).

Transplanted pancreas

PARATHYROIDECTOMY

GENERAL INFORMATION

DEFINITION—Removal of parathyroid tumors or the parathyroid glands.

BODY PARTS INVOLVED—Parathyroid glands (at least 4 glands, sometimes up to 7).

REASONS FOR SURGERY
- Hyperparathyroidism (see Illness section).
- Cancer or suspected cancer.

SURGICAL RISK INCREASES WITH
- Obesity; smoking; stress.
- Poor nutrition; alcoholism.
- Recent or chronic illness.
- Diabetes mellitus.
- Use of some prescription and nonprescription drugs. Inform your doctor of any drugs, medications, or vitamin and herb supplements you are using or have used in the last month.

WHAT TO EXPECT

WHO OPERATES—General surgeon.

WHERE PERFORMED—Hospital.

DIAGNOSTIC TESTS
- Before surgery: Blood and urine studies; x-rays of upper gastrointestinal tract; CT scan; ultrasound; fine needle biopsy; thyroid scan; (see Glossary for all).
- During surgery: Laboratory examination of removed tissue by frozen section (see Glossary).
- After surgery: Blood studies; laboratory examination of removed tissue.

ANESTHESIA—General anesthesia by injection and inhalation with an airway tube placed in the windpipe.

DESCRIPTION OF OPERATION
- An incision is made in the neck just under the Adam's apple.
- The parathyroid glands are located. A section of one is cut free, removed, frozen and examined.
- If cancer is found, all or part of the thyroid glands are removed.
- If the lymph glands on the neck are also involved, they will also be removed.
- If a benign tumor is detected, it is removed. If the tissue is an enlarged, overactive gland rather than a tumor, all except one of the other parathyroid glands are cut free and removed. One of the glands is left in place to help prevent hypoparathyroidism.

POSSIBLE COMPLICATIONS
- Excessive bleeding.
- Surgical-wound infection.
- Hypoparathyroidism.

- Inadvertent injury to thyroid gland or vocal-cord nerves.
- Kidney stones.

AVERAGE HOSPITAL STAY—1 to 3 days.

PROBABLE OUTCOME—Expect complete healing without complications. You will probably experience a sore throat and raspy voice following surgery; these are usually temporary symptoms and should diminish as you recover. Allow about 4 weeks for recovery from surgery.

POSTOPERATIVE CARE

GENERAL MEASURES
- A hard ridge should form along the incision. As it heals, the ridge will gradually recede.
- Use an electric heating pad, a heat lamp or a warm compress to relieve incisional pain.
- Bathe and shower as usual. You may wash the incision gently with mild, unscented soap. After bathing, replace any wet dressings with clean, dry ones.
- Move and elevate legs often while resting in bed to decrease the likelihood of deep-vein blood clots.

MEDICATION
- Your doctor may prescribe:
  Pain relievers. Don't take prescription pain medication longer than 4 to 7 days. Use only as much as you need.
  Stool softeners to prevent constipation.
  Antibiotics to fight or prevent infection.
- You may use nonprescription drugs, such as acetaminophen, for minor pain. Avoid aspirin.
- Don't take thiazide diuretics or antacids that contain calcium. These may cause a calcium, potassium or sodium imbalance.

ACTIVITY
- To help recovery and aid your well-being, resume daily activities, including work, as soon as you are able.
- Avoid vigorous activity for 6 weeks after surgery.
- Resume driving 2 weeks after returning home.

DIET—Your doctor will prescribe a diet.

CALL YOUR DOCTOR IF

- Pain, swelling, redness, drainage or bleeding increases in the surgical area.
- You develop signs of infection, including headache, muscle aches, dizziness or a general ill feeling and fever.
- You experience nausea, vomiting, constipation or abdominal swelling.
- You have numbness or tingling around the mouth or hands.
- New, unexplained symptoms develop. Drugs used in treatment may produce side effects.

PARATHYROIDECTOMY

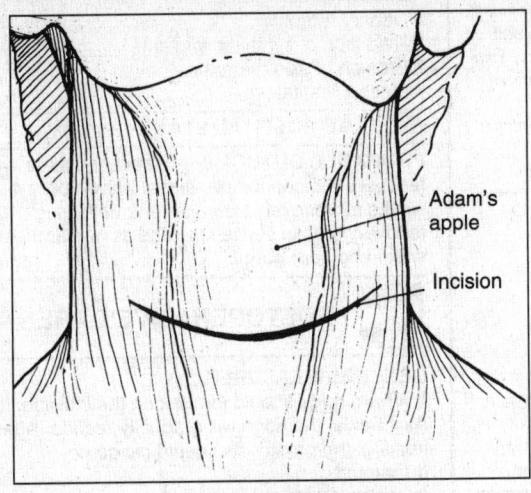

The incision site in the lower part of the neck below the protruding cartilage called the Adam's apple.

Adam's apple

Incision

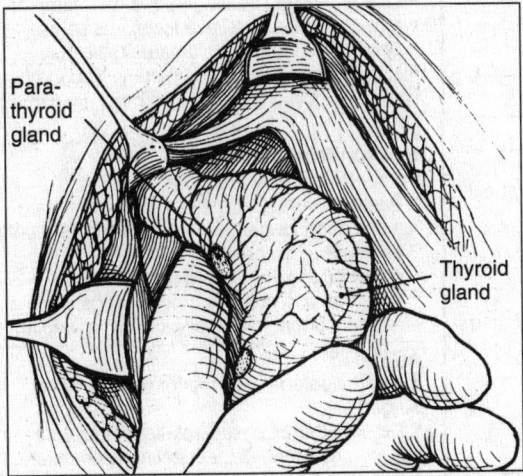

Parathyroid glands are located. Abnormal ones are removed. If the surgery is being performed because of overactivity of the parathyroid glands, rather than a tumor, all except one of the visualized parathyroid glands are cut free and removed.

Para-
thyroid
gland

Thyroid
gland

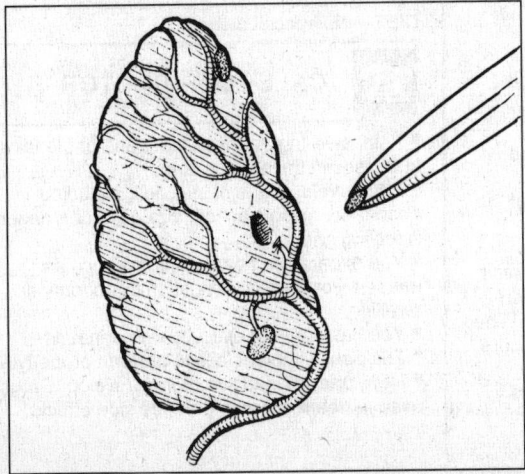

One parathyroid gland removed.
• After the surgery is finished, neck muscles are reapproximated, the tissue below the skin is closed with suture material and the skin is closed with clips.

PENILE IMPLANT

GENERAL INFORMATION

DEFINITION—Insertion of semiflexible plastic bars or an inflatable prosthesis in the penis. The former produces a permanent, partial erection. The latter can be inflated at will.

BODY PARTS INVOLVED—Penis.

REASONS FOR SURGERY—Impotence.

SURGICAL RISK INCREASES WITH
- Obesity.
- Smoking.
- Stress.
- Poor nutrition.
- Recent or chronic illness.
- Alcoholism.
- Diabetes mellitus.
- Use of some prescription and nonprescription drugs. Inform your doctor of any drugs, medications, or vitamin and herb supplements you are using or have used in the last month.

WHAT TO EXPECT

WHO OPERATES—Urologist.

WHERE PERFORMED—Hospital.

DIAGNOSTIC TESTS
- Before surgery: Blood and urine studies; chest x-ray; ultrasound (see Glossary).
- After surgery: Blood studies.

ANESTHESIA
- Spinal anesthesia by injection.
- General anesthesia by injection and inhalation with an airway tube placed in the windpipe.

DESCRIPTION OF OPERATION
Plastic Implant:
- An incision is made in the underside of the penis.
- The tissues on both sides of the urethra are expanded to allow placement of the implants.
- An implant is placed on each side of the urethra.
- The skin is closed with sutures that will be absorbed by the body.

Inflatable Prosthesis:
- Incisions are made in the underside of the penis, the side of the scrotum, and on the abdomen, several inches above the base of the penis.
- The penile tissue is stretched to allow placement of the prosthesis. The fluid reservoir for the prosthesis is implanted under the skin above the bladder at the base of the pelvis. The prosthesis can be inflated by applying pressure on the reservoir.
- The skin is closed with sutures that will be absorbed by the body.

POSSIBLE COMPLICATIONS
- Surgical-wound infection.
- Excessive bleeding.
- Urinary retention.
- Rejection of synthetic implants.
- Erosion of skin or urethra.
- Mechanical failure.

AVERAGE HOSPITAL STAY—1 to 2 days.

PROBABLE OUTCOME—Expect complete recovery without complications. Allow about 4 weeks for recovery from surgery. Following recovery, penile sensations and sexual arousal should be near normal.

POSTOPERATIVE CARE

GENERAL MEASURES
- A hard ridge should form along the incision. As it heals, the ridge will gradually recede. After healing, the prosthesis should cause no discomfort.
- Use an electric heating pad, a heat lamp or a warm compress to relieve incisional pain.
- Shower as usual. Avoid baths until the incisions have healed completely. You may wash the incisions gently with mild, unscented soap.

MEDICATION
- Your doctor may prescribe:
  Pain relievers. Don't take prescription pain medication longer than 4 to 7 days. Use only as much as you need.
  Antibiotics to fight or prevent infection.
- You may use nonprescription drugs, such as acetaminophen, for minor pain. Avoid aspirin.

ACTIVITY
- Avoid vigorous exercise for 6 weeks after surgery.
- Do not attempt sexual relations until your surgeon determines that healing is complete.
- Resume driving 1 week after returning home.

DIET—No special diet.

CALL YOUR DOCTOR IF
- Pain, swelling, redness, drainage or bleeding increases in the surgical area.
- You develop signs of infection, including headache, muscle aches, dizziness or a general ill feeling and fever.
- You experience new symptoms such as nausea, vomiting, constipation or abdominal swelling.
- You have pain or difficulty with urination.
- The penile implant fails to perform properly.
- New, unexplained symptoms develop. Drugs used in treatment may produce side effects.

PENILE IMPLANT

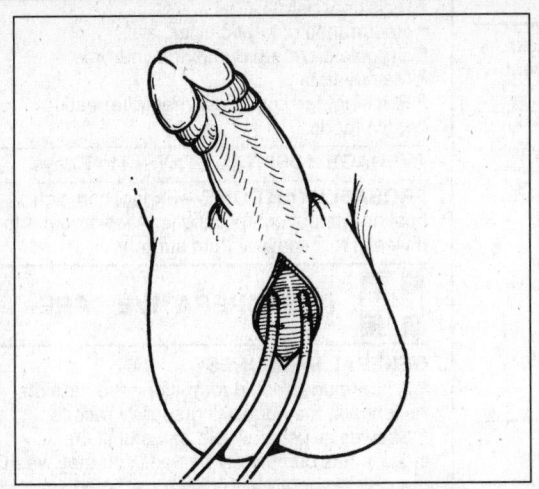

The incision for a penile implant, which may be either semi-rigid or an inflatable prosthesis. These drawings illustrate the inflatable form only. The equipment is different for a semi-rigid prosthesis but the principles and techniques for insertion are similar for both procedures.

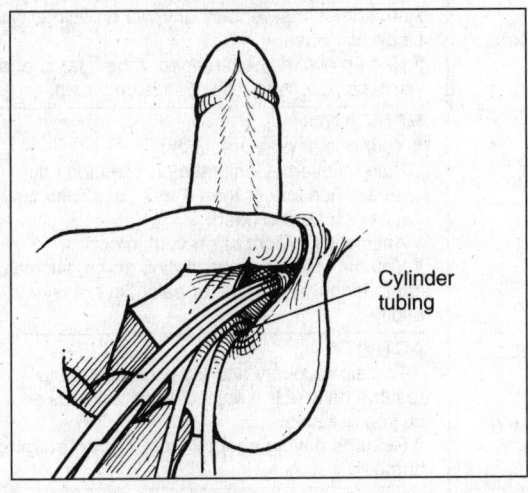

Cylinder tubing

After an incision has been made on the underside of the penis, the tissues on both sides of the urethra are expanded to allow placement of the implants.

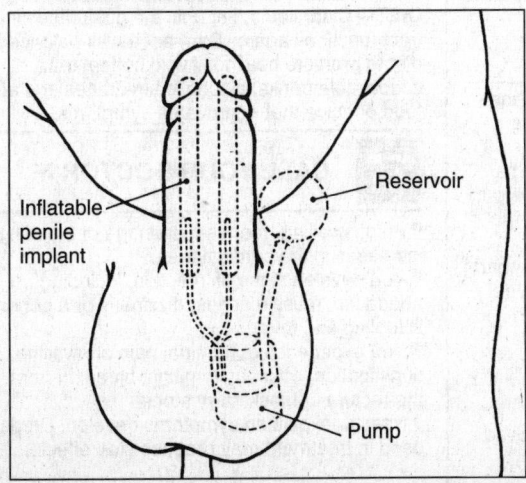

Inflatable penile implant

Reservoir

Pump

Implants in place, surgical incision closed with absorbable sutures.

PEPTIC ULCER SURGERY

 GENERAL INFORMATION

DEFINITION—Surgery to decrease the acid production in the stomach in order to prevent ulcer formation.

BODY PARTS INVOLVED—Esophagus; stomach; duodenum; jejunum; vagas nerves.

REASONS FOR SURGERY—Treatment of complications of peptic ulcers:
• Bleeding.
• Intolerable pain.
• Blockage of stomach contents from emptying.
• Perforation. If an ulcer perforates, the contents of the gastrointestinal tract are dumped into the abdominal cavity, causing peritonitis. This is a medical emergency requiring immediate surgery.

SURGICAL RISK INCREASES WITH
• Adults over 60.
• Chronic illness, especially pancreatitis, hepatitis, alcoholism or diabetes mellitus.
• Poor nutrition, especially vitamin and mineral deficiencies.
• Use of any drugs that irritate the stomach.
• Use of some prescription and nonprescription drugs. Inform your doctor of any drugs, medications, or vitamin and herb supplements you are using or have used in the last month.

 WHAT TO EXPECT

WHO OPERATES—General surgeon.

WHERE PERFORMED—Hospital.

DIAGNOSTIC TESTS
• Before surgery: Blood and urine studies; x-rays of abdomen; endoscopy (see Glossary).
• After surgery: Blood and urine studies; x-rays of abdomen.

ANESTHESIA—General anesthesia by injection and inhalation with an airway tube placed in the windpipe.

DESCRIPTION OF OPERATION—Any of the following procedures is used to perform this surgery:
• Vagotomy and pyloroplasty: The nerves that stimulate stomach-acid production are severed, and the outlet of the stomach that leads to the duodenum is enlarged.
• Gastric resection (antrectomy): The lower part of the stomach that produces acid is removed, and the remaining stomach is attached with sutures to the duodenum or the jejunum.
• Closure of perforated ulcer: The perforated ulcer is closed by various methods.
• Incisions that are made are closed with sutures or clips, which can usually be removed about 1 week after surgery.

POSSIBLE COMPLICATIONS
• Excessive bleeding; surgical-wound infection.
• Incisional hernia.
• Recurrence of peptic ulcer.
• Chronic diarrhea; dumping syndrome.
• Malnutrition.
• Flushing, fainting or diarrhea after eating certain foods.

AVERAGE HOSPITAL STAY—3 to 7 days.

PROBABLE OUTCOME—Expect complete healing without complications. Allow about 4 to 6 weeks for recovery from surgery.

 POSTOPERATIVE CARE

GENERAL MEASURES
• A hard ridge should form along the incision. As it heals, the ridge will gradually recede.
• Shower as usual. Avoid baths until the incision has completely healed. You may wash the incision gently with mild, unscented soap. After showering, replace any wet dressings with clean, dry ones.
• Use an electric heating pad, a heat lamp or a warm compress to relieve incisional pain.

MEDICATION
• Your doctor may prescribe:
  Pain relievers. Don't take prescription pain medication longer than 4 to 7 days. Use only as much as you need.
  Antibiotics to fight or prevent infection.
• You may use nonprescription drugs, such as acetaminophen, for minor pain. Do not take aspirin.

ACTIVITY
• To help recovery and aid your well-being, resume daily activities, including work, as soon as you are able.
• Resume driving about 2 weeks after returning home.

DIET—Clear liquid diet until the gastrointestinal tract functions again. Then eat a well-balanced diet to promote healing. Avoid coffee, tea, cocoa, cola drinks, alcoholic beverages and any food or spice that aggravates symptoms.

 CALL YOUR DOCTOR IF

• Pain, swelling, redness, drainage or bleeding increases in the surgical area.
• You develop signs of infection, including headache, muscle aches, dizziness or a general ill feeling and fever.
• You experience abdominal pain or swelling; constipation; nausea; vomiting; bleeding from the rectum or black, tarry stools.
• New, unexplained symptoms develop. Drugs used in treatment may produce side effects.

PEPTIC ULCER SURGERY

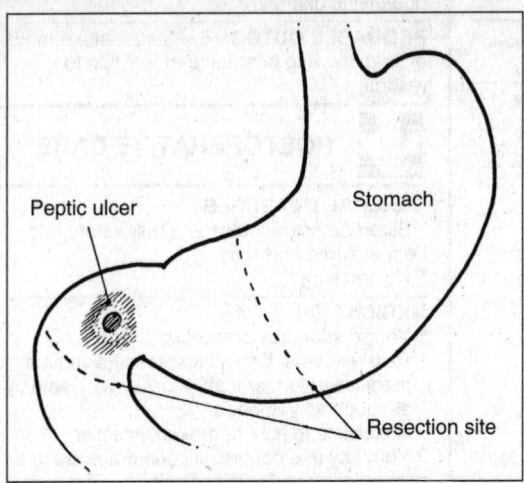

An illustration of the stomach with a peptic ulcer, the incision sites in the lower part of the stomach and the beginning portion of the duodenum.

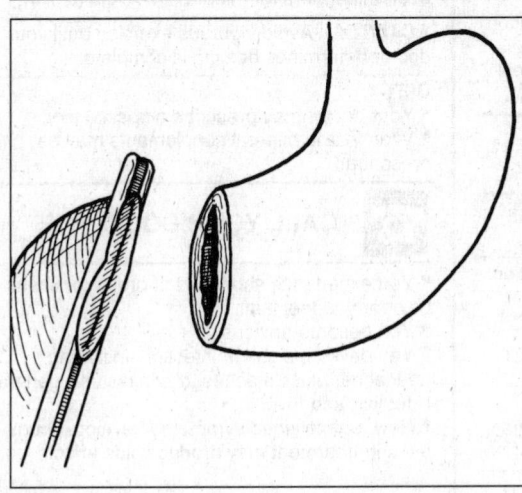

The part of the stomach that produces acid is removed along with the part of the stomach or duodenum that has a peptic ulcer or scarring from a healed or partially healed peptic ulcer.

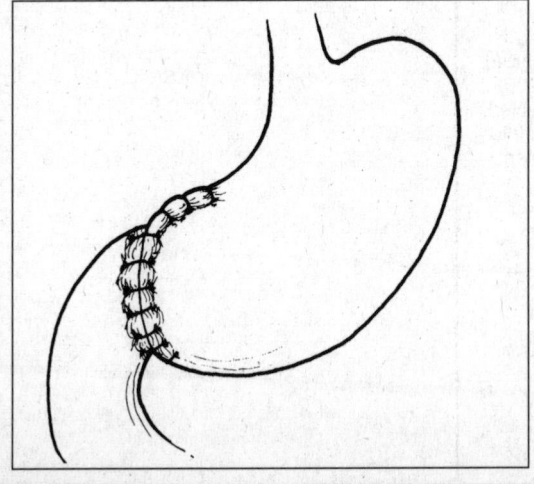

The remaining stomach is attached with sutures to the duodenum or sometimes to the jejunum located lower down in the small intestine.

SURGERIES

PERICARDIOCENTESIS

 GENERAL INFORMATION

DEFINITION—The needle aspiration of excess fluid from the pericardial sac.

BODY PARTS INVOLVED—Pericardium, a 2-layered membrane that surrounds the heart and the roots of the great blood vessels (aorta, pulmonary artery, pulmonary vein and vena cava).

REASONS FOR SURGERY—To remove abnormal fluid collections between the heart and the pericardium. The fluid may be there because the heart is inflamed, infected or injured (fluid may be blood).

SURGICAL RISK INCREASES WITH
- Obesity.
- Smoking.
- Excess alcohol consumption.
- Recent or chronic illness, especially chronic lung disease.
- Use of some prescription and nonprescription drugs. Inform your doctor of any drugs, medications, or vitamin and herb supplements you are using or have used in the last month.

 WHAT TO EXPECT

WHO OPERATES—Cardiothoracic surgeon; cardiologist (sometimes).

WHERE PERFORMED—Hospital or outpatient surgical facility.

DIAGNOSTIC TESTS
- Before surgery: Chest x-rays; CT scan; ECG (see Glossary for both).
- During surgery: Chest x-rays.
- After surgery: Chest x-rays; fluid examination; ECG (see Glossary).

ANESTHESIA—Local anesthesia.

DESCRIPTION OF OPERATION
- Patient lies down on back with upper torso elevated about 60 degrees with arms supported by pillows.
- An I.V. is started and local anesthetic injected.
- The pericardiocentesis needle is inserted into chest wall between the left rib margin adjacent to the breastbone, usually into the space between the 5th and 6th ribs.
- The needle is advanced until fluid can be aspirated.

POSSIBLE COMPLICATIONS
- Heartbeat irregularities.
- Inadvertent organ or artery puncture (rare).
- Hemothorax (see Glossary).
- Pneumothorax (see Glossary).

AVERAGE HOSPITAL STAY—0 to 1 day for procedure. Total time varies according to underlying disorder.

PROBABLE OUTCOME—Successful removal of fluid allowing normal heart function to resume.

 POSTOPERATIVE CARE

GENERAL MEASURES
- Blood pressure, pulse and respiratory rate will be measured and recorded.
- No smoking.

MEDICATION
- Your doctor may prescribe:
  Pain relievers. Don't take prescription pain medication longer than 4 to 7 days. Use only as much as you need.
  Antibiotics to fight or prevent infection.
- You may use nonprescription drugs, such as acetaminophen, for minor pain. Avoid aspirin.

ACTIVITY—Avoid vigorous exercise until your doctor determines healing is complete.

DIET
- Your doctor may prescribe a special diet.
- Vitamin and mineral supplements may be prescribed.

 CALL YOUR DOCTOR IF

- You experience shortness of breath or chest pain, or you feel faint.
- You become anxious.
- You develop signs of infection, including headache, muscle aches, dizziness or a general ill feeling and fever.
- New, unexplained symptoms develop. Drugs used in treatment may produce side effects.

PERICARDIOCENTESIS

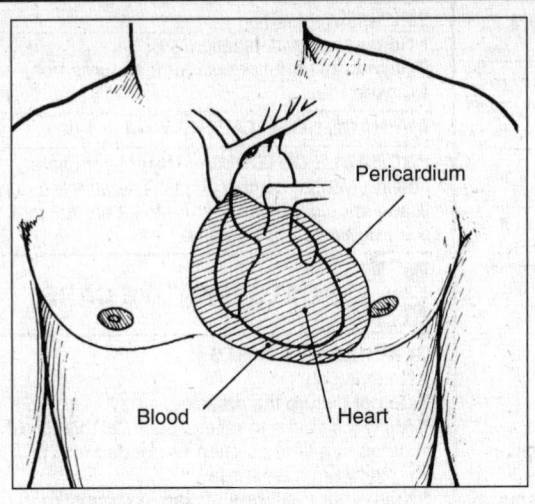

An illustration of the heart and surrounding structures.

Pericardium

Blood

Heart

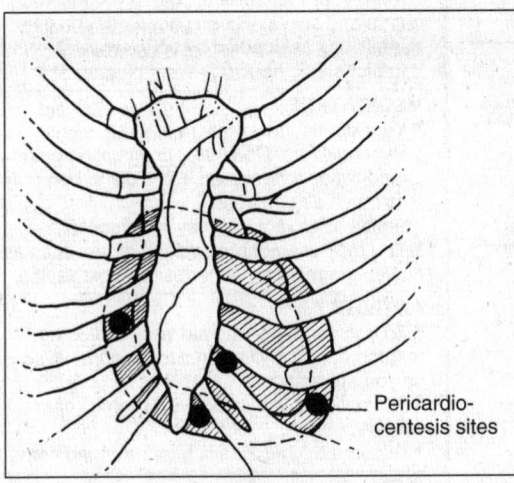

The muscles of the chest are pulled aside to illustrate possible sites for the pericardiocentesis needle to be placed into the pericardium.

Pericardio-centesis sites

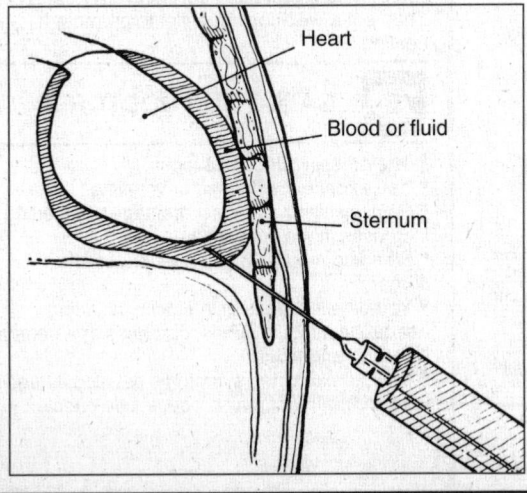

A needle attached to a syringe is advanced until the fluid can be aspirated. After fluid has been removed, the heart can function much more normally.

Heart

Blood or fluid

Sternum

PERIODONTAL SURGERY
(Pyorrhea Treatment)

 GENERAL INFORMATION

DEFINITION—Removal of infected tissue from the gums and reshaping of the bone underlying the gums.

BODY PARTS INVOLVED—Gums; surrounding bone.

REASONS FOR SURGERY—Prevention of the spread of gum infection.

SURGICAL RISK INCREASES WITH
- Adults over 60.
- Smoking.
- Excess alcohol consumption.
- Poor nutrition.
- Recent or chronic illness.
- Diabetes mellitus.
- Use of some prescription and nonprescription drugs. Inform your doctor of any drugs, medications, or vitamin and herb supplements you are using or have used in the last month.

 WHAT TO EXPECT

WHO OPERATES—Dentist or periodontist.

WHERE PERFORMED—Hospital, outpatient surgical facility or dentist's or periodontist's office.

DIAGNOSTIC TESTS
- Before surgery: Blood and urine studies; x-rays of the mouth.
- After surgery: Blood studies.

ANESTHESIA
- Local anesthesia by injection.
- General anesthesia (sometimes) by injection and inhalation with an airway tube placed in the windpipe.

DESCRIPTION OF OPERATION
- The diseased periodontal tissue is carefully cut free and removed.
- The gums are lifted or flapped away from the tooth and surrounding bone.
- The diseased root surfaces are cleaned or removed.
- The bone under the gum is reshaped, if necessary.
- A special type of fabric may be sewn around a tooth to cover a crater in the bone; the gum is then sewn over the fabric. After the bone and attachment to the root regenerate, the fabric is removed using a minor surgical procedure.
- Special dressings are applied that control bleeding and hasten healing. Your dentist will remove or replace dressings 5 to 10 days after surgery.

POSSIBLE COMPLICATIONS
- Excessive bleeding
- Surgical-wound infection.
- Sensitivity to hot or cold temperatures from exposed roots.

AVERAGE HOSPITAL STAY—0 to 1 day.

PROBABLE OUTCOME—Expect complete healing without complications. The affected gum tissue should heal and return to its normal pink color again in 2 to 3 weeks.

 POSTOPERATIVE CARE

GENERAL MEASURES
- No smoking.
- Do not disturb the dressing.
- Apply ice packs to relieve pain. Do this for 10 minutes at a time as often as needed for the first 24 hours after surgery.
- Keep your teeth free of plaque (germs, food debris and saliva). Brush your teeth and use dental floss as directed by your dentist. Mouth irrigations also help to prevent plaque.

MEDICATION
- Your dentist may prescribe:
  Pain relievers. Don't take prescription pain medication longer than 4 to 7 days. Use only as much as you need.
  Antibiotics to fight or prevent infection.
- You may use nonprescription drugs, such as acetaminophen, for minor pain. Avoid aspirin.

ACTIVITY
- To help recovery and aid your well-being, resume daily activities, including work, as soon as you are able.
- Avoid vigorous exercise for 3 weeks after surgery.
- Resume driving 2 days after returning home.

DIET—Clear liquid diet until healing occurs. Then eat a well-balanced diet to promote healing.

 CALL YOUR DOCTOR IF

- The dressing becomes loose.
- You experience nausea or vomiting.
- Pain, swelling, redness, drainage or bleeding increases in the surgical area.
- Bleeding recurs 48 hours or longer after surgery.
- You develop signs of infection, including headache, muscle aches, dizziness or a general ill feeling and fever.
- New, unexplained symptoms develop. Drugs used in treatment may produce side effects.

PERIODONTAL SURGERY
(Pyorrhea Treatment)

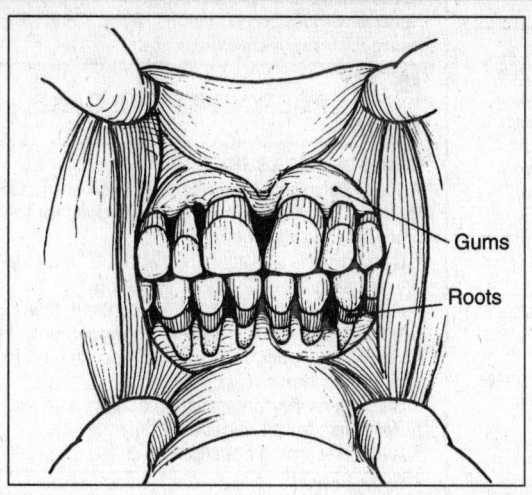

An illustration of the mouth, gums and roots of teeth.

Gums

Roots

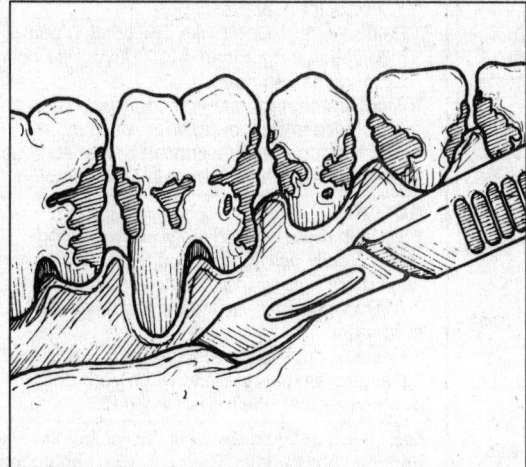

Periodontal tissue cut free and removed.

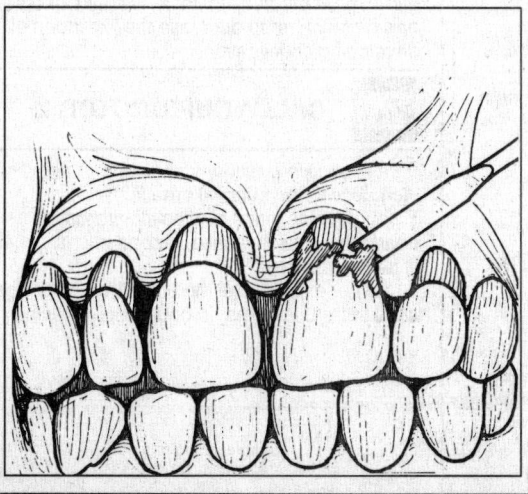

Special dressings are applied to control bleeding and hasten healing. These usually need to be removed or replaced 5 to 10 days after surgery.

SURGERIES

PILONIDAL CYST REMOVAL

GENERAL INFORMATION

DEFINITION—Removal of a pilonidal cyst, a cyst that is located in area of the sacrum. In a pilondial cyst, surface skin containing sweat glands, oil glands and hair follicles becomes trapped beneath the surface of the skin. The cyst often forms cavities, or openings to the outside, called sinuses. The cyst can also become infected, and an abscess can form.

BODY PARTS INVOLVED—Area over the tailbone.

REASONS FOR SURGERY—Relief of pain and prevention of the spread of infection.

SURGICAL RISK INCREASES WITH
• Obesity.
• Smoking.
• Recent or chronic illness.
• Diabetes mellitus.
• Use of some prescription and nonprescription drugs. Inform your doctor of any drugs, medications, or vitamin and herb supplements you are using or have used in the last month.

WHAT TO EXPECT

WHO OPERATES—General surgeon or proctologist.

WHERE PERFORMED—Hospital, outpatient surgical facility, doctor's office.

DIAGNOSTIC TESTS
• Before surgery: Blood and urine studies; chest x-ray; sigmoidoscopy (see Glossary).
• After surgery: Blood tests.

ANESTHESIA
• Local anesthesia by injection.
• General anesthesia by injection and inhalation with an airway tube placed in the windpipe.

DESCRIPTION OF OPERATION
• A variety of surgical treatments are available. One type is described here.
• The cyst and its cavities (also called sinuses) over the tailbone are identified with probes. An incision is made around the cyst.
• The cyst and all affected sinuses are removed.
• Bleeding is controlled with sutures or electrocauterization.
• The skin is usually left open to heal from the bottom out. This can take a period of 4 to 8 weeks.

POSSIBLE COMPLICATIONS
• Excessive bleeding.
• Surgical-wound infection.
• Slow healing.
• Recurrence of cyst.

AVERAGE HOSPITAL STAY—0 to 2 days.

PROBABLE OUTCOME—Expect complete healing without complications. Allow about 2 months for recovery from surgery.

POSTOPERATIVE CARE

GENERAL MEASURES
• Take warm baths to relieve discomfort. Do this for 15 to 20 minutes several times daily for the first week after surgery.
• Don't dry the surgical area with a towel. Drip dry or use a blow dryer after bathing.
• If the cyst is left open to heal by itself, it will drain and will require dressing changes until it is healed. Your doctor will instruct you on how to change the dressings.
• Sit on a rubber ring (available in drugstores) to relieve discomfort, if necessary.
• Avoid becoming constipated.

MEDICATION
• Your doctor may prescribe:
Pain relievers. Don't take prescription pain medication longer than 4 to 7 days. Use only as much as you need.
Stool softeners to prevent constipation.
Antibiotics to fight or prevent infection.
• You may use nonprescription drugs, such as acetaminophen, for minor pain. Avoid aspirin.

ACTIVITY
• To help recovery and aid your well-being, resume daily activities, including work, as soon as you are able.
• Avoid vigorous exercise for 6 weeks after surgery.
• Resume driving 1 week after returning home.
• Resume sexual relations when your doctor determines that healing is complete.

DIET—Clear liquid diet until the gastrointestinal tract functions again. Then eat a well-balanced diet to promote healing. Increase fluid intake and dietary fiber to decrease the likelihood of developing constipation.

CALL YOUR DOCTOR IF

• Pain, swelling, redness, drainage or bleeding increases in the surgical area.
• You develop signs of infection, including headache, muscle aches, dizziness or a general ill feeling and fever.
• New, unexplained symptoms develop. Drugs used in treatment may produce side effects.

PILONIDAL CYST REMOVAL

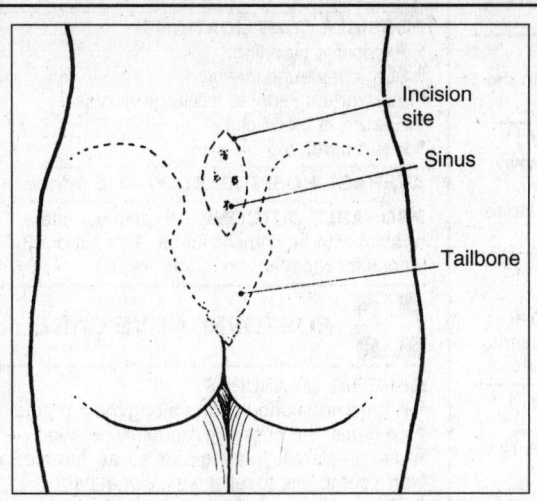

Incision
site

Sinus

Tailbone

An illustration of several sinuses that begin inside the lumen of the rectum and extend out through the skin.

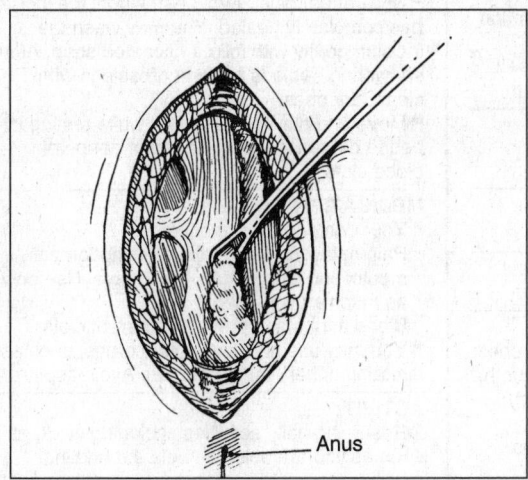

Anus

The cyst and all affected sinuses are identified and removed.

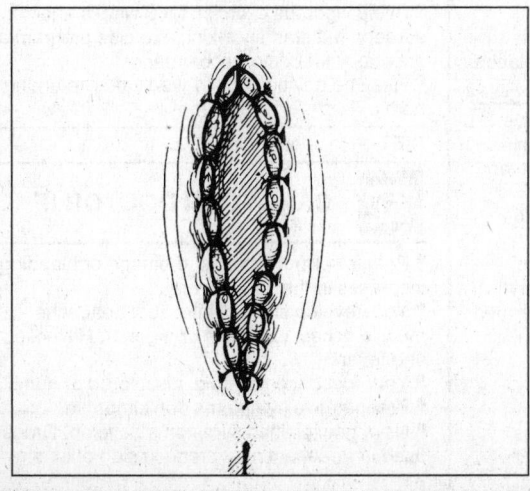

The skin is usually left open to heal slowly from the bottom. Some surgeons close the skin over the operative site at the time of surgery.

POPLITEAL ARTERY EMBOLECTOMY

GENERAL INFORMATION

DEFINITION—Removal of a blood clot (embolus) that has blocked blood supply to the leg and foot.

BODY PARTS INVOLVED—Blood vessel in the leg that is called the femoral artery below the groin and the popliteal artery behind the knee; the heart is the usual source of the blood clot.

REASONS FOR SURGERY—Restoration of normal blood circulation in the legs. Re-establishing blood flow can restore muscular function, prevent gangrene and enable patients to return to normal or almost normal activities.

SURGICAL RISK INCREASES WITH
- Obesity; smoking.
- Rheumatic heart disease or coronary artery disease.
- Diabetes mellitus.
- Use of some prescription and nonprescription drugs. Inform your doctor of any drugs, medications, or vitamin and herb supplements you are using or have used in the last month.

WHAT TO EXPECT

WHO OPERATES—General surgeon or vascular surgeon.

WHERE PERFORMED—Outpatient surgical facility or hospital.

DIAGNOSTIC TESTS
- Before surgery: Blood and urine studies; chest x-ray; ECG; arteriogram (see Glossary for both).
- During surgery: Arteriogram (see Glossary) after blood clot is removed.
- After surgery: Blood studies; heart studies, such as sonogram (see Glossary).

ANESTHESIA
- Spinal anesthesia by injection.
- General anesthesia by injection and inhalation with an airway tube placed in the windpipe.

DESCRIPTION OF OPERATION
- An incision is usually made over the artery where the clot is lodged. Sometimes, however, the incision is made in the groin.
- The artery is clamped above and below the blood clot.
- The artery is opened above the blood clot.
- A special catheter is passed into the artery beyond the blood clot. The catheter is expanded with air beyond the clot and then withdrawn, forcing the clot out of the artery.
- An anticoagulant is injected into the artery, and normal blood circulation is restored.
- The clamps are removed from the arteries. Muscles and connective tissue are sewn together in layers. The skin is closed with sutures or clamps, which usually can be removed about 1 week after surgery.

POSSIBLE COMPLICATIONS
- Excessive bleeding.
- Surgical-wound infection.
- Inadvertent injury to the large nerves.
- Recurrent blood clot.
- Heart problems.

AVERAGE HOSPITAL STAY—0 to 3 days.

PROBABLE OUTCOME—Expect complete healing without complications. Allow about 3 weeks for recovery from surgery.

POSTOPERATIVE CARE

GENERAL MEASURES
- A hard ridge should form along the incision. As it heals, the ridge will gradually recede.
- Use an electric heating pad, a heat lamp or a warm compress to relieve incisional pain.
- Shower as usual. Avoid baths until the incision has completely healed. You may wash the incision gently with mild, unscented soap. After showering, replace any wet dressings with clean, dry ones.
- Move and elevate legs often while resting in bed to decrease the likelihood of deep-vein blood clots.

MEDICATION
- Your doctor may prescribe:
  Pain relievers. Don't take prescription pain medication longer than 4 to 7 days. Use only as much as you need.
  Blood thinners to prevent recurrent clots.
- You may use nonprescription drugs, such as acetaminophen, for minor pain. Avoid aspirin.

ACTIVITY
- Resuming daily activities, including work, as soon as you are able can help the healing process.
- Avoid vigorous exercise for 3 weeks after surgery, but start a walking exercise program as soon as your doctor recommends.
- Resume driving about 1 week after returning home.

DIET—No special diet.

CALL YOUR DOCTOR IF

- Pain, swelling, redness, drainage or bleeding increases in the surgical area.
- You develop signs of infection: headache, muscle aches, dizziness or a general ill feeling and fever.
- Your foot becomes cold, discolored or numb.
- Preoperative symptoms don't improve.
- New, unexplained symptoms develop. Drugs used in treatment may produce side effects.

POPLITEAL ARTERY EMBOLECTOMY

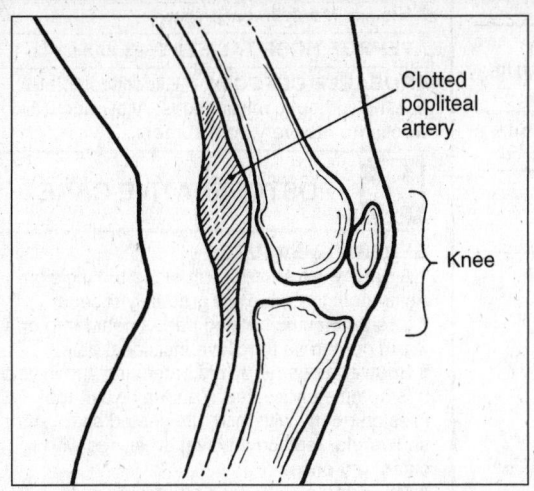

An illustration of a clot in the popliteal artery extending behind the knee.

Clotted popliteal artery

Knee

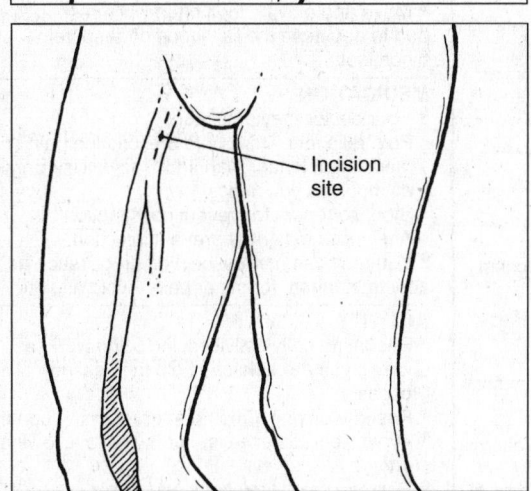

An incision for a special catheter is made inside the upper thigh at the inguinal level.

Incision site

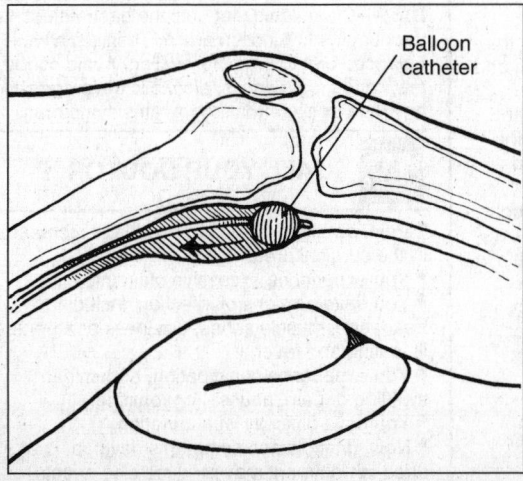

The catheter is passed into the artery beyond the blood clot. It is expanded with air and then withdrawn, forcing the clots out of the artery.

Balloon catheter

- After the clot has been removed, muscles and connective tissues are sewn together in layers. The skin is closed with sutures or clamps.

SURGERIES

PROSTATE GLAND REMOVAL, SUPRAPUBIC

 GENERAL INFORMATION

DEFINITION—Removal of part or all of an enlarged prostate gland through an opening in the lower abdomen.

BODY PARTS INVOLVED—Prostate gland; bladder; rectum; urethra.

REASONS FOR SURGERY
- Restoration of normal passage of urine.
- Cancer of the prostate.

SURGICAL RISK INCREASES WITH
- Adults over 60.
- Stress; smoking; obesity.
- Poor nutrition.
- Recent illness, especially upper-respiratory infection.
- Alcoholism or chronic illness.
- Diabetes mellitus.
- Use of some prescription and nonprescription drugs. Inform your doctor of any drugs, medications, or vitamin and herb supplements you are using or have used in the last month.

 WHAT TO EXPECT

WHO OPERATES—Urologist.

WHERE PERFORMED—Hospital.

DIAGNOSTIC TESTS
- Before surgery: Blood and urine studies; chest x-ray; kidney function studies; intravenous pyelogram; ultrasound; cystoscopy; ECG (see Glossary for all).
- After surgery: Blood studies.

ANESTHESIA
- Spinal anesthesia by injection.
- General anesthesia by injection and inhalation with an airway tube placed in the windpipe.

DESCRIPTION OF OPERATION
- An incision is made in the lower abdomen.
- The bladder and urethra are opened, and the enlarged parts of the prostate gland cut free and removed.
- Two catheters are placed in the bladder, and a tube to drain secretions is placed next to the bladder. The urethra and bladder are closed with sutures. One of the catheters will pass through the penis, and the other will be brought out through the incision along with the drain.
- The catheters and drains will usually remain in place for several days.
- The muscles are repositioned and sewn in place. The skin is closed with sutures or clips, which usually can be removed about 1 week after surgery.

POSSIBLE COMPLICATIONS
- Excessive bleeding.
- Surgical-wound infection.

- Inability to control urinary stream.
- Impotence.
- Sterility (sometimes).

AVERAGE HOSPITAL STAY—3 to 5 days.

PROBABLE OUTCOME—Expect complete healing without complications. Allow about 6 weeks for recovery from surgery.

 POSTOPERATIVE CARE

GENERAL MEASURES
- A hard ridge should form along the incision. As it heals the ridge will gradually recede.
- Use an electric heating pad, a heat lamp or a warm compress to relieve incisional pain.
- Shower as usual. Avoid baths until the incision has completely healed. You may wash the incision gently with mild, unscented soap. After showering, replace any wet dressings with clean, dry ones.
- Move and elevate legs often while resting in bed to decrease the likelihood of deep-vein blood clots.

MEDICATION
- Your doctor may prescribe:
  Pain relievers. Don't take prescription pain medication longer than 4 to 7 days. Use only as much as you need.
  Stool softeners to prevent constipation.
  Antibiotics to fight or prevent infection.
- You may use nonprescription drugs, such as acetaminophen, for minor pain. Avoid aspirin.

ACTIVITY
- Resuming daily activities, including work, as soon as you are able can help the healing process.
- Resume driving 1 month after returning home.
- Avoid vigorous exercise for 6 weeks following surgery.
- Resume sexual relations when able.

DIET—Clear liquid diet until the gastrointestinal tract begins to function again. Then eat a well-balanced diet to promote healing. Avoid coffee, tea, cocoa, cola drinks, alcoholic beverages and any food or spice that aggravates symptoms.

 CALL YOUR DOCTOR IF

- Pain, swelling, redness or drainage increases in the surgical area.
- You experience excessive bleeding.
- You develop signs of infection, including headache, muscle aches, dizziness or a general ill feeling and fever.
- You experience constipation, abdominal swelling or pain, nausea, or vomiting.
- You have difficulty with urination.
- New, unexplained symptoms develop. Drugs used in treatment may produce side effects.

PROSTATE GLAND REMOVAL, SUPRAPUBIC

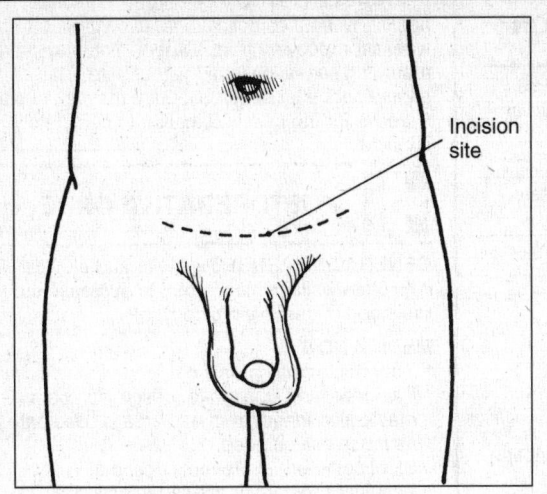

An illustration of the usual incision site for prostatectomy.

Incision site

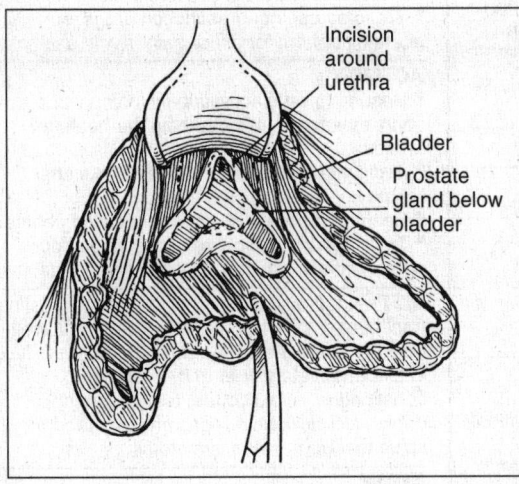

The bladder and urethra are opened and the enlarged parts of the prostate gland cut free and removed.

Incision around urethra

Bladder

Prostate gland below bladder

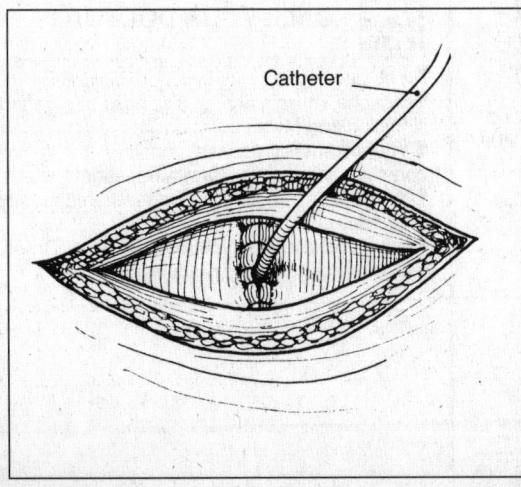

Two catheters are placed in the bladder and a tube to drain secretions is placed next to the bladder. The urethra and bladder are closed with sutures.

• One of the catheters will pass through the penis and the other will be brought out through the incision along with the drain (not illustrated).

Catheter

SURGERIES

PROSTATE GLAND REMOVAL, TRANSURETHRAL

GENERAL INFORMATION

DEFINITION—Removal of part or all of an enlarged prostate gland with a cystoscope, an instrument that is passed up through the urethra.

BODY PARTS INVOLVED—Penis; prostate gland; urethra; bladder.

REASONS FOR SURGERY—Restoration of normal passage of urine.

SURGICAL RISK INCREASES WITH
- Obesity; smoking.
- Poor nutrition.
- Recent or chronic illness.
- Alcoholism.
- Diabetes mellitus.
- Use of some prescription and nonprescription drugs. Inform your doctor of any drugs, medications, or vitamin and herb supplements you are using or have used in the last month.

WHAT TO EXPECT

WHO OPERATES—Urologist.

WHERE PERFORMED—Hospital.

DIAGNOSTIC TESTS
- Before surgery: Blood and urine studies; x-rays of kidneys and chest; kidney-function studies; ECG; intravenous pyelogram (IVP); ultrasound (see Glossary for all).
- After surgery: Blood studies.

ANESTHESIA
- Spinal anesthesia by injection.
- General anesthesia by injection and inhalation with an airway tube placed in the windpipe.

DESCRIPTION OF OPERATION
- A cystoscope (a thin, fiberoptic instrument with lenses and a light at its tip) is passed up through the urethra to the prostate gland.
- The prostate gland is examined for tumors and signs of infection.
- An electrosurgical loop is inserted through the cystoscope tip and cuts away the diseased parts of the prostate gland.
- The cystoscope is removed. A catheter may be placed in the bladder for a day or two.

POSSIBLE COMPLICATIONS
- Excessive bleeding.
- Inability to control urinary stream (incontinence).
- Urinary retention.
- Impotence (sometimes).
- Sterility.
- Epididymitis.

AVERAGE HOSPITAL STAY—2 to 3 days.

PROBABLE OUTCOME—Expect complete healing without complications. Allow about 3 weeks for recovery from surgery. You may have a burning sensation when you urinate. This should get better each day, but it may take up to 6 weeks for the painful urination to completely subside.

POSTOPERATIVE CARE

GENERAL MEASURES—Move and elevate legs often while resting in bed to decrease the likelihood of deep-vein blood clots.

MEDICATION
- Your doctor may prescribe:
  Pain relievers. Don't take prescription pain medication longer than 4 to 7 days. Use only as much as you need.
  Stool softeners to prevent constipation.
  Antibiotics to fight or prevent infection.
- You may use nonprescription drugs, such as acetaminophen, for minor pain. Avoid aspirin.

ACTIVITY
- Resuming daily activities, including work, as soon as you are able can help the healing process.
- Avoid vigorous exercise for 2 weeks after surgery.
- Resume driving 1 week after returning home.
- Try to resume sexual relations when your doctor determines that healing is complete.

DIET—Clear liquid diet until the gastrointestinal tract begins to function again. Then eat a well-balanced diet to promote healing. Increase fluid intake and dietary fiber to help prevent constipation. Avoid coffee, tea, cocoa, cola drinks, alcoholic beverages and any food or spice that aggravates symptoms.

CALL YOUR DOCTOR IF

- You develop signs of infection, including headache, muscle aches, dizziness or a general ill feeling and fever.
- You experience nausea, vomiting, constipation, or difficulty with urination.
- You remain impotent for longer than 3 months after surgery.
- New, unexplained symptoms develop. Drugs used in treatment may produce side effects.

PROSTATE GLAND REMOVAL, TRANSURETHRAL

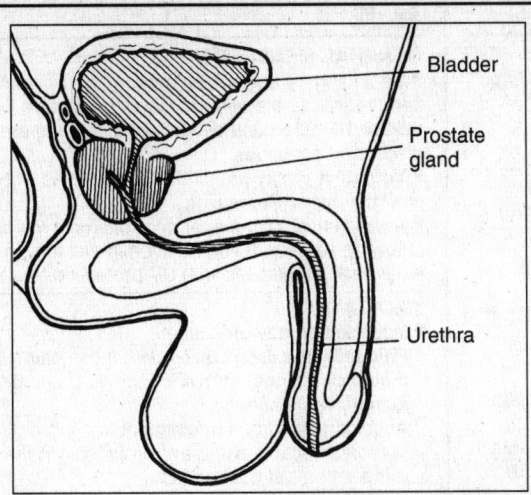

A side view of the bladder, urethra and prostate gland in the male.

Bladder

Prostate gland

Urethra

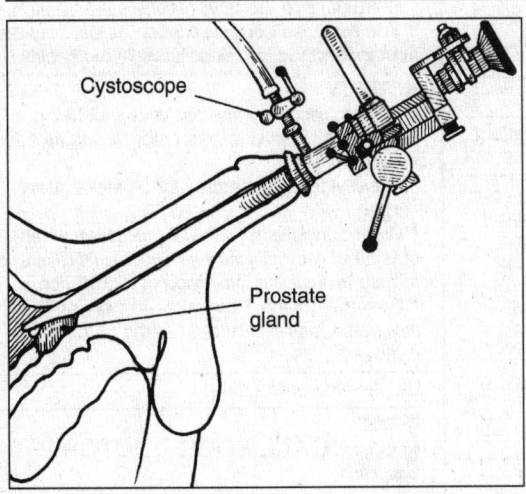

The cystoscope is passed through the urethra to the segment where the prostate gland is located.
- A miniature telescope and light inside the cystoscope make the prostate gland visible through the cystoscope.

Cystoscope

Prostate gland

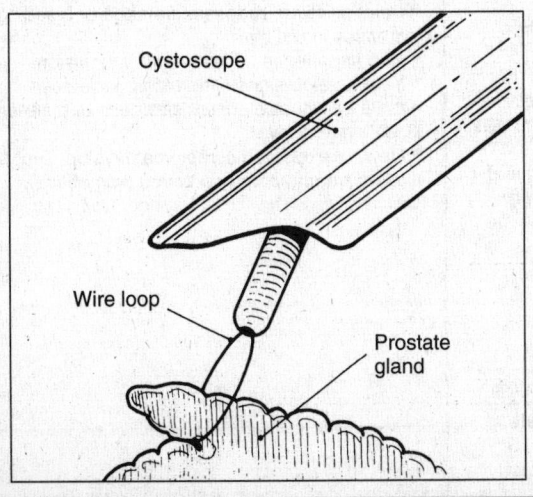

A wire snare is passed through the cystoscope tip to remove part of the diseased or enlarged prostate gland.

Cystoscope

Wire loop

Prostate gland

PTERYGIUM EXCISION

GENERAL INFORMATION

DEFINITION—Removal of a pterygium, an abnormal tissue that grows from the inner edge of the sclera (white outer coat enclosing the eyeball) and extends over a portion of the cornea.

BODY PARTS INVOLVED—Eye; cornea; conjunctiva (the membrane covering the eye).

REASONS FOR SURGERY
• Restoration or protection of normal vision.
• Improved appearance.

SURGICAL RISK INCREASES WITH
• Recent or chronic illness.
• Diabetes mellitus.
• Use of some prescription and nonprescription drugs. Inform your doctor of any drugs, medications, or vitamin and herb supplements you are using or have used in the last month.

WHAT TO EXPECT

WHO OPERATES—Ophthalmologist.

WHERE PERFORMED—Hospital or outpatient surgical facility.

DIAGNOSTIC TESTS
• Before surgery: Complete eye examination.
• After surgery: Complete eye examination.

ANESTHESIA
• Local anesthesia by topical application, usually accompanied by sedation.
• Local anesthesia by injection, usually accompanied by sedation.

DESCRIPTION OF OPERATION
• An incision is made in the conjunctiva around the pterygium.
• The pterygium is cut and brought upward, clear of the cornea.
• The lower edge of the pterygium is cut free and the entire pterygium is removed.
• A autograft is fashioned from an area of the conjunctiva underneath the eyelid and is placed to cover the area from where the pterygium was removed.
• Fine sutures are used to attach the graft and to close the membrane from where the graft was taken; the sutures will dissolve and will be absorbed by the body.

POSSIBLE COMPLICATIONS
• Surgical-wound infection.
• Recurrence of the pterygium.
• Scarring.

AVERAGE HOSPITAL STAY—Usually none.

PROBABLE OUTCOME—Expect complete healing without complications. Allow about 3 weeks for recovery from surgery.

POSTOPERATIVE CARE

GENERAL MEASURES
• Beginning 24 hours after surgery, apply warm compresses to the eye to relieve discomfort. Do this for 10 to 15 minutes each hour as long as discomfort continues.
• Your doctor may prescribe a patch to be worn over the eye while healing.
• Avoid sunlight whenever possible for 6 weeks following surgery. If you must be in the sun, wear dark sunglasses with UV protection.

MEDICATION
• Your doctor may prescribe:
  Pain relievers. Don't take prescription pain medication longer than 4 to 7 days. Use only as much as you need.
  Antibiotic eye drops or ointment to fight or prevent infection. Keep eye drops cold in the refrigerator, but not frozen.
  Steroidal eye drops to reduce inflammation.
• You may use nonprescription drugs, such as acetaminophen for minor pain. Avoid aspirin.

ACTIVITY
• To help recovery and aid your well-being, resume daily activities, including work, as soon as you are able.
• Avoid vigorous exercise for 3 weeks after surgery.
• Wear sunglasses with UV protection when outside to protect your eyes the sun's rays and to help reduce the likelihood of recurrence.
• Resume driving 1 day after surgery or, if an eye patch is prescribed, after the patch is removed.

DIET—No special diet.

CALL YOUR DOCTOR IF

• Pain, swelling, redness, drainage or bleeding increases in the eye.
• You experience difficulty with your vision.
• You develop signs of infection, including headache, muscle aches, dizziness or a general ill feeling and fever.
• New, unexplained symptoms develop. Drugs used in treatment may produce side effects.

PTERYGIUM EXCISION

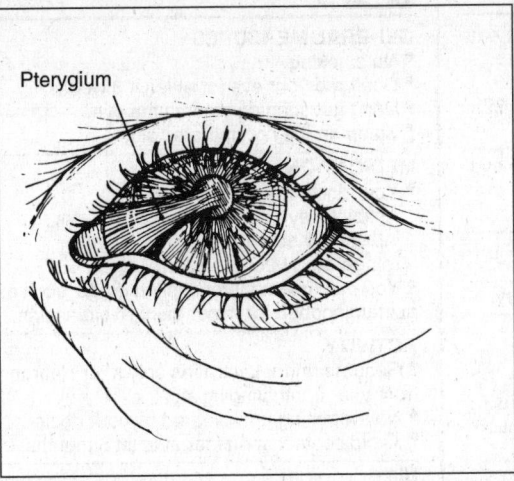

Pterygium

An illustration of a typical pterygium extending from the edge of the eye inward to attach to the cornea.

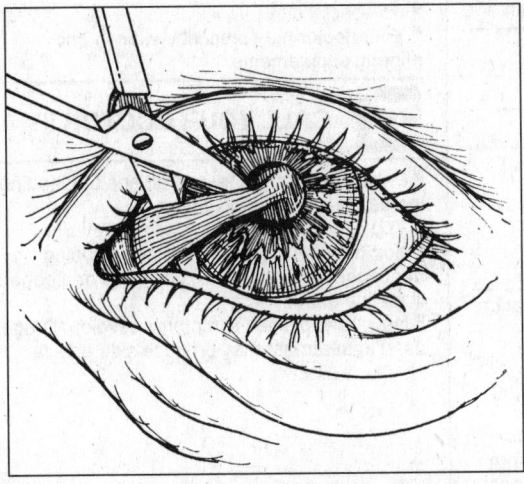

An incision is made in the conjunctiva around the pterygium.
- The pterygium is cut and brought upward clear of the cornea.

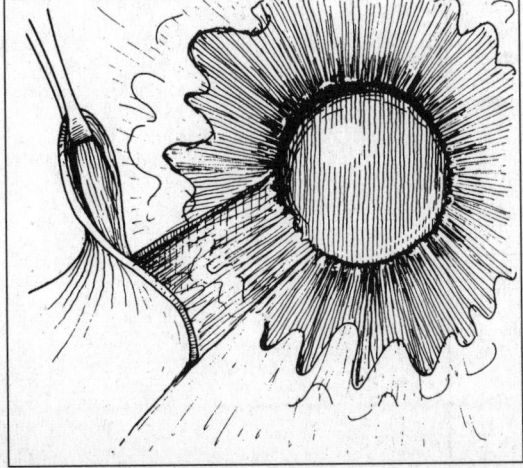

The lower edge of the pterygium is cut free and the entire growth is removed.
- Open areas in the membrane covering the eye are closed with fine sutures that will dissove and be absorbed by the body.

RADIAL KERATOTOMY

 GENERAL INFORMATION

DEFINITION—A surgical eye operation to treat nearsightedness or astigmatism. Surgery is performed on the cornea which, as it heals, flattens in the center changing the angle of light rays entering the eye.

BODY PARTS INVOLVED—Cornea of the eye (the rounded transparent tissue that covers the colored part [iris] and the pupil).

REASONS FOR SURGERY—Hope of curing nearsightedness or astigmatism so that corrective lenses will no longer be necessary.

SURGICAL RISK INCREASES WITH
- Adults over 60.
- Smoking.
- Chronic illness, especially diabetes mellitus.
- Use of some prescription and nonprescription drugs. Inform your doctor of any drugs, medications, or vitamin and herb supplements you are using or have used in the last month.

 WHAT TO EXPECT

WHO OPERATES—Ophthalmologist.

WHERE PERFORMED—Outpatient surgical facility.

DIAGNOSTIC TESTS
- Before surgery: Vision tests.
- After surgery: Vision tests.

ANESTHESIA—Local anesthesia with sedation.

DESCRIPTION OF OPERATION
- Head is positioned flat on operating table.
- A wire speculum is placed to prevent closing the eye during surgery.
- Under appropriate anesthesia, the surgeon makes 4 to 16 incisions radiating outward from the center of the cornea like spokes on a wheel. The incisions are about 90% deep into the cornea.
- One eye is operated on in 1 session, the other at another session.

POSSIBLE COMPLICATIONS
- Visual acuity fluctuations.
- Undercorrection; overcorrection.
- Infection.
- Immediate or future impairment of sight (rare).
- Glare at night; light sensitivity.

AVERAGE HOSPITAL STAY—None required.

PROBABLE OUTCOME—Uncertain. Total healing may require 2 or more years. Usually there is improvement in vision; sometimes vision is corrected to 20/20.

 POSTOPERATIVE CARE

GENERAL MEASURES
- No smoking.
- Don't rub your eye for at least 3 weeks.
- Don't get soap or water in the eye.
- Sleep on the nonoperated side.

MEDICATION
- Your doctor may prescribe:
  Antibiotic eye drops to fight or prevent infection. Keep eye drops cold in the refrigerator, but not frozen.
- You may use nonprescription drugs, such as acetaminophen for minor pain. Avoid aspirin.

ACTIVITY
- Resume normal activities only after clearance from your ophthalmologist.
- No swimming until cleared by your doctor.
- Avoid contact sports for at least 6 months.

DIET
- No special diet.
- Your doctor may prescribe vitamin and mineral supplements.

 CALL YOUR DOCTOR IF

- Pain, swelling, redness, drainage or bleeding increases in the surgical area.
- You experience difficulty with your vision.
- You develop signs of infection, including headache, muscle aches, dizziness or a general ill feeling and fever.
- New, unexplained symptoms develop. Drugs used in treatment may produce side effects.

RADIAL KERATOTOMY

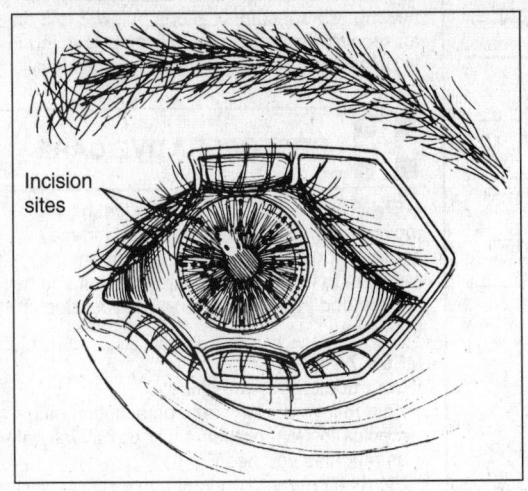

An illustration showing the proposed incisions into the cornea.

Incision sites

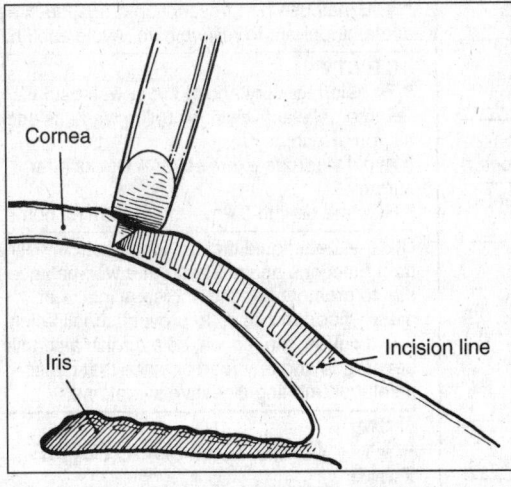

Surgical instrument that demonstrates the depth of the incision into the cornea.

Cornea

Incision line

Iris

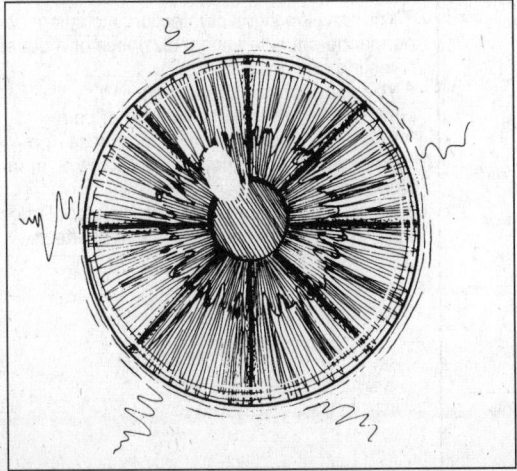

After healing, the incision lines are invisible and vision without glasses is usually improved.

RECTAL OR COLON POLYP REMOVAL
(Polypectomy)

 GENERAL INFORMATION

DEFINITION—Removal of a polyp from the membrane lining inside the rectum or colon.

BODY PARTS INVOLVED—Membrane lining of the rectum and colon.

REASONS FOR SURGERY
• Removal of a possible source of cancer.
• Removal of tissue to see if cancer is present.
• To remove the source of rectal bleeding.

SURGICAL RISK INCREASES WITH
• Obesity.
• Smoking.
• Poor nutrition.
• Recent or chronic illness.
• Diabetes mellitus.
• Use of some prescription and nonprescription drugs. Inform your doctor of any drugs, medications, or vitamin and herb supplements you are using or have used in the last month.

 WHAT TO EXPECT

WHO OPERATES—General surgeon; colon-rectal surgeon; gastroenterologist; family doctor.

WHERE PERFORMED—Hospital; outpatient surgical facility; doctor's office.

DIAGNOSTIC TESTS
• Before surgery: Blood and urine studies; x-rays of lower gastrointestinal tract; sigmoidoscopy; colonoscopy (see Glossary for both).
• After surgery: Blood studies; laboratory examination of removed tissue.

ANESTHESIA—Intravenous sedative and narcotic pain killer.

DESCRIPTION OF OPERATION
• The colon is cleansed the night before by drinking various solutions.
• A colonoscope or sigmoidoscope (see Glossary for both) is inserted through the rectum into the sigmoid colon. You may feel mild cramping.
• The polyp is located and removed with a wire snare.
• Bleeding is controlled with electric current or pressure applied with gauze soaked in epinephrine (see Glossary).

POSSIBLE COMPLICATIONS
• Excessive bleeding.
• Inadvertent perforation of the colon resulting in infection.

AVERAGE HOSPITAL STAY—Usually none.

PROBABLE OUTCOME—Expect complete healing without complications. Allow 2 to 3 days for recovery from surgery. If the polyp is found to be cancerous, treatment and outcome will vary.

 POSTOPERATIVE CARE

GENERAL MEASURES—Your first bowel movement may be red or maroon and may contain blood clots. If bowel movements continue to have this appearance, or if you have liquid blood in your stool, contact your doctor right away.

MEDICATION
• Your doctor may prescribe:
  Pain relievers. Don't take prescription pain medication longer than 4 to 7 days. Use only as much as you need.
  Stool softeners to prevent constipation.
• You may use nonprescription drugs, such as acetaminophen, to relieve pain. Avoid aspirin.

ACTIVITY
• To help recovery and aid your well-being, resume daily activities, including work, as soon as you are able.
• Avoid vigorous exercise for 4 weeks after surgery.
• Resume driving 3 days after returning home.

DIET—Clear liquid diet until the gastrointestinal tract functions again. Then eat a well-balanced diet to promote healing. Increase intake of dietary fiber and fluids to prevent constipation. Avoid coffee, tea, cocoa, cola drinks, alcoholic beverages and any food or spice that causes painful or irritating digestive symptoms.

 CALL YOUR DOCTOR IF

• You develop signs of infection, including headache, muscle aches, dizziness or a general ill feeling and fever.
• You experience nausea, vomiting, constipation, abdominal swelling or pain.
• You experience weakness, dizziness or a rapid pulse upon standing (symptoms of internal bleeding).
• New, unexplained symptoms develop. Drugs used in treatment may produce side effects.

RECTAL OR COLON POLYP REMOVAL
(Polypectomy)

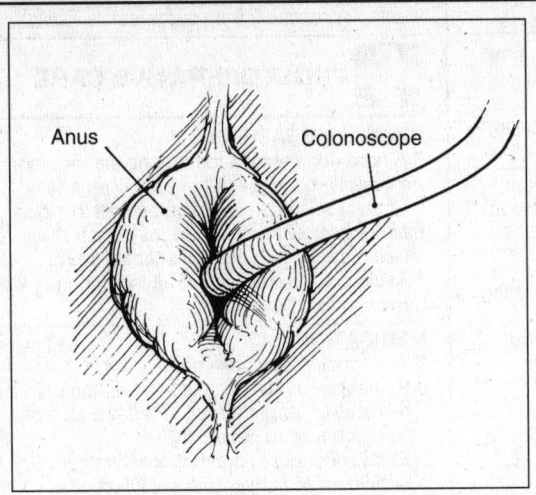

Anus

Colonoscope

An illustration of a flexible colonoscope inserted into the anus.

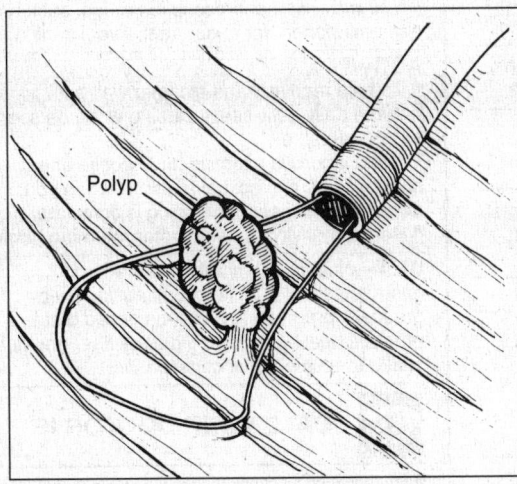

Polyp

The colonoscope or sigmoidoscope is advanced to reach the sigmoid colon where polyps (when present) are usually located.
- The polyp is removed with a wire snare.

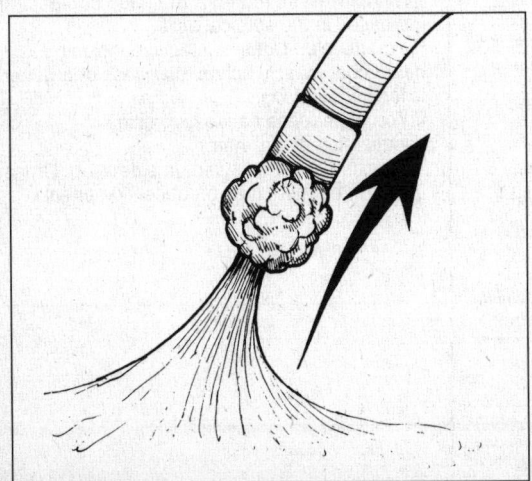

After the polyp has been removed, bleeding of the remaining stump is controlled with electric current.

SURGERIES

RECTOVAGINAL FISTULA REPAIR

GENERAL INFORMATION

DEFINITION—Repair of a fistula (an abnormal tract) between the rectum and vagina that usually results from diverticulitis, cervical cancer, inflammatory bowel disease, radiation therapy or surgical procedures.

BODY PARTS INVOLVED—Vagina; rectum; connective tissue; blood vessels and nerves in the perineum.

REASONS FOR SURGERY
- Prevention of fecal matter from contaminating the vagina or urinary tract.
- Discomfort and embarrassment caused by feces and gas passing through the vagina.

SURGICAL RISK INCREASES WITH
- Obesity; smoking.
- Poor nutrition; alcoholism.
- Recent or chronic illness.
- Diabetes mellitus.
- Use of some prescription and nonprescription drugs. Inform your doctor of any drugs, medications, or vitamin and herb supplements you are using or have used in the last month.

WHAT TO EXPECT

WHO OPERATES—Obstetrician-gynecologist, proctologist, colon-rectal surgeon or general surgeon.

WHERE PERFORMED—Hospital.

DIAGNOSTIC TESTS
- Before surgery: Blood and urine studies; x-rays of lower gastrointestinal tract and kidneys.
- After surgery: Blood studies.

ANESTHESIA—General anesthesia by injection and inhalation with an airway tube placed in the windpipe.

DESCRIPTION OF OPERATION
- An incision is made in the perineum.
- The abdomen is explored and the involved area of the colon is isolated. The colon is separated from the vaginal opening.
- The segment of colon involved is resected (removed) and the colon is sewn back together.
- Sometimes, a temporary colostomy (see in Surgery section) is necessary for proper healing. This is closed at a later time.
- The skin and muscles are closed with sutures. The skin sutures are removed in about a week.

POSSIBLE COMPLICATIONS
- Excessive bleeding.
- Surgical-wound infection.
- Failure to heal completely.

AVERAGE HOSPITAL STAY—5 to 7 days.

PROBABLE OUTCOME—Expect complete healing without complications. Allow about 6 weeks for recovery from surgery.

POSTOPERATIVE CARE

GENERAL MEASURES
- A hard ridge should form along the incision. As it heals, the ridge will gradually recede.
- Shower as usual. Avoid baths until the incision has completely healed. You may wash the incision gently with mild, unscented soap.
- Avoid constipation and straining during bowel movements.

MEDICATION
- Your doctor may prescribe:
  Pain relievers. Don't take prescription pain medication longer than 4 to 7 days. Use only as much as you need.
  Stool softeners to prevent constipation.
  Antibiotics to fight or prevent infection.
- You may use nonprescription drugs, such as acetaminophen, for minor pain. Avoid aspirin.

ACTIVITY
- To help recovery and aid your well-being, resume daily activities, including work, as soon as you are able.
- Avoid vigorous exercise for 6 weeks after surgery. Resume sexual relations when your doctor determines that healing is complete.
- Resume driving 3 weeks after returning home.

DIET—Nothing by mouth until the gastrointestinal tract functions again. Then, gradually progress to a well-balanced diet to promote healing. Increase dietary fiber and fluid intake to help prevent constipation.

CALL YOUR DOCTOR IF

- Pain, swelling, redness, drainage or bleeding increases in the surgical area.
- You develop signs of infection, including headache, muscle aches, dizziness or a general ill feeling and fever.
- You experience nausea, vomiting, constipation or diarrhea.
- New, unexplained symptoms develop. Drugs used in treatment may produce side effects.

RECTOVAGINAL FISTULA REPAIR

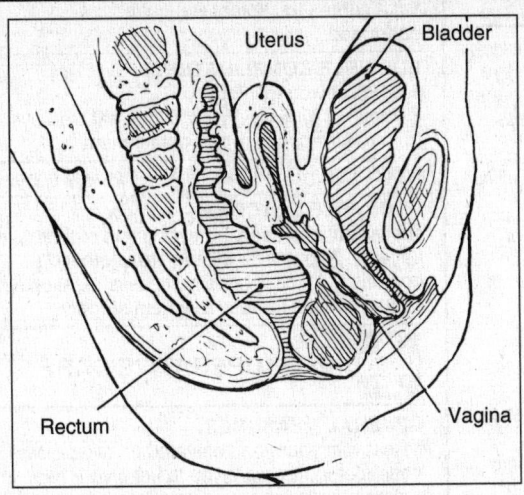

An illustration of the side view of the normal female urogenital tract.

Uterus

Bladder

Rectum

Vagina

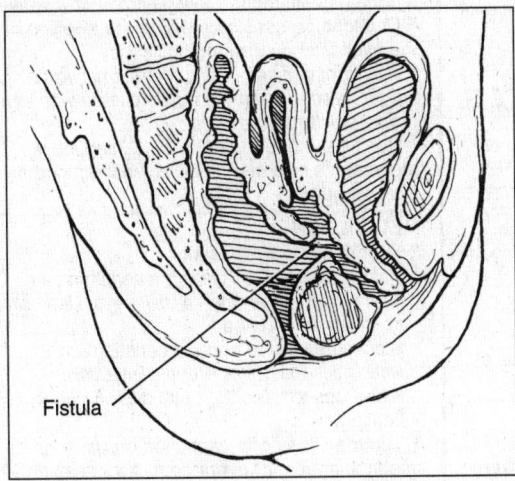

A view of a fistula (an abnormal tract) which has formed between the rectum and the vagina.

Fistula

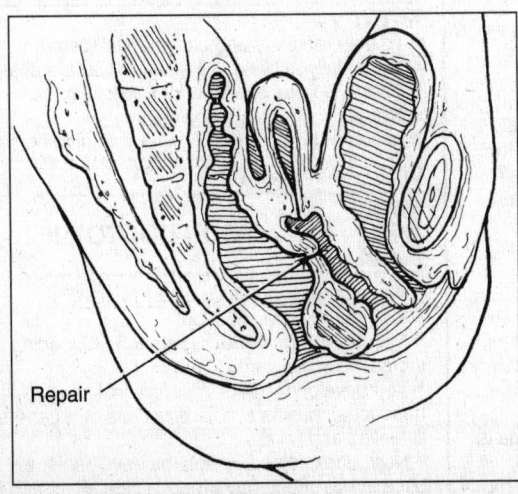

The involved area of the colon is isolated and separated from the vagina. The segment of the colon involved is removed and the colon is then sewn back together.

Repair

SURGERIES

RETINAL DETACHMENT REPAIR

GENERAL INFORMATION

DEFINITION—Reattachment of a retina that has become separated from the rest of the eye. The retina is the light-sensitive area at the back of the eye. See Retinal Detachment in Illness section.

BODY PARTS INVOLVED—The eye and all its parts.

REASONS FOR SURGERY—Prevention of vision loss.

SURGICAL RISK INCREASES WITH
- Obesity; smoking; alcoholism.
- Poor nutrition.
- Recent or chronic illness, especially diabetes mellitus.
- Use of some prescription and nonprescription drugs. Inform your doctor of any drugs, medications, or vitamin and herb supplements you are using or have used in the last month.

WHAT TO EXPECT

WHO OPERATES—Ophthalmologist.

WHERE PERFORMED—Hospital or outpatient surgical facility.

DIAGNOSTIC TESTS
- Before surgery: Complete eye examination.
- After surgery: Complete eye examination.

ANESTHESIA
- Local anesthesia by injection or topical application.
- General anesthesia by injection and inhalation with an airway tube placed in the windpipe.

DESCRIPTION OF OPERATION
Your doctor will choose one or more of the following procedures, depending on how severe the detachment is.
- Laser photocoagulation: Tears or holes in the retina are repaired with laser beams that coagulate the eye tissue and cause it to readjust to its normal position.
- Cryopexy: The membrane lining the eye is cut. A cryosurgical probe is placed around the detached retina. The probe applies extreme cold, causing eye tissue to coagulate and to adhere to its normal position.
- Diathermy: Heat from an electric current is applied to seal a tear in the retina.
- Pneumatic retinopexy: If the tear or tears which caused the retina to detach are in the upper part of the eye, a gas can be injected into the eye to push the retina back into place. The tears can then be repaired with laser photocoagulation or cryopexy.
- Scleral buckling: If a large area of the retina is detached, it is often necessary to drain fluid from under the retina and then place a silicone band or sponge on the outside of the eye to push it against the retina.
- If a cornea transplant is required, it is performed.

POSSIBLE COMPLICATIONS
- Surgical-wound infection.
- Partial or total vision loss in the affected eye from recurrence of retinal detachment.

AVERAGE HOSPITAL STAY—Usually none.

PROBABLE OUTCOME—Surgery is successful in preserving eyesight in over 90% of patients. About 10% will require another operation, which is usually successful. Allow about 2 weeks for recovery from surgery.

POSTOPERATIVE CARE

GENERAL MEASURES
- Rest with your head elevated on two pillows. Your doctor may want you to keep your head in a certain position for a few days to a few weeks.
- Cool compresses can reduce the swelling of the eyelids and surrounding tissue.
- Use dark glasses in bright light until you no longer need to keep the pupils dilated with eye drops. Don't rub the eyes.
- Don't bend over or strain with lifting, bowel movements or urination for at least 6 months after surgery.

MEDICATION
- Your doctor may prescribe:
  Pain relievers. Don't take prescription pain medication longer than 4 to 7 days. Use only as much as you need.
  Stool softeners to prevent constipation.
  Antibiotics to fight or prevent infection.
  Eye drops to keep the pupil dilated during healing.
- You may use nonprescription drugs, such as acetaminophen for minor pain. Avoid aspirin.

ACTIVITY
- To help recovery and aid your well-being, resume daily activities as soon as you are able.
- Avoid vigorous exercise for 6 weeks after surgery.
- Resume driving 4 weeks after returning home.

DIET—No special diet.

CALL YOUR DOCTOR IF

- You experience any change in vision.
- You develop constipation.
- Pain, swelling, redness, drainage or bleeding increases in the surgical area.
- You develop signs of infection, including headache, muscle aches, dizziness or a general ill feeling and fever.
- New, unexplained symptoms develop. Drugs used in treatment may produce side effects.

RETINAL DETACHMENT REPAIR

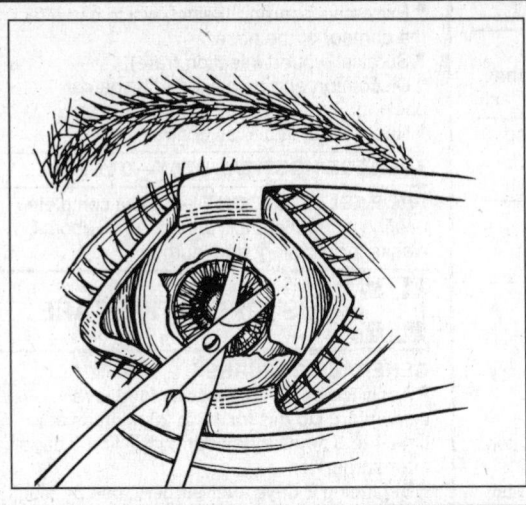

An illustration of the relationship of parts of the eye.
- Scissors cutting the sclera (the membrane lining the eye).

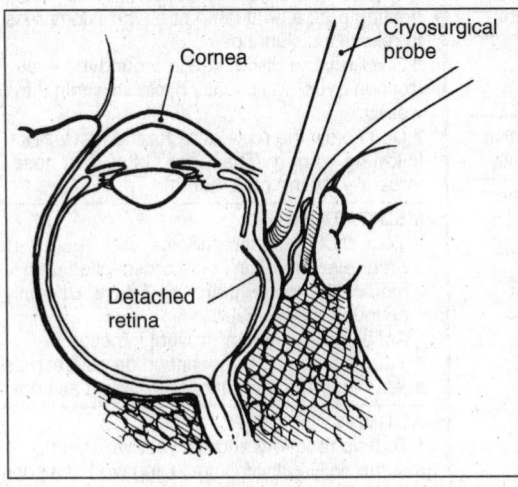

Cornea

Cryosurgical probe

Detached retina

Cyrosurgical probe is placed around the detached retina. The probe applies extreme cold causing eye tissue to coagulate and adhere to its normal position.

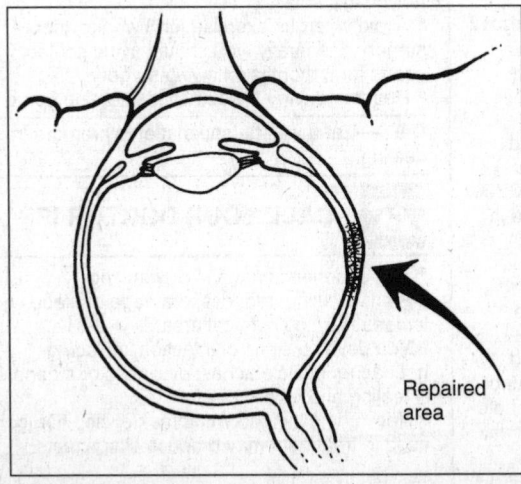

Repaired area

The retina returned to normal position after the detached retina has been secured in its proper position.

RHINOPLASTY & SEPTOPLASTY

GENERAL INFORMATION

DEFINITION—Reconstruction of the nose (rhinoplasty) and removal of deformities of the septum (septoplasty).

BODY PARTS INVOLVED—Nose, including nasal cartilage and bone and mucous membrane of the septum.

REASONS FOR SURGERY
- Opening of blocked nasal passages.
- Improved appearance.

SURGICAL RISK INCREASES WITH
- Obesity; smoking.
- Poor nutrition.
- Excess alcohol consumption.
- Recent or chronic illness.
- Diabetes mellitus.
- Use of some prescription and nonprescription drugs. Inform your doctor of any drugs, medications, or vitamin and herb supplements you are using or have used in the last month.

WHAT TO EXPECT

WHO OPERATES—Plastic and reconstructive surgeon or an ear, nose and throat specialist.

WHERE PERFORMED—Hospital or outpatient surgical facility.

DIAGNOSTIC TESTS
- Before surgery: Blood and urine studies; x-rays of facial bones.
- After surgery: Blood studies.

ANESTHESIA
- Local anesthesia by injection.
- General anesthesia by injection and inhalation with an airway tube placed in the windpipe.

DESCRIPTION OF OPERATION
- The nostril is held open with a speculum.
- An incision is made in the nose. To minimize visual scarring, the incision is usually made from within the nostrils; external cuts may be made if the shape of the nostrils is being changed.
- The bone or cartilage is fractured, trimmed and molded into the desired shape. If the goal is to increase the length of the nose, or to elevate the bridge, cartilage or bone from elsewhere in the body may be used as an implant. A synthetic material may also be used for the implant.
- The mucous membrane is closed with fine sutures, which usually can be removed about 10 days after surgery. Bandages are applied.
- For some procedures, petroleum-jelly-coated packing gauze or plastic splints are used to hold the septum in place during healing (up to 2 weeks).

POSSIBLE COMPLICATIONS
- Excessive bleeding.
- Excessive scarring (keloid) which can affect the contour of the nose.
- Surgical-wound infection (rare).
- Discomfort and pain caused by gauze packing.
- Recurrence of airway obstruction.

AVERAGE HOSPITAL STAY—0 to 1 day.

PROBABLE OUTCOME—Expect complete healing without complications. Allow about 3 weeks for recovery from surgery.

POSTOPERATIVE CARE

GENERAL MEASURES
- Apply ice packs to the nose to relieve discomfort. Do this for 10 to 20 minutes at a time 4 to 8 times a day during the first 2 days after surgery.
- Beginning 2 days after surgery, use an electric heating pad, a heat lamp or a warm compress to relieve incisional pain.
- Swelling and discoloration around the eyes (racoon eyes) will usually diminish within 2 to 3 weeks.
- Don't blow the nose at all for the first week following surgery. Then, don't blow your nose forcefully for the next month.

MEDICATION
- Your doctor may prescribe:
  Pain relievers. Don't take prescription pain medication longer than 4 to 7 days. Use only as much as you need.
  Antibiotics to fight or prevent infection.
- You may use nonprescription drugs, such as acetaminophen, for minor pain. Avoid aspirin.

ACTIVITY
- To help recovery and aid your well-being, resume daily activities, including work, as soon as you are able.
- Avoid vigorous exercise for 3 weeks after surgery. Generally, you should avoid contact sports for 6 months following surgery.
- Resume driving 1 week after returning home.

DIET—Eat a well-balanced diet to promote healing.

CALL YOUR DOCTOR IF

- You experience nausea or vomiting.
- Pain, swelling, redness, drainage or bleeding increases in the surgical area.
- You develop signs of infection, including headache, muscle aches, dizziness or a general ill feeling and fever.
- New, unexplained symptoms develop. Drugs used in treatment may produce side effects.

RHINOPLASTY & SEPTOPLASTY

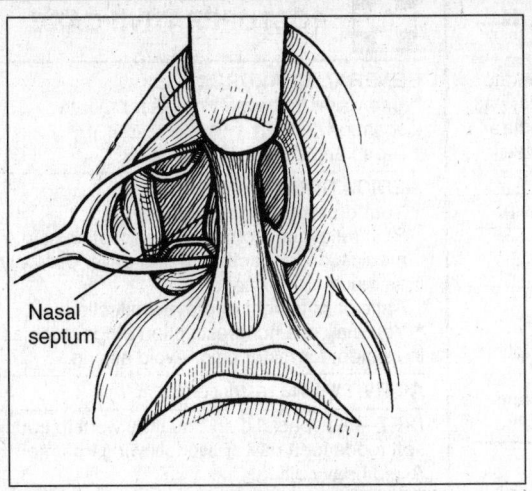

Nasal septum

An illustration of the mouth and nose with a speculum opening one side of the nose.

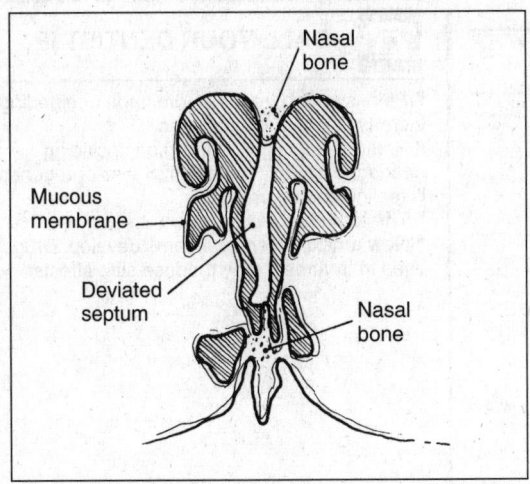

Nasal bone

Mucous membrane

Deviated septum

Nasal bone

An incision is made inside the nose. The bone or cartilage is fractured, trimmed and molded into the desired shape.

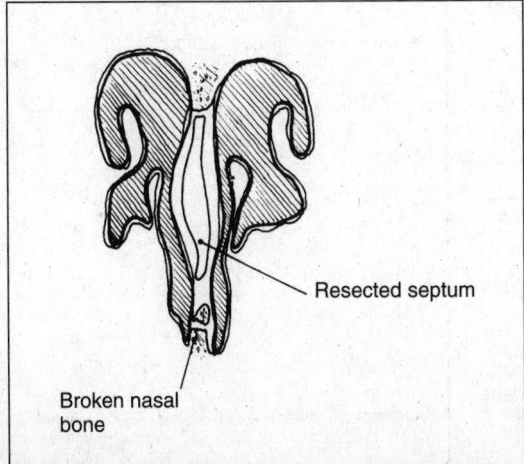

Resected septum

Broken nasal bone

Resected septum closed with fine sutures that usually can be removed about 10 days after surgery.

SURGERIES

ROOT CANAL TREATMENT
(Endodontic Therapy)

 GENERAL INFORMATION

DEFINITION—A dental procedure designed to save a tooth in which the living tissue (pulp) has died or is chronically diseased. The procedure cleans out dead or dying nerve tissue, as well as any infection, from the inside of a tooth.

BODY PARTS INVOLVED—Teeth and pulp.

REASONS FOR SURGERY—To avoid extraction of the affected tooth.

SURGICAL RISK INCREASES WITH
- Diabetes mellitus.
- Use of some prescription and nonprescription drugs. Inform your doctor of any drugs, medications, or vitamin and herb supplements you are using or have used in the last month.

 WHAT TO EXPECT

WHO OPERATES—Endodonist; general dentist.

WHERE PERFORMED—Dentist's office.

DIAGNOSTIC TESTS
- Before surgery: X-rays.
- During surgery: X-rays.
- After surgery: X-rays.

ANESTHESIA—Local anesthetic.

DESCRIPTION OF OPERATION
- Root canal therapy is usually done in 1 to 2 appointments.
- A hole is drilled into the pulp so that any infected matter can be removed.
- The root canals are enlarged and shaped with long, fine-tipped instruments.
- Medicated cotton and a temporary filling are placed in the cavity.
- After a week, or at the next appointment, the filling is removed and the cavity is filled with special material, gutta percha, and the root is sealed.

POSSIBLE COMPLICATIONS
- Pain and swelling.
- Surgical-wound infection.
- Persistent or recurring abscess.

AVERAGE HOSPITAL STAY—Usually none.

PROBABLE OUTCOME—Expect complete healing without complications. Allow about 2 weeks for recovery from surgery. Complete healing may take several months, but there should be no symptoms or discomfort. The tooth should function as long as a normal tooth would. Teeth that undergo root canal treatment usually require a crown.

 POSTOPERATIVE CARE

GENERAL MEASURES
- Use warm, salt-water rinses for mouth discomfort.
- Brush and floss teeth as usual.

MEDICATION
- Your dentist may prescribe:
  Pain relievers. Don't take prescription pain medication longer than 2 or 3 days. Use only as much as you need.
  Antibiotics to fight or prevent infection.
- You may use nonprescription drugs, such as ibuprofen, for minor pain. Avoid aspirin.

ACTIVITY—No restrictions.

DIET—No special diet. You may want to eat soft foods for a day or two following treatments. Avoid heavy biting.

 CALL YOUR DENTIST IF

- Pain, swelling, redness, drainage or bleeding increases in the surgical area.
- You develop signs of infection, including headache, muscle aches, dizziness or a general ill feeling and fever.
- The tooth feels loose.
- New, unexplained symptoms develop. Drugs used in treatment may produce side effects.

ROOT CANAL TREATMENT
(Endodontic Therapy)

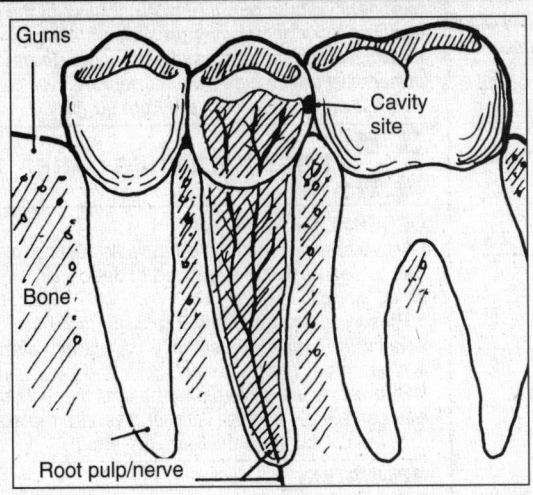

Gums

Cavity site

Bone

Root pulp/nerve

Cavity site is identified.

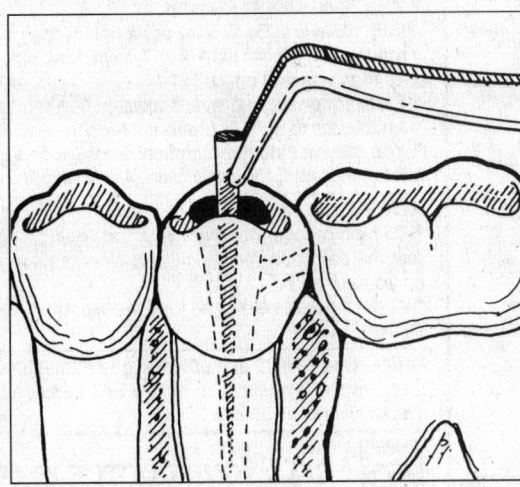

Cavity is drilled and root canal is enlarged.

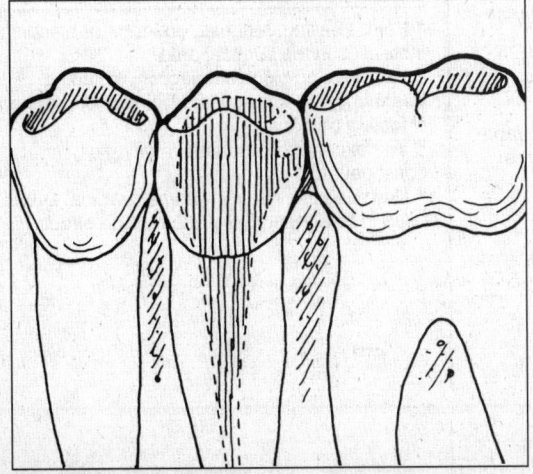

Canal is filled with special material to seal it off.

SALIVARY GLAND TUMOR REMOVAL

 GENERAL INFORMATION

DEFINITION—Removal of a cancerous tumor of the salivary glands.

BODY PARTS INVOLVED—Salivary glands under the tongue (sublingual) or under the jawbone (submaxillary).

REASONS FOR SURGERY—Cancer or suspected cancer of the sublingual or submaxillary salivary glands.

SURGICAL RISK INCREASES WITH
- Adults over 60.
- Obesity.
- Smoking.
- Excess alcohol consumption.
- Stress.
- Poor nutrition.
- Recent or chronic illness.
- Diabetes mellitus.
- Use of some prescription and nonprescription drugs. Inform your doctor of any drugs, medications, or vitamin and herb supplements you are using or have used in the last month.

 WHAT TO EXPECT

WHO OPERATES—Ear, nose and throat specialist (otolaryngologist) or general surgeon.

WHERE PERFORMED—Hospital.

DIAGNOSTIC TESTS
- Before surgery: Blood and urine studies; x-rays of the head, neck, upper gastrointestinal tract and chest.
- After surgery: Blood studies.

ANESTHESIA—General anesthesia by injection and inhalation with an airway tube placed in the windpipe.

DESCRIPTION OF OPERATION
- Incisions are made in the mucous membrane or skin over the tumor.
- The tumor is isolated, cut free and removed.
- The tissue is examined to determine if the tumor is benign or cancerous.
- If the tumor is benign, the mucous membrane over the tumor is closed with fine silk sutures.
- A plastic drain tube may be placed in the incision and left for several days.
- If the tumor is cancerous, a radical neck dissection (see in Surgery section) is usually performed.

POSSIBLE COMPLICATIONS
- Excessive bleeding.
- Surgical-wound infection.
- Facial nerve injury.
- Fistula (see Glossary) from salivary gland.

AVERAGE HOSPITAL STAY—1 to 2 days.

PROBABLE OUTCOME—Expect complete healing without complications. You may experience some permanent numbness of the earlobe. Your doctor may prescribe further treatment with radiation and anticancer drugs depending on findings from surgery. Allow about 3 months for recovery from surgery.

 POSTOPERATIVE CARE

GENERAL MEASURES
- Move and elevate legs often while resting in bed to decrease the likelihood of deep-vein blood clots.
- Rinse your mouth every 2 to 3 hours with a solution of 1 teaspoon salt in 8 oz. warm water. A clean mouth heals faster.
- Shower as usual. Avoid baths until the incision has completely healed. After showering, replace any wet dressings with clean, dry ones.

MEDICATION
- Your doctor may prescribe:
  Pain relievers. Don't take prescription pain medication longer than 4 to 7 days. Use only as much as you need.
  Stool softeners to prevent constipation.
  Antibiotics to fight or prevent infection.
- You may use nonprescription drugs, such as acetaminophen, for minor pain. Avoid aspirin.

ACTIVITY
- To help recovery and aid your well-being, resume daily activities, including work, as soon as you are able.
- Avoid vigorous exercise for 3 weeks after surgery.

DIET—Clear liquid diet until the gastrointestinal tract functions again. Then eat a well-balanced diet to promote healing.

 CALL YOUR DOCTOR IF

- Pain, swelling, redness, drainage or bleeding increases in the surgical area.
- You develop signs of infection, including headache, muscle aches, dizziness or a general ill feeling and fever.
- You experience nausea, vomiting or constipation.
- New, unexplained symptoms develop. Drugs used in treatment may produce side effects.

SALIVARY GLAND TUMOR REMOVAL

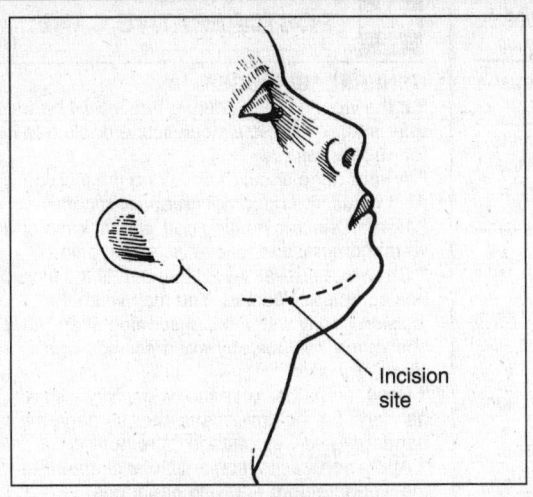

An illustration of the submaxillary area with the dotted line indicating the incision site for submaxillary gland removal.

Incision site

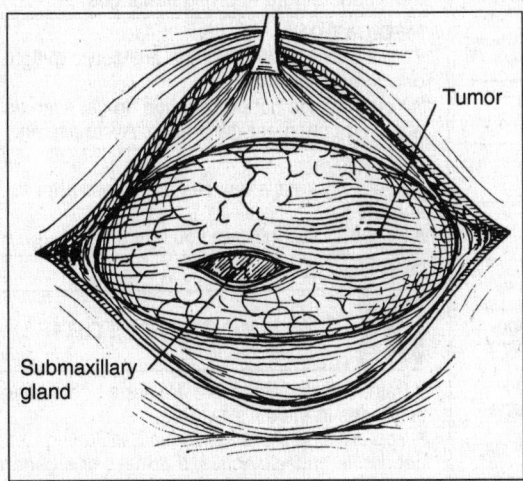

Incisions are made through the skin and tissues under the skin to expose the tumor.

Tumor

Submaxillary gland

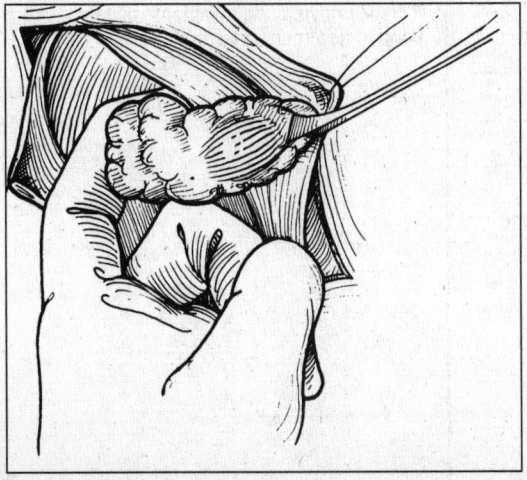

The tumor is isolated, cut free and scooped out with a finger or surgical instrument.

SEBACEOUS CYST REMOVAL
(Epidermoid Cyst Removal)

 GENERAL INFORMATION

DEFINITION—Removal of benign sebaceous cysts, sometimes called epidermoid cysts.

BODY PARTS INVOLVED—Sebaceous cysts, usually occurring on the skin of the trunk, face, scalp and neck. They often appear behind the ear.

REASONS FOR SURGERY
- Prevention of infections.
- Improved appearance.

SURGICAL RISK INCREASES WITH
- Any bleeding disorder.
- Diabetes mellitus.
- Use of some prescription and nonprescription drugs. Inform your doctor of any drugs, medications, or vitamin and herb supplements you are using or have used in the last month.

 WHAT TO EXPECT

WHO OPERATES—Family doctor, general surgeon or dermatologist.

WHERE PERFORMED—Doctor's office or outpatient surgical facility.

DIAGNOSTIC TESTS
- Before surgery: Usually none.
- After surgery: Laboratory examination of removed tissue.

ANESTHESIA—Local anesthesia by injection.

DESCRIPTION OF OPERATION
- An incision is made over the cyst, with care taken not to rupture its confining wall. Leakage from the cyst can cause inflammation and delayed healing.
- The cyst and its contents are removed intact.
- The skin is closed with sutures or clips, which usually can be removed about 1 week after surgery.

POSSIBLE COMPLICATIONS
- Excessive bleeding.
- Surgical-wound infection.
- Recurrence of the cyst, if the cyst wall is not completely removed.

AVERAGE HOSPITAL STAY—Usually none.

PROBABLE OUTCOME—Expect complete healing without complications. Allow about 2 to 3 weeks for healing to be fairly complete.

 POSTOPERATIVE CARE

GENERAL MEASURES
- If the wound bleeds during the first 24 hours after surgery, press a clean tissue or cloth to it for 10 minutes.
- A hard ridge should form along the incision. As it heals, the ridge will gradually recede.
- Use an electric heating pad, a heat lamp or a warm compress to relieve incisional pain.
- Shower as usual. Avoid baths until the incision has completely healed. You may wash the incision gently with mild, unscented soap. After showering, replace any wet dressings with clean, dry ones.
- Between baths, keep the wound dry with a bandage for the first 2 days after surgery. If a bandage gets wet, change it promptly.
- Apply nonprescription antibiotic ointment to the wound before applying bandages.

MEDICATION
- Your doctor may prescribe antibiotics to fight or prevent infection.
- You may use nonprescription drugs, such as acetaminophen, for minor pain. Avoid aspirin.

ACTIVITY
- Avoid vigorous exercise for 2 weeks after surgery.
- Resume driving when you feel well enough to.

DIET—No special diet.

 CALL YOUR DOCTOR IF

- Pain, swelling, redness, drainage or bleeding increases in the surgical area.
- You develop signs of infection, including headache, muscle aches, dizziness or a general ill feeling and fever.
- New, unexplained symptoms develop. Drugs used in treatment may produce side effects.

SEBACEOUS CYST REMOVAL
(Epidermoid Cyst Removal)

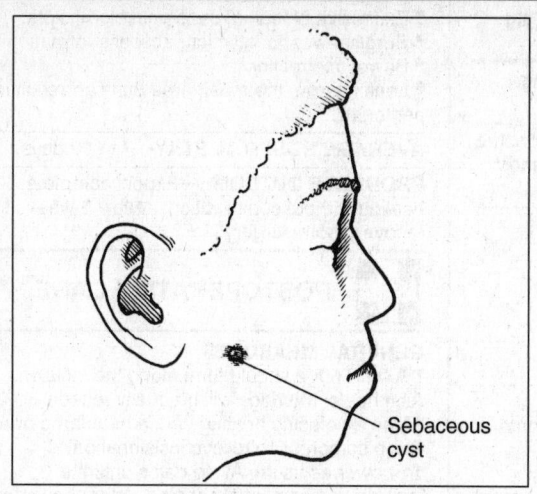

An illustration of a typical sebaceous cyst. In this case, on the side of the face.

Sebaceous cyst

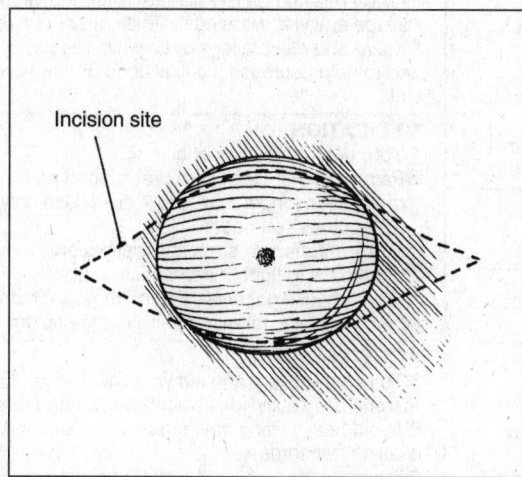

An incision is made over the cyst with care taken not to rupture its capsule (soft tissue lining the surface of the cyst).

Incision site

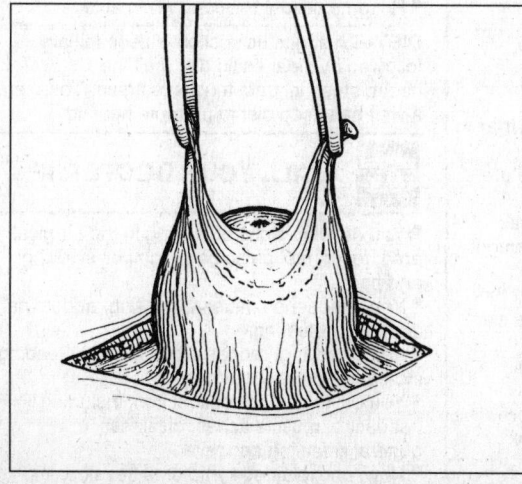

The cyst and its contents are removed intact.

SURGERIES

SIGMOID COLON REMOVAL
(Sigmoid Colectomy)

GENERAL INFORMATION

DEFINITION—Removal of part or all of the sigmoid colon.

BODY PARTS INVOLVED—Sigmoid colon, the part of the large intestine (colon) that extends from the descending colon to the rectum.

REASONS FOR SURGERY
- Diverticulitis with bleeding or infection.
- Cancer or precancerous polyps.
- Volvulus (see Glossary).
- Colon stricture.
- Rectovaginal fistula.
- Prolapse of rectum.

SURGICAL RISK INCREASES WITH
- Adults over 60 years; newborns and infants.
- Obesity; smoking; stress.
- Poor nutrition.
- Excess alcohol consumption.
- Chronic illness; recent illness such as acute, recurrent diverticulitis.
- Diabetes mellitus.
- Use of some prescription and nonprescription drugs. Inform your doctor of any drugs, medications, or vitamin and herb supplements you are using or have used in the last month.

WHAT TO EXPECT

WHO OPERATES—General surgeon.

WHERE PERFORMED—Hospital.

DIAGNOSTIC TESTS
- Before surgery: Blood and urine studies; x-rays of upper and lower gastrointestinal tract; ECG; endoscopy; proctoscopy; colonoscopy (see Glossary for all).
- After surgery: Blood studies.

ANESTHESIA—General anesthesia by injection and inhalation with an airway tube placed in the windpipe.

DESCRIPTION OF OPERATION
- An incision is made in the abdomen, and the abdominal muscles are opened.
- The sigmoid colon is isolated and clamps are placed at each end.
- All of the diseased sigmoid colon is cut free and removed. The two healthy ends are brought back together and joined.
- The abdominal contents are replaced into the abdomen, and the muscles are closed. The skin is closed with sutures or skin clips, which usually can be removed about 1 week after surgery.
- If surgery is performed to treat infection or tumor, a temporary colostomy (see Surgery section) may be necessary.

POSSIBLE COMPLICATIONS
- Excessive bleeding; deep-vein blood clots.
- Surgical-wound infection; abscess formation.
- Bowel obstruction.
- Leaking from the repair area that can result in peritonitis.

AVERAGE HOSPITAL STAY—7 to 10 days.

PROBABLE OUTCOME—Expect complete healing without complications. Allow 6 weeks for recovery from surgery.

POSTOPERATIVE CARE

GENERAL MEASURES
- A hard ridge should form along the incision. As it heals, the ridge will gradually recede.
- Use an electric heating pad, a heat lamp or a warm compress to relieve incisional pain.
- Shower as usual. Avoid baths until the incision has completely healed. After showering, replace any wet dressings with clean, dry ones.
- Move and elevate legs often while resting in bed to help decrease the likelihood of deep-vein clots.

MEDICATION
- Your doctor may prescribe:
  Pain relievers. Don't take prescription pain medication longer than 4 to 7 days. Use only as much as you need.
  Stool softeners to prevent constipation.
  Antibiotics to fight or prevent infection.
- You may use nonprescription drugs, such as acetaminophen, for minor pain. Avoid aspirin.

ACTIVITY
- To help recovery and aid your well-being, resume daily activities as soon as you are able.
- Avoid heavy lifting or vigorous exercise for 6 weeks after surgery.
- Resume driving 3 weeks after returning home.
- Resume sexual relations when able.

DIET—Nasogastric suction is used initially, followed by clear liquid diet until the gastrointestinal tract functions again. Then, eat a well-balanced diet to promote healing.

CALL YOUR DOCTOR IF

- You develop signs of leaking in the surgical area: fever, fast pulse or abdominal swelling and pain.
- You experience nausea, vomiting, abdominal cramps or bloating.
- Pain, swelling, redness, drainage or bleeding increases in the surgical area.
- You develop signs of infection, including headache, muscle aches, dizziness, or a general ill feeling and fever.
- New, unexplained symptoms develop.

SIGMOID COLON REMOVAL
(Sigmoid Colectomy)

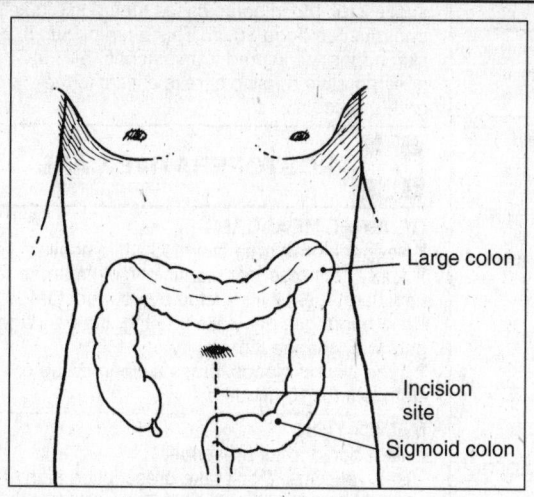

An illustration of the large intestine, sigmoid colon and the usual incision site for this surgical procedure.

Large colon

Incision site

Sigmoid colon

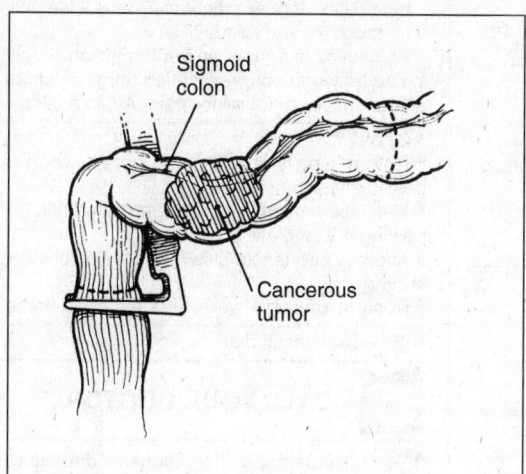

Sigmoid colon

Cancerous tumor

The sigmoid colon is isolated and clamps are placed at each end.
• All of the diseased sigmoid colon is cut free and removed.

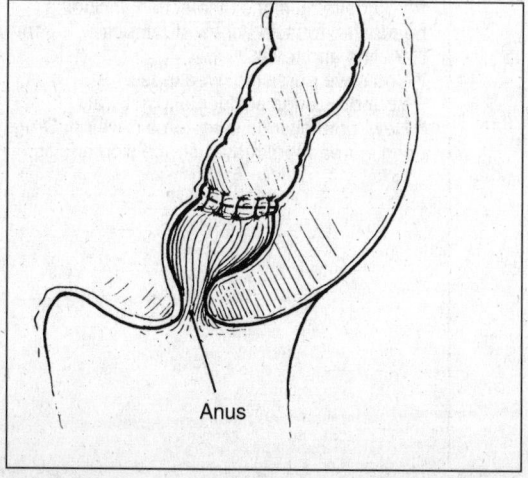

Anus

The two healthy ends of the colon are repositioned and joined whenever possible.

SKIN GRAFT

GENERAL INFORMATION

DEFINITION—Taking skin from one area of the body and attaching it to another area where no skin exists.

BODY PARTS INVOLVED—Skin (donor sites and recipient sites).

REASONS FOR SURGERY—Extensive wounds, burns or certain surgeries may require skin grafts for healing to occur.

SURGICAL RISK INCREASES WITH
- Adults over 60.
- Newborns and infants.
- Obesity; smoking.
- Poor nutrition.
- Anemia.
- Recent or chronic illness.
- Diabetes mellitus.
- Use of some prescription and nonprescription drugs. Inform your doctor of any drugs, medications, or vitamin and herb supplements you are using or have used in the last month.

WHAT TO EXPECT

WHO OPERATES—General surgeon or plastic and reconstructive surgeon.

WHERE PERFORMED—Hospital, outpatient surgical facility or emergency room (rarely).

DIAGNOSTIC TESTS
- Before surgery: Blood and urine studies.
- After surgery: Blood studies.

ANESTHESIA
- Local anesthesia by injection.
- General anesthesia by injection and inhalation with an airway tube placed in the windpipe.

DESCRIPTION OF OPERATION
- Skin is removed from a donor site. The donor site is covered with gauze.
- Debris is cleared from the recipient site.
- The skin from the donor site is placed on the recipient site and fastened at each corner with sutures. Bandages are applied. New blood vessels begin growing from the recipient area into the transplanted skin within 36 hours.

POSSIBLE COMPLICATIONS
- Excessive bleeding.
- Surgical-wound infection.
- Collection of serum under recipient site that prevents growth of new blood vessels.
- Loss of grafted skin.

AVERAGE HOSPITAL STAY—2 to 12 days, depending on extent of surgery.

PROBABLE OUTCOME—Allow about 6 weeks for recovery from surgery. Most skin grafts are successful, but in some cases they don't "take" and must be done again. This often occurs if skin edges are injured from stitches. Skillful postoperative nursing care is critical to the graft's success.

POSTOPERATIVE CARE

GENERAL MEASURES
- Keep the graft area elevated while healing.
- Apply nonprescription antibiotic ointment to new bandages, if instructed by your doctor. Keep bandages dry while bathing. If a bandage gets wet, change it promptly.
- If the wound bleeds, press a clean tissue or cloth to it for 10 minutes.

MEDICATION
- Your doctor may prescribe:
  Pain relievers. Don't take prescription pain medication longer than 4 to 7 days. Use only as much as you need.
  Antibiotics to fight or prevent infection.
- You may use nonprescription drugs, such as acetaminophen, for minor pain. Avoid aspirin.

ACTIVITY
- Return to daily activities and work as soon as possible to promote healing.
- Minimize movement of the graft site until healing is complete.
- Avoid vigorous exercise for 6 weeks following surgery.
- Resume driving 1 week after returning home.

DIET—No special diet.

CALL YOUR DOCTOR IF

- You have pain, swelling, redness, drainage, bleeding or odor in the surgical area.
- You develop signs of infection, including headache, muscle aches, dizziness or a general ill feeling and fever.
- You have persistent weakness.
- Your dressings accidentally get wet.
- New, unexplained symptoms develop. Drugs used in treatment may produce side effects.

SKIN GRAFT

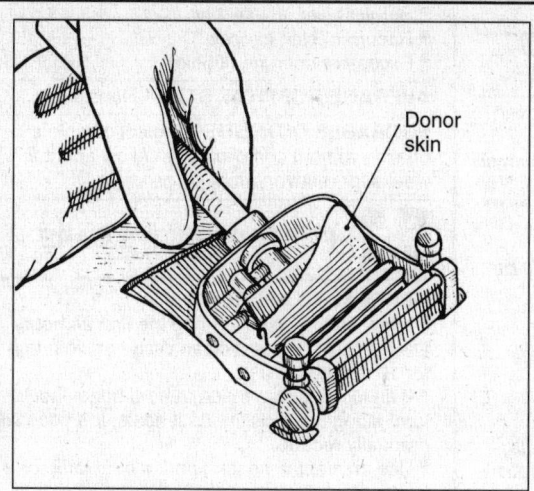

A thin layer of skin to be used for skin grafting is removed with a dermatoma (skin cutting instrument).

Donor skin

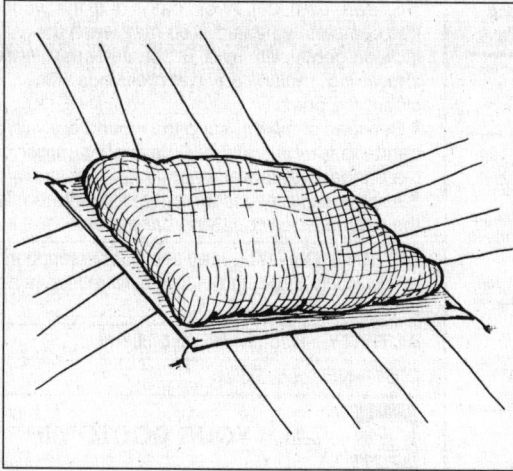

After skin has been removed from donor site, it is placed over the recipient site and fastened to normal skin at each corner.

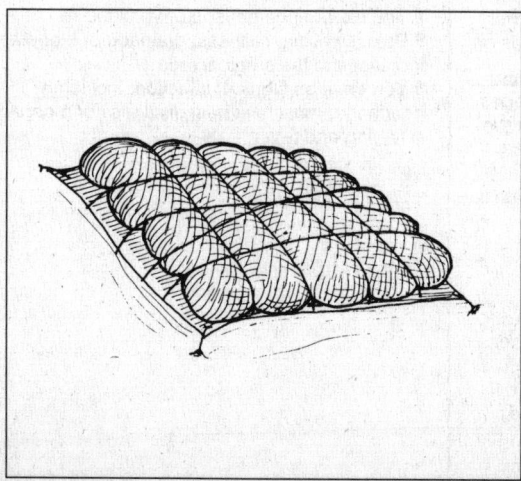

Pressure bandages are applied over the skin graft. The new blood vessels begin growing from the recipient area into the transplanted skin within 36 hours.

SKIN LESION REMOVAL

 GENERAL INFORMATION

DEFINITION—Removal or ablation of any benign or cancerous lesion on the skin.

BODY PARTS INVOLVED—Abnormal growth on the skin. The most common are warts, moles, skin cancers, molluscum contagiosum or senile keratoses.

REASONS FOR SURGERY
● Diagnosis of the abnormal growth.
● Removal of any abnormality suspected to be cancerous.
● Concern about appearance.
● Irritation of the lesion due to clothing.

SURGICAL RISK INCREASES WITH
● Adults over 60.
● Obesity; poor nutrition; anemia.
● Recent or chronic illness; diabetes mellitus.
● Use of some prescription and nonprescription drugs. Inform your doctor of any drugs, medications, or vitamin and herb supplements you are using or have used in the last month.

 WHAT TO EXPECT

WHO OPERATES—Family doctor, dermatologist, general surgeon or plastic and reconstructive surgeon.

WHERE PERFORMED—Hospital, emergency room, doctor's office or outpatient surgical facility.

DIAGNOSTIC TESTS
● Before surgery: Blood and urine studies.
● After surgery: Laboratory examination of removed tissue.

ANESTHESIA
● Local anesthesia by injection.
● General anesthesia by injection and inhalation with an airway tube placed in the windpipe (for large excisions, skin grafts, or for procedures on young children).

DESCRIPTION OF OPERATION—Techniques to remove or ablate abnormal growths from the skin include:
● Scraping the abnormality away (curettement).
● Cutting with scissors, especially if the lesion is on a stalk.
● Freezing warts and benign superficial keratoses (cryotherapy).
● Using heat (electrosurgery).
● Incising the skin with a cold scalpel, removing the lesion and sewing the skin edges together.
● The technique chosen depends on the nature of the lesion and the condition of the patient. If sutures or clips are used to close the wound, they can usually be removed about 1 week after surgery.
● Skin grafting is sometimes required.

POSSIBLE COMPLICATIONS
● Excessive bleeding.
● Surgical-wound infection.
● Recurrent skin cancer.
● Excessive scarring (keloid).

AVERAGE HOSPITAL STAY—None.

PROBABLE OUTCOME—Expect complete healing without complications. Allow about 2 weeks for recovery from surgery.

 POSTOPERATIVE CARE

GENERAL MEASURES
● If the wound bleeds during the first 24 hours after surgery, press a clean tissue or cloth to it for 10 minutes.
● If an incision was made, a hard ridge should form along the incision. As it heals, the ridge will gradually recede.
● Use an electric heating pad, a heat lamp or a warm compress to relieve incisional pain.
● Shower as usual. Avoid baths until the wound has completely healed. You may wash the incision gently with mild, unscented soap. After showering, replace any wet dressings with clean, dry ones.
● Between showers, keep the wound dry with a bandage for the first 2 or 3 days after surgery. If the bandage gets wet, change it promptly.
● Apply a nonprescription antibiotic ointment to the wound before applying bandages.

MEDICATION—You may use nonprescription drugs, such as acetaminophen, to relieve minor pain. Avoid aspirin.

ACTIVITY—Usually, no restrictions.

DIET—No special diet.

 CALL YOUR DOCTOR IF

● You experience nausea or vomiting.
● Pain, swelling, redness, drainage or bleeding increases in the surgical area.
● You develop signs of infection, including headache, muscle aches, dizziness or a general ill feeling and fever.

SKIN LESION REMOVAL

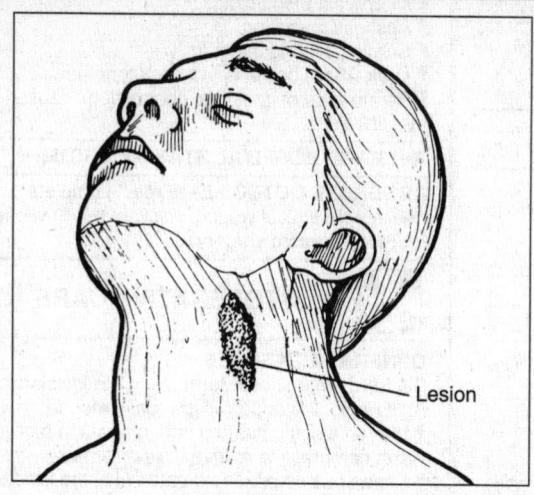

An illustration of a skin lesion on the neck to be treated with cryosurgery (very low temperature).

Lesion

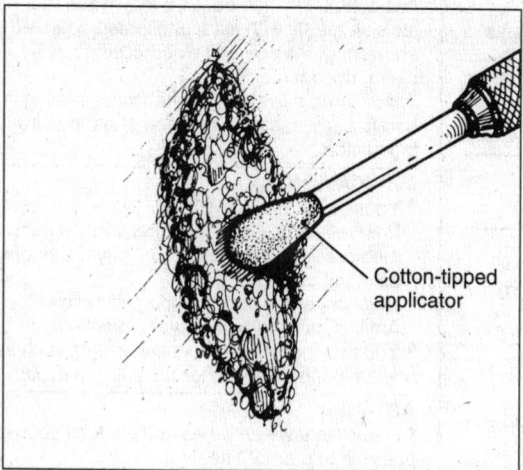

A cotton-tipped applicator that has been dipped in liquid nitrogen is held against the lesion to destroy abnormal tissue.

Cotton-tipped applicator

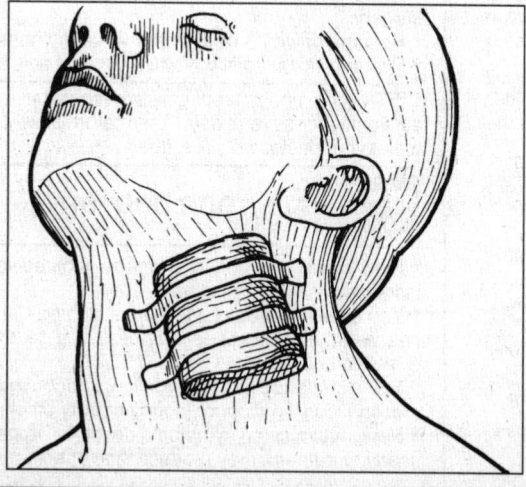

Large treated areas should be covered with bandages until healing is complete.

SURGERIES

SMALL-BOWEL RESECTION

GENERAL INFORMATION

DEFINITION—Removal of diseased, injured, or abnormal section of the small bowel (small intestine).

BODY PARTS INVOLVED—Small intestine, including the mesentery (blood supply) around it.

REASONS FOR SURGERY
- Tumor, gangrene, narrowing or obstruction in the small intestine.
- Trauma, such as from a wound.

SURGICAL RISK INCREASES WITH
- Adults over 60.
- Obesity.
- Smoking.
- Poor nutrition.
- Previous abdominal surgery.
- Recent or chronic illness.
- Diabetes mellitus.
- Use of some prescription and nonprescription drugs. Inform your doctor of any drugs, medications, or vitamin and herb supplements you are using or have used in the last month.

WHAT TO EXPECT

WHO OPERATES—General surgeon.

WHERE PERFORMED—Hospital.

DIAGNOSTIC TESTS
- Before surgery: Blood and urine studies; x-rays of chest and gastrointestinal tract; CT; MRI; colonoscopy (see Glossary for all).
- After surgery: Blood studies.

ANESTHESIA
- Spinal anesthesia by injection.
- General anesthesia by injection and inhalation with an airway tube placed in the windpipe.

DESCRIPTION OF OPERATION
- Operative procedures will vary depending on the cause.
- An incision is made in the abdomen.
- The muscles are separated or cut, and the abdominal cavity is entered.
- The intestine is examined for disease.
- The small intestine is clamped above and below the diseased section. The diseased section between the clamps is cut free and removed.
- The two open ends of the remaining small bowel are fastened together with sutures or staples. Occasionally, a temporary ileostomy (see Surgery section) is necessary.
- The peritoneum and muscles are closed with sutures. The skin is closed with sutures or clips, which usually can be removed about 1 week after surgery.

POSSIBLE COMPLICATIONS
- Excessive bleeding.
- Deep-vein blood clots.
- Abscess formation.
- Surgical-wound infection.
- Leak where bowel is put back together.
- Recurrence of intestinal obstructions caused by adhesions.

AVERAGE HOSPITAL STAY—7 to 10 days.

PROBABLE OUTCOME—Expect complete healing of surgical wound. Allow about 6 weeks for recovery from surgery.

POSTOPERATIVE CARE

GENERAL MEASURES
- A hard ridge should form along the incision. As it heals, the ridge will gradually recede.
- Use an electric heating pad, a heat lamp or a warm compress to relieve incisional pain.
- Shower as usual. Avoid baths until the incision has completely healed. You may wash the incision gently with mild, unscented soap. After showering, replace any wet dressings with clean, dry ones.
- Move and elevate legs often while resting in bed to decrease the likelihood of deep-vein blood clots.

MEDICATION
- Your doctor may prescribe:
  Pain relievers. Don't take prescription pain medication longer than 4 to 7 days. Use only as much as you need.
  Stool softeners to prevent constipation.
  Antibiotics to fight or prevent infection.
- You may use nonprescription drugs, such as acetaminophen, for minor pain. Avoid aspirin.

ACTIVITY
- Return to daily activities and work as soon as possible to promote healing.
- Avoid vigorous exercise for 6 weeks after surgery.
- Resume driving 3 weeks after returning home.
- Resume sexual relations when you feel able to.

DIET—Intravenous feeding with nasogastric suctioning for several days, then return slowly to a diet your doctor will prescribe.

CALL YOUR DOCTOR IF

- Pain, swelling, redness, drainage or bleeding increases in the surgical area.
- You develop signs of infection, including headache, muscle aches, dizziness or a general ill feeling and fever.
- You experience nausea, vomiting, abdominal swelling, constipation, or bloody or tarry stools.
- New, unexplained symptoms develop. Drugs used in treatment may produce side effects.

SMALL-BOWEL RESECTION

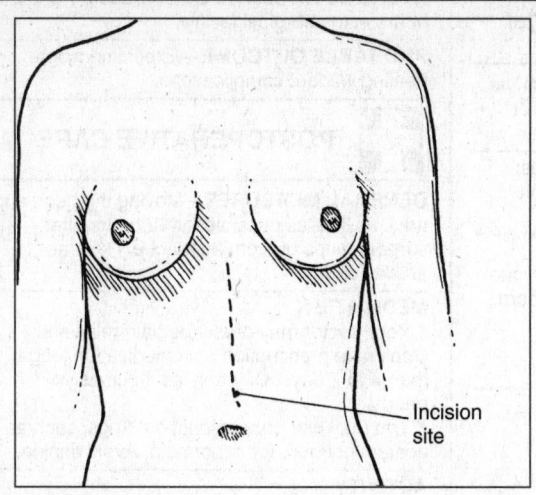

An illustration of a typical incision site for small bowel removal.

Incision site

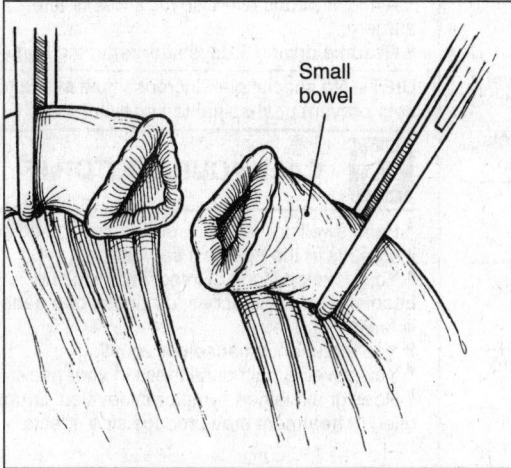

Small bowel

After the abdominal muscles are separated, the abdominal cavity is entered and the intestinal tract is examined for disease.
• The small intestine is clamped above and below the diseased section. The diseased section between the clamps is cut free and removed.

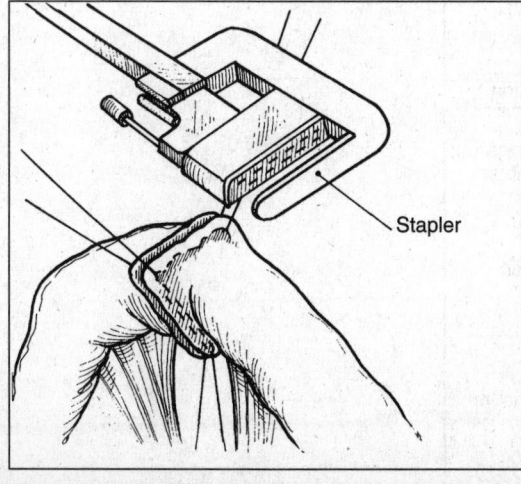

The 2 open ends of the remaining small bowel are fastened together with sutures or staples.

Stapler

SURGERIES

SPINAL TAP
(Lumbar Puncture)

GENERAL INFORMATION

DEFINITION—Removal of spinal fluid from the spinal canal, either for laboratory analysis or prior to surgery with spinal anesthesia.

BODY PARTS INVOLVED—Skin; muscles; covering of spinal cord (meninges); vertebral column.

REASONS FOR PROCEDURE
- Diagnosis of disorders of the central nervous system that may involve the brain, spinal cord, or their coverings.
- Injection of spinal anesthesia.
- Myelogram (see Glossary).

SURGICAL RISK INCREASES WITH
- Recent or chronic illness.
- Alcoholism.
- Increased intracranial pressure due to any cause.
- Central nervous system infection.
- Severe arthritis in spine.
- Diabetes mellitus.
- Use of some prescription and nonprescription drugs. Inform your doctor of any drugs, medications, or vitamin and herb supplements you are using or have used in the last month.

WHAT TO EXPECT

WHO OPERATES—General surgeon, family doctor, neurologist, neurosurgeon, anesthesiologist or internist.

WHERE PERFORMED—Hospital, outpatient surgical facility or emergency room.

DIAGNOSTIC TESTS
- Before surgery: Blood and urine studies.
- During surgery: Pressure of spinal fluid measured with a manometer (see Glossary).
- After surgery: Laboratory examination of removed fluid.

ANESTHESIA—Local anesthesia by injection.

DESCRIPTION OF OPERATION
- The patient is positioned on his side with the knees drawn as close to the chest as possible.
- A hollow needle is inserted in the back between the 2nd and 3rd lumbar vertebrae.
- The spinal canal is penetrated with the needle. Fluid pressure is measured and then fluid is removed.
- The surgical wound will heal by itself.

POSSIBLE COMPLICATIONS
- Surgical wound infection.
- Headaches (common during the first 24 hours after the procedure).
- Meningitis (rare).

AVERAGE HOSPITAL STAY—Usually 6 to 24 hours in the surgical facility.

PROBABLE OUTCOME—Expect complete healing without complications.

POSTOPERATIVE CARE

GENERAL MEASURES—Moving the head and neck as little as possible for 12 hours after surgery helps prevent headache. Resume activity slowly.

MEDICATION
- Your doctor may prescribe pain relievers. Don't take prescription pain medication longer than 4 to 7 days. Use only as much as you need.
- You may use nonprescription drugs, such as acetaminophen, for minor pain. Avoid aspirin.

ACTIVITY
- Avoid vigorous exercise for 2 weeks after surgery.
- Resume driving 3 days after returning home.

DIET—No special diet. Increase fluid intake to help prevent post-spinal-tap headaches.

CALL YOUR DOCTOR IF

- Pain, swelling, redness, drainage or bleeding increases in the needle insertion area.
- You develop signs of infection, including headache, muscle aches, dizziness or a general ill feeling and fever.
- You experience nausea or vomiting.
- You develop pain or stiffness in your neck.
- New, unexplained symptoms develop. Drugs used in treatment may produce side effects.

SPINAL TAP
(Lumbar Puncture)

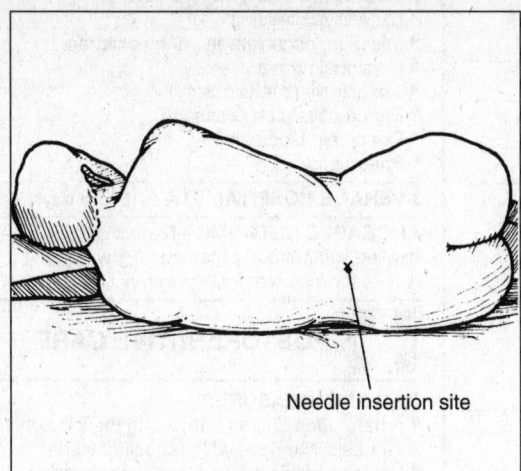

An illustration of a typical needle insertion site and the mid-spine.

Needle insertion site

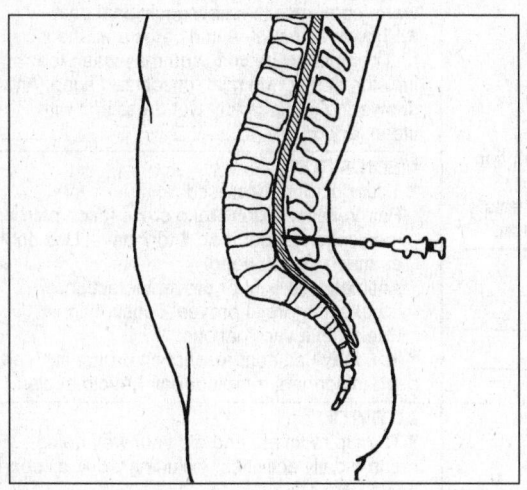

The needle is inserted between sinus processes of the bone into the cavity of the spinal canal, which surrounds the spine and is filled with fluid.

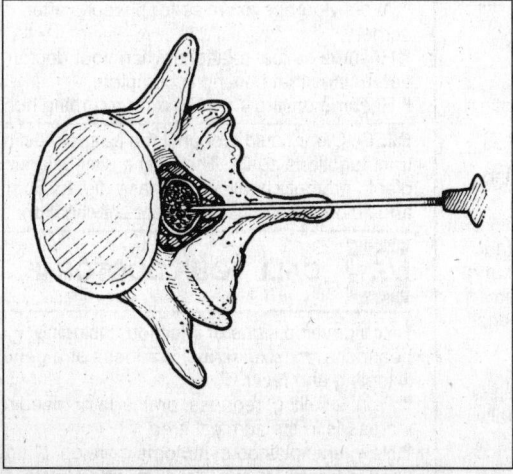

The spinal canal is penetrated with the needle. The fluid pressure is measured, then fluid is removed for laboratory examination.

SURGERIES

SPLEEN REMOVAL
(Splenectomy)

 GENERAL INFORMATION

DEFINITION—Removal of the spleen.

BODY PARTS INVOLVED—The spleen, a large organ on the left side of the upper abdominal cavity next to the stomach.

REASONS FOR SURGERY
* Injury to the spleen causing rupture and bleeding.
* Various blood diseases, including spherocytosis, thrombocytopenia or lymphatic leukemia (see Glossary for all).
* Splenic-vein thrombosis caused by esophageal varices (see Glossary).
* Benign or cancerous tumors.

SURGICAL RISK INCREASES WITH
* Adults over 60.
* Newborns and infants.
* Obesity.
* Smoking.
* Excess alcohol consumption.
* Poor nutrition.
* Recent or chronic illness.
* Diabetes mellitus.
* Use of some prescription and nonprescription drugs. Inform your doctor of any drugs, medications, or vitamin and herb supplements you are using or have used in the last month.

 WHAT TO EXPECT

WHO OPERATES—General surgeon.

WHERE PERFORMED—Hospital.

DIAGNOSTIC TESTS
* Before surgery: Blood and urine studies; x-rays of abdomen; CT scan (see Glossary).
* After surgery: Blood studies.

ANESTHESIA—General anesthesia by injection and inhalation with an airway tube placed in the windpipe.

DESCRIPTION OF OPERATION
* An incision is made in the abdomen.
* The spleen is located and isolated.
* Blood vessels to the spleen are cut and tied off.
* The spleen is rotated and removed from its bed where it is attached to the coverings of the stomach, kidney and diaphragm (see Glossary).
* If the spleen has been ruptured, the abdomen is explored to identify any other injured organs or blood vessels. Other surgeries may be performed at this time.
* The muscles are closed in layers. The skin is closed with sutures or skin clips, which usually can be removed in about 1 week.

POSSIBLE COMPLICATIONS
* Excessive bleeding.
* Infection, especially in young children.
* Incisional hernia.
* Atelectasis (see Glossary).
* Pancreatitis (see Glossary).
* Deep-vein blood clots.
* Pneumonia.

AVERAGE HOSPITAL STAY—3 to 5 days.

PROBABLE OUTCOME—Expect complete healing without complications. Allow about 4 weeks for recovery from surgery.

 POSTOPERATIVE CARE

GENERAL MEASURES
* A hard ridge should form along the incision. As it heals, the ridge will gradually recede.
* Use an electric heating pad, a heat lamp or a warm compress to relieve incisional pain.
* Shower as usual. Avoid baths until the incision has completely healed. You may wash the incision gently with mild, unscented soap. After showering, replace any wet dressings with clean, dry ones.

MEDICATION
* Your doctor may prescribe:
  Pain relievers. Don't take prescription pain medication longer than 4 to 7 days. Use only as much as you need.
  Antibiotics to fight or prevent infection.
  Stool softeners to prevent constipation.
  Pneumonia vaccinations.
* You may use nonprescription drugs, such as acetaminophen, for minor pain. Avoid aspirin.

ACTIVITY
* To help recovery and aid your well-being, resume daily activities, including work, as soon as you are able.
* Avoid vigorous exercise for 6 weeks after surgery.
* Resume sexual relations when your doctor determines that healing is complete.
* Resume driving 4 weeks after returning home.

DIET—Clear liquid diet until the gastrointestinal tract functions again. Then eat a well-balanced diet to promote healing. Increase dietary fiber and fluid intake to help prevent constipation.

 CALL YOUR DOCTOR IF

* You develop signs of infection, including headache, muscle aches, dizziness or a general ill feeling and fever.
* Pain, swelling, redness, drainage or bleeding increases in the surgical area.
* New, unexplained symptoms develop. Drugs used in treatment may produce side effects.

SPLEEN REMOVAL
(Splenectomy)

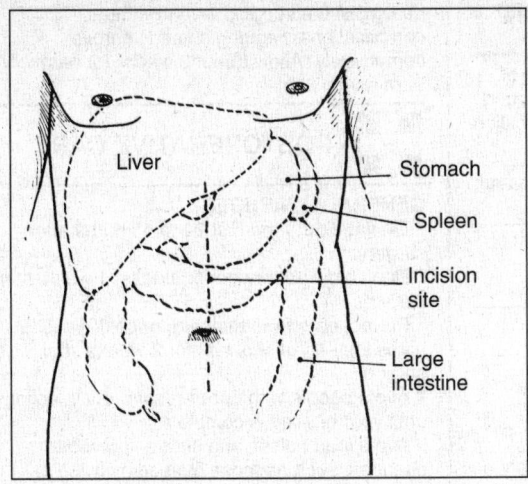

An illustration of the spleen, other internal organs and the usual incision site for a spleen removal.

Liver

Stomach

Spleen

Incision site

Large intestine

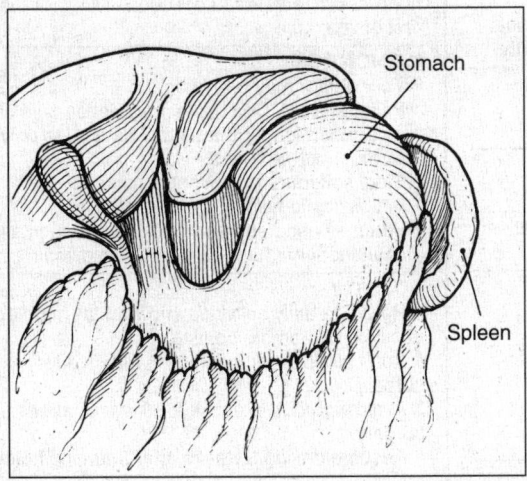

The spleen is rotated and removed from its bed where it's attached to the coverings of the stomach, kidney and diaphragm.

Stomach

Spleen

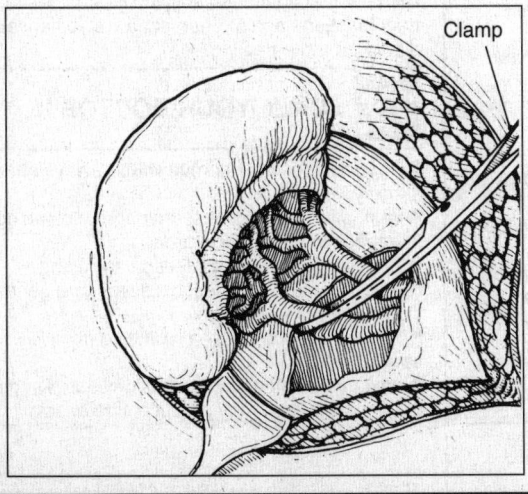

Blood vessels that supply the spleen are clamped and tied and the spleen is removed.

Clamp

STAPES REMOVAL
(Stapedectomy)

GENERAL INFORMATION

DEFINITION—Removal of the stapes, one of the bones in the middle ear that transmit sound waves to the inner ear. The stapes is also called the stirrup.

BODY PARTS INVOLVED—External ear canal; eardrum; middle ear; stapes.

REASONS FOR SURGERY—Improvement of hearing ability or prevention of continued hearing loss, usually due to otosclerosis.

SURGICAL RISK INCREASES WITH
- Obesity.
- Smoking.
- Poor nutrition.
- Recent or chronic illness.
- Diabetes mellitus.
- Use of some prescription and nonprescription drugs. Inform your doctor of any drugs, medications, or vitamin and herb supplements you are using or have used in the last month.

WHAT TO EXPECT

WHO OPERATES—Ear, nose and throat specialist (otolaryngologist).

WHERE PERFORMED—Hospital or outpatient surgical facility.

DIAGNOSTIC TESTS
- Before surgery: Blood and urine studies; hearing tests.
- After surgery: Hearing tests.

ANESTHESIA—General anesthesia by injection and inhalation with an airway tube placed in the windpipe.

DESCRIPTION OF OPERATION
- If both ears are affected, surgery is usually done on separate occasions.
- The operating microscope is positioned, and an incision is made in the middle ear.
- The small bones in the ear are identified, and the stapes is isolated and removed.
- Sometimes, a prosthesis made of stainless steel wire and cellulose sponge is inserted to replace the stapes.
- Blood and fluid are suctioned gently from the ear.
- The wound is closed with fine sutures, which can usually be removed about 1 week after surgery.

POSSIBLE COMPLICATIONS
- Excessive bleeding.
- Surgical-wound infection.

AVERAGE HOSPITAL STAY—3 to 5 days.

PROBABLE OUTCOME—Expect complete healing of the surgical wound without complications. Hearing should improve immediately. Allow about 3 weeks for recovery from surgery.

POSTOPERATIVE CARE

GENERAL MEASURES
- Lie flat during the first 24 to 48 hours after surgery.
- Don't blow your nose for at least 1 week after surgery.
- Protect ears from moisture or cold. Take tub baths instead of showers for 2 weeks after surgery.
- Avoid people with upper-respiratory infections until your healing is complete.
- Avoid loud noises and sudden pressure changes, such as those caused by flying in nonpressurized aircraft or scuba diving, for the rest of your life.

MEDICATION
- Your doctor may prescribe:
  Pain relievers. Don't take prescription pain medication longer than 4 to 7 days. Use only as much as you need.
  Stool softeners to prevent constipation.
  Antibiotics to fight or prevent infection.
- You may use nonprescription drugs, such as acetaminophen, for minor pain. Avoid aspirin.

ACTIVITY
- Return to daily activities and work as soon as possible to promote healing.
- Don't strain, bend or lift for 3 weeks after surgery.
- Avoid vigorous exercise for 6 weeks after surgery.
- Resume driving 3 weeks after returning home.

DIET—Clear liquid diet until the gastrointestinal tract functions again. Then eat a well-balanced diet to promote healing.

CALL YOUR DOCTOR IF

- Hearing does not improve within 2 days after surgery.
- Pain, swelling, redness, drainage or bleeding increases in the surgical area.
- You develop signs of infection, including headache, muscle aches, dizziness or a general ill feeling and fever.
- You experience nausea, vomiting or constipation.
- New, unexplained symptoms develop. Drugs used in treatment may produce side effects.

STAPES REMOVAL
(Stapedectomy)

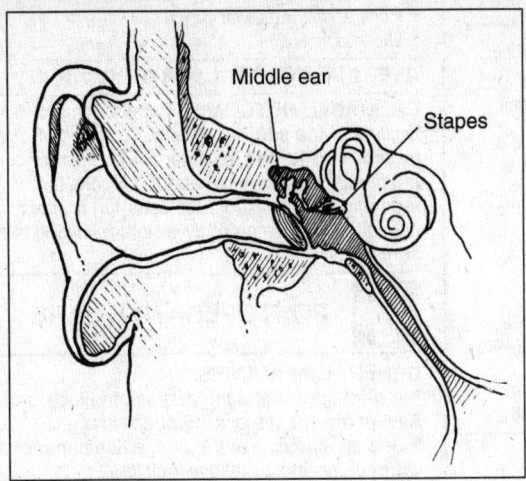

An illustration of the outer ear, middle ear and the stapes (one of the bones in the middle ear that transmits sound waves to the inner ear). The stapes is also called the stirrup.

Middle ear

Stapes

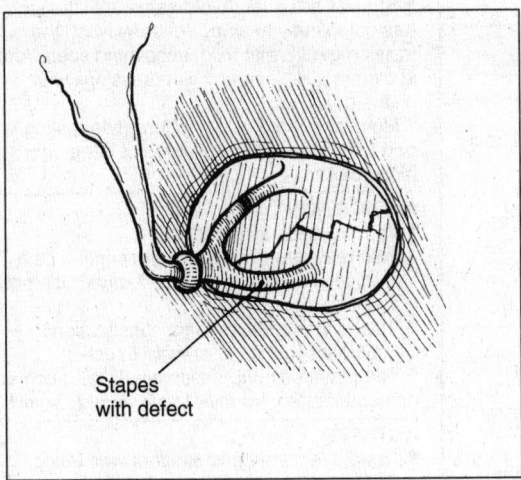

Appearance of the middle ear structure as seen through an operating microscope. Small bones in the ear are identified and the stapes is isolated and removed.

Stapes
with defect

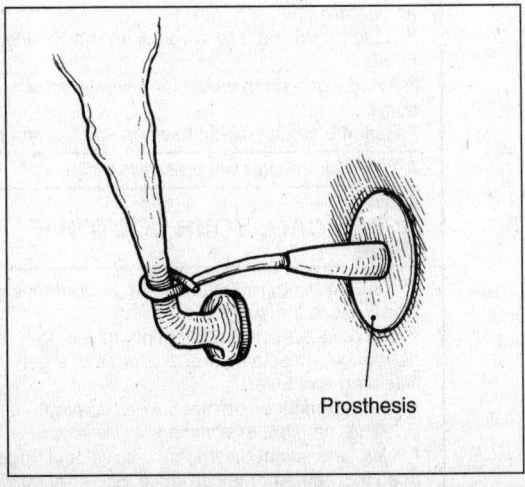

Sometimes a prosthesis made of stainless steel wire and cellulose sponge is inserted to replace the defective stapes.

Prosthesis

STOMACH CANCER SURGERY

 GENERAL INFORMATION

DEFINITION—Removal of cancerous tissue (gastric carcinoma) in the stomach.

BODY PARTS INVOLVED—Stomach; small intestine; esophagus (sometimes).

REASONS FOR SURGERY—Cancer of the stomach.

SURGICAL RISK INCREASES WITH
- Adults over 60.
- Obesity; poor nutrition; smoking.
- Alcoholism.
- Recent or chronic illness; diabetes mellitus.
- Use of some prescription and nonprescription drugs. Inform your doctor of any drugs, medications, or vitamin and herb supplements you are using or have used in the last month.

 WHAT TO EXPECT

WHO OPERATES—General surgeon.

WHERE PERFORMED—Hospital.

DIAGNOSTIC TESTS
- Before surgery: X-rays of gastrointestinal tract and chest; blood and urine studies; ECG; endoscopy; CT scan; (see Glossary for all).
- During surgery: Laboratory examination of removed tissue by frozen section (see Glossary).
- After surgery: Blood studies; laboratory examination of removed tissue.

ANESTHESIA—General anesthesia by injection and inhalation with an airway tube placed in the windpipe.

DESCRIPTION OF OPERATION
- An incision is made below the ribs.
- Abdominal muscles are cut or retracted, the peritoneum is opened and the stomach is isolated.
- Usually, the entire stomach is removed. The esophagus is attached to a pouch made of small intestine, to create a new "stomach". The nearby lymph nodes and omentum (see Glossary) are removed; sometimes the spleen is also removed.
- If any stomach is left the remaining stump of stomach is joined to a loop of small intestine (usually the jejunum) to allow normal digestive flow.
- The peritoneum is closed and the muscles are sewn together. The skin is closed with sutures or clips, which usually can be removed about 10 days after surgery.

POSSIBLE COMPLICATIONS
- Excessive bleeding.
- Surgical-wound infection.
- Incisional hernia.

- Chronic diarrhea; dumping syndrome.
- Malnutrition.
- Poor emptying of stomach.
- Ulcer disease.

AVERAGE HOSPITAL STAY—10 to 14 days.

PROBABLE OUTCOME—Expect complete healing of the surgical wound. Your doctor may recommend further treatment with radiation and anticancer drugs. Allow about 6 weeks for recovery from surgery. It is common to have difficulty maintaining body weight following this surgery.

 POSTOPERATIVE CARE

GENERAL MEASURES
- A hard ridge should form along the incision. As it heals, the ridge will gradually recede.
- Use an electric heating pad, a heat lamp or a warm compress to relieve incisional pain.
- Shower as usual. Avoid baths until the incision has completely healed. You may wash the incision gently with mild, unscented soap. After showering, replace any wet dressings with clean, dry ones.
- Move and elevate legs often while resting in bed to decrease the likelihood of deep-vein blood clots.

MEDICATION
- Your doctor may prescribe:
  Pain relievers. Don't take prescription pain medication longer than 4 to 7 days. Use only as much as you need.
  Stool softeners to prevent constipation.
  Antibiotics to fight or prevent infection.
- You may use nonprescription drugs, such as acetaminophen, for minor pain. Avoid aspirin.

ACTIVITY
- To help recovery and aid your well-being, resume daily activities, including work, as soon as you are able.
- Resume driving 3 to 4 weeks after returning home.
- Avoid vigorous exercise for 6 weeks after surgery.
- Resume sexual relations when you feel able.

DIET—Your doctor will prescribe a diet.

 CALL YOUR DOCTOR IF

- Pain, swelling, redness, drainage or bleeding increases in the surgical area.
- You develop signs of infection, including headache, muscle aches, dizziness or a general ill feeling and fever.
- You experience constipation, abdominal swelling, nausea, or vomiting.
- New, unexplained symptoms develop. Drugs used in treatment may produce side effects.

STOMACH CANCER SURGERY

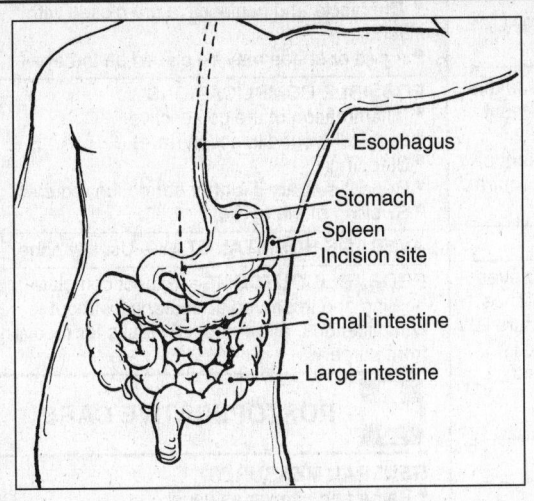

An illustration of the digestive system which shows the esophagus, stomach, spleen, large and small intestines, and a typical incision site for stomach cancer surgery.

Esophagus

Stomach

Spleen

Incision site

Small intestine

Large intestine

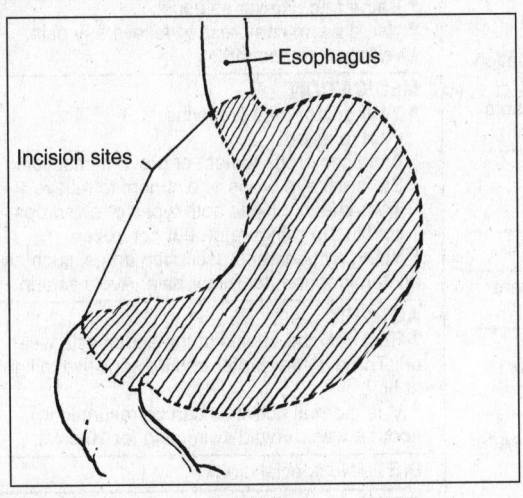

The abdominal muscles are cut and retracted; the peritoneum is opened and the stomach is isolated (not shown).
- Incisions are made in the lower part of the esophagus and the top of the small intestine, and the entire stomach is removed.

Esophagus

Incision sites

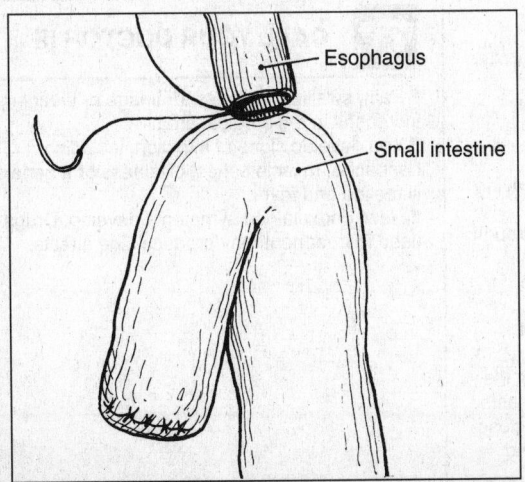

The esophagus is attached to a pouch made of small intestine, to create a new "stomach".
- Not shown: The peritoneum is closed and the muscles are sewn together. The skin is closed with sutures or clips which usually can be removed about 10 days after surgery.

Esophagus

Small intestine

SURGERIES

STRABISMUS SURGERY
(Squint Repair)

 GENERAL INFORMATION

DEFINITION—Surgery to strengthen or weaken the muscles that regulate horizontal movement of the eyeball (see Strabismus in Illness section). The surgery will vary with the extent of the deviation of the movement, and may require more than one operation.

BODY PARTS INVOLVED—Eyes.

REASONS FOR SURGERY—Realign the eyes to restore single binocular vision and a balance in the appearance of the eyes. The procedure is usually performed in children while the eye is still developing to save vision in the affected eye. In adults, the surgery is for cosmetic reasons only.

SURGICAL RISK INCREASES WITH
- Poor nutrition.
- Recent or chronic illness.
- Diabetes mellitus.
- Use of some prescription and nonprescription drugs. Inform your doctor of any drugs, medications, or vitamin and herb supplements you are using or have used in the last month.

 WHAT TO EXPECT

WHO OPERATES—Ophthalmologist.

WHERE PERFORMED—Hospital, outpatient surgical facility.

DIAGNOSTIC TESTS
- Before surgery: Special eye examinations to determine the amount of deviation. Tests performed will depend on the age of the patient; usually an older child or an adult can cooperate with instructions for visual testing, while an infant cannot.
- After surgery: Eye examinations may be repeated as necessary.

ANESTHESIA—General anesthesia by injection and inhalation with an airway tube placed in the windpipe.

DESCRIPTION OF OPERATION
- The head is wrapped in sterile towels, leaving the eyes exposed.
- The eye muscle is exposed by cutting through the conjunctiva and fascia and a special instrument (called a squint hook) holds the whole width of the muscle.
- If the muscle is to be lengthened, it is cut close to its root and reattached with non-absorbable stitches to the surface layers of the eye at a distance determined by the initial tests.
- If the muscle is to be shortened, it is cut close to its root and a section is removed. The two ends are then stitched together.

- The fascia and conjunctiva are closed with stitches.
- A pad or shade may be placed on the eye.

POSSIBLE COMPLICATIONS
- Inflammation of the conjunctiva.
- Surgical-wound infection (rare).
- Bleeding.
- Repeat surgery if further correction required.
- Swelling of the eyelid.

AVERAGE HOSPITAL STAY—Usually none.

PROBABLE OUTCOME—Expect complete healing and improved appearance without complications. Allow about 2 weeks for recovery from surgery.

 POSTOPERATIVE CARE

GENERAL MEASURES
- Bathe and shower as usual.
- Use a warm compress to relieve any pain, swelling or discomfort.

MEDICATION
- Your doctor may prescribe:
  Pain relievers.
  Antibiotic drops to fight or prevent infection.
  Steroidal eye drops or ointment to relieve inflammation. Keep both types of eye drops cold in the refrigerator, but not frozen.
- You may use nonprescription drugs, such as acetaminophen, for minor pain. Avoid aspirin.

ACTIVITY
- Rest until the effects of the anesthesia wear off. The eye may water and be sensitive to light at first.
- Most normal activities can be resumed in about a week. Avoid swimming for 10 days.

DIET—No special diet.

 CALL YOUR DOCTOR IF

- Pain, swelling, redness, drainage or bleeding increases in the surgical area.
- You develop signs of infection, including headache, muscle aches, dizziness or a general ill feeling and fever.
- New, unexplained symptoms develop. Drugs used in treatment may produce side effects.

STRABISMUS SURGERY
(Squint Repair)

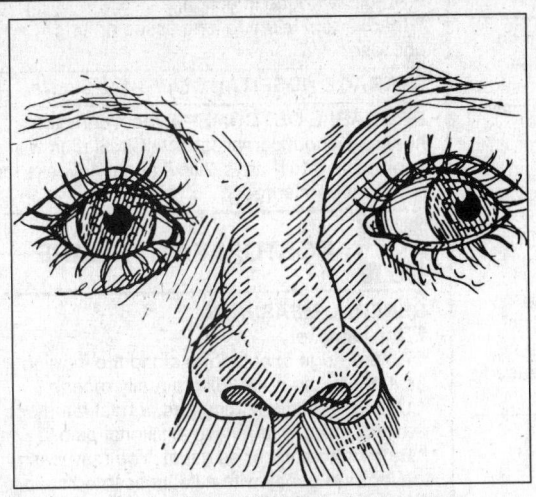

An infant's left eye demonstrates an external deviation.

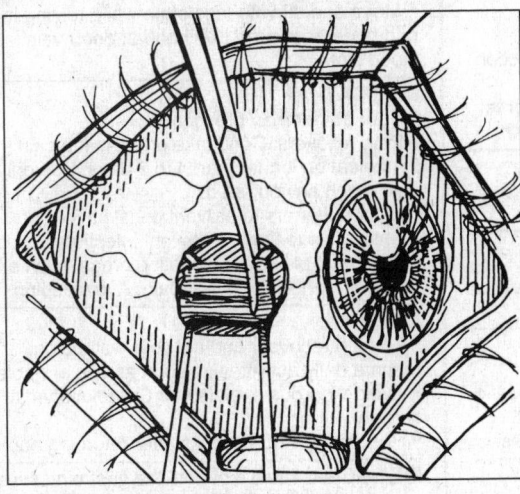

The eye muscle is surgically exposed and cut.

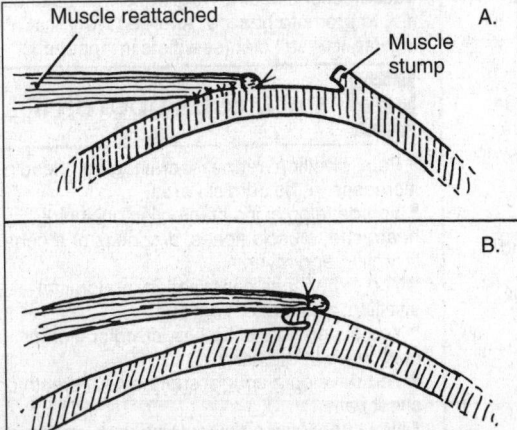

Muscle reattached

Muscle stump

A.

B.

A. Muscle shortening.

B. Muscle lengthening.

SYMPATHECTOMY, CERVICODORSAL

GENERAL INFORMATION

DEFINITION—Interruption of the sympathetic nerve chain at the base of the neck near the spine.

BODY PARTS INVOLVED—Cervicodorsal sympathetic nerves (part of the autonomic nervous system) that control contraction and expansion of small arteries in the arms; lungs; upper ribs.

REASONS FOR SURGERY
- Relieve post-traumatic pain complex.
- Restoration of normal blood supply to the arms. Removing part of the sympathetic nervous system stops spasms in the blood vessels that can cause or aggravate decreased circulation.

SURGICAL RISK INCREASES WITH
- Obesity; smoking; alcoholism.
- Recent or chronic illness.
- Atherosclerosis.
- Diabetes mellitus.
- Use of some prescription and nonprescription drugs. Inform your doctor of any drugs, medications, or vitamin and herb supplements you are using or have used in the last month.

WHAT TO EXPECT

WHO OPERATES—General surgeon, neurosurgeon or vascular surgeon.

WHERE PERFORMED—Hospital.

DIAGNOSTIC TESTS
- Before surgery: Blood and urine studies; x-rays of chest; ECG (see Glossary); diagnostic sympathetic nerve block.
- After surgery: Blood studies; x-rays of chest.

ANESTHESIA—General anesthesia by injection and inhalation with an airway tube placed in the windpipe.

DESCRIPTION OF OPERATION
- An incision is made in the armpit.
- The muscles are divided, and part of the 3rd rib is removed.
- One lung is allowed to collapse temporarily to allow easier entry into the chest cavity.
- The cervical and dorsal sympathetic nerve chains are identified and divided.
- The lung is re-expanded. The muscles and skin edges are closed with sutures or clips, which usually can be removed about 1 week after surgery.
- This procedure can now be done via a thoracoscope (an optical instrument with a lighted tip).

POSSIBLE COMPLICATIONS
- Excessive bleeding.
- Surgical-wound infection.
- Inadvertent injury to lung tissue or lung collapse.

AVERAGE HOSPITAL STAY—1 to 3 days.

PROBABLE OUTCOME—Expect complete healing without complications. Circulation will improve in 3 to 4 days. Allow about 4 weeks for recovery from surgery.

POSTOPERATIVE CARE

GENERAL MEASURES
- Don't smoke.
- A hard ridge should form along the incision. As it heals, the ridge will gradually recede.
- Use an electric heating pad, a heat lamp or a warm compress to relieve incisional pain.
- Bathe and shower as usual. You may wash the incision gently with mild, unscented soap.
- Move and elevate legs often while resting in bed to decrease the likelihood of deep-vein blood clots.

MEDICATION
- Your doctor may prescribe:
  Pain relievers. Don't take prescription pain medication longer than 4 to 7 days. Use only as much as you need.
  Stool softeners to prevent constipation.
  Antibiotics to fight or prevent infection.
- You may use nonprescription drugs, such as acetaminophen, for minor pain. Avoid aspirin.

ACTIVITY
- To help recovery and aid your well-being, resume daily activities as soon as you are able.
- Avoid vigorous exercise for 6 weeks after surgery.
- Resume driving 2 weeks after returning home.

DIET—Clear liquid diet until the gastrointestinal tract functions again. Then eat a well-balanced diet to promote healing. After recovery, eat a low-fat, low-salt diet (see diets in Appendix).

CALL YOUR DOCTOR IF

- Pain, swelling, redness, drainage or bleeding increases in the surgical area.
- You develop signs of infection, including headache, muscle aches, dizziness or a general ill feeling and fever.
- You experience constipation, abdominal swelling, nausea, or vomiting.
- You experience coldness, discoloration or numbness in the hand.
- You develop a cough, shortness of breath or chest pain.
- New, unexplained symptoms develop. Drugs used in treatment may produce side effects.

SYMPATHECTOMY, CERVICODORSAL

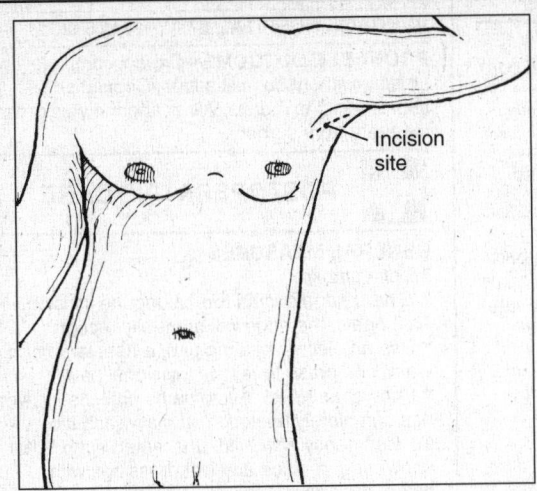

An illustration of the usual incision site for a cervicodorsal sympathectomy.

Incision site

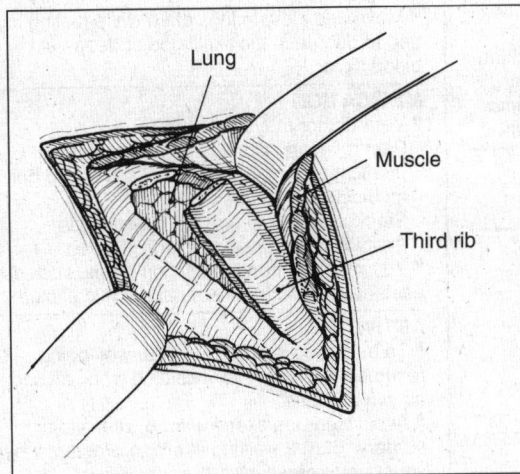

Muscles attached to ribs are divided and part of the 3rd rib is removed. One portion of the lung is allowed to temporarily collapse to allow easier entry into the chest cavity.

Lung

Muscle

Third rib

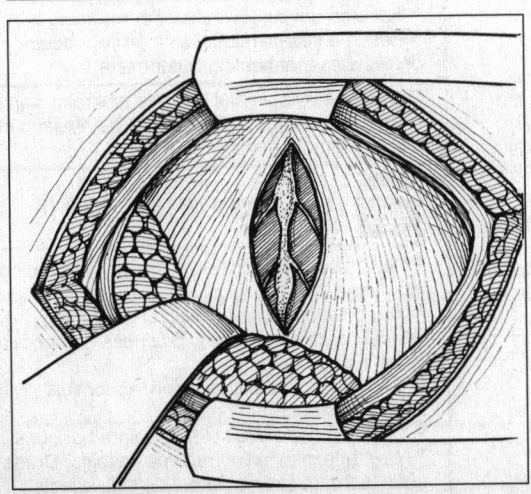

The cervical and dorsal sympathetic nerve chains are identified and divided.
 • Following the operation, the ribs are reconstructed and held in place with heavy sutures. The lung is re-expanded and the muscles and skin edges are closed with sutures or clips (not illustrated).

SURGERIES

SYMPATHECTOMY, LUMBAR

 GENERAL INFORMATION

DEFINITION—Removing a section of the sympathetic nerves located near the spinal cord in the lower back.

BODY PARTS INVOLVED—The lumbar sympathetic nerves (part of the autonomic nervous system) that control contraction and expansion of small arteries in the legs.

REASONS FOR SURGERY
- Improve blood flow to the legs. Removing part of the sympathetic nervous system stops spasms in the blood vessels that can cause or aggravate decreased blood flow and cause severe pain.
- Relieve symptoms of reflex sympathetic dystrophy.
- Nonhealing ulcers in legs or feet.

SURGICAL RISK INCREASES WITH
- Obesity; smoking.
- Recent or chronic illness.
- Atherosclerosis.
- Diabetes mellitus.
- Use of some prescription and nonprescription drugs. Inform your doctor of any drugs, medications, or vitamin and herb supplements you are using or have used in the last month.

 WHAT TO EXPECT

WHO OPERATES—General surgeon, neurosurgeon or vascular surgeon.

WHERE PERFORMED—Hospital.

DIAGNOSTIC TESTS
- Before surgery: Blood and urine studies; lumbar sympathetic nerve block.
- After surgery: Blood studies.

ANESTHESIA—General anesthesia by injection and inhalation with an airway tube placed in the windpipe.

DESCRIPTION OF OPERATION
- A short, horizontal incision is made on the abdomen slightly above and to the side of the navel. The muscles are separated.
- The lumbar sympathetic chain of nerves is located, cut free, and a short segment is removed.
- The muscles are sewn together with large sutures.
- The skin is closed with sutures or clips, which usually can be removed about 1 week after surgery.

POSSIBLE COMPLICATIONS
- Excessive bleeding.
- Surgical-wound infection.
- Incisional hernia (rare).
- Inadvertent injury to the ureter (rare).
- May result in impotence.

- Incomplete resection of nerves due to accessory fibers.

AVERAGE HOSPITAL STAY—3 to 5 days.

PROBABLE OUTCOME—Expect complete healing without complications. Circulation will improve in 3 to 4 days. Allow about 4 weeks for recovery from surgery.

 POSTOPERATIVE CARE

GENERAL MEASURES
- Don't smoke.
- A hard ridge should form along the incision. As it heals, the ridge will gradually recede.
- Use an electric heating pad, a heat lamp or a warm compress to relieve incisional pain.
- Shower as usual. Avoid baths until the incision has completely healed. You may wash the incision gently with mild, unscented soap. After showering, replace any wet dressings with clean, dry ones.
- Move and elevate legs often while resting in bed to decrease the likelihood of deep-vein blood clots.

MEDICATION
- Your doctor may prescribe:
  Pain relievers. Don't take prescription pain medication longer than 4 to 7 days. Use only as much as you need.
  Stool softeners to prevent constipation.
  Antibiotics to fight or prevent infection.
- You may use nonprescription drugs, such as acetaminophen, for minor pain. Avoid aspirin.

ACTIVITY
- To help recovery and aid your well-being, resume daily activities, including work, as soon as you are able.
- Avoid vigorous exercise for 6 weeks after surgery. Start a walking exercise program when your doctor prescribes it.
- Resume driving 2 weeks after returning home.
- Resume sexual relations when your doctor determines that healing is complete.

DIET—Clear liquid diet until the gastrointestinal tract functions again. Then eat a well-balanced diet to promote healing.

 CALL YOUR DOCTOR IF

- Pain, swelling, redness, drainage or bleeding increases in the surgical area.
- You develop signs of infection, including headache, muscle aches, dizziness or a general ill feeling and fever.
- You experience constipation, abdominal swelling, nausea or vomiting.
- Your foot becomes cold, discolored or numb.
- New, unexplained symptoms develop. Drugs used in treatment may produce side effects.

SYMPATHECTOMY, LUMBAR

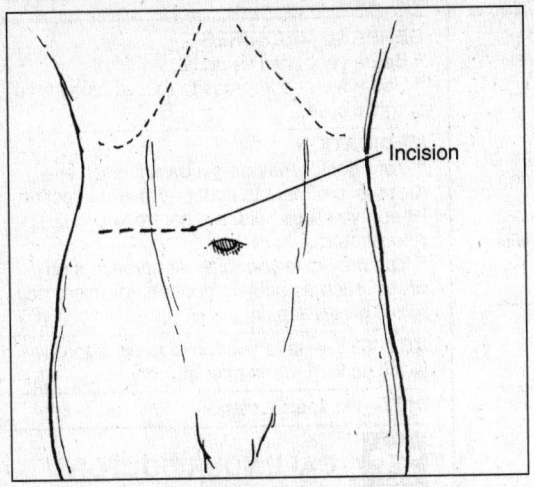

An illustration of a typical incision site to allow access to the sympathetic chain.

Incision

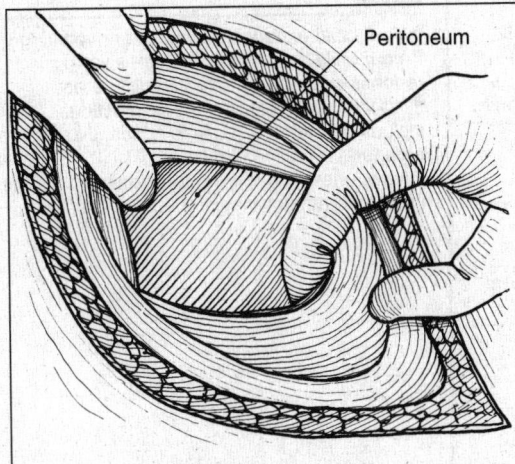

Peritoneum

Muscles overlying the spine are separated.

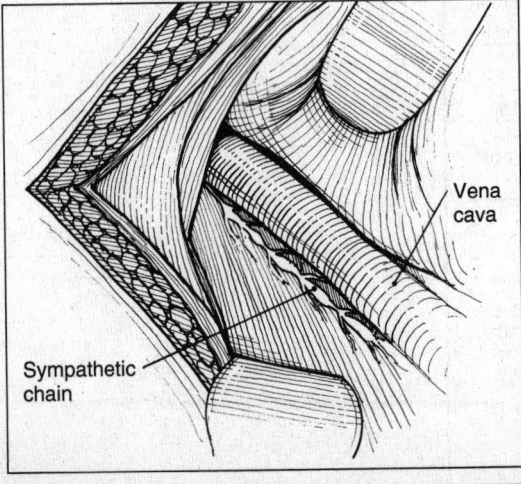

The lumbar sympathetic chain of nerves is located, cut free and removed.

Vena cava

Sympathetic chain

TEAR DUCT, OPENING OF

GENERAL INFORMATION

DEFINITION—Opening of tear ducts (also called lacrimal ducts) in the corners of the eyes closer to the nose. They may be blocked by infection or foreign material, or may be incompletely open in newborns. This is a common problem, affecting 6% of newborns. In 90% of these cases, however, the ducts open spontaneously by 1 year of age.

BODY PARTS INVOLVED—Tear glands and tear ducts, usually in newborns, infants or young children.

REASONS FOR SURGERY—Infection or complete blockage that does not respond to simple treatment.

SURGICAL RISK INCREASES WITH
- Obesity.
- Poor nutrition.
- Recent or chronic illness.
- Diabetes mellitus.
- Use of some prescription and nonprescription drugs. Inform your doctor of any drugs, medications, or vitamin and herb supplements your child is using or has used in the last month.

WHAT TO EXPECT

WHO OPERATES—Ophthalmologist or pediatric surgeon.

WHERE PERFORMED—Hospital or outpatient surgical facility.

DIAGNOSTIC TESTS
- Before surgery: Blood and urine studies.
- After surgery: Blood studies.

ANESTHESIA
- Local anesthesia by injection or topical application (sometimes).
- General anesthesia by injection and inhalation with an airway tube placed in the windpipe.

DESCRIPTION OF OPERATION
- The tear duct is expanded, probed and irrigated until fluid flows freely through it. The procedure is repeated on the other tear duct.
- Sutures are not needed. Bleeding should not be a problem.

POSSIBLE COMPLICATIONS—Surgical-wound infection.

AVERAGE HOSPITAL STAY—0 to 1 day.

PROBABLE OUTCOME—Expect complete healing without complications. Allow about 10 days for recovery from surgery.

POSTOPERATIVE CARE

GENERAL MEASURES
- Bathe your child as usual.
- Use a warm compress to relieve pain in the surgical area.

MEDICATION
- Your doctor may prescribe antibiotic eye drops or ointment to fight or prevent infection. Keep eye drops cold, but not frozen, in the refrigerator.
- You may give your child nonprescription drugs, such as acetaminophen, for minor pain. Avoid giving aspirin.

ACTIVITY—Have your child avoid vigorous exercise for 1 week after surgery.

DIET—No special diet.

CALL YOUR DOCTOR IF

- Your child experiences nausea or vomiting.
- Your child has increased pain, swelling, redness or drainage in the surgical area.
- Your child develops signs of infection, including headache, muscle aches, dizziness or a general ill feeling and fever.
- New, unexplained symptoms develop. Drugs used in treatment may produce side effects.

TEAR DUCT, OPENING OF

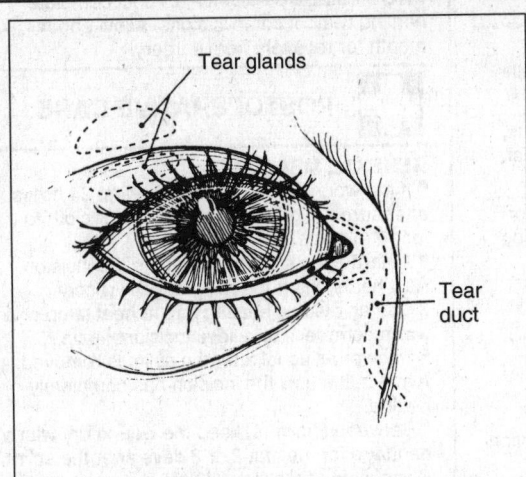

An illustration of tear glands, tear duct and other parts of the eye.

Tear glands

Tear duct

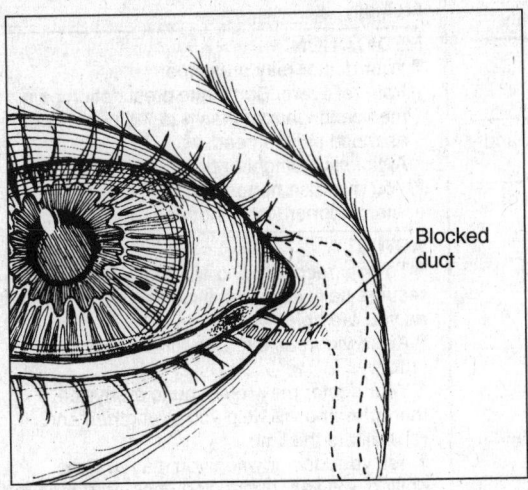

The blocked tear duct is identified.

Blocked duct

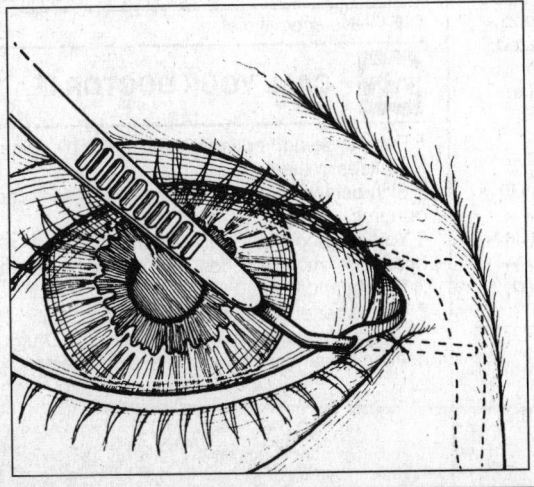

The blocked duct is expanded, probed and irrigated until fluid freely flows through it.

TENDON REPAIR

GENERAL INFORMATION

DEFINITION—Reattaching tendons (see Glossary) to their connective tissue, or sewing sections of cut or torn tendons together.

BODY PARTS INVOLVED—Injured tendons, most frequently in the hand, foot, ankle, wrist, shoulder, hip, knee and elbow.

REASONS FOR SURGERY—Restoration of normal function of joints or tissue surrounding tendons.

SURGICAL RISK INCREASES WITH
- Adults over 60.
- Obesity; smoking; alcoholism.
- Poor nutrition.
- Recent or chronic illness.
- Diabetes mellitus.
- Use of some prescription and nonprescription drugs. Inform your doctor of any drugs, medications, or vitamin and herb supplements you are using or have used in the last month.

WHAT TO EXPECT

WHO OPERATES—Orthopedic surgeon, hand surgeon or general surgeon.

WHERE PERFORMED—Hospital, outpatient surgical facility or emergency room.

DIAGNOSTIC TESTS
- Before surgery: Blood and urine studies; x-rays of the injured part.
- After surgery: Blood studies.

ANESTHESIA
- Local anesthesia by injection.
- Spinal anesthesia by injection.
- General anesthesia by injection and inhalation with an airway tube placed in the windpipe.

DESCRIPTION OF OPERATION
- An incision is made over the injured tendon.
- The severed ends of the tendon are located and sewn together. If the tendon has been destroyed, a tendon graft may be required to bridge the gap.
- If necessary, tendons are reattached to surrounding connective tissue.
- The surgical area is examined for injuries to nerves and blood vessels.
- The skin is closed with sutures, which usually can be removed about 10 days after surgery.
- Usually, the injured part is kept rigid with a splint or plaster cast.

POSSIBLE COMPLICATIONS
- Excessive bleeding.
- Surgical-wound infection.
- Partial loss of function in joint served by the injured tendon(s).
- Repeat rupture of tendon.

AVERAGE HOSPITAL STAY—0 to 1 day.

PROBABLE OUTCOME—Expect complete healing without complications. Allow about 1 month for recovery from surgery.

POSTOPERATIVE CARE

GENERAL MEASURES
- If the wound bleeds during the first 24 hours after surgery, press a clean tissue or cloth to it for 10 minutes.
- A hard ridge should form along the incision. As it heals, the ridge will gradually recede.
- Use an electric heating pad, a heat lamp or a warm compress to relieve incisional pain.
- Shower as usual after the splint is removed. Avoid baths until the incision has completely healed.
- Between showers, keep the wound dry with a bandage for the first 2 or 3 days after the splint is removed. If a bandage gets wet, change it promptly.

MEDICATION
- Your doctor may prescribe:
  Pain relievers. Don't take prescription pain medication longer than 4 to 7 days. Use only as much as you need.
  Antibiotics to fight or prevent infection.
- You may use nonprescription drugs, such as acetaminophen, for minor pain. Avoid aspirin.

ACTIVITY
- To help recovery and aid your well-being, resume daily activities, including work, as soon as you are able.
- Avoid vigorous exercise for 6 weeks after surgery.
- Your doctor may refer you to a physical therapist who will help you strengthen and rehabilitate the limb.
- Ask your doctor when you may resume driving; will vary depending upon area repaired.

DIET—No special diet.

CALL YOUR DOCTOR IF

- Pain, swelling, redness, drainage or bleeding increases in the surgical area.
- Skin below the cast becomes cold, discolored or numb.
- You develop signs of infection, including headache, muscle aches, dizziness or a general ill feeling and fever.
- You experience nausea or vomiting.
- New, unexplained symptoms develop. Drugs used in treatment may produce side effects.

TENDON REPAIR

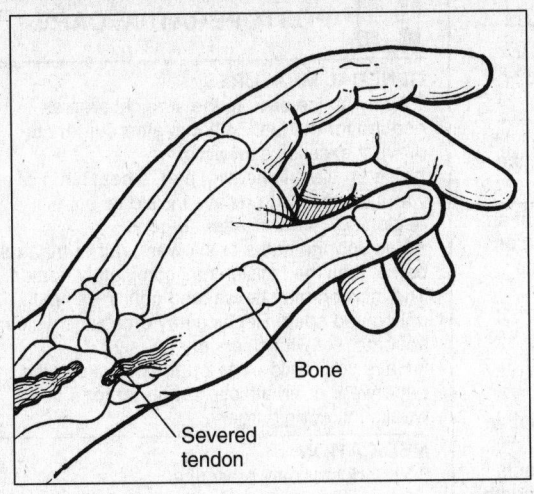

An illustration of a typical severed tendon in the wrist.

Bone

Severed
tendon

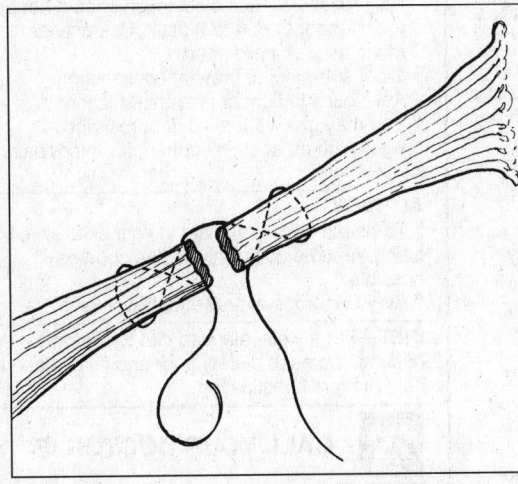

Severed ends of a tendon are located and sewn together.

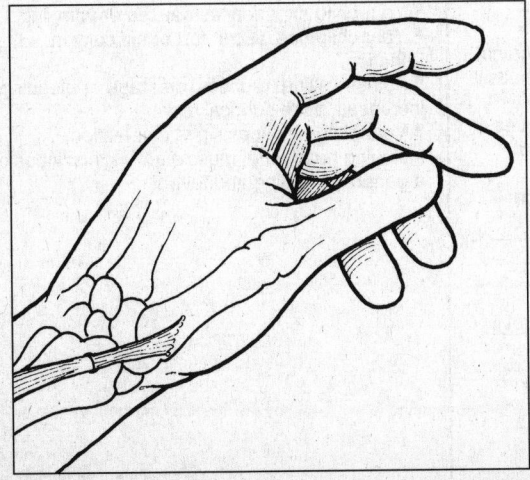

If necessary, tendons are reattached to surrounding connective tissue.

TESTICLE FIXATION
(Orchiopexy)

 GENERAL INFORMATION

DEFINITION—Fastening an undescended or twisted testicle in its normal position.

BODY PARTS INVOLVED—Scrotum; testicle; vas deferens; blood vessels and nerves in the scrotum.

REASONS FOR SURGERY—Placement of an undescended testicle in its normal position, or correction of a twisted testicle. Usually done before a boy is age 5.

SURGICAL RISK INCREASES WITH
- Congenital disorders.
- Chronic illness.
- Diabetes mellitus.
- Use of some prescription and nonprescription drugs. Inform your doctor of any drugs, medications, or vitamin and herb supplements your child is using or has used in the last month.

 WHAT TO EXPECT

WHO OPERATES—Urologist or general surgeon.

WHERE PERFORMED—Hospital.

DIAGNOSTIC TESTS
- Before surgery: Blood and urine studies; ultrasound (see Glossary).
- After surgery: Blood studies.

ANESTHESIA
- Spinal anesthesia by injection.
- Local anesthesia by injection.

DESCRIPTION OF OPERATION
- An incision is made in the scrotum or groin area.
- The blood supply and nerves leading to the testicle are located and carefully preserved.
- If the testicle has not descended from the abdomen, the surgeon reaches into the inguinal canal with special instruments and gently pulls it down.
- The testicle and its blood supply and nerves are pulled to the bottom of the scrotum and sewn in place.
- The skin is closed with sutures that will be absorbed by the body.

POSSIBLE COMPLICATIONS
- Excessive bleeding.
- Surgical-wound infection.
- Damage to blood supply to the testicle; death of the testicle.

AVERAGE HOSPITAL STAY—0 to 2 days.

PROBABLE OUTCOME—Expect complete healing without complications. Allow about 3 weeks for recovery from surgery.

 POSTOPERATIVE CARE

GENERAL MEASURES
- Apply an ice pack to the surgical area as needed for the first 24 hours after surgery to prevent excessive swelling.
- Use an electric heating pad, a heat lamp or a warm compress to relieve incisional pain beginning 24 hours after surgery.
- Use sponge baths or showers, rather than tub baths, until the incision has completely healed. The incision may be washed gently with mild, unscented soap. Replace any dressings which become wet with clean, dry ones.
- Have your child wear 2 pairs of jockey type underwear or an athletic supporter for 4 to 6 weeks following surgery.

MEDICATION
- Your doctor may prescribe:
  Pain relievers. Pain medication should not be used longer than 4 to 7 days. Use only as much as your child need.
  Stool softeners to prevent constipation.
  Antibiotics to fight or prevent infection.
- You may give your child nonprescription drugs, such as acetaminophen, for minor pain. Avoid aspirin.

ACTIVITY
- To help recovery and aid in your child's well-being, resume daily activities as soon as possible.
- Avoid vigorous exercise for 6 weeks.

DIET—Eat a well-balanced diet to promote healing. Increase dietary fiber and fluid intake to help prevent constipation.

 CALL YOUR DOCTOR IF

- Your child experiences nausea or vomiting.
- Your child has discomfort or difficulty in urination.
- Pain, swelling, redness, drainage or bleeding increases in the surgical area.
- Your child develops signs of infection, including headache, muscle aches, dizziness or a general ill feeling and fever.

TESTICLE FIXATION
(Orchiopexy)

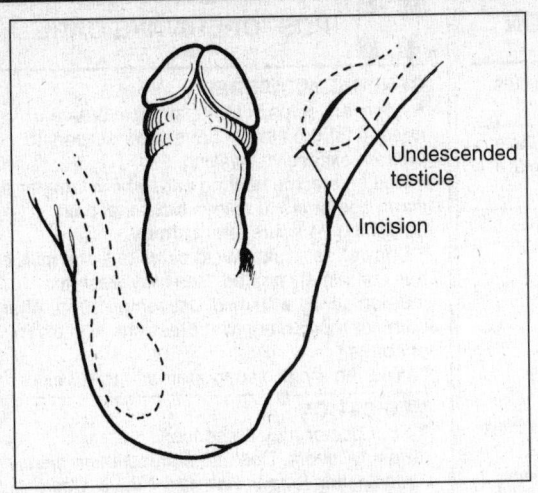

An illustration of an undescended testicle on the patient's left side and a typical incision site into the scrotum.

Undescended testicle

Incision

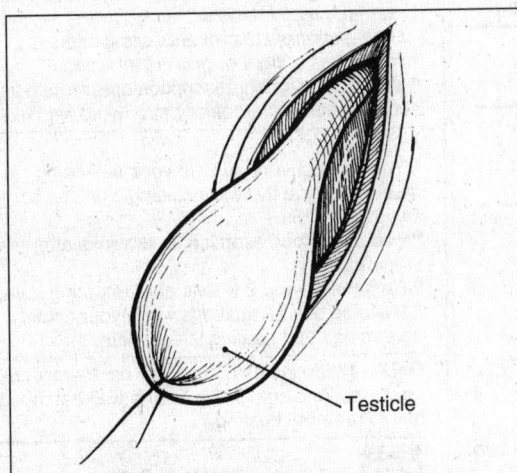

The blood supply and nerves leading to the testicle are carefully preserved.
• The surgeon reaches into the inguinal canal with special instruments and gently pulls the testicle down into the scrotum.

Testicle

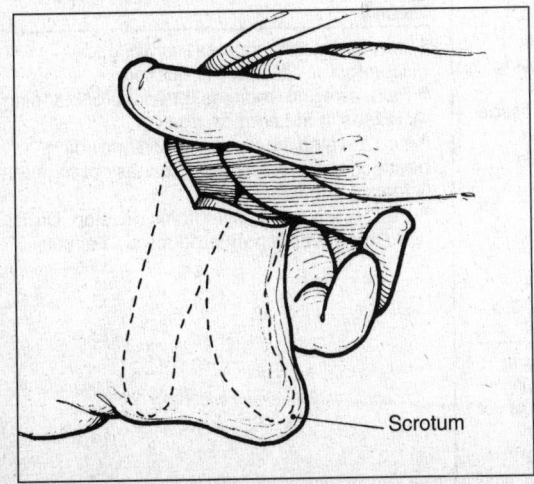

The testicle, its blood supply and nerves are pulled to the bottom of the scrotum and sewn into place.

Scrotum

SURGERIES

TESTICLE REMOVAL
(Orchiectomy)

 GENERAL INFORMATION

DEFINITION—Removal of one of the testicles (orchiectomy).

BODY PARTS INVOLVED—Scrotum; testicle; vas deferens; blood vessels and nerves in the scrotum.

REASONS FOR SURGERY
- Cancer or gangrene of the testicle.
- Prostate cancer.

SURGICAL RISK INCREASES WITH
- Adults over 60.
- Smoking.
- Recent or chronic illness.
- Diabetes mellitus.
- Use of some prescription and nonprescription drugs. Inform your doctor of any drugs, medications, or vitamin and herb supplements you are using or have used in the last month.

 WHAT TO EXPECT

WHO OPERATES—Urologist or general surgeon.

WHERE PERFORMED—Hospital.

DIAGNOSTIC TESTS
- Before surgery: Blood and urine studies; x-rays; CT scan; ultrasound; ECG (see Glossary for all).
- After surgery: Blood studies; laboratory studies of the removed testicle.

ANESTHESIA
- Local anesthesia by injection.
- Spinal anesthesia by injection.
- General anesthesia by injection and inhalation with an airway tube placed in the windpipe.

DESCRIPTION OF OPERATION
- An incision is made in the inguinal region or scrotum. The blood supply and nerves leading to the testicle are located and cut free.
- The testicle is cut free from surrounding tissue and removed.
- The skin is closed with sutures that will be absorbed by the body.

POSSIBLE COMPLICATIONS
- Excessive bleeding.
- Surgical-wound infection.
- Urinary retention.

AVERAGE HOSPITAL STAY—0 to 2 days.

PROBABLE OUTCOME—Expect complete healing without complications. Allow about 3 weeks for recovery from surgery. Removal of one testicle should not interfere with normal sexual function or the ability to have children.

 POSTOPERATIVE CARE

GENERAL MEASURES
- Apply an ice pack to the surgical area as needed for the first 24 hours after surgery to prevent excessive swelling.
- Use an electric heating pad, a heat lamp or a warm compress to relieve incisional pain beginning 24 hours after surgery.
- Shower as usual. Avoid baths until the incision has completely healed. You may wash the incision gently with mild, unscented soap. After bathing, replace any wet dressings with clean, dry ones.
- Wear an athletic supporter for 4 to 6 weeks.

MEDICATION
- Your doctor may prescribe:
  Pain relievers. Don't take prescription pain medication longer than 4 to 7 days. Use only as much as you need.
  Stool softeners to prevent constipation.
  Antibiotics to fight or prevent infection.
- You may use nonprescription drugs, such as acetaminophen, for minor pain. Avoid aspirin.

ACTIVITY
- To help recovery and aid your well-being, resume daily activities, including work, as soon as you are able.
- Avoid vigorous exercise for 6 weeks after surgery.
- Resume driving 2 weeks after returning home.
- Resume sexual relations when your doctor determines that healing is complete.

DIET—Clear liquid diet until the gastrointestinal tract functions again. Then eat a well-balanced diet to promote healing.

 CALL YOUR DOCTOR IF

- You experience nausea, vomiting, or discomfort or difficulty in urination.
- Pain, swelling, redness, drainage or bleeding increases in the surgical area.
- You develop signs of infection, including headache, muscle aches, dizziness or a general ill feeling and fever.
- New, unexplained symptoms develop. Drugs used in treatment may produce side effects.

TESTICLE REMOVAL
(Orchiectomy)

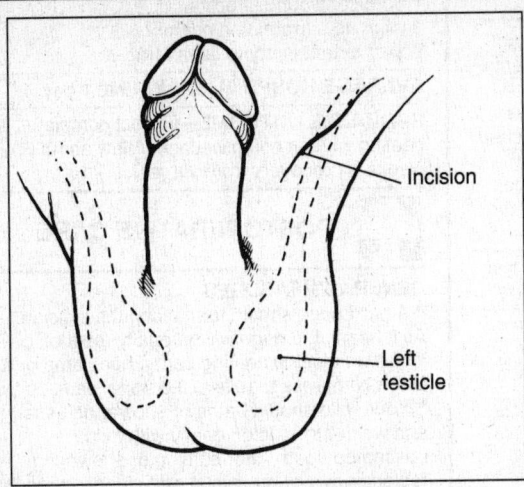

An illustration of the penis, scrotum, testicle and incision site for removal of a testicle.
- Sometimes the incision for this operation is made higher up in the groin.

Incision

Left testicle

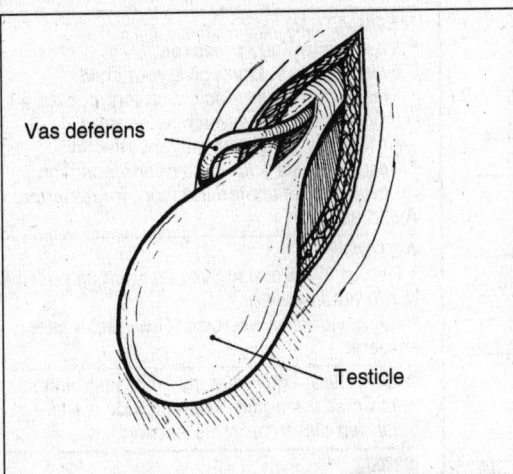

The blood supply, vas deferens (carries sperm for testicle) and nerves leading to the testicle are located and cut free. The testicle is then cut free from surrounding tissue.

Vas deferens

Testicle

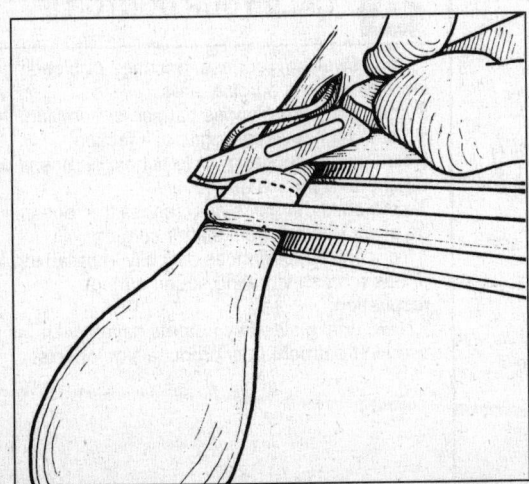

The excised testicle is removed.
- The skin is closed with sutures that will be absorbed by the body.

SURGERIES

THYROGLOSSAL DUCT & CYST REMOVAL

 ## GENERAL INFORMATION

DEFINITION—Removal of a thyroglossal duct that has a cyst. The cyst results from remnants of the thyroid gland that do not descend normally during early fetal development. The cyst usually appears during childhood, attached to the hyoid bone by the duct. The duct then passes upward to its origin at the base of the tongue. Surgery is usually performed when the patient is between 6 and 10 years old.

BODY PARTS INVOLVED—Thyroglossal cyst; remnants of the thyroglossal duct; hyoid bone.

REASONS FOR SURGERY
- Prevention of infections.
- Relief of pressure on the airway that causes difficulty in breathing or swallowing.

SURGICAL RISK INCREASES WITH
- Obesity.
- Poor nutrition.
- Recent or chronic illness.
- Other congenital disorders.
- Diabetes mellitus.
- Use of some prescription and nonprescription drugs. Inform your doctor of any drugs, medications, or vitamin and herb supplements you are using or have used in the last month.

 ## WHAT TO EXPECT

WHO OPERATES—General surgeon or ear, nose and throat specialist (otolaryngologist).

WHERE PERFORMED—Hospital.

DIAGNOSTIC TESTS
- Before surgery: Blood and urine studies; ultrasound; CT scan (see Glossary).
- After surgery: Blood studies.

ANESTHESIA—General anesthesia by injection and inhalation with an airway tube placed in the windpipe.

DESCRIPTION OF OPERATION
- An incision is made in the neck over the thyroglossal cyst.
- The cyst is cut free of muscle and connective tissue. The part of the hyoid bone to which the cyst is attached is cut, and the cyst and bone are removed.
- The thyroglossal duct is located, tied, cut and removed.
- The neck muscles are closed with fine sutures.
- The skin is closed with either sutures or clips, which usually can be be removed about 4 to 7 days after surgery.

POSSIBLE COMPLICATIONS
- Excessive bleeding.
- Surgical-wound infection.
- Injury to surrounding nerves.
- Inadvertent injury to larynx (rare).

AVERAGE HOSPITAL STAY—0 to 1 day.

PROBABLE OUTCOME—Expect complete healing without complications. Allow about 6 weeks for recovery from surgery.

 ## POSTOPERATIVE CARE

GENERAL MEASURES
- A hard ridge should form along the incision. As it heals, the ridge will gradually recede.
- Use an electric heating pad, a heat lamp or a warm compress to relieve incisional pain.
- Your child should bathe or shower as usual, and wash the incision gently with mild, unscented soap. After bathing or showering, replace any wet dressings with clean, dry ones.

MEDICATION
- Your doctor may prescribe:
  Pain relievers. Don't give your child prescription pain medication longer than 4 to 7 days. Use only as much as needed.
  Antibiotics to fight or prevent infection.
- You may give your child nonprescription drugs, such as acetaminophen, for minor pain. Avoid aspirin.

ACTIVITY
- Return to normal activity as soon as possible to promote healing.
- Avoid vigorous exercise for 3 weeks after surgery.

DIET—Clear liquid diet until the gastrointestinal tract functions again. Then provide a well-balanced diet to promote healing.

 ## CALL YOUR DOCTOR IF

- Pain, swelling, redness, drainage or bleeding increases in the surgical area.
- Your child experiences nausea or vomiting.
- Your child develops signs of infection, including headache, muscle aches, dizziness or a general ill feeling and fever.
- Your child develops hoarseness that doesn't go away within 2 weeks after surgery.
- Your child experiences difficulty in breathing or has a harsh vibrating sound during respiration.
- New, unexplained symptoms develop. Drugs used in treatment may produce side effects.

THYROGLOSSAL DUCT & CYST REMOVAL

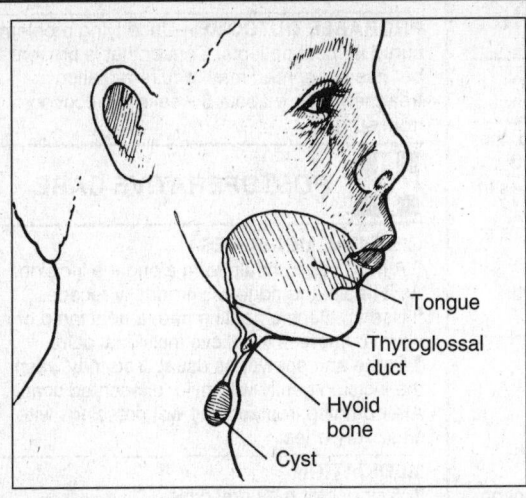

An illustration of the tongue, thyroglossal duct, hyoid bone and a cyst in the thyroglossal duct.

Tongue

Thyroglossal duct

Hyoid bone

Cyst

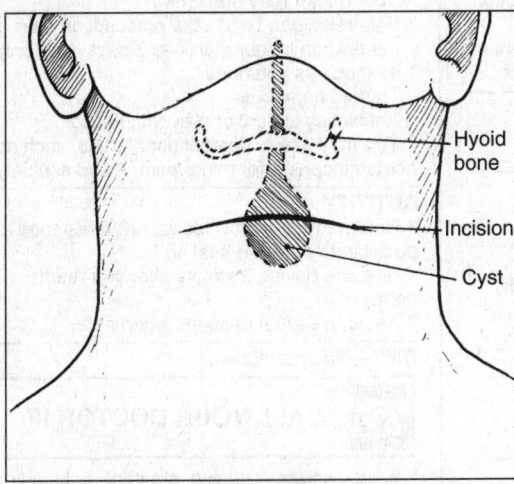

The skin is incised directly over the cyst.

Hyoid bone

Incision

Cyst

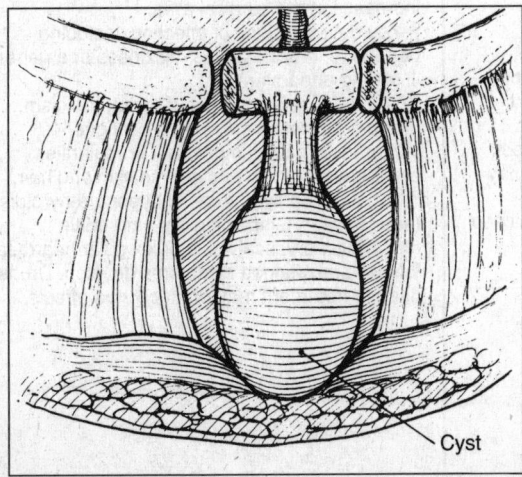

The cyst is cut free of muscle, connective tissue and part of the hyoid bone to which the cyst is attached. The cyst and bone are removed.
- Muscles and connective tissue are returned to their normal positions (not illustrated).

Cyst

THYROID GLAND REMOVAL
(Thyroidectomy)

GENERAL INFORMATION

DEFINITION—Removal of part or all of the thyroid gland.

BODY PARTS INVOLVED—Thyroid gland, the organ in the neck below the Adam's apple that controls the body's metabolism; lymph nodes in the neck.

REASONS FOR SURGERY
- Hyperthyroidism.
- Benign or cancerous tumors of the thyroid.
- Goiter (see Glossary).

SURGICAL RISK INCREASES WITH
- Adults over 60.
- Obesity; poor nutrition.
- Smoking.
- Untreated hyperthyroidism (see Glossary).
- Diabetes mellitus.
- Use of some prescription and nonprescription drugs. Inform your doctor of any drugs, medications, or vitamin and herb supplements you are using or have used in the last month.

WHAT TO EXPECT

WHO OPERATES—General surgeon.

WHERE PERFORMED—Hospital.

DIAGNOSTIC TESTS
- Before surgery: Blood studies; ultrasound; CT scan; needle biopsy; radioactive-iodine uptake and scan (see Glossary for all).
- After surgery: Blood studies.

ANESTHESIA—General anesthesia by injection and inhalation with an airway tube placed in the windpipe.

DESCRIPTION OF OPERATION
- An incision is made in the neck following natural skin lines.
- Neck muscles are cut or retracted.
- Blood supply to the thyroid gland is clamped.
- The thyroid gland is cut free and removed, and a drain is left in place. In certain cases, some normal thyroid gland tissue is left intact.
- If cancer is present, some lymph nodes may be removed around the thyroid.
- The muscles are closed and the skin is closed with sutures or clips, which can usually be removed in 2 to 10 days after surgery.

POSSIBLE COMPLICATIONS
- Hoarseness or loss of voice, if vocal-cord nerves are damaged during surgery.
- Hypothyroidism (see Glossary).
- Hypoparathyroidism (see Glossary).
- Excessive bleeding.
- Surgical-wound infection.

AVERAGE HOSPITAL STAY—1 to 3 days.

PROBABLE OUTCOME—Underlying problem cured in most patients. Cancer that is present but has not spread may require radiation treatment. Allow about 6 weeks for recovery from surgery.

POSTOPERATIVE CARE

GENERAL MEASURES
- A hard ridge should form along the incision. As it heals, the ridge will gradually recede.
- Use an electric heating pad, a heat lamp or a warm compress to relieve incisional pain.
- Bathe and shower as usual. You may wash the incision gently with mild, unscented soap. After bathing, replace any wet dressings with clean, dry ones.

MEDICATION
- Your doctor may prescribe:
  Pain relievers. Don't take prescription pain medication longer than 4 to 7 days. Use only as much as you need.
  Thyroid hormones.
  Antibiotics to fight or prevent infection.
- You may use nonprescription drugs, such as acetaminophen, for minor pain. Avoid aspirin.

ACTIVITY
- Return to daily activities and work as soon as possible to promote healing.
- Resume driving 2 weeks after you return home.
- Resume sexual relations when able.

DIET—No special diet.

CALL YOUR DOCTOR IF

- Pain, swelling, redness, drainage or bleeding increases in the surgical area.
- You develop signs of infection, including headache, muscle aches, dizziness or a general ill feeling and fever.
- You develop symptoms of hypothyroidism, including excessive weakness, fatigue, intolerance to cold, menstrual irregularities, constipation, or dry and coarse skin and hair.
- You develop symptoms of hypoparathyroidism (see Glossary), including dry hair, brittle fingernails; dry, scaly skin or irregular heartbeat.
- New, unexplained symptoms develop. Drugs used in treatment may produce side effects.

THYROID GLAND REMOVAL
(Thyroidectomy)

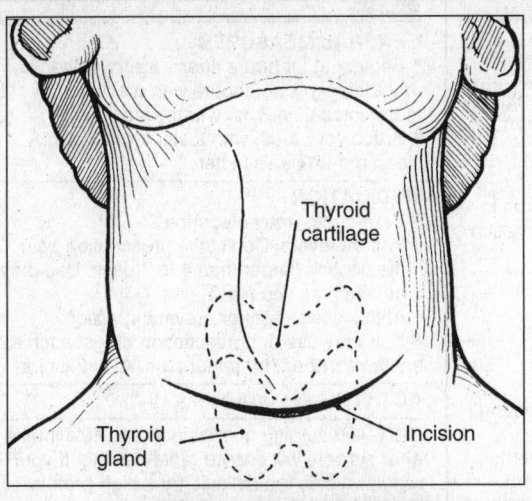

An illustration of structures in the neck and the typical incision site for thyroid gland removal.

Thyroid cartilage

Thyroid gland

Incision

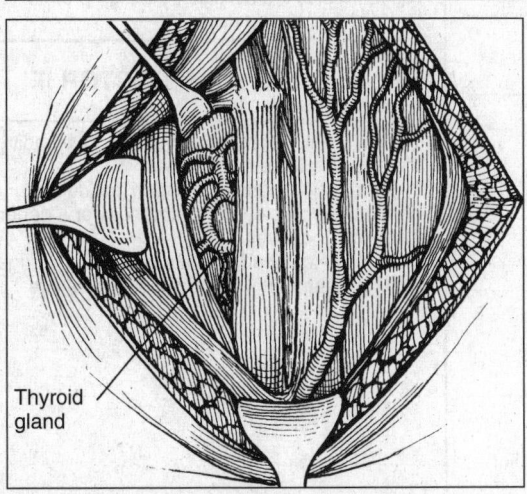

Muscles and connective tissue are retracted revealing the thyroid gland.

Thyroid gland

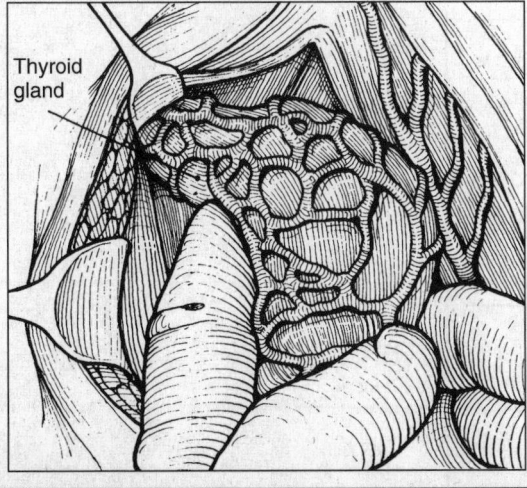

Thyroid gland

The blood supply to the thyroid gland is clamped and all or part of the gland is cut free and removed.
- The remaining tissue is replaced in its normal position. The skin is closed with sutures or clips (not illustrated).

SURGERIES

TONGUE, CHEEK OR GUM BIOPSY

 GENERAL INFORMATION

DEFINITION—Removal of tissue from the oral cavity.

BODY PARTS INVOLVED—Tongue; cheek; gums; roof of mouth; salivary glands under the tongue.

REASONS FOR SURGERY—Usually performed to determine if any unusual lesion in the mouth is cancerous. Laboratory examination of the removed tissue aids in diagnosis.

SURGICAL RISK INCREASES WITH
- Adults over 60.
- Smoking.
- Excess alcohol consumption.
- Diabetes mellitus.
- Use of some prescription and nonprescription drugs. Inform your doctor of any drugs, medications, or vitamin and herb supplements you are using or have used in the last month.

 WHAT TO EXPECT

WHO OPERATES—Dentist, oral surgeon, general surgeon or ear, nose and throat specialist.

WHERE PERFORMED—Hospital, outpatient surgical facility or doctor's, dentist's or oral surgeon's office.

DIAGNOSTIC TESTS
- Before surgery: Blood and urine studies; CT scan; MRI (see Glossary for both).
- After surgery: Laboratory examination of removed tissue.

ANESTHESIA
- Local anesthesia by injection.
- General anesthesia (sometimes) by injection and inhalation with an airway tube placed in the windpipe.

DESCRIPTION OF OPERATION
- The area where the tissue is to be gathered is numbed with a local anesthetic.
- Abnormal tissue and a small amount of healthy surrounding tissue is removed.
- Small stitches may be needed to close the incision. These usually can be removed in 3 to 5 days after surgery.

POSSIBLE COMPLICATIONS
- Excessive bleeding.
- Surgical-wound infection.

AVERAGE HOSPITAL STAY—None.

PROBABLE OUTCOME—Tissue obtained successfully without complications in virtually all cases. Allow about 2 weeks for recovery from surgery.

 POSTOPERATIVE CARE

GENERAL MEASURES
- Beginning 24 hours after surgery, rinse your mouth every 1 or 2 hours with a solution of 1/2 teaspoon salt in 8 oz. warm water.
- Brush your teeth with a soft toothbrush. A clean mouth heals faster.

MEDICATION
- Your doctor may prescribe:
  Pain relievers. Don't take prescription pain medication longer than 4 to 7 days. Use only as much as you need.
  Antibiotics to fight or prevent infection.
- You may use nonprescription drugs, such as acetaminophen, for minor pain. Avoid aspirin.

ACTIVITY—No restrictions.

DIET—Resuming normal food and fluid intake after surgery will ensure rapid healing. If your regular diet is too difficult, try a high-protein liquid diet for 2 or 3 days.

 CALL YOUR DOCTOR IF

- Pain, swelling, redness, drainage or bleeding increases in the surgical area.
- You develop signs of infection, including headache, muscle aches, dizziness or a general ill feeling and fever.
- New, unexplained symptoms develop. Drugs used in treatment may produce side effects.

TONGUE, CHEEK OR GUM BIOPSY

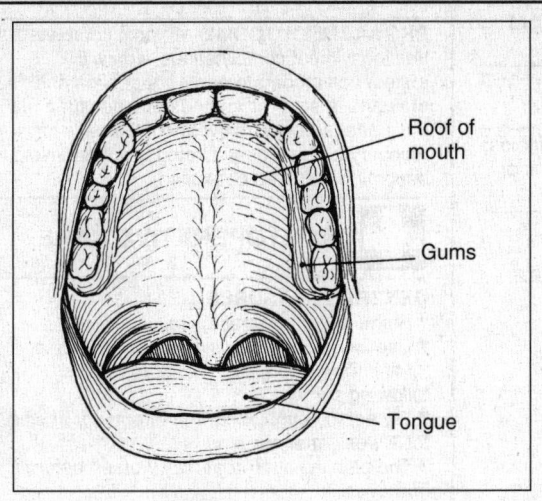

An illustration of the roof of the mouth, gums, teeth and tongue.

Roof of mouth

Gums

Tongue

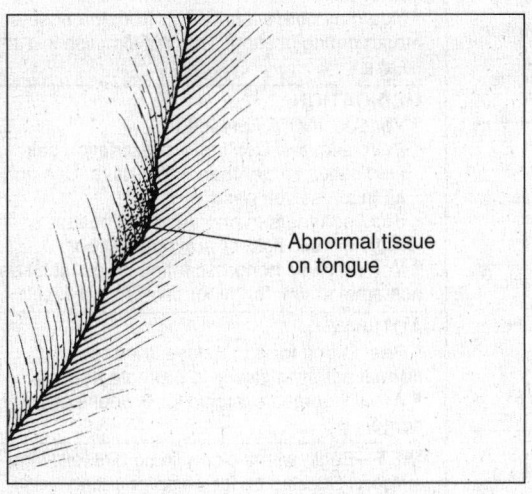

The abnormal tissue on the edge of the tongue illustrated here.

Abnormal tissue on tongue

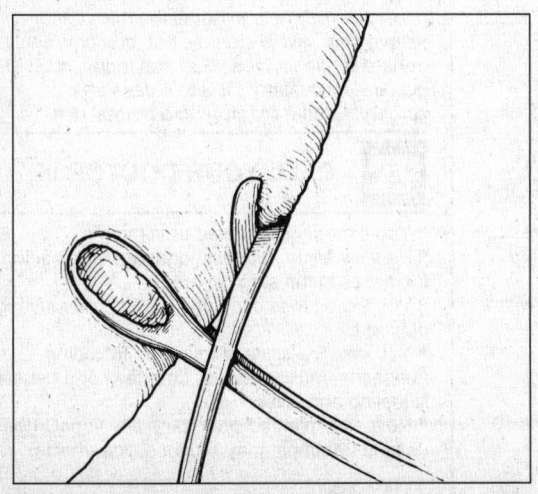

After injecting a local anesthetic, the abnormal tissue and a small amount of healthy surrounding tissue is removed.
- Small stitches may be needed to close the incision. If so, they usually can be removed in 3 to 5 days after surgery (not illustrated).

TONSIL & ADENOID REMOVAL
(Tonsillectomy & Adenoidectomy)

 GENERAL INFORMATION

DEFINITION—Removal of the tonsils and adenoids.

BODY PARTS INVOLVED—Tonsils; adenoids; opening from the nose into the throat; back of the throat.

REASONS FOR SURGERY
In tonsils:
- More than 5 attacks of tonsillitis in 1 year.
- Peritonsillar abscess (see Glossary).
In adenoids:
- Obstruction of air through the nose.
- Infections in the middle ear.

SURGICAL RISK INCREASES WITH
- Obesity; smoking.
- Poor nutrition.
- Recent or chronic illness.
- Diabetes mellitus.
- Use of some prescription and nonprescription drugs. Inform your doctor of any drugs, medications, or vitamin and herb supplements you are using or have used in the last month.

 WHAT TO EXPECT

WHO OPERATES—Ear, nose and throat specialist or general surgeon.

WHERE PERFORMED—Hospital or outpatient surgical facility.

DIAGNOSTIC TESTS
- Before surgery: Blood and urine studies.
- After surgery: Laboratory examination of removed tissue; blood studies.

ANESTHESIA—General anesthesia by injection and inhalation with an airway tube placed in the windpipe.

DESCRIPTION OF OPERATION
- Several techniques are available; one is described here.
- The mouth is held open to expose the tonsils.
- The tonsils are grasped with clamps and pulled toward the middle of the mouth. The tonsils are cut free of surrounding membrane and removed.
- Bleeding is controlled by pressure, sutures or clamps and ties or with use of electrocautery (see Glossary).
- The adenoids are located and removed with a special instrument.

POSSIBLE COMPLICATIONS
- Excessive bleeding, sometimes requiring reoperation.
- Adenoid-tissue regrowth.
- Nausea and dehydration.

AVERAGE HOSPITAL STAY—0 to 2 days.

PROBABLE OUTCOME—Expect complete healing without complications. You will experience moderate nasal congestion and drainage, a sore throat and earaches for a few days after surgery. Allow about 3 weeks for recovery from surgery. During this time, avoid becoming hot, tired or excited.

 POSTOPERATIVE CARE

GENERAL MEASURES
- Bathe and shower as usual.
- Use ice packs or popsicles to relieve pain.
- Minimize talking in the first 2 to 3 days following surgery.
- Try not to cough, clear the throat, cry or sing for 1 week after surgery.
- The pain in your throat may worsen before it improves.
- You may notice a bad odor from the nose or mouth during healing. This will diminish in 1 to 2 weeks.

MEDICATION
- Your doctor may prescribe:
  Pain relievers. Don't take prescription pain medication longer than 4 to 7 days. Use only as much as you need.
  Stool softeners to prevent constipation.
  Antibiotics to fight or prevent infection.
- You may use nonprescription drugs, such as acetaminophen, for minor pain. Avoid aspirin.

ACTIVITY
- Rest in bed for 2 to 3 days, then resume normal activities slowly to promote healing.
- Avoid vigorous exercise for 6 weeks after surgery.

DIET—Begin with a clear, liquid diet following surgery. Sucking on ice chips or eating popsicles may help to numb the throat and relieve pain. Avoid steamy, hot, crunchy, spicy, or hard-to-digest foods. Eat soft foods, such as gelatin and custard, for 3 to 4 days after surgery. Gradually return to a normal diet.

 CALL YOUR DOCTOR IF

- You experience nausea or vomiting.
- Pain, swelling, redness, drainage or bleeding increases in the surgical area.
- You experience coughing, spitting or vomiting of blood.
- You develop signs of infection, including headache, muscle aches, dizziness or a general ill feeling and fever.
- New, unexplained symptoms develop. Drugs used in treatment may produce side effects.

TONSIL & ADENOID REMOVAL
(Tonsillectomy & Adenoidectomy)

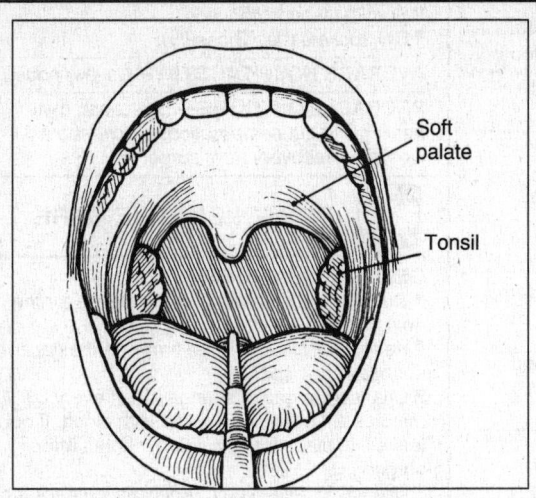

Soft palate

Tonsil

An illustration of the roof of the mouth, tongue (pushed downward by a retractor), the soft and hard palate, and tonsils.

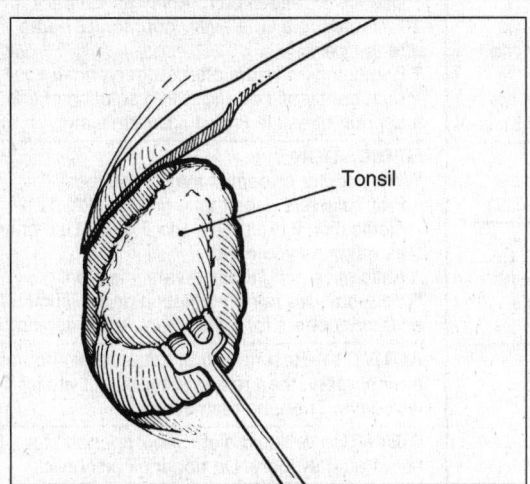

Tonsil

The tonsils are grasped with clamps and pulled toward the middle of the mouth. The tonsils are cut free of surrounding membrane and tension is applied to the base of the tonsil.

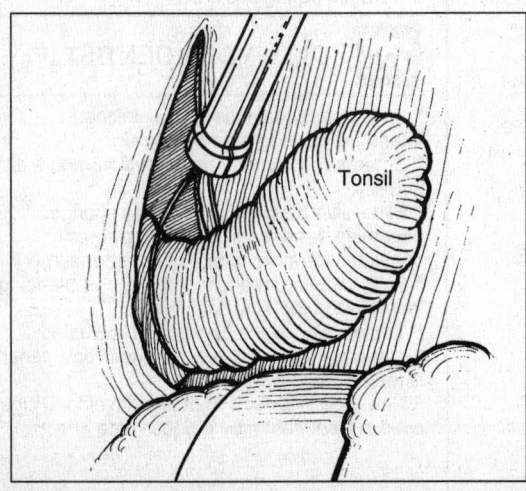

Tonsil

The base of the tonsil is generally reached with a wire snare that cuts through the tonsil allowing easy removal.

- Bleeding is controlled by pressure sutures, electrocautery or clamps and ties.
- Frequently, the adenoids will be removed at the same time (which are not shown in this illustration). Adenoids are tissues similar anatomically to tonsillar tissue and are located in the back of the throat up behind the hard palate toward the rear opening into the nose.

TOOTH EXTRACTION

GENERAL INFORMATION

DEFINITION—Removal (extraction) of a tooth.

BODY PARTS INVOLVED—Teeth; gums; bones in jaw.

REASONS FOR SURGERY
Routine removals:
- Loss of supporting tissue, bone or gums.
- Infection of the nerve in the tooth.
- Fractured teeth that cannot be restored.

Impacted-tooth removals:
- Infection and pain around the lower wisdom teeth.
- Pain upon closing the jaws.
- Destruction or erosion of nearby teeth and bone due to growth of surrounding tissue.
- Lack of space for normal tooth growth.

SURGICAL RISK INCREASES WITH
- Smoking.
- Poor nutrition.
- Diabetes mellitus.
- Use of some prescription and nonprescription drugs. Inform your doctor of any drugs, medications, or vitamin and herb supplements you are using or have used in the last month.

WHAT TO EXPECT

WHO OPERATES—Dentist or oral surgeon.

WHERE PERFORMED—Hospital, outpatient surgical facility or dentist's or oral surgeon's office.

DIAGNOSTIC TESTS
- Before surgery: Blood and urine studies; x-rays of mouth.

ANESTHESIA
- Local anesthesia by injection.
- General anesthesia by injection and inhalation with an airway tube placed in the windpipe.

DESCRIPTION OF OPERATION
- For impacted teeth, the gum is incised over the tooth to be removed.
- For all extractions, the tooth is grasped with special instruments, rotated and elevated from the surrounding gum and bone.
- A gauze sponge is packed into the space left by the extracted tooth.
- Sometimes, sutures are used to close the gum edges. They usually come out by themselves, but may need removal in 3 or 4 days after surgery.

POSSIBLE COMPLICATIONS
- Excessive bleeding.
- Surgical-wound infection.
- Dry sockets (see Glossary).

AVERAGE HOSPITAL STAY—Usually none.

PROBABLE OUTCOME—Expect complete healing without complications. Allow about 3 weeks for recovery from surgery.

POSTOPERATIVE CARE

GENERAL MEASURES
- Do not smoke or use drinking straws for the next 24 hours.
- Keep your mouth closed firmly on the gauze sponge. Don't spit.
- Change the gauze sponge about every 30 minutes if it becomes soaked with blood. If not, leave it in place for about 3 to 4 hours after surgery.
- Use ice to relieve pain. Apply an ice pack for 10 minutes at a time every hour for 12 hours after surgery.
- Beginning 24 hours after surgery, rinse your mouth gently as needed with a solution of 1/2 teaspoon of salt in 8 oz. lukewarm water.

MEDICATION
- Your doctor or dentist may prescribe:
  Pain relievers. Don't take prescription pain medication longer than 4 to 7 days. Use only as much as you need.
  Antibiotics to fight or prevent infection.
- You may use nonprescription drugs, such as acetaminophen, for minor pain. Avoid aspirin.

ACTIVITY—Rest quietly at home for 24 hours after surgery, then resume limited activity for 1 or 2 days. Then, no restrictions.

DIET—Soft or liquid diet (See Appendix) for 24 hours after surgery. Do not drink alcoholic beverages during this time.

CALL YOUR DENTIST IF

- You experience nausea or vomiting.
- Medication does not relieve pain.
- Sutures drop out during the first 48 hours after surgery.
- Excessive bleeding (one gauze sponge becoming deep red in 10 to 15 minutes) continues for more than 4 hours after surgery.
- Pain, swelling, redness, drainage or bleeding increases in the surgical area.
- You develop signs of infection, including headache, muscle aches, dizziness or a general ill feeling and fever.
- New, unexplained symptoms develop. Drugs used in treatment may produce side effects.

TOOTH EXTRACTION

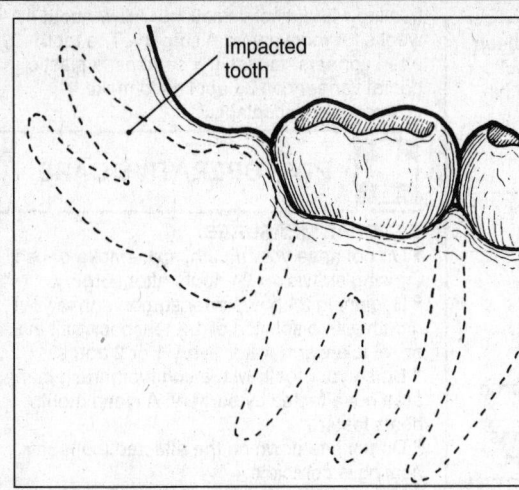

A bony impacted tooth.

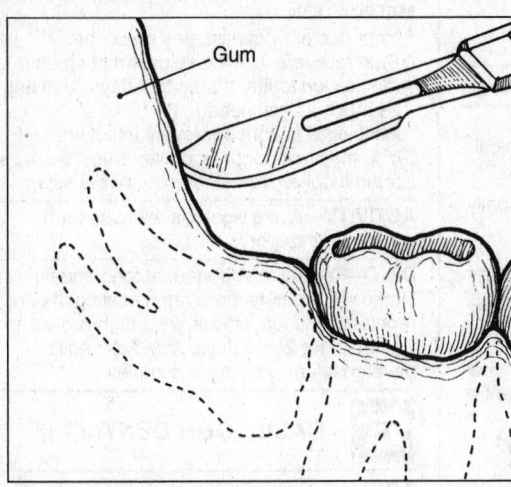

The gum is incised over the tooth to be removed.

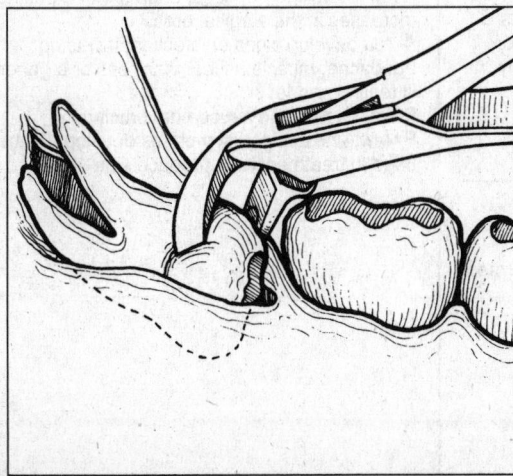

Tooth to be extracted is grasped with special instruments, rotated and elevated from the gum and bone. If sutures are used to close the surgical site, they may need removal 3 to 4 days after surgery.

TOOTH REPLANTATION

 GENERAL INFORMATION

DEFINITION—Replanting a tooth that has been knocked out of its normal position. Best results are obtained when the tooth is replanted within 2 hours after injury.

BODY PARTS INVOLVED—Mouth; teeth; gums.

REASONS FOR SURGERY—Prevention of permanent loss of a tooth.

SURGICAL RISK INCREASES WITH
- Smoking; poor nutrition.
- Recent or chronic illness.
- Poor dental hygiene or gum disease.
- Diabetes mellitus.
- Use of some prescription and nonprescription drugs. Inform your doctor of any drugs, medications, or vitamin and herb supplements you are using or have used in the last month.

 WHAT TO EXPECT

WHO OPERATES—Oral surgeon or dentist.

WHERE PERFORMED—Hospital, oral surgeon's or dentist's office, outpatient surgical facility, doctor's office or emergency room.

DIAGNOSTIC TESTS—Before surgery: Usually none, because of the need for immediate surgery.

ANESTHESIA—Local anesthesia by injection.

DESCRIPTION OF OPERATION
- If you or your child has a tooth knocked out, try to find the tooth, wash it and replace it in the socket as quickly as possible. Go to your dentist as soon as possible.
- If you cannot replace the tooth in its socket, wash it and keep it wet. Go to your dentist immediately.
- Usually the root canal nerve of the tooth is removed and filled with plastic material before the tooth is reinserted. Some dentists simply place the tooth back into the socket immediately.
- The replanted tooth is anchored to neighboring teeth with wire or plastic.

POSSIBLE COMPLICATIONS
- Excessive bleeding.
- Surgical-wound infection.
- Rejection of tooth (rare if surgery is performed within 2 hours after injury).

AVERAGE HOSPITAL STAY—0 to 1 day.

PROBABLE OUTCOME—Expect complete healing without complications. Allow about 4 weeks for recovery from surgery. The tooth often appears normal. If it darkens, a plastic dental veneer can be applied to make it cosmetically acceptable.

 POSTOPERATIVE CARE

GENERAL MEASURES
- Do not rinse your mouth, spit, smoke or use drinking straws for 24 hours after surgery.
- Beginning 24 hours after surgery, rinse your mouth with a solution of 1/2 teaspoon salt in 8 oz. of lukewarm water every 1 or 2 hours.
- Brush your teeth with a soft toothbrush in the area not affected by surgery. A clean mouth heals faster.
- Do not bite down on the affected tooth until healing is complete.

MEDICATION
- Your doctor or dentist may prescribe:
  Pain relievers. Don't take prescription pain medication longer than 4 to 7 days. Use only as much as you need.
  Antibiotics to fight or prevent infection.
- You may use nonprescription drugs, such as acetaminophen, for minor pain. Avoid aspirin.

ACTIVITY—Avoid vigorous exercise for 6 weeks after surgery.

DIET—Resuming your normal food and fluid intake will promote more rapid healing. If your regular diet is too difficult, try a high-protein liquid diet for 2 or 3 days. Avoid alcoholic beverages until healing is complete.

 CALL YOUR DENTIST IF

- Pain, swelling, redness, drainage or bleeding increases in the surgical area.
- You develop signs of infection, including headache, muscle aches, dizziness or a general ill feeling and fever.
- You experience nausea or vomiting.
- New, unexplained symptoms develop. Drugs used in treatment may produce side effects.

TOOTH REPLANTATION

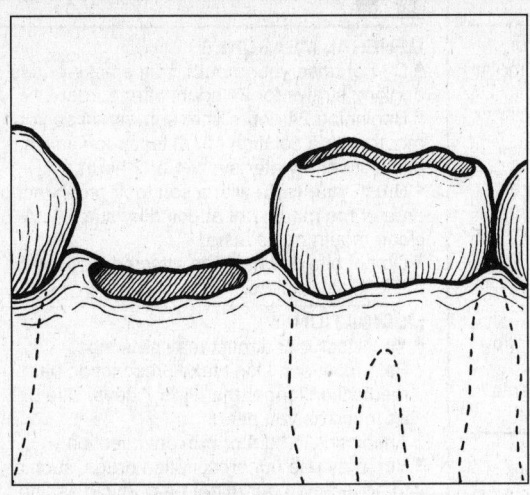

An illustration of teeth, gums and a socket left by a missing tooth.

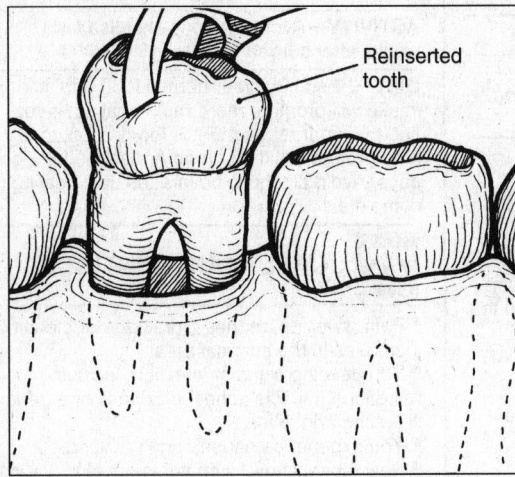

Reinserted tooth

The root canal nerve of the tooth is removed and filled with plastic material before the tooth is reinserted.

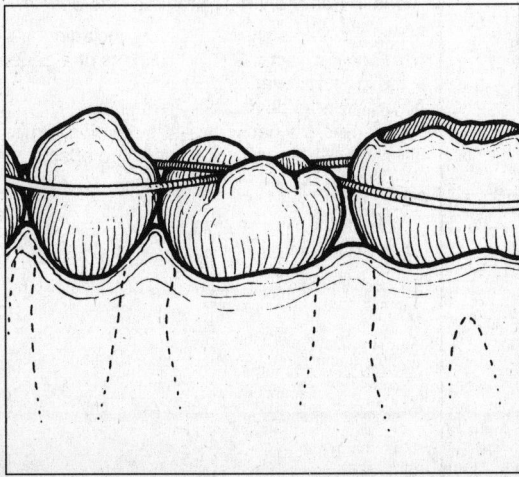

The replanted tooth is anchored to neighboring teeth with wire or plastic.

TOOTH TRANSPLANTATION

 GENERAL INFORMATION

DEFINITION—Replacement of an injured or diseased first or second molar with a third molar (wisdom tooth).

BODY PARTS INVOLVED—Mouth; teeth; gums.

REASONS FOR SURGERY—Restoration of normal tooth function.

SURGICAL RISK INCREASES WITH
- Recent or chronic illness.
- Smoking.
- Diabetes mellitus.
- Use of some prescription and nonprescription drugs. Inform your doctor of any drugs, medications, or vitamin and herb supplements you are using or have used in the last month.

 WHAT TO EXPECT

WHO OPERATES—Dentist or oral surgeon.

WHERE PERFORMED—Dentist's or oral surgeon's office, outpatient surgical facility or hospital.

DIAGNOSTIC TESTS
- Before surgery: Blood and urine studies.
- After surgery: Blood studies.

ANESTHESIA
- Local anesthesia by injection.
- General anesthesia (sometimes) by injection and inhalation, with an airway tube placed in the windpipe.

DESCRIPTION OF OPERATION
- A wisdom tooth is pulled.
- Sometimes, the root of the pulled tooth may be shortened for better fit.
- The socket where the tooth will be transplanted is enlarged.
- The wisdom tooth is inserted in the socket and secured to neighboring teeth. This provides support during healing.

POSSIBLE COMPLICATIONS
- Excessive bleeding.
- Surgical-wound infection.
- Rejection of transplanted tooth (rare).

AVERAGE HOSPITAL STAY—0 to 1 day.

PROBABLE OUTCOME—Expect complete healing without complications. Allow about 1 month for recovery from surgery.

 POSTOPERATIVE CARE

GENERAL MEASURES
- Do not rinse your mouth, spit, smoke or use drinking straws for 24 hours after surgery.
- Beginning 24 hours after surgery, rinse your mouth with a solution of 1/2 teaspoon salt in 8 oz. lukewarm water every 1 or 2 hours.
- Brush your teeth with a soft toothbrush in the area of the mouth not affected by surgery. A clean mouth heals faster.
- Do not bite down on the affected tooth until healing is complete.

MEDICATION
- Your doctor or dentist may prescribe:
  Pain relievers. Don't take prescription pain medication longer than 4 to 7 days. Use only as much as you need.
  Antibiotics to fight or prevent infection.
- You may use nonprescription drugs, such as acetaminophen, for minor pain. Avoid aspirin.

ACTIVITY—Avoid vigorous exercise for 3 weeks after surgery.

DIET—Resuming your normal food and fluid intake will promote more rapid healing. If you find that your regular diet is too difficult, try a high-protein liquid diet (see Appendix) for 2 or 3 days. Avoid alcoholic beverages until healing is complete.

 CALL YOUR DENTIST IF

- Pain, swelling, redness, drainage or bleeding increases in the surgical area.
- You develop signs of infection, including headache, muscle aches, dizziness or a general ill feeling and fever.
- You experience nausea and vomiting.
- New, unexplained symptoms develop. Drugs used in treatment may produce side effects.

TOOTH TRANSPLANTATION

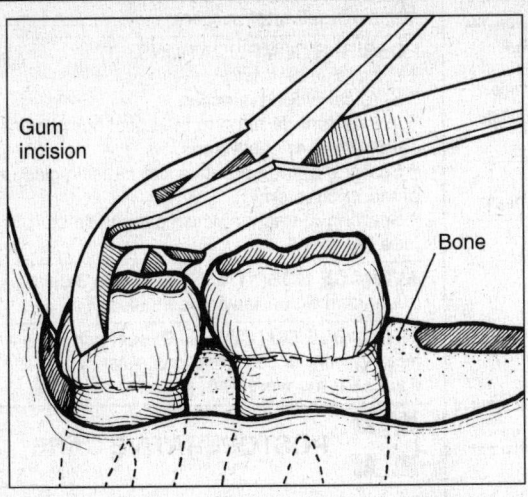

Shown here are the gums, bones and lower teeth, with forceps grasping the tooth to be transplanted.

Gum incision

Bone

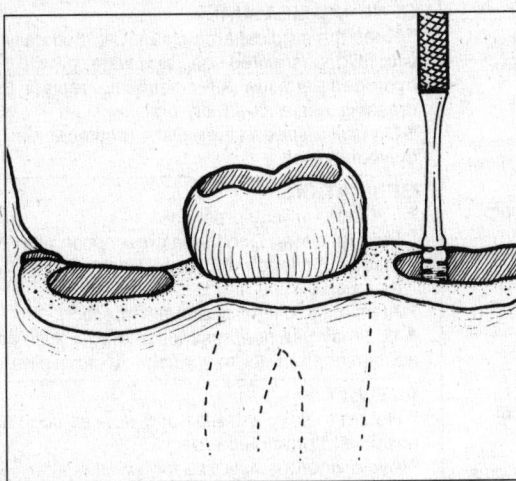

The socket where the tooth will be transplanted is enlarged.

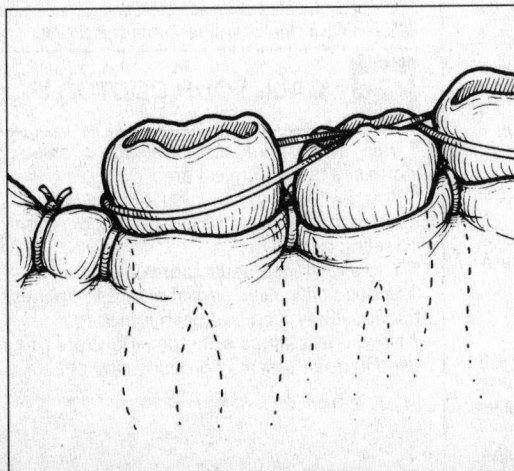

In this example, the wisdom tooth, having been removed, is inserted in the socket and secured to neighboring teeth to provide support during healing.

SURGERIES

TRACHEOSTOMY

GENERAL INFORMATION

DEFINITION—Creation of an opening in the windpipe (trachea) that will function as an airway either temporarily or permanently. The opening bypasses obstructions that prevent air from being inhaled or exhaled.

BODY PARTS INVOLVED—Windpipe; muscles, blood vessels and nerves in the neck.

REASONS FOR SURGERY
- Restoration of normal breathing.
- Control of secretions from the nose and throat, particularly in patients who are unconscious.
- Creation of an open airway in patients who require prolonged breathing assistance.
- Creation of an airway in patients whose larynx is removed.

SURGICAL RISK INCREASES WITH
- Newborns and infants.
- Adults over 75.
- Obesity; smoking; poor nutrition.
- Recent illness, especially upper-respiratory infection.
- Alcoholism or chronic illness.
- Diabetes mellitus.
- Use of some prescription and nonprescription drugs. Inform your doctor of any drugs, medications, or vitamin and herb supplements you are using or have used in the last month.

WHAT TO EXPECT

WHO OPERATES—Ear, nose and throat specialist or general surgeon.

WHERE PERFORMED—Hospital, outpatient surgical facility or emergency room.

DIAGNOSTIC TESTS—Blood and urine studies and x-rays of chest before and after surgery if necessary.

ANESTHESIA
- Local anesthesia (in emergencies) by injection.
- General anesthesia (when time allows) by injection and inhalation with an airway tube placed in the windpipe.

DESCRIPTION OF OPERATION
- An incision is made in the neck. The muscles and connective tissue around the windpipe are divided.
- A section at the front of the windpipe is cut free and removed.
- A tracheostomy tube is fitted into the opening in the windpipe to function as an airway. The patient will breathe through this tube as long as it is in place. Supplemental oxygen and mechanical assisted breathing can be supplied if necessary.

- The skin is closed around the tube with sutures or clips, which usually can be removed about 1 week after surgery.

POSSIBLE COMPLICATIONS
- Excessive bleeding.
- Surgical-wound infection.
- Inadvertent damage to the vocal cords, vocal-cord nerves or esophagus.
- Scarring at the operative site causing closure of the tracheotomy.
- Scarring of trachea which causes stricture (see Glossary).

AVERAGE HOSPITAL STAY—1 to 3 days, depending on underlying condition.

PROBABLE OUTCOME—Expect complete healing without complications. Allow about 2 weeks for recovery from surgery.

POSTOPERATIVE CARE

GENERAL MEASURES
- Keep the surgical area clean. Cleanse daily with mild, unscented soap and water or with hydrogen peroxide. After cleansing, replace the dressing with a clean, dry one.
- Consult a speech therapist if recommended by your doctor.

MEDICATION
- Your doctor may prescribe:
  Pain relievers. Don't take prescription pain medication longer than 4 to 7 days. Use only as much as you need.
  Antibiotics to fight or prevent infection.
- You may use nonprescription drugs, such as acetaminophen, for minor pain. Avoid aspirin.

ACTIVITY
- Return to daily activities and work as soon as possible to promote healing.
- Avoid vigorous exercise for 6 weeks after surgery.

DIET—Your doctor will recommend a diet.

CALL YOUR DOCTOR IF

- Pain, swelling, redness, drainage or bleeding increases in the surgical area.
- You develop signs of infection, including headache, muscle aches, dizziness or a general ill feeling and fever.
- You experience nausea or vomiting.
- Speech difficulties persist after a temporary tracheostomy tube has been removed.
- New, unexplained symptoms develop. Drugs used in treatment may produce side effects.

TRACHEOSTOMY

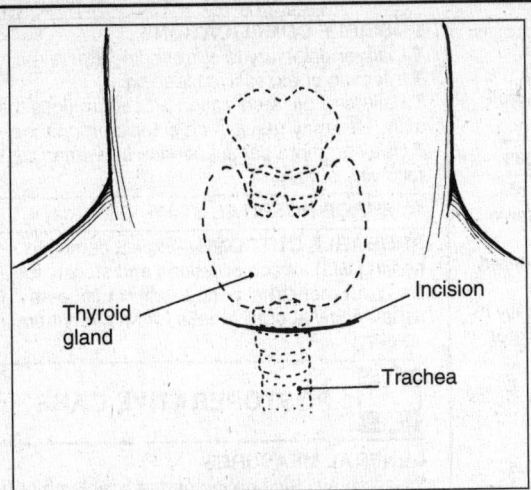

An illustration of structures in the neck and the usual incision site through the skin.

Thyroid gland

Incision

Trachea

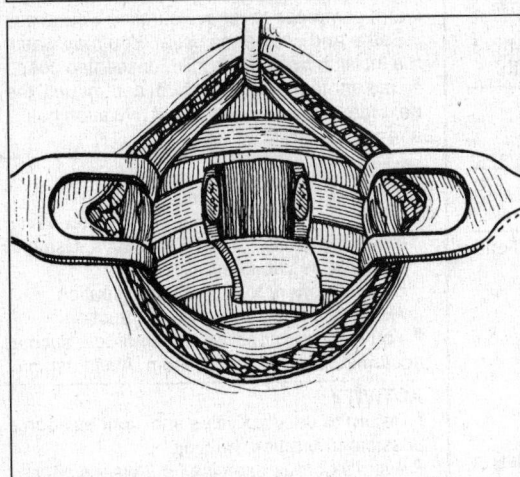

A section at the front of the windpipe is incised and widened.

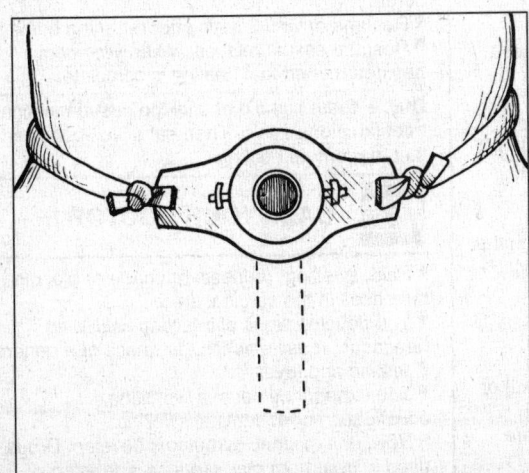

A tracheostomy tube is fitted into the opening in the windpipe to function as an airway. As long as the tracheostomy tube is in place and open, the patient will breathe through it instead of through the mouth or nose.

TUBAL LIGATION

GENERAL INFORMATION

DEFINITION—A method of sterilization that involves blocking the Fallopian tubes in such a way that the ovum (egg) becomes inaccessible for fertilization.

BODY PARTS INVOLVED—Fallopian tubes.

REASONS FOR SURGERY—Prevention of unwanted pregnancy. It is important to receive professional counseling before deciding to undergo this surgery. Sterilization is considered a permanent form of birth control. In some cases, it can be surgically reversed, generally at a considerable cost and with increased risk for subsequent pregnancies (e.g., ectopic pregnancy).

SURGICAL RISK INCREASES WITH
- Obesity; smoking; poor nutrition.
- Recent or chronic illness; diabetes mellitus.
- Use of some prescription and nonprescription drugs. Inform your doctor of any drugs, medications, or vitamin and herb supplements you are using or have used in the last month.

WHAT TO EXPECT

WHO OPERATES—Obstetrician-gynecologist or general surgeon.

WHERE PERFORMED—Hospital or outpatient surgical facility.

DIAGNOSTIC TESTS
- Before surgery: Blood and urine studies.
- After surgery: Blood studies.

ANESTHESIA
- Local anesthesia by injection.
- Spinal anesthesia by injection.
- General anesthesia by injection and inhalation with an airway tube placed in the windpipe.

DESCRIPTION OF OPERATION
- One of several techniques is used to expose the Fallopian tubes for surgery. The most common is laparoscopy, which involves two small incisions, and the use of a telescopic instrument with a fiberoptic light. Other methods used are: minilaparotomy, which involves a vaginal approach and an incision just at or above the pubic hairline; laparotomy, which requires a standard surgical incision through the abdomen; and posterior colpotomy (rare) which utilizes an approach through the rear of the vagina.
- Once the Fallopian tubes are exposed, a small section of each tube is cut free and removed. The severed ends are tied (ligated) or blocked completely by coagulation using an electric current. In some cases, the tubes are clamped using a clip or band.

- The skin is closed with sutures or clips, which can usually be removed 1 week after surgery.

POSSIBLE COMPLICATIONS
- Inadvertent injury to surrounding structures.
- Infection or excessive bleeding.
- Failure of the sterilization procedure (less than 1%). This may result in an ectopic pregnancy.
- Heavier, more painful periods or ovarian cysts following surgery.

AVERAGE HOSPITAL STAY—0 to 1 day.

PROBABLE OUTCOME—Expect complete healing without complications and sterility for life. Your menstrual periods will continue as usual. Allow about 2 weeks for recovery from surgery.

POSTOPERATIVE CARE

GENERAL MEASURES
- Use an electric heating pad, a heat lamp or a warm compress to relieve surgical-wound pain.
- Bathe and shower as usual. You may wash the incision gently with mild, unscented soap.
- Use another method of birth control until the next menstrual period in case ovulation has already occurred.

MEDICATION
- Your doctor may prescribe:
  Pain relievers. Don't take prescription pain medication longer than 4 to 7 days. Use only as much as you need.
  Stool softeners to prevent constipation.
  Antibiotics to fight or prevent infection.
- You may use nonprescription drugs, such as acetaminophen, for minor pain. Avoid aspirin.

ACTIVITY
- Return to daily activities and work as soon as possible to promote healing.
- Avoid vigorous exercise for 2 weeks after surgery.
- Resume driving 3 days after returning home.
- Resume sexual relations when your doctor has determined that healing is complete.

DIET—Clear liquid diet until the gastrointestinal tract functions again. Then eat a well-balanced diet to promote healing.

CALL YOUR DOCTOR IF

- Pain, swelling, redness, drainage or bleeding increases in the surgical area.
- You develop signs of infection, including headache, muscle aches, dizziness or a general ill feeling and fever.
- You experience nausea, vomiting, constipation or abdominal swelling.
- New, unexplained symptoms develop. Drugs used in treatment may produce side effects.

TUBAL LIGATION

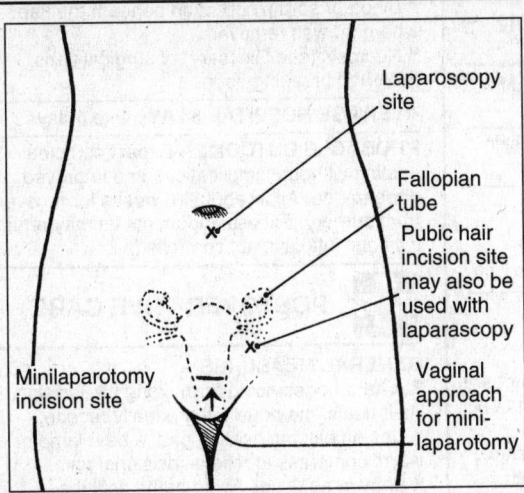

An illustration of structures of the female abdomen and pelvis showing 3 possible sites for a tubal ligation. One is a laparoscopy site, the other a vaginal approach, the third an incision at about the top of the pubic hairline.

Laparoscopy site

Fallopian tube

Pubic hair incision site may also be used with laparascopy

Vaginal approach for mini-laparotomy

Minilaparotomy incision site

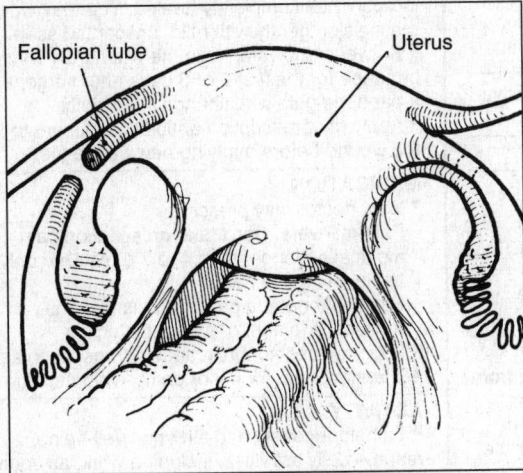

Once the fallopian tubes are exposed, a small section of each tube is cut free and removed.

Fallopian tube

Uterus

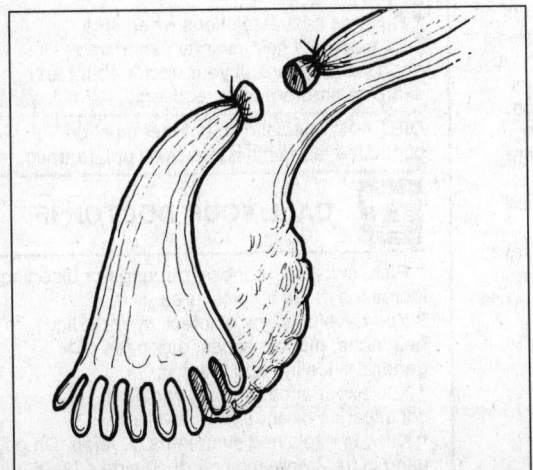

The severed ends are tied.

TUMMY TUCK
(Abdominoplasty)

 GENERAL INFORMATION

DEFINITION—Removal of excess skin and fat from the abdomen.

BODY PARTS INVOLVED—Fat between skin and muscles in abdomen; skin.

REASONS FOR SURGERY
- Improved appearance.
- Reduce incidence of fungal infections in overlapping tissue.

SURGICAL RISK INCREASES WITH
- Smoking; alcoholism; poor nutrition.
- Previous abdominal surgery.
- Recent or chronic illness, especially diabetes.
- Use of some prescription and nonprescription drugs. Inform your doctor of any drugs, medications, or vitamin and herb supplements you are using or have used in the last month.

 WHAT TO EXPECT

WHO OPERATES—Plastic and reconstructive surgeon.

WHERE PERFORMED—Hospital.

DIAGNOSTIC TESTS
- Before surgery: Blood and urine studies.
- After surgery: Blood studies.

ANESTHESIA—General anesthesia by injection and inhalation with an airway tube placed in the windpipe.

DESCRIPTION OF OPERATION
- A large, elliptical incision, usually running from hip to hip, is made in the abdomen. Another incision is usually made around the navel so that it can be moved to a new position after the excess skin has been removed.
- Excessive skin and the underlying apron of excess fat are cut free and removed. Liposuction may also be performed to remove some of the excess fat.
- The navel is reattached in its new location.
- Drains are left under the operative site to prevent accumulation of blood and fluid from tissue drainage.
- Both edges of the skin are gently stretched and carefully sewn together with sutures. Bandages and a firm, elastic dressing similar to a girdle may be placed over the abdomen and buttocks to help hold the stitches together while healing takes place.
- Sutures can usually be removed in 10 to 14 days.

POSSIBLE COMPLICATIONS
- Wide or excessive scars (keloid).
- Excessive bleeding.
- Surgical-wound infection.
- Blood or serum collection beneath the flap where fat was removed.
- Necrosis (see Glossary) of surgical flaps.
- Wound breaking open.

AVERAGE HOSPITAL STAY—2 to 5 days.

PROBABLE OUTCOME—Expect complete healing without complications and improved appearance. Allow about 10 weeks for recovery from surgery. Excess abdominal fat may return if caloric intake is not controlled.

 POSTOPERATIVE CARE

GENERAL MEASURES
- A hard ridge should form along the incision. As it heals, the ridge will gradually recede.
- Use an electric heating pad, a heat lamp or a warm compress to relieve incisional pain.
- Shower as usual. Avoid baths until the incision has completely healed. You may wash the incision gently with mild, unscented soap.
- Between showers, keep the wound dry with a bandage for the first 2 or 3 days after surgery. If a bandage gets wet, change it promptly.
- Apply nonprescription antibiotic ointment to the wound before applying new bandages.

MEDICATION
- Your doctor may prescribe:
  Pain relievers. Don't take prescription pain medication longer than 4 to 7 days. Use only as much as you need.
  Stool softeners to prevent constipation.
  Antibiotics to fight or prevent infection.
- You may use nonprescription drugs, such as acetaminophen, for minor pain. Avoid aspirin.

ACTIVITY
- To help recovery and aid your well-being, resume daily activities, including work, as soon as you are able.
- Resume sexual relations when able.
- Exercise will help maintain improved appearance. Consult your doctor about an exercise program after recovery.

DIET—No special diet, but diet must be controlled to maintain improved appearance.

 CALL YOUR DOCTOR IF

- Pain, swelling, redness, drainage or bleeding increases in the surgical area.
- You develop signs of infection, including headache, muscle aches, dizziness or a general ill feeling and fever.
- You experience nausea, vomiting, constipation or abdominal swelling.
- New, unexplained symptoms develop. Drugs used in treatment may produce side effects.

TUMMY TUCK
(Abdominoplasty)

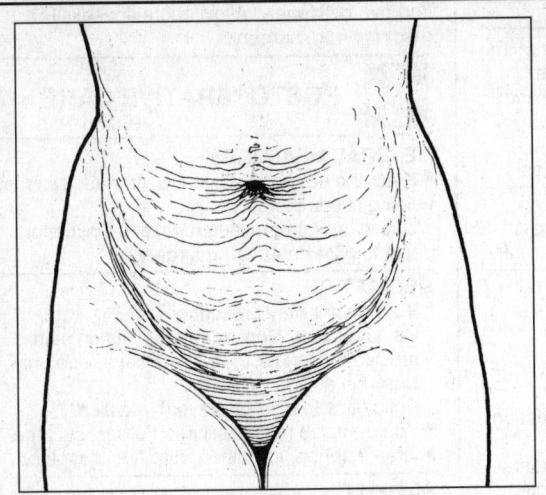

An illustration of typical distribution of excess skin and fat in the lower abdomen.

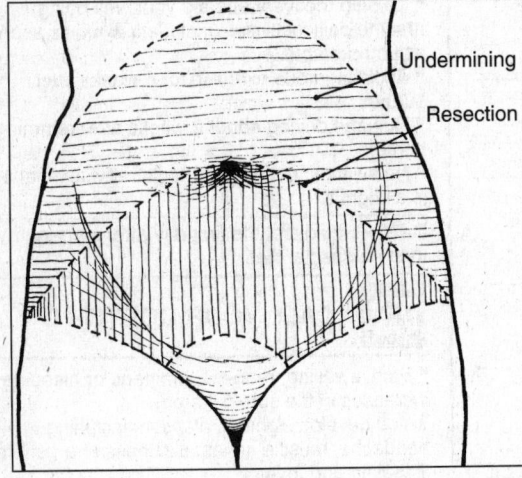

Undermining

Resection

A large elliptical incision is made in the lower abdomen.
- Excessive skin and the underlying apron of excess fat are cut and removed.

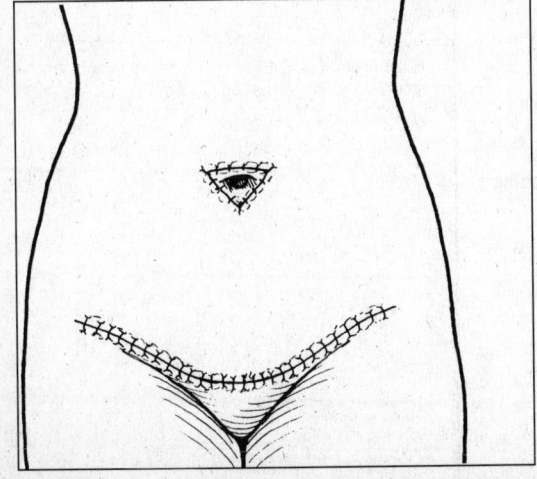

Drains are usually left under the operative site to prevent accumulation of blood and fluid from tissue drainage.
- Both edges of the skin are gently stretched and carefully sewn together with sutures, which can usually be removed in 10 to 14 days.

SURGERIES

TYMPANOPLASTY

 GENERAL INFORMATION

DEFINITION—Repair, removal or bypass of an obstruction or defect in the middle ear that prevents sound waves from reaching the inner ear. This is called conductive hearing loss, which can be total or partial. Usually, it is caused by chronic infection in the middle ear.

BODY PARTS INVOLVED—Eardrum (tympanic membrane); middle ear cavity; skin separating middle ear from inner ear; inner ear.

REASONS FOR SURGERY—Restoration of, or improvement in, hearing ability.

SURGICAL RISK INCREASES WITH
- Recent or chronic illness.
- Diabetes mellitus.
- Use of some prescription and nonprescription drugs. Inform your doctor of any drugs, medications, or vitamin and herb supplements you are using or have used in the last month.

 WHAT TO EXPECT

WHO OPERATES—Ear, nose and throat specialist (otolaryngologist).

WHERE PERFORMED—Hospital.

DIAGNOSTIC TESTS
- Before surgery: Blood and urine studies; hearing tests.
- After surgery: Hearing tests.

ANESTHESIA—General anesthesia by injection and inhalation with an airway tube placed in the windpipe.

DESCRIPTION OF OPERATION
- An instrument called an ear speculum is placed in the external ear canal, and the operating microscope is positioned.
- The middle ear is entered through an incision in the eardrum.
- Depending on the type of defect, one of the following procedures is performed:
Repair of a defect in the eardrum.
Closure of the defect in the eardrum with a graft.
Fenestration, which is the creation of a new opening into a part of the inner ear. This method is used to treat otosclerosis (see Illness section).

POSSIBLE COMPLICATIONS
- Excessive bleeding.
- Surgical-wound infection.
- Recurrence of hole in the eardrum.

AVERAGE HOSPITAL STAY—0 to 2 days.

PROBABLE OUTCOME—Expect complete healing without complications. Hearing should improve noticeably. Allow about 4 weeks for recovery from surgery.

 POSTOPERATIVE CARE

GENERAL MEASURES
- Keep the ear dry until your doctor advises that healing is complete.
- Use warm compresses to relieve discomfort beginning 24 hours after surgery.

MEDICATION
- Your doctor may prescribe:
Pain relievers. Don't take prescription pain medication longer than 4 to 7 days. Use only as much as you need.
Antibiotics to fight or prevent infection.
- You may use nonprescription drugs, such as acetaminophen, for minor pain. Avoid aspirin.

ACTIVITY
- To help recovery and aid your well-being, resume daily activities, including work, as soon as you are able.
- Avoid vigorous exercise for 4 weeks after surgery.
- Resume driving about 2 weeks after returning home.
- No swimming until your doctor advises that it is all right to do so.

DIET—Liquid diet the first day after surgery, then no special diet.

 CALL YOUR DOCTOR IF

- Pain, swelling, redness, drainage or bleeding increases in the surgical area.
- You develop signs of infection, including headache, muscle aches, dizziness or a general ill feeling and fever.

TYMPANOPLASTY

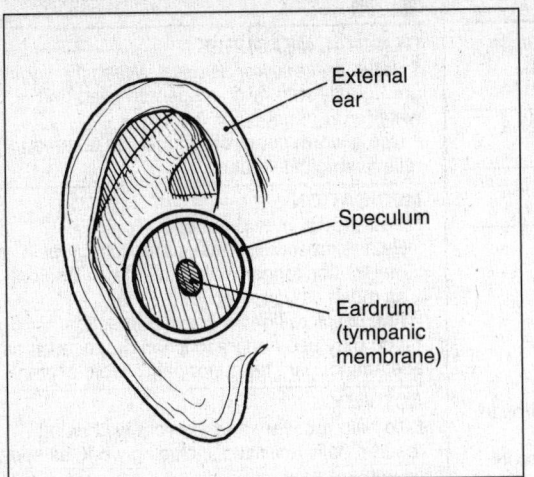

External
ear

Speculum

Eardrum
(tympanic
membrane)

An illustration of the external ear with
a speculum in place showing the
appearance of the eardrum through
the ear speculum.

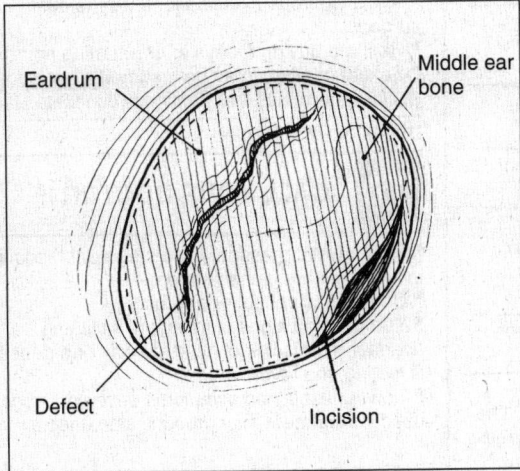

Eardrum

Middle ear
bone

Defect

Incision

The middle ear is entered through an
incision in the eardrum.

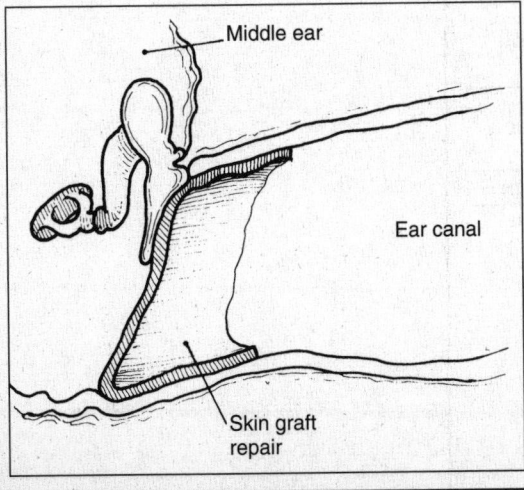

Middle ear

Ear canal

Skin graft
repair

A graft repair of the defect once again
seals off the middle and inner ear
from air and debris in the ear canal.

URETHRAL CARUNCLE REMOVAL

 GENERAL INFORMATION

DEFINITION—Removal of a urethral caruncle, a small benign tumor that develops at the opening of the female urethra.

BODY PARTS INVOLVED—Urethra; vagina (route for surgery).

REASONS FOR SURGERY—Treatment of excessive bleeding or discomfort.

SURGICAL RISK INCREASES WITH
- Adults over 60.
- Obesity; smoking.
- Poor nutrition.
- Recent or chronic illness.
- Alcoholism.
- Diabetes mellitus.
- Use of some prescription and nonprescription drugs. Inform your doctor of any drugs, medications, or vitamin and herb supplements you are using or have used in the last month.

 WHAT TO EXPECT

WHO OPERATES—Urologist or obstetrician-gynecologist.

WHERE PERFORMED—Hospital, outpatient surgical facility or doctor's office.

DIAGNOSTIC TESTS
- Before surgery: Pap smear (see Glossary); pelvic examination; blood and urine studies.
- After surgery: Pelvic examination.

ANESTHESIA—Local anesthesia by injection and topical application.

DESCRIPTION OF OPERATION
- The vagina is held open with a speculum. The caruncle is located, cleansed and anesthetized with local anesthesia.
- The caruncle is then removed with electrocauterization or a scalpel.
- Bleeding is controlled with pressure or electrocauterization.

POSSIBLE COMPLICATIONS
- Excessive bleeding.
- Surgical-wound infection.

AVERAGE HOSPITAL STAY—Usually none.

PROBABLE OUTCOME—Expect complete healing without complications. Allow about 2 weeks for recovery from surgery.

 POSTOPERATIVE CARE

GENERAL MEASURES
- Bathe and shower as usual. Wash the vaginal area gently with mild, unscented soap and water after urination.
- Use a warm compress in the genital area to relieve surgical-wound pain.

MEDICATION
- Your doctor may prescribe:
  Pain relievers. Don't take prescription pain medication longer than 4 to 7 days. Use only as much as you need.
  Antibiotics to fight or prevent infection.
- You may use nonprescription drugs, such as acetaminophen, for minor pain. Avoid aspirin.

ACTIVITY
- To help recovery and aid your well-being, resume daily activities, including work, as soon as you are able.
- Avoid vigorous exercise for 2 weeks after surgery.
- Resume driving 3 days after returning home.
- Sexual relations may be resumed when your doctor determines that healing is complete.

DIET—No special diet.

 CALL YOUR DOCTOR IF

- Pain, swelling, redness, drainage or bleeding increases in the surgical area.
- Urination is painful or difficult.
- You develop signs of infection, including headache, muscle aches, dizziness or a general ill feeling and fever.
- New, unexplained symptoms develop. Drugs used in treatment may produce side effects.

URETHRAL CARUNCLE REMOVAL

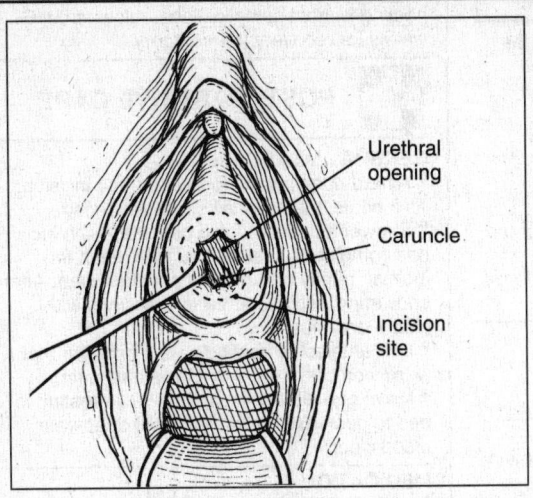

Urethral opening

Caruncle

Incision site

View of the vagina, held open with a speculum, showing the caruncle to be removed and the usual incision site.

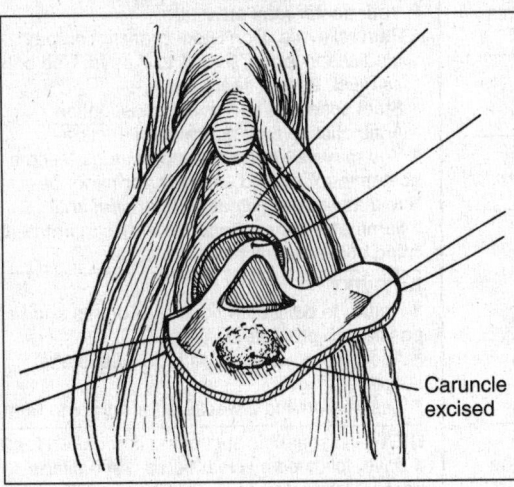

Caruncle excised

Caruncle is removed with electrocauterization or by cutting with a scalpel.

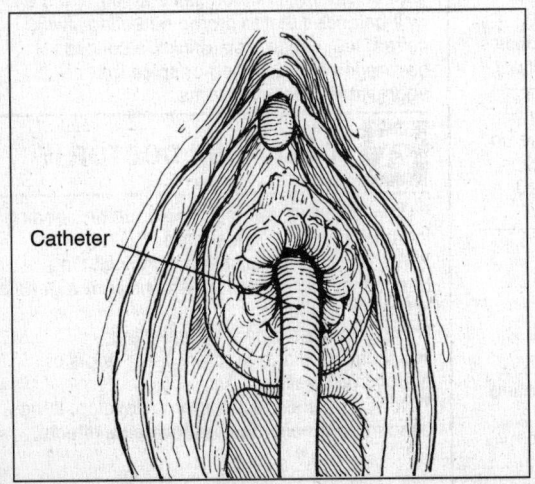

Catheter

After repair, a catheter may be left inside the bladder until healing begins.

VAGOTOMY

GENERAL INFORMATION

DEFINITION—Disconnecting branches of the vagus nerve to slow acid production in the stomach. Usually, this surgery is performed before other surgeries such as gastroenterostomy (see in Surgery section).

BODY PARTS INVOLVED—Stomach; branches of the vagus nerve.

REASONS FOR SURGERY—Treatment of the complications of peptic ulcers such as: obstruction of digestive flow; ulcer perforation; bleeding of an ulcer; or intolerable pain.

SURGICAL RISK INCREASES WITH
- Obesity; smoking; stress.
- Poor nutrition.
- Recent or chronic illness.
- Diabetes mellitus.
- Use of some prescription and nonprescription drugs. Inform your doctor of any drugs, medications, or vitamin and herb supplements you are using or have used in the last month.

WHAT TO EXPECT

WHO OPERATES—General surgeon.

WHERE PERFORMED—Hospital.

DIAGNOSTIC TESTS
- Before surgery: Blood and urine studies; x-rays of gastrointestinal tract; gastroscopy; gastroduodenoscopy; ECG (see Glossary).
- After surgery: Blood studies; tissue studies.

ANESTHESIA—General anesthesia by injection and inhalation with an airway tube placed in the windpipe.

DESCRIPTION OF OPERATION
- An incision is made in the abdomen, and the abdominal muscles are separated.
- The vagus nerve is identified, and the branches that control stomach-acid production are isolated, divided and clipped. Segments of the vagus nerve are removed for laboratory study.
- The abdominal muscles are sewn together in layers. The skin is closed with sutures or clips, which usually can be removed about 7 to 10 days after surgery.

POSSIBLE COMPLICATIONS
- Excessive bleeding.
- Surgical-wound infection.
- Incisional hernia.
- Dumping syndrome.
- Diarrhea.
- A sensation of flushing or fainting after eating some foods.
- Recurrent ulcer due to incomplete vagotomy.

AVERAGE HOSPITAL STAY—3 to 5 days.

PROBABLE OUTCOME—Expect complete healing without complications. Allow about 6 weeks for recovery from surgery.

POSTOPERATIVE CARE

GENERAL MEASURES
- A hard ridge should form along the incision. As it heals, the ridge will gradually recede.
- Shower as usual. Avoid baths until the incision has completely healed. You may wash the incision gently with mild, unscented soap. After showering, replace any wet dressings with clean, dry ones.
- Use an electric heating pad, a heat lamp or a warm compress to relieve incisional pain.
- Move and elevate legs often while resting in bed to decrease the likelihood of deep-vein blood clots.

MEDICATION
- Your doctor may prescribe:
  Pain relievers. Don't take prescription pain medication longer than 4 to 7 days. Use only as much as you need.
  Stool softeners to prevent constipation.
  Antibiotics to fight or prevent infection.
- You may use nonprescription drugs, such as acetaminophen and antacids, for minor pain. Avoid aspirin and other nonsteroidal anti-inflammatory drugs because they can irritate the lining of the stomach.

ACTIVITY
- Return to daily activities and work as soon as possible to promote healing.
- Avoid vigorous exercise for 6 weeks after surgery.
- Resume driving 2 weeks after returning home.

DIET—Nasogastric suctioning is required for 3-4 days, followed by clear liquid diet until the gastrointestinal tract functions again. Then eat a well-balanced diet to promote healing. Avoid coffee, tea, cocoa, cola drinks, alcoholic beverages and any food or spice that aggravates ulcer symptoms.

CALL YOUR DOCTOR IF

- Pain, swelling, redness, drainage or bleeding increases in the surgical area.
- You develop signs of infection, including headache, muscle aches, dizziness or a general ill feeling and fever.
- You experience nausea, vomiting, constipation, diarrhea, black tarry stools or abdominal swelling.
- New, unexplained symptoms develop. Drugs used in treatment may produce side effects.

VAGOTOMY

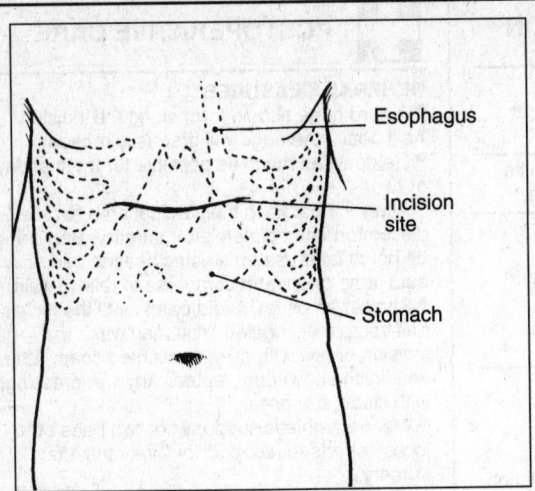

An illustration of the esophagus, stomach, rib cage and a typical incision site.

- Esophagus
- Incision site
- Stomach

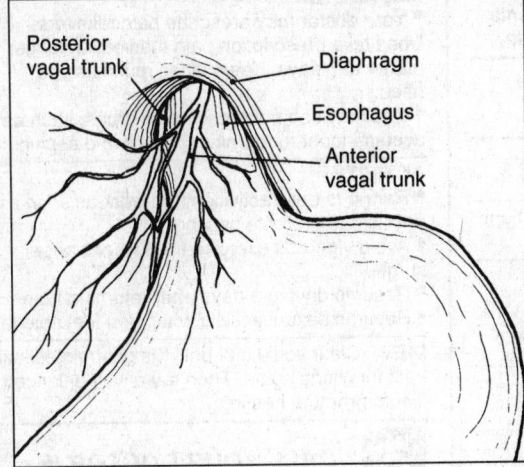

The vagas nerve is identified.
- The branches that control stomach acid production are isolated, divided and clipped.

- Posterior vagal trunk
- Diaphragm
- Esophagus
- Anterior vagal trunk

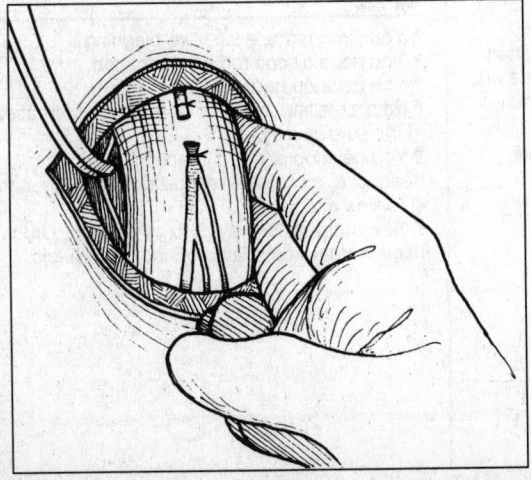

The abdominal muscles that were opened to gain access to the vagas nerve are repaired in layers.
- The overlying muscles and skin are repaired with sutures or clips (not illustrated).

SURGERIES

VARICOCELE REMOVAL
(Varicocelectomy)

 GENERAL INFORMATION

DEFINITION—Removal of a varicocele, a swelling in the scrotum caused by veins that have become distended and twisted.

BODY PARTS INVOLVED—Scrotum and its contents (usually the left testis); varicocele.

REASONS FOR SURGERY
- Relief of discomfort in the scrotum.
- Reduced congestion of the venous system around the testicles.
- Improved quality and quantity of sperm production (sometimes).

SURGICAL RISK INCREASES WITH
- Recent or chronic illness.
- Obesity.
- Diabetes mellitus.
- Use of some prescription and nonprescription drugs. Inform your doctor of any drugs, medications, or vitamin and herb supplements you are using or have used in the last month.

 WHAT TO EXPECT

WHO OPERATES—General surgeon or urologist.

WHERE PERFORMED—Hospital or outpatient surgical facility.

DIAGNOSTIC TESTS
- Before surgery: Blood and urine studies; ultrasound (see Glossary).
- After surgery: Blood studies.

ANESTHESIA
- Local anesthesia by injection.
- Spinal anesthesia by injection.

DESCRIPTION OF OPERATION
- An incision is made in the scrotum.
- The spermatic cord is identified.
- Abnormal veins are cut and tied. The twisted, dilated vein or veins that form the varicocele are cut free and removed. The artery and normal-appearing veins are protected.
- The skin is closed with sutures that will be absorbed by the body.
- A snug bandage is placed over the incision.

POSSIBLE COMPLICATIONS
- Excessive bleeding.
- Surgical-wound infection.
- Difficulty with urination.
- Inadvertent injury to the spermatic cord.

AVERAGE HOSPITAL STAY—0 to 1 day.

PROBABLE OUTCOME—Expect complete healing without complications. Allow about 1 week for recovery from surgery.

 POSTOPERATIVE CARE

GENERAL MEASURES
- A hard ridge should form along the incision. As it heals, the ridge will gradually recede.
- Lie down as much as possible for the first day or two.
- Apply ice packs to the surgical area to relieve discomfort immediately after surgery. Beginning 24 hours later use an electric heating pad, a heat lamp or a warm compress to relieve pain.
- Shower as usual. Avoid baths until the incision has completely healed. You may wash the incision gently with mild, unscented soap. After you finish showering, replace any wet dressings with clean, dry ones.
- Wear an athletic supporter or two pairs of jockey shorts for support for 2 months after surgery.

MEDICATION
- Your doctor may prescribe pain relievers. Don't take prescription pain medication longer than 4 to 7 days. Use only as much as you need.
- You may use nonprescription drugs, such as acetaminophen, for minor pain. Avoid aspirin.

ACTIVITY
- Return to daily activities and work as soon as possible to promote healing.
- Avoid vigorous exercise for 6 weeks after surgery.
- Resume driving 3 days after returning home.
- Resume sexual activity when you feel able to.

DIET—Clear liquid diet until the gastrointestinal tract functions again. Then eat a well-balanced diet to promote healing.

 CALL YOUR DOCTOR IF

- You experience excessive bleeding.
- You have discomfort with urination.
- You develop nausea or vomiting.
- Pain, swelling, redness or drainage increases in the surgical area.
- You develop signs of infection, including headache, muscle aches, dizziness or a general ill feeling and fever.
- New, unexplained symptoms develop. Drugs used in treatment may produce side effects.

VARICOCELE REMOVAL
(Varicocelectomy)

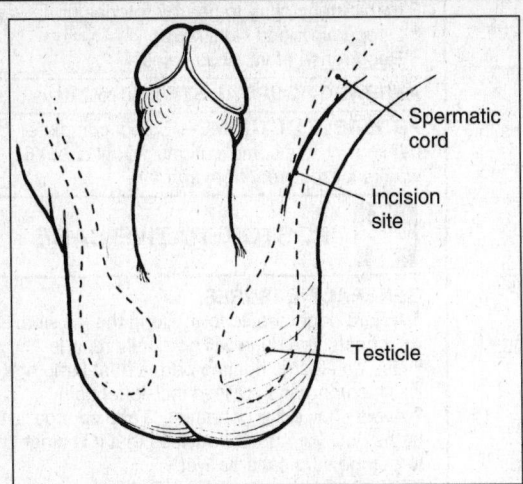

An illustration of the penis, scrotum, spermatic cord, testicle and a typical incision site.

Spermatic cord

Incision site

Testicle

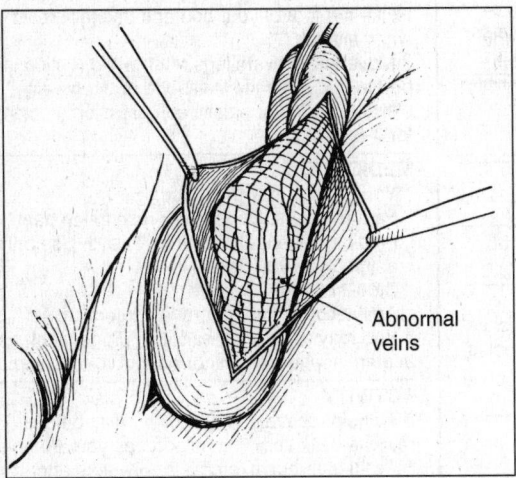

The open cord revealing the abnormal veins.

Abnormal veins

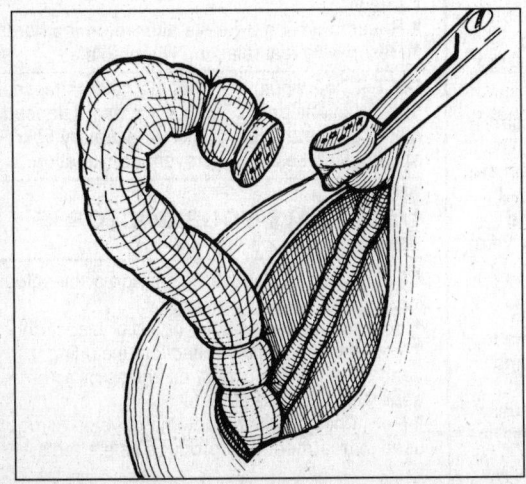

Abnormal veins are cut and tied. The twisted, dilated vein or veins that form the varicocele are cut free and removed.
- The skin is closed with sutures that will be absorbed by the body (not illustrated).

SURGERIES

VARICOSE VEIN REMOVAL

GENERAL INFORMATION

DEFINITION—Removal of varicose veins, which are veins in the leg that have become abnormally swollen or dilated.

BODY PARTS INVOLVED—Diseased veins in the legs, usually in the greater and lesser saphenous veins.

REASONS FOR SURGERY
- Improvement of appearance.
- Relief of pain or pressure symptoms.
- Treatment of recurrent superficial phlebitis (see Glossary).
- Help heal venous statis ulcers (see Glossary).

SURGICAL RISK INCREASES WITH
- Stress; obesity; smoking; poor nutrition.
- Excess alcohol consumption.
- Adults over 60.
- History of phlebitis (blood clots); diabetes.
- Use of some prescription and nonprescription drugs. Inform your doctor of any drugs, medications, or vitamin and herb supplements you are using or have used in the last month.

WHAT TO EXPECT

WHO OPERATES—Vascular or general surgeon; plastic surgeon.

WHERE PERFORMED—Outpatient surgical facility or hospital.

DIAGNOSTIC TESTS
- Before surgery: Blood and urine studies; chest x-ray; ultrasound; ECG; doppler venous studies (see Glossary for all).
- After surgery: Blood studies.

ANESTHESIA
- Local anesthesia by injection.
- Spinal anesthesia by injection.
- General anesthesia by injection and inhalation with an airway tube placed in the windpipe.

DESCRIPTION OF OPERATION
- An incision is made over the top of the saphenous-femoral vein system (see Glossary).
- The large, diseased veins are identified. The upper and lower ends of each diseased vein are cut and tied. A thin wire instrument is passed through the vein, beginning at the ankle and extending upward through the inside of the vein; the wire is used to strip (remove) the entire vein.
- After the main veins have been removed, smaller veins are identified; incisions are made and the smaller veins are tied individually and removed.
- The skin is closed with sutures, which usually can be removed about 1 week after surgery.
- The legs are wrapped snugly in elastic bandages.

POSSIBLE COMPLICATIONS
- Excessive bleeding; surgical-wound infection.
- Inadvertent injury to nearby arteries or nerves.
- Deep-vein blood clots (rare).
- Recurrence of varicose veins.

AVERAGE HOSPITAL STAY—0 to 2 days.

PROBABLE OUTCOME—Expect complete healing without complications. Allow about 6 weeks for recovery from surgery.

POSTOPERATIVE CARE

GENERAL MEASURES
- A hard ridge should form along the incision. As it heals, the ridge will gradually recede.
- Use an electric heating pad, a heat lamp or a warm compress to relieve incisional pain.
- Avoid showering or bathing. Take sponge baths until your doctor advises that it is alright to get the surgical area wet.
- Keep your legs elevated whenever possible. Raise the foot of your bed and use foot rests when sitting.
- Move and elevate legs often while resting in bed to decrease the likelihood of deep-vein blood clots. Wear elastic compression stockings for 4-6 weeks.

MEDICATION
- Your doctor may prescribe:
  Pain relievers. Don't take prescription pain medication longer than 4 to 7 days. Use only as much as you need.
  Stool softener laxatives.
  Antibiotics to fight or prevent infection.
- You may use nonprescription drugs, such as acetaminophen, for minor pain. Avoid aspirin.

ACTIVITY
- To help recovery and aid your well-being, resume daily activities as soon as you are able.
- Avoid vigorous exercise for 6 weeks after surgery.
- Resume driving 3 weeks after returning home.
- Resume sexual relations when able.

DIET—Clear liquid diet until the gastrointestinal tract functions again. Then eat a well-balanced diet to promote healing. Increase dietary fiber and fluid intake to help prevent constipation.

CALL YOUR DOCTOR IF

- Pain, swelling, redness, drainage or bleeding increases in the surgical area.
- Your foot becomes cold, numb or discolored.
- You develop signs of infection, including headache, muscle aches, dizziness or a general ill feeling and fever.
- New, unexplained symptoms develop. Drugs used in treatment may produce side effects.

VARICOSE VEIN REMOVAL

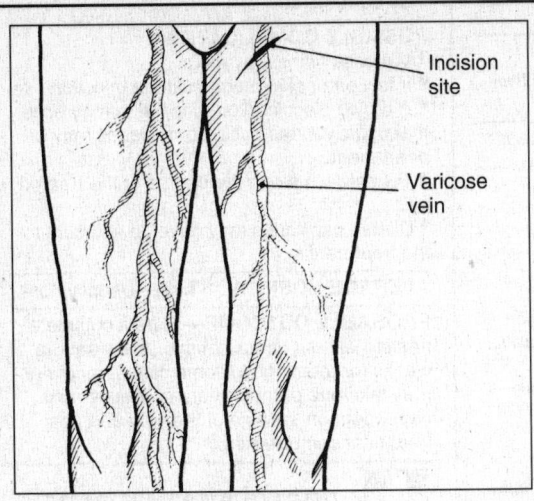

Incision site

Varicose vein

An illustration of diseased veins in the legs, usually the greater and lesser saphenous veins.

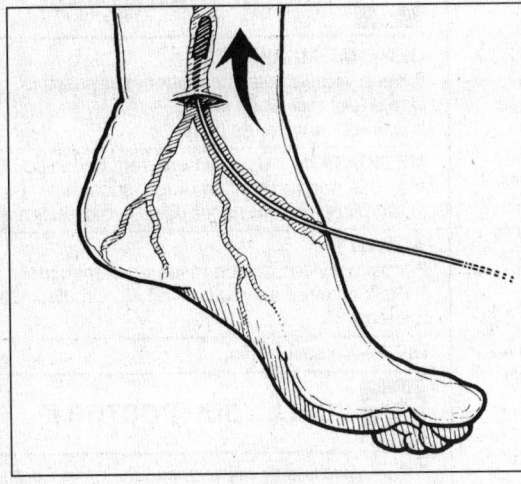

The large diseased veins are identified.
- The upper and lower ends of each diseased vein are cut and tied and a thin wire instrument is passed through the inside of the vein; the wire is used to strip (remove) the entire vein.

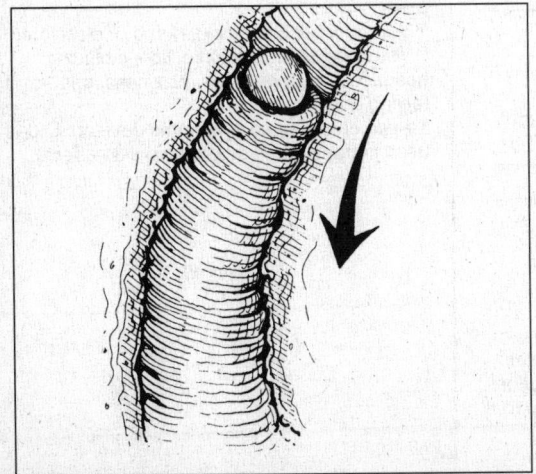

- After the main veins have been removed, smaller veins are identified, incisions are made into the skin and smaller veins are tied individually and removed.
- After surgery, the legs are wrapped snugly in elastic bandages.

VARICOSE VEIN SCLEROTHERAPY

GENERAL INFORMATION

DEFINITION—Use of a special injected chemical solution to collapse veins so that they no longer carry blood.

BODY PARTS INVOLVED—Veins in the legs, usually on the backs of the calves or on the insides of the leg. Spider veins (superficial, small veins in skin) usually form a linear, discrete or grouped pattern.

REASONS FOR SURGERY
• To relieve symptoms of varicose veins (swelling, distortion or twisting of a vein) such as pain, aching, fatigue or swelling of feet and ankles.
• As a follow-up treatment following varicose vein removal (see in Surgery section).
• As an early treatment to prevent the development of larger varicose veins.
• To improve cosmetic appearance of the legs.

SURGICAL RISK INCREASES WITH
• Obesity; smoking.
• Excess alcohol consumption.
• Adults over 60.
• History of thrombophlebitis, deep-vein thrombosis or pulmonary embolism.
• Diabetes mellitus.
• Use of some prescription and nonprescription drugs. Inform your doctor of any drugs, medications, or vitamin and herb supplements you are using or have used in the last month.

WHAT TO EXPECT

WHO OPERATES—General surgeon, family doctor, dermatologist, vascular surgeon or plastic surgeon.

WHERE PERFORMED—Outpatient surgical facility, doctor's office.

DIAGNOSTIC TESTS
• Before surgery: Normally a physical examination is sufficient, but your doctor may perform a tourniquet test to evaluate the problem or special x-rays (venography).
• After surgery: None expected.

ANESTHESIA—None required.

DESCRIPTION OF OPERATION
• A special solution (called a sclerosant) is injected into the vein or veins. This causes inflammation in the lining of the vein, and eventual fibrosis (scar tissue formation), which leads to the vein's obliteration. The blood is forced to reroute itself through healthier veins. Complete treatment may take several injections.
• After injection, firm pressure is applied so that the walls of the vein are pressed together.

• In severe cases, a comprehension bandage may be required.

POSSIBLE COMPLICATIONS
• Varicose veins may recur.
• Infection or skin reaction at the injection site.
• A brown discoloration of the skin may occur that usually fades but in some cases may be permanent.
• Tenderness along the course of the treated vein.
• Dilated capillaries may develop adjacent to the treatment site.

AVERAGE HOSPITAL STAY—Usually none.

PROBABLE OUTCOME—Expect complete healing without complications. Allow several weeks for recovery; in some cases, recovery may take one or more months. Recovery is dependent on the size of the vein and post-treatment compression.

POSTOPERATIVE CARE

GENERAL MEASURES
• Keep your leg elevated whenever possible. Use a foot rest when sitting.
• Bathe or shower as usual.

MEDICATION—Usually none required. You may use nonprescription drugs, such as acetaminophen, for minor pain. Avoid aspirin.

ACTIVITY
• Most activities can be resumed immediately.
• Walk as often as you can to help circulation in the legs.

DIET—No special diet.

CALL YOUR DOCTOR IF

• Pain, swelling or redness occurs in the treated area.
• Your foot becomes cold, numb or discolored.
• You develop signs of infection, including headache, muscle aches, dizziness, general ill feeling and fever.
• New, unexplained symptoms develop. Drugs used in treatment may produce side effects.

VARICOSE VEIN SCLEROTHERAPY

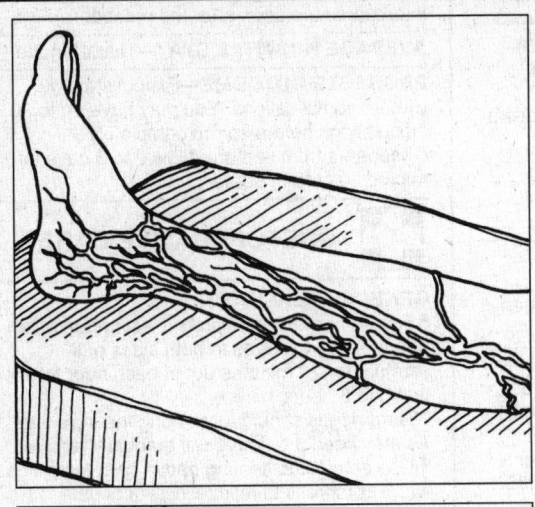

Leg is prepared and positioned for treatment.

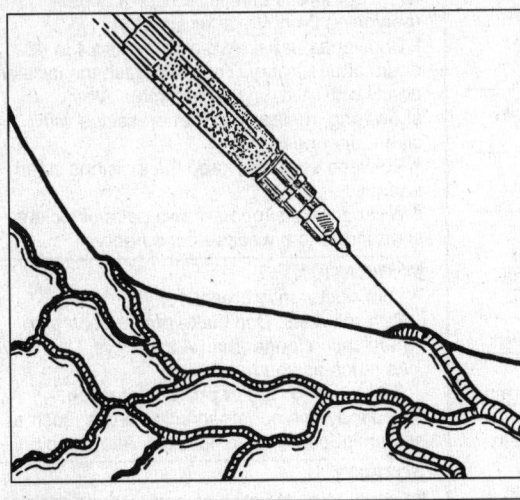

A special solution is injected into a vein.

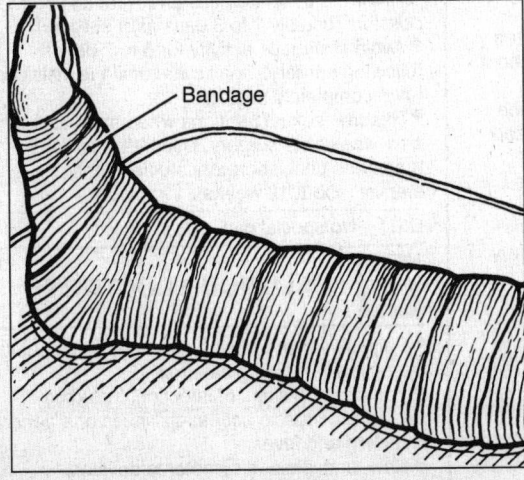

In severe cases, a compression bandage may be required.

Bandage

VASECTOMY

GENERAL INFORMATION

DEFINITION—A method of sterilization that involves cutting and tying the vas deferens (sperm channels inside the scrotum). The surgery stops the flow of sperm and provides a safe, effective form of birth control without affecting sexual desire or ability.

BODY PARTS INVOLVED—Scrotum; vas deferens.

REASONS FOR SURGERY
• Voluntary sterilization.
• Recurrent epididymitis (see Glossary) when caused by chronic prostate infection.

SURGICAL RISK INCREASES WITH
• Recent or chronic illness; diabetes mellitus.
• Use of some prescription and nonprescription drugs. Inform your doctor of any drugs, medications, or vitamin and herb supplements you are using or have used in the last month.

WHAT TO EXPECT

WHO OPERATES—General surgeon, family doctor, or urologist.

WHERE PERFORMED—Doctor's office, outpatient surgical facility or hospital.

DIAGNOSTIC TESTS
• Before surgery: None required.
• After surgery: Sperm studies, at least twice during 10 weeks after surgery.

ANESTHESIA—Local anesthesia by injection.

DESCRIPTION OF OPERATION
• The scrotum is shaved at home before surgery.
• Incisions are made on both sides of the scrotum. The vas deferens is identified, tied in two places and cut between the ties.
• The divided vas deferens is returned to the scrotum.
• The edges of incised skin are reconstructed with fine sutures, which usually fall out in about 7 days.
• Another method for vasectomy is called the no-scalpel technique. It requires 2 specialized instruments and avoids the usual surgical incisions. It requires no sutures to close the surgical site, and may result in fewer complications. Some men may not be appropriate candidates for this type of surgery because of differences in scrotal anatomy.

POSSIBLE COMPLICATIONS
• Collection of blood in scrotum.
• Excessive bleeding; surgical-wound infection.
• Epididymitis (see Glossary).
• Sperm granuloma (benign lump in the surgical area).
• Small possibility of re-establishing fertility.

• Pregnancy may still occur in about 1% of cases (often as a result of unprotected intercourse too soon after the procedure).

AVERAGE HOSPITAL STAY—Usually none.

PROBABLE OUTCOME—Expect sterility without complications. You may have up to 30 ejaculations before sperm completely disappears from semen. Allow 2 to 3 days for full recovery from surgery.

POSTOPERATIVE CARE

GENERAL MEASURES
• Return home immediately. Rest in bed for 24 hours. Apply ice bags to both sides of the scrotum for 20 minutes out of each hour for the first 6 to 8 hours.
• Hard ridges should form along the incisions. As they heal, the ridges will gradually recede.
• Use an electric heating pad, a heat lamp or a warm compress to relieve incisional pain (beginning 24 hours after surgery).
• Shower as usual. Avoid baths for 24 to 48 hours after surgery. You may wash the incisions gently with mild, unscented soap. After showering, replace any wet dressings with clean, dry ones.
• Between showers, keep the incisions clean and dry.
• Wear scrotal support or two pairs of jockey shorts for 4 to 6 weeks after surgery.

MEDICATION
• Your doctor may prescribe:
  Pain relievers. Don't take prescription pain medication longer than 4 to 7 days. Use only as much as you need.
  Antibiotics to fight or prevent infection.
• You may use nonprescription drugs, such as acetaminophen, for minor pain. Avoid aspirin.

ACTIVITY
• Return to daily activities and work as soon as possible (usually 2 to 3 days after surgery).
• Avoid strenuous activity for 5 to 7 days following surgery. Don't swim until the incisions have completely healed.
• Resume sexual relations when able, as soon as 1 week after surgery. Use birth-control measures until laboratory studies confirm sterility (about 12 weeks).

DIET—No special diet.

CALL YOUR DOCTOR IF

• Pain, swelling, redness, drainage or bleeding increases in the surgical area.
• You develop signs of infection, including headache, muscle aches, dizziness or a general ill feeling and fever.
• New, unexplained symptoms develop.

VASECTOMY

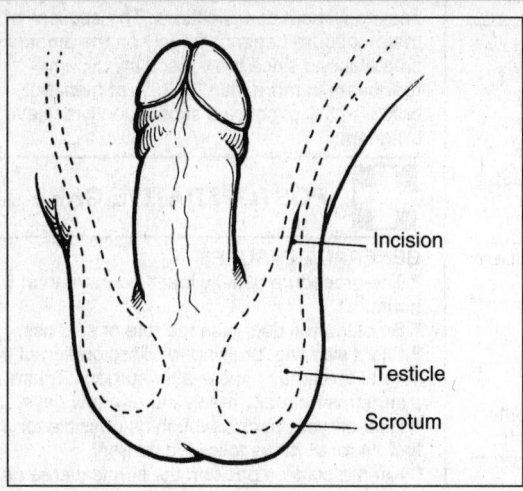

The penis, scrotum and testicles showing a typical incision site for a vasectomy.

Incision

Testicle

Scrotum

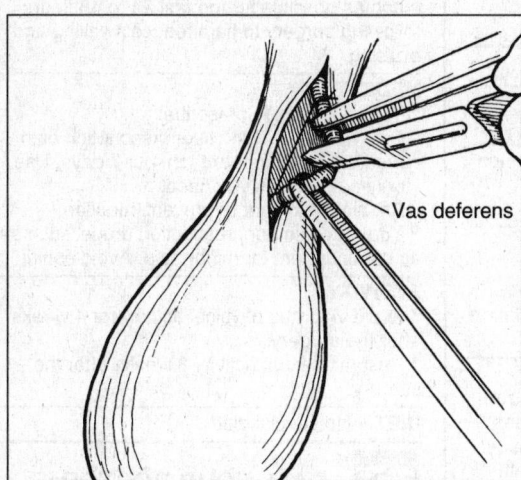

The vas deferens is identified, tied in 2 places and cut between the ties.

Vas deferens

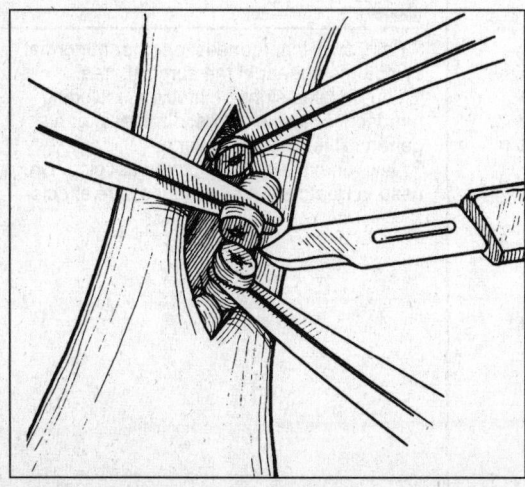

The divided vas deferens is returned to the scrotum and the edges of incised skin are reconstructed with fine sutures that usually fall out in about 7 days (not illustrated).

VASECTOMY REVERSAL

GENERAL INFORMATION

DEFINITION—A procedure to restore the flow of sperm through the vas deferens (the tubes that carry the sperm from the testicle to the urethra). There are two types of vasectomy reversal: a vasovasostomy and a vasoepididymostomy.

BODY PARTS INVOLVED—Scrotum; vas deferens.

REASONS FOR SURGERY—Restores male reproduction ability (fertility).

SURGICAL RISK INCREASES WITH
• Diabetes mellitus.
• Use of some prescription and nonprescription drugs. Inform your doctor of any drugs, medications, or vitamin and herb supplements you are using or have used in the last month.

WHAT TO EXPECT

WHO OPERATES—Urologist.

WHERE PERFORMED—Doctor's office, outpatient surgical facility, or a hospital.

DIAGNOSTIC TESTS—Usually none. For men over 40, an ECG (see Glossary) may be performed.

ANESTHESIA
• Local anesthesia by injection.
• Regional anesthesia by injection.
• General anesthesia by injection and inhalation with an airway tube placed in the windpipe.

DESCRIPTION OF OPERATION
• The area around the scrotum is anesthetized.
• The previously cut ends of the vas deferens are located and trimmed back to normal tissue.
• The ends are then sewn back together with very fine sutures.
• When too much scarring or inflammation has occurred in the epididymis, sperm can be blocked from getting to the vas deferens. If this blockage has occurred, connecting the two ends of the vas deferens will not prove successful, and bypassing the blockage via a vasoepididymostomy must be performed.
• A vasoepididymostomy is performed by connecting the vas deferens directly to the epididymis.

POSSIBLE COMPLICATIONS
• Infection.
• Scrotal hematoma (black and blue bruised scrotum).
• Scarring where the ends are connected, causing continued blockage.
• Epididymitis (see Glossary).
• Urinary retention.

AVERAGE HOSPITAL STAY—0 to 1 day.

PROBABLE OUTCOME—Expect complete healing without complications. The success of the procedure depends largely on the amount of time elapsed since the vasectomy. Sperm reappears in more than 80-95% of men, but only 50-75% of couples subsequently achieve pregnancy.

POSTOPERATIVE CARE

GENERAL MEASURES
• The procedure usually takes no more than 5 hours.
• Smoking will decrease the rate of success.
• Slight swelling, bruising, or discoloration of the scrotal area may appear after surgery. These symptoms normally resolve after a few days.
• Rest on your back as much as possible for the first 24 to 48 hours following surgery.
• Keep a cold ice pack on the surgical area as much as possible for the first 24 to 48 hours following surgery to help reduce swelling and bruising.

MEDICATION
• Your doctor may prescribe:
  Pain relievers. Don't take prescription pain medication for longer than 4 to 7 days. Use only as much as you need.
  Antibiotics to fight or prevent infection.
• You may use nonprescription drugs, such as acetaminophen, for minor pain. Avoid aspirin.

ACTIVITY
• Avoid vigorous physical activity for 4 weeks after the surgery.
• Resume sexual activity 3 weeks after the surgery.

DIET—No special diet.

CALL YOUR DOCTOR IF

• Pain, swelling, redness, or other abnormal symptoms appear in the surgical area.
• You develop signs of infection, including headache, muscle aches, dizziness, or a general ill feeling and fever.
• New, unexplained symptoms develop. Drugs used in treatment may produce side effects.

VASECTOMY REVERSAL

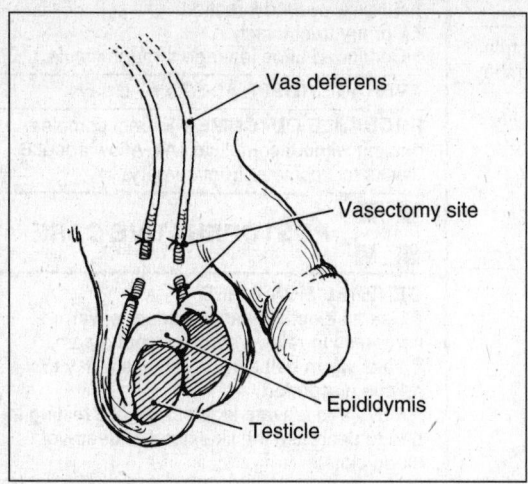

Vas deferens

Vasectomy site

Epididymis

Testicle

An illustration showing the site of a previous vasectomy. The vas deferens has previously been cut and tied to prevent the flow of sperm from the testicles to the urethra.

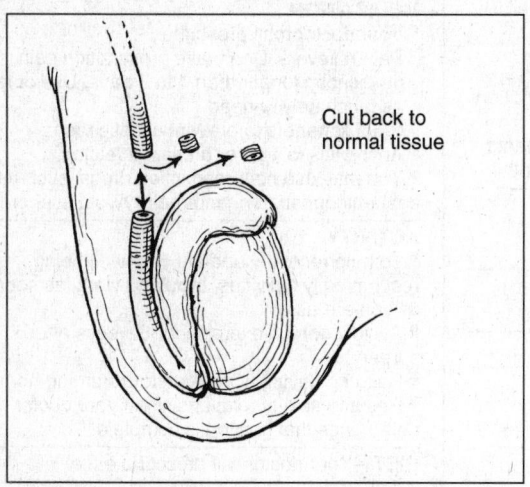

Cut back to normal tissue

The previously cut ends of the vas deferens have been located and trimmed back to reveal normal tissue.

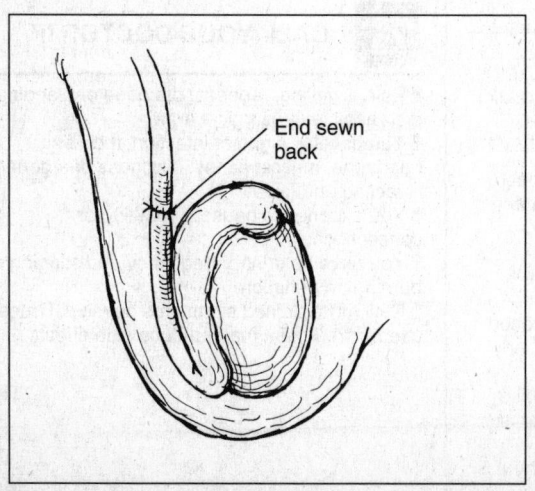

End sewn back

The ends are sewn back together with very fine sutures.

VESICOVAGINAL FISTULA REPAIR

GENERAL INFORMATION

DEFINITION—Repair of a vesicovaginal fistula, an abnormal tract between the bladder and the vagina that usually results from tearing in childbirth, as a complication of cervical uterine surgery (e.g., vaginal hysterectomy), or as a complication of cervical cancer (particularly when radiation therapy is used).

BODY PARTS INVOLVED—Vagina and bladder.

REASONS FOR SURGERY
- Control of urine flow from the bladder.
- Prevention of vaginal and urinary tract infections.

SURGICAL RISK INCREASES WITH
- Adults over 60.
- Obesity; smoking; stress.
- Poor nutrition.
- Recent or chronic illness.
- Alcoholism.
- Previous pelvic surgery.
- Diabetes mellitus.
- Use of some prescription and nonprescription drugs. Inform your doctor of any drugs, medications, or vitamin and herb supplements you are using or have used in the last month.

WHAT TO EXPECT

WHO OPERATES—Obstetrician-gynecologist, urologist or general surgeon.

WHERE PERFORMED—Hospital.

DIAGNOSTIC TESTS
- Before surgery: Blood and urine studies; pelvic exam; cystoscopy (see Glossary) with biopsy (sometimes).
- After surgery: Blood studies; laboratory examination of removed tissue.

ANESTHESIA
- Spinal anesthesia by injection.
- General anesthesia by injection and inhalation with an airway tube placed in the windpipe.

DESCRIPTION OF OPERATION
- A speculum is used to hold the vagina open.
- Scar tissue around the fistula is cut free and removed; this tissue is often sent to the laboratory for examination.
- Healthy tissue is interposed between the 2 layers of the fistula.
- The bladder wall and vaginal wall are closed with sutures that will be absorbed by the body.
- The bladder is filled with sterile water to search for leaks. If leaks exist, further repairs are made. If no leaks are found, a catheter is placed in the bladder.
- The catheter usually can be removed about 5 to 7 days after surgery.

POSSIBLE COMPLICATIONS
- Excessive bleeding.
- Surgical-wound infection.
- Urinary tract infection.
- Continued urine leakage through fistula.

AVERAGE HOSPITAL STAY—6 days.

PROBABLE OUTCOME—Expect complete healing without complications. Allow about 6 weeks for recovery from surgery.

POSTOPERATIVE CARE

GENERAL MEASURES
- Use an electric heating pad, or a warm compress to relieve surgical-wound pain.
- Take warm baths several times a day to relieve discomfort.
- Move and elevate legs often while resting in bed to decrease the likelihood of deep-vein blood clots.

MEDICATION
- Your doctor may prescribe:
  Pain relievers. Don't take prescription pain medication longer than 4 to 7 days. Use only as much as you need.
  Stool softeners to prevent constipation.
  Antibiotics to fight or prevent infection.
- You may use nonprescription drugs, such as acetaminophen, for minor pain. Avoid aspirin.

ACTIVITY
- To help recovery and aid your well-being, resume daily activities, including work, as soon as you are able.
- Avoid vigorous exercise for 6 weeks after surgery.
- Resume driving 3 weeks after returning home.
- Resume sexual relations when your doctor determines that healing is complete.

DIET—Your doctor will prescribe a diet.

CALL YOUR DOCTOR IF

- Pain, swelling, redness, drainage or bleeding increases in the surgical area.
- You develop signs of infection, including headache, muscle aches, dizziness or a general ill feeling and fever.
- You experience nausea, vomiting or constipation.
- You develop urinary frequency and stinging or burning on urination.
- New, unexplained symptoms develop. Drugs used in treatment may produce side effects.

VESICOVAGINAL FISTULA REPAIR

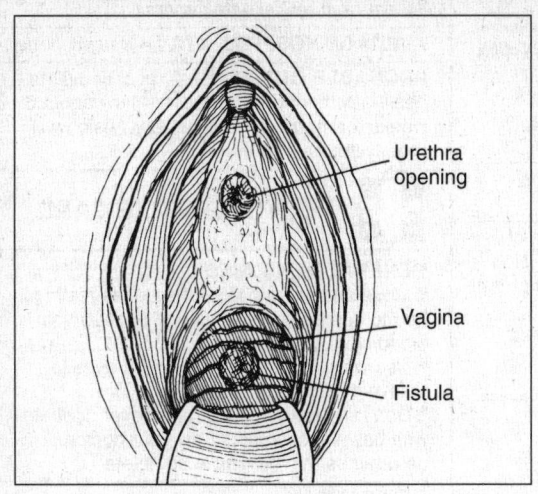

Urethra opening

Vagina

Fistula

The vagina with a retractor in place to expose the fistula, an abnormal tract between the bladder and the vagina that usually results from tearing in childbirth, as a complication of cervical uterine surgery (e.g., vaginal hysterectomy), or as a complication of cervical cancer (particularly when radiation therapy is used).

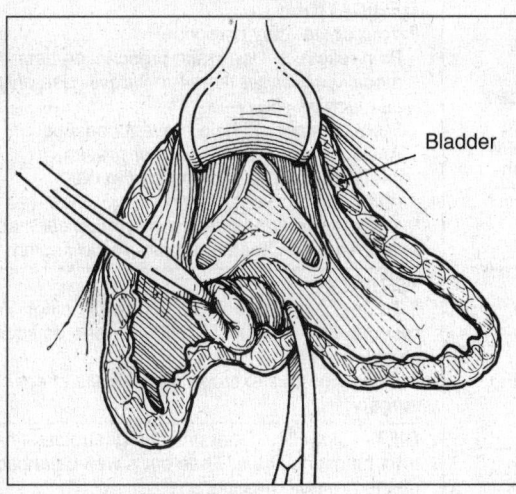

Bladder

Scar tissue around the fistula is cut free and removed. Healthy tissue is interposed between the 2 layers of the fistula.
 • The bladder wall and vaginal wall are both closed with absorbable sutures.

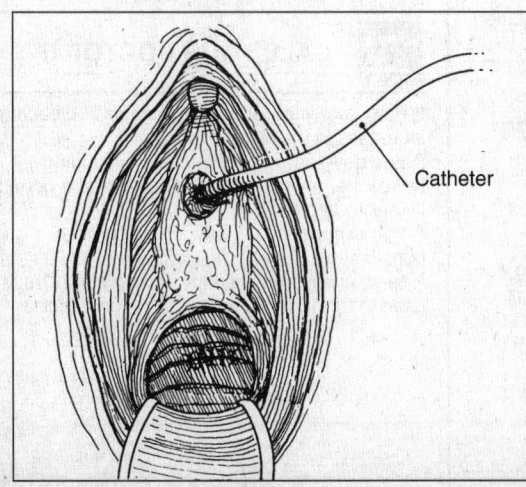

Catheter

The bladder is filled with sterile water to search for leaks. If leaks exist, further repairs are made. If no leaks are found, a catheter is placed in the bladder and the opening closed with sutures.

SURGERIES

VITRECTOMY

GENERAL INFORMATION

DEFINITION—Removal of fluid from the eyeball that has clouded and blocked light from reaching the retina, causing loss of vision. A chemical solution is injected to replace the removed fluid.

BODY PARTS INVOLVED—Eye and all its parts.

REASONS FOR SURGERY—Restoration of normal vision or prevention of continued vision loss resulting from disease that blocks light from reaching the retina. These include: bleeding, injury or infection inside the eyeball; diabetes mellitus; sickle-cell disease; complications of cataract surgery; or glaucoma.

SURGICAL RISK INCREASES WITH
- Adults over 60.
- Obesity; smoking; stress.
- Poor nutrition.
- Recent or chronic illness.
- Alcoholism.
- Diabetes mellitus.
- Use of some prescription and nonprescription drugs. Inform your doctor of any drugs, medications, or vitamin and herb supplements you are using or have used in the last month.

WHAT TO EXPECT

WHO OPERATES—Ophthalmologist.

WHERE PERFORMED—Hospital.

DIAGNOSTIC TESTS
- Before surgery: Eye examination; blood and urine studies.
- After surgery: Eye examination.

ANESTHESIA
- Local anesthesia by injection.
- General anesthesia by injection and inhalation with an airway tube placed in the windpipe.

DESCRIPTION OF OPERATION
- A small instrument is inserted behind the cornea. The instrument is used to cut free and remove the clouded vitreous fluid and scar tissue.
- This surgery often causes a retinal detachment. Usually this is corrected by injecting gas into the vitreous cavity.
- A chemical solution that promotes healing and stimulates normal vitreous fluid production is injected.
- If sutures are needed to close the surgical wound, they will be absorbed by the body.

POSSIBLE COMPLICATIONS
- Surgical-wound infection in the eye.
- Recurrent retinal detachment.

AVERAGE HOSPITAL STAY—Usually none.

PROBABLE OUTCOME—Expect complete healing without complications. Allow about 6 weeks for recovery from surgery. Vision will greatly improve by then.

POSTOPERATIVE CARE

GENERAL MEASURES
- Move and elevate legs often while resting in bed to decrease the likelihood of deep-vein blood clots.
- Use warm compresses over the eyes to relieve discomfort.
- Don't lift heavy objects, bend over or strain with bowel movements until your doctor determines that healing is complete.

MEDICATION
- Your doctor may prescribe:
  Pain relievers. Don't take prescription pain medication longer than 4 to 7 days. Use only as much as you need.
  Stool softeners to help prevent constipation. Antibiotic eye drops to fight or prevent infection. Keep eye drops cold in the refrigerator; do not freeze.
- You may use nonprescription drugs, such as acetaminophen, for minor pain. Avoid aspirin.

ACTIVITY
- To help recovery and aid your well-being, resume daily activities, including work, as soon as you are able.
- Avoid vigorous exercise for 6 weeks after surgery.

DIET—Clear liquid diet until the gastrointestinal tract functions again. Then eat a well-balanced diet to promote healing.

CALL YOUR DOCTOR IF

- Pain, swelling, redness, drainage or bleeding increases in the surgical area.
- You develop signs of infection, including headache, muscle aches, dizziness or a general ill feeling and fever.
- You experience nausea, vomiting or constipation.
- New, unexplained symptoms develop. Drugs used in treatment may produce side effects.

VITRECTOMY

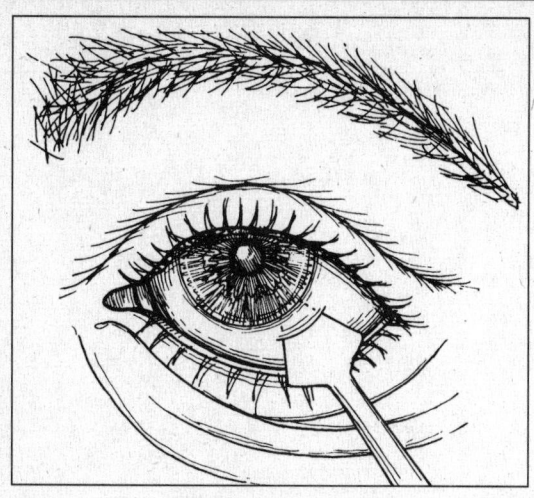

An illustration of the various structures of the eye.

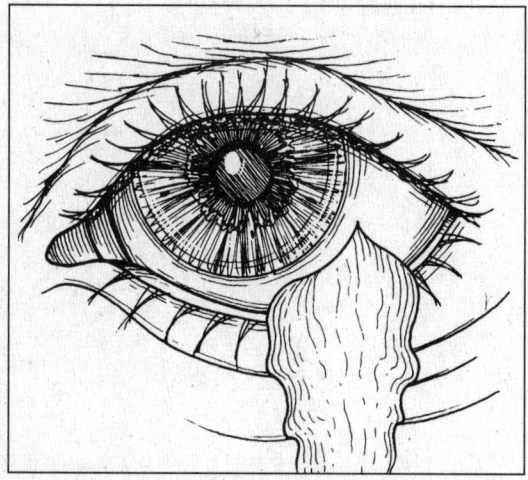

A small instrument is inserted behind the cornea to cut free and remove the clouded vitreous fluid and scar tissue.
  • Occasionally gas is injected into the vitreous cavity to help prevent the complication of retinal detachment.

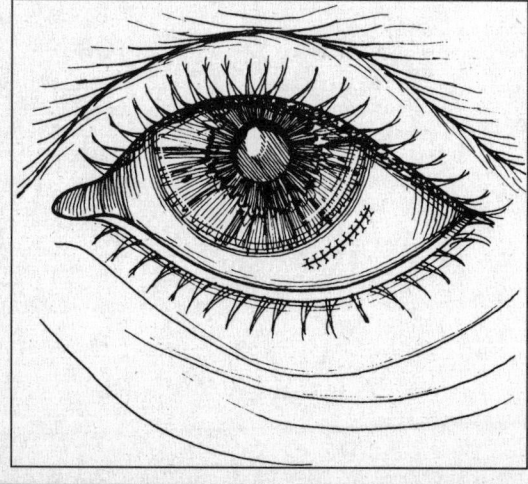

Sutures to close the incision can be removed in 4 to 6 days.

SURGERIES

Appendix

ADULT DIET, STANDARD

This diet is designed to promote optimum health through good nutrition. It is to be used for those individuals requiring no special dietary modification or restrictions.

Foods from all basic food groups are included with the addition of other foods to meet energy needs and provide essential nutrients. The diet is planned to promote the prevention of chronic diseases such as heart disease, cancer and diabetes.

The Dietary Guidelines for Americans outline what people should eat to stay healthy. The guidelines include:

- Eat a variety of foods.
- Maintain healthy weight.
- Choose a diet low in fat, saturated fat and cholesterol.
- Use sugars only in moderation.
- Choose a diet with plenty of vegetables, fruits, and grain products.
- Use salt and sodium only in moderation.
- If you drink alcoholic beverages, do so in moderation.

The United States Department of Agriculture (USDA) Food Guide Pyramid is a diet plan to help individuals meet the dietary guidelines. Each of these food groups provides some, but not all, of the nutrients that people need. Foods in one group can not replace those in another. For good health all are needed.

The Food Guide Pyramid emphasizes foods from these food groups:

- **Bread, Cereal, Rice and Pasta** (6-11 Servings Daily)
All of these foods are from grains. Individuals need the most of these foods each day.

- **Vegetables** (3-5 Servings daily) & Fruits (2-4 Servings Daily)
All of these foods are from plants. Most people need to eat more of these foods for the vitamins, minerals and fiber they supply. Examples of a serving are 1 orange, 1/2 cup juice, 1/2 medium cantaloupe, 1/2 cup vegetable or fruit. Good sources of vitamin A (beta carotene) are dark green or dark yellow vegetables. Good sources of vitamin C are citrus fruits, tomatoes, peppers, potatoes and various greens.

- **Milk, Yogurt, Cheese** (2-3 Servings Daily) & Meat, Poultry, Fish, Dry Beans, Eggs and Nuts (2-3 Servings Daily)
Most of these foods come from animals. These foods are important for protein, calcium, iron and zinc.

- **Fats, Oils, & Sweets** (Use Sparingly)
These foods provide calories and little else nutritionally. People should use these foods sparingly.

Suggested meal plan and sample menu

BREAKFAST
Fruit Juice (orange juice)
Cereal (oatmeal)
Meat/Meat Substitute (scrambled egg)
Bread (whole wheat toast; jelly; margarine*)
Milk (skim milk)
Beverage (coffee or tea)

LUNCH (can be noon or evening meal)
Meat/Meat Substitute (baked chicken)
Potato/Potato Substitute (sweet potatoes)
Vegetable (green beans)
Salad (coleslaw)
Bread (whole wheat roll; margarine*)
Dessert (strawberries)
Beverage (coffee or tea)

DINNER (can be evening or noon meal)
Soup or Juice (vegetable-bean soup)
Meat/Meat Substitute
  (meatballs & tomato sauce)
Potato/Potato Substitute (spaghetti)
Vegetable (broccoli)
Salad (spinach & salad dressing*)
Bread (garlic bread)
Beverage (skim milk)
Dessert (rice pudding)
*To reduce the fat in your diet, omit margarine, use nonfat salad dressing.

Adapted from Arizona Diet Manual (revised 1992)

ALLERGY/FOOD SENSITIVITY DIET
(continued on next page)

The diet is is a preliminary step in omitting some of the foods that cause an allergic reaction, either immediate or delayed.

Common signs and symptoms of food allergies include skin reactions (itching, erythema, hives, eczema, edema) or reactions of the gastrointestinal tract (vomiting, diarrhea, abdominal pain). Systemic anaphylactic reactions could include sneezing, wheezing, conjunctivitis, palpitations, cardiac arrhythmia, shock, or collapse. Reactions can be immediate, or take up to 72 hours to appear.

The following information describes some of the more common food allergies (wheat, egg, milk, corn). Other common food allergens include: Seafood, nuts, legumes, chocolate, cola, citrus fruit, beef, white potatoes, pork, chicken, oatmeal, rye, mustard, garlic, tomatoes and cucumbers. The wheat-, egg-, corn- and milk-free diets commonly use an "elimination" approach to assess potential food allergens and intolerances. Elimination diets must be planned carefully and monitored regularly by your doctor.

WHEAT SENSITIVITY
Avoid foods containing wheat and wheat products. These include:
- Beverages: Flavored milk drinks (malted, chocolate, etc.), instant coffee unless 100% coffee, coffee substitutes, beer, gin, and whiskey.
- Breads: Commercial breads including rye unless 100% rye, soy, cracked wheat, graham, whole wheat, many corn breads, matzo, pretzels, melba toast, zwieback, etc.
- Cereals: All dry or cooked wheat cereals, wheat germ, wheat bran, graham flour.
- Crackers/Cookies: All commercial products.
- Desserts: Cakes, doughnuts, pastries, cones, commercial ice cream, prepared cake and cookie mixes, commercial pie fillings, custards, and puddings thickened with wheat flour.
- Gravies, Sauces, and Cream Soups: Commercially prepared products are usually thickened with wheat flour.
- Macaroni, Noodles, Spaghetti, Vermicelli: Avoid all, except specially made wheat-free products.
- Meats: Breaded or prepared with wheat flour, cold cuts such as wieners, sausage, and bologna, canned meat dishes with sauce.
- Miscellaneous: Cream cheese dips, seasoned potato chips, soy sauce, salad dressing (thickened with wheat), and commercial baked beans.

EGG SENSITIVITY
Avoid foods containing egg. These include:
- Beverages: Eggnog, root beer, malted drinks, any drinks made with egg.
- Breads: Any breads and rolls with glazed crust, sweet rolls, pancakes, waffles, doughnuts, pretzels, French toast, etc.
- Broth or consomme: Avoid all.
- Cookies and Cakes: Check labels of all commercial mixes and products. Frostings must be egg-free.
- Desserts: Cream pies, meringues, custards, ice cream, sherbet, candy (almond paste, cream, chocolate, fondant, marshmallow, etc.).
- Noodles: Egg noodles.
- Meats: Any meat containing eggs such as meat loaf, meatballs, croquettes, breaded meats, etc.
- Dressings: Salad dressings and mayonnaise unless egg-free. Egg sauces such as hollandaise.
- Other: Egg substitutes containing egg.

MILK SENSITIVITY
Avoid all products containing milk. These include:
- Beverages: Cow's milk in all forms, fresh, buttermilk, dry, evaporated, condensed, yogurt, and whey. Chocolate milk, cocoa, or any beverage made with milk.
- Breads: Commercial breads or rolls with milk or milk products added to ingredients list. Check prepared mixes.
- Fats: Avoid butter.
- Cheese: All kinds.
- Cookies and Cakes: Check labels on all commercial products and mixes.
- Desserts: Cream pies, custards, ice cream, sherbet, chocolate, and caramel.
- Creams: Cream, whipped cream, and sour cream.
- Meats: Meat loaf, cold cuts, frankfurters, etc.
- Miscellaneous: Mashed potatoes (made with milk), cream sauces, cream soups, creamed vegetables, milk gravy, and milk chowder.

ALLERGY/FOOD SENSITIVITY DIET
(continued from previous page)

CORN SENSITIVITY

Avoid food containing corn. (This includes corn syrup and corn starch). These include:
* Beverages: Ale, beer, coffee lightener, gin, grape juice, instant tea, milk substitutes, soy milk, and whiskey.
* Breads: Corn bread, muffins, or rolls, enchiladas, English muffins, corn chips, tacos, corn tortillas, graham crackers.
* Cereals: Hominy, many ready-to-eat such as corn flakes.
* Desserts: Cakes, candied fruits, canned or frozen fruit juice, cream pie, ice cream, pastries, pudding mixes, sherbet.
* Fats: Corn oil, corn oil margarine, gravies, salad dressings thickened with cornstarch, and shortenings unless source of oil is specified.
* Meats: Bacon, ham, luncheon meats, sausage.
* Soups: All commercial soups, homemade soup thickened with cornstarch.
* Sweets: Candy, cane sugar, corn syrup, imitation maple syrup, jam, jelly, and preserves.
* Vegetables: Harvard beets, corn, mixed vegetables, succotash.
* Miscellaneous: Baking powder, catsup, chewing gum, cheese spreads, Chinese foods, commercial mixes of all types, confectioner's sugar, distilled vinegar, MSG, peanut butter, popcorn, vitamin capsules, and yeast.

WHEAT, EGG, MILK, CORN-FREE DIET — SAMPLE MENU

	Suggested Meal Plan	Suggested Foods and Beverages
BREAKFAST		
	Fruit juice	orange juice
	Cereal	oatmeal
	Bread and spread	rice cake
	Beverage	coffee
LUNCH (can be noon or evening meal)		
	Meat/Meat substitute	tuna salad (nonegg mayo)
	Bread	Rye-Krisp crackers
	Vegetable and/or salad	tossed salad
	Dessert	fresh fruit
	Beverage	iced tea
DINNER (can be evening or noon meal)		
	Soup or Juice	turkey rice soup
	Meat/Meat substitute	baked chicken
	Potato/Potato substitute	rice
	Vegetable and/or salad	peas
	Dessert	fresh fruit
	Beverage	coffee
SNACK		
	Fruit or juice	fresh orange
	Bread	rice cake

Adapted from Arizona Diet Manual (revised 1992)

BLAND DIET
(continued on next page)

PURPOSE
This diet is designed to provide adequate nutrition during treatment of inflammatory or ulcerative conditions of the esophagus, stomach, and intestines. It is intended to decrease irritation of the mucosa and aid in physical comfort.

DESCRIPTION
The basic food groups are used for planning nutritionally adequate meals. The diet may vary due to individual food intolerances and the patient's lifestyle. Active gastric irritants are avoided. These include caffeine, coffee, decaffeinated coffee, tea, cocoa, carbonated beverages containing caffeine, alcohol, chocolate, pepper, chili powder, and any other foods that cause individual discomfort. Most foods stimulate gastric secretions and are therefore not useful as buffers. Three meals per day are recommended, if tolerated, since additional meals stimulate acid secretion. Avoid bedtime snacks that can stimulate acid production during the night.

There is no scientific evidence that foods other than those listed above will contribute to the formation or continuation of ulcerative disease.

NUTRITIONAL ADEQUACY
The bland diet will meet the requirements for all essential nutrients. Food intolerances or habits that limit variety and quantity of food selection may cause some deficiencies. Patients on this diet will need to be individually assessed to determine if nutritional supplementation is necessary. Blood loss may lead to iron deficiency.

FOOD LISTS

Food Group	Foods Allowed	Foods to Avoid
Milk & Dairy	Whole, low fat or skim milk, dry or instant milk, evaporated milk, butter or margarine, buttermilk, yogurt, cheese.	Chocolate milk or cocoa.
Meats & Meat Substitutes	Lean with fat trimmed: beef, veal, lamb, fresh pork, cooked medium to well-done. Turkey, chicken, cornish game hen. Fish or shellfish. Or substitute eggs.	Fried or smoked meats, processed ham, sausage, spiced or highly seasoned meats.
Potatoes & Substitutes	Plain or buttered white rice; macaroni; noodles; spaghetti; white potato, baked, served without skin, boiled, mashed, diced or creamed. Sweet potato and yams.	Fried or seasoned potatoes.
Breads & Grains	Enriched breads. Cooked or ready-to-eat cereals. Tortillas, dinner rolls, English muffins, melba toast, rusks, zwieback, saltines, crackers.	None.
Fruits & Vegetables	All fruit and fruit juices except citrus. All vegetables & vegetable juices.	Citrus fruits, gas forming vegetables.
Desserts & Sweets	Custard, vanilla or fruit puddings. Tapioca, sherbet, ice milk or ice cream, except chocolate or peppermint. Pies, pastries. Gelatins. Junket. Plain or iced cakes, sponged, angel food or pound cakes, cookies without chocolate or peppermint. Sugar, jam, jelly, honey, syrup.	Chocolate, cocoa.

BLAND DIET
(continued from previous page)

FOOD LISTS (Continued)

Food Group	Foods Allowed	Foods to Avoid
Beverages	Decaffeinated tea. Cereal beverages such as Postum and Pero. Juices as allowed. Caffeine-free carbonated beverages	Coffee, tea, decaffeinated coffee, chocolate drinks.
Miscellaneous	Salt, lemon and lime juice, vanilla and other extracts and flavorings. Sage, cinnamon, thyme, mace, allspice, paprika, vinegar, prepared mustard.	Pepper, chili powder, cocoa or chocolate.

SAMPLE MENU

Suggested Meal Plan	Suggested Foods and Beverages
BREAKFAST	
Fruit juice	Apple juice
Cereal with milk	Oatmeal (strained) with milk
Meat/meat substitute	Soft cooked egg
Bread/margarine	Toast, jelly
Beverage	Milk, decaffeinated tea
DINNER (noon or evening meal)	
Soup	Cream soup & crackers
Meat/meat substitute	Meat loaf without gravy
Vegetable	Buttered green beans
Fruit juice	Apricot juice
Dessert	Lemon sponge pudding
Bread/margarine	Bread & margarine
Beverage	Milk
SUPPER (noon or evening meal)	
Juice	Tomato Juice
Meat/meat substitute	Sliced baked chicken & noodles
Vegetable	Peas
Dessert	Applesauce
Bread/margarine	Bread, butter or margarine
Beverage	Milk, decaffeinated tea

Adapted from Arizona Diet Manual (revised 1992)

HIGH-FIBER DIET
(continued on next page)

This diet is designed to provide foods containing indigestible fiber as a part of preventive and/or therapeutic nutrition.

The high fiber diet is based on the basic food groups with a greater emphasis on fiber-rich foods such as fruits, legumes, vegetables, whole-grain breads, and high fiber cereals. The Daily Reference Value for fiber is 25 grams (based on 2000 calorie per day diet). The American Diabetes Association has reported that up to 40 gm fiber daily or 25 gm per 1000 Kcal may be beneficial (National Cancer Institute recommends 25-30 gm).

Dietary fiber is the component found in many foods that cannot be digested by the intestinal tract. Adequate fluid intake is important when following a high fiber diet due to the water binding capacity of fiber. Fiber should be increased in the diet slowly to avoid unpleasant side effects (gas, abdominal bloating/cramps). Dietary fiber can be divided into two separate categories: Water insoluble fiber and water soluble fiber.

Water Insoluble Fiber
Water insoluble components, such as cellulose, hemicellulose and lignin, remain essentially unchanged during digestion. Foods containing water insoluble fiber include: fruits, vegetables, cereals, and whole grain products. Research suggests that insoluble fiber may be beneficial in the prevention and/or treatment of constipation and diverticular disease and may decrease the risk of colon cancer.

Water Soluble Fiber
Water soluble fiber, such as gum, pectin and mucilages, does dissolve in water and is found in oats, beans, barley and some fruits and vegetables. Some studies showed that this type of fiber may improve blood glucose and cholesterol levels.

DIETARY FIBER CONTENT OF FOODS IN COMMONLY SERVED PORTIONS

FOOD GROUP

	Breads (1 slice)	Cereals (1 oz.)	Pasta (1 cup)	Rice (1/2 cup)	Legumes (1/2 cup)
Less 1 gm	bagel, white French	Rice-Krispies, Special K, Cornflakes	None	Trace	None
1-1.9 gm	whole-wheat	oatmeal, Nutri-Grain, Cheerios	macaroni, spaghetti	Trace	None
2-2.9 gm	bran muffin	Wheaties, Shredded-Wheat	None	Trace	None
3-3.9 gm	None	Most, Honey-Bran	whole-wheat spaghetti	Trace	lentils
4-4.9 gm	None	Bran Chex, 40% Bran-Flakes, Raisin Bran	None	Trace	lima beans, dried peas
5-5.9 gm	None	Corn Bran	None	Trace	None
More 6 gm	None	All-Bran, Bran Buds, 100% Bran			kidney beans, baked beans, navy beans

HIGH-FIBER DIET
(continued from previous page)

DIETARY FIBER CONTENT OF FOODS IN COMMONLY SERVED PORTIONS

FOOD GROUP

	Vegetables (1/2 cup)	Fruits (medium)
Less 1 gm	cucumber, lettuce (1 cup)	grapes (20), watermelon (1 cup)
1-1.9 gm	asparagus, green beans, cabbage, cauliflower, potato (no skin), celery, green pepper	apricots (3), grapefruit (1/2), peach with skin, pineapple (1/2 cup)
2-2.9 gm	broccoli, spinach, Brussels sprouts, carrots, corn, potato (with skin)	apple without skin, banana, orange
3-3.9 gm	peas	apple with skin, pear with skin, raspberries (1/2 cup)
4-4.9 gm	None	None
5-5.9 gm	None	None
More 6 gm	None	None

SAMPLE MENU

	Suggested Meal Plan	Suggested Foods and Beverages
BREAKFAST		
	Fruit juice	prune juice
	Cereal	All Bran cereal
	Meat/Meat substitute	egg
	Bread and spread	whole grain toast & margarine
	Beverage	1% milk & coffee or tea
LUNCH (can be noon or evening meal)		
	Meat/Meat substitute	meat loaf
	Potato/Potato substitute	baked potato
	Vegetable and/or salad	lima beans, tossed salad with dressing
	Bread and spread	rye bread & margarine
	Dessert	fig cookie
	Beverage	coffee or tea
DINNER (can be evening or noon meal)		
	Soup or juice	lentil soup
	Meat/Meat substitute	baked chicken
	Vegetable and/or salad	banana squash, tossed salad & dressing
	Bread and spread	rye bread & margarine
	Dessert	baked apple with cinnamon
	Beverage	1% milk & coffee or tea

Adapted from Arizona Diet Manual (revised 1992)

LACTOSE INTOLERANCE DIET
(continued on next page)

This diet is designed to minimize gastrointestinal (GI) disturbances associated with ingestion of the carbohydrate lactose such as abdominal cramps, bloating, flatulence, increased GI motility and diarrhea. This diet can be individualized to provide the appropriate amount of lactose that a lactose-intolerant individual may tolerate. Milk and milk products are limited.

Current research indicates that most lactose-intolerant individuals can consume 15-30 grams of lactose without experiencing severe symptoms. Tolerance level is highly individualized.

FOOD LISTS

Food Groups	Foods Allowed	Foods to Avoid
Milk/Dairy	Milk substitutes and nondairy products. Milk treated with lactose reducing enzymes.	Milk or milk products in excess of allowed amounts. Avoid or decrease intake with development of intolerance.
Meats/Meat substitute	Any meat, fish and poultry except those listed to avoid, peanut butter. The following cheeses contain no detectable lactose and may be used if tolerated: brick, Swiss, Camembert, cheddar, colby, mozzarella, muenster, provolone. Eggs without milk.	All other cheese and cheese products. Creamed meats. Casseroles made with foods to avoid. Breaded meats, fish or poultry. Eggs made with milk, souffles, quiche with milk or cream.
Breads/Grains	Breads, cereals, crackers. Quick breads such as muffins, biscuits, etc., in moderation if made with milk. Broth-type soups.	Excessive use of commercial products with added milk or lactose. Milk or cream-based soups.
Fruits/Vegetables	Any fresh, canned or frozen.	Artificial fruit juice containing lactose and dietetic fruits with added lactose. Creamed vegetables or vegetables in cheese sauce.
Desserts/Sweets	Sugar, honey, jelly, jams. Plain sugar candies such as gumdrops, jelly beans, marshmallows. Angel food cake, fruit ices, gelatin. Commercial mixes or baked products containing milk in moderation. Nondairy frozen desserts.	Cream candies, tablet candies containing lactose. Cream pies. Products with cream fillings, cream cheese or sour cream. Commercial puddings.
Beverages	Coffee, tea, carbonated beverages, cereal beverages, alcoholic beverages if allowed by your doctor. Isomil, Pregestimil, Prosobee.	Cocoa, ovaltine, cocoa malt, cocoa mixes, beverages containing cream.

LACTOSE INTOLERANCE DIET
(continued from previous page)

FOOD LISTS (continued)

Food Groups	Foods Allowed	Foods to Avoid
Miscellaneous	Condiments, pure flavorings, popcorn, nuts, salt, vinegar, spices, lactate, lactic acid, lactalbumin, citric acid, MSG, margarine, butter, bacon, lard, mayonnaise, vegetable oils, vegetable shortenings. Most oil based salad dressings. Nondairy whipped cream.	Cream sauces, milk gravies, gum, ascorbic acid tablets, spice blends with lactose added, peppermints, whey. Salad dressing with added milk or cheese not allowed. Sour cream, alone, or in spreads and dips, cream cheese, whipped cream.

SAMPLE MENU

	Suggested Meal Plan	Suggested Foods/Beverages
BREAKFAST		
	Fruit juice	orange juice w/calcium
	Cereal	Shredded Wheat
	Meat/Meat substitute	soft cooked egg
	Bread and spread	wheat toast with margarine
	Milk	lactose free milk
	Beverage	coffee
LUNCH (can be noon or evening meal)		
	Meat/Meat Substitute	baked chicken
	Potato/Potato Substitute	brown rice
	Vegetable and/or Salad	spinach, sliced tomato salad
	Bread and spread	wheat bread with margarine
	Dessert	angel food cake, strawberries
	Beverage	coffee
DINNER (can be evening or noon meal)		
	Soup or juice	apple juice
	Meat/Meat substitute	lean roast beef
	Vegetable and/or salad	cooked carrots, three bean salad
	Bread and spread	rye bread
	Dessert	fruit sorbet
	Beverage	coffee or tea

Adapted from Arizona Diet Manual (revised 1992)

LIQUID DIET, CLEAR

This diet is often used to minimize digestion within the gastrointestinal tract. The diet consists of clear liquids or foods which are fluid at body temperature.

Due to the extremely restrictive nature of this diet, use should be limited to three days or less. For prolonged use, consult your doctor.

This diet is extremely inadequate in nutrition and is planned for brief use only. Specific items and amounts depend upon patient tolerance and should be offered frequently.

FOOD LISTS

Food Groups	Foods Allowed	Foods to Omit
Milk/Dairy	None	All
Meat/Meat Substitute	None	All
Breads/Grains	None	All
Fruits/Vegetables	Clear fruit juices, such as: apple, grape or cranberry or strained juices such as orange, lemonade or grapefruit, pulp-free fruit ices.	All others
Desserts/Sweets	Clear, flavored gelatin, Popsicles, clear fruit ices, sugar, honey, sugar substitute, hard candy.	All others
Beverages	Clear coffee or tea, carbonated beverages, sports drinks.	All others including milk, nectars, cream, juices with pulp.
Miscellaneous	High-protein broth or gelatin, iodized salt, clear broth or bouillon.	All others

SAMPLE MENU

Breakfast	Dinner or lunch	Supper or lunch
Grape juice	Apple juice	Cranberry juice
Clear broth	Clear beef broth	Clear chicken broth
Flavored gelatin	Flavored gelatin	Flavored gelatin
Black coffee	Clear tea	Clear tea

Adapted from Arizona Diet Manual (revised 1992)

LIQUID DIET, FULL

This diet is intended for the patient who cannot chew or swallow solid foods or as a transition from the clear liquid to soft or general diet. This diet is a modification in the consistency or texture of the normal diet. It contains foods which are liquid or will become liquid at body temperature. Milk-based foods make up a large proportion of this diet.

FOOD LISTS

Food Groups	Foods Allowed	Foods to Avoid
Milk & Dairy	All milk and milk drinks such as milk shakes and eggnogs made from commercial mix; yogurt, plain or flavored (no seeds or fruit pieces). All beverages including high-protein, high-calorie oral supplements.	Cheese, cottage cheese.
Meat/Meat Substitutes	Eggnogs, custards.	All others.
Breads / Grains	Thin, cooked cereal such as farina, grits, oatmeal.	All others.
Fruits / Vegetables	Vitamin C sources (daily): Strained citrus and tomato juices. Vitamin A sources (alternate days): Strained carrot juice.	All others.
Desserts and Sweets	Custards, puddings, plain gelatin, plain ice cream, ice milk, sherbet, sugar, hard candy, honey, Popsicles, syrup, frozen yogurt.	All others.
Miscellaneous	Butter, margarine, cream, nondairy creamer.	All others.

SAMPLE MENU

	Suggested Meal Plan	Suggested Foods and Beverages
BREAKFAST		
	Fruit juice	orange juice, strained
	Cereal	Farina
	Meat/Meat substitute	custard
	Milk/Dairy	2% Milk
	Beverage	coffee
LUNCH (can be noon or evening meal)		
	Soup	strained cream soup
	Juice	tomato juice
	Salad	lime gelatin
	Dessert	ice cream
	Beverage	ginger ale
SNACK	Milk/Dairy	1 milk shake
DINNER (can be evening or noon meal)		
	Soup	strained cream soup
	Juice	peach nectar
	Dessert	Popsicle
	Beverage	chocolate milk
SNACK	Juice	cranberry juice
	Milk/Dairy	vanilla pudding, 2% milk

Adapted from Arizona Diet Manual (revised 1992)

LOW-FAT/LOW-CHOLESTEROL DIET
(continued on next page)

Most diet experts agree that Americans eat too much fat. A low-fat diet can help prevent obesity and the dangers it causes to health. Use the diet suggestions below for general good health or for dietary treatment of your condition as recommended by your doctor.

Fat and Cholesterol Information

The National Cholesterol Education Program (NCEP) Guidelines indicate that a serum total cholesterol should be measured in all adults over the age of 20 at least once every 5 years. Levels below 200 mg/dl are classified as "desirable blood cholesterol," those 200-239 mg/dl as "borderline high cholesterol" and those 240 mg/dl as "high blood cholesterol."

- Cholesterol is found only in animal products.
- Saturated fats are often solid at room temperature and are usually found in animal products such as meats, poultry, butter, cheese and ice cream. Plant sources of saturated fats include palm oil, palm kernel oil and coconut oil.
- Monounsaturated fats are found in products such as olive oil, peanuts, flaxseed oil and canola (rapeseed) oil.
- Polyunsaturated fats are usually liquid at room temperature and are found in safflower, sunflower, corn, soybean and cottonseed oils.

FOOD LISTS

Milk/Dairy (Limit to 2-4 servings a day)
- Allowed: Skim (nonfat) or 1% fat milk (liquid, powdered, evaporated), nonfat or low-fat yogurt, low-fat cottage cheese (2% fat or less), low-fat cheese (labeled 6 grams of fat or less per ounce); nonfat sour cream; nonfat cream cheese.
- Avoid: Whole milk (4% fat) (liquid, evaporated, condensed), 2% milk, cream, half and half, imitation milk products, most nondairy creamers, whipped toppings; whole milk yogurt; regular cottage cheese (4% fat); natural cheeses made from whole milk (cheddar, Swiss, blue, Camembert, etc.); cream cheese; goat's milk cheese; sour cream; low-fat cream cheese; low-fat sour cream. NOTE: If 2% milk is used, decrease added fat by 1 teaspoon for each cup of milk.

Meat/Meat Substitute (Limit to 5 oz a day from animal products; limit 4 egg yolks a week)
- Allowed: Dried beans, split peas, lentils, pinto beans cooked without salt; poultry without the skin; fish; tuna packed in water; lean beef (extra lean ground beef, eye of round, sirloin, round tip, round, top round, tenderloin, top loin); lean pork (fresh not cured, tenderloin, leg, shoulder); lamb (arm, leg, loin, rib); shrimp or lobster (limit 3 oz per week); luncheon meats (1 gram fat or less per ounce); egg whites (2 egg whites = 1 whole egg); low cholesterol egg substitutes.
- Avoid: Fried meats or meat substitutes; fatty cuts of beef, pork or lamb. Goose, duck, liver, kidney, brains, or other organ meats; hot dogs, sausages, bacon; regular luncheon meats; peanut butter; egg yolks.

Breads & Grains (6-11 servings a day)
- Allowed: Whole-grain breads (oatmeal, whole wheat, rye, bran, multigrain, etc.); rice; pasta; homemade baked goods low in fat; low-fat crackers (ricecakes, popcorn cakes, Rye Krisp, melba toast, pretzels, breadsticks); hot or cold cereals (with 1 to 2 grams of fat or less per serving).
- Avoid: High fat baked goods (pies, cakes, doughnuts, croissants, pastries, muffins, biscuits); high fat crackers; egg noodles; granola type cereals; cereals with more than 2 grams of fat per serving; pasta and rice prepared with cream, butter or cheese sauces.

Vegetables (3-5 servings per day or more)
- Allowed: Any fresh, frozen, canned or dried.
- Avoid: Vegetables prepared in butter, cream or other sauces; fried vegetables.

Fruits (4 servings per day or more)
- Allowed: Any fresh, frozen, canned or dried.
- Avoid: Coconuts, avocados, and olives except as allowed under miscellaneous.

Desserts & Sweets (Limit to control calories)
- Allowed: Sugar, jelly, jam, honey, molasses; low-fat frozen desserts (like sherbet, sorbet, ices, nonfat frozen yogurt, Popsicles); angel food cake; low-fat cakes and cookies (like vanilla wafers, graham crackers, ginger snaps); baking cocoa; low-fat candy (like jelly beans, hard candy).
- Avoid: Ice cream; high-fat cakes, pies and cookies (most commercially made); chocolate.

LOW-FAT/LOW-CHOLESTEROL DIET
(continued from previous page)

FOOD LISTS (continued)

Beverages
- Allowed: Juices, tea, coffee, decaffeinated coffee, carbonated drinks, most alcoholic beverages.
- Avoid: Milk shakes; ice cream floats; eggnog; alcoholic beverages containing milk, cream or coconut; commercially softened water as beverage or in food preparation.

Miscellaneous Foods
- Allowed: Limit fat based on total number of calories consumed. Generally no more than 6-8 servings/day of added fat such as margarine and salad dressing should be eaten; overweight, sedentary or elderly individuals may need less.

Limit: (1 tsp per serving) Unsaturated vegetable oils (corn, olive, canola, flaxseed, safflower, sesame, soybean, sunflower); margarine or shortening made from unsaturated vegetable oils; mayonnaise and salad dressings made from unsaturated oils (1 Tbsp); diet margarine (2 tsp); avocado (1/8 medium or 2 Tbsp); salt-free seeds and nuts (1 Tbsp seeds, 6 almonds, 20 small peanuts); salt-free peanut butter (2 tsp).

No Limit: Vegetable oil sprays; fat-free salad dressings, fat-free sour cream; herbs, spices, pepper, salt substitute with physician approval; mustard; vinegar; lemon and lime juice; cream sauces made with allowed ingredients.

- Avoid: Butter; coconut oil; palm oil; palm kernel oil; lard; bacon fat; salad dressings made with egg yolk; fried snack foods (potato chips, cheese curls, tortilla chips); olives; avocados; regular cream sauces.

Suggested Meal Plan	Suggested Foods and Beverages
BREAKFAST	
Fruit juice	grapefruit half
Cereal	bran flake cereal
Meat/Meat substitute	low-cholesterol egg substitute
Bread and spread	2 slices whole wheat toast; 1 tsp jelly
Milk	1 cup skim milk
Beverage	coffee
LUNCH (can be noon or evening meal)	
Meat/Meat substitute	3 oz skinless chicken breast
Potato/Potato substitute	sweet potato
Vegetable and/or salad	green beans
Bread and spread	whole wheat bread; margarine
Dessert	strawberries
Beverage	iced tea
DINNER (can be evening or noon meal)	
Soup or Juice	1/2 cup vegetable juice
Meat/Meat Substitute	3 oz low-fat meatballs in tomato sauce
Potato/Substitute	spaghetti
Vegetable and/or Salad	broccoli
Bread and spread	garlic bread; 1 tsp margarine*
Dessert	fruit sorbet
Beverage	1 cup skim milk; coffee or tea

Adapted from Arizona Diet Manual (revised 1992)

LOW-SALT DIET
(continued on next page)

The estimated average daily intake of sodium in the American diet ranges from 4 to 5.8 grams per day. The American Heart Association recommends that sodium intake should not exceed 3 grams per day. The National Heart, Lung and Blood Institute recommends a maximum of 3.3 grams of sodium for healthy adults.

Sodium controlled diets are used to reduce blood pressure in hypertension and to promote the loss of excess fluids in edema due to cardiovascular or kidney disease and other disorders. Sodium controlled diets may also enhance the action of some medications. This diet allows approximately 2.5 grams of salt a day.

Foods high in sodium content are omitted. One-fourth teaspoon of salt is allowed in the preparation of food or may be used at the table. Since sodium is widely distributed in foods, portions and number of servings are restricted according to the sodium content.

Salt substitutes should be approved by your doctor. Salt-free herbs and spices may be used freely. Carefully reading labels is important as some salt-replacement seasonings contain sodium chloride. "Light" salts which are a mixture of potassium chloride and sodium chloride are also limited on sodium controlled diets.

Approximately 75% of the sodium Americans consume is added to foods during processing. The following list will help you interpret sodium information on food labels:
- Sodium free — 5 mg or less of sodium per serving
- Very low sodium — 35 mg or less of sodium per serving
- Low sodium — 140 mg or less of sodium per serving
- Reduced sodium — 75% less sodium than the original version of the product
- No added salt or unsalted — no salt is added during processing (but this does not guarantee the food product is naturally low in sodium)

Water Supply
Water supplies vary in natural sodium content. For the sodium content in your water supply, call your city's water department. Water softeners may add large amounts of sodium to the water. The sodium content of softened water ranges between 7 and 220 milligrams per quart. The company that installed your softener can tell you how much sodium is in your system. Distilled drinking water may be used for cooking and drinking when water supplies more than 120 mg sodium per liter and the diet is below 2.5 grams.

FOOD LISTS

Milk and Dairy Products (1-4 servings/day)
- Allowed: Any milk - white, low-fat, skim, chocolate and cocoa; yogurt; eggnog, ice cream, sherbet, natural cheese (limit 1 oz per day). Substitute for 8 oz of milk: 4 oz evaporated milk, 4 oz condensed milk, 1/3 cup dry milk powder.
- Avoid: Buttermilk, malted milk.

Meats and Meat Substitutes (6 ounces/day)
- Allowed: Fresh or fresh frozen: beef, lamb, pork, veal and game; chicken, turkey, cornish hen or other poultry; any fresh-water or fresh-frozen unbreaded fish and shellfish; low-sodium canned tuna or salmon; low-sodium peanut butter; eggs, dried beans and peas.
- Avoid: Any meat, fish or poultry that is smoked, cured, salted or canned such as bacon, dried beef, corned beef, cold cuts, ham, turkey ham, hot dogs, sausages, sardines, anchovies, pickled herring or pickled meats; pickled eggs.

Breads and Grains (6 or more servings/day)
- Allowed: Enriched white, wheat, rye and pumpernickel bread; hard rolls, bagels, English muffins, cooked cereal without salt; dry low-sodium cereals; unsalted crackers and breadsticks; corn or flour tortillas; biscuits, muffins, cornbread, pancakes, and waffles all made with low-sodium baking powder; low-sodium or homemade bread crumbs; rice, noodles, barley, spaghetti, macaroni and other pastas; homemade bread stuffing.
- Avoid: Breads and rolls with salted tops; quick breads; instant hot cereals; dry cereals with added salt; crackers with salted tops; pancakes, waffles, muffins, biscuits, and cornbread with salt, baking powder, self-rising flour or instant mixes; regular bread crumbs or cracker crumbs; instant rice and pasta mixes; commercial stuffing; commercial casserole mixes.

LOW-SALT DIET
(continued from previous page)

FOOD LISTS (continued)

Vegetables (3 or more servings/day)
- Allowed: Fresh, frozen and low-sodium canned vegetables; regular canned, drained vegetables (limit to 1/2 cup serving per day); low-sodium vegetable juice; regular vegetable juice (limit 1/2 cup per day); white or sweet potatoes; salt-free potato chips.
- Avoid: Regular canned vegetables (over 1/2 cup per day); vegetable juices; sauerkraut; pickled vegetables and others prepared in brine; potato casserole mixes; potato chips; frozen vegetables in sauce.

Fruits (3-4 or more servings a day)
- Allowed: All fruits and juices.
- Avoid: None except salted prunes (saladitos).

Desserts/Sweets
- Allowed: Any sweets like sugar, honey, jam, jelly, syrup, marmalade, hard candy; limit regular baked products (cake, pie, cookies) to 1 serving per day.
- Avoid: None.

Beverages
- Allowed: Coffee, tea, soft drinks, Postum, alcoholic beverages (with medical approval).
- Avoid: Commercially softened water as beverage or in food preparation.

Miscellaneous
- Allowed: Limit added salt to 1/4 teaspoon per day, may be used in cooking or at the table; limit 3 tsp salted butter or margarine per day; salt-free butter or margarine; vegetable oils, shortening and mayonnaise; salt-free salad dressings; salt substitute with physician's approval; pepper, herbs and spices; flavorings; vinegar and lemon or lime juice; salt-free seasonings; low-sodium condiments: catsup, chili sauce, mustard, and pickles; fresh-ground horseradish; Tabasco sauce; homemade or salt-free soups; low-sodium baking powder; unsalted snacks: nuts, seeds, pretzels and popcorn.
- Avoid: Added salt in excess of 1/4 tsp per day; light-salt; garlic salt, celery salt, onion salt and seasoned salt; sea salt, rock salt and kosher salt; seasonings containing salt and sodium compounds; monosodium glutamate (MSG, Accent); regular catsup, chili sauce, mustard, pickles, relishes, olives and horseradish; Kitchen Bouquet; gravy and sauce mixes; barbecue sauce, soy and teriyaki sauce; Worcestershire and steak sauce; salted snack foods: nuts, seeds, pretzels and popcorn; commercially prepared convenience foods; regular canned or dried soups.

	Suggested Meal Plan	Menu (may use 1/4 teaspoon added salt)
BREAKFAST		
	Fruit juice	1/2 grapefruit
	Cereal	1 oz cornflake cereal
	Meat/Meat substitute	1 egg (optional)
	Bread and spread	2 slices whole wheat toast;1 tsp margarine
	Beverage	1 cup 2% milk; coffee or tea
LUNCH (can be noon or evening meal)		
	Meat/Meat substitute	3 oz salt-free hamburger patty
	Potato/Potato substitute	salt-free oven fries
	Vegetable or salad	tomato slices & 1 cup lettuce
	Soup	1 cup salt-free vegetable beef soup
	Bread and spread	hamburger bun; 1 Tbsp salt-free catsup
	Dessert	2 oatmeal raisin cookies, 1/2 cup fresh fruit
	Beverage	coffee or tea
DINNER (can be evening or noon meal)		
	Soup or juice	1/2 cup salt-free tomato juice
	Meat/Meat substitute	3 oz salt-free herbed baked chicken
	Potato/Potato substitute	1/2 cup salt-free brown rice
	Vegetable and/or salad	1/2 cup carrot-raisin salad; 1 tsp dressing
	Bread and spread	1 slice whole wheat bread; 1 tsp margarine
	Dessert	4 oz strawberry frozen yogurt
	Beverage	1 cup 1 or 2% milk; coffee or tea
SNACK		1/2 cup apple juice; 2 squares graham cracker

Adapted from Arizona Diet Manual (revised 1992)

WEIGHT LOSS DIET
(continued on next page)

This is a simple "exchange list" diet for individuals who want to lose weight. The goal of diet therapy is to reduce caloric intake to a level that can be safely and comfortably tolerated. Usually diets that provide 1200 to 1500 calories a day are acceptable for most people. However, you and your doctor should determine the appropriate amount of calories required for your weight, height, activity level and general health. The example shown is for a 1200 calories per day menu. It may be modified by adding more food portions.

Plan your breakfast, lunch and dinner meals by selecting items from the appropriate food list. This sample diet allows you one fruit portion, one starch and one milk for breakfast. You may choose cereal with banana and milk. Coffee or tea are "free" items. Amounts of each portion are indicated in each food list. Portions can be interchanged among breakfast, lunch and dinner as long as the total for the day doesn't exceed those indicated. For example, you can eat all your fruits for breakfast if desired, but don't exceed 4 portions for the day.

SUGGESTED MEAL PLANS FOR 1200 CALORIES PER DAY DIET
DAILY PORTIONS FROM FOOD LISTS
(See lists below and following page)

BREAKFAST	LUNCH	DINNER	SNACK
1 Fruit	2 Meats	2 Meats	1 Starch
1 Starch/Bread	1 Vegetable	1 Fat	1 Fruit
1 Milk	1 Fat	2 Starch/Bread	1 Milk
	2 Starch/Bread	1 Vegetable	
	1 Fruit	1 Fruit	
	(raw vegetable	(raw vegetable	
	as desired)	as desired)	

FRUIT LIST (60 calories, 15 grams carbohydrates)
(A portion is 1 small piece or 1/2 cup unless listed)

Apples (juice or sauce)	Fruit cocktail	Plums (2)
Apricots (4)	Grapefruit or juice	Prunes (3)
Apricots, dried (7 halves)	Grapes (15)	Prune juice (1/4 cup)
Banana (1/2)	Grape juice	Raspberries (1 cup)
Blackberries (3/4 cup)	Lemon	Raisins (2 Tbsp)
Blueberries (3/4 cup)	Orange/orange juice	Rhubarb
Cantaloupe (1/3)	Peach	Strawberries (10)
Cherries	Pear	Tangerine
Dates (2)	Pineapple	Watermelon (1 cup)

VEGETABLE LIST (25 calories, 5 grams carbohydrates, 2 grams protein)
(A portion is 1 cup raw or 1/2 cup cooked)

Artichoke	Celery	Peppers
Asparagus	Cucumber	Peas
Beans (green, wax or sprouts)	Eggplant	Pumpkin
Beets	Endive	Radish
Broccoli	Mixed Vegetables	Rutabaga
Brussels Sprouts	Mushrooms	Spinach
Cabbage or Sauerkraut	Okra	Squash
Cauliflower	Onions	Tomato
Carrot	Parsnips	Turnips

Note: Some vegetables are shown in the Starch List.

APPENDIX

WEIGHT LOSS DIET
(continued from previous page)

BREAKFAST	LUNCH	DINNER	SNACK

STARCH LIST (80 calories, 15 grams carbohydrates, 2-3 grams protein, 1-2 grams fat)
(A portion is 1/4 cup or as listed)

Angel Food Cake (1 oz)	Cornbread (1 in. cube)	Popcorn, fat free (3 cups)
Bagel (small or 1 oz)	Cornstarch (2 Tbsp)	Potato, white (1/2 cup)
Beans, canned (1/3 cup)	English Muffin (1/2)	Potato, sweet (1/3 cup)
Biscuit (1)	Gelatin (1/2 cup)	Pretzels (5 small)
Bread (1 slice)	Graham Crackers (2)	Rice (1/3 cup)
Bun (1/2)	Lentils, canned (1/3 cup)	Ricecakes (2)
Cereal (3/4 cup, dry;	Matzo crackers (3/4 oz)	Saltines (6)
1/2 cup, hot)	Pancakes (1)	Taco Shell (1)
Corn (1/2 cup)	Pasta (1/2 cup)	Tortilla (one 6-inch)
Cookies (fat-free,1 or 2 small)	Pita bread (1/2)	

MEAT OR MEAT SUBSTITUTE LIST (55-70 calories, 7 grams protein, 3-5 grams fat)
(A portion is 1 ounce or 1/4 cup or as listed)

Beef (lean cuts)	Eggs (3 per week)	Pork (chops, ham, roast)
Cheese (skim milk types)	Fish (all types)	Shellfish
Cold Cuts or Frankfurters	Lamb (leg, roasted)	Soybeans, cooked (1/3 cup)
(95% fat-free)	Peanut Butter (1 Tbsp)	Veal
Cottage Cheese (1/3 cup)	Poultry (no skin)	

FAT LIST (45 calories, 5 grams fat)
(Use nonfat or low-fat products when they are available.)

Bacon, crisp (1 slice)	Gravy (2 Tbsp)	Oils (1 teaspoon)
Cheese, cream (1 Tbsp)	Margarine* (1 teaspoon)	Olives (5 small)
Coconut (1 Tbsp)	Mayonnaise* (1 teaspoon)	Salad Dressings* (1 Tbsp)
Cream, light (2 Tbsp)	Nuts (6 to 10)	Seeds (1 Tbsp)

* Portion amounts may be increased if using nonfat products (e.g., mayonnaise, 2 Tbsp)

MILK LIST (80 calories, 12 grams carbohydrates, 8 grams protein)
Skim milk (1 cup)   Yogurt (1 cup plain, nonfat, unsweetened except with sugar substitute)

FREE ITEMS (you may have these as desired)

Beverages: Coffee, tea, sugar-free beverages	Sugar-free gelatin
Pickles, except sweet pickles	Salad greens
Bouillon and consommés	Nonstick pan spray
All spices, herbs, flavorings and artificial sweeteners	Sugar substitutes
Catsup, mustard, soy sauce, vinegars	Lemon or lime juice
Worcestershire sauce	

ADDITIONAL INFORMATION

- Purchase fruits fresh, fresh-frozen or canned unsweetened, or in natural juices. All juices should be unsweetened.
- Vegetable and fruit portions are for the edible amounts of the item.
- Allowed amounts of meats are after cooking; amounts shown are for edible parts only (excluding bones). Be sure to trim all extra fat away from meat prior to cooking. Remove skin from all poultry. Roasting or broiling of meats is preferred.
- If salt intake is limited, avoid foods high in sodium (pickles) and don't use salt at the table.
- Even though the diet should meet your nutritional needs, a vitamin and mineral supplement may be recommended by your doctor.
- Everyone on a diet will experience an occasional setback. This doesn't mean failure. Long-term success is still possible.
- Combine your diet with behavior modification to help you maintain the weight loss.

WEIGHT LOSS SUGGESTIONS

Weight control diets are designed to provide a specific calorie level calculated to meet an individual's requirement to attain optimal body weight. An exercise program is also highly recommended. Weight loss of 1-2 pounds per week is generally optimal.

The U.S. Department of Agriculture's Food Guide Pyramid diet plan can be used as a guide to healthy eating and is likely to produce desired weight loss. Weight loss diets of greater than 1200 calories per day are generally adequate in all nutrients except iron, as long as the diet is planned to include a variety of foods from all food groups.

FOOD GUIDE PYRAMID — DAILY SERVINGS
- Fats, Oils, & Sweets (Use Sparingly): These foods provide calories and little else nutritionally. Most people should use these foods sparingly.
- Milk, Yogurt, Cheese (2-3 Servings) & Meat, Poultry, Fish, Dry Beans, Eggs, Nuts (2-3 Servings): Most of these foods come from animals. These foods are important for protein, calcium, iron and zinc.
- Vegetables (3-5 Servings) & Fruits (2-4 Servings): All of these foods are from plants. Most people need to eat more of these foods for the vitamins, minerals and fiber they supply.
- Bread, Cereal, Rice and Pasta (6-11 Servings): All of these foods are from grains. Individuals need the most of these foods each day.

BEHAVIORAL STRATEGIES IN MANAGEMENT OF WEIGHT CONTROL
Individuals seeking to make a lifetime commitment to improve their eating and exercise habits can succeed at long-term weight loss. Most of the successful long-term weight-loss programs include several components; behavior modification; exercise; nutrition; social support; and cognitive changes, including goal setting, assertiveness training, and coping with mistakes and motivation. Emphasis should be placed on slow, progressive weight loss.

The following is a list of behavior modification techniques which can be used to promote healthy eating, lifestyle and in turn, weight loss.

BEHAVIOR MODIFICATION TECHNIQUES
- Evaluate what behaviors, activities or feelings trigger eating.
- Don't use food as a reward for desired behavior.
- Drink plenty of noncaloric fluids, including water daily.
- Change usual eating places, avoid eating while involved in other activities.
- Make an effort to eat breakfast and small, frequent meals.
- Eat fresh fruits and raw vegetables at least 4 times daily.
- Exercise along with television exercise programs or during commercials when watching television.
- Eat slowly, putting your utensil down between bites.
- Weight should be checked on a weekly basis only.
- Clean high-calorie, low-nutrient foods out of cupboards.
- Keep busy so the focus is not food.
- Shop from a healthy food list and not when hungry.
- Leave the table soon after eating and don't feel a need to finish everything.
- Trim fat off meat and skin off poultry.
- Place a photo of a thinner you on the mirror.
- Plan ahead, especially when attending social events.
- Keep records of intake and/or weight loss progress.
- When weight drops, give away clothes that no longer fit.
- Break the habit of nibbling while cooking or cleaning up from meals.
- Try low-fat and low-calorie food items (the taste keeps improving).

Adapted from Arizona Diet Manual (revised 1992)

APPENDIX

BREAST SELF-EXAMINATION

WHY SHOULD YOU EXAMINE YOUR BREASTS MONTHLY?

Most breast cancer is first discovered by women themselves. Since breast cancer found early and treated promptly has an excellent chance for cure, learning how to examine your breasts properly can help save your life. Use the simple 3-step breast self-examination (BSE) procedure described below.

WHEN TO EXAMINE YOUR BREASTS

• Follow the same procedure once a month about 1 week after your period, when your breasts are usually not tender or swollen.

• After menopause, check your breasts on the first day of each month. After a hysterectomy, consult with your doctor or clinic for an appropriate time of the month.

• Doing a monthly self-exam will give you peace of mind, and seeing your doctor once a year will reassure you there is nothing wrong.

This simple 3-step procedure could save your life by finding breast cancer early when it is most curable. For each procedure, think of your breast as an imaginary clock face. Begin at the outermost top of your right breast for 12 o'clock, then move to 1 o'clock, and so on around the circle back to 12.

1. IN THE SHOWER

Examine your breasts during a bath or shower—hands glide easier over wet skin. With the fingers flat, move the hand gently over every part of each breast. Use your right hand to examine the left breast, left hand for the right breast. Check for any lump, hard knot or thickening.

2. IN FRONT OF A MIRROR

Inspect your breasts with arms at your sides. Next, raise your arms high overhead. Look for any changes in contour of each breast (swelling, dimpling or changes in the nipple).

3. LYING DOWN ON YOUR BACK

• To examine your right breast, put a pillow or folded towel under your right shoulder. Place your right hand under your head—this distributes breast tissue more evenly on the chest.

• With the left hand, fingers flat, press gently in small circular motions around an imaginary clock face. A ridge of firm tissue in the lower curve of each breast is normal. Then move in an inch, toward the nipple, and keep circling to examine every part of your breast, including the nipple. This requires at least three more circles. Now slowly repeat the procedure on your left breast with a pillow under your left shoulder and the left hand under your head. Notice how your breast structure feels.

• Check the area under each arm (with your elbow slightly bent). Your lymph glands are located in this area and they may become swollen if you are sick. If you feel a small lump that moves freely, check it daily for a few days. If it doesn't go away, call the doctor.

• Squeeze the nipple of each breast gently between thumb and index finger. Any discharge, clear or bloody, should be reported to your doctor immediately.

WHAT TO DO IF YOU FIND A LUMP OR THICKENING

• If a lump, dimple or discharge is discovered during a self-exam, it is important to see your doctor as soon as possible. Don't be frightened. Most breast lumps or changes are not cancer, but only your doctor can make the diagnosis.

• Remember, however, that your monthly breast exam is not a substitute for an examination by a medical professional. See your doctor once a year (more often if you are in a risk group) and get a mammogram as recommended. The American Cancer Society recommendations: Ages 35-39, one baseline mammogram; ages 40-49, one every 1-2 years; over age 50, one every year.

CONDOM USAGE
(continued on next page)

WHO SHOULD USE A CONDOM?
- Because condoms are used for both birth control and reducing the risk of disease, some people think that other forms of birth control will also protect them against disease. This is not true. Even if you use another form of birth control you need a condom to reduce the risk of getting STD's (sexually transmitted diseases).
- Condoms do not make sex 100 percent safe, but, if properly used, they can reduce the chance of contracting STD's, including AIDS. This can mean protection not only for you and your partner, but also for any children you may have in the future.

CHOOSING A CONDOM
Read the label and look for the following:
- The condoms should be made of latex (rubber) or made of polyurethane (a new condom product).
- It should say that the condoms are to prevent disease, and if used properly, latex condoms help reduce risk of HIV transmission and many other STD's. If the package doesn't say anything about preventing disease, the condoms may not provide the protection you want. Novelty condoms, for example, will not be labeled for either disease- or pregnancy-prevention. Condoms that don't cover the entire penis are not labeled for disease prevention and should not be used for this purpose. For proper protection, a condom must unroll to cover the entire penis.
- Check the expiration date (EXP followed by date). The condom should not be purchased or used after that date.
- Condoms are available in many stores and from vending machines. If purchasing condoms from vending machines, check for proper labeling. Do not purchase condoms from a vending machine located where it may be subject to extreme temperatures or direct sunlight.
- Condoms should be stored in a cool, dry place out of direct sunlight. Closets or drawers usually make good storage places. Condoms should not be kept in a pocket, wallet or purse for more than a few hours at a time because they may be exposed to extreme temperatures.

HOW TO USE A CONDOM
- When opening a condom, handle the package gently. Don't use teeth, sharp fingernails, scissors, or other sharp instruments as these may damage the condom. And make sure you can see what you're doing!
- After you open the package, inspect the condom. If the material sticks to itself or is gummy, the condom is no good. Check the condom top for other obvious damage such as brittleness, tears and holes, but don't unroll the condom to check it because this could damage it.
- Use a new condom for every act of intercourse and oral sex.
- Put the condom on after the penis is erect and before any contact is made between the penis and any part of the partner's body.
- If using a spermicide (see spermicide below), put some inside the condom tip.
- If the condom does not have a reservoir top, pinch the tip enough to leave a half-inch space for semen to collect. Make sure to eliminate any air in the tip to help keep the condom from breaking.
- Holding the condom by the rim (and pinching the half-inch tip, if necessary) place the condom on top of the penis. Then, continuing to hold it by the rim, unroll it all the way to the base of the penis. If you are using water-based lubricant, you can put more on the outside of the condom.
- If you feel the condom break, stop immediately, withdraw and put on a new condom.
- After ejaculation and before the penis gets soft, grip the rim of the condom and carefully withdraw.
- To remove the condom, gently pull it off the penis, being careful the semen doesn't spill out.
- Wrap the used condom in a tissue and throw it in the trash. Because condoms may cause problems in sewers, don't flush them down the toilet. Afterwards, wash your hands with soap and water.

PRECAUTION
Although condoms afford good protection for vaginal and oral sex (where the penis is in contact with the mouth), the protection they give for anal sex is questionable. The Surgeon General of the Public Health Service has said, "Condoms provide some protection, but anal intercourse is simply too dangerous a practice." Condoms may be more likely to break during anal intercourse than during other types of sex because of the greater amount of friction and other stresses involved. Even if the condom doesn't break, anal intercourse is very risky because it can cause rectal tissue to tear and bleed, allowing disease germs to pass more easily from one partner to another.

CONDOM USAGE
(continued from previous page)

SPERMICIDES

Spermicides, which kill sperm, are used for birth control either alone or with barrier contraceptives such as the diaphragm or cervical cap. Scientists have observed that, in test tubes, a spermicide called nonoxynol-9 kills organisms that cause STD's. Although it has not been scientifically proven, it is possible that nonoxynol-9 may reduce the risk of transmission of the AIDS virus during intercourse as well. Using a spermicide along with a latex condom is therefore advisable, and is an added precaution in case the condom breaks. Some condoms come with nonoxynol-9 already added. Their packages are required to be labeled with the expiration date of the spermicide, and they should not be used after that date.

Some experts think that even if a condom with spermicide is used, additional spermicide in the form of a jelly, cream or foam should be added. These are sold over the counter in pharmacies and some supermarkets. (Although swallowing small amounts of spermicide has not proven harmful in animal tests, it is not known if this is true for humans. For that reason, and because spermicides have a bitter taste, for oral sex it may be best to use a condom without spermicide.)

LUBRICANTS

Lubricants may help prevent condoms from breaking during use and may prevent irritation that might increase the chance of infection. Some condoms come lubricated with dry silicone, jelly or cream or you can add water-based lubricants specifically made for this purpose (for example, K-Y Lubricating Jelly). If you use a separate lubricant, never use a product that contains oils, fats or greases such as a petroleum based jelly (for example, Vaseline), baby oil or lotion, hand or body lotion, cooking shortenings, or oily cosmetics such as cold creams. These can seriously weaken latex, causing a condom to tear easily. If you use a spermicide, you do not need to use a lubricant because spermicide acts as a lubricant.

ADDITIONAL RESOURCES FOR INFORMATION:
- National AIDS Hotline (800) 342-AIDS
- Sexually Transmitted Diseases Hotline (800) 227-8922

EXERCISE AND PHYSICAL FITNESS BENEFITS

Regular exercise can play a key role in staying healthy or getting healthier. Exercise can be an important part of treating many medical problems, such as hypertension, sleep disorders, depression, anxiety, diabetes mellitus and high blood-fat levels (especially high levels of low-density cholesterol).

Regular exercise also can help improve your body image and increase your energy level. It can help control weight, reduce stress and help protect you from heart and blood-vessel disease.

EXERCISE COMPONENTS
There are four components for exercise:

Type of Exercise
Popular ones include brisk walking, swimming, bike riding, jogging.

Frequency of Exercise
It's best to start at about three exercise sessions per week, then increase gradually to four, five or more.

Duration of Exercise
The ideal duration is 30 minutes of continuous activity. It's best to begin with 10 or 15 minutes and increase as your tolerance for exercise improves.

Intensity of Exercise
This component varies greatly depending on your age, sex and medical condition. You may require specific instructions that apply uniquely to you after your physical checkup.

KEYS TO SUCCESS OF AN EXERCISE PROGRAM
- Fit exercise into your normal daily schedule and lifestyle.
- Exercise regularly—increase your pace gradually.
- Recruit a spouse or a friend to make exercise fun.
- Vary your activity. Alternate forms of exercise to avoid boredom.
- Increase exercise in easy, day-by-day activities. For example, park your car far enough away from a destination to allow a good walk, walk up a flight of stairs, use manual rather than power tools.

AEROBIC EXERCISE
- An exercise is aerobic if it provides:
  1. Sustained physical activity that uses major muscle groups of the body.
  2. Regulated intensity, long-duration exercise for 20 minutes or more.

Medical experts recommend aerobic exercise as a good program for achieving and maintaining cardiopulmonary vascular fitness—strong and healthy heart, lungs and blood vessels.

- Proper aerobic benefit is based on sufficient exercise to accelerate the heart rate to a prescribed level and keep it there a certain length of time. Most exercise routines call for aerobic sessions three to five times per week for maximum benefit.

- Best forms of aerobic exercise include brisk walking, swimming, bike riding, jogging, rope jumping and rowing. Sports such as tennis and golf have good recreational effects, but they do not require enough effort to reach sustained aerobic levels.

See your doctor prior to starting a fitness program, especially if you are male and over age 40, or if you have any risk factors for coronary artery disease (hypertension, cigarette smoking, obesity, sedentary lifestyle, high cholesterol or low high-density lipoprotein [HDL], high stress, or family history of early coronary artery disease.)

IMMUNIZATIONS, CHILDHOOD

Immunizations protect children and adults from serious diseases that can be fatal. The schedule below is adapted from the current recommendation of the Immunization Practices Advisory Committee, American Academy of Pediatrics and American Academy of Family Physicians.

Don't consider the recommended ages as absolute. For example, "2 months" can mean a range of 6 to 10 weeks. Also, certain amounts of time are needed between dosages. Immunizations may not be a good idea at the recommended time if your child is ill or taking certain medications (immunosuppressants or cortisone). Rely on the judgment of informed professionals.

CHILDHOOD IMMUNIZATION SCHEDULE
Age and recommended vaccines:

Birth (first visit)
- Hepatitis B vaccine 1

1-2 months
- Hepatitis B vaccine 2 (or vaccine 1 if not given previously)

2 months
- DTP 1 (diphtheria, tetanus and pertussis)
- HbCV 1 (Haemophilus influenza type b conjugate vaccine) or one vaccine that combines DTP and HbCV (Tetramune)
- TOPV 1 (trivalent oral poliovirus vaccine)

4 months
- Hepatitis B vaccine 2 (if 1 given late)
- DTP 2 (diphtheria, tetanus and pertussis)
- HbCV 2 (Haemophilus influenza type b conjugate vaccine) or one vaccine that combines DTP and HbCV (Tetramune)
- TOPV 2 (trivalent oral poliovirus vaccine)

6 months
- DTP 3 (diphtheria, tetanus and pertussis)
- HbCV 3 (Haemophilus influenza type b conjugate vaccine, if HbOC* used in 1 & 2) or one vaccine that combines DTP and HbCV (Tetramune)

6-18 months
- Hepatitis B vaccine 3 (if vaccine 2 given late, 3 will be delayed)
- TOPV 3 (trivalent oral poliovirus vaccine)

12-15 months
- HbCV 3 (Haemophilus influenza type b conjugate vaccine, if PRP-OMP* used in 1 & 2)
- HbCV 4 (Haemophilus influenza type b conjugate vaccine, if HbOC* used for 1 & 2) or one vaccine that combines DTP and HbCV (Tetramune)
- MMR 1 (measles, mumps and rubella [German measles])

15 months
- DTP 4 (diphtheria, tetanus and pertussis)

4-6 years
- DTP 5 (diphtheria, tetanus and pertussis)
- TOPV 4 (trivalent oral poliovirus vaccine)
- MMR 2 (measles, mumps and rubella [German measles])

14-16 years
- Td 1 (tetanus and diphtheria; every 10 years after last dose)
- MMR 2 (if missed at 4-6 years)

* HbOC and PRP-OMP are 2 types of Haemophilus b conjugate vaccine.

Vaccines are also available to protect against pneumococcal pneumonia, rabies, typhoid fever and other diseases. These vaccines are given only under special circumstances.

Ask the doctor, health department or travel agent about vaccinations required or recommended before travel in another country. Inquire several months before your expected departures.

R.I.C.E. THERAPY

R.I.C.E. is an acronym (a word formed from the first letters of a term) for the most important elements—rest, ice, compression, and elevation—in first aid for many injuries. This acronym appears repeatedly in medical literature in reference to athletic injuries. Use the word R.I.C.E. to jog your memory when you are faced with such injuries as contusions, sprains, strains, dislocations, or uncomplicated fractures.

REST
Stop using the injured part and rest it as soon as you realize an injury has taken place. Continued exercise or other activity could cause further injury, delay healing, increase pain, and stimulate bleeding. Use crutches to avoid bearing weight on injuries of the foot, ankle, knee, or leg. Use splints for injuries of the hand, wrist, elbow, or arm. After medical treatment, the injured part may require immobilization with splints or a cast to keep the area at rest until it heals.

ICE
Ice helps stop bleeding from injured blood vessels and capillaries. Sudden cold causes small blood vessels to contract. This contraction of blood vessels decreases the amount of blood that can collect around the wound. The more blood that collects, the longer the healing time.

Ice can be safely applied in several ways:
• For injuries to small areas, such as a finger, toe, foot, or wrist, immerse the injured area for 15 to 35 minutes in a bucket of ice water. Use ice cubes to keep the water cold, adding more as ice cubes dissolve.
• For injuries to larger areas, use ice packs. Avoid placing ice directly on the skin. Before applying the ice, place a towel, cloth, or one or two layers of an elasticized compression bandage on the skin to be iced. To make the ice pack, put ice chips or ice cubes in a plastic bag or wrap them in a thin towel. Place the ice pack over the cloth. The pack may sit directly on the injured part, or it may be wrapped in place.
• Ice the injured area for about 30 minutes (no matter what form of ice treatment you are using).
• Remove the ice to allow the skin to warm for 15 minutes.
• Reapply the ice.
• Repeat the icing and warming cycles for 3 hours. Follow the instructions below for compression and elevation. If pain and swelling persist after 3 hours call your doctor. You may need to change the icing schedule after the first 3 hours. Regular ice treatment is often discontinued after 24 to 48 hours. At that point, heat is sometimes more comfortable.

COMPRESSION
Compression decreases swelling by slowing bleeding and limiting the accumulation of blood and plasma near the injured site. Without compression, fluid from adjacent normal tissue seeps into the injured area. The more blood and fluid that accumulate around an injury, the slower the healing.

To apply compression safely to an injury:
• Use an elasticized bandage (Ace bandage) for compression, if possible. If you do not have one available, any kind of cloth will suffice for a short time.
• Wrap the injured part firmly, wrapping over the ice. Begin wrapping below the injury site and extend above the injury site.
• Be careful not to compress the area so tightly that the blood supply is impaired. Signs of deprivation of the blood supply include pain, numbness, cramping, and blue or dusky nails. Remove the compression bandage immediately if any of these symptoms appears. Leave the bandage off until all signs of impaired circulation disappear. Then rewrap the area—less tightly this time.

ELEVATION
Elevating the injured part above the level of the heart is another way to decrease swelling and pain at the injury site. Elevate the iced, compressed area in whatever way is most convenient. Prop an injured leg on a solid object or pillows. Elevate an injured arm by lying down and placing pillows under the arm or on the chest with the arm folded across. The whole upper part of the body may be elevated gently with pillows, with a reclining chair, or by raising the top of the bed on blocks.

APPENDIX

SAFE USE OF MEDICINE

These suggestions for wise, safe use of medicine apply to all medicines.

INFORMATION YOU SHOULD PROVIDE
Always give the information listed in 1 and 2 below to your physician, dentist or other health-care professional so that they can prescribe medications properly:

1. YOUR COMPLETE MEDICAL HISTORY
Tell the important facts of your medical history dealing with medicines. Include allergic reactions, side effects or adverse reactions you have experienced in the past. Describe the allergic problems you have, such as hay fever, asthma, eye watering and itching, throat irritation and reactions to food. People who have allergies to common substances are more likely to develop side effects or adverse reactions to drugs.

2. MEDICINES YOU ARE TAKING NOW
List all prescription and nonprescription drugs. Don't forget common ones such as laxatives; vitamin or mineral supplements; skin, rectal or vaginal medicines; antacids; antihistamines; cold and cough remedies; aspirin and aspirin-containing pain pills; motion sickness remedies; weight-loss aids; salt and sugar substitutes; caffeine (in coffee, tea, cola drinks and cocoa); oral contraceptives; sleeping pills; or "tonics."

KNOW THIS INFORMATION BEFORE TAKING ANY MEDICINE
- Generic names and brand names of all the medicines you take. Write them down to help you remember. If a drug is a mixture of two or more generic ingredients, learn the names of each.
- Uses for each medicine you take.
- How to take each medicine—for example, with or without water, or with food.
- When to take.
- What to do if you forget a dose.
- How each drug works in your body.
- Time lapse before drug works.
- Symptoms and treatment of overdose.
- Possible adverse reactions and side effects and what to do if they occur.
- Interactions with other drugs and other substances such as alcohol, food, beverages, cocaine, marijuana and tobacco. When mixed with some medicines, these substances can sometimes cause life-threatening interactions.
- Know all warnings and precautions that apply to special circumstances, such as:
  1. Reasons not to take the drug in the presence of some medical conditions. These reasons are called contraindications.
  2. Special considerations for elderly patients, pregnant or breast-feeding women, infants and children.
  3. Implications for prolonged use, exposure to sun and sunlight, driving, piloting aircraft, hazardous work, flying in airplanes.
  4. Instructions before discontinuing the drug.

OTHER SAFETY TIPS
- Before taking any prescribed medicine, discuss with your doctor plans that you may have for elective surgery, pregnancy, and breast-feeding.
- Don't hesitate to ask questions about a drug.
- Never take medicine in the dark! It is always possible to take the wrong one. Recheck the label before each drug use.
- Notify your doctor about any new or unexpected symptoms you develop while taking medicine. You may need to change medicines or have a dose adjustment.
- Store all medicines out of children's reach. Keep drugs in a cool, dry place, such as a kitchen cabinet or bedroom. Avoid medicine cabinets in bathrooms—they get too moist and warm at times. Keep medicine in its original container, tightly closed. Don't remove the label! If directions call for refrigeration, keep cool but don't freeze.
- Don't save leftover oral or injectable medicine to use later. Discard it before or on the expiration date shown on the container. Dispose of it safely to protect children and pets.
- Study any information you can find about the specific drugs you take.
- Don't take any drug prescribed for someone else.
- Prior to any surgery (including oral surgery or simple dental procedures), tell the doctor or dentist about all medicines you take or have taken in the past few weeks.
- If you become pregnant while taking any medicine, including birth-control pills, tell the doctor immediately. Avoid all drugs when you are pregnant, if possible.

SEXUALLY TRANSMITTED DISEASES

STD FACTS
- Sexually transmitted diseases affect more than 12 million men and women in the United States each year. Many are teenagers or young adults.
- Using drugs or alcohol increases your chances of getting STD's because these substances can interfere with your judgment and your ability to use a condom properly.
- Intravenous (IV) drug use puts a person at higher risk for HIV and hepatitis B because IV drug users usually share needles.
- The more sexual partners you have, the higher your chance of being exposed to HIV or other STD's. This is because it is difficult to know whether a person is infected, or has had sex with people who are more likely to be infected due to intravenous drug use or other risk factors.
- Sometimes, early in the infection, there may be no symptoms, or symptoms may be easily confused with other illnesses.
- You cannot tell by looking at someone whether he or she is infected with HIV or another STD.
- Sexually transmitted diseases include HIV, chancroid, chlamydial infections, trichomoniasis, genital herpes, pubic lice, genital warts, gonorrhea, lymphogranuloma venereum, syphilis, viral hepatitis, scabies, candidiasis, molluscum contagiosum and others.

STD's CAN CAUSE:
- Pelvic inflammatory disease (PID) which can damage a woman's Fallopian tubes and result in pelvic pain and sterility.
- Tubal pregnancies (where the fetus grows in the Fallopian tube instead of the womb), sometimes fatal to the mother and always fatal to the fetus.
- Death or severe damage to a baby born to all infected women.
- Sterility—the inability to have children—in both men and women.
- Cancer of the cervix in women.
- Damage to major organs, such as the heart, kidney and brain, if STD's go untreated.
- Death, especially with HIV infection.

RISKS
High-risk behaviors include having sex — vaginal, anal or oral — with:
- A person who has an STD. This is the riskiest behavior. If you know your partner is infected, avoid intercourse (including oral sex). If you do decide to have sex with an infected person, always be sure to use a condom from start to finish, every time.
- Someone who has shared needles to inject drugs with an infected person.
- Someone whose past partner(s) was infected. Because the AIDS virus can be in the body a long time before a person feels sick, if your partner had intercourse with a person infected with HIV, he or she could pass it on to you even if the sexual contact was a long time ago–even as long as 10 years–and even if your partner seems perfectly healthy.

PREVENTION
- To lessen the chance of being infected with AIDS or other STD's, people who take part in risky sexual behavior should always use a condom.
- Use of a condom is also important for an uninfected pregnant woman because it can help protect her and her unborn child from STD's.

SEE A DOCTOR IF YOU HAVE ANY OF THESE STD SYMPTOMS
- Discharge from the vagina, penis or rectum.
- Pain or burning during urination or intercourse.
- Pain in the abdomen (women), testicles (men), and buttocks and legs (both men and women).
- Blisters, open sores, warts, rash, or swelling in the genital or anal area, or mouth.
- Persistent flu-like symptoms—including fever, headache, aching muscles, or swollen glands—which may precede STD symptoms.

ADDITIONAL RESOURCES FOR INFORMATION
- National AIDS Hotline (800) 342-AIDS
- Sexually Transmitted Diseases Hotline (800) 227-8922

SKIN SELF-EXAMINATION

Performing your own examination of your skin is important as most physical exams do not include an overall check of your skin on a regular basis. Your skin exam should be performed monthly and may take about 10-15 minutes. Two types of skin cancer (basal cell carcinoma and squamous cell carcinoma) are almost always cured once correctly diagnosed. With melanoma (the most serious type of skin cancer) early diagnosis is essential to start treatment before it spreads. Along with your self-exam, always practice sun-protection care by using an effective sunscreen (SPF of 15 or higher), wearing protective clothing, and limiting exposure time to the sun.

Get to know your skin, so you know what is normal for you. The first time you do the self-examination, locate all moles, warts, birthmarks, scars, spots, bumps, lumps, or other skin markings. It may be difficult to remember the color, shape and size of each, so you may want to write down the information or draw a sketch of each area and abnormality.

MONTHLY EXAMINATION ROUTINE
After undressing completely, look at your body in a full length mirror in a well-lighted room. Have a spouse help you to check the parts of your body that are difficult to see or use a large hand mirror (a magnifying hand mirror may be helpful).

VISUAL EXAM
• Look for any changes in the size, shape, or color of moles, warts, birthmarks, scars, or other skin markings; and look for new moles or sores.
• Lift your scalp hair and look at the skin underneath.
• Look at your face, neck and ears closely in the mirror. This area is prone to skin damage from the sun. Men with facial hair should look at the skin underneath.
• Look at your arms and hands (backs and fronts), including fingernails. Dark spots under the nail can be an early sign of melanoma.
• Examine buttocks, legs, feet and toenails. Use the hand mirror to view the areas not easily seen. Be sure you look at the bottom of the feet and between your toes.
• Look at your chest, abdomen.

TOUCH EXAM
• Run your fingers over your whole body including your scalp (hair and bald spots). Feel for any lumps, bumps, or rough spots.
• Feel the back of your arms and shoulders carefully (these are areas susceptible to sun damage).
• Notice particularly if there is any bleeding, itching, tenderness or pain in or near a mole.

CALL YOUR DOCTOR IF
• You find any noticeable change in a mole or wart, or other skin marking.
• You have a new or unexplained skin lump, ulcer, or unhealed sore that has appeared since your last examination.
• You have an unusual or changing skin spot in an area of irritation or sun-damaged skin.

STRESS, HOW TO COPE

CAUSES OF STRESS
Changes in lifestyle and disruptions in your normal routine can bring about stress.

Some of the common causes of stress are:
- Recent death of a loved one—spouse, child, friend.
- Loss of anything valuable to you.
- Injuries or severe illnesses.
- Getting fired or changing jobs.
- Recent move to a new home.
- Sexual difficulties between you and your partner.
- Business or financial reverses, or taking on a large debt, such as purchasing a new home.
- Regular conflict between you and a family member, close friend or business associate.
- Constant fatigue brought about by inadequate rest, sleep or recreation.

STRESS-RELATED DISORDERS
A certain amount of stress is not always bad. It varies from person to person how much stress one can handle easily. Sometimes, stress can push us on to greater achievement. But excessive stress can be self-defeating. Too much stress can be a risk factor for any of the following disorders:
- Mental and emotional upheavals.
- Skin eruptions, such as eczema and neurodermatitis.
- Digestive system problems, including peptic ulcers, colitis and irritable colon.
- Endocrine disorders, including overactive thyroid, adrenal- or pituitary-gland overactivity or underactivity, changes in menstrual patterns, impotence and premature ejaculation in men, or orgasmic dysfunction in women.
- Lung disorders associated with spasm of the bronchial tubes, such as in asthma.
- Pain syndromes, such as chronic or recurrent disabling headaches or back pain.

Many doctors believe that stress has a role in almost any disorder. Practically no one doubts that stress can complicate an illness by preventing normal recovery, prolonging pain and sustaining disability.

TIPS FOR COPING
Here are some tips that may help you reduce stress:
- Learn a meditation technique and practice it regularly—daily if possible. There are many methods available. Most of them include "tuning in to" and giving complete attention to a word, sound, sentence or concept that you silently repeat to yourself. Don't try to banish other thoughts that enter your mind during your period of concentration, but don't focus on them enough to stop you from meditating. The purpose of meditation is to empty your mind of all disturbing thoughts for a given period of time to encourage mental relaxation. Mental relaxation, in turn, will help reduce stress.
- Take a short period of time away from any stressful situation you encounter during a day. Practice a muscle-tensing and muscle-relaxing technique. Close your eyes. Take a series of deep breaths. Then start with the muscle groups in your face. Consciously tense them and hold the contraction for a few seconds. Then consciously relax them. Continue through all major muscle groups in the body: neck, shoulders, hands, abdomen, back and legs. When you become skillful, you can use this technique to produce relaxation quickly any time you need to and in almost any environment.
- Adopt an exercise program. People in good physical condition are less likely to suffer the negative effects of stress, anxiety or depression.
- Avoid taking your problems to bed with you. At the end of the day, spend a few minutes reviewing your entire day's experiences, event by event, as if you're replaying a tape. Release all negative emotions you have harbored (anger, feelings of insecurity or anxiety). Relish all good energy or emotion (loving thoughts, praise, feeling good about your work or yourself). Reach a decision about unfinished events, and release mental or muscular tension. Now you're ready for a relaxing and emotionally healing sleep.

TESTICULAR SELF-EXAMINATION

You should examine your testicles once a month in order to help detect abnormalities early. Each male is different and it may take a few self-examinations to know what is normal for you. Eventually, you'll become familiar with how your testicles feel and appear and will be able to recognize anything abnormal.

Remove your clothes and stand in front of a mirror. After a warm bath or shower is a good time because the scrotal skin is relaxed. With one hand, lift your penis and check your scrotum (the sac containing your testicles) for any change in shape or size and for red, distended veins. The scrotum's left side may hang slightly lower than the right.

Then, feel your testicles for lumps, nodules, swelling or a change of consistency. To examine your right testicle, place your right thumb on the front of the testicle and your index and middle fingers behind it. Gently press your thumb and fingers together; they should meet. Make sure you check your entire testicle. Then, use your left hand to examine your left testicle in the same manner. Your testicles should feel smooth, rubbery and slightly tender, and you should be able to move them.

Locate the ropelike structure at the back of your testicles. This is called the epididymis. Your spermatic cord extends upward from the epididymis. Gently squeeze the spermatic cord above your right testicle between the thumb and first two fingers of your right hand. Then, using the thumb and first two fingers of your left hand, examine the spermatic cord above your left testicle. Check for lumps and masses by squeezing along the entire length of the cords.

If you notice any lumps, nodules, swelling or changes, call your doctor.

Glossary

A

Abdominal Aorta—Section of the aorta that passes through the abdomen to supply blood to the lower part of the body.

Abscess—Swollen, inflamed, tender area of infection containing pus.

Accident Proneness—Tendency of some persons to have more accidents than normal. It may be due to a risk factor such as poor vision, but unconscious factors are often the cause.

Acetaminophen—Nonprescription medication used to relieve minor pain and to reduce fever. Its analgesic effects are similar to aspirin, but it does not reduce inflammation or swelling. It is less irritating to the stomach than aspirin.

Achalasia—Condition of the esophagus that disrupts normal swallowing.

Acquired Immune Deficiency Syndrome, Acquired Immunodeficiency Syndrome, AIDS—A disease of the human immune system that is caused by infection with HIV (human immunodeficiency virus).

Acupuncture—Method of anesthesia and treatment of pain developed by the Chinese. Needles are inserted through the skin to stimulate precise areas.

Acute—Beginning suddenly; also severe, but of short duration.

Addiction—Intense craving for substances such as alcohol, tobacco or narcotics, or a compulsive behavior such as gambling.

Adenoids—Infection-fighting tissue (part of the lymphatic system) in the upper throat, near the tonsils.

Adenoids, Enlarged—Adenoids that have swollen and impaired speech.

Adenovirus—Group of viruses that cause certain respiratory and eye infections.

Adhesions—Small strands of fibrous tissue that cause organs in the abdomen and pelvis to cling together abnormally, creating a risk of intestinal obstruction.

Adolescence—Time of life from the beginning of puberty until maturity.

Adrenal Glands—Two glands attached to the kidneys. Each has an outer layer (cortex) that produces steroid hormones and an inner layer (medulla) that produces adrenalin.

Adrenalin—Hormone produced by the adrenal glands that increases heart rate and prepares the body for crisis. Also called epinephrine.

Aging—The normal process of gradual physical and mental decline.

AIDS—*See Acquired Immune Deficiency Syndrome.*

Airways—Tubular passages that air passes through to the lungs: the trachea (windpipe), bronchi and bronchioles.

Alcoholic Cirrhosis—Widespread destruction of normal liver tissue caused by excessive intake of alcohol.

Alveoli—Lung cells at ends of the airways where oxygen enters the blood and waste gases leave the blood.

Ambulatory Medical Center—A health-care facility for patients who do not require prolonged bed rest or hospitalization.

Amniocentesis—The extraction and examination of a small amount of amniotic fluid in order to determine genetic and other disorders in the unborn child.

Amniotic Sac—The thin, transparent membrane filled with fluid in which the fetus lives until born.

Amphetamine Drugs—Habit-forming drugs that stimulate the brain and central nervous system, increase blood pressure, reduce nasal stuffiness or suppress appetite.

Amyloid Deposits—Abnormal protein material deposited in tissues, usually caused by diseases. These deposits cause impairment of certain organs.

Analgesics—Medications that relieve pain.

Anemia—Condition in which red blood cells or hemoglobin (oxygen-carrying substance in blood) is inadequate.

Anesthesia, General—Causing temporary loss of consciousness and inability to feel pain by use of inhaled gases or injected anesthetics.

Anesthesia, Local (Nerve Block)—Injection of the local anesthetic near the nerves of the surgical area.

Anesthesia, Local—Temporary prevention of pain by injecting medication (local anesthetic).

Aneurysm—Abnormal swelling or ballooning of a blood vessel.

Angina—Pain or pressure beneath the breastbone caused by inadequate blood supply to the heart.

Angiogram, Angiography—Study of arteries and veins by injecting material into them that x-rays can outline.

Anoscopy—Visual examination of the anus by means of a short tube called an anoscope, an optical instrument with lenses and a lighted tip.

Antacid—Medicine taken orally that reduces or neutralizes stomach acid.

Anti-inflammatory Drugs—Medications used to control inflammation not caused by infection.

Anti-arrhythmics—Medications used to treat heartbeat irregularities (arrhythmias).

Antibiotics—Medications that attack germs and fight infection.

Antibiotics, Cephalosporin—Class of antibiotics related to penicillin, capable of destroying more kinds of germs than penicillin.

Antibiotics, Erythromycin—Class of antibiotics that destroys germs similar to those destroyed by penicillin. Often used to treat infections in patients who are allergic to penicillin.

Antibodies—Proteins created in blood and body tissue by the immune system to neutralize or destroy sources of disease.

Anticancer Drugs—Medications that weaken or destroy cancerous tissues without harming healthy tissues.

Anticholinergic Drugs—Medications that reduce nerve impulses in the parasympathetic nervous system. They control some activities of the gastrointestinal system, heart, bladder and other organs.

Anticoagulants—Medications that slow or delay blood clotting.

Anticonvulsants—Medications that control seizures (convulsions), pain or conditions in which the brain or nerves are overly sensitive.

Antidepressants—Medications that help control depression.

Antiemetic Drugs—Medications that prevent or stop nausea and vomiting.

Antifungal Drugs—Medications used to treat fungus diseases.

Antigens—Germs or other sources of disease that antibodies (produced by the immune system) neutralize or destroy.

Antihelmintic Drugs—Medications used to treat worms in the intestines.

Antihistamines—Medications used to treat allergies.

Antihyperlipidemic Drugs—Medications that reduce fat (cholesterol) in the blood. They help prevent blood-vessel disease.

Antihypertensives—Medications used to reduce blood pressure.

Antimalarial Drugs—Medications used to prevent or treat malaria.

Antimetabolite Drugs—Medications that are used to treat some cancers and autoimmune diseases.

Antimicrobial Drugs—Same as *Antibiotics*.

Antinuclear Antibody—Substance that appears in the blood, indicating presence of an autoimmune disease.

Antiparkinsonian Drugs—Medications used to treat Parkinson's disease.

Antiprotozoal Drugs—Medications used in treatment of single-celled parasites (protozoa).

Antipruritic Drugs—Medications that reduce itching.

Antispasmodic Drugs—Medications that improve digestion and relieve intestinal cramps.

Antistreptococcal Titer—Blood test that measures body's response to infection by streptococcal bacteria.

Antithyroid Drugs—Medications used to counter the effects of an overactive thyroid gland.

Antiviral Drugs—Medications used to treat infections caused by viruses.

Anus—A muscular band at the end of the rectum that opens and expands to allow passage of feces.

Anus, Imperforate—Congenital abnormality of newborn infants in which the anus cannot pass feces.

Anxiety—Uncomfortable feeling that something unpleasant or dangerous will happen.

Aorta—Body's largest blood vessel, arising from the top of the heart. It carries blood from the heart to all parts of the body.

Aphrodisiac—Substance claimed to increase sexual arousal or pleasure.

Appendage—Body part that has a minor role (or no role at all) in normal body function. For example, the appendix is an appendage to the colon that seems to have no function.

Arteriogram, Arteriography—Studying arteries by injecting material into them that x-rays can outline.

Arteriosclerosis—Hardening of the arteries.

Arterial Doppler Studies—Measurement of blood flow through the arteries by means of doppler ultrasound.

Artery—Blood vessels that carry blood from the heart to the body.

Arthrograms—X-rays of the joints taken with an arthroscope.

Arthroscope—Slender optical instrument with a lighted tip that allows direct visual examination of some joints. It can also be used to correct some defects in joints.

Artificial Limbs—Mechanical substitutions for amputated arms or legs.

Ascending Colon—First part of the large colon (intestine) extending from the lower end of the small intestine.

Aspiration—1) Removal of accumulated pus or fluid with a needle. 2) Accidental inhalation of objects or fluids into the lungs.

Astigmatism—Visual impairment caused by abnormal eye shape.

Asymmetrical—Uneven in size, shape or position.

Atelactasis—Collapse of the expanded lung.

Atriums—Small chambers in the heart that pump blood into the ventricles. Also called auricles.

Atropine—Medication used to treat diseases of the eye, heart, gastrointestinal system and nervous system.

Audiogram, Audiometry—Test of hearing ability.

Autism—Mental illness of children in which they seem unaware of their surroundings.

Autoimmune Assays (ANA Tests)—Blood tests to identify autoimmune disease.

Autoimmune Disorder—Disease in which the immune system produces antibodies that attack the body's own tissues.

Autoimmune, Autoimmunity—Disease in which a person's immune system attacks its own tissues.

Autonomic Nervous System—Part of the nervous system that controls organs that function involuntarily, such as the heart, lungs, digestive system and blood vessels.

B

Bacteria—One-celled micro-organisms that can sometimes cause disease.

Balloon Angioplasty—Treatment for obstructed arteries, especially those supplying blood to the heart and brain. A small uninflated balloon is passed up the artery to the obstruction, and then expanded to release the obstruction.

Barium Enema—See *Barium X-rays*.

Barium X-Rays—Examining the gastrointestinal system by filling it with a barium solution that is detected by x-rays. Common barium tests are the barium swallow (upper GI series) and the barium enema (lower GI series).

Bartholin's Glands—Small glands in the lips of the vagina that secrete a lubricating fluid, especially during sexual arousal.

Behavior Therapy—Psychotherapy that focuses on ways to change the undesired behavior.

Belladonna—Medication derived from a plant used to treat some diseases of the gastrointestinal system. It is similar to atropine.

Benign—1) Tumor or growth that is neither cancerous nor located where it might impair normal function. 2) Harmless.

Beta-Adrenergic Blockers (Beta-Blockers)—Medications that reduce heart or blood-vessel overactivity to improve blood circulation. Also used to prevent migraine headaches, high blood pressure and angina.

Bile Duct—A small tube that allows bile to pass from the gallbladder into the intestines.

Bile—A digestive juice produced in the liver and stored in the gallbladder. Bile empties into the small intestine for digestive processes.

Biliary Cirrhosis— Cirrhosis of the liver due to inflammation or obstruction of the bile ducts.

Bilirubin—A yellowish, red-blood-cell waste product in bile that the blood carries to the liver. It contributes to urine's yellowish color and can cause jaundice if it builds up in the blood.

Biopsy—Removal of a small amount of tissue or cells (such as fluid from a cyst) for laboratory examination that aids in diagnosis. The tissue sample may be removed by a variety of methods depending on the site to be biopsied.

Biopsy Needle—Instrument often used to perform a biopsy.

Biopsy, Skin—Removal of a sample of skin tissue for laboratory examination that aids in diagnosis. Skin biopsy is often required to confirm a clinical (visual) diagnosis. Removal techniques include shave excision, punch excision and elliptical excision.

Birth Canal—Passageway through the cervix and the vagina through which the baby passes during childbirth.

Bladder—An organ that holds fluids such as urine (urinary bladder) or bile (gallbladder).

Blood Cells, Red—Microscopic cells in the blood that carry oxygen to tissues of the body. One drop of blood contains about 200 million red cells.

Blood Cells, White—Microscopic cells in the blood that help fight infection by destroying germs. One drop of blood contains about 400,000 white cells.

Blood Chemistries—Tests that measure chemicals in the blood.

Blood Count—Counting red and white blood cells to aid in diagnosis of many diseases.

Blood Platelets—See *Platelet Count*.

Blood Studies—Examination of a blood sample to measure white blood cells, red blood cells, hemoglobin, hematocrit and chemical substances. See **Blood Chemistries**.

Blood Vessels—Arteries, veins and capillaries; the tubes in which blood circulates through the body.

Bone Bank—Facility where human bone is stored and made available for transplantation.

Bone Scan—Method of studying the bone structure or function by injecting into the bloodstream a medication that can be detected by a special scanning camera.

Bone Spurs—Abnormal and sometimes painful protrusions of bone with sharp points near joints or tendons.

Bronchial Tubes (Bronchi)—Hollow air passageways that branch from the windpipe (trachea) into the lungs. They carry oxygen into the lungs and pass waste gases (mostly carbon dioxide) out of the body.

Bronchioles—Small air passageways that serve the same purpose as bronchial tubes. Bronchioles are the smallest parts of the respiratory system.

Bronchodilator Drugs—Medications used to treat diseases of the bronchi that cause shortness of breath, such as asthma. The medicines help constricted tubes to relax.

Bronchogram—Diagnosing lung diseases by placing a material in the lung that x-rays can outline.

Bronchoscope, Bronchoscopy—An optical instrument with a lighted tip that is passed into the windpipe, then into the bronchi.

Bruising—Discoloration under the skin caused by injury or bleeding.

C

Calcification—A process in which calcium from the blood is deposited abnormally into tissues due to injury,

infection or aging. Often it is part of healing and not a sign of active disease.

Calcium-Channel Blocker Drugs—Medication used to treat angina, hypertension and heartbeat irregularities.

Cancerous Growths—Extensions of cancerous tissues that invade nearby healthy tissues.

Cancers—Destructive tumors that can arise in almost all parts of the body. Cancer can destroy nearby healthy tissue and may spread to distant organs.

Capillaries—Microscopic vessels that supply all body cells and tissues with blood.

Carbohydrates, Complex—Starches, sugars, cellulose and gums. Complex carbohydrates are those contained in whole grains, fresh fruits and fresh vegetables. These are considered more nutritious than simple carbohydrates.

Carbohydrates, Simple—Refined carbohydrates (sugars) that have lower molecular weights than complex carbohydrates. They produce a quick rise in blood-sugar levels. Most nutrition counselors recommend that daily diets contain minimal amounts of refined sugars. So-called "junk foods" are frequently very high in simple carbohydrates.

Cardiac Catheter—A slender tube that is inserted into an artery or vein and then passed into the heart. It is used to examine the heart and nearby blood vessels by injecting material into the heart that x-rays can detect.

Cardiac Catheterization—Studying heart function with a cardiac catheter.

Cardiac Monitoring—see ECG

Cardiac Ouput—The volume of blood ejected from the left side of the heart in a one minute period.

Cardiopulmonary Resuscitation (CPR)—Emergency treatment for a patient whose heart has stopped (cardiac arrest).

Cardiovascular—Relating to the heart and blood vessels.

Cardiovascular Surgeon—Doctor specially trained to operate on the heart and blood vessels.

Cardiovascular System—System that supplies the body with blood. It consists of the heart and blood vessels (arteries, capillaries, veins).

Carotid Arteries—Large arteries that supply much of the blood to the brain.

Cartilage—Rubbery, dense connective tissue that permits smooth movement of joints. It also helps shape flexible parts of the nose and external ear.

Caruncle—Small, red protrusion of tissue near a body opening. The most common caruncles arise from the urethra or cervix.

CAT Scan—See *CT Scan*.

Catheter—A hollow tube used to introduce fluids into the body or to drain fluids away.

Catheterization—Any procedure in which a small flexible tube is inserted into the body for the purpose of withdrawing or introducing substances. It most often involves the passage of a small catheter through a vein in the arm or leg or the neck and into the heart for securing blood samples or to detect problems.

Caudal Anesthesia—Form of local (low-spinal) anesthesia used to reduce pain during childbirth and surgery on pelvic areas.

Cauterant—Chemical used to destroy abnormal or diseased cells on the skin.

Cauterization—Destruction of tissue by burning or searing it with a red-hot instrument, caustic chemicals or electricity.

Cautery—Destroying small areas of diseased tissue by burning with an electric needle or laser beam, freezing with low-temperature instruments or using a chemical that destroys tissue.

Cecum—The part of the intestinal tract at the beginning of the large colon (intestine).

Central Nervous System—System that controls the body's voluntary acts. It consists of the brain and spinal cord.

Cervical Spine—Bones in the neck at the top of the spinal column.

Cervix—Lower third of the uterus, which protrudes into the vagina.

Cesarean Section—Delivery of a baby through incisions in the mother's abdomen and uterus. It is performed when normal vaginal delivery would be dangerous for the mother or baby.

Chancre—Hard, slightly ulcerated, painless lesion that forms where syphilis enters the body, usually on the genital lips.

Chemocautery—Destruction of abnormal tissue by means of acids, caustics or poisons.

Chemotherapy—Treatment of cancer by injecting medications that kill cancer cells without harming healthy tissue. It is used to treat cancers that cannot be completely cured or treated with surgery or radiation.

Chiggers—Small red biting insects. Also called "red bugs."

Child—Person in the first 10 years of life.

Chiropractor—Practitioner of chiropractic treatment of disease, which involves massage and manipulations to restore normal body functions.

Chokes—Severe breathing difficulty experienced by scuba divers and others who go from high to normal air pressure too rapidly. Bubbles of nitrogen develop in the blood stream and obstruct blood supply to vital organs, sometimes resulting in severe injury or death.

Cholangiogram, Cholangiography—X-ray procedures to diagnose diseases of the bile system (liver, gallbladder, bile ducts). Special medications are used to make the bile system visible on x-rays.

Cholecystectomy—Surgical removal of the gallbladder.

Cholecystography—An x-ray of the gallbladder.

Cholera—Acute, severe, infectious disease causing extreme diarrhea and dehydration.

Choroiditis—Inflammation of the part of the eye that supports the retina and supplies blood to it.

Chromosome—Structures inside the nucleus of living cells that contain hereditary information. Defects in chromosomes cause many birth defects and inherited diseases.

Chronic—Long-term, continuing. Chronic illnesses are usually not curable, but they can often be prevented from worsening. Symptoms usually can be controlled.

Cinematography—Form of motion-picture photography used to record a fast-moving series of x-ray images.

Circulatory System—The system that provides blood to the body, consisting of the heart, arteries, veins and lymphatic system.

Cirrhosis—Chronic scarring of the liver, leading to loss of normal liver function.

Clinician—Health-care professional who has direct contact with patients. The word literally means "someone who is at the patient's bedside."

Clips—See *Skin Clips*.

Clot Retraction Test—Measurement of the time necessary for a tube of blood to form a clot. Abnormal results often indicate a defect in blood platelets, cells important in blood coagulation.

Clotting—Activity of the blood and blood vessels that cause blood to form a jellylike clot, usually near an injury. Clotting helps stop bleeding. The body's clotting mechanism is slowed or reduced ("thinning the blood") with anticoagulants to treat certain diseases.

Coagulation—Same as *Clotting*.

Cocaine—Medication applied directly to mucous membranes to control pain in the nose and throat. Used illegally as a mind-altering drug, it is addicting and dangerous.

Cognitive Therapy—Psychotherapy that is based on the idea that the way we think about the world and ourselves affects our emotions and behavior.

Colic, Colicky—A pain that recurs in a regular pattern every few seconds or minutes.

Collagen—A gelatinous protein from which body tissues are formed.

Colon—The last major portion of the gastrointestinal tract, where waste material is formed into feces and held for elimination. It is also known as the large intestine.

Colonoscope, Colonoscopy—Method of diagnosing diseases of the colon by visual examination of the inside of the colon through a flexible colonoscope, a fiber-optic instrument with a lighted tip.

Color-Blindness—Inability to recognize red and green, which appear to be gray. It is usually hereditary.

Colposcopy—Visual examination of the cervix by means of a colposcope, a slender optical instrument with a lighted tip.

Combined Immunodeficiency Disease—Serious inherited disease in which the immune system of infants is unable to defend against disease.

Complication—Undesirable event during disease or treatment that causes further symptoms and delay in recovery.

Compress—Cloth, sometimes soaked in warm water or coated with medication. It is applied to the skin to relieve discomfort.

Compression—Applying pressure to the surface of the body, usually to stop bleeding.

Compulsion, Compulsive—Intense, irrational urge to perform some action.

Condom—A thin sheath, usually of latex, applied to the penis before sexual intercourse. It is used to help prevent disease of the genitals and as a contraceptive.

Congenital—Abnormality of the body, present at birth, usually meaning a defect. Congenital defects may be inherited or caused by conditions occurring while the fetus grows in the uterus.

Congenital Hypoplastic Anemia—See *Hypoplastic Anemia*.

Conization of the Cervix—Removal of a cone of tissue from the cervix. Laboratory examination of the removed tissue identifies possible cancer.

Conjunctiva—The mucous membrane lining the outermost surface of the eye (white of the eye).

Connective Tissue—Body's supporting framework of tissue consisting of strands of collagen, elastic fibers and simple cells.

Contact Lenses—Small plastic lenses worn on the eyes to correct nearsightedness, farsightedness or astigmatism.

Contagious—Disease or condition that spreads from one person to another.

Convalescence—Recovery from an illness or surgery.

Copious—Large in amount.

Cornea—Clear thickened surface of the eye through which light passes. It has no blood supply and can be transplanted without danger of rejection.

Coronary—Referring to the blood vessels supplying the heart. Sometimes, it refers to a heart attack resulting from coronary-artery obstruction.

Coronary-Care Unit (CCU)—Area of a hospital equipped to care for patients who have suffered a heart attack or other life-threatening heart conditions.

Cortisone Drugs—Medications similar to natural hormones produced by the central core of the adrenal glands.

Cosmetic Surgery—Surgery to improve appearance.

Coxsackie Viruses—Group of viruses causing infections such as poliomyelitis, aseptic meningitis, herpangina and myocarditis.

CPR—See *Cardiopulmonary Resuscitation*.

Cranium—Bones that make up the skull.

Cryosurgery—Destruction of abnormal tissue by applying freezing temperatures, usually with liquid nitrogen.

Cryotherapy—The use of cold (below -200F) temperatures in treatment.

CT Scan, CAT Scan (Computerized Axial Tomography)—A computerized x-ray procedure that provides exceptionally clear images of parts of the body. It aids in diagnosis of diseases that cannot be diagnosed by ordinary x-ray methods.

Culdocentesis—Piercing of the space deep in the vagina under the cervix, to obtain fluid. Laboratory examination of the removed fluid aids in diagnosis of ectopic pregnancy and other disorders.

Culdoscopy—Visual examination of the female pelvic organs by means of a slender instrument brought into the pelvic cavity by penetrating through the space deep in the vagina under the cervix.

Culture—Identification of bacteria, fungi and viruses. Material (pus, blood or urine) from an infected area is collected, placed on nutrient material, and kept warm (usually in an incubator) until the infecting agent has grown. The resulting growth is examined with a microscope.

Curettage—Scraping process frequently used to obtain tissue from the lining of the uterus for laboratory examination that aids in diagnosis.

Curette—Instrument with a sharp end used to scrape tissue from the inner lining of the uterus and to scrape away skin lesions.

Cyst—Sac or cavity filled with fluid or diseased matter.

Cyst Aspiration—Removal of cyst contents for examination, or drainage for relief of symptoms.

Cystography—An x-ray of the urinary bladder that is obtained by injecting a solution visible on x-rays into the bladder.

Cystoscopy—Visual examination of the inside of the urinary bladder by means of a cystoscope, a slender optical instrument with a lighted tip.

Cystourethroscope, Cystourethroscopy—An instrument used for examination of the posterior urethra and bladder.

Cytotoxic Drugs—Medications used to destroy cancerous cells with minimal harm to healthy cells.

D

DC Cardioversion—The restoration of normal rhythm of the heart by a brief electrical shock via two metal plates placed on the wall of the chest.

D & C—Same as *Dilatation and Curettage.*

Debilitating—Causing a general weakening or deterioration in health.

Defibrillation, Cardiac—Applying an electric current to the chest over the heart to interrupt fibrillation, a disturbance of heartbeat.

Dehydration—Loss of essential fluids from the tissues and blood of the body.

Dependence—Condition in which a person requires substances such as narcotics or alcohol to remain comfortable. If the substances are not used, withdrawal symptoms develop.

Dermatome—Area of the skin to which feeling (sensation) is provided by a nerve to the spinal cord.

Descending Colon—The part of the colon in the left side of the abdomen that stores feces until they are passed from the body.

Desensitization—1) Reduction or prevention of allergic (hypersensitivity) reactions by administration of graded doses of allergen. 2) Treatment for phobias and other psychological disorders. A patient gradually increases the exposure to the source of fear while simultaneously learning to relax.

Diabetic Retinopathy—Degeneration of the retina that develops in patients with diabetes mellitus. It may cause vision impairment or blindness.

Diagnosis—Identifying disease. A complete diagnosis names the part of the body affected, the disease process (such as inflammation, cancer or allergy) and the cause of disease.

Dialysis—Removal of natural wastes from the bloodstream. It is used to treat patients with kidney failure.

Diaphragm—Thin, broad sheet of muscle separating the chest cavity from the abdominal cavity.

Diathermy—Treatment in which mild heat is generated within the body by high-frequency radio waves.

Digestive System—Organs in which food is processed for absorption into the blood stream. The major digestive organs are the mouth, esophagus, stomach, duodenum, small bowel (small intestine), colon (large intestine), and rectum. The liver, gallbladder and pancreas are also considered parts of the digestive system.

Digitalis—A drug used to treat congestive heart failure and some other heart diseases.

Dilatation and Curettage—A gynecological treatment or diagnostic procedure that involves the stretching (dilatation) of the cervix so that a spoon-shaped instrument (curet) can be inserted into the uterus to scrape away the lining (endometrium). The scrapings may be examined under a microscope to assess the condition of the uterus.

Dilate, Dilation, Dilatation—To widen, expand or open up.

Dilator—Instrument used to widen organs that have narrowed because of disease.

Discolored Teeth—A yellowish-brown discoloration of the teeth frequently occurring in infants whose mothers took tetracycline while pregnant. Children may also be affected if they take tetracycline before they have their permanent teeth.

Discomfort—Unpleasant physical or mental sensation.

Disease—Adverse change in health; sickness or ailment. A disease can be defined by the body part involved (for example, the heart or liver), by the abnormality present (cancer, infection, allergy, degeneration, etc.) or by its cause (bacteria, poisons, injury, etc.).

Disk—Same as *Intervertebral Disk*.

Disorder—Same as *Disease*.

Diuretics—Medications that force the kidneys to excrete more urine, sodium and potassium than normal, which helps eliminate excessive body fluid.

Diverticulum—Small pouch or sac that develops in the wall of tubular organs such as the esophagus or colon.

Dizziness—Sensation of faintness, lightheadedness or spinning (vertigo).

Donor—Person who gives to someone else. In transplantation surgery, the donor gives up an organ (such as a kidney) to be transplanted into the recipient.

Doppler Ultrasound—See *Ultrasound*; this is one of several methods of ultrasound.

Doppler Venous Studies—Measurement of blood flow through the veins by means of doppler ultrasound.

Dormant—Sleeping or inactive state of living things. Also, an inactive state of a disease.

Drainage—Passage of fluids out of the body through an opening or incision.

Dry Socket—A tooth socket in which after extraction a blood clot fails to form; a condition marked by pain associated with the occurrence of a dry socket.

Ductus Arteriosus—Small blood vessel connecting the aorta and the pulmonary artery, which is the main artery to the lung. The vessel is open during the time the fetus is in the uterus, but normally closes at birth.

Duodenum—First 12 inches of the small intestine.

Dupuytren's Contracture—Chronic condition in which scar tissue forms in the palms. In severe cases, it can impair use of the fingers.

Dwarfism—Condition of being undersized for one's age. It may be due to endocrine disorders, malnutrition or an inherited defect.

Dyspnea—Difficult or painful breathing.

E

Ear Canal—Passageway extending from the outer ear inward to the eardrum.

Ear, Nose and Throat (ENT) Specialist—A physician specially trained to treat diseases of the ears, nose and throat.

ECG (Electrocardiography)—Method of diagnosing heart diseases by measuring electrical activity of the heart with an electrocardiograph. The record produced is called an electrocardiogram.

Echocardiogram, Echocardiography—Studying the heart by examining sound waves created by an instrument placed on the chest. The waves reflected from the heart form an image (echocardiogram) on a monitor, aiding in diagnosis of heart diseases.

Echography—The use of ultrasound as a diagnostic aid.

Eclampsia—Convulsions or coma late in pregnancy in an individual affected with preeclampsia.

Ectopic Pregnancy—A gestation which occurs elsewhere than in the uterus, usually in a Fallopian tube or the peritoneal cavity.

Edema—Accumulation of fluid under the skin, in the lungs or elsewhere.

EEG (Electroencephalography)—Studying the brain by measuring electric activity ("brain waves") with an electroencephalograph. The record produced is the electroencephalogram.

EKG—See *ECG*.

Electrocardiography—See *ECG*.

Electrocautery—Destruction of tissue by heat applied with a controlled electric current.

Electroencephalography—See *EEG*.

Electrolyte—A chemical that is dissolved in the blood and all other body fluids. Electrolytes play an essential role in all body functions. The major electrolytes are: sodium, potassium, chloride, calcium, phosphorus, magnesium and carbon dioxide. Electrolytes come from food. They are regulated mostly by the kidneys and lungs.

Electrolyte Measurement—Laboratory test on blood or urine to identify and measure the electrolytes present.

Electrolyte Supplements—Electrolytes taken to correct or to prevent body-fluid or electrolyte imbalance.

Electromyography—Studying nerve and muscle disorders by recording electrical activity of muscles with an electromyograph. The record produced is the electromyogram.

Electroneuronography—A diagnostic procedure in which the nerve of a muscle under study is stimulated by application of an electric current.

Endemic—Disease that is constantly present in a community or group of people. Endemic disease may affect only a few people at any one time.

Endocrine System—System of organs that secrete hormones into the blood to regulate basic functions of cells and tissues. The endocrine organs are the anterior and posterior pituitary glands, thyroid and parathyroid glands, pancreas, adrenal glands, ovaries (in women) and testicles (in men).

Endocrinologist—Doctor specially trained in diagnosis and treatment of endocrine disorders.

Endometritis—Inflammation of the endometrium.

Endometrium—The mucous membrane lining of the uterus.

Endoscopy—Method of diagnosing diseases in hollow organs. An endoscope (an optical instrument with a lighted tip) is inserted into the organ, which allows visual examination of the cavity. Used in the abdomen, pelvis, lumen of the bronchial tubes or intestines.

Endotracheal Tube—Tube temporarily placed in the trachea (windpipe) of patients who are unable to breathe normally because of disease or surgery.

Enteric—Relating to the small intestine. Enteric-coated medicine is coated with a hard shell that dissolves when it reaches the small intestine.

Enteroscopy—Examination of the inside of the intestines with an endoscope, an optical instrument.

Enterostomy—Surgically created artificial opening for elimination of feces.

Enterostomy Nurse, Enterostomy Specialist—a professional who teaches patients how to care for an enterostomy.

Enzymes—Proteins manufactured by the body that regulate the rate of essential life processes (metabolism).

Epididymis—A system of ducts at the rear of the testes which holds sperm during maturation.

Epididymitis—Inflammation of the epididymis.

Epinephrine—Same as *Adrenalin*.

Episcleritis—Inflammation of tissues on the sclera (the white of the eye).

Epithelial Horn—Thick, rough lesion protruding from the skin. It may become cancerous if not removed.

Equine Virus—Virus that causes a serious form of encephalitis in horses and humans.

Ergot—Medication derived from a fungus that grows on rye plant. It is used to treat migraine headache and to increase strength of uterine contractions during and immediately after childbirth.

Esophageal Varices—Enlarged veins on the lining of the esophagus. They are subject to severe bleeding and often appear in patients with severe liver disease.

Esaphagogram, Esophagoscopy—Method of diagnosing diseases of the esophagus by means of an esophagoscope, an optical instrument with lenses and a lighted tip.

Esophagus—Muscular tube connecting the throat and stomach.

Estrogen—Female sex hormone, primarily secreted by the ovaries. It can also be produced synthetically for use in estrogen replacement therapy.

Estrogen Receptor Value—Used in the study of breast-cancer cells to determine the best treatment.

Etiology—Cause or causes of a disease.

Eustachian Tubes—Slender passages between the throat and the middle ear that maintain normal air pressure in the middle ear.

Excise—To remove by cutting out.

Exploratory Laparotomy—Diagnosing abdominal disease by surgically opening the abdomen and examining its contents.

Extremities—Arms and legs.

Eye Bank—Facility where living corneas are stored and made available for transplantation.

Eyes, Crossed—Condition in which muscles controlling the eyes are unbalanced. The eyes point in different directions. Also called squint or strabismus.

F

Fallopian Tubes—Organs of the female reproductive tract through which an egg (ovum) passes from the ovary to the uterus. Tying these tubes (tubal ligation) accomplishes sterility.

Familial Polyposis—Inherited condition in which the lining of the intestines contains many polyps, some of which may become cancerous.

Family History—Information about illnesses that tend to occur within a family. This information is used to determine the likelihood of diseases occurring in other members of the family.

Farsightedness—Same as *Hypermetropia*.

Fascia—Sheet or band of tough, fibrous tissue that covers muscles and other body organs.

Fecal—Relating to feces, waste products eliminated through the lower intestinal tract.

Fecal-Oral—Pathway by which some fecal germs gain entry into the bloodstream. Sewage in drinking water, hand-to-mouth transmission after bowel movements or sexual contact can cause infection.

Feces—Body waste formed of undigested food that has passed through the gastrointestinal system to the colon. Feces are and stored in the colon until eliminated.

Fetal Monitoring—Measuring the heart rate of the fetus during labor.

Fetal-Scalp Electrodes—Fine wires attached to the scalp of a fetus to measure heart rate and rhythm during labor.

Fetal-Scalp Monitoring—Measuring the well-being of the fetus during labor by obtaining blood from the scalp or by measuring the heart rate of the fetus or contraction strength of the uterus.

Fever—Above-normal body temperature. Normal mouth temperature is 98.6F (37C). Normal rectal temperature is 99.6F (37.6C).

Fiber Optics—System of transmitting light and images through thread-like strands of glass. Fiber-optic instruments make some examinations and surgical procedures simple, safe and effective.

Fiber—A non-nutritious ingredient of many complex carbohydrates. Fiber increases bulk in the diet. Many nutritionists recommend including ample fiber in the diet. Experimental studies and clinical studies show that people who eat high-fiber diets are less likely to develop colon cancer, diverticulitis, atherosclerosis and gallbladder disease.

Fibrin—Protein formed by the action of blood clotting on fibrinogen.

Fibrinogen—Protein in the blood needed for blood clotting.

Fibrositis—Inflammatory conditions affecting connective tissue of muscles, joints, ligaments and tendons.

Fine Needle Biopsy—The use of a fine needle to remove cells or fluid from the body for microscopic laboratory examination.

First Molars—First permanent flat teeth, used for grinding food, which appear at about age 6 to 7.

Fissure—Break in the skin or inner lining of organs.

Fistula—Abnormal passage between two organs or between the body and the outside.

Flank—Area on the side of the body below the ribs and above the hip.

Fleas—Tiny biting insects. Most cause minor skin irritation; some carry and transmit serious diseases such as plague and typhus.

Flooding—A drastic form of psychotherapy used for treatment of phobias. A patient is suddenly confronted with the feared object or placed in the feared situation with no chance of escape. Having experienced the phobia at its fullest intensity, a person comes to realize that the dreaded thing is not dangerous.

Only a competent therapist should subject a phobic person to it.

Fluorescein-Dye Test—Method of diagnosis using fluorescein, a dye, to study tissues and germs. When these dyed tissues are exposed to ultraviolet light, they glow. Substances to which the dye does not cling do not glow.

Fluorescent Antibody Studies—Tests used to study some allergic and infectious conditions. When antibodies created by these conditions are present in the blood, they can be made to glow by using a dye and a microscope with ultraviolet light.

Fluoroscopy—Method of x-ray diagnosis in which moving organs (such as the heart or intestinal tract) can be studied in action.

Foley Catheter—Slender, flexible tube used to drain urine from the bladder of patients who are unable to urinate normally.

Forceps—Instrument with two blades and handles. It is used to grasp tissue, body parts or sterile materials. Also used to deliver babies when progress of labor is slow.

Fracture—Break; usually used to refer to a bone or tooth.

Frei Test—Test used to make a precise diagnosis of lymphogranuloma, a sexually transmitted disease.

Friedreich's Ataxia—Rare, inherited nervous-system disease that causes loss of balance and coordination, awkward walking, speech difficulty and tremors.

Frozen Section—A study in a pathology laboratory of fresh tissue that was removed during surgery. The purpose is to determine if a suspicious area is or is not cancerous.

Fungus—Mold or yeast that may infect skin, internal surfaces (mouth, vagina) or tissues.

Fungus Infection—Infection caused by fungus.

Fusiform Bacteria—Bacteria shaped like slender rods.

G

Galactorrhea—1) Continued breast-milk flow after weaning. 2) Excess breast-milk flow during nursing.

Galactosemia—Inherited disease of infants in which milk cannot be digested. Milk should be eliminated from the infant's diet to prevent malnutrition, liver and kidney disease and mental retardation.

Gallbladder—Small organ under the liver that stores bile. For digestion, the gallbladder contracts to empty bile into the intestines.

Gamma Globulin—Protein in the blood manufactured by the immune system to help destroy or neutralize infection-causing germs. Gamma globulin derived and concentrated from blood of other humans is used to help create temporary immunity to some diseases.

Gammaglobulinemia—Extremely low levels in the blood of gamma globulin brought about by a disease of the immune system. The deficiency causes increased susceptibility to many infections by bacteria, viruses and fungi. Also called hypogammaglobulinemia.

Gangrene—Death of tissue, usually due to partial or total loss of blood supply.

Gastrectomy—Removal of part or all of the stomach.

Gastroduodenoscopy—Examination of the stomach and duodenum by means of a gastroscope.

Gastroenterologist—Doctor who specializes in the diagnosis and treatment of diseases of the gastrointestinal system.

Gastrointestinal Series (Upper GI Series)—X-rays of the upper digestive system (esophagus, stomach and duodenum).

Gastrointestinal Tract—See *Digestive System.*

Gastroscope, Gastroscopy—Visual examination of the inside of the stomach by means of a gastroscope, an optical instrument with a lighted tip.

Gene—Basic unit of protein molecules in chromosomes of cells. Genes transmit inherited characteristics such as eye color, blood type, gender or body shape. Defective genes cause many kinds of birth defects and inborn diseases.

Gene, Dominant or Recessive—Dominant gene, if present in either the mother's egg or father's sperm, will transmit its characteristics to the newborn child. Recessive gene must be present in both parents before its characteristic will be transmitted.

General Surgeon—A doctor specially trained to perform operations.

Genetic Counseling—Counseling to help couples decide whether to have children or not when there is a risk of genetic disease being transmitted to the child.

Genetics—Science of determining inherited factors that result in the unique make-up of every human being; also, science that traces the appearance patterns to genetic (inherited) disease.

Genitourinary Tract—Body system that forms, stores and eliminates urine. Also has a role in male and female reproductive functions. Organs include the kidneys, ureters, bladder, urethra, uterus, Fallopian tubes, ovaries, vagina, cervix, penis, scrotum and testicles.

Germs—Organisms that cause infection such as bacteria, viruses or fungi.

Gestation—Time spent in the mother's uterus by the fetus. Average gestation time for the human infant, from conception to delivery, is approximately 39 weeks.

Gigantism—Condition in which the body or a body part grows excessively, sometimes due to an overactive pituitary gland.

Glucagon—Hormone secreted by the pancreas that increases blood sugar. A synthetic form is sometimes used as emergency treatment for patients with diabetes who have temporarily low blood sugar.

Glucose—Major form of sugar in the blood, stored primarily in the liver. It provides energy to most tissues, organs and systems.

Glucose-Tolerance Test—Method of diagnosing diabetes mellitus or functional hypoglycemia. The patient drinks a measured amount of glucose (sugar). The blood and urine are tested at measured intervals for glucose content.

Gluten—Protein found in wheat and other foods that cannot be digested by some persons because of genetic disease. A gluten-free diet allows persons with the disorder to digest food and grow normally.

Glycosuria—Sugar in the urine.

Goiter—An enlargement of the thyroid gland that is visible as a swelling in the neck.

Gonads—Parts of the reproductive system that produce and release female eggs (ovaries) or male sperm (testes).

Growth Disorders—Conditions in children that result in underdevelopment or overdevelopment of the body. Diseases of the endocrine glands, nutritional problems or genetic abnormalities are frequently the causes.

Gynecologist—Doctor specially trained to treat diseases of the female reproductive system.

H

H-2 Blocker Drugs—Class of antihistamines that reduce the production of stomach acid for treatment of peptic ulcers.

Hallucinogens—Substances that produce hallucinations, apparent sights, sounds or other experiences that do not actually exist.

Hand Surgeon—Surgeon specially trained to treat hand diseases, injuries, infections and arthritic conditions.

Hangover—Unpleasant aftereffects of excessive consumption of alcoholic beverages. Symptoms include irritability, headache and nausea. Sometimes, the same feelings result from using certain medications.

Hashimoto's Thyroiditis—One of several kinds of inflammation of the thyroid gland.

Heart Catheterization—Same as *Cardiac Catheterization*.

Heart Tumors—Rare tumors that grow in the heart wall or in the heart chambers, interfering with normal heart function.

Heart-Lung Machine—Complex mechanical device that provides artificial function of a patient's heart and lungs for a short time during open-heart surgery and heart or lung transplantation.

Hematocrit—Blood test used to detect anemia and other blood disorders. It is expressed as the percentage of blood made up of red blood cells (remainder of the blood is made up of serum or plasma). Normal hematocrit range is approximately 35 to 45%, but it varies with age and sex.

Hematologist—Doctor specially trained to diagnose and treat diseases of the blood and blood-forming organs.

Hemochromatosis—Disease in which excessive iron accumulates in the liver, pancreas and skin, resulting in liver disease, diabetes mellitus and a bronzed skin color.

Hemoglobin, Hemoglobin Range—1) Component that carries oxygen to body tissues. 2) Blood test used to detect anemia and other blood disorders, expressed in grams per 100 cubic centimeters. The normal hemoglobin range is approximately 12 to 18 grams per 100 cubic centimeters and varies according to age and sex.

Hemothorax—blood in the pleural cavity.

Hepatitis—A disease or condition marked by inflammation of the liver.

Hirschsprung's Disease—Congenital defect of infants in which the colon cannot eliminate feces, resulting in severe constipation.

Histamine—Chemical in body tissues that dilates the smallest blood vessels, constricts the muscle around the bronchial tubes, stimulates stomach secretions and produces an allergic response.

HIV—*See Human Immunodeficiency Virus.*

Holter Monitor—Instrument that detects heartbeat-rhythm abnormalities 24 hours or longer. The device is portable for patients to carry wherever they go.

Hormones—Powerful substances manufactured by the endocrine glands and carried by the blood to body tissues and organs. Hormones determine growth and structure of many organs (such as during growth and maturation) and also control many vital body functions.

Host—Person or animal with an infection that has been received from another person, animal or plant, or the environment.

Human Immunodeficiency Virus—Any of a group of retroviruses that infect and destroy helper T cells of the immune system and weaken the body's natural abilities to fight infections and cancer. Also called the AIDS virus.

Hyaline-Membrane Disease—Serious condition of premature infants in which the lungs can't expand normally. Cause is unknown.

Hydatidiform Mole—Disease occurring during early pregnancy resulting in death of the fetus and an overgrowth of tissue within the uterus.

Hydramnios and Polyhydramnios—Condition in which amniotic fluid (fluid in the uterus that surrounds the fetus until birth) becomes excessive.

Hygiene—Personal self-care and cleanliness that reduces the risk of infections and diseases.

Hyoid Bone—V-shaped bone located just above the larynx.

Hyperalimentation—Method of supplying total nutritional needs of patients unable to eat normally. The method (usually intravenous or by tube through the nose into the stomach) provides nutrients containing essential proteins, fats, carbohydrates and vitamins.

Hyperbaric Chamber—Large, sealed room in which air pressure can be raised above normal levels. It is used primarily to treat patients with either decompression sickness or severe burns (sometimes).

Hypercalcemia—Presence of excessive calcium in the blood, occasionally a sign of malignancy.

Hyperlipoproteinemia—Condition in which excessive lipoproteins (cholesterol and other fatty materials) accumulate in the blood.

Hypermetropia—Seeing distant objects clearly while nearby objects appear blurred; also called farsightedness.

Hypersensitivity—Extreme sensitivity to any agent (drugs, pollens, chemicals, etc.) that causes allergic reactions. Some reactions can be life-threatening, but most are less serious.

Hyperthyroidism—Excessive activity of the thyroid gland marked by increased metabolic rate, enlargement of the thyroid gland, rapid heart rate and high blood pressure.

Hypnotics—Medications that produce sleep.

Hypochondriasis—Mental illness in which a person is convinced that serious disease is present, despite examination that proves otherwise. The symptoms of the imagined disease seem real to the patient (often called a hypochondriac).

Hypogammaglobulinemia—An immunologically deficient state characterized by an abnormally low level of all classes of gamma globulin in the blood.

Hypoparathyroidism—Deficiency of parathyroid hormone in the body.

Hypoplastic Anemia (Aplastic Anemia)—Group of anemias that decrease blood-producing bone marrow. This can be life-threatening.

Hypothalamus—Part of the brain that regulates body functions such as temperature, blood pressure, appetite and thirst.

Hypothyroidism—Deficient activity of the thyroid gland, marked by decreased metabolic rate and loss of vigor.

Hysteria—1) Condition in which a person becomes anxious and excitable and experiences impaired sensory and motor abilities. Sometimes, hysterical persons simulate conditions of diseases such as deafness or blindness. 2) Outbreak of uncontrolled emotions, such as fits of laughing or crying.

Hysterogram—An x-ray of the uterus.

Hysterosalpingography—Studying the uterus and Fallopian tubes by injecting material into the uterus that x-rays can detect. It is used primarily to determine if the passageway for the ovum (egg) is open all the way to the uterus. The x-ray image is the hysterosalpingogram.

Hysteroscope—An instrument with lens system and lighted tip used in direct visual examination of the cervix and cavity of the uterus.

Hysterotomy—Incision of the uterus to prepare for cesarean section delivery of a baby.

I

I-131 Uptake—Measuring thyroid activity with radioactive iodine and radiation emission counters.

Idiopathic—Condition caused by unknown factors.

Ileum—Part of the small intestine just above the large intestine (colon).

Ileus—Condition of the small intestine in which either an obstruction or paralysis prevents material from passing through the intestine.

Iliac Arteries—Large arteries in the inner pelvis that supply blood to the legs.

Immune System—Body's system of defense against infection.

Immune, Immunity—Resistance or protection against infection by the body's natural defenses. A person may be immune to one kind of infection but not immune to another. Some infections, such as measles, chickenpox or mumps, cause the body to become immune permanently to that infection.

Immunization—Producing immunity by giving a vaccine (orally or by injection) of germs that have been altered so they cannot produce significant disease. The vaccine causes the body's immune system to produce antibodies that create immunity.

Immunosuppressants—Drugs used in immunosuppression treatment to weaken the immune system and to inhibit immune response.

Immunosuppression—Prevention of the body from forming a normal immune response. It is used to treat diseases (especially when organs must be transplanted) where certain antibodies must be inactivated.

Impotence—Male's inability to achieve or to sustain an erection or to ejaculate sperm during sexual intercourse.

Incise, Incision—To cut open or cut into.

Incomplete Spontaneous Miscarriage—Naturally occurring miscarriage in which the fetus is expelled, but part of the placenta remains in the uterus. Excessive bleeding and infection can result unless the uterus is emptied, usually by dilatation and curettage of the uterus (D & C) or suction curettage.

Incubation Period—The time between exposure to an infecting germ and the appearance of symptoms indicating an infection. Also describes the period of bacterial growth in laboratory cultures.

Infant—Child between the ages of 2 weeks and 1 year.

Infection, Infectious—Disease caused by germs (bacteria, viruses, fungi) that enter the body and cause inflammation or other processes that have an adverse effect on health.

Inflammation, Inflammatory Process—Process by which the body attempts to overcome illness-producing causes such as germs, injuries such as burns, or diseases such as arthritis. The process causes increased body heat (fever or local warmth), swelling, pain and tenderness. If the inflammation is near the skin, redness results.

Inhalation—Breathing air into the lungs.

Inherited—Body characteristic that is transmitted from one generation to the next by chromosomes in the mother's egg and father's sperm. Some inherited characteristics such as brown eyes are normal; others such as Down's syndrome are disorders.

Ingestion—Taking in food, medicine, etc., by mouth.

Inoculation—Injection of infected material such as pus into a nutrient medium where the germs will grow, or incubate. They are then stained and analyzed through a microscope. Also describes any kind of immunization.

Insufflation Test—See *Rubin's Insufflation Test*.

Insulin—Hormone produced by the pancreas that helps regulate sugar in the blood and helps produce energy.

Intensive Care Unit (ICU)—Area of a hospital where patients who are seriously ill or recovering from serious surgery are given more care than is available in other hospital units. As soon as the condition improves, the patient is transferred from the ICU to a regular hospital unit.

Intermittent—Happening only occasionally or under certain conditions.

Internist—Doctor specially trained in nonsurgical diagnosis and treatment of diseases in adults.

Intervertebral Disk—Cartilage that connects adjacent vertebrae in the spinal column.

Intestinal Tract—All parts of the gastrointestinal tract except the mouth, esophagus and stomach. The intestinal tract organs are: duodenum, small bowel, ileum, cecum, appendix, ascending colon, transverse colon, descending colon, sigmoid colon, rectum and anus.

Intestine, Large—Last major portion of the gastrointestinal tract located just under the small intestine. It is also called the colon or large bowel. It processes waste material into feces, which are stored until eliminated from the body.

Intestine, Small—Longest section of the gastrointestinal tract, located just under the stomach and duodenum. It absorbs digested food into the bloodstream and passes waste material into the large intestine.

Intracardiac Pressures—Pressures occurring within the heart.

Intrauterine Death—Death of a fetus while inside the mother's uterus.

Intrauterine Device (IUD)—Birth-control method in which a small device placed permanently in the uterus prevents growth of fertilized eggs.

Intravenous—Within the vein. Fluids, medications and nutrients that cannot be taken orally are given intravenously by a needle placed in a large vein near the surface of the skin.

Intravenous Pyelogram (IVP)—See *Pyelogram, Intravenous*.

Intravenous Urography—Method of studying the kidneys and urinary tract by injecting into the bloodstream a medication that x-rays can detect.

IQ (Intelligence Quotient)—Supposedly a measure of a person's intelligence, rather than what one has learned. Recent research on intelligence raises questions about the accuracy and meaning of the I.Q. test.

Iridectomy—Surgery performed to treat some kinds of glaucoma.

Irrigation—Flooding with water or other liquid. It is used frequently to clean wounds or areas of the body that will undergo surgery.

**Isolation, Reverse
Isolation**—Procedures to prevent spread of infection in a hospital. Isolation protects hospital staff and visitors from contracting a contagious disease from a patient. Reverse isolation protects a patient susceptible to infection because of immunosuppression from contracting infection from hospital staff or visitors.

IUD—See *Intrauterine Device*.

IVP— See *Pyelogram, Intravenous*.

J

Jaundice—Yellow skin and whites of the eyes, dark urine and light stools, symptoms of diseases of the liver and blood.

Joint—Structure that enables two or more bones to move easily in relation to each other. A joint consists of ligaments and cartilage that hold bones together.

Joint Capsule—Tough, fibrous tissue that surrounds a joint.

Joint Replacement—Replacement of diseased joints with mechanical joints. The wrist, hip and knee joints are among the most common joints replaced.

K

Ketoacidosis—Serious complication of diabetes mellitus in which the body produces acids that cause fluid and electrolyte disorders, dehydration and sometimes coma.

Klinefelter's Syndrome—Inherited disease of young males in which secondary sex characteristics are underdeveloped. The condition does not become evident until puberty. Mental deficiency and some female characteristics are present.

L

Laceration—Wound with jagged edges.

Lactiferous Ducts—Network of tubes in the female breast that collects milk and delivers it to the nipple.

Laminaria—Freeze-dried seaweed sometimes used to dilate the cervix when performing an abortion.

**Laparoscope,
Laparoscopy**—Exploratory examination of the organs inside the abdominal cavity with a laparoscope, an optical instrument with a lighted tip. The laparoscope is inserted into the abdomen through a small incision. Visual examination can then be made of many abdominal organs.

Laparotomy—Exploratory surgery in the abdomen performed to diagnose and sometimes treat abdominal disease.

Laryngeal Nerve—Nerve located in the neck that controls the vocal cords and enables a person to speak.

Laryngoscopy—Examination of the inside of the larynx with a laryngoscope, an optical instrument.

Larynx—Structure of muscle and cartilage in the upper neck. It contains the vocal cords. Air passes through the larynx into the windpipe and then into the lungs. The "Adam's apple" is part of the larynx.

Laser Therapy—Using a laser beam to treat many diseases. Sharply focused laser light creates intense heat and is valuable in cutting tissue, destroying unwanted tissue and joining tissue together. It is most often used to treat retinal detachment, endometriosis or atherosclerosis.

Latent—Present but inactive; something that exists in an undeveloped form.

Laxatives—Medications used to treat constipation.

Lesion—General term for injury or damage to an organ or tissue.

Lethargy—Fatigue or lack of usual physical or mental energy.

Libido—Sexual desire.

Life Cycle—Growth and development from birth to death.

Ligaments—Strong, flexible cords of tissue near joints that hold bones together and permit bone motion.

Lipoproteins (High Density and Low Density)—Components of the fluid in blood that are measured to help predict the likelihood of atherosclerosis (hardening of the arteries).

Liquid Nitrogen—Nitrogen that has been cooled until it becomes a liquid. It is used most often in cryosurgery.

Local Anesthesia—See *Anesthesia, Local*.

Low-Residue Diet—Diet consisting of foods that are digested almost entirely, leaving minimal material to form feces.

Low-Spinal Anesthesia—Also called "saddle-block" anesthesia. An injection into the lower spinal canal provides anesthesia to the lower body.

Lower GI Series—Same as *Barium-Enema X-rays*.

Lumbar Puncture (Spinal Tap)—A diagnostic procedure in which a needle is inserted between 2 bones (vertebra) of the lower spine to collect spinal fluid for laboratory examination.

Lumbar Spine—Lower part of the spine, from the lowest ribs to the bottom of the spine.

Lung Function Studies—Tests to determine the effectiveness of a patient's respiration.

Lymph (or Lymphatic) System—Lymph channels and lymph glands considered as a single body system.

Lymph Channels—Tubes of tissue that carry lymph fluid away from tissues and back to the bloodstream. Lymph fluid is composed of proteins and water, varying in composition in different parts of the body.

Lymph Glands—Small collections of tissue (nodes) located along lymph channels in areas such as the elbow, armpit or groin. When infection is present, nearby lymph glands enlarge, become tender and destroy germs that enter lymph channels. Lymph glands also manufacture antibodies to help fight infection.

Lymphangiogram, Lymphangiography—Diagnostic method of studying the lymphatic system by infecting a material into the lymph channels that x-rays can detect. The image on x-ray film is the lymphangiogram.

Lymphatic Leukemia—Class of leukemias, involving primarily lymphatic cells, affecting children and adults.

Lymphedema—Painful swelling of soft tissues, caused by edema due to faulty lymphatic drainage. Swelling is often accompanied by decreased mobility in the affected limb, and by increased risk of infection.

Lymphocytes—One of several types of white blood cells that help fight infection.

Lymphosarcoma—Class of cancers of the lymphatic system.

M

Macular Degeneration of the Eye—Condition of the macula (area on the retina that provides detailed vision) in which impaired blood supply causes gradual vision loss.

Macule—General term for any discolored spot or patch on the skin, such as a freckle.

Malignant—Capable of causing great harm, including death. It usually refers to cancerous growth.

Magnetic Resonance Imaging—See *MRI*.

Mammogram, Mammography—Diagnostic method of studying the female breast by an x-ray technique that detects cancerous growths while they are still treatable. The image on x-ray film is the mammogram.

Manic-Depressive Illness—Mental illness in which behavior alternates between unrealistic enthusiasm and deep depression.

Manometer, Manometry—The measuring of pressure (of either liquid or gas) by means of a manometer.

MAO Inhibitors—See *Monoamine Oxidase Inhibitors.*

Marijuana—Mood-altering substance that is usually taken into the body by smoking. It is derived from Indian hemp or Cannabis leaves, stems and seed pods.

Marrow—Core of many bones, where most of the body's blood cells are produced.

Mastoiditis—Infection of the mastoid (bony area just behind the ear).

Mediators—Substances that: 1) help nerve impulses travel from one cell to the next; 2) participate in the allergic process.

Medic Alert—Nonprofit agency that maintains a medical-record system. Subscribers receive a bracelet or pendant that states their medical condition and provides a toll-free number for more information. The service can save the life of a person with a major medical condition who may not be able to provide medical history. For information write: Medic Alert Foundation, P.O. Box 1009, Turlock, CA 95381, (800) 344-3226.

Medical History—Essential facts about past and present medical conditions. Knowing your medical history enables your doctor to plan the best possible health care. Carry a card stating essential health details in your purse or wallet, and consider joining the Medic-Alert program (see above).

Meibomian Glands—Small glands on the inner eyelid. They secrete a fluid that helps the eyelids move easily over the surface of the eye.

Membrane—Thin tissue lining a body cavity, covering an internal organ or dividing a space.

Meninges—Three-layered membrane covering the brain.

Mental System (Mind)—Functions of the brain that provide the abilities to perceive surroundings, to have emotions, imagination, memory, will, and to process information.

Metastases—Cancerous cells or infectious germs that spread from their original location to other parts of the body.

Metatarsal Bones—Bones in the middle of the foot.

Midwife—Nurse with special training and experience in childbirth.

Mole—Skin lesion, often dark-brown or black.

Monoamine Oxidase (MAO) Inhibitors—Medications used to treat some forms of depression.

Motor Nerve—Nerve that transmits the stimulus that causes muscles to contract.

MRI (Magnetic Resonance Imaging)—A method of studying the body's internal structures that employs a strong magnetic field (rather than x-rays) and a computer to produce detailed pictures.

Mucous Membrane—Thin tissue lining internal cavities (nose, mouth, vagina) and tubular systems (respiratory and gastrointestinal) that produce mucus.

Mucus—Slippery liquid produced by the lining of internal cavities and tubular systems to protect tissue.

Muscle—Tissue that contracts, often with considerable force, when stimulated by the motor-nerve impulses.

Muscle Relaxants—Medications that relieve muscle spasms. They also can have significant side effects.

Muscle Tumors—Benign or cancerous tumors arising from muscle tissue.

Musculo-Skeletal System—The system of bones, muscles, ligaments and tendons that enable the body to move.

Myelogram, Myelography—Special x-ray of the spinal canal and spinal cord, requiring a spinal tap and injection of dye that is visible on x-ray film. Myelograms frequently are used to identify the location of ruptured disks.

Myoma—Tumor of the muscle.

Myopia—Disease of the eye in which close objects are clearly visible while distant objects are blurred. Also called nearsightedness.

Myringotomy—A surgical opening made through the eardrum to allow drainage of the middle ear cavity. It is usually performed on children.

N

Narcotics—Medications used to control severe pain. Narcotics should be used only when necessary because of their serious side effects: addiction; reduced breathing; nausea and vomiting; low blood pressure; reduced cough reflex; and constipation.

Nasogastric Tube—Slender tube passed through the nose into the stomach. It is used to drain away stomach secretions or to feed patients unable to eat normally.

Naturopathy—Health-care system relying on diet, sunshine, exercises, herbs and other nonmedicinal treatment.

Nausea—Unpleasant sensation of being about to vomit.

Nearsightedness—Same as *Myopia*.

Nebulizer—Device for administering medications used to treat asthma and similar conditions. It converts medication into a fine mist that is inhaled deeply into the lungs.

Necrosis—Death of living tissue.

Nerve-Block Local Anesthesia—See *Anesthesia, Nerve Block or Local*.

Nerve-Conduction Studies, Nerve Conduction Test—Diagnostic test that measures the rate at which an electrical impulse moves along a nerve. It is used to diagnose disorders of the peripheral nerves and muscle.

Nervous Breakdown—Nontechnical term for mental illness serious enough to interfere with daily activities.

Neuralgia—Severe, sharp pain along a nerve.

Neuritis—Inflammation of a nerve.

Neuro-Muscular System—Nerves and muscles acting together as a system to control body movements.

Neurological—Relating to the body's nervous system.

Neurologist—Doctor specially trained to diagnose and treat diseases of the nervous system.

Neuroma—Tumor arising from nerve tissue.

Neurosis—Mental illness in which anxiety is controlled by avoidance, blaming others, developing bodily complaints or other mechanisms.

Neurosurgeon—Doctor specially trained to diagnose and surgically treat diseases of the brain, spinal cord and nerves.

Nodes—See *Lymph Glands*.

Nodule—Small, rounded lump or firm swelling underneath the skin.

Nonsteroidal Anti-Inflammatory Drugs—Medications that control inflammation other than that caused by infection. Usually used to treat conditions of the joints and muscles and pain such as menstrual cramps or headache. "Nonsteroidal" means they are not steroid hormones such as cortisone, prednisone, dexamethasone and others.

Norwalk Virus—A type of virus that commonly causes epidemics of acute gastroenteritis with diarrhea and vomiting that lasts from 24 to 48 hours.

Nuclear Imaging—See *Radionuclide Scans*.

Nurse Practitioner (NP)—Registered nurse with additional medical training who can diagnose and treat common illness. Nurse practitioners usually work closely with a doctor, although in some states the practitioner can prescribe medicine and work independently of a physician.

Nutrient—Food or material containing elements needed to promote growth and development or to support life.

O

Obsessions—Unpleasant, frightening, senseless thoughts that won't go away despite reasoning.

Obstetrician-Gynecologist—Doctor specially trained to treat diseases of the female reproductive system and provide health care for pregnant mothers.

Occlusion—Closing or obstruction. Usually used to describe blockage in blood vessels. In dentistry, it means the way the teeth come together when the mouth is closed.

Occupational Therapy—Treatment for people disabled by accident or illness to relearn muscular control and coordination to cope with daily living tasks (dressing, eating, bathing, etc.) and if possible, to resume some form of employment.

Omentum—A fold of peritoneum which supports or connects abdominal structures.

Oncologist—Doctor specially trained to diagnose and treat cancer.

Operative Death Rate—Percentage of patients who die as a result of a certain surgery. It provides general measure of the risk of a surgery.

Ophthalmologist—Doctor specially trained to diagnose and treat diseases of the eyes.

Optic Neuritis—Inflammation of the nerve that conducts vision impulses from the eye to the brain.

Oral—Relating to the mouth.

Oral-Fecal—See *Fecal-Oral*.

Organic—Conditions or diseases resulting from change in body organs that can be measured or seen. Organic diseases are distinct from functional diseases in which no change can be observed in an organ that is not functioning normally.

Organic Psychosis—Mental illness that results from disease in the brain.

Orthodontia—Straightening teeth by applying temporary braces.

Orthopedic Surgeon (Orthopedist)—Doctor specially trained to diagnose and treat diseases of the muscles, bones and joints using surgical or mechanical means. A rheumatologist is an internist who diagnoses and treats similar conditions primarily with medications and other nonsurgical means.

Osteogenesis Imperfecta—Inherited condition in which the bones are brittle and easily broken.

Otolaryngologist—See *Ear, Nose and Throat Specialist*.

Ovary—Female sexual gland where eggs mature and ripen for fertilization.

Ovulation—Monthly process in which an egg leaves the ovary for possible fertilization by a sperm cell.

Ovum—Egg produced by the ovary.

P

Pain—Unpleasant sensation arising from stimulation of sensory nerves located in almost every part of the body. Disease, injury and strenuous activity can all cause pain.

Palate—Roof of the mouth, consisting of a bony front portion (hard palate) and a soft back portion (soft palate).

Palpitations—Irregular rapid heartbeat, noticeable to the patient.

Pancreas—Organ located on the back abdominal wall that produces and secretes digestive juices into the small intestine. It also produces and secretes insulin into the bloodstream to regulate the level of sugar and other nutrients.

Pancreatitis—Inflammation of the pancreas.

Pap Smear, Papanicolaou Smear—Test routinely done to screen for cancer of the cervix and uterus in an early and treatable stage.

Papule—Small, raised skin lesion. Papules may be red, brown, yellow, white or skin-colored. They may be flat-topped, pointed or dome-shaped.

Paranoia—Mental illness in which a person believes that he or she is being talked about or plotted against.

Parasite—Organism that lives within, upon or at the expense of another living organism. Human parasites include disease-causing agents such as amoebas or worms that infect the digestive system, or fungi that live on the skin.

Parasympathetic Nervous System—System of nerves that controls digestion, heartbeat, and relaxation or contraction of small muscles.

Parathyroid Glands—Small glands that control calcium levels in the blood and bones. They are located within or next to the thyroid glands at the base of the neck.

Passive Exercises—Exercises in which a therapist moves the arms and legs of a patient while the patient relaxes. These exercises keep the joints limber until the patient is able to move without assistance.

Patency—Blood vessels or any hollow organs that clog or become blocked are said to lose their patency.

Pathogenic—Disease-producing.

Pathological—Relating to an abnormal condition.

Pathological Examination—Laboratory study of abnormal tissue to establish or confirm a diagnosis.

Pediatrician—Doctor specially trained to care for children and adolescents, especially to foster normal growth and development.

Pediculicide—Medication that cures body lice (pediculosis). Usually applied to the skin.

Pelvic Examination—Examination of a woman's reproductive organs to diagnose pregnancy or detect diseases.

Pelvic Ultrasonography—Examination of a woman's reproductive organs that uses high-frequency sound waves to create an image. It is used to determine the age, size and position of a fetus in the uterus or to diagnose disease of the pelvic organs.

Pelvis—Lower part of the trunk of the body.

Penis—Male organ used for urination and sexual intercourse.

Perforation—Abnormal hole or opening.

Perforation, Intestinal—Complication of conditions such as ulcers, cancers, or injury to the digestive system. When this occurs, intestinal contents enter the abdominal cavity, causing severe inflammation.

Perfusionist—Medical professional who controls the heart-lung machine to sustain a patient's life during open-heart and lung-transplant surgery.

Perineum—Area between the vulva and anus in females and between the scrotum and anus in males.

Peripheral Nervous System—Nerves that connect to all parts of the body and carry information via electrical impulses to and from the brain and spinal cord.

Peripheral Vascular System—Network of arteries, veins and lymphatic channels supplying the head, arms and legs.

Perirectal—Skin and underlying tissue around the rectum.

Peristalsis—Rhythmic movements of hollow muscular organs (such as the intestines) that move contents (such as digestive material) in one direction.

Peritoneal Cavity—Space enclosed by the peritoneum.

Peritoneum—Very thin, two-layered tissue. One layer lines the outer surface of all the abdominal organs. The other layer lines the abdominal wall.

Peritonitis—Inflammation of the peritoneum.

Peritonsillar Abscess—Abscess forming in the back of the throat near the tonsils.

Pessary—Small ring-shaped device that is inserted into the vagina to help maintain the uterus in a normal position.

PET Scan—A sectional view of the body constructed by positron-emission tomography, which uses integrated x-ray and computing equipment.

pH Balance—Measure of blood's acidity or alkalinity. The pH is controlled by body fluids and electrolytes. Body tissues cannot function normally if the pH varies from a limited range.

Phallus—Penis.

Phenothiazine Drugs—Medications used to slow and regulate mental-system activity. Usually used to treat anxiety and other mental conditions; also useful in producing sleep.

Phlebitis—Inflammation of a vein.

Phlebotomy—Removing blood from the blood vessels. This was once believed to cure many diseases; today, it is done to remove blood for diagnostic testing.

Phobia—Fear that cannot be overcome by reason.

Photochemotherapy—A treatment for some skin disorders that combines oral medication with exposure to ultraviolet light rays for set periods of time.

Physical Therapy—Treatment of diseases of the bone, muscular and nervous systems to help restore normal function after disease or injury.

Physician's Assistant (PA)—Someone trained to do some of the simpler tasks ordinarily performed by a doctor. The PA works under the direction of the doctor.

Pilocarpine—Medication used principally in eye drops to treat glaucoma.

Pituitary Gland—Small endocrine gland at the base of the brain that controls growth and regulates other endocrine glands.

Placenta—Disk-shaped organ that attaches and grows inside the uterus during pregnancy. It enables the fetus to receive nutrients from and transfer natural wastes to the mother's bloodstream. The umbilical cord connects the placenta to the fetus.

Placenta previa—An abnormal placement of the placenta in the lower uterine segment, so that it covers or adjoins the internal opening of the uterine cervix.

Plaque—1) Small raised area of abnormal material on a surface such as the skin or lining of a blood vessel. 2) Mixture of bacteria and calcium deposited on the teeth that can cause cavities and gum diseases.

Plasma—Liquid part of blood that remains when blood cells are removed.

Plastic and Reconstructive Surgeon (Plastic Surgeon)—Doctor specially trained to perform plastic and reconstructive surgery.

Plastic and Reconstructive Surgery—Special surgery to repair and change body parts to improve function or appearance. The face, hands, breasts and skin are areas most frequently treated.

Platelet Count—Platelets are blood cells (much smaller than red or white blood cells) that assist in the blood-clotting process. A drop of blood contains about 12.5 million platelets. A platelet count determines if the number of platelets is normal.

Plethysmography—A study that estimates the amount of blood flowing in vessels by measuring changes in the size of a body part.

Pleura—Thin tissue lining the lungs and chest cavity. Inflammation of the pleura (pleurisy) is a painful condition caused by lung diseases.

Pleural Effusion (Pleural Fluid Effusion)—Fluid that collects around the lungs, usually caused by inflammation of the lungs and pleura or congestive-heart failure.

Pneumonia—Infection and inflammation of the lungs.

Pneumothorax—A collection of air or gas in the lung which causes collapse of all or part of a lung.

Podiatrist—Health-care professional trained in the medical and surgical treatment of foot diseases.

Polyp—A growth, often on a stalk arising from dry mucous membranes, such as in the nose, cervix or colon.

Portal-Vein System—Veins that drain blood from the gastrointestinal system. The smaller veins empty into the portal vein, which transports blood into the liver.

Postmature Infant—Infant that spends 3 weeks or more beyond the normal 39 weeks of pregnancy in the womb.

Postoperative—Period of recuperation and return to normal health after surgery.

Postural Drainage—Exercises and body positions that promote drainage of fluid and secretions that collect in the lungs and airways.

Potassium—Electrolyte present in all body cells, blood and body fluids. Potassium is important in maintaining normal heart contractions and the strength and contractions of all muscles. Foods high in potassium include: dried apricots and peaches; whole-grain cereals; plain cocoa, dried lentils and peas; bananas; and molasses.

Precancerous—Characteristic of a growth that has the potential to become cancerous.

Predisposition—Tendency. For example, a person who gets many infections has a predisposition to infection.

Preeclampsia—A toxic condition of late pregnancy characterized by a sudden rise in blood pressure, excessive weight gain, generalized edema, protein in the urine, severe headache and visual disturbances.

Premature Labor—Labor beginning before the usual 39 weeks of pregnancy.

Presbyopia—Form of nearsightedness that normally accompanies aging.

Primary Disorder—Basic disease that may result in complications. Diabetes mellitus, for example, is a primary disorder that often causes secondary complications involving the kidneys, blood vessels and eyes.

Proctoscope, Proctoscopy—Method of examining the rectum and lower part of the colon with a proctoscope, an optical instrument with a lighted tip.

Prolapse—Pushing or falling out of a part or an organ from its normal position.

Prolapsed (Dropped) Uterus—Uterus that has moved from its normal position because of loose pelvic muscles and ligaments. In severe cases, it can protrude completely outside the vagina.

Prophylaxis—Measures taken to prevent an illness.

Prophylaxis, Dental—Regular care (including cleaning) of the teeth and gums that helps prevent tooth decay and gum inflammation.

Prostaglandins—Natural substances found in semen, menstrual fluid and many body tissues. They are involved in basic body functions such as inflammation, immune response and activities of the lungs, heart, kidneys, uterus and digestive system.

Prostate (Prostate Gland)—Male sex gland located at the base of the urinary bladder. It produces a fluid that is added to sperm to produce semen.

Prosthesis—Artificial device used as a substitute for a missing or badly functioning part of the body.

Prothrombin Time—Test to measure one of the components of the body's blood-clotting mechanism. It is used to diagnose clotting diseases and to control blood-thinning (anticoagulation) in treatment of some diseases of the heart and blood vessels.

Protozoa—One-celled organisms, the smallest type of animal life. Amoeba are protozoa. Some protozoa can cause disease.

Psychiatrist—Doctor specially trained to diagnose and treat mental illnesses.

Psychoanalysis—Treatment of some mental illness that involves a detailed understanding of how past events in a person's life may have resulted in mental disturbances.

Psychogenic—A symptom with an emotional origin instead of an organic one.

Psychologist—Health-care professional specially trained to diagnose and treat some kinds of mental illness.

Psychopathy—Psychological or mental illness.

Psychosis—Mental illness characterized by deranged personality, loss of contact with reality, and possible delusions, hallucinations or illusions.

Psychosocial—Influences of society on growth and development.

Psychosomatic Illness—Illness in which thoughts and emotions play an important role.

Psychotherapist—Professional specially trained to diagnose and treat some mental illnesses.

Puberty—Period in early adolescence when hormonal changes bring about full sexual maturity and capacity to reproduce.

Pubic Bone—One of the bones of the pelvis located above the genitals in both sexes.

Pulmonary—Relating to the lungs and breathing.

Pulmonary Angiography—Studies of the arteries and veins in the lungs.

Pulmonary Hypertension—Increased pressure in the blood vessels of the lungs.

Pulse—Heartbeat (contraction of the heart) as felt in an artery. Heart rate is often measured by counting the pulse felt in the artery in the wrist.

Pus—Thick fluid, usually green or yellow, that forms to fight local infection. Pus often collects in an enclosed sac, an abscess, at the site of an infection.

PUVA—A type of phototherapy used to treat some skin conditions. It combines the use of a psoralen drug that sensitizes the skin to sunlight with a controlled dose of ultraviolet light.

Pyelogram, Intravenous—Method of studying the kidneys and urinary tract by injecting into the bloodstream a medication that x-rays can detect.

Pyelogram, Retrograde—Method of studying the kidneys, similar to an intravenous pyelogram, but in which the medication detected by x-rays is placed in the urinary system by a catheter inserted through the bladder into the ureters.

R

Radiation Therapy or Treatment—Use of high-energy waves (generated by special x-ray machines, cobalt machines and other devices) to treat some forms of cancer. Radiation destroys cancerous tissue but does little harm to healthy tissue.

Radioactive Chromium Studies—Diagnostic method used to measure total blood in the body.

Radioactive Iodine Uptake and Scan—Same as *Thyroid Scan*.

Radioactive Studies—Same as *Radioisotope Studies*.

Radioactive Technetium 99 Scan—Radioisotope scan method used to diagnose some disorders of the heart, liver, spleen and other organs.

Radioisotope—Radioactive form of chemicals normally present in the body.

Radioisotope Scan—Scan of radioisotopes given orally or intravenously to a patient that become concentrated in organs such as the heart, lungs or brain. Instruments measure the radiation given off by the radioisotopes and create a photographic image of the organ being studied.

Radioisotope Studies—Radioisotopes are chemical elements that give off radiation. A radioisotope of a chemical element normally present in the body (such as carbon), if injected into the body, will mix with the nonisotopes. The body doesn't know the difference, but radiation from the isotopes can be detected with special instruments. Determining where radioisotopes go in the body allows diagnosis of diseases that cannot be detected otherwise.

Radioisotope Therapy—Treatment of some cancers with radioisotopes.

Radiologist—Doctor specially trained to use x-rays and other kinds of radiation in diagnosis and treatment.

Radionuclide Scan—Method of studying various body functions by means of photographs or videotape taken by special camera or a scanner after intravenous injection of radioactive chemical.

Rebound Phenomenon—A reversed response to the withdrawal of a stimulus. A common rebound phenomenon occurs when nose drops, which decrease congestion, wear off. The nasal congestion that develops on the rebound is greater than that which existed before the drops were administered.

Recovery Room—Specially equipped and staffed area of a hospital for observing and caring for a patient who has just undergone surgery. Postoperative patients usually remain in the recovery room until they are awake and their vital signs (blood pressure, pulse and respiration) are satisfactory.

Rectum—End of the large intestine, located in the pelvis below the sigmoid colon and above the anus.

Regenerate—Ability of some parts of the body to grow back to normal after being damaged.

Regurgitate—To vomit.

Relapse—Stage of illness in which the patient gets worse after having improved.

Remission—Stage of a chronic illness when the patient's condition improves.

Renal—Having to do with the kidneys.

Renal Dialysis—Mechanical and chemical method of removing normal wastes from the body of a patient whose kidneys cannot function adequately. It is also used to remove harmful poison or a drug overdose from the bloodstream.

Reproductive Organs, Female—Organs of a woman's body that enable her to become pregnant and deliver a baby. The major organs are the vagina, uterus, Fallopian tubes and ovaries.

Reproductive Organs, Male—Organs of a man's body that enable him to produce sperm and impregnate the woman. The major organs are the penis, testicles, seminal vesicles and prostate gland.

Reproductive System—Body system enabling impregnation and delivery of a baby. It also provides characteristic male or female appearance.

Resect—Surgical removal of a part of the body.

Respiratory-Distress Syndrome—A condition of newborn infants (often born prematurely) in which the lungs cannot supply adequate oxygen to the body.

Retained Placenta—Condition occurring immediately after childbirth in which part of the placenta remains attached to the uterus, creating a risk of serious bleeding or infection.

Retina—Light-sensitive part of the eye at the back of the eyeball on which the lens focuses images. The retina converts the image to impulses that go to the brain.

Retinal-Vein Occlusion—Condition in which a clot forms in the vein supplying the retina with blood.

Retinoblastoma—Cancerous tumor that forms in the eye of an infant.

Retrograde Pyelography—See *Pyelogram, Retrograde.*

Retrovirus—Group of viruses that cause HIV (human immunodeficiency virus) and some types of lymphoma and leukemia.

Rh Negative Blood—A subtype of red blood cells. Blood subtypes are inherited. The major subtypes are types A, B, O and Rh negative.

Rheumatologist—A specialist in internal medicine who subspecializes in medical diagnosis and treatment of rheumatic and arthritic disorders.

Rhinitis—Swelling of the nasal passages.

Rinne Test—Test using a tuning fork to diagnose hearing disorders.

Rotavirus—A type of virus that is often responsible for acute gastroenteritis in infants and for diarrhea in young children.

Rubin's Insufflation Test—Test used in diagnosing fertility problems in women. A harmless gas is introduced into the uterus to determine if there is a blockage in the Fallopian tubes.

S

Sacroiliac Region—Area of the lower back where the spine meets the pelvic bone.

Saline—Salt-containing solution similar to normal body fluid that is given intravenously to help correct fluid and electrolyte imbalances.

Salivary Glands—Glands located inside the mouth around the jaw that secrete saliva into the mouth.

Saphenous-Femoral Vein System—Network of large veins in the legs that helps return blood from the leg to the inferior vena cava, then to the heart.

Scale, Scaling—Flakes of dried skin that form as whitish skin lesions.

Schizophrenia—Mental illness characterized by a distorted sense of reality, bizarre behavior and fragmentation of the personality.

Sciatic Nerve—Large nerve that begins at the base of the spine and passes through the buttocks down the back side of the thigh and down the leg.

Sciatica—Painful condition resulting from irritation of the sciatic nerve.

Scleritis—Inflammation of the sclera (the white of the eye).

Scopolamine—Medication used to treat hyperactive or spastic conditions of the digestive system and to prevent motion sickness.

Scrotum—Organ of the male reproductive system that contains the testicles, blood vessels and the vas deferens.

Scurvy—Disease of bones, gums and blood vessels that is caused by a deficiency of vitamin C.

Second Molars—Permanent grinding teeth that appear at about age 11 to 13.

Secondary Infection—Infection that results from some other problem. It may occur after surgery or develop during antibiotic treatment of another infection.

Sedative—Medication used to produce relaxation or sleep.

Sedative-Hypnotics—Class of medications that help relieve anxiety and promote sleep.

Sedimentation Rate—Blood test measuring the rate that blood settles in a test tube. It identifies infection, inflammation or tissue damage.

Self-Care—Treatment that patients can administer for themselves.

Seminal Vesicles—Small sacs next to the prostate that help make and store seminal fluid and contract to eject semen.

Senile Dementia—Permanent loss of mental functions of older persons, resulting from conditions such as Alzheimer's disease and atherosclerosis (hardening of the arteries).

Senile Keratosis—Same as *Seborrheic Keratoses*. (See *Illness section*.)

Sensitivity Studies (Antibiotics)—Laboratory method of determining which antibiotic will most likely be successful in treating infections caused by bacteria.

Sensory—Ability to feel or experience sensations such as sound, light or pain.

Septic—Infected.

Serological Tests—Tests of serum (blood without cells) used to diagnose a variety of diseases, especially infections and autoimmune conditions.

Serum—Liquid portion of blood that remains after blood cells and blood clots have been removed.

Serum Alkaline Phosphatase—Material present in excessive amounts in the blood of patients with some bone and liver diseases.

Serum Electrolytes—Same as *Electrolytes*.

Sesamoid Bones—Small oval-shaped bones in the tendons of the hands and feet.

Sever's Disease—Painful condition of the heel bone of growing children.

Sexual Dysfunction—Inability to participate in sexual relations that are satisfactory for both partners.

Shave Biopsy—Procedure to diagnose skin disorders in which a thin layer of tissue from under a skin lesion is shaved away for laboratory examination.

Shock—Condition in which the blood pressure falls below the level needed to supply blood to the body. Signs and symptoms include weakness, paleness, rapid heartbeat, dry mouth, cold sweat and feelings of doom.

Sick-Sinus Syndrome—Form of heart-rhythm disorder (arrhythmia).

Sigmoid Colon—Lower part of the large colon (intestine) located in the pelvis just above the rectum.

Sigmoidoscope, Sigmoidoscopy—Same as *Proctoscope, Proctoscopy*.

Signs—Evidence of disease that can be observed and measured, in contrast to symptoms, which only patients can experience. For example, blood-pressure measurement or red tonsils are signs; headache or nausea are symptoms.

Silicone—Artificial compound used by plastic and reconstructive surgeons to reshape parts of the body, such as the breast.

Silver Nitrate—Chemical used for cautery.

Sims-Huhner Test—Test used in diagnosis of reasons for infertility in women in which the mucus from the cervix is examined, especially for presence of sperm after sexual intercourse.

Skin Clips—Small U-shaped metal strips used instead of stitches to close skin that has been incised during surgery.

Skin Tests for Allergy—Diagnostic method used to determine whether a particular substance is causing allergic reactions. The test is carried out by introducing a small amount of the suspected material, such as pollen or dust, under the skin or on the skin. If inflammation results, the patient is allergic to the material.

Sleep Inducers—Medications used to produce sleep.

Sleep-Study Laboratory—Laboratory where persons are studied with sensitive instruments while asleep. Information from sleep study aids in diagnosis of sleep disorders.

Slow Viruses—Group of viruses that infect the brain but do not cause disease until many years afterward.

Small-Bowel Series—A test used to look for blockage in the small bowel, in which the patient swallows a radiopaque fluid (barium), which allows intermittent x-rays to be taken to follow the flow of the fluid through the eposhagus, stomach, duodenum and then through the entire small intestine to the colon.

Soaks—Applying moisture—either plain water or water with dissolved medicines—to an inflamed area of the skin.

Soft Palate—Fleshy part of the roof of the mouth close to the throat.

Sonogram, Sonography—See *Ultrasound*.

Spasmodic—Sudden intermittent symptom, or intermittent muscle spasm.

Spastic, Spasticity—A description of muscles that are continuously contracting and in a state of excessive tension.

Speculum—Instrument used to examine the interior of openings such as the vagina, nose, ear or rectum.

Sperm—Male reproductive cells manufactured in testicles and ejaculated in semen.

Spherocytosis—Abnormally shaped red blood cells caused by some anemias. These cells are sphere-shaped, in contrast to the doughnut shape of normal red blood cells.

Spikes, Temperature—High but brief episodes of fever.

Spina Bifida—Congenital (inherited) disorder in which the base of the spine remains open, sometimes exposing the spinal cord and nerves.

Spinal Anesthesia—Method to provide anesthesia to the lower body by injecting an anesthetic into the fluid in the space that surrounds the lower spinal cord.

Spirometry—Test of lung (pulmonary) function.

Spleen—A large organ in the upper abdomen on the left side, located close to the left side of the stomach. It is the largest structure of the lymph system. The spleen causes disintegration of old red blood cells in adults, manufactures red blood cells in the fetus and newborn, and serves as an important reservoir of blood.

Splenic-Vein Thrombosis—Clot in the major vein that carries blood away from the spleen.

Splints—Rigid supports, made of metal, plastic or plaster, used to immobilize an injured or inflamed part of the body. Splints are used temporarily in the case of injury, following some surgical procedures on joints or ligaments, or occasionally in the case of arthritis.

Spore—Microscopic seed form of fungi. Spores are extremely hardy and survive extremes of temperature. If they enter the body of a susceptible person, they can cause fungal disease.

Sputum—Secretion of the lungs, coughed up in large amounts in some lung diseases.

Staphylococcus—Bacteria which frequently cause boils, abscesses, pneumonias, bone infections and infections in other tissues or organs.

Staples—Small U-shaped metal wires used in place of stitches to close incised skin after some surgeries, especially in the digestive system. Also used to close off some portions of the stomach during operations for extreme obesity.

Stenosis—Constriction or narrowing of a passage or opening.

Sterilized—1) Made completely free of all germs, usually by steam heat, toxic gas or chemicals. All instruments used in surgeries are sterilized, as is most other medical equipment. 2) Made unable to conceive children.

Steroids—Medications that resemble hormones produced by the cortex of the adrenal glands, ovaries and testicles.

Stethoscope—Instrument used to listen to the sounds produced by the heart, lungs, blood vessels and pregnant uterus.

Still's Disease—Form of arthritis in children similar to rheumatoid arthritis in adults.

Stimulant Drugs—Medications that increase the activity of the brain and nervous system.

Stomatitis—Inflammation of the mouth.

Stool—Feces.

Streptococcus—Bacteria that cause illnesses such as laryngitis, cellulitis of the skin, pneumonia, meningitis and others. If not treated, streptococcal infections may also cause serious heart and kidney diseases as complications that appear after the original infection has cleared.

Stricture—An abnormal narrowing of a bodily passage.

Subcutaneous—Under the skin.

Sublingual Salivary Glands—Small glands near the base of the tongue that secrete saliva into the mouth.

Submaxillary Salivary Glands—Small glands near the jaw that secrete saliva into the mouth.

Sulfonamides (Sulfa Drugs)—Class of drugs used to fight infections.

Sulfonurea Drugs—Medications taken orally to treat some forms of diabetes mellitus.

Surgery—Treatment in which the body is restored to a healthy condition by physical methods (or operations) such as cutting, removing, replacing, straightening, repairing or joining.

Surgical Suite—Group of rooms used to perform surgery. In addition to operating rooms, where surgery takes place, there are supply areas, a recovery room, administrative rooms and a lounge for the staff to rest between surgeries.

Suture—Thread-like material used to hold tissues or skin edges together.

Symmetry, Symmetrical—Refers to the arrangement of the body in pairs, such as two arms, legs, kidneys, lungs, etc.

Sympathomimetics—Medications similar to adrenalin in their actions.

Symptoms—Effects of disease that only the patient can experience, such as pain, nausea, dizziness, anxiety, depression and others.

Synovial Membranes—Delicate tissue that lines the inside of joints.

Systemic—Conditions that affect most or all of the body, in contrast to conditions that affect only a limited area. For example, diabetes mellitus is a systemic condition; an abscess is a local condition.

T

Tartar—Hard deposit that forms on the teeth and causes inflammation of the gums.

Temperature Spike—See *Spikes, Temperature*.

Temporomandibular Joint—Joint that joins the jaw to the other head bones.

Tenderness—Condition that causes pain when pressure is applied.

Tendon—Tough cord of tissue at the end of muscles that attach to bone. Tendons transmit the force of muscle contraction to cause movement.

Testes or Testicles—Male sex glands that produce sex hormones and sperm.

Therapeutic Trial—Form of diagnosis and treatment where medication is used even though the diagnosis is not firmly established. If the patient improves after treatment with a medication known to be useful in treating a specific condition, the improvement suggests that the specific disease was present. Therapeutic trials are somewhat risky and are used only when other forms of diagnosis and treatment have failed.

Therapist—Health-care professional specially trained to provide therapy.

Thermogram, Thermography—Method of diagnosis that measures body heat. The area being studied is scanned by a heat-sensitive instrument capable of producing an image (thermogram) of areas of increased heat. They are useful in studying female breast tumors and some blood-vessel conditions.

Thiazide Diuretics—Class of medications that promote excretion of excess fluids by the kidneys.

Third Molars—Permanent grinding teeth that appear at about age 17 to 25.

Thoracic Duct—The largest channel of the lymphatic system, through which lymph fluid enters the vena cava.

Thoracic Spine—That part of the spinal column below the neck and above the back. Ribs attach to the thoracic spine.

Thoracic Surgeon—A surgeon who specializes in surgical treatment of disorders of the organs in the thorax (chest), including lungs, pericardium, heart, pleura (covering of lungs), bronchial tubes and large blood vessels.

Thyroglossal Duct—Small passageway, normally closed, located in the upper neck. It extends from the back of the tongue to just above the larynx. If an abnormally open duct becomes filled with fluid, a thyroglossal cyst results.

Thyroid Cartilage—Larynx (also called the voice box, or Adam's apple), made of semi-hard cartilage.

Thyroid Gland—Endocrine gland located in the lower neck next to the trachea that produces hormones that regulate the rate at which all body cells function. Thyroid hormones are also essential for normal growth and development.

Thyroid Scan—Method of examination of the thyroid gland in which a small amount of radioactive iodine introduced into the body collects in the thyroid gland. An instrument passed over the thyroid produces an image of the gland based on the concentration of the radioactive iodine.

Thrombocytopenia—A persistent decrease in the number of blood platelets, often associated with hemmorhaging.

TIA—See Transient Ischemic Attack.

Ticks—Small biting insects that may cause inflammation of the skin or serious infections such as Rocky Mountain spotted fever.

Tics—Brief, uncontrollable muscle spasms. Tics usually involve the face and the shoulders.

Tissue—Building blocks of body organs; living cells all of one type.

Tonsils—Lymphatic tissues that help fight infection located at the entrance of the throat. They frequently become infected, especially in children.

Topical—Medications applied to the skin, conjunctiva, or mucous membrane of the mouth, nose, vagina or rectum.

Tourette's Syndrome—A rare disorder of movement. It involves repetitive grimaces and tics, usually of the head and neck, sometimes arms, legs and trunk. Involuntary noises and foul language may occur.

Tourniquet—Cord or band wrapped around an arm or leg tightly enough to stop blood circulation temporarily.

Toxic, Toxicity—Harmful; capable of causing body damage.

Toxin—Poison. Usually refers to the chemicals produced by some living organisms that harm the human body.

Tracheostomy Tube—A tube which is connected to an artificial opening into the trachea through the neck, and through which breathing is performed.

Traction—Method of treating some conditions of bones, muscles and ligaments by exerting a steady pull on the affected parts. Some bone fractures and back pain due to a ruptured disk are treated this way.

Tranquilizer—Medication used to help diminish anxiety and to produce calmness.

Tranquilizers, Benzodiazepine—Class of tranquilizers commonly used to treat anxiety, nervousness or tension.

Transfuse—To give a patient blood, necessary in treatment of some conditions.

Transfusion—Process of introducing blood through a needle placed in the patient's vein.

Transfusion Reaction—Undesirable symptom or condition resulting from a blood transfusion.

Transient Ischemic Attack, TIA—A temporary decrease in the blood supply to part of the brain which temporarily interferes with normal brain function.

Transmission, Transmit—Passing a disease to another person.

Transplant, Transplantation—Living organ (such as kidney, cornea, heart, bone marrow or skin), removed from one person (donor), and placed in the body of another (recipient).

Transverse Colon—Middle part of the colon (intestine), lying horizontally in the middle or upper abdomen.

Trauma—Force that injures or damages any part of the body.

Tricyclic Antidepressant Drugs (Tricyclics)—Class of medications used to treat depression.

Trophoblastic Tumors—See *Hydatidiform Mole*.

Tube Feeding—Providing nutrients through a small tube placed in the stomach of patients who are unable to eat. The tube may pass through the nose to the stomach or be inserted through an incision in the stomach.

Tuberous Sclerosis—Rare inherited condition of the skin, nervous system and other organs of the body.

Tumor—Literally, a swelling; usually used to refer to a benign or cancerous growth.

Tympanogram—A test which measures the function of the tympanic membrane in the middle ear.

U

Ulceration—Wearing away of the surface or lining of an organ, exposing underlying tissue. Ulceration of the lining of the stomach exposes blood vessels, which may bleed. Ulceration may erode through the wall of an organ (perforation). Ulceration frequently affects the skin, if rubbed excessively or if diseased.

Ultrasonography, Ultrasound—Diagnostic method in which high-frequency (ultrasound) sound waves are transmitted into the body. Their reflections create images of body organs.

Ultrasound Treatment—Method of treatment in which high-energy sound waves are focused on the affected area, producing mild heat that helps relieve inflammation. It is especially useful in treatment of muscular symptoms.

Underlying—Beneath, below or more basic. Thus, losing weight may result from an underlying condition such as diabetes mellitus or cancer.

Upper Gastrointestinal Series—X-ray examination of the esophagus, stomach and duodenum accomplished by having the patient swallow barium solution that x-rays can detect.

Upper Respiratory System—Upper part of the breathing system, consisting of the nose, throat, larynx, trachea and bronchial tubes.

Uremia—A serious condition associated with kidney failure in which body wastes build up in the blood and body tissues.

Ureters—Slender muscular tubes that carry urine from the kidneys to the urinary bladder, where it is stored until eliminated from the body.

Urethra—Tubular passageway extending from the urinary bladder to the outside of the body.

Uric Acid—Chemical normally produced in the body from metabolism or breakdown of protein and eliminated in the urine. If the level of uric acid rises in the body as a result of disease, gout or kidney stones may result.

Urinalysis—Laboratory test performed on a urine sample that helps diagnose diseases of the kidney and other parts of the body.

Urinary Bladder—Muscular sac in the lower abdomen that stores urine brought to it from the kidneys by the ureters. The bladder stores urine until it can be eliminated through the urethra by contractions of the bladder muscles.

Urinary Studies—Laboratory or x-ray tests of the urinary tract.

Urinary Tract—Organs that produce, store and eliminate urine. The organs are the kidneys, ureters, urinary bladder and urethra.

Urography—See *Intravenous Urography*.

Uterus—Organ of the female reproductive system on the wall of which the fertilized egg (ovum) attaches and develops to form a fetus.

Uveitis—Inflammation of the parts of the eyes that make up the iris (the colored tissue encircling the clear center, the pupil).

Uvula—Soft tissue hanging down from the soft palate at the back of the throat.

V

Vaccination—Method of providing protection against disease (immunity) by giving a patient a small amount of the disease-causing germ that is weakened, killed or otherwise modified so that it cannot itself cause disease. Same as *Immunization*.

Vaccine—Medication used to provide immunity by vaccination. Vaccines are given mostly by injection or by mouth.

Vagus Nerve—Long cranial nerve, arising in the base of the brain and passing to the chest and abdomen. It helps regulate heart rate, breathing, swallowing, digestion and many other body functions.

Varicose—Swollen and twisting; usually used to describe varicose veins.

Vas Deferens—Tube that carries sperm manufactured by the testicles toward the prostate gland and seminal vesicles.

Vasculitis—Inflammation of blood vessels, the basis of many illnesses.

Vasoconstrictor Drugs—Medications that cause blood vessels to contract, tighten or become smaller.

Vasodilator Drugs—Medications that cause small arteries to widen, providing more blood to an area of the body where the blood vessels are constricted by spasm, narrowed or obstructed.

Vector—1) An imaginary line that represents both direction and quantity used to study electrocardiograms (ECG's). 2) An agent that transmits infectious germs from one organism to another.

Veins—Blood vessels that return blood from body organs to the heart and lungs. Veins are much thinner than arteries. Veins carry blood at a much lower pressure than do arteries.

Vena Cava—Largest vein in the body. It collects blood from the venous system and carries it to the heart.

Vena Cavography—Method of studying the vena cava by injecting into the bloodstream a medication that x-rays can detect.

Venereal—Related to sexual intercourse or sexual contact. Venereal diseases such as genital herpes, gonorrhea or syphilis are now usually referred to as sexually transmitted diseases (STD's).

Venography—Method of studying the veins by injecting into the bloodstream a medication that x-rays can detect.

Venous Stasis Ulcer—An open sore on the skin of the lower extremities, caused when normal outflow of blood in the legs is obstructed (as in deep venous thrombosis). The resulting pressure from the back-up of blood causes leaking and weeping of fluid into the surrounding tissues (edema), which then stretches the arteries and deprives the skin of oxygen. The skin then breaks down into open sores which leak serum and are prone to infection.

Venous System—Network of veins that extend from all body organs and transport blood back to the heart.

Ventricles—Chambers containing fluid. The ventricles of the heart pump blood; ventricles of the brain contain cerebrospinal fluid.

Ventricular Aneurysm—Ballooning of the wall of the heart resulting from a weakening of the heart muscle, a complication of scarring from a previous heart attack.

Vertebrae—Bones of the spine that form the vertebral column (backbone).

Vertebral Column—The spine; the bones of the back.

Virulent—Extremely dangerous or harmful. Virulent bacteria are ones capable of causing diseases.

Viruses—Small germs responsible for a variety of infectious illnesses. Viruses are not alive until they enter cells of the body, where they grow and reproduce, causing viral illnesses.

Visual Acuity—Clarity with which objects are seen.

Vitamins—Chemical substances found in food that are necessary for healthy body growth, function and tissue repair.

Vitreous—Clear fluid that fills much of the eye.

Vocal Cords—Two narrow bands of fibrous and muscular tissue in the larynx that vibrate to create the sounds of the voice.

Volvulus—Twisting of loops of intestines, which become closed off (obstructed) and may lose their blood supply.

Vulva—The external genitalia of the female including the clitoris and vaginal lips.

W

Warts—Small, often hard and rough skin growths caused by viruses that infect the skin.

Wasting of Body or Muscles—Severe loss of body tissues (other than surplus fat), especially muscles and vital organs, resulting in weakness, susceptibility to infection, bone fractures and sometimes death.

Weber Test—Hearing test performed with a tuning fork.

Wheezes—High-pitched sounds and whistles produced in the lungs where secretions have partially blocked air passages.

Wheal—A temporary skin elevation usually a result of an allergic reaction.

Whirlpool Treatment—Method of treating minor blood-vessel and musculo-skeletal diseases by immersion in a pool where jets of warm water enter and swirl under high pressure.

Wisdom Teeth—Same as *Third Molars*.

X

X-Rays—High energy, invisible waves capable of penetrating the body and creating shadows on photographic film. The shadows provide images of the body tissues through which the x-rays pass.

Xeroradiogram—Method of x-ray diagnosis, usually of the female breast, which uses a process similar to that used to produce photocopies.

Xerosis—Abnormal dryness.

Y

Yellow Fever—An acute disease caused by a virus spread by insect bites. Usually seen in Africa and South America.

Yersinia Infection—A type of foodborne bacteria that can cause gastroenteritis and diarrhea.

Z

Zoster—"Girdle," used to describe a form of virus infection (herpes zoster, shingles) that often produces bands of inflammation across the chest or abdomen.

Zygote—The fertilized egg before division.

RESOURCES FOR ADDITIONAL INFORMATION

The following list provides names of organizations and support groups that offer medical information and assistance by phone, mail or the internet. If you are unable to find a listing for your disorder or problem, call the National Health Information Center at (800) 336-4797 or the National Organization for Rare Disorders information line, (800) 999-NORD.

Many of the national organizations listed below have local chapters. Check your telephone directory for telephone numbers and addresses.

Acne Rosacea
National Rosacea Society
220 S. Cook St., Suite 201
Barrington, IL 60010
(708) 382-8971
www.rosacea.org

Aging
National Council on the Aging
409 Third St., S.W., 2nd Flr.
Washington, DC 20024
(202) 479-1200

AIDS
National AIDS Hotline
(800) 342-2437
(800) 342-7432 (Spanish)

Alcoholism
Alcoholics Anonymous
475 Riverside Dr., 11th Flr.
New York, NY 10115
(212) 870-3400
www.alcoholics-anonymous.org

National Council on Alcoholism
12 W. 21st St.
New York, NY 10010
(800) 622-2255

Allergies
American Academy of Allergy and
  Immunology
611 Wells St.
Milwaukee, WI 53202
(800) 822-ASMA

Alopecia Areata
National Alopecia Areata Foundation
714 C St., Suite 216
San Rafael, CA 94901
(415) 456-4644
www.alopeciaareata.com

Alzheimer's
Alzheimer's Disease and Related Orders
  Association
5252 N. Western Ave.
Chicago, IL 60601
(800) 621-0379
(800) 572-6037 (IL only)

Alzheimer's Association
919 N. Michigan Ave., Suite 1000
Chicago, IL 60611-1676
(800) 272-3900
www.alz.org

Amyotrophic Lateral Sclerosis
Amyotrophic Lateral Sclerosis Society
  of America
15300 Ventura Blvd., Suite 315
P. O. Box 5951
Sherman Oaks, CA 91403
(800) 782-4747

Anorexia Nervosa
Anorexia Nervosa & Related Eating
  Disorders
P.O. Box 5102
Eugene, OR 97405
(503) 344-1144
www.anred.com

Anxiety
Anxiety Disorders Association of
  America
6000 Executive Blvd., Suite 513
Rockville, MD 20852
(301) 231-9350
www.adaa.org

National Institute of Mental Health
(NIMH)
National Anxiety Awareness Program
9000 Rockville Pike
Bethesda, ND 20892.
(800) 64-PANIC
www.nimh.nih.gov

Arthritis
Arthritis Foundation
1314 Spring St. N.W.
Atlanta, GA 30309
(800) 283-7800
www.arthritis.org

Asbestosis
Asbestos Victims of America
P.O. Box 559
Capitola, CA 95010
(408) 476-3646

American Lung Association
1740 Broadway
New York, NY 10019
(800) 586-4872
www.lungusa.org

Asthma
Asthma & Allergy Foundation of
America
1717 Massachusetts Ave., Suite 305
Washington, DC 20036
(800) 7-ASTHMA
www.aafa.org

National Asthma-Center Lung Line
1400 Jackson St.
Denver, CO 80206
(800) 222-LUNG

Atelectasis—See Lung Disorders

Atherosclerosis—See Heart Disorders

Atrial Fibrillation—See Heart Disorders

Bed Wetting
American Academy of Child and
Adolescent Psychology
(202) 966-7300

American Sleep Disorders
1610 14th St., Suite 300
Rochester, MN 55901
(507) 287-6006
www.asda.org

Birth Control & Family Planning
Planned Parenthood Federation of
America
810 Seventh Ave.
New York, NY 10019
(212) 541-7800
www.plannedparenthood.org

Birth Defects
National Foundation March of Dimes
1275 Mamaroneck Ave.
White Plains, NY 10605
(914) 428-7100

Blindness
American Foundation for the Blind (AFB)
15 W. 16th St.
New York, NY 10011
(800) 232-5463
www.igc.org/afb

American Council of the Blind
(800) 424-8666
(202) 393-3666 (DC only)
www.acb.org

Brain Tumor
American Brain Tumor Association
2720 River Rd Ste 146
Des Plaines, IL 60018
(800) 886-2282

Brain Disorders
Brain Research Foundation
208 S. LaSalle St., Suite 1426
Chicago, IL 60604
(312) 782-4311

Breast Cancer
Y-ME National Organization for Breast
Cancer
18220 Harwood Ave.
Homewood, IL 60430
(800) 221-2141
www.y-me.org

Bronchiectasis—See Lung Disorders

Bronchitis—See Lung Disorders

Bulimia
Anorexia Nervosa & Related Eating
  Disorders
P.O. Box 5102
Eugene, OR 97405
(503) 344-1144
www.anred.org

Burns
National Burn Victim Foundation
32-34 Scotland Rd.
Orange, NJ 07050
(201) 676-7700

Cancer
American Cancer Society
1599 Clifton Rd.
Atlanta, GA 30329
(800) ACS-2345
www.cancer.org

National Cancer Institute Cancer
  Information Service
(800) 4-CANCER

Celiac Disease
American Celiac Society/Dietary Support
  Coalition
58 Musano Ct.
West Orange, NJ 07052
(201) 325-8837

Cerebral Palsy
United Cerebral Palsy Association
(800) 872-5827

Cholecystitis or Cholangitis—See
Digestive Diseases

Chronic Fatigue Syndrome
Chronic Fatigue and Immune Dysfunction
  Syndrome (CFIDS) Association
P.O. Box 220398
Charlotte, NC 28222-0398
(800) 442-3437
www.cfids.org

Chronic Obstructive Pulmonary
Disease—See Lung Disorders

Cirrhosis of the Liver—See Liver
Disorders

Colitis, Ulcerative
Crohn's and Colitis Foundation of
  America
11th Flr., Park Ave. S.
New York City, NY 10016
(800) 343-3637
www.ccfa.org

Cor Pulmonale—See Heart Disorders

Coronary Artery Disease—See Heart
Disorders

Crohn's Disease
Crohn's and Colitis Foundation of
  America
11th Flr., Park Ave. S.
New York City, NY 10016
(800) 343-3637
www.ccfa.org

Cystic Fibrosis
Cystic Fibrosis Foundation
6931 Arlington Rd., Suite 2000
Bethesda, MD 20814
(800) 344-4823
www.cff.org/default.htm

Dementia—See Alzheimer's Disease

Dental Problems
American Dental Association
211 E. Chicago Ave.
Chicago, IL 60611
(312) 440-2500

Depression
National Foundation for Depressive
  Illness
245 7th Ave.
New York, NY 10001
(800) 248-4344

National Institute of Mental Health
  (NIMH)
National Anxiety Awareness Program
9000 Rockville Pike
Bethesda, MD 20892
(800) 64-PANIC
www.nimh.nih.gov

Diabetes
American Diabetes Association
P.O. Box 25757
1660 Duke St.
Alexandria, VA 22314
(800) 232-3472
www.diabetes.org

Digestive Diseases
National Digestive Diseases
    Information Clearinghouse
Box NDDIC
Bethesda, MD 20892
(301) 654-3810

Diverticular Disease—See Digestive
Diseases

Down Syndrome
National Down Syndrome Congress
1800 Dempster St.
Park Ridge, IL 60068-1146
(800) 232-NDSC

National Down Syndrome Society
666 Broadway
New York, NY 10012
(800) 221-4602

Drug Abuse
Cocaine Abuse Hotline
(800) COCAINE

Do It Now Foundation
6423 S. Ash Ave.
Tempe, AZ 85283
(602) 257-0797

Dysthymia—See Depression or Mental
Health

**Endocrine Disorders (Thyroid,
Parathyroid, Pituitary, Sex Glands,
Adrenals)**
National Institute of Metabolic Disease
9650 Rockville Pike
Bethesda, MD 20205

Endometriosis
Endometriosis Association
8585 N. 76th Pl.
Milwaukee, WI 53223
(800) 992-ENDO
www.endometriosisassn.org

Fertility Problems
Fertility Research Foundation
1430 Second Ave., Suite 103
New York, NY 10021
(212) 744-5500
www.frfbaby.com

Food Allergy
Food Allergy Network
4744 Holly Ave.
Fairfax, VA 22030-5647
(703) 691-3179
www.foodallergy.org

Foot Disorders
American Podiatry Association
9312 Old Georgetown Rd.
Bethesda, MD 20814-1621
(800) FOOTCARE

Gallstones—See Digestive Diseases

Glaucoma
Foundation for Glaucoma Research
490 Post St., Suite 830
San Francisco, CA 94102
(415) 986-3162

Glomerulonephritis—See Kidney
Disorders

Gonorrhea—See Sexually Transmitted
Diseases

Guillain-Barré
Guillain-Barré Syndrome Foundation
P.O. Box 262
Wynnewood, PA 19096
(610) 667-0131
www.webmast.com/gbs

Head Injury
National Head Injury Foundation
1776 Massachusetts Ave. N.W.
Washington, DC 20026
(800) 444-6443

Headache
National Headache Foundation
5252 N. Western Ave.
Chicago, IL 60625
(800) 843-2256
(800) 523-88658 (IL only)
www.headaches.org

Hearing Disorders
National Association of the Deaf
814 Thayer Ave.
Silver Spring, MD 20910
(301) 587-1788
www.nad.org

American Speech-Language-Hearing
    Association
10801 Rockville Pike
Rockville, MD 20852
(800) 638-8255

Dial a Hearing Test
(800) 222-EARS
(800) 345-EARS (PA only)

National Hearing Aid Helpline
20361 Middlebelt Rd.
Livonia, MI 48152
(800) 521-5247

Heart Disorders
American Heart Association
7320 Greenville Ave.
Dallas, TX 75231
(800) 242-8721
www.amhrt.org

American Heart Institute & Foundation
2632 N. 20th St.
Phoenix, AZ 85006
(800) 345-HART

National Heart, Lung & Blood Institute
Building 31, Room 41-21
9000 Rockville Pike
Bethesda, MD 20892
(301) 251-1222

Hemophilia
National Hemophilia Foundation
110 Green St., Room 406
New York, NY 10012
(800) 424-2643
www.hemophilia.org

Herpes
Herpes Resource Center
P.O. Box 13827
Research Triangle Park, NC 27709
(919) 361-8488

HIV—See AIDS

Hypertension
American Heart Association
7320 Greenville Ave.
Dallas, TX 75231
(800) 242-8721
www.amhrt.org

Immunodeficiency Disease
Immune Deficiency Foundation
P.O. Box 586
Columbia, MD 21045
(410) 461-3127
www.primaryimmune.org

Impotence, Male Sexual
Recovery of Male Potency
(313) 357-1314

Incontinence
Help for Incontinent People
P.O. Box 544
Union, SC 29379
(803) 579-7900

Simon Foundation
P.O. Box 815
Wilmette, IL 60091
(800) 23-SIMON
www.continence-fdn.ca

Irritable Bowel Syndrome
National Foundation for Ileitis and Colitis
444 Park Ave. S., 11th Flr.
New York, NY 10016-7374
(800) 343-3637

Kidney Disorders
American Kidney Fund
6100 Executive Blvd., Suite 1010
Rockville, MD 20852
(800) 638-8299

National Kidney Foundation
30 E. 33rd St., Suite 1100
New York, NY 10016
(800) 622-9010
www.kidney.org

Lead Poisoning
Environmental Protection Agency (EPA)
(800) 424-9346
www.epa.gov

Leukemia
Leukemia Society of America
733 3rd Ave.
New York, NY 10017
(212) 573-8484
www.leukemia.org

Lice
National Pediculosis Association
P.O. Box 149
Newton, MA 02161
(617) 449-NITS
www.headlice.org

Liver Disorders
American Liver Foundation
1425 Pompton Ave.
Cedar Grove, NJ 07009
(800) 223-0179
(201) 857-2626 (NJ only)
www.liverfoundation.org

Lung Disorders
American Lung Association
1740 Broadway
New York, NY 10019
(800) 586-4872
www.lungusa.org

National Asthma-Center Lung Line
1400 Jackson St.
Denver, CO 80206
(800) 222-LUNG
(303) 355-Lung (Denver only)

Lupus
Lupus Foundation of America, Inc.
4 Research Pl., Suite 180
Rockville, MD 20850-3226
(800) 558-0121
www.lupus.org

Lyme Disease
Lyme Borreliosis Foundation
P.O. Box 462
Tolland, CT 06084
(203) 525-2000

Marfan Syndrome
National Marfan Foundation
(800) 862-7326
www.marfan.org

Medical Identification
Medic Alert Foundation International
P.O. Box 1009
Turlock, CA 95381
(800) 344-3226

Menopause
National Institute on Aging Information
  Center
(800) 222-2225

Mental Health
National Mental Health Association
1800 N. Kent St.
Arlington, VA 22209
(800) 969-6642

National Institute of Mental Health
  (NIMH)
National Anxiety Awareness Program
9000 Rockville Pike
Bethesda, MD 20892
(800) 64-PANIC
www.nimh.nih.gov

Multiple Sclerosis
National Multiple Sclerosis Society
205 E. 42nd St.
New York, NY 10017
(800) 532-7667
www.nmss.org

Multiple Sclerosis Association
601-05 White Horse Pike
Oaklyn, NJ 08107
(800) 822-4672

Muscular Dystrophy
Muscular Dystrophy Association
3561 E Sunrise Dr.
Tucson, AZ 85718
(800) 572-1717
www.mdausa.org

Myasthenia Gravis
Myasthenia Gravis Foundation
53 W. Jackson, Suite 1352
Chicago, IL 60604
(800) 541-5454
www.myasthenia.org

Myocarditis—See Heart Disorders

Narcolepsy
Narcolepsy Institute
(718) 920-6799

Nephrosis—See Kidney Disorders

Nutrition and Dietetics
Center for Nutrition and Dietetics
    National Consumer Hotline
(800) 366-1655

Meat & Poultry Hotline
Dept. of Agriculture
Room 1165-S
Washington, DC 20205
(800) 535-4555

Obsessive-Compulsive Disorder
Obsessive-Compulsive Anonymous
P.O. Box 215
New Hyde Park, NY 11040
(516) 741-4901

Osteoporosis
National Osteoporosis Foundation
2100 M St. N.W., Suite 602
Washington, DC 20037
(800) 223-9994
www.nof.org

Otosclerosis—See Hearing Problems

Pancreatitis—See Digestive Diseases

Parkinson's Disease
American Parkinson Disease Association
60 Bay St., Suite 401
Staten Island, NY 10301
(800) 223-2732

National Parkinson Foundation
1501 N.W. 9th Ave.
Miami, FL 33136
(800) 327-4545
(800) 433-7022 (FL only)
www.parkinson.org

Parkinson's Education Program
3900 Birch St., Suite 105
Newport Beach, CA 92660
(800) 344-7872

Pericarditis, Acute—See Heart
Disorders

Phobias
Anxiety Disorders Association of
    America
6000 Executive Blvd., Suite 513
Rockville, MD 20852
(301) 231-9350
www.adaa.org

Pneumonia—See Lung Disorders

Porphyria
American Porphyria Foundation
P.O. Box 11163
Montgomery, AL 36111
www.enterprise.net/apf

Premenstrual Syndrome
PMS Access
P.O. Box 9326
Madison, WI 53715
(800) 222-4767
(608) 833-4767 (WI only)

Polyarteritis Nodosa—See Arthritis

**Polymyalgia Rheumatica or Temporal
Arteritis**—See Arthritis

Polymyositis—See Muscular Dystrophy

Prostate Disorders
Prostate Information Hot Line
(800) 543-9632

Psoriasis
National Psoriasis Foundation
6415 S.W. Canyon Ct., Suite 200
Portland, OR 97221
(503) 244-7404
www.psoriasis.org

Rape Crisis Syndrome
Women Organized Against Rape
P. O. Box 64
Harrisburg, PA 17108
(800) 692-7445

Rare Disorders
National Organization for Rare
    Disorders
(800) 999-NORD

Renal Failure—See Kidney Disorders

Reye's Syndrome
National Reye's Syndrome Foundation
426 N. Lewis
P.O. Box 829
Bryan, OH 43506
(800) 233-7393
(800) 231-7393 (OH only)

Rheumatic Fever—See Heart Disorders

Scleroderma
Scleroderma Federation
P.O. Box 910
Lynnfield, MA 01940
(508) 535-6600

Scoliosis
Scoliosis Association, Inc.
(800) 800-0669

Seasonal Affective Disorder
National Organization for Seasonal
    Affective Disorder
P.O. Box 40133
Washington, DC 20016

Seizure Disorders
Epilepsy Foundation of America
4351 Garden City Dr.
Landover, MD 20785
(800) EFA-1000
www.efa.org

Sexually Transmitted Diseases
Sexually Transmitted Diseases Hotline
(800) 227-8922

Sickle Cell Anemia
National Association for Sickle Cell
    Disease
3345 Wilshire Blvd., Suite 1106
Los Angeles, CA 90010-1880
(800) 421-8453

Silicosis—See Lung Disorders

Sjögren's Syndrome
Sjögren's Syndrome Foundation
382 Main St.
Port Washington, NY 11050
(516) 767-2866
www.sjogrens.com

Skin Cancer
Skin Cancer Foundation
245 5th Ave., Suite 2402
New York, NY 10016
(212) 725-5176
www.skincancer.org

Skin Disorders
American Academy of Dermatology
930 N. Meacham Rd.
P.O. Box 4014
Schaumber, IL 60168
(708) 330-0230
www.aad.org

Sleep Disorders
American Sleep Disorders
1610 14th St., Suite 300
Rochester, MN 55901
(507) 287-6006
www.asda.org

National Sleep Foundation
122 S. Robertson Blvd., Suite 201
3rd Flr., Dept. FC
Los Angeles, CA 90048
(312) 288-0466

Stroke
National Stroke Association
1565 Clarkson St.
Denver, CO 80218
(800) STROKES

American Heart Association
7320 Greenville Ave.
Dallas, TX 75231
(800) 242-8721
www.amhrt.org

Syphilis—See Sexually Transmitted
Diseases

Tay-Sachs Disease
National Tay-Sachs and Allied Disease
Association
2001 Beacon St., Suite 204
Brookline, MA 02146l
(617) 277-4463

Thyroid Disorders
Thyroid Foundation of America
630 Ambulatory Care Center
Massachusetts General Hospital
Boston, MA 02114
(800) 832-8321

Tinnitus
American Tinnitus Association
P.O. Box 5
Portland, OR 97207
(503) 248-9985

Tooth Problems
American Dental Association
211 E. Chicago Ave.
Chicago, IL 60611
(800) 621-8099
www.ada.org

Travel and Health
The International Association for
    Medical Assistance to Travelers
736 Center St.
Lewiston, NY 20402
(716) 754-4883

Tuberculosis—See Lung Disorders

Tumors, Malignant—See Cancer

Ulcer, Peptic—See Digestive Diseases

Urinary Calculi—See Kidney Disorders

Vision
American Council of the Blind
(800) 424-8666
(202) 393-3666 (DC only)
www.acb.org

Wilm's Tumor—See Cancer

EMERGENCY FIRST AID

ANAPHYLAXIS (Severe allergic reaction)
Symptoms
Itching, rash, hives, runny nose, wheezing, paleness, cold sweats, dizziness, low blood pressure, coma, cardiac arrest. Symptoms usually occur within 30 minutes after an insect sting or ingestion of certain foods or drugs.

Treatment
If Victim is Unconscious, Not Breathing
1. Yell for help. Don't leave victim.
2. Call or have someone call 911 (or your local emergency number) for an ambulance or medical help.
3. Clear the victim's mouth of foreign material, tilt jaw forward without moving the neck, pinch nose shut, cover victim's mouth with your mouth and begin mouth-to-mouth breathing. Give one slow breath every 5 seconds.
4. If there is no pulse, give cardiopulmonary resuscitation (CPR). Place hands on center of breastbone, press down 15 times and then do rescue breathing, giving 2 slow breaths.
5. Keep alternating between chest compressions and rescue breathing until help arrives or the victim is breathing on his or her own and there is a pulse.

If Victim is Unconscious and Breathing
1. Call or have someone call 911 (or your local emergency number) for an ambulance or medical help.
2. If you can't get help immediately, take patient to nearest emergency room or other facility with adequate equipment and personnel to care for medical emergencies.

BLEEDING
Symptoms
Bleeding caused by any serious injury should be treated in an emergency facility. There is usually a lot of bright-red blood pumping from an injured artery, or darker blood if a large vein has been injured.

Treatment
1. Call or have someone call 911 (or your local emergency number) for an ambulance or medical help. In the meantime, render first aid yourself.
2. Cover the injured area with the cleanest cloth you can find, or bare hands if no cloth is available.
3. Apply strong pressure directly on injured area with the heel of your hand until the bleeding stops or medical help arrives.
4. If possible, raise a bleeding arm or leg (if not broken) above the level of the victim's heart.

BURNS

Symptoms

First- and second-degree burns are not usually life-threatening.
First-degree burns cause only red skin and mild swelling.
Second-degree burns cause blisters, pain and oozing.
Third-degree burns can be life-threatening if extensive. Skin turns white or appears charred.

Treatment for first- and most second- degree burns

1. Place the victim's burned area under cold running water for 15 to 20 minutes. Don't put ice directly on the burn and don't apply butter.
2. Cover the burn area with clean, moist bandages and seek medical assistance.

Treatment for more extensive burns

1. Keep victim lying flat and lightly covered to prevent shock. Elevate the feet and legs if possible. Wrap or cover the burned area with a clean, moist cloth. Call or have someone call 911 (or your local emergency number) for an ambulance or medical help.
2. Remove clothes and jewelry unless they are sticking to burned skin. Do not immerse the victim in a cold bath or apply any type of ointment.

Special instructions

Electrical Burns— Turn off the source of electricity if possible. If not, use a non-conductive material, such as a board or wooden chair, to pull the victim away from the electrical source. Don't use your bare hands. If the victim is not breathing, begin mouth-to-mouth breathing.

Chemical Burns of the Eye or Skin— Hold the victim's head or other burned area beneath a faucet. Turn on cool water at medium pressure. Rinse for at least 15 minutes, directing the water away from the unaffected area.

For Burns of Large Areas— Prepare a solution for the victim to drink on the way to the emergency room. Mix 1 quart of water with 1 teaspoon of salt and 1/2 teaspoon of baking soda. This may help prevent kidney failure.

CHOKING
Symptoms

Clutching at throat and is unable to speak. Has trouble breathing or is unable to breathe; skin may turn blue, white or gray. Loss of consciousness.

Treatment

1. If the victim can still talk, breathe and cough, don't intervene.
2. If the victim is unable to breathe, cough and talk, perform the Heimlich Maneuver as follows:

Heimlich Maneuver

1. Stand behind person, place both arms around his abdomen and clasp your hands just below the ribcage and above the naval. Make a fist with one hand, thumb side in. Grasp the fist with your other hand.
2. Give 3 or 4 quick forceful squeezes, pushing in and up until the object is coughed up.
3. If victim becomes unconscious, call for emergency help. If necessary, perform rescue breathing and CPR as described above until help arrives.

Note: If you are alone and are choking, lean forward on your abdomen against back of a chair and push forcefully.

FRACTURES OR DISLOCATIONS
Symptoms

Extreme pain and tenderness in any injured area; change in appearance of injured part, such as swelling, protruding bone or blood under skin. Extremity, such as finger, arm or leg, may be bent out of normal alignment.

Treatment

1. Immobilize any injured area and don't move a broken limb unless absolutely necessary. Keep victim as warm and comfortable as possible. Control any bleeding. Call or have someone call 911 (or your local emergency number) for an ambulance or medical help.
2. If you must move a victim, improvise a splint from stiff rolled-up paper, scrap wood or metal. Pad the splint with clothing or blankets. The splint should extend beyond the joint on either end of the injury. Attach splint firmly to injured extremity with strips of cloth, twine or similar material to prevent movement (don't cut off the blood flow).
3. If leg, back or neck is severely injured and possibly fractured or dislocated, keep patient warm and still until ambulance arrives. Don't move the victim.

HEART ATTACK

Symptoms

Chest pain lasting more than 10 minutes that radiates into jaw or arm. Heavy sweating without obvious other cause. Weakness, nausea, pale skin. Irregular pulse.

Treatment

If Victim is Unconscious, Not Breathing

1. Yell for help. Don't leave victim.
2. Call or have someone call 911 (or your local emergency number) for an ambulance or medical help.
3. Clear the victim's mouth of foreign material, tilt jaw forward without moving the neck, pinch nose shut, cover victim's mouth with your mouth and begin mouth-to-mouth breathing. Give one slow breath every 5 seconds.
4. If there is no pulse, give cardiopulmonary resuscitation (CPR). Place hands on center of breastbone, press down 15 times and then do rescue breathing, giving 2 slow breaths.
5. Keep alternating between chest compressions and rescue breathing until help arrives or the victim is breathing on his or her own and there is a pulse.

If Victim is Unconscious and Breathing

1. Call or have someone call 911 (or your local emergency number) for an ambulance or medical help.
2. If you can't get help immediately, take patient to nearest emergency room or other facility with adequate equipment and personnel to care for medical emergencies.

Index

INDEX

INDEX

INDEX

INDEX

INDEX

INDEX

INDEX

INDEX

INDEX

INDEX

INDEX